MAGILL'S

MEDICAL GUIDE

MAGILL'S

MEDICAL GUIDE

Third Revised Edition

Volume II
Down syndrome — Laser use in surgery

Medical Consultants

Anne Chang, M.D.
University of California, San Francisco

Laurence M. Katz, M.D.
University of North Carolina, Chapel Hill

H. Bradford Hawley, M.D.
Wright State University

Nancy A. Piotrowski, Ph.D.
University of California, Berkeley

Karen E. Kalumuck, Ph.D.
The Exploratorium, San Francisco

Connie Rizzo, M.D.
Columbia University

Project Editor
Tracy Irons-Georges

SALEM PRESS, INC.
Pasadena, California   Hackensack, New Jersey

Editor in Chief: Dawn P. Dawson
Project Editor: Tracy Irons-Georges
Copy Editor: Sarah M. Hilbert
Photograph Editor: Philip Bader
Production Editor: Joyce I. Buchea
Page Design: James Hutson
Layout: Eddie Murillo
Cover Design: Moritz Design

Illustrations: Hans & Cassady, Inc., Westerville, Ohio

Magill's Medical Guide: Health and Illness, 1995
Supplement, 1996
Magill's Medical Guide, revised edition, 1998
Second revised edition, 2002
Third revised edition, 2005

∞ The paper used in these volumes conforms to the American National Standard for Permanence of Paper for Printed Library Materials, Z39.48-1992 (R1997).

Note to Readers
The material presented in *Magill's Medical Guide* is intended for broad informational and educational purposes. Readers who suspect that they suffer from any of the physical or psychological disorders, diseases, or conditions described in this set should contact a physician without delay; this work should not be used as a substitute for professional medical diagnosis or treatment. This set is not to be considered definitive on the covered topics, and readers should remember that the field of health care is characterized by a diversity of medical opinions and constant expansion in knowledge and understanding.

Library of Congress Cataloging-in-Publication Data
Magill's medical guide. — 3rd rev. ed. / medical consultants, Anne Chang . . . [et al.].
    p.   ;   cm.
  Includes bibliographical references and index.
    ISBN 1-58765-159-9 (set : alk. paper) — ISBN 1-58765-160-2 (vol. 1 : alk. paper) — ISBN 1-58765-161-0 (vol. 2 : alk. paper) — ISBN 1-58765-162-9 (vol. 3 : alk. paper) — ISBN 1-58765-163-7 (vol. 4 : alk. paper)
1. Medicine—Encyclopedias.
  [DNLM: 1. Medicine—Encyclopedias—English. W 13 M194 2005] I. Title: Medical Guide. II. Chang, Anne.
  RC41.M34   2005
  610′.3—dc22
                                                                        2004011759

First Printing

TABLE OF CONTENTS

MAGILL'S
MEDICAL GUIDE

DOWN SYNDROME

DISEASE/DISORDER

ANATOMY OR SYSTEM AFFECTED: Brain, nervous system, psychic-emotional system

SPECIALTIES AND RELATED FIELDS: Embryology, genetics, obstetrics, pediatrics

DEFINITION: A congenital abnormality characterized by moderate to severe mental retardation and a distinctive physical appearance caused by a chromosomal aberration, the result of either an error during embryonic cell division or the inheritance of defective chromosomal material.

KEY TERMS:

chromosomes: small, threadlike bodies containing the genes that are microscopically visible during cell division

gametes: the egg and sperm cells that unite to form the fertilized egg (zygote) in reproduction

gene: a segment of the DNA strand containing instructions for the production of a protein

homologous chromosomes: chromosome pairs of the same size and centromere position that possess genes for the same traits; one homologous chromosome is inherited from the father and the other from the mother

meiosis: the type of cell division that produces the cells of reproduction, which contain one-half of the chromosome number found in the original cell before division

mitosis: the type of cell division that occurs in nonsex cells, which conserves chromosome number by equal allocation to each of the newly formed cells

translocation: an aberration in chromosome structure resulting from the attachment of chromosomal material to a nonhomologous chromosome

CAUSES AND SYMPTOMS

Down syndrome is an example of a genetic disorder, that is, a disorder arising from an abnormality in an individual's genetic material. Down syndrome results from an incorrect transfer of genetic material in the formation of cells. Genetic information is contained in large "library" molecules of deoxyribonucleic acid (DNA). DNA molecules are formed by joining together units called nucleotides which come in four different varieties: adenosine, thymine, cytosine, and guanine (identified by their initials A, T, C, and G). These nucleotides store hereditary information by forming "words" with this four-letter alphabet. In a gene, a section of DNA which contains the chemical message controlling an inherited trait, three consecutive nucleotides combine to specify a particular amino acid. This word order forms the "sentences" of a recipe telling cells how to construct proteins, such as those coloring the hair and eyes, from amino acids.

In living systems, tissue growth occurs through cell division processes in which an original cell divides to form two cells containing duplicate genetic material. Just before a cell divides, the DNA organizes itself into distinct, compact bundles called chromosomes. Normal human cells, diploid cells, contain twenty-three pairs (or a total of forty-six) of these chromosomes. Each pair is a set of homologues containing genes for the same traits. These chromosomes are composed of two DNA strands, chromatids, joined at a constricted region known as the centromere. The bundle is similar in shape to the letter X. The arms are the parts above and below the constriction, which may be centered or offset toward one end (giving arms of equal or different lengths, respectively). During mitosis, the division of nonsex cells, the chromatids separate at the centromere, forming two sets of single-stranded chromosomes, which migrate to opposite ends of the cell. The cell then splits into two genetically equivalent cells, each containing twenty-three single-stranded chromosomes that will duplicate to form the original number of forty-six chromosomes.

In sexual reproduction, haploid egg and sperm cells, each containing twenty-three single-stranded chromosomes, unite in fertilization to produce a zygote cell with forty-six chromosomes. Haploid cells are created through a different, two-step cell division process termed meiosis. Meiosis begins when the homologues in a diploid cell pair up at the equator of the cell. The attractions between the members of each pair then break, allowing the homologues to migrate to opposite ends of the cell, each twin to a different pole, without splitting at the centromere. The parent cell then divides once to

---

INFORMATION ON DOWN SYNDROME

CAUSES: Genetic defect

SYMPTOMS: Mental retardation, characteristic facial appearance, lack of muscle tone, increased risk for heart malformations, increased disease susceptibility

DURATION: Lifelong

TREATMENTS: None

give two cells containing twenty-three double-stranded chromosomes, and then divides again through the process of mitosis to form cells that contain only twenty-three single-stranded chromosomes. Thus, each cell contains half of the original chromosomes.

Although cell division is normally a precise process, occasionally an error called nondisjunction occurs when a chromosome either fails to separate or fails to migrate to the proper pole. In meiosis, the failure to move to the proper pole results in the formation of one gamete having twenty-four chromosomes and one having twenty-two chromosomes. Upon fertilization, zygotes of forty-seven or forty-five chromosomes are produced, and the developing embryo must function with either extra or missing genes. Since every chromosome contains a multitude of genes, problems result from the absence or excess of proteins produced. In fact, the embryos formed from most nondisjunctional fertilizations die at an early stage in development and are spontaneously aborted. Occasionally, nondisjunction occurs in mitosis, when a chromosome migrates before the chromatids separate, yielding one cell with an extra copy of the chromosome and no copy in the other cell.

Down syndrome is also termed trisomy 21 because it most commonly results from the presence of an extra copy of the smallest human chromosome, chromosome 21. Actually, it is not the entire extra chromosome 21 that is responsible, but rather a small segment of the long arm of this chromosome. Only two other trisomies occur with any significant frequency: trisomy 13 (Patau's syndrome) and trisomy 18 (Edwards' syndrome). Both of these disorders are accompanied by multiple severe malformations, resulting in death within a few months of birth. Most incidences of Down syndrome are a consequence of a nondisjunction during meiosis. In about 75 percent of these cases, the extra chromosome is present in the egg. About 1 percent of Down syndrome cases occur after the fertilization of normal gametes from a mitosis nondisjunction, producing a mosaic in which some of the embryo's cells are normal and some exhibit trisomy. The degree of mosaicism and its location will determine the physio-

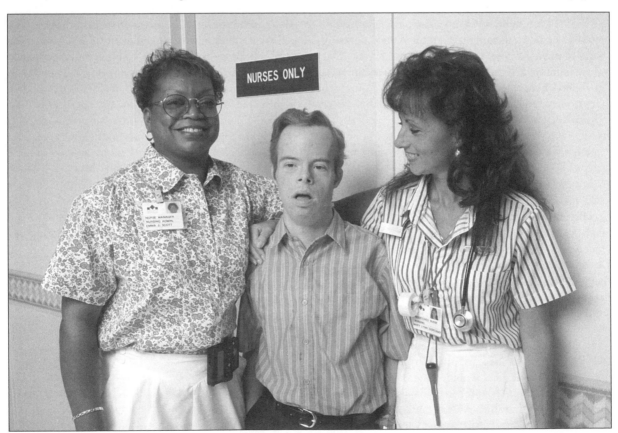

Nurses and other health care professionals can offer both medical and emotional support to people with Down syndrome. (PhotoDisc)

logical consequences of the nondisjunction. Although mosaic individuals range from apparent normality to completely affected, typically the disorder is less severe.

In about 4 percent of all Down syndrome cases, the individual possesses not an entire third copy of chromosome 21 but rather extra chromosome 21 material, which has been incorporated via a translocation into a nonhomologous chromosome. In translocation, pieces of arms are swapped between two nonrelated chromosomes, forming "hybrid" chromosomes. The most common translocation associated with Down syndrome is that between the long arm (Down gene area) of chromosome 21 and an end of chromosome 14. The individual in whom the translocation has occurred shows no evidence of the aberration, since the normal complement of genetic material is still present, only at different chromosomal locations. The difficulty arises when this individual forms gametes. A mother who possesses the 21/14 translocation, for example, has one normal 21, one normal 14, and the hybrid chromosomes. She is a genetic carrier for the disorder, because she can pass it on to her offspring even though she is clinically normal. This mother could produce three types of viable gametes: one containing the normal 14 and 21; one containing both translocations, which would result in clinical normality; and one containing the normal 21 and the translocated 14 having the long arm of 21. If each gamete were fertilized by normal sperm, two apparently normal embryos and one partial trisomy 21 Down syndrome embryo would result. Down syndrome that results from the passing on of translocations is termed familial Down syndrome and is an inherited disorder.

The presence of an extra copy of the long arm of chromosome 21 causes defects in many tissues and organs. One major effect of Down syndrome is mental retardation. The intelligence quotients (IQs) of affected individuals are typically in the range of 40-50. The IQ varies with age, being higher in childhood than in adolescence or adult life. The disorder is often accompanied by physical traits such as short stature, stubby fingers and toes, protruding tongue, and an unusual pattern of hand creases. Perhaps the most recognized physical feature is the distinctive slanting of the eyes, caused by a vertical fold (epicanthal fold) of skin near the nasal bridge which pulls and tilts the eyes slightly toward the nostrils. For normal Caucasians, the eye runs parallel to the skin fold below the eyebrow; for Asians, this skin fold covers a major portion of the up-

per eyelid. In contrast, the epicanthal fold in trisomy 21 does not cover a major part of the upper eyelid.

It should be noted that not all defects associated with Down syndrome are found in every affected individual. About 40 percent of Down syndrome patients have congenital heart defects, while about 10 percent have intestinal blockages. Affected individuals are prone to respiratory infections and contract leukemia at a rate twenty times that of the general population. Although Down syndrome children develop the same types of leukemia in the same proportions as other children, the survival rates of the two groups are markedly different. While the survival rate for patients without Down syndrome after ten years is about 30 percent, survival beyond five years is negligible in those with Down syndrome. It appears that the extra copy of chromosome 21 not only increases the risk of contracting the cancer but also exerts a decisive influence on the disease's outcome. Reproductively, males are sterile while some females are fertile. Although many Down syndrome infants die in the first year of life, the mean life expectancy is about thirty years. This reduced life expectancy results from defects in the immune system, causing a high susceptibility to infectious disease. Most older Down syndrome individuals develop an Alzheimer's-like condition, and less than 3 percent live beyond fifty years of age.

TREATMENT AND THERAPY

Trisomy 21 is one of the most common human chromosomal aberrations, occurring in about 0.5 percent of all conceptions and in one out of every seven hundred to eight hundred live births. About 15 percent of the patients institutionalized for mental deficiency suffer from Down syndrome.

Even before the chromosomal basis for the disorder was determined, the frequency of Down syndrome births was correlated with increased maternal age. For mothers at age twenty, the incidence of Down syndrome is about 0.05 percent, which increases to 0.9 percent by age thirty-five and 3 percent at age forty-five. Studies comparing the chromosomes of the affected offspring with those of both parents have shown that the nondisjunction event is maternal about 75 percent of the time. This maternal age effect is thought to result from the different manner in which the male and female gametes are produced. Gamete production in the male is a continual, lifelong process, while it is a one-time event in females. Formation of the female's gametes begins early in embryonic life, somewhere between the eighth and twentieth weeks. During this time, cells in the developing ovary divide rapidly by mitosis, forming cells called primary oocytes. These cells then begin meiosis by pairing up the homologues. The process is interrupted at this point, and the cells are held in a state of suspended animation until needed in reproduction, when they are triggered to complete their division and form eggs. It appears that the frequency of nondisjunction events increases with the length of the storage period. Studies have demonstrated that cells in a state of meiosis are particularly sensitive to environmental influences such as viruses, X rays, and cytotoxic chemicals. It is possible that environmental influences may play a role in nondisjunction events. Up to age thirty-two, males contribute an extra chromosome 21 as often as do females. Beyond this age, there is a rapid increase in nondisjunctional eggs, while the number of nondisjunctional sperm remains constant. Where the maternal age effect is minimal, mosaicism may be an important source of the trisomy. An apparently normal mother who possesses undetected mosaicism can produce trisomy offspring if gametes with an extra chromosome are produced. In some instances, characteristics such as abnormal fingerprint patterns have been observed in the mothers and their Down syndrome offspring.

Techniques such as amniocentesis, chorionic villus sampling, and alpha-fetoprotein screening are available for prenatal diagnosis of Down syndrome in fetuses. Amniocentesis, the most widely used technique for prenatal diagnosis, is generally performed between the fourteenth and sixteenth weeks of pregnancy. In this technique, about one ounce of fluid is removed from the amniotic cavity surrounding the fetus by a needle inserted through the mother's abdomen. Although some testing can be done directly on the fluid (such as the assay for spina bifida), more information is obtained from the cells shed from the fetus that accompany the fluid. The mixture obtained in the amniocentesis is spun in a centrifuge to separate the fluid from the fetal cells. Unfortunately, the chromosome analysis for Down syndrome cannot be conducted directly on the amount of cellular material obtained. Although the majority of the cells collected are nonviable, some will grow in culture. These cells are allowed to grow and multiply in culture for two to four weeks, and then the chromosomes undergo karyotyping, which will detect both trisomy 21 and translocational aberration.

In karyotyping, the chromosomes are spread on a microscope slide, stained, and photographed. Each type of chromosome gives a unique, observable banding pattern when stained, which allows it to be identified. The chromosomes are then cut out of the photograph and arranged in homologous pairs, in numerical order. Trisomy 21 is easily observed, since three copies of chromosome 21 are present, while the translocation shows up as an abnormal banding pattern. Termination of the pregnancy in the wake of an unfavorable amniocentesis diagnosis is complicated, because the fetus at this point is usually about eighteen to twenty weeks old, and elective abortions are normally performed between the sixth and twelfth weeks of pregnancy. Earlier sampling of the amniotic fluid is not possible because of the small amount of fluid present.

An alternate testing procedure called chorionic villus sampling became available in the mid-1980's. In this procedure, a chromosomal analysis is conducted on a piece of placental tissue that is obtained either vaginally or through the abdomen during the eighth to eleventh week of pregnancy. The advantages of this procedure are that it can be done much earlier in the pregnancy and that enough tissue can be collected to conduct the chromosome analysis immediately, without the cell culture step. Consequently, diagnosis can be completed during the first trimester of the pregnancy, making therapeutic abortion an option for the parents. Chorionic villus sampling does have some negative aspects. One disadvantage is the slightly higher incidence of test-induced miscarriage as compared to amniocentesis—around 1 percent (versus less than 0.5 percent). Also, because tissue of both the mother and the fetus are obtained in the sampling process, they must be carefully separated, complicating the analysis. Occasionally, chromosomal abnormalities are observed in the tested tissue that are not present in the fetus itself.

Prenatal maternal alpha-fetoprotein testing has also been used to diagnose Down syndrome. Abnormal levels of a substance called maternal alpha-fetoprotein are often associated with chromosomal disorders. Several research studies have described a high correlation between low levels of maternal alpha-fetoprotein and the occurrence of trisomy 21 in the fetus. By correlating alpha-fetoprotein levels, the age of the mother, and specific female hormone levels, between 60 percent and 80 percent of fetuses with Down syndrome can be detected. Although techniques allow Down syndrome to be detected readily in a fetus, there is no effective intrauterine therapy available to correct the abnormality.

The care of a Down syndrome child presents many challenges for the family unit. Until the 1970's, most of these children spent their lives in institutions. With the increased support services available, however, it is now common for such children to remain in the family environment. Although many Down syndrome children have happy dispositions, a significant number have behavioral problems that can consume the energies of the parents, to the detriment of the other children. Rearing a Down syndrome child often places a large financial burden on the family: Such children are, for example, susceptible to illness; they also have special educational needs. Since Down syndrome children are often conceived late in the parents' reproductive period, the parents may not be able to continue to care for these children throughout their offspring's adult years. This is problematic because many Down syndrome individuals do not possess sufficient mental skills to earn a living or to manage their affairs without supervision.

All women in their mid-thirties have an increased risk of producing a Down syndrome infant. Since the resultant trisomy 21 is not of a hereditary nature, the abnormality can be detected only by the prenatal screening, which is recommended for all pregnancies of women older than age thirty-four.

For parents who have produced a Down syndrome child, genetic counseling can be beneficial in determining their risk factor for future pregnancies. The genetic counselor determines the specific chromosomal aberration that occurred utilizing chromosome studies of the parents and affected child, along with additional information provided by the family history. If the cause was nondisjunction and the mother is young, the recurrence risk is much less than 1 percent; for mothers over the age of thirty-four, it is about 5 percent. If the cause was translocational, the Down syndrome is hereditary and risk is much greater—statistically, a one-in-three chance. In addition, there is a one-in-three chance that clinically normal offspring will be carriers of the syndrome, producing it in the next generation. It is suggested that couples who come from families having a history of spontaneous abortions, which often result from lethal chromosomal aberrations, and/or incidence of Down syndrome, undergo chromosomal screening to detect the presence of a Down syndrome translocation.

PERSPECTIVE AND PROSPECTS

English physician John L. H. Down is credited with the first clinical description of Down syndrome, in 1886.

Since the distinctive epicanthic fold gave Down children an appearance that John Down associated with Asians, he called the condition "mongolism"—an unfortunate term implying that those affected with the condition are throwbacks to a more "primitive" racial group. Today, the inappropriate term has been replaced with the name Down syndrome.

A French physician, Jérôme Lejeune, suspected that Down syndrome had a genetic basis and began to study the condition in 1953. A comparison of the fingerprints and palm prints of affected individuals with those of unaffected individuals showed a high frequency of abnormalities in the prints of those with Down syndrome. These prints appear very early in development and serve as a record of events that take place early in embryogenesis. The extent of the changes in print patterns led Lejeune to the conclusion that the condition was not a result of the action of one or two genes but rather of many genes or even an entire chromosome. Upon microscopic examination, he observed that Down syndrome children possess forty-seven chromosomes instead of the forty-six chromosomes found in normal children. In 1959, Lejeune published his findings, showing that Down syndrome is caused by the presence of the extra chromosome which was later identified as a copy of chromosome 21. This first observation of a human chromosomal abnormality marked a turning point in the study of human genetics. It demonstrated that genetic defects not only were caused by mutations of single genes but also could be associated with changes in chromosome number. Although the presence of an extra chromosome allows varying degrees of development to occur, most of these abnormalities result in fetal death, with only a few resulting in live birth. Down syndrome is unusual in that the affected individual often survives into adulthood.

—*Arlene R. Courtney, Ph.D.*

See also Amniocentesis; Birth defects; Chorionic villus sampling; DNA and RNA; Genetic diseases; Genetics and inheritance; Leukemia; Mental retardation; Mutation.

FOR FURTHER INFORMATION:

Cohen, William, et al., eds. *Down Syndrome: Visions for the Twenty-first Century.* New York: Wiley, 2002. Reviews the medical and research advances in the clinical, educational, developmental, psychosocial, and vocational aspects of Down syndrome.

Hassold, Terry J., and David Patterson, eds. *Down Syndrome: A Promising Future, Together.* New York:

John Wiley & Sons, 1999. Discusses clinical, educational, developmental, psychosocial, and vocational issues relevant to people with Down syndrome.

Miller, Jon F., Mark Leddy, and Lewis A. Leavitt, eds. *Improving the Communication of People with Down Syndrome*. Baltimore: Paul H. Brookes, 1999. Discusses how to assess and treat speech, language, and communication problems in children and adults with Down syndrome.

Moore, Keith L., and T. V. N. Persaud. *The Developing Human*. 7th ed. Philadelphia: W. B. Saunders, 2003. An outstanding textbook on human embryonic development, with specific information about the causes of congenital malformations and common defects occurring in each of the body's systems.

National Down Syndrome Society. http://www.ndss .org/. An excellent organization that focuses on research, advocacy, and education. The Web site promotes virtual communities and provides up-to-date information about upcoming events.

Pueschel, Siegfried. *A Parent's Guide to Down Syndrome*. 2d ed. Baltimore: Paul H. Brookes, 2000. An informative guide highlighting the important developmental stages in the life of a child with Down syndrome.

Rondal, Jean A., et al., eds. *Down's Syndrome: Psychological, Psychobiological, and Socioeducational Perspectives*. San Diego, Calif.: Singular, 1996. An academic text on issues surrounding Down syndrome. Includes references and an index.

DRUG ADDICTION. *See* ADDICTION.

DRUG RESISTANCE
DISEASE/DISORDER

ANATOMY OR SYSTEM AFFECTED: All

SPECIALTIES AND RELATED FIELDS: Bacteriology, microbiology, pharmacology, public health, virology

DEFINITION: The ability of a pathogen, formerly susceptible to a particular medication, to change in such a way that it is no longer affected by it.

KEY TERMS:

antibiotic: a substance that kills or prevents the growth of a pathogen

bacteria: microscopic single-celled organisms

bacterial chromosome: a circular cell component in bacteria that contains deoxyribonucleic acid (DNA)

bacteriophage: a virus that attaches itself to bacteria

conjugation: the direct exchange of genetic material between bacteria

nosocomial infection: a disease or organism that is acquired in a hospital

pathogen: a living organism that causes disease

plasmids: circular pieces of DNA within bacteria; these are much smaller than bacterial chromosomes

transduction: the indirect transfer of genetic material between bacteria by a bacteriophage

transposons: pieces of DNA that can be transferred between plasmids and chromosomes

virus: a microscopic organism consisting of DNA or ribonucleic acid (RNA) within a protein coating

CAUSES AND SYMPTOMS

Drug resistance occurs whenever pathogens—disease-causing organisms such as bacteria, viruses, or fungi—that have been successfully eradicated with a certain chemical agent develop the ability to resist that agent. The most clinically important form of drug resistance is the ability of bacteria to develop resistance to antibiotics.

An antibiotic attacks a bacterial cell by interfering with a vital biochemical process needed by the organism. Antibiotics are generally engineered to kill bacteria, while leaving body cells unharmed. This bacteria-specific approach creates a safe way of killing pathogens with strong chemicals, while keeping the affected person safe from harm.

Bacteria can develop resistance to an antibiotic in several ways, but the spread of that resistance may be blamed on one primary phenomenon related to evolution: selection. Selection is the "weeding out" of individuals in a population, leaving a smaller number of "tougher" individuals. If environmental pressure (such as an antibiotic treatment) is placed on any population of organisms, the only individuals that will survive and reproduce are those resistant to that pressure.

Resistance to a particular antibiotic arises in a bacterial cell by random genetic mutation. Because a particular cell is genetically altered and survives the antibiotic treatment that destroys other bacteria of the same kind, it is able to survive, unlike its susceptible relatives. The small, resistant population that is left grows rapidly and cannot be halted.

Even if an antibiotic is completely successful in eradicating a particular type of bacteria, problems with drug resistance can still arise. The human body contains billions of bacteria of many different kinds. These bacteria fill large and small environmental niches in the microflora that human beings carry in and on their bodies. When one or more of these susceptible bacteria types are eliminated by an antibiotic, their niches are left empty. This leaves room for the resistant bacteria that are left to multiply in greater numbers. This is not generally a problem because most of the resistant bacteria are harmless, but even if they are, they may have the ability to genetically transfer antibiotic resistance to pathogenic bacteria.

Use of multiple antibiotics or broad spectrum antibiotics that attack many kinds of bacteria can cause other problems. By eliminating a large number of the bacteria normally present and emptying essentially all the environmental niches, powerful antibiotics encourage the growth of fungi such as *Candida albicans*. Fungal infections are not affected by bacterial antibiotics and require special antifungal drugs.

The ability to resist a particular antibiotic is encoded as genetic information in deoxyribonucleic acid (DNA) molecules. Bacterial DNA is located in a special bacterial chromosome found in the cytoplasm of a bacterial cell. Additionally, bacterial DNA may be found on small, circular fragments of DNA called plasmids. These plasmids are separate from the bacterial chromosome and carry special information needed for the bacteria to survive under adverse environmental conditions. Plasmids carry "mating" genes, which allow the bacteria to transfer a plasmid from one bacteria to another. They also carry genes that make a bacteria resistant to a particular antibiotic. Consequently, plasmids are of particular importance because they allow antibiotic resistance to be transferred between bacteria.

Two bacterial cells may exchange plasmids by direct contact in a process known as conjugation. Not all plasmids can be exchanged in this way, but the genetic information that encodes for resistance may be transferred from a plasmid that cannot be exchanged to one that can. This occurs when a small piece of DNA known as a transposon breaks away from one plasmid and attaches itself to another. A transposon may also break away from a bacterial chromosome and attach itself elsewhere on the chromosome or onto a plasmid.

Antibiotic resistance may also be transferred between bacteria indirectly by a bacteriophage in transduction. A bacteriophage is a virus that attaches itself to a bacterial cell. The virus sometimes incorporates DNA from the invaded bacterial cell into its own DNA. The virus may then transfer this DNA to the next bacterial cell to which it attaches. In this way, it can transfer drug resistance between bacteria that are unable to undergo conjugation.

The various ways in which genetic information can be exchanged between bacteria may result in organisms with resistance to multiple drugs. Some bacteria are known to be resistant to at least ten different antibiotics. They carry a series of genes on their plasmids able to make enzymes that can degrade and destroy antibiotics. For example, bacteria able to resist penicillin treatments carry an enzyme called penicillinase that destroys penicillin, thus protecting the bacteria.

An important factor in the emergence of antibiotic resistance is the misuse of antibiotics. For example, antibiotics have no effect on viruses but are often used against viral illnesses. A study published in 1997 revealed that at least half of all patients in the United States who visited doctors' offices with colds, upper respiratory tract infections, and bronchitis received antibiotics, even though 90 percent of these illnesses are caused by viruses. The same study showed that almost a third of all antibiotic prescriptions written in doctors' offices were used for these kinds of illnesses. Similar problems are also seen in hospitals. This misuse or overuse of antibiotics has been one of the strongest forces pushing selection of antibiotic-resistant bacteria. Even if doctors stopped overprescribing antibiotics today, there are other factors at work. In 2000, an estimated fifty million pounds of antibiotics were used in the United States; half that amount was used for veterinary and agricultural purposes. Antibiotics are administered in huge doses to farm animals to keep them healthy and allow them to grow larger. These drugs are even being used in the petroleum industry for cleaning pipelines. The World Health Organization (WHO) noted a sharp decrease in the incidence of antibiotic-resistant bacterial strains in Denmark after antibiotic use was all but eliminated from livestock in 1998.

A final factor in the increase in antibiotic resistance is the use and overuse of substandard and counterfeit antimicrobial agents in developing countries. In Nigeria, for example, WHO estimates that there are twenty thousand unlicensed medical stands scattered throughout the country. These street vendors do not require prescriptions to dose patients. Additionally, the common use of antibiotics in developing nations to "sterilize" households risks the development of cross-resistant bacterial strains.

Several public health concerns have arisen as a result of drug resistance. One of the earliest problems occurred in Japan in 1955, when an outbreak of dysentery was caused by bacteria resistant to four antibiotics. For the last fifty years multiple antibiotic resistance has emerged in bacteria causing pneumonia, gonorrhea, meningitis, and other serious illnesses.

In the 1980's, drug-resistant tuberculosis emerged as a public health concern. In 1991, in New York City, for example, 33 percent of all tuberculosis infections were resistant to at least one drug, and 19 percent were resistant to both of the most effective drugs used to treat the disease. Because of resistance, many tuberculosis patients now require treatment with four drugs for several months. Some patients are required to be directly observed by a health care worker every time they take a dose of medication to ensure compliance. The use of multiple drugs and the need for increased numbers of health care workers greatly increase the cost of treating tuberculosis.

A new challenge appeared in 1997, when patients in Japan and the United States developed infections caused by bacteria known as *Staphylococcus aureus*. This bacteria is an ordinarily harmless organism found on human skin, but it can cause potentially fatal infections when it enters the bloodstream. The most pathogenic strain is known as the multiresistant *Staphylococcus aureus* (MRSA). Since 1997, vancomycin-resistant *Staphylococcus aureus* (VRSA) has emerged, causing major public health problems.

TREATMENT AND THERAPY

The antibiotic vancomycin is one of a small group of "glycopeptide" antibiotics. At one time, its administration was considered a last resort. Vancomycin is toxic to humans in the wrong dosage, so it must be dispensed carefully by a physician. The drug eradicates bacteria by inhibiting the synthesis of their outer protective wall. Without this outer cell wall, bacteria become sensitive to minor environmental changes and die. Vancomycin has been a valuable antibiotic because it is so important in the fight against bacteria that are resistant to penicillin. The VRSA-type bacteria have nullified this valuable antibiotic and made it much less useful.

The most common sites for MRSA and VRSA invasion and growth are wounds, the nasal cavities, and surgical incisions. Both these strains generally arise as nosocomial infections, that is, infections contracted in a hospital.

The *Enterococcus* bacteria are the second most common nosocomial infection found in hospitals. These bacteria often give rise to infections in the urinary tracts of patients, but they are also the cause of meningitis, septicemia, and endocarditis. Most frequently, *Enterococcus* is found in children, the elderly, HIV-infected individuals, or the immunologically compromised, whose immune systems are not fully functioning. *Enterococcus* bacteria are now resistant to vancomycin. This means that vancomycin-resistant *Enterococcus* (VRE) can spread vancomycin resistance to other organisms, producing major medical problems.

Another problem bacteria is pneumococcus. This bacterial species was once completely sensitive to penicillin, but now, according to bacteriologist Perry Dickinson, up to 55 percent of the pneumococcal strains are penicillin-resistant. The group most at risk for infection with the drug-resistant *Streptococcus pneumoniae* (DRSP) is children age six or younger. Adult pneumococcal strains seem not to be as generally antibiotic resistant. The resistant strains are becoming quite a serious threat among children, but pneumococcus is still vancomycin-sensitive and amoxicillin is still effective at high dosages.

One of the most promising new superdrugs, linezolid (Zyvox), developed to combat antibiotic resistance, falls into a new category of antibiotics called oxazolidinones. These drugs act at an early stage in the synthesis of protein by bacteria. Without protein production, bacteria cannot multiply, and they die. The antibiotic linezolid acts strongly against many bacteria, including MRSA, VRSA, VRE, and penicillin-resistant pneumococci. In hospital trials involving patients with MRSA infections, linezolid produced clinical success in more than 83 percent of the patients. The drug can be taken orally or injected, making it quite versatile. Robert Moellering of Harvard University Medical School suggests that this versatility is convenient for patients because they can complete their therapy at home. This drug has also been shown to have few side effects.

A whole series of promising new antibiotics are presently being examined by the Food and Drug Administration for use against the variously resistant superbugs. GlaxoWellcome has at least three new antibiotics that are effective against VRE, MRSA, and VRSA infections. These include Sanfetrinem, GV143253, and Grepafloxacin. The company Microcide, Incorporated, has recently developed MC02479, a cephalosporin-type antibiotic that works in a fashion similar to penicillin and is strongly active against VRE, MRSA, and VRSA. As long as these drugs and others like them are used and prescribed responsibly, they may offer a therapeutic benefit for decades to come.

PERSPECTIVE AND PROSPECTS

Several different strategies have been suggested for handling the problem of antibiotic resistance. In general, these strategies involve educating the public and health care workers, monitoring antibiotic use, and promoting research into methods to deal with resistant bacteria.

The general public should be aware of the proper use of antibiotics. Many patients expect to be given antibiotics for illnesses that do not respond to them, such as viral infections. They may pressure physicians into prescribing antibiotics even when physicians are aware that these drugs are useless. Patients must learn to understand the difference between a bacterial and a viral infection and how each is treated. Patients must also be educated not to use another person's antibiotics or an old supply of antibiotics that they have saved from previous illnesses. Finally, patients must learn to take the entire course of antibiotics. Often, when antibiotics are properly prescribed, patients who begin to feel better may fail to take the entire amount prescribed. This leads to an increased risk of drug-resistant infection if they do not completely eliminate the original infection.

All health care workers should be aware of the importance of avoiding the spread of resistant pathogens from one patient to another. In the late 1990's, about two million Americans per year acquired nosocomial infections. These infections were responsible for about eighty thousand deaths per year. The most important factors in reducing the rate of nosocomial infections are frequent and thorough hand washing, glove changes, and disinfectant applications.

Children should be immunized at a young age against pneumococcal infections. Children who are immunized do not get the infections; hence no antibiotics are needed, and no extra antibiotics enter into the general population. Additionally, children who are ill should be kept home from day care centers. Day care centers are becoming dangerous incubators, where disease may potentially run rampant. In these places, children spread bacterial infections among themselves, often amplifying pathogenicity and drug resistance. This can be avoided by isolating sick children at home.

Physicians need to be aware of the proper ways to use antibiotics. Microbiologists have suggested better instruction in antibiotic use in medical schools, more continuing education on the subject for practicing physicians, and the development of computer programs to aid physicians in selecting antibiotics. Some have suggested that all physicians prescribing antibiotics in hospitals be required to consult with physicians who specialize in infectious diseases. Standardized order forms that include guidelines for proper use of each antibiotic have also been proposed. Additionally, doctors who have been thoroughly educated must learn not to accede to patient demands for antibiotics, and they must defer antibiotic use in self-limiting infections that will heal on their own. They must also avoid prescribing antibiotics over the phone.

Unfortunately, overall antibiotic prescription rates still seem to be rising, despite warnings of increased antimicrobial resistance. Since 1992, yearly prescriptions have increased by more than thirty million. The most commonly prescribed antibiotic has been amoxicillin, which represents more than 25 percent of the total prescriptions. Erythromycin use has fallen to less than 7 percent, while penicillin and tetracycline use have fallen as well. The new broad-spectrum antibiotics called macrolides have replaced these drugs and make up more than 10 percent of antibiotic use. Despite the overall increases, the proportion of antibiotic prescriptions for the common cold has decreased to 40 percent from a high of 52 percent in 1994.

Researchers agree that monitoring antibiotic use is critical in fighting drug resistance. A study published in 1997 demonstrated the effectiveness of education and monitoring in reducing resistance. Physicians in Finland were educated in the proper use of the antibiotic erythromycin, and use of the drug was monitored. In 1992, 16.5 percent of bacteria known as group A *Streptococci* were resistant to erythromycin. In 1996, only 8.6 percent were resistant. Some experts have proposed using computers to share information about antibiotic use and resistance among as many health care facilities as possible.

Faster development of new antibiotics for use on multiply resistant bacteria is another improvement. Researchers stress, however, that these new antibiotics must be used only when necessary, in order to avoid promoting resistance to them. Consequently, linezolid and other new antibiotics are being used sparingly.

Other methods have been proposed for minimizing antibiotic resistance. Because patients often expect or demand prescriptions when they visit physicians, some experts have suggested that the physician write a lifestyle prescription when drug use is not appropriate. Such a prescription would explain why antibiotics should not be used in a particular situation and would give the patient specific instructions on how to treat the illness without them.

Eliminating the routine use of antibiotics in farm animals would be of great help. As the Danish study suggests, the risk of resistant bacterial strains in livestock could be reduced, making human lives safer as well.

International concerns over antibiotic resistance are at such a height that in 2000, eight international medical societies gathered to spend a full day discussing the problem. They called this event Global Resistance Day, and the medical professionals discussed the dilemma and solutions for global antibiotic resistance.

—Rose Secrest;
updated by James J. Campanella, Ph.D.
See also Antibiotics; Bacterial infections; Bacteriology; Epidemiology; Fungal infections; Hospitals; Iatrogenic disorders; Infection; Microbiology; Mutation; Pharmacology; Pharmacy; Viral infections.

FOR FURTHER INFORMATION:

Fisher, Jeffrey A. *The Plague Makers: How We Are Creating Catastrophic New Epidemics and What We Must Do to Avert Them.* 3d ed. New York: Continuum International, 2002. A discussion of antibiotic resistance and steps that can be taken to prevent it. Includes discussions of biological warfare, anthrax, and West Nile virus.

Harrison, Polly F., et al., eds. *Antimicrobial Resistance: Issues and Options.* Washington, D.C.: National Academy Press, 1998. An excellent, up-to-date text describing the problems that society faces with antibiotic resistance, and possible solutions.

Levy, Stuart B. *The Antibiotic Paradox: How the Misuse of Antibiotics Destroys Their Curative Powers.* Cambridge, Mass.: Perseus, 2001. A leading researcher in molecular biology explores a modern-day massive evolutionary change in bacteria due to misuse of antibiotics. He argues that a buildup of new antibiotic-resistant bacteria in individuals and in the environment is leading medicine into a dangerous territory where "miracle" drugs may be obsolete.

Murray, Barbara E. "Can Antibiotic Resistance Be Controlled?" *New England Journal of Medicine* 330, no. 17 (April 28, 1994): 1229-1230. An editorial that outlines the future consequences of increasing drug resistance and offers several suggestions for fighting it.

Rosen, Barry P. and Shahriar Mobashery, eds. *Resolving the Antibiotic Paradox: Progress in Understanding Drug Resistance and Development of New Antibiotics.* New York: Plenum, 1998. A more technical book than some others. It addresses the issue of bacterial resistance, highlighting both conventional and new drug discovery approaches.

Shnayerson, Michael. *The Killers Within: The Deadly Rise of Drug Resistant Bacteria.* New York: Little, Brown, 2002. Traces the evolution of drug-resistant bacteria and how physicians are trying to combat it.

Smaglik, Paul. "Proliferation of Pills." *Science News* 151, no. 20 (May 17, 1997): 310-311. An account of the frequent misuse of antibiotics, with opinions from several experts.

Walsh, Christopher. *Antibiotics: Actions, Origins, Resistance.* Washington, D.C.: ASM Press, 2003. Examines such topics as how antibiotics block specific proteins, how the molecular structure of drugs enables such activity, the development of bacterial resistance, and the molecular logic of antibiotic biosynthesis.

DRUG THERAPY. *See* ANTIBIOTICS; ANTIDEPRESSANTS; ANTIHISTAMINES; ANTI-INFLAMMATORY DRUGS; APHRODISIACS; CHEMOTHERAPY; DECONGESTANTS; NARCOTICS; STEROIDS.

DWARFISM
DISEASE/DISORDER

ANATOMY OR SYSTEM AFFECTED: Back, bones, brain, endocrine system, glands, hips, legs, musculoskeletal system, nervous system

SPECIALTIES AND RELATED FIELDS: Endocrinology, genetics, orthopedics, pediatrics

DEFINITION: Underdevelopment of the body, most often caused by a variety of genetic or endocrinological dysfunctions and resulting in either proportionate or disproportionate development, sometimes accompanied by other physical abnormalities and/or mental deficiencies.

KEY TERMS:

amino acid: the building blocks of protein

autosomal: refers to all chromosomes except the X and Y chromosomes (sex chromosomes) that determine body traits

cleft palate: a gap in the roof of the mouth, sometimes present at birth and frequently combined with harelip

collagen: protein material of which the white fibers of the connective tissue of the body are composed

hypoglycemia: low blood sugar

laminae: arches of the vertebral bones

spondylosis: a condition characterized by restriction of movement of the vertebral bones; occurs naturally as a child grows

stenosis: any narrowing of a passage or orifice of the body

CAUSES AND SYMPTOMS

A person of unusually small stature is generally termed a "dwarf." Dwarfism in humans may be caused by a number of conditions that occur either before birth or in early childhood. When short stature is the only observable feature, growth—though abnormal relative to height—is proportionate. Short stature is nearly always blamed on endocrinological dysfunction, but few cases are actually the result of endocrinopathy. If shortness is caused by endocrinopathy, it is often attributable to a deficiency in one or two glands: the pituitary gland (which produces growth hormone) and the thyroid gland. Those who are unusually short but have no other obvious disease are divided into two categories: those who were afflicted prenatally and those who were afflicted postnatally. Many of those born "growth-retarded" are actually the result of chromosomal aberrations and skeletal abnormalities; other events that may cause prenatal growth retardation might include magnesium deficiency (which would prohibit ribosome synthesis and, in turn, halt protein synthesis) or a uterus that is too small. Postnatal growth retardation may be caused by heredity if both parents are short; there is no skeletal abnormality at fault. Other short-statured children may simply mature at a much slower rate, yet grow normally. Typically, one of the parents may have had a late onset of puberty; such children may reach normal height in their late teens.

Unusually short-statured males are those who are shorter than five feet tall; in females, fifty-eight inches and below is short-statured. Children are classified as dwarfs if their height is below the third percentile for their age. When this is the case, doctors will look primarily to four major causes of dwarfism: an underactive or inactive pituitary gland, achondroplasia (failure of normal development in cartilage), emotional or nutritional deprivation, or Turner syndrome (the possession of a single, X, chromosome). If the answer is not found in one of these alternatives, then it may be found in rarer causes, either genetically based or disease-induced.

Growth hormone, also called somatotropin, determines a person's height. Growth hormone does not affect brain growth but may influence the brain's functions. In addition, it may enhance the growth of nerves

---

> **INFORMATION ON DWARFISM**
>
> **CAUSES:** Genetic or endocrinological dysfunctions
>
> **SYMPTOMS:** Short stature, higher-than-average body fat, high forehead, wrinkled skin, high-pitched voice, episodic hypoglycemia during childhood, late onset of puberty
>
> **DURATION:** Lifelong
>
> **TREATMENTS:** Growth hormone

---

radiating from the brain so that they can reach their targets. Growth hormone elevates the appetite, increases metabolic rate, maintains the immune system, and works in coordination with other hormones to regulate carbohydrate, protein, lipid, nucleic acid, water, and electrolyte metabolism. Target areas for growth hormone include cell membranes, as well as other cell organelles, in bone, cartilage, bone marrow, adipose tissue, and the liver, kidney, heart, pancreas, mammary glands, ovaries, testes, thymus gland, and hypothalamus. Fetuses not producing growth hormone still grow normally until birth; they may even weigh more than average at birth. These babies may thrive at first, but if no growth hormone is administered, they will be "miniature" adults with a maximum height of two and a half feet. Other telltale physical attributes include higher-than-average body fat, a high forehead, wrinkled skin, and a high-pitched voice. During childhood, there may be episodic hypoglycemia attacks. If the endocrine system is functioning properly, puberty may be delayed but still will occur. Complete reproductive maturity will be reached, and there is great likelihood that the afflicted person will develop his or her complete intellectual potential. When it is inherited, growth hormone deficiency occurs as an autosomal recessive trait. Yet the genetic basis for growth hormone deficiency may not simply be caused by a gene. The condition could, in theory, be the result of a structural defect in the pituitary gland or the hypothalamus, or in the secretory mechanisms of growth hormone itself.

Prenatal thyroid dysfunction that goes untreated results in cretinism. Cretins do not undergo nervous, skeletal, or reproductive maturation; they may not grow over thirty inches tall. Before two months of age, treatment can cause a complete reversal of symptoms. Delayed treatment, however, cannot reverse brain damage, although growth and reproductive organs can be dramatically affected.

Achondroplasia is inherited as an autosomal dominant form of short-limb dwarfism. Only when one dominant gene is inherited is achondroplasia expressed; when an offspring inherits the dominant gene from both parents, the condition is lethal. Incidence of achondroplasia increases with parental age and is more closely related to the father's age. Mutations may account for a majority of cases of achondroplasia, since in only 15 to 20 percent of cases is there an afflicted parent. Achondroplasia results from abnormal embryonic development that affects bone growth; metaphyseal development is prevented, which means that cartilaginous bone growth is impaired. This impairment is accompanied by unusually small laminae of the spine, resulting in spinal stenosis. The spinal cord may become compressed during the normal process of spondylosis. These individuals may experience slowly progressing spastic weakness of the legs as a result of the spinal cord compression. The torso may be normal, but the head will be disproportionately large and the limbs may be dwarfed and curved. In addition, there will be a prominent forehead and a depressed nasal bridge. A shallow thoracic cage and pelvic tilt may cause a protuberant abdomen. Bowlegs are caused by overly long fibulae. Many infants so affected are stillborn. Those surviving to adulthood are typically three feet to five feet tall and have unusual muscular strength; reproductive and mental development are not affected, and neither is longevity.

Marasmus, severe emaciation resulting from malnutrition prenatally or in early infancy, may be considered a form of dwarfism. It is caused by extremely low caloric and protein intake, which causes a wasting of body tissues. Usually marasmus is found in babies either weaned very early or never breast-fed. All growth is retarded, including head circumference. If the area housing the brain fails to grow, then it cannot house a normal-sized brain, and some degree of retardation will occur. Not only is growth stunted, but such infants will be apathetic and hyperirritable as well. As they lie in bed, they are completely unresponsive to their environment and are irritable when moved or handled. Although the symptoms are treatable and may disappear, the growth failure is permanent.

Occasionally, dwarfism may be induced by emotional starvation. This type of child abuse causes extreme growth retardation, inhibition of skeletal growth, and delayed psychomotor development. Fortunately, it can be reversed by social and dietary changes. These children are extremely small but perfectly proportioned; however, they have distended abdomens.

The height achieved in females with Turner syndrome is typically between four and a half and five feet. Turner syndrome results when an egg has no X chromosome and is fertilized by an X-bearing sperm. The offspring are females with only one X; their ovaries never develop and are unable to function. These individuals cannot undergo puberty; physical manifestations of Turner syndrome include short stature, stocky build, and a webbed neck.

Another cause of short stature may be as a consequence of chronic disease. Children suffering from chronic renal (kidney) failure nearly always experience growth retardation because of hormonal, metabolic, and nutritional abnormalities, effects seen in 35 to 65 percent of children with renal failure. The failure to grow occurs more often in children with congenital renal disease than in those with acquired renal disease.

With congenital heart disease, several factors may prohibit growth. Growth failure may be a direct result of the disease or an indirect result of other problems associated with heart disease. These babies experience stress, with periods of cardiac failure, and either caloric or protein deficiency. These inadequacies grossly slow the multiplication of cells and hence growth. If surgery corrects the condition, some catching up can be expected, but normal growth is dependent on how much time has elapsed without treatment.

Treatment and Therapy

In the United States population in 1992, there were roughly five million people of short stature, with 40 percent of this number under the age of twenty-one. The more a child is below the average stature, the greater is the likelihood of determining the cause. A child who is short-statured should be evaluated so that, if an endocrine disorder is the root, the child can be treated. Time is an important consideration with hypothyroidism especially, since the longer it goes untreated, the more likely it is that mental development will be arrested.

Children born with congenital growth hormone deficiency are sometimes small for their gestational age; however, the majority of growth hormone-deficient children acquire the disorder after birth. The first year or two, the children grow normally; then growth dramatically decreases. Diagnosis of growth hormone deficiency requires numerous tests and sampling. If bone age appears the same as the child's age, then growth hormone deficiency can be eliminated. A test for normal growth hormone secretion is done by measuring a blood sample for growth hormone twenty minutes after exercise in a fasting child. If this test shows a hormone deficiency, then growth hormone therapy may help the child overcome the obstacles of being labeled "short."

At first, growth hormone was harvested from human pituitary glands after persons' deaths. This process was so expensive, however, that few children with hormone deficiency could be treated. Even worse, some of those who did get this treatment were inadvertently infected with a slow-acting virus that proved fatal. In the mid-1980's, it was found that some men who had received human growth hormone died at an early age of a neurological disorder called Creutzfeldt-Jakob disease (CJD). These men were found to have been given the disease via a growth hormone that had been obtained from pituitary glands during autopsies. Once the relationship was determined, more victims were traced. CJD is a nervous disorder caused by a slow-acting, viruslike particle. Its symptoms include difficulty in balance while walking, loss of muscular control, slurred speech, impairment of vision, and other muscular disorders including spasticity and rigidity. Behavioral changes and mental incapacities may also occur (memory loss, confusion, dementia). The symptoms appear, progress rapidly over the next months, and usually cause death in less than a year. There is no treatment or cure.

These unfortunate circumstances led to the development of a synthetic growth hormone. It is made by encoding bacterial deoxyribonucleic acid (DNA) with the sequence of human growth hormone; the bacteria used are those that grow normally in the human intestinal tract. The bacteria synthesize human growth hormone using the preprogrammed human sequence of DNA; it is then purified so that no bacteria remain in the hormone that is used for treatment. The Food and Drug Administration (FDA) approved the biosynthetic hormone in 1985. The sole difference between the synthetic and the naturally produced growth hormone was one amino acid; in 1987, a new synthetic form without the extra amino acid became available. This synthetic hormone works exactly as natural growth hormone does. Moreover, it does not carry the danger of contamination attributed to human growth hormone. In most cases, the patient's immune system fails to interfere with the synthetic growth hormone's effectiveness. In fact, no major health-threatening side effects have surfaced in using artificial growth hormone. In 1992, more than 150,000 growth hormone-deficient children

in the United States were receiving growth hormone therapy.

Those children suffering from various forms of chondrodystrophies (cartilage disorders), such as achondroplasia, are diagnosed by using skeletal measurements, clinical manifestations, X rays, laboratory study and analysis of cartilage, and observed abnormalities of the body's proteins, such as collagen and cell membranes. In chondrodystrophies, skeletal growth is disproportionate, with shortened limbs more common than a shortened trunk. If visual examination is not confirmation enough, the diagnosis may be assured through X rays. Although histological studies do not necessarily enhance diagnosis, making an analysis of the patient's cartilage may lead to a better understanding of the disease. Biochemical studies of abnormal proteins in chondrodystrophies actually have little diagnostic value, but they too may lead to better understanding. Because achondroplasia is genetically inherited, prevention of the affliction involves genetic counseling before conception.

A child so affected may be treated symptomatically; surgery on the fibulae to correct bowlegs may be desirable, either for cosmetic reasons or for functional reasons. Laminectomies or skull surgery may be indicated for neurological problems. If hearing loss occurs because of recurrent ear infections, then corrective surgery may be necessary. Achondroplasiacs generally enjoy a normal life span, barring complications.

Other chondrodystrophies that cause dwarfism may have more severe symptoms than achondroplasia. Cockayne syndrome, a type of progeria, is the sudden onset of premature old age in extremely young children. It is the result of inheritance of an autosomal recessive gene. Physical signs of the disease begin after a normal first year of life. In the second year, growth begins to falter, and psychomotor development becomes abnormal. As time passes, dwarfism, and sometimes mental retardation, becomes evident. Other observable characteristics that develop are a shrunken face with sunken eyes and a thin nose, optic degeneration, cavities of the teeth, a photosensitive skin rash that produces scarring, disproportionately long limbs with large hands and feet, and hair loss. The life span for children with this disease is very short.

Another chondrodystrophy inherited through autosomal recessive genes is thanotophoric dwarfism. All known cases have died during the first four weeks of life as a result of respiratory distress; most are stillborn. Postnatal death occurs as a result of an extremely small thoracic cage with only eleven pairs of ribs present. Other physical characteristics of the disease are that the infant has a large skull relative to its face, which is often elongated with a prominent forehead. The eyes are widely spaced, and there is a broad, flat nasal bridge. Frequently, cleft palate is present. The ears are low-set and poorly formed, and the neck is short and fleshy. The limbs, particularly the legs, are bowed; clubfoot is common, as are dislocated hip joints.

A small percentage of short-statured individuals may be unusually short because of social and psychological factors. This condition is called psychosocial dwarfism. This type of nongrowth is secondary to emotional deprivation and is representative of a type of child abuse. The behavior of such children is characterized by apathy and inadequate interpersonal relationships, with retarded motor and language development. They generally do not gain weight in spite of their extraordinary appetite and excessive thirst; such a child may steal and hoard food yet have the distended abdomen of a starving child. Diagnosis generally identifies a growth hormone deficiency, and when these children are moved to stimulating and accepting environments, their behavior becomes more normal. Their caloric intake decreases as their growth hormone secretion becomes normal, and their growth undergoes a dramatic catch-up.

Perspective and Prospects

Dwarfism is certainly not a new phenomenon. Two well-known Egyptian deities, Bes and Ptah, are represented as dwarfs. At one time, short-statured individuals were attractions in the royal courts. Jeffery Hudson, a favorite of Charles I of England, is said to have been only eighteen inches high at the age of thirty, and Bébé, the celebrated dwarf in the court of Stanisław I of Poland, was thirty-three inches tall. More recently, perfectly proportioned dwarfs have made a living by working in circuses and sideshows. It is likely that the best known of these individuals was P. T. Barnum's General Tom Thumb (Charles Stratton), who at twenty-five was thirty-one inches tall.

Today, because of the negative consequences of being short-statured, counseling should begin early. Counseling would be preceded by a physical examination to determine the nature of the affliction. If it is ascertained that the short stature cannot be treated, both patient and parents should be informed of the nature of the disease. The patient should be assured that intelligence will not be affected, even if the head is somewhat large. Ear infections are common, and the child should be closely watched to avoid hearing loss. Normal fertility is the rule, but giving birth will necessitate a cesarean section. These characteristics of a majority of dwarfism cases should assure families that, as the child matures, he or she will not be limited physically or mentally. The problems that the patients may face usually deal with social and emotional consequences. Short-statured children will usually be thought younger than their age; finding appropriate clothes and shoes may be difficult. Children are often cruel, and as afflicted individuals are highly noticeable, they may be the butt of jokes and teasing and will experience discrimination on many fronts. Seeking affiliation with support groups may aid in coping with the difficulties that a short-statured person will undoubtedly meet.

The rate at which those diagnosed with dwarfism develop psychologically is directly related to two components: if their parents treat them according to their age rather than their size, and if they can cope with the notoriety that their size brings them. It is common for such children to lag in development; personality traits often exhibited with delayed maturation are withdrawal, inhibition, dissociation, and learning problems. There have been no observed tendencies toward aggression or acting out. Inhibition and withdrawal are likely if affected children are appalled by their notoriety; if they use it to measure popularity, they may act the clown to minimize their size difference.

—*Iona C. Baldridge*

See also Congenital heart disease; Cornelia de Lange syndrome; Endocrine disorders; Endocrinology; Endocrinology, pediatric; Gigantism; Growth; Hormones; Rubinstein-Taybi syndrome.

For Further Information:

Brooks, S. J., and Robert S. Bar. *Early Diagnosis and Treatment of Endocrine Disorders.* Totowa, N.J.: Humana Press, 2003. Reviews the early signs and symptoms of common endocrine diseases, surveys the clinical testing needed for a diagnosis, and presents recommendations for therapy.

Juul, Anders, and Jens O. L. Jorgensen, eds. *Growth Hormone in Adults: Physiological and Clinical Aspects.* 2d ed. New York: Cambridge University Press, 2000. This book examines the use of somatotropin on adults to treat dwarfism.

Kelly, Thaddeus E. *Clinical Genetics and Genetic Counseling.* 2d ed. Chicago: Year Book Medical, 1986. This text of genetic disorders and their treatment was written to aid medical students and physicians. Aside from the sometimes difficult medical terminology, the case illustrations and discussions of genetic counseling are interesting.

Little People of America. http://www.lpaonline.org/. A nonprofit organization that provides support and information to people of short stature and their families. Web site offers a research library, FAQs, chatrooms, and information on local chapters.

Morgan, Brian L. G., and Roberta Morgan. *Hormones: How They Affect Behavior, Metabolism, Growth, Development, and Relationships*. Los Angeles: Price, Stern, Sloan, 1989. A book written for use by the general reader as a resource on hormones and their roles in the human body. Very readable, it also contains sections about hormonal diseases and includes a bibliography.

Shaw, Michael, ed. *Everything You Need to Know About Diseases*. Springhouse, Pa.: Springhouse Press, 1996. This well-illustrated consumer reference, compiled by more than one hundred doctors and medical experts, describes five hundred illnesses and conditions, their causes, symptoms, diagnosis, treatment, and prevention. Of particular interest is chapter 21, "Genetic Disorders."

Wilson, Jean D. *Wilson's Textbook of Endocrinology*. 10th ed. New York: Elsevier, 2003. Text that covers the spectrum of information related to the endocrine system, including dwarfism, thyroid disorders, diabetes, and endocrine hypertension.

DYSENTERY. *See* DIARRHEA AND DYSENTERY.

DYSLEXIA

DISEASE/DISORDER

ANATOMY OR SYSTEM AFFECTED: Brain, ears, eyes, nervous system, psychic-emotional system

SPECIALTIES AND RELATED FIELDS: Audiology, neurology, psychology, speech pathology

DEFINITION: Severe reading disability in children with average to above-average intelligence.

KEY TERMS:

auditory dyslexia: the inability to perceive individual sounds that are associated with written language

cognitive: relating to the mental process by which knowledge is acquired

computed tomography (CT) scan: a detailed X-ray picture that identifies abnormalities of fine tissue structure

dysgraphia: illegible handwriting resulting from impaired hand-eye coordination

electroencephalogram: a graphic record of the brain's electrical activity

imprinting: training that overcomes reading problems by use of repeated, exaggerated language drills

kinesthetic: related to sensation of body position, presence, or movement, resulting mostly from the stimulation of sensory nerves in muscles, tendons, and joints

phonetics: the science of speech sounds; also called phonology

visual dyslexia: the inability to translate observed written or printed language into meaningful terms

CAUSES AND SYMPTOMS

Nearly 25 percent of the individuals in the United States and in many other industrialized societies who otherwise possess at least average intelligence cannot read well. Many such people are viewed as suffering from a neurological disorder called dyslexia. This term was first introduced by the German ophthalmologist Rudolf Berlin in the nineteenth century. Berlin defined it as designating all those individuals who possessed average or above-average intelligence quotients (IQs) but who could not read adequately because of their inability to process language symbols. At the same time as Berlin and later, others reported on dyslexic children. These children saw everything perfectly well but acted as if they were blind to all written language. For example, they could see a bird flying but were unable to identify the written word "bird" seen in a sentence.

The problem involved in dyslexia has been defined and redefined many times, since its introduction. The modern definition of the disorder, which is close to Berlin's definition, is based on long-term, extensive studies of dyslexic children. These studies have identified dyslexia as a complex syndrome composed of a large number of associated behavioral dysfunctions that are related to visual-motor brain immaturity and/or brain dysfunction. These problems include a poor memory for details, easy distractibility, poor motor skills, visual letter and word reversal, and the inability to distinguish between important elements of the spoken language.

Understanding dyslexia in order to correct this reading disability is crucial and difficult. To learn to read well, an individual must acquire many basic cognitive and linguistic skills. First, it is necessary to pay close attention, to concentrate, to follow directions, and to understand the language spoken in daily life. Next, one must develop an auditory and visual memory, strong sequencing ability, solid word decoding skills, the ability to carry out structural-contextual language analysis, the capability to interpret the written language, a solid vocabulary which expands as quickly as is needed, and speed in scanning and interpreting written language. These skills are taught in good developmental reading programs, but some or all are found to be deficient in dyslexic individuals.

Two basic explanations have evolved for dyslexia. Many physicians propose that it is caused by brain damage or brain dysfunction. Evolution of the problem is attributed to accident, disease, and/or hereditary faults in body biochemistry. Here, the diagnosis of dyslexia is made by the use of electroencephalograms (EEGs), computed tomography (CT) scans, and related neurological technology. After such evaluation is complete, medication is often used to diminish hyperactivity and nervousness, and a group of physical training procedures called patterning is used to counter the neurological defects in the dyslexic individual.

In contrast, many special educators and other researchers believe that the problem of dyslexia is one of dormant, immature, or undeveloped learning centers in the brain. Many proponents of this concept strongly encourage the correction of dyslexic problems by the teaching of specific reading skills. While such experts agree that the use of medication can be of great value, they attempt to cure dyslexia mostly through a process called imprinting. This technique essentially trains dyslexic individuals and corrects their problems via the use of exaggerated, repeated language drills.

Another interesting point of view, expressed by some experts, is the idea that dyslexia may be the fault of the written languages of the Western world. For example, Rudolf F. Wagner notes that Japanese children exhibit an incidence of dyslexia that is less than 1 percent. The explanation for this, say Wagner and others, is that unlike Japanese, the languages of Western countries require both reading from left to right and phonetic word attack. These characteristics—absent in Japanese—may make the Western languages either much harder to learn or much less suitable for learning.

A number of experts propose three types of dyslexia. The most common type and the one most often identified as dyslexia is called visual dyslexia, the lack of ability to translate the observed written or printed language into meaningful terms. The major difficulty is that afflicted people see certain words or letters backward or upside down. The resultant problem is that—to the visual dyslexic—any written sentence is a jumble of many letters whose accurate translation may require five or more times as much effort as is needed by an unafflicted person. The other two problems viewed as dyslexia are auditory dyslexia and dysgraphia. Auditory dyslexia is the inability to perceive individual sounds of spoken language. Despite having normal hearing, auditory dyslexics are deaf to the differences between certain vowel and/or consonant sounds, and what they cannot hear they cannot write. Dysgraphia is the inability to write legibly. The basis for this problem is a lack of the hand-eye coordination that is required to write clearly.

Many children who suffer from visual dyslexia also exhibit elements of auditory dyslexia. This complicates the issue of teaching many dyslexic students because only one type of dyslexic symptom can be treated at a time. Also, dyslexia appears to be a sex-linked disorder, being much more common in boys than in girls. Estimates vary between three and seven times as many boys having dyslexia as girls.

Treatment and Therapy

The early diagnosis and treatment of dyslexia is essential to its eventual correction. Many experts agree that if a treatment begins before the third grade, there is an 80 percent probability that the dyslexia can be corrected. If the disorder remains undetected until the fifth grade, however, success at treating dyslexia is cut in half. If treatment does not begin until the seventh grade, the

---

INFORMATION ON DYSLEXIA

Causes: Unknown; possibly neurological disorder from accident, disease, or hereditary faults in body biochemistry; dormant, immature, or undeveloped learning centers in the brain

Symptoms: Poor written schoolwork, easy distractibility, clumsiness, poor coordination, poor spatial orientation, confused writing and/or spelling, poor left-right orientation

Duration: Often long term

Treatments: Medication, patterning, teaching of specific reading skills and repeated language drills (imprinting)

b   d

p   q

on   no

Dyslexia may make it difficult to distinguish letters and words that are mirror images of each other, thus making it difficult for an otherwise intelligent child to learn to read.

probability of successful treatment drops below 5 percent.

The preliminary identification of a dyslexic child can be made from symptoms that include poor written schoolwork, easy distractibility, clumsiness, poor coordination, poor spatial orientation, confused writing and/or spelling, and poor left-right orientation. Because numerous nondyslexic children also show many of these symptoms, a second step is required for such identification: the use of written tests designed to identify dyslexics. These tests include the Peabody Individual Achievement Test, the Halstead-Reitan Neuropsychological Test Battery, and the SOYBAR Criterion Tests.

Electroencephalograms and CT scans are often performed in the hope of pinning down concrete brain abnormalities in dyslexic patients. There is considerable disagreement, however, over the value of these techniques, beyond finding evidence of tumors or severe brain damage—both of which may indicate that the condition observed is not dyslexia. Most researchers agree that children who seem to be dyslexic but who lack tumors or damage are no more likely to have EEG or CT scan abnormalities than nondyslexics. An interesting adjunct to EEG use is a technique called brain electrical activity mapping (BEAM). BEAM converts an EEG into a brain map. Viewed by some workers in the area as a valuable technique, BEAM is contested by many others.

Once conclusive identification of a dyslexic child has been made, it becomes possible to begin corrective treatment. Such treatment is usually the preserve of special education programs. These programs are carried out by the special education teacher in school resource rooms. They also involve special classes limited to children with reading disabilities and schools that specialize in treating learning disabilities.

An often-cited method used is that of Grace Fernald, which utilizes kinesthetic imprinting, based on combined language experience and tactile stimulation. In this popular method or adaptations of it, a dyslexic child learns to read in the following way. First, the child tells a spontaneous story to the teacher, who transcribes it. Next, each word that is unknown to the child is written down by the teacher, and the child traces its letters repeatedly until he or she can write the word without using the model. Each word learned becomes part of the child's word file. A large number of stories are handled this way. Though the method is quite slow, many reports praise its results. Nevertheless, no formal studies of its effectiveness have been made.

A second common teaching technique used by special educators is the Orton-Gillingham-Stillman method, which was developed in a collaboration between two teachers and a pediatric neurologist, Samuel T. Orton. The method evolved from Orton's conceptualization of language as developing from a sequence of processes in the nervous system that ends in its unilateral control by the left cerebral hemisphere. He proposed that dyslexia arises from conflicts between this cerebral hemisphere and the right cerebral hemisphere, which is usually involved in the handling of nonverbal, pictorial, and spatial stimuli.

Consequently, the corrective method that is used is a multisensory and kinesthetic approach, like that of Fernald. It begins, however, with the teaching of individual letters and phonemes. Then, it progresses to dealing with syllables, words, and sentences. Children taught by this method are drilled systematically, to imprint them with a mastery of phonics and the sounding out of unknown written words. They are encouraged to learn how the elements of written language look, how they sound, how it feels to pronounce them, and how it feels to write them down. Although the Orton-Gillingham-Stillman method is as laborious as that of Fernald, it is widely used and appears to be successful.

Another treatment aspect that merits discussion is the use of therapeutic drugs in the handling of dyslexia. Most physicians and educators propose the use of these drugs as a useful adjunct to the special education training of those dyslexic children who are restless and easily distracted and who have low morale because of continued embarrassment in school in front of their peers. The drugs that are utilized most often are amphetamine, Dexedrine, and methylphenidate (Ritalin).

These stimulants, given at appropriate dose levels, will lengthen the time period during which certain dyslexic children function well in the classroom and can also produce feelings of self-confidence. Side effects of their overuse, however, include loss of appetite, nausea, nervousness, and sleeplessness. Furthermore, there is also the potential problem of drug abuse. When they are administered carefully and under close medical supervision, however, the benefits of these drugs far outweigh any possible risks.

A proponent of an entirely medical treatment of dyslexia is psychiatrist Harold N. Levinson. He proposes that the root of dyslexia is in inner ear dysfunction and that it can be treated with the judicious application of proper medications. Levinson's treatment includes amphetamines, antihistamines, drugs used against motion sickness, vitamins, health food components, and nutrients mixed in the proper combination for each patient. He asserts that he has cured more than ten thousand dyslexics and documents many cases. Critics of Levinson's work pose several questions, including whether the studies reported were well controlled and whether the patients treated were actually dyslexics. A major basis for the latter criticism is Levinson's statement that many of his cured patients were described to him as outstanding students. The contention is that dyslexic students are never outstanding students and cannot work at expected age levels.

An important aspect of dyslexia treatment is parental support of these children. Such emotional support helps dyslexics to cope with their problems and with the judgment of their peers. Useful aspects of this support include a positive attitude toward an afflicted child, appropriate home help that complements efforts at school, encouragement and praise for achievements, lack of recrimination when repeated mistakes are made, and positive interaction with special education teachers.

PERSPECTIVE AND PROSPECTS

The identification of dyslexia by German physician Rudolf Berlin and England's W. A. Morgan began the efforts to solve this unfortunate disorder. In 1917, Scot-

tish eye surgeon James Hinshelwood published a book on dyslexia, which he viewed as being a hereditary problem, and the phenomenon became much better known to many physicians.

Attempts at educating dyslexics were highly individualized until the endeavors of Orton and his coworkers and of Fernald led to more standardized and widely used methods. These procedures, their adaptations, and several others not mentioned here had become the standard treatments for dyslexia by the late twentieth century.

Interestingly, many famous people—including Hans Christian Andersen, Winston Churchill, Albert Einstein, General George Patton, and Woodrow Wilson—had symptoms of dyslexia, which they subsequently overcame. This was fortunate for them, because adults who remain dyslexic are very often at a great disadvantage. In many cases in modern society, such people are among the functionally illiterate and the poor. Job opportunities open to dyslexics of otherwise adequate intelligence are quite limited.

Furthermore, with the development of a more complete understanding of the brain and its many functions, better counseling facilities, and the conceptualization and actualization of both parent-child and parent-counselor interactions, the probability of success in dyslexic training has improved greatly. Moreover, while environmental and socioeconomic factors contribute relatively little to the occurrence of dyslexia, they strongly affect the outcome of its treatment.

The endeavors of special education have so far made the greatest inroads in the treatment of dyslexia. It is hoped that many more advances in the area will be made as the science of the mind grows and diversifies, and the contributions of psychologists, physicians, physiologists, and special educators mesh even more effectively. Perhaps BEAM or the therapeutic methodology suggested by Levinson may provide or contribute to definitive understanding of and treatment of dyslexia.

—Sanford S. Singer, Ph.D.
See also Learning disabilities.

FOR FURTHER INFORMATION:

Huston, Anne Marshall. *Understanding Dyslexia: A Practical Approach for Parents and Teachers.* Rev. ed. Lanham, Md.: Madison Books, 1992. Explains dyslexia, describes its three main types, identifies causes and treatments, and covers useful teaching techniques. A bibliography, a useful glossary, appendices, and teaching materials are valuable additions.

International Dyslexia Association. http://www.interdys.org/index.jsp. Web site includes a bookstore and information on new assistive technology. Site is divided into sections for children, teens, college students, adults, educators, and parents.

Jordan, Dale R. *Overcoming Dyslexia in Children, Adolescent, and Adults*. Austin, Tex.: Pro-Ed, 2002. Examines the role of genetics and brain development in relation to learning disabilities and explains the perceptual and emotional nature of dyslexia. Eight "success stories," strategies for improving academic performance and social skills, and assessment checklists are included.

Levinson, Harold N. *Smart but Feeling Dumb*. Rev. ed. New York: Warner Books, 2003. Argues that the basis of dyslexia and other disorders is an inner ear dysfunction that can be cured with judicious application of the correct medications. Also discusses adults and families with dyslexia, speech disorders, and attention deficit disorders.

Reid, Gavin, and Jane Kirk. *Dyslexia in Adults*. New York: John Wiley & Sons, 2001. Offers a comprehensive guide for professionals to working with adults with dyslexia in the learning and working environment.

Routh, Donald K. "Disorders of Learning." In *The Practical Assessment and Management of Children with Disorders of Development and Learning*, edited by Mark L. Wolraich. Chicago: Year Book Medical, 1987. This succinct article summarizes salient facts about learning disorders, including etiology, assessment, management, and outcome.

Snowling, Margaret. *Dyslexia: A Cognitive Developmental Perspective*. 2d ed. New York: Basil Blackwell, 2000. Covers aspects of dyslexia, including its identification, associated cognitive defects, the basis for language skill development, and the importance of phonetics.

DYSMENORRHEA
DISEASE/DISORDER

ANATOMY OR SYSTEM AFFECTED: Reproductive system, uterus

SPECIALTIES AND RELATED FIELDS: Gynecology

DEFINITION: A common menstrual disorder characterized by painful menstrual flow that is more severe than the usual cramps experienced by women with menstruation.

CAUSES AND SYMPTOMS

Dysmenorrhea is classified into primary and secondary dysmenorrhea. In primary dysmenorrhea, no organic cause of the menstrual pain is found, although multiple theories exist in the medical literature as to why pain occurs. Dysmenorrhea is associated with a number of psychological symptoms, including depression, irritability, and insomnia, although it is not clear whether these psychological symptoms are causes or effects.

Secondary dysmenorrhea is painful menstruation that occurs in the setting of known pelvic disease, such as endometriosis, adenomyosis, infection such as endometritis or pelvic inflammatory disease (PID), or anatomic abnormalities such as uterine fibroids or developmental abnormalities of the uterus, cervix, or vagina.

The symptoms of dysmenorrhea involve dull lower abdominal pain or cramping at the midline. The discomfort may radiate to the lower back or thighs. It can be associated with a number of other symptoms, most commonly nausea and vomiting or fatigue. Dysmenorrhea can occur up to one to two days before the onset of menstrual flow and usually lasts for forty-eight to seventy-two hours. The most severe pain usually occurs on the first day of menstrual flow.

TREATMENT AND THERAPY

Treatment is recommended if dysmenorrhea interferes with activities of daily living. The two most common treatments are hormones and prostaglandin synthetase inhibitors. In women who do not desire pregnancy, oral

---

INFORMATION ON DYSMENORRHEA

CAUSES: Primary type unknown but associated with psychological symptoms (depression, irritability, insomnia); secondary type caused by pelvic disease (endometriosis or adenomyosis), infection (endometritis or pelvic inflammatory disease), or anatomic abnormalities (uterine fibroids or developmental abnormalities of uterus, cervix, or vagina)

SYMPTOMS: Dull lower abdominal pain or cramping radiating to lower back or thighs; associated with nausea, vomiting, fatigue

DURATION: Two or three days

TREATMENTS: Hormones, prostaglandin synthetase inhibitors, treatment of underlying condition

contraceptive pills are an effective method of controlling dysmenorrhea, as they can reduce the volume of blood flow and the number of menstrual periods a woman has, if the pills are taken in continuous fashion.

In women nearing the menopause, hormones that artificially induce the menopause can serve as a bridge until natural menopause occurs. In women with primary dysmenorrhea whose symptoms do not improve after six to twelve months of medical treatment, laparoscopy may be considered to search for organic causes of pain.

In secondary dysmenorrhea, the treatment of any underlying pelvic disease may ameliorate the symptoms. For instance, any anatomic abnormalities may be amenable to surgery. Endometriosis may be treated with hormones or removal procedures.

Pain from either primary or secondary amenorrhea is often responsive to prostaglandin synthetase inhibitors, such as ibuprofen. These drugs decrease the levels of prostaglandins (which cause uterine cramping) in the menstrual blood. Patients with psychological symptoms accompanying their dysmenorrhea may benefit from psychological counseling and therapy. In cases of dysmenorrhea that resist standard treatment, a number of alternate treatments have been tried, with varying levels of success. They include nonspecific analgesics (such as opioids), acupuncture, and even surgical procedures such as presacral neurectomy, the interruption of the nerves going to the uterus.

—*Anne Lynn S. Chang, M.D.*

See also Endometriosis; Gynecology; Hormones; Menstruation; Pain; Pain management; Pelvic inflammatory disease (PID); Premenstrual syndrome (PMS); Reproductive system.

FOR FURTHER INFORMATION:

Braunwald, Eugene, et al., eds. *Harrison's Principles of Internal Medicine*. 15th ed. New York: McGraw-Hill, 2001.

Stenchever, Morton A, ed. *Comprehensive Gynecology*. 4th ed. St. Louis: Mosby, 2001.

Tierney, Lawrence M., Stephen J. McPhee, and Maxine A. Papadakis, eds. *Current Medical Diagnosis and Treatment 2004*. 43d ed. Stamford, Conn.: Appleton & Lange, 2003.

DYSPHASIA. *See* APHASIA AND DYSPHASIA.

E. COLI INFECTION
DISEASE/DISORDER

ANATOMY OR SYSTEM AFFECTED: Blood, cells, gastrointestinal system, immune system, intestines, nervous system, urinary system

SPECIALTIES AND RELATED FIELDS: Bacteriology, cytology, epidemiology, gastroenterology, internal medicine, microbiology, neonatology, nephrology, public health, urology

DEFINITION: Infection with a rod-shaped, anaerobic, self-propelling bacterium of the family Enterobacteriaceae. It normally inhabits mammal intestines without ill effect, but some strains can cause life-threatening illness.

KEY TERMS:

intestines: the bowel, a two-part tube (the small intestine and the large intestine, or colon) connecting the stomach and anus; it absorbs nutrients from food

mucosa: a mucus-secreting membrane lining the bowel wall

strain: a subgroup in a species

toxin: a substance, usually a protein made by a cell, that causes injury

CAUSES AND SYMPTOMS

Escherichia coli (*E. coli*), the organism most often used for experiments in microbiology, is the best understood type of cell. These bacteria dwell in large numbers in the colons of mammals and constitute a major part of normal feces. More than 250 strains of *E. coli* are known, nearly all harmless to humans, although some may sicken other mammals. Scientists classify those strains that are toxic to humans according to the manner in which they cause disease (pathogenesis). People infected with the bacteria do not always develop symptoms.

Enterotoxigenic *E. coli* (ETEC) strains are the most common source of "travelers' diarrhea" in the United States and Europe. They colonize the small intestine and make it secrete fluid rather than absorb fluid. The result may be watery diarrhea. The afflicted person does not have a fever or inflammation of the bowel wall, which is not damaged by the bacteria.

Enteropathogenic *E. coli* (EPEC) strains attack the lower section of the small intestine, the ileum. Binding tightly to the mucosa cells, they damage the bowel wall. The infected person may feel cramps and have bloody diarrhea (dysentery).

Enterohemorrhagic *E. coli* (EHEC) strains can inflame the colon, damaging the mucosa and causing bleeding and severe cramps, a condition known as hemorrhagic colitis. In some cases, toxins absorbed through the bowel wall enter the bloodstream and travel to the kidneys. There, the glomeruli are attacked and red blood cells are destroyed, a condition called hemolytic-uremic syndrome (HUS). The infected person will have difficulty urinating, and the urine will contain blood products such as hemoglobin. Fever may ensue, and the kidneys may fail, potentially a fatal condition. A related condition, thrombotic thrombocytopenic purpura, in which platelets and red blood cells are destroyed, produces high fever, vomiting, cramps, and damage to one or more organs. Untreated, it is almost always fatal.

Enteroinvasive *E. coli* (EIEC) strains penetrate the mucosa of the colon. The result is intense inflammation and moderate dysentery. A related set of strains afflict infants less than six months of age; the diarrhea may persist for weeks, and the resulting malnutrition and dehydration can be fatal. These strains are rare in the United States.

E. coli strains that enter the bloodstream can cause inflammation when they lodge and multiply in a localized part of the body: meningitis in the spine, prostatitis in the prostate gland, or cystitis in the bladder. After infection, people with depressed immune systems, such as those with acquired immunodeficiency syndrome (AIDS), may develop septicemia—blood poisoning throughout the body that can harm organs and cause sudden fevers, vomiting, skin eruptions, diarrhea, and, if persistent, death.

TREATMENT AND THERAPY

There is no specific treatment for *E. coli* infection. Medical research recommends managing the symptoms and providing supportive therapy while waiting

---

INFORMATION ON *E. COLI* INFECTION

CAUSES: Bacterial infection

SYMPTOMS: Stomach cramping, fever, watery or bloody diarrhea, bowel wall inflammation, difficulty urinating, platelet and red blood cell destruction, organ damage

DURATION: Acute

TREATMENTS: None; symptom management and supportive therapy

for the body's immune system to clear the disease on its own. Thus, doctors seek to reduce fever, stop diarrhea, and ensure that the patient gets nourishment and enough fluid to prevent dehydration. Bed rest is often necessary in moderate and severe cases.

If the infection leads to a secondary disease, such as HUS, then doctors treat symptoms vigorously. Dialysis can support patients during kidney failure. Infusions of plasma can amend anemia from blood loss. A variety of medications can be taken to reduce the inflammation in such disorders as meningitis and prostatitis.

Most studies do not recommend antibiotics for killing E. coli bacteria. Clinical trials have not shown that such treatments help the patient. On the contrary, antibacterial medications appear to increase the patient's chance of developing a secondary condition, particularly HUS. Use of antidiarrheal drugs may also foster HUS.

PERSPECTIVES AND PROSPECTS

German biochemist Theodor Escherich (1857-1911) first isolated *Escherichia coli* in 1884; the species is named after him. The bacteria were best known as the "laboratory rats" of microbiologists until several outbreaks of the O157:H7 EHEC strain attracted public attention in the 1990's. *E. coli* bacteria spread most often from food or beverages contaminated by feces of cattle and humans. Hamburger was the usual culprit, although deer jerky, unpasteurized apple juice, milk, and bean sprouts have also been linked to outbreaks. Many secondary infections arose in people who had contact with those infected from foods. Dozens died, nearly all of them children or the elderly.

Proper food handling is the best defense against *E. coli:* Making sure that foods and liquids do not touch feces prevents the bacteria from spreading. If they do spread, the bacteria are relatively easy to kill. Pasteurization cleanses liquids; thorough cooking purifies meats and vegetables.

Studies in the mid-1990's found, unexpectedly, that some strains of *E. coli*—O157:H7, for example— mutate at an extremely high rate. Most mutations are harmless, but the chance of a new toxic variety is appreciable. Additionally, some types of *E. coli* have shown increasing resistance to antibiotics; however, epidemiologists deny that an *E. coli* strain such as O157:H7 could be an epidemic-causing "superbug." *E. coli* of all types cause less sickness in the United States than *Campylobacter*, *Salmonella*, and *Shigella* bacteria.

—*Roger Smith, Ph.D.*

See also Antibiotics; Bacterial infections; Bacteriology; Centers for Disease Control and Prevention (CDC); Colitis; Diarrhea and dysentery; Drug resistance; Food poisoning; Gastroenterology; Gastroenterology, pediatric; Gastrointestinal disorders; Gastrointestinal system; Infection; Intestinal disorders; Intestines; Meningitis; Microbiology; Mutation; Renal failure.

FOR FURTHER INFORMATION:

Biddle, Wayne. *Field Guide to Germs*. 2d ed. New York: Anchor Books, 2002. This comprehensive book is easily accessible to the nonspecialist and includes a discussion of nearly every virus, bacterium, and fungus known to cause human and nonhuman animal disease. The history of the microbe and the treatment of diseases are included.

Dixon, Bernard. *Power Unseen: How Microbes Rule the World*. New York: W. H. Freeman, 1996. This book portrays the many, diverse and often unexpected activities of microbes through a series of seventy-five vignettes, each focusing on one particular organism and its characteristic behavior. Dixon leaves the reader in no doubt that microbes, not macrobes, rule the world.

Lederberg, Joshua, ed. *Encyclopedia of Microbiology*. 2d ed. San Diego, Calif.: Academic Press, 2000. This encyclopedic reference source covers all aspects of microbiology. Includes bibliographical references and an index.

Parker, James N., and Philip M. Parker, eds. *The Official Patient's Sourcebook on E. Coli*. San Diego, Calif.: Icon Health, 2002. Draws from public, academic, government, and peer-reviewed research to provide a wide-ranging handbook for patients with *E. coli*.

Snyder, Larry, and Wendy Champness. *Molecular Genetics of Bacteria*. Rev. ed. Washington, D.C.: ASM Press, 2002. A text that introduces the field of bacterial molecular genetics and describes the mechanisms of mutations and gene exchange in bacteria and phages. Concentrates specifically on the bacterium *E. coli* while using examples from other bacteria as appropriate.

Sussman, Max, ed. *The Virulence of "Escherichia coli": Reviews and Methods*. London: Academic Press, 1985. This work is based on the Society for General Microbiology's Symposium "Virulence Markers of *Escherichia coli*," which took place in Newcastle-upon-Tyne, England, in January, 1983. Includes bibliographical references and an index.

Wilson, Michael, Brian Henderson, and Rod McNab. *Bacterial Virulence Mechanisms*. New York: Cambridge University Press, 2002. Basing their discussion on research advances in microbiology, molecular biology, and cell biology, the authors describe the interactions that exist between bacteria and human cells both in health and during infection.

EAR INFECTIONS AND DISORDERS
DISEASE/DISORDER

ANATOMY OR SYSTEM AFFECTED: Ears

SPECIALTIES AND RELATED FIELDS: Audiology, neurology, otorhinolaryngology

DEFINITION: Infections or disorders of the outer, middle, or inner ear, which may result in hearing impairment or loss.

KEY TERMS:

conductive loss: a hearing loss caused by an outer-ear or middle-ear problem which results in reduced transmission of sound

frequency: the number of vibrations per second of a source of sound, measured in hertz; correlates with perceived pitch

intensity of sound: the physical phenomenon that correlates approximately with perceived loudness; measured in decibels

otitis: any inflammation of the outer or middle ear

sensorineural loss: a hearing loss caused by a problem in the inner ear; this impairment is caused by a hair cell or nerve problem and is usually not amenable to surgical correction

CAUSES AND SYMPTOMS

The hearing mechanism, one of the most intricate and delicate structures of the human body, consists of three sections: the outer ear, the middle ear, and the inner ear. The outer ear converts sound waves into the mechanical motion of the eardrum (tympanic membrane), and the middle ear transmits this mechanical motion to the inner ear, where it is transformed into nerve impulses sent to the brain.

The outer ear consists of the visible portion, the ear canal, and the eardrum. The middle ear is a small chamber containing three tiny bones—the auditory ossicles, termed malleus (hammer), incus (anvil), and stapes (stirrup)—which transmit the vibrations of the eardrum (attached to the hammer) into the inner ear. The chamber is connected to the back of the throat by the Eustachian tube, which allows equalization with the external air pressure. The inner ear, or cochlea, is a fluid-filled cavity containing the complex structure necessary to convert the mechanical vibrations of the cochlear fluid into nerve pulses. The cochlea, shaped something like a snail's shell, is divided lengthwise by a slightly flexible partition into upper and lower chambers. The upper chamber begins at the oval window, to which the stirrup is attached. When the oval window is pushed or pulled by the stirrup, vibrations of the eardrum are transformed into cochlear fluid vibrations.

The lower surface of the cochlear partition, the basilar membrane, is set into vibration by the pressure difference between the fluids of the upper and lower ducts. Lying on the basilar membrane is the organ of Corti, containing tens of thousands of hair cells attached to the nerve transmission lines leading to the brain. When the basilar membrane vibrates, the cilia of these cells are bent, stimulating them to produce electrochemical impulses. These impulses travel along the auditory nerve to the brain, where they are interpreted as sound.

Although well protected against normal environmental exposure, the ear, because of its delicate nature, is subject to various infections and disorders. These disorders, which usually lead to some hearing loss, can occur in any of the three parts of the ear.

The ear canal can be blocked by a buildup of waxy secretions or by infection. Although earwax serves the useful purpose of trapping foreign particles that might otherwise be deposited on the eardrum, if the canal becomes clogged with an excess of wax, less sound will reach the eardrum, and hearing will be impaired.

Swimmers' ear, or otitis externa, is an inflammation caused by contaminated water which has not been completely drained from the ear canal. A moist condition in a region with little light favors fungal growth. Symp-

---

INFORMATION ON EAR INFECTIONS AND DISORDERS

CAUSES: Infection, buildup of earwax, fluid retention, injury, fungal growth, allergies, exposure to loud noise, sudden change in air pressure, certain drugs

SYMPTOMS: Hearing impairment or loss, itchiness, pain, inflammation, discharge, tinnitus

DURATION: Temporary to chronic

TREATMENTS: Wide ranging; can include flushing ear with a warm solution under pressure, antibiotics, surgery

Otitis Externa

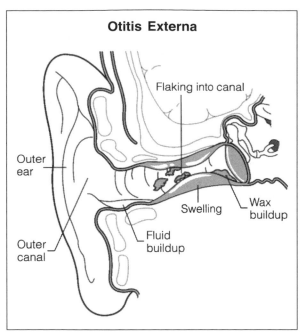

Otitis externa (swimmers' ear) results when the outer ear is inflamed by contaminated water that has not been completely drained from the ear canal.

toms of swimmers' ear include an itchy and tender ear canal and a small amount of foul-smelling drainage. If the canal is allowed to become clogged by the concomitant swelling, hearing will be noticeably impaired.

A perforated eardrum may result from a sharp blow to the side of the head, an infection, the insertion of objects into the ear, or a sudden change in air pressure (such as a nearby explosion). Small perforations are usually self-healing, but larger tears require medical treatment.

Inflammation of the middle ear, acute otitis media, is one of the most common ear infections, especially among children. Infection usually spreads from the throat to the middle ear through the Eustachian tube. Children are particularly susceptible to this problem because their short Eustachian tubes afford bacteria in the throat easy access to the middle ear. When the middle ear becomes infected, pus begins to accumulate, forcing the eardrum outward. This pressure stretches the auditory ossicles to their limit and tenses the ligaments so that vibration conduction is severely impaired. Untreated, this condition may eventually rupture the eardrum or permanently damage the ossicular chain. Furthermore, the pus from the infection may invade nearby structures, including the facial nerve, mastoid bones, the inner ear, or even the brain. The most common symptom of otitis is a sudden severe pain and an impairment of hearing resulting from the reduced mobility of the eardrum and the ossicles.

Secretory otitis media is caused by occlusion of the Eustachian tube as a result of conditions such as a head cold, diseased tonsils and adenoids, sinusitis, improper blowing of the nose, or riding in unpressurized airplanes. People with allergic nasal blockage are particularly prone to this condition. The blocked Eustachian tube causes the middle-ear cavity to fill with a pale yellow, noninfected discharge which exerts pressure on the eardrum, causing pain and impairment of hearing. Eventually, the middle-ear cavity is completely filled with fluid instead of air, impeding the movement of the ossicles and causing hearing impairment.

A mild, temporary hearing impairment resulting from airplane flights is termed aero-otitis media. This disorder results when a head cold or allergic reaction does not permit the Eustachian tube to equalize the air pressure in the middle ear with atmospheric pressure when a rapid change in altitude occurs. As the pressure outside the eardrum becomes greater than the pressure within, the membrane is forced inward, while the opening of the tube into the upper part of the throat is closed by the increased pressure. Symptoms are a severe sense of pressure in the ear, pain, and hearing impairment. Although the pressure difference may cause the eardrum to rupture, more often the pain continues until the middle ear fills with fluid or the tube opens to equalize pressure.

Chronic otitis media may result from inadequate drainage of pus during the acute form of this disease or from a permanent eardrum perforation that allows dust, water, and bacteria easy access to the middle-ear cavity. The main symptoms of this disease are fluids discharging from the outer ear and hearing loss. Perforations of the eardrum result in hearing loss because of the reduced vibrating surface and a buildup of fibrous tissue which further induces conductive losses. In some cases, an infection may heal but still cause hearing loss by immobilizing the ossicles. There are two distinct types of chronic otitis, one relatively harmless and the other quite dangerous. An odorless, stringy discharge from the mucous membrane lining the middle ear characterizes the harmless type. The dangerous type is characterized by a foul-smelling discharge coming from a bone-invading process beneath the mucous lining. If neglected, this process can lead to serious complications, such as meningitis, paralysis of the facial nerve, or complete sensorineural deafness.

The ossicles may be disrupted by infection or by a jarring blow to the head. Most often, a separation of the linkage occurs at the weakest point, where the anvil joins the stirrup. A partial separation results in a mild hearing loss, while complete separation causes severe hearing impairment.

Disablement of the mechanical linkage of the middle ear may also occur if the stirrup becomes calcified, a condition termed otosclerosis. The normal bone is resorbed and replaced by very irregular, often richly vascularized bone. The increased stiffness of the stirrup produces conductive hearing loss. In extreme cases, the stirrup becomes completely immobile and must be surgically removed. Although the exact cause of this disease is unknown, it seems to be hereditary. About half of the cases occur in families in which one or more relatives have the same condition, and it occurs more frequently in females than in males. There is also some evidence that the condition may be triggered by a lack of fluoride in drinking water and that increasing the intake of fluoride may retard the calcification process.

Tinnitus is characterized by ringing, hissing, or clicking noises in the ear that seem to come and go spontaneously without any sound stimulus. While technically tinnitus is not a disease of the ear, it is a common symptom of various ear problems. Possible causes of tinnitus are earwax lodged against the eardrum, a perforated or inflamed eardrum, otosclerosis, high aspirin dosage, or excessive use of the telephone. Tinnitus is most serious when caused by an inner-ear problem or by exposure to very intense sounds, and it often accompanies hearing loss at high frequencies.

Ménière's disease is caused by production of excess cochlear fluid, which increases the pressure in the cochlea. This condition may be precipitated by allergy, infection, kidney disease, or any number of other causes, including severe stress. The increased pressure is exerted on the walls of the semicircular canals, as well as on the cochlear partition. The excess pressure in the semicircular canals (the organs of balance) is interpreted by the brain as a rapid spinning motion, and the victim experiences abrupt attacks of vertigo and nausea. The excess pressure in the cochlear partition has the same effect as a very loud sound and rapidly destroys hair cells. A single attack causes a noticeable hearing loss and could result in total deafness without prompt treatment.

Of all ear diseases, damage to the hair cells in the cochlea causes the most serious impairment. Cilia may be destroyed by high fevers or from a sudden or prolonged exposure to intensely loud sounds. Problems include destroyed or missing hair cells, hair cells which fire spontaneously, and damaged hair cells that require unusually strong stimuli to excite them. At the present time, there is no means of repairing damaged cilia or of replacing those which have been lost.

Viral nerve deafness is a result of a viral infection in one or both ears. The mumps virus is one of the most common causes of severe nerve damage, with the measles and influenza viruses as secondary causes.

Ototoxic (ear poisoning) drugs can cause temporary or permanent hearing impairment by damaging auditory nerve tissues, although susceptibility is highly individualistic. A temporary decrease of hearing (in addition to tinnitus) accompanies the ingestion of large quantities of aspirin or quinine. Certain antibiotics, such as those of the mycin family, may also create permanent damage to the auditory nerves.

Repeated exposure to loud noise (in excess of 90 decibels) will cause a gradual deterioration of hearing by destroying cilia. The extent of damage, however, depends on the loudness and the duration of the sound. Rock bands often exceed 110 decibels; farm machinery averages 100 decibels.

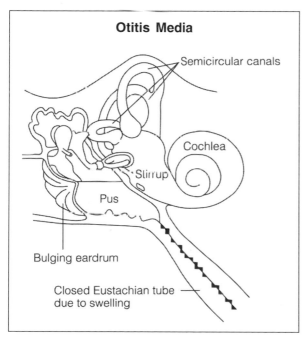

Otitis Media

Semicircular canals

Cochlea

Stirrup

Pus

Bulging eardrum

Closed Eustachian tube due to swelling

Otitis media occurs when infection spreads from the throat to the middle ear via the Eustachian tube; it is a serious condition which, left untreated, may lead to permanent ear damage and even infection of the brain.

Presbycusis (hearing loss with age) is the inability to hear high-frequency sounds because of the increasing deterioration of the hair cells. By age thirty, a perceptible high-frequency hearing loss is present. This deterioration progresses into old age, often resulting in severe impairment. The problem is accelerated by frequent unprotected exposure to noisy environments. The extent of damage depends on the frequency, intensity, and duration of exposure, as well as on the individual's predisposition to hearing loss.

TREATMENT AND THERAPY

The simplest ear problems to treat are a buildup of earwax, swimmers' ear, and a perforated eardrum. A large accumulation of wax in the ear canal is best removed by having a medical professional flush the ear with a warm solution under pressure. One should never attempt to remove wax plugs with a sharp instrument. A small accumulation of earwax may be softened by a few drops of baby oil left in the ear overnight, then washed out with warm water and a soft rubber ear syringe. Swimmers' ear can usually be prevented by thoroughly draining the ears after swimming. The disease can be treated by an application of antibiotic eardrops after the ear canal has been thoroughly cleaned. A small perforation of the eardrum will usually heal itself. Larger tears, however, require an operation, tympanoplasty, that grafts a piece of skin over the perforation.

Fortunately, the bacteria that usually cause acute otitis respond quickly to antibiotics. Although antibiotics may relieve the symptoms, complications can arise unless the pus is thoroughly drained. The two-part treatment—draining the fluid from the middle ear and antibiotic therapy—resolves the acute otitis infection within a week. Secretory otitis is cured by finding and removing the cause of the occluded Eustachian tube. The serous fluid is then removed by means of an aspirating needle or by an incision in the eardrum so as to inflate the tube by forcing air through it. In some cases, a tiny polyethylene tube is inserted through the eardrum to aid in reestablishing normal ventilation. If the Eustachian tube remains inadequate, a small plastic grommet may be inserted. The improvement in hearing is often immediate and dramatic. The pain and hearing loss of aero-otitis is usually temporary and disappears of its own accord. If, during or immediately after flight, yawning or swallowing does not allow the Eustachian tube to open and equalize the pressure, medicine or surgical puncture of the eardrum may be required. The harmless form of chronic otitis is treated with applied

medications to kill the bacteria and to dry the chronic drainage. The eardrum perforation may then be closed to restore the functioning of the ear and to recover hearing. The more dangerous chronic form of this disease does not respond well to antibacterial agents, but careful X-ray examination allows diagnosis and surgical removal of the bone-eroding cyst.

Ossicular interruption can be surgically treated to restore the conductive link by repositioning the separated bones. This relatively simple operation has a very high success rate. Otosclerosis is treated by operating on the stirrup in one of several ways. The stirrup can be mechanically freed by fracturing the calcified foot plate, or by fracturing the foot plate and one of the arms. Although this operation is usually successful, recalcification often occurs. Alternatively, the stirrup can be completely removed and replaced by a prosthesis of wire or silicon, yielding excellent and permanent results.

Since tinnitus has many possible, and often not readily identifiable, causes, only about 10 percent of the cases are treated successfully. The tinnitus masker has been invented to help sufferers live with this annoyance. The masker, a noise generator similar in appearance to a hearing aid, produces a constant, gentle humming sound which masks the tinnitus.

Ménière's disease, usually treated by drugs and a restricted diet, may also require surgical correction to relieve the excess pressure in severe cases. If this procedure is unsuccessful, the nerves of the inner ear may be cut. In drastic cases, the entire inner ear may be removed.

Presently there is no cure for damaged hair cells; the only treatment is to use a hearing aid. It is more advantageous to take preventive measures, such as reducing noise at the source, replacing noisy equipment with quieter models, or using ear protection devices. Recreational exposure to loud music should be severely curtailed, if not completely eliminated.

PERSPECTIVE AND PROSPECTS

For many centuries, treatment of the ear was associated with that of the eye. In the nineteenth century, the development of the laryngoscope (to examine the larynx) and the otoscope (to examine the ears) enabled doctors to examine and treat disorders such as croup, sore throat, and draining ears, which eventually led to the control of these diseases. As an offshoot of the medical advances made possible by these technological devices, the connection between the ear and throat became known, and otologists became associated with laryngologists.

The study of ear diseases did not develop scientifically until the early nineteenth century, when Jean-Marc-Gaspard Itard and Prosper Ménière made systematic investigations of ear physiology and disease. In 1853, William R. Wilde of Dublin published the first scientific treatise on ear diseases and treatments, setting the field on a firm scientific foundation. Meanwhile, the scientific investigation of the diseased larynx was aided by the laryngoscope, invented in 1855 by Manuel Garcia, a Spanish singing teacher who used his invention as a teaching aid. During the late nineteenth century, this instrument was adopted for detailed studies of larynx pathology by Ludwig Türck and Jan Czermak, who also adapted this instrument to investigate the nasal cavity, which established the link between laryngology and rhinology. Friedrich Voltolini, one of Czermak's assistants, further modified the instrument so that it could be used in conjunction with the otoscope. In 1921, Carl Nylen pioneered the use of a high-powered binocular microscope to perform ear surgery. The operating microscope opened the way for delicate operations on the tiny bones of the middle ear. With the founding of the American Board of Otology in 1924, otology (later otolaryngology) became the second medical specialty to be formally established in North America.

Prior to World War II, the leading cause of deafness was the various forms of ear infection. Advances in technology and medicine have now brought ear infections under control. Today the leading type of hearing loss in industrialized countries is conductive loss, which occurs in those who are genetically predisposed to such loss and who have had lifetime exposure to noise and excessively loud sounds. In the future, ear protection devices and reasonable precautions against extensive exposure to loud sounds should reduce the incidence of hearing loss to even lower levels.

—*George R. Plitnik, Ph.D.*

See also Altitude sickness; Audiology; Balance disorders; Decongestants; Ear surgery; Ears; Hearing loss; Hearing tests; Ménière's disease; Motion sickness; Myringotomy; Nasopharyngeal disorders; Neurology; Neurology, pediatric; Otoplasty; Otorhinolaryngology; Sense organs; Sinusitis; Speech disorders; Tonsillitis.

FOR FURTHER INFORMATION:

Canalis, Rinaldo, and Paul R. Lambert. *The Ear: Comprehensive Otology.* Philadelphia: Lippincott Williams & Wilkins, 2000. A text covering all aspects of otology.

Dugan, Marcia B. *Living with Hearing Loss.* Washington, D.C.: Gallaudet University Press, 2003. Offers a range of practical advice for those with hearing loss, including strategies for dealing with everyday situations and emergencies, speechreading, oral interpreters, and assertive communication.

Ferrari, Mario. *Ear, Nose, and Throat Disorders.* New York: Elsevier, 2002. A clinical yet accessible reference text that provides a comprehensive list of disorders, with a summary of the condition, background, diagnosis, treatment, outcomes, prevention, and resources.

Friedman, Ellen M., and James M. Barassi. *My Ear Hurts! A Complete Guide to Understanding and Treating Your Child's Ear Infections.* New York: Simon & Schuster, 2001. Reviews current research on ear infections and reviews a range of treatment approaches from both conventional and alternative medicine.

Greene, Alan R. *The Parent's Complete Guide to Ear Infections.* Reprint. Allentown, Pa.: People's Medical Society, 1999. Every parent who has ever had a child with recurrent otitis will appreciate this book. It explains the anatomy of normal ears, causes of infections, prevention, symptoms, evaluation, initial and ongoing treatment, antibiotics, the pros and cons of surgical intervention, hearing loss, tubes, and complications.

Jerger, James, ed. *Hearing Disorders in Adults: Current Trends.* San Diego, Calif.: College-Hill Press, 1984. A reliable and readable introductory treatise on common hearing disorders.

Kemper, Kathi J. *The Holistic Pediatrician: A Pediatrician's Comprehensive Guide to Safe and Effective Therapies for the Twenty-five Most Common Ailments of Infants, Children, and Adolescents.* New York: HarperCollins, 2002. Integrates mainstream and alternative medicine to aid parents in dealing with the most common childhood health problems such as diaper rash, ear infections, and allergies.

"Lack of Consensus About Surgery for Ear Infections." *Health News* 18, no. 3 (June/July, 2000): 11. Children who suffer from recurrent otitis media, or ear infections, may be candidates for a surgical procedure called "myringotomy," which involves the insertion of tiny tubes into the ear drums. The goal of the surgery is to prevent future infections and reduce the chances of hearing loss.

Pender, Daniel J. *Practical Otology.* Philadelphia: J. B. Lippincott, 1992. A well-illustrated text on diseases of the ear and their surgical correction.

Roland, Peter S., Bradley F. Marple, and William L. Meyerhoff, eds. *Hearing Loss.* New York: Thieme, 1997. Provides information on hearing disorders and discusses the anatomy and physiology of the ear.

EAR, NOSE, AND THROAT MEDICINE. *See* OTORHINOLARYNGOLOGY.

EAR SURGERY

PROCEDURE

ANATOMY OR SYSTEM AFFECTED: Bones, ears, musculoskeletal system, nervous system

SPECIALTIES AND RELATED FIELDS: Audiology, general surgery, otorhinolaryngology, speech pathology

DEFINITION: An invasive procedure to correct structural problems of the ear that produce some degree of hearing loss.

KEY TERMS:

cochlea: a structure in the inner ear that receives sound vibrations from the ossicles and transmits them to the auditory nerve

myringotomy: incision of the tympanic membrane used to drain fluid and reduce middle-ear pressure

ossicles: tiny bones located between the eardrum and the cochlea

otosclerosis: a condition in which the stapes becomes progressively more rigid, and hearing loss results

stapedectomy: a surgical procedure in which the stapes is replaced with an artificial substitute

stapes: the ossicle that makes contact with the cochlea

tympanic membrane: the eardrum, which separates the external ear canal from the middle ear and ossicles and which transmits sound vibration to the ossicles

tympanoplasty: a surgical procedure to repair the tympanic membrane

INDICATIONS AND PROCEDURES

Humans are able to detect sound because of the interaction between the ears and the brain. When sound waves strike the tympanic membrane (eardrum), it vibrates. The movement of the tympanic membrane then causes the movement of the ossicles, the three tiny bones within the middle ear (malleus, incus, and stapes). These moving bones transfer the vibrations to the cochlea of the inner ear, which stimulates the auditory nerve and eventually the brain.

Hearing problems may result when any part of the ear is damaged. Hearing difficulties can be categorized into two main areas: conductive and sensorineural hearing loss. In conductive hearing loss, the ear loses its ability to transmit sound from the external ear to the cochlea. Common causes include earwax buildup in the outer ear canal; otosclerosis, in which the stapes loses mobility and cannot stimulate the cochlea effectively; and otitis media, in which the middle ear becomes infected and a sticky fluid is produced which causes the ossicles to become inflexible. Otitis media is the most common cause of conductive hearing loss and typically occurs in children. If antibiotics such as amoxicillin or ampicillin fail to clear the ear of infection, surgery may be required. Sensorineural hearing loss results from damage to the cochlea or auditory nerve. Common causes include loud noises, rubella (a type of viral infection) during embryonic development, and certain drugs such as gentamicin and streptomycin. Occasionally, a tumor (neuroma) of the auditory nerve may cause sensorineural hearing loss.

Myringotomy is a surgical procedure in which an incision is made in the tympanic membrane to allow drainage of fluid (effusion) from the middle ear to the external ear canal. The surgeon usually performs this operation to treat recurrent otitis media, a condition in which pressure builds in the middle ear and pushes outward on the tympanic membrane. The patient, usually a child, is given general anesthesia. An incision is made in the eardrum so that a small tube can be inserted to allow continuous drainage of the pus. The tube usually falls out in a few months, and the tympanic membrane heals rapidly.

Otosclerosis, the overgrowth of bone that impedes the movement of the stapes, can be treated by stapedectomy (surgical removal of the stapes). General anesthesia is used to prevent pain or movement when an incision is made in the ear canal and the tympanic membrane is folded to access the ossicles. The stapes can then be removed and a metal or plastic prosthesis inserted in its place. The eardrum is then repaired.

Tympanoplasty is an operation to repair the tympanic membrane or ossicles. Sudden pressure changes in an airplane or during deep-sea diving may perforate the tympanic membrane (barotrauma) and require tympanoplasty. The procedure is similar to stapedectomy. With the patient under general anesthesia, an incision is made next to the eardrum to provide access to the tympanic membrane and ossicles. The tympanic membrane may need to be repaired if the perforated eardrum does not heal on its own. An operating microscope is employed for optimal visualization of the middle ear. If the tympanoplasty involves the ossicles, microsurgical instruments are used to reposition, repair, or replace the damaged bones. They are then reset in their natural positions, and the eardrum is repaired.

Auditory neuromas are benign tumors of the supporting cells surrounding the auditory nerve. Although rare, these tumors can cause deafness. Once neuromas are confirmed by computed tomography (CT) scanning, surgical removal is necessary. With the patient under general anesthesia, the surgeon must make a hole in the skull and attempt to remove the tumor carefully without damaging the auditory nerve or adjacent nerves.

Uses and Complications

More than 90 percent of the patients undergoing stapedectomy experience improved hearing. Approximately 1 percent, however, show deterioration of hearing or total hearing loss postoperatively. For this reason, most surgeons perform stapedectomy on one ear at a time.

Occasionally, the surgical removal of auditory neuromas causes total deafness because of damage to the auditory nerve itself. In rare cases, damage to nearby nerves may cause weakness and/or numbness in that part of the face. Depending on the extent of nerve damage, the symptoms may or may not lessen with time.

Perspective and Prospects

Improvements in technology promise new methods of treating hearing loss. For example, cochlear implants have been developed for the treatment of total sensorineural hearing loss. These implants are surgically inserted into the inner ear. Electrodes in the cochlea receive sound signals transmitted to them from a miniature receiver implanted behind the skin of the ear. Directly over the implant, the patient wears an external transmitter which is connected to a sound processor and microphone. As the microphone picks up sound, the sound is eventually conducted to the electrodes within the cochlea.

—*Matthew Berria, Ph.D.,*
and Douglas Reinhart, M.D.

See also Audiology; Ear infections and disorders; Ears; Hearing loss; Ménière's disease; Myringotomy; Neurology; Neurology, pediatric; Otoplasty; Otorhinolaryngology; Plastic surgery; Sense organs.

For Further Information:

Clayman, Charles B., ed. *The American Medical Association Encyclopedia of Medicine.* New York: Random House, 1994. A concise presentation of numerous medical terms and illnesses. A good general reference.

Ferrari, Mario. *Ear, Nose, and Throat Disorders.* New York: Elsevier, 2002. A clinical yet accessible reference text that provides a comprehensive list of disorders, with a summary of the condition, background, diagnosis, treatment, outcomes, prevention, and resources.

Jackler, Robert, and Michael Kaplan. "Ear, Nose, and Throat." In *Current Medical Diagnosis and Treatment: 2001,* edited by Lawrence M. Tierney, Jr., et al. 38th ed. New York: McGraw-Hill, 2000. A chapter in a text which is the point of reference for physicians and other health care practitioners. It incorporates each year's biomedical research discoveries that have immediate, relevant, and applicable use for the patient.

Nadol, Joseph, and Michael J. McKenna. *Surgery of the Ear and Temporal Bone.* Philadelphia: Lippincott Williams & Wilkins, 2003. Written by specialists at the Massachusetts Eye and Ear Infirmary, details surgical techniques that have been found reproducible and effective, as well as surgical decision making, including discussions of indications, contraindications, complications, and therapeutic alternatives.

Pender, Daniel J. *Practical Otology.* Philadelphia: J. B. Lippincott, 1992. A well-illustrated text on diseases of the ear and their surgical correction.

Schwartz, Seymour I., ed. *Principles of Surgery.* 7th ed. New York: McGraw-Hill, 1999. A standard textbook on the topic. Intended for practicing surgeons, but valuable to general readers for its details.

Ears

Anatomy

Anatomy or system affected: Bones, musculoskeletal system, nervous system

Specialties and related fields: Audiology, neurology, otorhinolaryngology, speech pathology

Definition: The organs responsible for both hearing and balance.

Key terms:

auditory nerve: the nerve that conducts impulses originating in hair cells of cochlea to the brain for processing as the sensation of sound

cochlea: the fluid-filled coil of the inner ear containing hair cells that change vibrations in the fluid into nerve impulses

eardrum: the membrane separating the outer ear canal from the middle ear that changes sound waves into movements of the ossicles; also called the tympanic membrane

Eustachian tube: the tube connecting the middle ear to the back of the throat; air exchange through this tube equalizes air pressure in the middle ear with the outside air pressure

inner ear: an organ that includes the cochlea (for detection of sound) and the labyrinth (for detection of movement)

labyrinth: a structure consisting of three fluid-filled, semicircular canals at right angles to one another in the inner ear; they monitor the position and movement of the head

middle ear: the air-filled cavity in which vibrations are transmitted from the eardrum to the inner ear via the ossicles

ossicles: three small bones in the middle ear that transmit vibrations from the eardrum to the fluid of the inner ear

otoscope: an instrument for viewing the ear canal and the eardrum

outer ear: the visible, fleshy part of the ear and the ear canal; transmits sound waves to the eardrum

tympanic membrane: another term for the eardrum

STRUCTURE AND FUNCTIONS

The ear is composed of three parts: the outer ear, the middle ear, and the inner ear. All three parts are involved in hearing, while only the inner ear is involved in balance.

Sound can be thought of as pressure waves that travel through the air. These waves are collected by the fleshy part of the outer ear and are funneled down the ear canal to the eardrum. The eardrum, being a thin membrane, vibrates as it is hit by the sound waves. Attached to the eardrum is the first of the ossicles (the hammer or malleus), which moves when the eardrum moves. The second ossicle (the anvil or incus) is attached to the first, and the third to second. Therefore, as the first bone moves, the others move also. The base of the third bone (the stirrup or stapes) is in contact with the oval window at the beginning of the inner ear. Movement of the oval window sets up vibrations in the fluid of the cochlea. These vibrations are detected by hair cells. Depending on their position in the cochlea, the hair cells are sensitive to being moved by vibrations of different frequencies. When the hair of a hair cell is bent by the fluid, an impulse is generated. The impulses are transmitted to the brain via the auditory nerve. The nerve impulses are processed in the brain, and the result is the sensation of sound, in particular the sense of pitch. Thus the three parts of the ear turn sound waves into "sound" by changing air vibrations into eardrum vibrations, then ossicle movement, then fluid vibrations, and finally nerve impulses.

DISORDERS AND DISEASES

Each of the three parts of the ear can be affected by diseases that can lead to temporary or, in some cases, permanent hearing loss. Damage to the eardrum, ossicles, or any part of the ear before the cochlea results in conductive hearing loss, as these structures conduct the sound or vibrations. Damage to the hair cells or to the auditory nerve results in sensorineural hearing loss. Sound may be conducted normally but cannot be detected by the hair cells or transmitted as nerve impulses to the brain.

Disorders of the outer ear include cauliflower ear, blockage by earwax, otitis externa, and tumors. Cauliflower ear is a severe hematoma (bruise) to the outer ear. In some cases, the blood trapped beneath the skin does not resorb and instead turns into fibrous tissue that may become cartilaginous or even bonelike.

Earwax is secreted by the cells in the lining of the ear canal. Its function is to protect the eardrum from dust and dirt, and it normally works its way to the outer opening of the ear. The amount secreted varies from person to person. In some people, or in people who are continually exposed to dusty environments, excessive amounts of wax may be secreted and may block the ear canal sufficiently to interfere with its transmission of sound waves to the eardrum.

Otitis externa can take two forms, either localized or generalized. The localized form, a boil or abscess, is a bacterial infection that results from breaks in the lining of the ear canal and is often caused by attempts to scratch an itch in the ear or to remove wax. The generalized form can be a bacterial or fungal infection, known as otomycosis. Generalized otitis externa is also called swimmers' ear because it often results from swimming in polluted waters or from chronic moisture in the ear canal.

Tumors of the ear can be benign (noncancerous) or malignant (cancerous) growths of either the soft tissues or the underlying bone. Bony growths, or osteomas, can cause sufficient blockage, by themselves or by leading to the buildup of earwax, to result in hearing loss.

The middle ear consists of the eardrum, three small bones called the ossicles, and the Eustachian tube. The bones of the middle ear move in an air-filled cavity. Air pressure within this cavity is normally the same as the outside air pressure because air is exchanged between the middle ear and the outside world via the Eustachian tube. When this tube swells and closes, as it often does with a head cold, one experiences a stuffy feeling, decreased hearing, mild pain, and sometimes ringing in the ears (tinnitus) or dizziness. The middle ear is susceptible to infection, such as otitis media, because bacteria and viruses can sometimes enter via the Eustachian tube. Young children are especially prone to middle-ear infections because a child's Eustachian tubes are shorter and more directly in line with the back of the throat than those of adults. Untreated ear infections can sometimes spread into the surrounding bone (mastoiditis) or into the brain (meningitis).

Fluid in the middle ear during an ear infection interferes with the free movement of the ossicles, causing hearing loss that, although significant while it lasts, is temporary. In other instances, there is the prolonged presence of clear fluid in the middle ear, resulting from a combination of infection or allergy and Eustachian tube dysfunction, which itself can result from swelling caused by allergy. This condition, known as "glue ear" or persistent middle-ear effusion, can last long enough to cause detrimental effects on speech, particularly in young children. Middle-ear infections can sometimes become chronic, as in chronic otitis media; permanent damage to the hearing can result from the ossicles being dissolved away by the pus from these chronic infections.

During a middle-ear infection, fluid can build up and increase pressure within the middle-ear cavity sufficiently to rupture (perforate) the eardrum. Very loud noises are another form of increased pressure, in this case from the outside. If a loud noise is very sudden, such as an explosion or gunshot, then pressure cannot be equalized fast enough and the eardrum can rupture. Scuba diving without clearing one's ears (that is, getting the Eustachian tube to open and allow airflow) can also result in ruptured eardrums. Other causes of ruptured eardrums include puncture by a sharp object in-

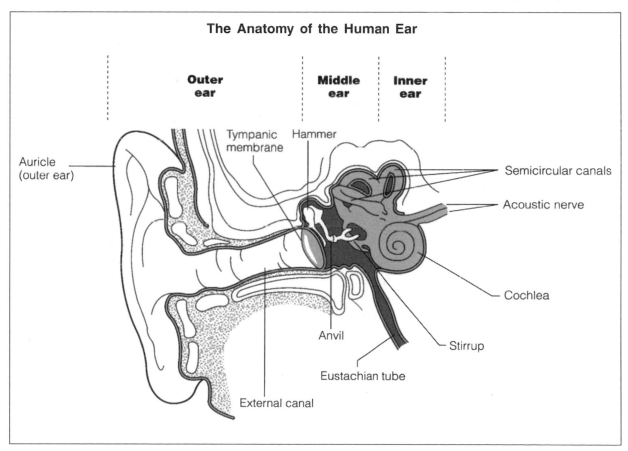

The Anatomy of the Human Ear

Outer ear

Middle ear

Inner ear

Tympanic membrane

Hammer

Auricle (outer ear)

Semicircular canals

Acoustic nerve

Cochlea

Anvil

Stirrup

Eustachian tube

External canal

serted into the ear canal to remove wax or relieve itching, a blow to the ear, or a fractured skull. Some hearing is lost when the eardrum is ruptured, but if the damage is not too severe, the eardrum heals itself and hearing returns.

The middle ear does not always fill with fluid if the Eustachian tube is blocked. In some instances, the middle-ear cavity remains filled with trapped air. This trapped air is taken up by the cells lining the middle-ear cavity, decreasing the air pressure inside the middle ear and allowing the eardrum to push inward. Cells that are constantly shed from the eardrum collect in this pocket and form a ball that can become infected. This infected ball, or cholesteatoma, produces pus, which can erode the ossicles. If left untreated, the erosion can continue through the roof of the middle-ear cavity (causing brain abscesses or meningitis) or through the walls (causing abscesses behind the ear). The symptoms of a cholesteatoma go beyond the symptoms of an earache to include headache, dizziness, and weakness of the facial muscles.

Permanent conductive hearing loss can also result from calcification of the ossicles, a condition called osteosclerosis. Abnormal spongy bone can form at the base of the stirrup bone, interfering with its normal movement against the oval window. Hearing loss caused by osteosclerosis occurs gradually over ten to fifteen years, although it may be accelerated in women by pregnancy. There is a hereditary component.

The inner ear begins at the oval window, which separates the air-filled cavity at the middle ear from the fluid-filled cavities of the inner ear. The inner ear consists of the cochlea, which is involved in hearing, and the labyrinth, which maintains balance.

Disorders of the cochlea result in permanent sensorineural hearing loss. Hair cells can be damaged by the high fever accompanying some diseases such as meningitis. They may also be damaged by some drugs. The largest, and most preventable, sources of damage to the hair cells are occupational and recreational exposure to loud sounds, particularly if they are prolonged. In some occupations, the hearing loss from working without ear protection may be confined to certain frequencies of sounds, while other occupations lead to general loss at all sound frequencies. Prolonged exposure to over-amplified music will likewise cause permanent hearing loss at all frequencies. This is more severe and has much earlier onset than presbycusis—the progressive loss of hearing, particularly in the high frequencies, that occurs with normal aging.

The labyrinth is the part of the ear that maintains one's balance; therefore the major system of disorders of the labyrinth is vertigo (dizziness). Labyrinthitis is an infection, generally viral, of the labyrinth. The vertigo can be severe but is temporary.

With Ménière's disease, there is an increase in the volume of fluid in the labyrinth and a corresponding increase in internal pressure, which distorts or ruptures the membrane lining. The symptoms, which include vertigo, noises in the ear, and muffled or distorted hearing especially of low tones, flare up in attacks that may last from a few hours to several days. The frequency of these attacks varies from one individual to another, with some people having episodes every few weeks and others having them every few years. This condition, which may be accompanied by migraine headaches, usually clears spontaneously but in some people may result in deafness.

DIAGNOSTIC AND TREATMENT TECHNIQUES

The most common ear disorders, outer-ear or middle-ear infections, are diagnosed visually with an otoscope. This handheld instrument is a very bright light with a removable tip. Tips of different sizes can be attached so that the doctor can look into ear canals of various sizes. Infections or obstructions in the outer ear are readily visible. Middle-ear infections can often be discerned by the appearance of the eardrum, which may appear red and inflamed. Fluid in the middle ear can sometimes be seen through the eardrum, or its presence can be surmised if the eardrum is bulging toward the ear canal. In other cases, the eardrum will be seen to be retracted or bulging inward toward the middle-ear cavity. Holes in the eardrum can also be seen, as can scars from previous ruptures that have since healed.

Impedance testing may be used in addition to the otoscope for diagnosis of middle-ear problems. Impedance testing is based on the fact that, when sound waves hit the eardrum, some of the energy is transmitted as vibrations of the drum, while some of the energy is reflected. If the eardrum is stretched tight by fluid pushing against it or by being retracted, it will be less mobile and will reflect more sound waves than a normal eardrum. In the simplest form, the mobility of the eardrum is tested with a small air tube and bulb attached to an otoscope. The doctor gently squeezes a puff of air into the ear canal while watching through the otoscope to see how well the eardrum moves.

A far more quantitative version of impedance testing can be done in cases of suspected hearing loss. This type of impedance testing is generally administered by an audiologist, a professional trained in administering and interpreting hearing tests. The ear canal is blocked with an earplug containing a transmitter and receiver. The transmitter releases sound of known frequency and intensity into the ear canal while also changing the pressure in the ear canal by pumping air into it. The receiver then measures the amount of energy reflected back. The machine analyzes the efficiency of reflection at various pressures and prints out a graph. By comparison of the graph to that from an eardrum with normal mobility, conclusions can be drawn about the degree of immobility and, consequently, about the stage of the middle-ear infection. Many pediatricians or family practice doctors have handheld versions of this instrument, which resembles an otoscope but is capable of transmitting sound and measuring reflected sound intensity.

When an ear infection has been diagnosed, the treatment is generally with antibiotics. For outer-ear infections, drops containing antibiotic or antifungal agents are prescribed. For middle-ear infections, antibiotics are prescribed that can be taken by mouth. The patient is rechecked in about three weeks to ensure that the ear has healed.

In some cases, the ear does not heal, or the fluid in the middle ear does not go away. This can occur if a new infection starts before the ear is fully recovered or if the infecting microorganisms are resistant to the antibiotic used for treatment. In cases of chronic or repeated otitis media, a surgical procedure called a myringotomy can be performed in which a small slit is made in the eardrum to release fluid from the middle ear. Often, a small tube is inserted into the slit. These ear tubes, or tympanostomy tubes, keep the middle ear ventilated, allowing it to dry and heal. In most cases, these tubes are spontaneously pushed out by the eardrum as healing takes place, usually within three to six months. Patients must be cautious to keep water out of their ears while the tubes are in place.

A permanently damaged eardrum—from an explosion, for example—can be replaced by a graft. This procedure is called tympanoplasty, and the tissue used for the graft is generally taken from a vein from the same person. If the ossicles are damaged, they too can be replaced, in this case by metal copies of the bones. For example, when otosclerosis has damaged the stapes (stirrup) bone, hearing can often be restored by replacing it with a metal substitute.

Tumors, osteomas in the ear canal, or cholesteatomas on the eardrum may need to be removed surgically. Surgery may also be needed if infections have spread into the surrounding bone. Bone infections or abnormalities of the inner ear are diagnosed by X rays or by computed tomography (CT) scans.

For some persons who have complete sensorineural hearing loss, some awareness of sound can be restored with a cochlear implant. This electronic device is surgically implanted and takes the place of the nonexistent hair cells in detecting sound and generating nerve impulses.

Problems of balance may sometimes be treated successfully with drugs to limit the swelling in the labyrinth. Ringing in the ears (tinnitus) is usually resolved when the underlying condition is resolved. In some cases, tinnitus is caused by drugs (large doses of aspirin, for example) and will cease when the drugs are stopped.

Doctors who specialize in diagnosis and treatment of disorders of the ear and who do these surgeries are called otorhinolaryngologists (ear, nose, and throat doctors). They are medical doctors who have several years of training beyond medical school in surgery and in problems of the ear, nose, and throat.

PERSPECTIVE AND PROSPECTS

The basic anatomy of the ear has been known for some time. Bartolommeo Eustachio (1520-1574), an Italian anatomist, first described the Eustachian tube as well as a number of the nerves and muscles involved in the functioning of the ear. An understanding of how the ear functions to discriminate the pitch of sounds, however, was not arrived at until the twentieth century. Georg von Békésy won the Nobel Prize in Physiology or Medicine in 1961 for his work on the acoustics of the ear and how it functions to analyze sounds of varying frequencies (pitch).

Treatment of diseases of the ear has been radically changed by the advent of antibiotics. Older texts describe rupture of the eardrum by middle-ear fluid as a desired outcome of middle-ear infection, one which would ensure that the infection drained and healed, rather than becoming chronic.

Chronic ear infections used to be associated with diseases such as tuberculosis, measles, and syphilis, which themselves became far less common with the widespread use of antibiotics or vaccines. In the past, chronic ear infections were much more likely to result in mastoiditis, or infection of the air spaces of the mastoid bone, requiring surgical removal of the infected portions of the mastoid bone.

Adenoids and tonsils were frequently removed from patients with recurrent ear infections, as these were thought to be the source of the reinfection. It is now known that these tissues are involved in the formation of immunity to infectious bacteria and viruses. Their removal is not advocated in most circumstances—except, for example, when they are large enough to block the opening of the Eustachian tube.

Reconstructive surgery began in the 1950's with the development by Samuel Rosen and others of the operation to free up the calcified stapes bone in cases of otosclerosis. Today virtually all the components of the middle ear can be replaced.

While ear infections used to be much more dangerous, perhaps there is an equal danger today of taking threats to the ears too lightly. Chronic ear infections can still cause permanent hearing loss and even become life-threatening infections if left untreated. Damage involving the inner ear remains untreatable, as do many cases of tinnitus and loss of balance. Because the largest source of inner ear damage is prolonged exposure to noise, the prevention of damage is far more effective than treatment.

—Pamela J. Baker, Ph.D.

See also Altitude sickness; Anatomy; Audiology; Balance disorders; Biophysics; Dyslexia; Ear infections and disorders; Ear surgery; Hearing loss; Hearing tests; Ménière's disease; Motion sickness; Myringotomy; Nervous system; Neurology; Neurology, pediatric; Otoplasty; Otorhinolaryngology; Plastic surgery; Sense organs; Speech disorders; Systems and organs.

FOR FURTHER INFORMATION:

Clayman, Charles B., ed. *The American Medical Association Family Medical Guide.* New York: Random House, 1994. Includes a nondetailed, readable description of the anatomy of the ear and a complete listing of common ailments, each with a section on treatment that includes "self-help" and "professional help." Good illustrations and some photographs are provided.

Gelfand, Stanley A. *Essentials of Audiology.* 2d ed. New York: Thieme, 2001. Undergraduate text covering a wide range of relevant topics, including acoustics, anatomy and physiology, sound perception, auditory disorders and the nature of hearing impairment.

Katz, Jack, ed. *Handbook of Clinical Audiology.* 5th ed. Philadelphia: Lippincott Williams & Wilkins, 2002. Text that examines advances in the scientific, clinical, and philosophical understanding of audiology. Sections of the book cover behavioral tests, physiologic tests, special populations, and the management of hearing disorders.

Mendel, Lisa Lucks, Jeffrey L. Danhauer, and Sadanand Singh. *Singular's Illustrated Dictionary of Audiology.* San Diego, Calif.: Singular, 1999. A comprehensive reference guide to the field that includes numerous photographs, charts, and diagrams. Appendixes cover acronyms, illustrations, topic categories, and physical quantities.

Pender, Daniel J. *Practical Otology.* Philadelphia: J. B. Lippincott, 1992. A well-illustrated text on diseases of the ear and their surgical correction.

Suddarth, Doris S., ed. *The Lippincott Manual of Nursing Practice.* 7th ed. Philadelphia: J. B. Lippincott, 2000. Presents hearing problems and other problems of the ear, each in outline form, with sections including clinical manifestations, management, and patient education. Contains an extensive bibliography.

Zuckerman, Barry S., and Pamela A. M. Zuckerman. *Child Health: A Pediatrician's Guide for Parents.* New York: Hearst Books, 1986. A very readable description of the ear ailments and treatments most common to children. Includes sections on swimmers' ear, otitis media, glue ear, ear tubes, hearing tests, and other topics.

EATING DISORDERS
DISEASE/DISORDER

ANATOMY OR SYSTEM AFFECTED: Endocrine system, gastrointestinal system, glands, intestines, psychicemotional system, reproductive system, stomach

SPECIALTIES AND RELATED FIELDS: Nutrition, psychiatry, psychology

DEFINITION: A set of emotional disorders centering on body image that lead to misuse of food in a variety of ways—through overeating, overeating and purging, or undereating—that severely threaten the physical and mental well-being of the individual.

KEY TERMS:

amenorrhea: the cessation of menstruation

anorexia nervosa: a disorder characterized by the phobic avoidance of eating, the relentless pursuit of thinness, and fear of gaining weight

arrythmia: irregularity or loss of rhythm, especially of the heartbeat

bulimia: a disorder characterized by binge eating followed by self-induced vomiting

electrolytes: ionized salts in blood, tissue fluid, and cells, including salts of potassium, sodium, and chloride

CAUSES AND SYMPTOMS

The presence of an eating disorder in a patient is defined by an abnormal mental and physical relationship between body image and eating. While obesity is considered an eating disorder, the most prominent conditions are anorexia nervosa and bulimia nervosa. Anorexia nervosa (the word "anorexia" comes from the Greek for "loss of appetite") is an illness characterized by the relentless pursuit of thinness and fear of gaining weight. Bulimia nervosa (the word "bulimia" comes from the Greek for "ox appetite") refers to binge eating followed by self-induced vomiting. These conditions are related in intimate, yet ill-defined ways.

Anorexia nervosa affects more women than men by the overwhelming ratio of nineteen to one. It most often begins in adolescence and is more common among the upper and middle classes of the Western world. According to most studies, its incidence increased severalfold from the 1970's to the 1990's. Prevalence figures vary from 0.5 to 0.8 cases per one hundred adolescent girls. A familiar pattern of anorexia nervosa is often present, and studies indicate that 16 percent of the mothers and 23 percent of the fathers of anorectic patients had a history of significantly low adolescent weight or weight phobia.

The criteria for anorexia nervosa include intense fear of becoming obese, which does not diminish with the progression of weight loss; disturbance of body image, or feeling "fat" even when emaciated; refusal to maintain body weight over a minimal weight for age and height; the loss of 25 percent of original body weight or being 25 percent below expected weight based on standard growth charts; and no known physical illness that would account for the weight loss. Anorexia nervosa is also classified into primary and secondary forms. The primary condition is the distinct constellation of behaviors described above. In secondary anorexia nervosa, the weight loss results from another emotional or organic disorder.

The most prominent symptom of anorexia nervosa is a phobic avoidance of eating that goes beyond any reasonable level of dieting in the presence of striking thinness. Attending this symptom is the characteristic distorted body image and faulty perceptions of hunger and satiety, as well as a pervasive sense of inadequacy.

> ## INFORMATION ON EATING DISORDERS
>
> **CAUSES:** Psychological disorder
> **SYMPTOMS:** Intense preoccupation with food and weight, disordered eating; may include ingestion of laxatives, depression and suicidal feelings, nutritional deficiencies, dehydration, hormonal changes, gastrointestinal problems, changes in metabolism, heart disorders, persistent sore throat, teeth and gum damage
> **DURATION:** Chronic
> **TREATMENTS:** Psychotherapy, nutritional counseling, medication

The distortion of body image renders patients unable to evaluate their body weight accurately, so that they react to weight loss by intensifying their desire for thinness. Patients characteristically describe themselves as "fat" and "gross" even when totally emaciated. The degree of disturbance in body image is a useful prognostic index. Faulty perception of inner, visceral sensations, such as hunger and satiety, extends also to emotional states. The problem of nonrecognition of feelings is usually intensified with starvation.

Other cognitive distortions are also common in anorectic patients. Dichotomous reasoning—the assessment of self or others—is either idealized or degraded. Personalization of situations and a tendency to overgeneralize are common. Anorectics display an extraordinary amount of energy, directed to exercise and schoolwork in the face of starvation, but may curtail or avoid social relationships. Crying spells and complaints of depression are common findings and may persist in some anorectic patients even after weight is gained.

Sleep disturbances have also been reported in anorectics. Obsessive and/or compulsive behaviors, usually developing after the onset of the eating symptoms, abound with anorexia. Obsession with cleanliness and house cleaning, frequent handwashing, compulsive studying habits, and ritualistic behaviors are common.

As expected, the most striking compulsions involve food and eating. Anorectics' intense involvement with food belies their apparent lack of interest in it. The term "anorexia" is, in fact, a misnomer because lack of appetite is rare until late in the illness. Anorectics often carry large quantities of sweets in their purses and hide candies or cookies in various places. They frequently collect recipes and engage in elaborate meal preparation for others. Anorectics' behavior also includes refusal to eat with their families and in public places. When unable to reduce food intake openly, they may resort to such subterfuge as hiding food or disposing of it in toilets. If the restriction of food intake does not suffice for losing weight, the patient may resort to vomiting, usually at night and in secret. Self-induced vomiting then becomes associated with bulimia. Some patients also abuse laxatives and diuretics.

Commonly reported physical symptoms include constipation, abdominal pain, and cold intolerance. With severe weight loss, feelings of weakness and lethargy replace the drive to exercise. Amenorrhea (cessation of menstruation) occurs in virtually all cases, although it is not essential for a diagnosis of anorexia. Weight loss generally precedes the loss of the menstrual cycle. Other physical symptoms reveal the effects of starvation. Potassium depletion is the most frequent serious problem occurring with both anorexia and bulimia. Gastrointestinal disturbances are common, and death may occur from either infection or electrolyte imbalance.

Bulimia usually occurs between the ages of twelve and forty, with greatest frequency between the ages of fifteen and thirty. Unlike anorectics, bulimics usually are of normal weight, although some have a history of anorexia or obesity. Like anorectics, however, they are not satisfied by normal food intake. The characteristic symptom of bulimia is episodic, uncontrollable binge eating followed by vomiting or purging. The binge eating, usually preceded by a period of dieting lasting a few months or more, occurs when patients are alone at home and lasts about one hour. In the early stages of the illness, patients may need to stimulate their throat with a finger or spoon to induce vomiting, but later they can vomit at will. At times, abrasions and bruises on the back of the hand are produced during vomiting. The binge-purge cycle is usually followed by sadness, self-deprecation, and regret. Bulimic patients have troubled interpersonal relationships, poor self-concept, a high level of anxiety and depression, and poor impulse control. Alcohol and drug abuse are not uncommon with bulimia, in contrast to their infrequency with anorexia.

In the News: Genetic Links to Eating Disorders

A study published in the April, 2003, volume of the *International Journal of Eating Disorders* revealed substantial heritability for obesity and moderate heritability for binge eating among 2,163 female twins. The study also showed that obesity and binge eating share a moderate genetic correlation. Another study published in the same volume demonstrated that some genetic influences may be activated during puberty, suggesting that age-related development may be an important factor to consider in the study of eating disorders. This study used 530 twins who were eleven years of age and 602 twins who were seventeen years of age from the Minnesota Twins Family Study. The genetic contribution was zero in the eleven-year-olds but 55 percent in the seventeen-year-olds. The correlation of developmental stage with eating disorders was also highlighted in a 2001 issue of *Aging and Mental Health*, which reported on anorexia and the elderly.

The February, 2003, issue of *Clinical Psychology Review* presented a review of relevant literature suggesting that disorders such as anorexia nervosa and bulimia nervosa may also share relationships with other conditions that have genetic contributions. For instance, both disorders may be associated with depression, and anorexia has been associated with obsessive-compulsive disorder.

Similarly, a study of 256 female twins reported in a 2002 issue of *Journal of Abnormal Psychology* suggested that eating disorders might be related to inherited personality characteristics. In this study, the results indicated that phenotypic associations between the Multidimensional Personality Questionnaire and the Eating Disorders Inventory were more likely to be genetic; however, their shared genetic variance was limited. Thus, personality may play a role in the expression of eating disorders, but this role may be limited.

Together, these studies suggest that genetics and environment play roles in the development of various eating disorders. They also suggest that more than one mechanism may account for these contributions related to factors such as psychiatric conditions (depression or anxiety), personality factors, and even age-related development.

—*Nancy A. Piotrowski, Ph.D.*

From the medical perspective, bulimia is nearly as damaging to its practitioners as anorexia. Dental problems, including discoloration and erosion of tooth enamel and irritation of gums by highly acidic gastric juice, are frequent. Electrolyte imbalance, such as metabolic alkalosis or hypokalemia (low potassium levels) caused by the self-induced vomiting, is a constant threat. Parotid gland enlargement, esophageal lacerations, and acute gastric dilatation may occur. Cardiac irregularities may also result. The chronic use of emetics such as ipecac to induce vomiting after eating may result in cardiomyopathy (disease of the middle layer of the walls of the heart, the myocardium), occasionally with a fatal outcome. While their menstrual periods are irregular, these patients are seldom amenorrheic.

Another eating disorder, obesity, is the most prevalent nutritional disorder of the Western world. Using the most commonly accepted definition of obesity—a body weight greater than 20 percent above an individual's normal or desirable weight—approximately 35 percent of adults in the United States were considered obese in the early 1990's. This figure represents twice the proportion of the population that was obese in 1900. Evidently, more sedentary lifestyles strongly contributed to this increase, since the average caloric intake of the population decreased by 5 percent since 1910. Although the problem affects both sexes, obesity is found in a larger portion of women than men. In the forty- to forty-nine-year-old age group, 40 percent of women, while only 30 percent of men, were found to meet the criterion for obesity. Prevalence of obesity increases with both age and lower socioeconomic status.

While results of both animal and human studies suggest that obesity is genetically influenced to some degree, most human obesity is reflective of numerous influences and conditions. Evidence indicates that the relationship between caloric intake and adipose tissue is not as straightforward as had been assumed. In the light of this evidence, the failure to lose unwanted pounds and the failure to maintain hard-won weight loss experienced by many dieters seem much more understandable. In the past, obese individuals often were viewed pejoratively by others and by themselves. They were seen as having insufficient willpower and self-discipline. It was incorrectly assumed that it is no more difficult for most obese individuals to lose fat by decreasing caloric intake than it is for individuals in a normal weight range and that it would be just as easy for the obese to maintain normal weight as it is for those who have never been obese.

Treatment and Therapy

The management of anorectic patients, in either hospital or outpatient settings, may include individual psychotherapy, family therapy, behavior modification, and pharmacotherapy. Many anorectic patients are quite physically ill when they first consult a physician, and medical evaluation and management in a hospital may be necessary at this stage. A gastroenterologist or other medical specialist familiar with this condition may be required to evaluate electrolyte disturbance, emaciation, hypothermia, skin problems, hair loss, sensitivity to cold, fatigue, and cardiac arrhythmias. Starvation may cause cognitive and psychological disturbances that limit the patient's cooperation with treatment.

Indications for hospitalization are weight loss exceeding 30 percent of ideal body weight or the presence of serious medical complications. Most clinicians continue the hospitalization until 80 percent to 85 percent of the ideal body weight is reached. The hospitalization makes possible hyperalimentation (intravenous infusion of nutrients) when medically necessary. Furthermore, individual and family psychiatric evaluations can be performed and a therapeutic alliance established more rapidly with the patient hospitalized.

Most programs utilize behavior modification during the course of hospitalization, making increased privileges such as physical and social activities and visiting contingent on weight gain. A medically safe rate of weight gain is approximately one-quarter of a pound a day. Patients are weighed daily, after the bladder is emptied, and daily fluid intake and output are recorded. Patients with bulimic characteristics may be required to stay in the room two hours after each meal without access to the bathroom to prevent vomiting. Some behavior modification programs emphasize formal contracting, negative contingencies, the practice of avoidance behavior, relaxation techniques, role-playing, and systematic desensitization.

The goal of dynamic psychotherapy is to achieve patient autonomy and independence. The female anorectic patient often uses her body as a battleground for the separation or individuation struggle with her mother. The cognitive therapeutic approach begins with helping the patient to articulate beliefs, change her view of herself as the center of the universe, and render her expectations of the consequences of food intake less catastrophic. The therapist acknowledges the patient's beliefs as genuine, particularly the belief that her self-worth is dependent on achieving and maintaining a low weight. Through a gradual modification of self-assessment, the deficits in the patient's self-esteem are remedied. The therapist also challenges the cultural values surrounding body shape and addresses behavioral and family issues such as setting weight goals and living conditions.

The behavioral management of bulimia includes an examination of the patient's thinking and behavior toward eating and life challenges in general. The patient is made fully aware of the extent of her binging by being asked to keep a daily record of her eating and vomiting practices. A contract is then established with the patient to help her restrict her eating to three or four planned meals per day. The second stage of treatment emphasizes self-control in eating as well as in other areas of the patient's life. In the final stage of treatment, the patient is assisted in maintaining her new, more constructive eating behaviors.

Almost all clinicians work intensively with the families of anorectic patients, particularly in the initial stage of treatment. Family treatment begins with the current family structure and later addresses the early family functioning that can influence family dynamics dramatically. Multigenerational sources of conflict are also examined.

Family therapy with bulimics explores the sources of family conflicts and helps the family to resolve them. Particular attention is directed toward gender roles in the family, as well as the anxiety of the parents in allowing their children autonomy and self-sufficiency. The roots of impulsive and depressive behaviors and the role of parental satisfaction in the patients' lives and circumstances are often explored and addressed.

In the treatment of obesity, the use of a reduced-calorie diet regimen alone does not appear to be an effective approach for many patients, and it is believed that clinicians may do more harm than good by prescribing it. In addition to the high number of therapeutic failures and possible exacerbation of the problem, negative emotional responses are common side effects. Depression, anxiety, irritability, and preoccupation with food appear to be associated with dieting. Such responses have been found to occur in as many as half of the general obese population while on weight-loss diets and are seen with even greater frequency in the severely obese. Some researchers conclude that some cases are better off with no treatment. Their reasoning is based not only on the ineffectiveness of past treatments and the evidence of biological bases for differences in body size but also on the fact that mild to moderate obesity does not appear to put women (or

men) at significant health risk. Moreover, an increase in the incidence of serious eating disorders in women has accompanied the increasingly stringent cultural standards of thinness for women. Given the present level of knowledge, it may be that some individuals would benefit most by adjusting to a weight that is higher than the culturally determined ideal.

When an individual of twenty-five to thirty-four years of age is more than 100 percent above normal weight level, however, there is a twelvefold increase in mortality, and the need for treatment is clear. Although much of the increased risk is related to the effects of extreme overweight on other diseases (such as diabetes, hypertension, and arthritis), these risks can decrease with weight loss. Conservative treatments have had very poor success rates with this group, both in achieving weight reduction and in maintaining any reductions accomplished. Inpatient starvation therapy has had some success in reducing weight in the severely obese but is a disruptive, expensive, and risky procedure requiring very careful medical monitoring to avoid fatality. Furthermore, for those patients who successfully reduce their weight by this method, only about half will maintain the reduction.

Severe obesity seems to be treated most effectively by surgical measures, which include wiring the jaws to make oral intake nearly impossible, reducing the size of the stomach by suturing methods, or short-circuiting a portion of the intestine so as to reduce the area available for uptake of nutrients. None of these methods, however, is without risk.

Perspective and Prospects

The apparent increase in the incidence of anorexia and bulimia in the 1980's and the interest that they have generated both within the scientific community and among the general public have created the impression that these are new diseases. Although scientific writings on the two disorders were uncommon before the early 1960's, eating disorders are by no means recent developments.

Many early accounts of what might have been the condition of anorexia nervosa exist. The clearest and most detailed account is probably the treatise by Richard Morton, a London physician, in his *Phthisiologica: Or, A Treatise of Consumptions* (1694), first published in Latin. In the book, he described several conditions of consumption, devoting one section to the condition of "nervous consumption" in which the emaciation occurred without any remarkable fever, cough, or shortness of breath. He believed the illness to be the result of violent "passions of the mind," the intemperate drinking of alcohol, and an "unwholesome air." He then described two cases, an eighteen-year-old woman who subsequently died following a "fainting fit" and a sixteen-year-old boy who made a partial recovery.

The term "anorexia nervosa" was first used by Sir William Gull (1816-1890), a physician at Guy's Hospital in London, in a paper published in 1874 in which he described the case histories of four women, including one for whom the illness was fatal. He had first mentioned the illness, briefly calling it "apepsia hysterica," in a lengthy address on diagnosis in medicine that he delivered in Oxford, England, in 1868. By 1874, however, he believed that the term "anorexia" would be more correct, and he preferred the more general term "nervosa," since the disease occurs in males as well as females. As part of the clinical picture of the illness, he emphasized the presence of amenorrhea, constipation, bradycardia, loss of appetite, emaciation, and in some cases low body temperature, edema in the legs, and cyanotic peripheries. He commented particularly on the remarkable restlessness and "mental perversity" of the patients and was convinced that the loss of appetite was central in origin. He found the illness to occur mainly in young females between the ages of sixteen and twenty-three.

Ernest Charles Laseque (1816-1883), a professor of clinical medicine in Paris, published an article in 1873 in which he reported on eight patients. He found the illness to occur mostly in young women between the ages of fifteen and twenty, with the onset precipitated by some emotional upset. He also described the occurrence of diminished food intake, constipation, increased activity, amenorrhea, and the patient's contentment with her condition despite the entreaties and threats of family members.

Despite these promising beginnings, the concept of anorexia nervosa was not clearly established until modern times. The main reason for the conceptual confusion was the overgeneralized interpretation of the nature of the patient's refusal to eat. A second source of confusion was the erroneous view that severe emaciation was a frequent, if not primary, feature of hypopituitarism, a condition first described in 1914. That anorexia nervosa was not related to hypopituitarism was finally clarified by researchers in 1949, but the overgeneralized interpretation of the nature of the food refusal persisted into the early 1960's.

If anorexia is taken to mean a loss of the desire to eat,

then there is no doubt that the term "anorexia nervosa" is a misnomer. Anorectic patients refuse to eat not because they have no appetite, but because they are afraid to eat; the food refusal or aversion to eating is the result of an implacable and distorted attitude toward weight, shape, and fatness. The idea that this characteristic attitude is the primary feature of the disorder was not clearly formulated until the early 1960's. Once the concept took hold, the illness of anorexia nervosa became distinguishable from other illnesses that led to similar malnutrition. Thus, for example, a person with hysteria may refuse to eat because of a genuine loss of appetite but does demonstrate the characteristic pursuit of thinness. In the 1980's, there was a revival of the idea that the eating disorders are merely variants of an affective illness.

After occurrences of vomiting and binge eating in a context of anorexia nervosa were described, other investigators proposed two subgroups of anorectic patients: the restrictors and the vomiters. This idea was taken further in 1980 by researchers who divided anorexia nervosa into the restrictor and the bulimic subgroups. The occurrence of binge eating in the context of obesity was described as early as 1959, and in 1970, one investigator described the condition as the "stuffing syndrome." Meanwhile, in 1977, several researchers in Japan proposed that *kibarashigui* (binge eating with an orgiastic quality) be delineated as a separate syndrome from anorexia nervosa. The confusion produced by using a symptom (bulimia) to describe a syndrome (also bulimia) is considerable, and in the English-speaking world the terms "bulimarexia," "dietary chaos syndrome," and "abnormal normal weight control syndrome" have been proposed for the binge-eating syndrome in patients with a normal or near-normal weight.

In 1980, the American Psychiatric Association (APA) distinguished bulimia as a syndrome from anorexia nervosa, and in 1987, the APA replaced the term with "bulimia nervosa." Doubts still persisted, however, regarding the identification of the eating disorders. On one hand, the boundary between the disorders and "normal" dieting behavior seems blurred. On the other hand, the eating disorders are sometimes considered to be variants of other psychiatric illnesses, previously schizophrenia, obsessive-compulsive disorder, and in the 1980's, the mood disorders. A discussion of the eating disorders is necessary if researchers are to agree on definitions so that the disorders are distinguishable from a major depression or from each other.

—Genevieve Slomski, Ph.D.

See also Addiction; Amenorrhea; Anorexia nervosa; Anxiety; Bariatric surgery; Depression; Hyperadiposis; Malnutrition; Nutrition; Obesity; Obsessive-compulsive disorder; Psychiatric disorders; Psychiatry; Psychiatry, child and adolescent; Puberty and adolescence; Sports medicine; Stress; Vitamins and minerals; Weight loss and gain; Weight loss medications.

FOR FURTHER INFORMATION:

Abraham, Suzanne, and Derek Llewellyn-Jones. *Eating Disorders: The Facts.* 5th ed. New York: Oxford University Press, 2002. Examines eating disorders from psychological, sociocultural, and biological perspectives. This edition includes new information on eating disorders and pregnancy and the impact of eating disorders on families.

Brownell, Kelly D., and Christopher G. Fairburn, eds. *Eating Disorders and Obesity: A Comprehensive Handbook.* 2d ed. New York: Guilford Press, 2001. This text addresses all eating disorders, particularly obesity. Includes references and an index.

Field, Howard L., and Barbara B. Domangue, eds. *Eating Disorders Throughout the Life Span.* New York: Praeger, 1987. This collection of essays, intended for the layperson as well as the professional, offers insight into eating disorders of infancy and childhood, adolescent and adult eating disorders, and eating disturbances in the elderly. Includes a bibliography.

Garner, David M., and Paul E. Garfinkel, eds. *Handbook of Treatment for Eating Disorders.* 2d ed. New York: Guilford Press, 1997. This is an updated source on the diagnosis, assessment, and treatment of eating disorders, as well as key issues associated with developing eating disorders.

Herrin, Marcia, and Nancy Matsumoto. *The Parent's Guide to Childhood Eating Disorders: A Nutritional Approach to Solving Eating Disorders.* New York: Henry Holt, 2002. An excellent guide to children's eating disorders, covering early warning signs; dealing with school, friends, sports, and camp; knowing when to seek professional help; and avoiding a relapse.

Hsu, L. K. George. *Eating Disorders.* New York: Guilford Press, 1990. The work provides a summary of the knowledge about the eating disorders of anorexia and bulimia, a historical development of the concepts, their clinical features, methods of diagnostic evaluation, and various treatment options.

Maj, Mario, et al., eds. *Eating Disorders.* New York: Wiley, 2003. Combines research and clinical evidence to inform diagnosis and treatment options.

Moe, Barbara. *Understanding the Causes of a Negative Body Image.* New York: Rosen, 1999. Designed for students in grades seven and above, who are bombarded by misinformation and media images of the perfect young adult. Looks at the causes behind a negative body image and stresses that self-esteem is more important than personal size.

National Association of Anorexia Nervosa and Associated Disorders. http://www.altrue.net/site/anadweb/ A site that provides hotline counseling, a national network of free support groups, referrals to health care professionals, and education and prevention programs to promote self-acceptance and healthy lifestyles.

Parker, James M., and Philip M. Parker, eds. *The 2002 Official Patient's Sourcebook on Binge Eating Disorder.* San Diego, Calif.: Icon Health, 2002. Draws from public, academic, government, and peer-reviewed research to provide a wide-ranging handbook for patients with eating disorders.

EBOLA VIRUS

DISEASE/DISORDER

ANATOMY OR SYSTEM AFFECTED: Blood, circulatory system, gastrointestinal system, muscles, skin

SPECIALTIES AND RELATED FIELDS: Epidemiology, public health, virology

DEFINITION: A virus responsible for a severe and often fatal hemorrhagic fever.

KEY TERMS:

Filoviridae: the family to which the Ebola virus belongs

maculopapular rash: a discolored skin rash observed in patients with Ebola fever.

CAUSES AND SYMPTOMS

The Ebola virus is named after the Ebola River in northern Zaire, Africa, where it was first detected in 1976, when hundreds of deaths were recorded there as well as in neighboring Sudan. A fatal disease among cynomolgus laboratory monkeys that were imported from the Philippines showed symptoms similar to those of the Ebola virus in 1989, but that disease is possibly attributed to the closely related Marburg virus. An equally devastating outbreak among humans took place again in early 1995 in Kirkwit, 500 kilometers east of Kinshasha, Zaire; the disease claimed the lives of 244 pa-

INFORMATION ON EBOLA VIRUS

Causes: Viral infection
Symptoms: Severe blood clotting and hemorrhaging, fever, lethargy, appetite loss, headaches, muscle aches, skin rash
Duration: Acute
Treatments: None

tients out of 315 reported cases, a 77 percent fatality rate. It is interesting to note that the epidemic ended within a few months, as suddenly as it began; this puzzled scientists, who are still unaware of the causes and nature of this so-called hot virus. Despite the dreadful speed with which the disease killed its victims, scientists were happy that they contained it with a relatively small number of fatalities. Recently obtained historical documentation suggests the possibility that the Athenian plague at the beginning of the Peloponnesian War around 430 B.C.E. could be attributed to the Ebola virus.

The Ebola virus appears to have an incubation period of four to sixteen days, after which time the impact is devastating. The patient develops appetite loss, increasing fever, headaches, and muscle aches. The next stage involves disseminated intravascular coagulation (DIC), a condition characterized by both blood clots and hemorrhaging. The clots usually form in vital internal organs such as the liver, spleen, and brain, with subsequent collapse of the neighboring capillaries. Other symptoms include vomiting, diarrhea with blood and mucus, and conjunctivitis. An unusual type of skin irritation known as maculopapular rash first appears in the trunk and quickly covers the rest of the body. The final stages of the disease involve a spontaneous hemorrhaging from all body outlets, coupled with shock and kidney failure and often death within eight to seventeen days.

TREATMENT AND THERAPY

The Ebola virus is classified as a ribonucleic acid (RNA) virus and is closely related to the Marburg virus, first discovered in 1967. The Marburg and the Ebola viruses make up the only two members of the Filoviridae family, which was first established in 1987. Electron microscope studies show the Ebola virus as long filaments, 650 to 14,000 nanometers in length, that are often either branched or intertwined. Its virus part, known as the virion, contains one single noninfectious minusstrand RNA molecule and an endogenous RNA poly-

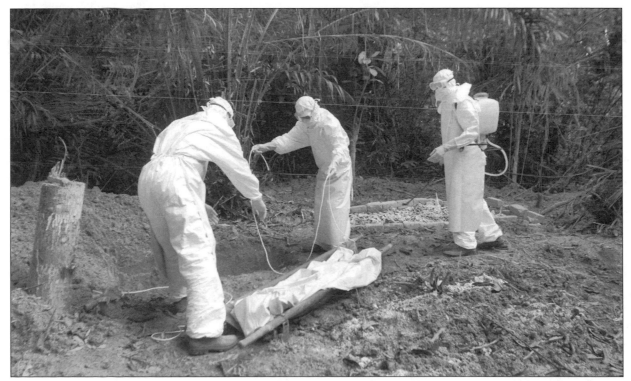

Workers wear protective clothing when burying a young victim of the Ebola virus in Gabon in 2001. (AP/Wide World Photos)

merase. The lipoprotein envelope contains a single glycoprotein, which behaves as the type-specific antigen. Spikes are approximately 7 nanometers in length, are spaced at approximately 10-nanometer intervals, and are visible on the virion surface. It is believed that once in the body, the virus produces proteins that suppress the organism's immune system, thus allowing its uninhibited reproduction. In 2002, researchers announced a new discovery about how Ebola makes entry into and subverts human cells. Findings show that the virus targets a "lipid raft," tiny fat platforms that float atop the membranes of human cells. These rafts act as gateways for the virus, the assembly platform for making new virus particles, and the exit point where new particles bud. This research is a significant step toward one day creating drugs that would stop viruses from replicating.

The Ebola virus can be transmitted through contact with body fluids, such as blood, semen, mucus, saliva, and even urine and feces.

The level of infectivity of the Ebola virus is quite stable at room temperature. Its inactivation is accomplished via ultraviolet or gamma irradiation, 1 percent formalin, beta propiolactone, and an exposure to phenolic disinfectants and lipid solvents, such as deoxycholase and ether. The virus isolation is usually achieved from acute-phase serum of appropriate cell cultures, such as the Ebola-Sudan virus MA-104 cells from a fetal rhesus monkey kidney cell line. Satisfactory results have been accomplished using tissues from the liver, spleen, lymph nodes, kidneys, and heart during autopsy. The virus isolation from brain and other nervous tissues, however, has been rather unsuccessful so far. Neutralization tests have been inconsistent for all filoviruses. Ebola strains, however, show cross-reactions in tests of immunofluorescence assays.

There appears to be no known or standard treatment for Ebola fever. No chemotherapeutic or immunization strategies are available, and no antiviral drug has been shown to provide positive results, even under in vitro conditions. Human interferon, human convalescent plasma, and anticoagulation therapy have been used with unconvincing results.

At this stage, therapy involves sustaining the desired fluid and electrolyte balance by the fre-

---

In the News:
Congo Outbreak of Ebola in 2003

In December, 2002, reports that gorillas and chimpanzees were dying in remote forests within the northern region of the Republic of Congo alarmed Congolese authorities. In January, 2003, word spread of a possible outbreak of Ebola virus in the country's Cuvette-Ouest district. At that point in time, twelve people had died of apparent hemorrhagic fever in the town of Kelle, and four more persons had died at Mbomo. The previous year, in the same area, a similar episode had resulted in the deaths of forty-three people in the Republic of Congo and fifty-three residents of neighboring Gabon.

At the peak of the epidemic, most of the population of Kelle fled into the forest in the attempt to hide from the deadly virus. Volunteers from the Congolese Red Cross, clad in protective suits, cared for the sick and the elderly who were left behind. Few villagers believed that the epidemic was a natural disease brought about by eating infected primate meat—rather, they suspected witchcraft. Four teachers, accused of causing the outbreak, were reportedly killed by a mob.

Medical teams from the United Nations World Health Organization (WHO), the Red Cross, and Médecins Sans Frontières set up makeshift hospital wards in the affected area. The United States Centers for Disease Control (CDC) sent an expert epidemiologist. The European Commission's Humanitarian Aid Office appropriated 500,000 euros to support the relief work.

Aid workers began a public awareness campaign to halt the spread of the disease. The WHO held meetings with local leaders to assure them they could limit the outbreak by avoiding primate meat and by not touching the bodies of those sick with the disease. Heads of families were urged to refrain from washing deceased family members, a ritual required by traditional burial practices.

By late April, the epidemic appeared to be under control, and people began to return to their homes. Fears that the returning villagers might start a new series of infections after eating the meat of dead gorillas while hiding in the forest proved unfounded. Out of 144 reported cases, the disease claimed 126 lives, a death rate approaching 90 percent.

—Milton Berman, Ph.D.

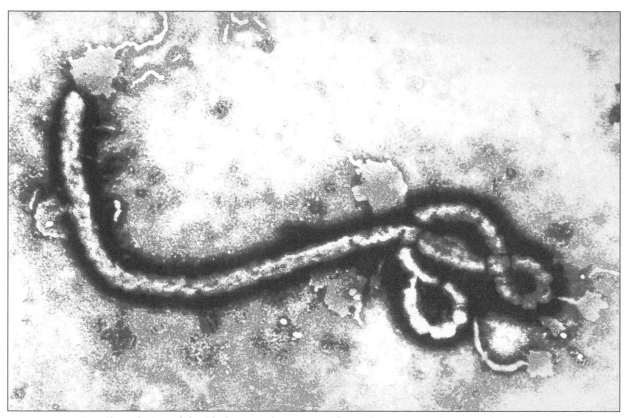

An enlarged view of the Ebola virus that causes African hemorrhagic fever. (Digital Stock)

quent administration of fluids. Bleeding may be fought off with blood and plasma transfusion. Sanitary conditions to avoid further contact with the disease are required. Proper decontamination of medical equipment, isolation of the patients from the rest of the community, and prompt disposal of infected tissues, blood, and even corpses limit the spread of the disease.

PERSPECTIVE AND PROSPECTS

The puzzling characteristics of the Ebola virus are the location of its primary natural reservoir, its sudden eruption and the unknown reason for its quick end, and the unusual discovery of the virus in the organs of people who have survived it.

In the past, experimental work on the virus has been slow because of its high pathogenicity. The progress of recombinant deoxyribonucleic acid (DNA) technology has shed the first light on the molecular structure of this virus. It is hoped that further work using this technique as well as the results of viruses of lower pathogenicity (such as the Reston virus) will provide the desired information on replication and virus-host interactions. Finally, the improvement of the various diagnostic tools will allow more accurate virus identification and assessment of transmission modes.

In 1995, the World Health Organization (WHO) investigators and epidemiologists captured about three thousand birds, rodents, and other animals and insects that are suspected of spreading the disease in order to investigate the source of the virus. The results, however, were obscure and inconclusive, and the main facts about the disease are still a mystery, with the exception of the established link between primates and Ebola virus infection in humans. This conclusion was reached after the fatal infection of a French researcher in Ivory Coast who performed an autopsy on a chimpanzee that had died from a disease with the same symptoms as Ebola fever. Yet, the human outbreaks in Zaire and the Sudan have not been traced to monkeys. As long as these puzzling questions linger, the disease should be contained, with particular emphasis on the improvement of sanitary conditions and the control of body fluid contact.

—Soraya Ghayourmanesh, Ph.D.

See also Bleeding; Centers for Disease Control and Prevention (CDC); Epidemiology; Tropical medicine; Viral infections; Zoonoses.

For Further Information:

Balter, Michael. "On the Trail of Ebola and Marburg Viruses." *Science* 290, no. 5493 (November 3, 2000): 923-925. Researchers are making headway on understanding hemorrhagic fever viruses. Perplexing to researchers is how Marburg and Ebola viruses cause such devastating symptoms as shock and massive bleeding.

Biddle, Wayne. *Field Guide to Germs.* 2d ed. New York: Anchor Books, 2002. This comprehensive book is easily accessible to the nonspecialist and includes a discussion of nearly every virus, bacterium, and fungus known to cause human and nonhuman animal disease. The history of the microbe and the treatment of diseases are included.

Dyer, Nicole. "Killers Without Cures." *Science World* 57, no. 3 (October 2, 2000): 8-12. In the last thirty years, more than fifty lethal viruses once found only in animals have infected humans. A look at how virus hunters on a 1995 mission worked to stop a deadly outbreak of the Ebola virus in the Congo.

"Ebola." In *McGraw-Hill Encyclopedia of Science and Technology.* 8th ed. Vol. 5. New York: McGraw-Hill, 1997. A chapter in a complete reference for the nonspecialist, which offers thousands of articles written by world-renowned scientists and engineers. It includes many new and revised articles and extensive cross-references and bibliographies and is fully illustrated.

Jaax, Nancy. *Lethal Viruses, Ebola, and the Hot Zone: Worldwide Transmission of Fatal Viruses.* Lincoln: University of Nebraska Foundation, 1996. This text is based on a forum on world issues sponsored by the Cooper Foundation and the University of Nebraska at Lincoln. Illustrated.

Jahrling, P. B. "Filoviruses and Arenaviruses." In *Manual of Clinical Microbiology*, edited by Patrick R. Murray. 7th ed. Washington, D.C.: American Society of Microbiology, 1999. A chapter in a text devoted to medical and diagnostic microbiology. Includes bibliographical references and an index.

Peters, C. J., and J. W. LeDuc. "An Introduction to Ebola: The Virus and the Disease." *The Journal of Infectious Diseases* 179, supp. 1 (1999): ix-xvi. This paper is sponsored by the World Health Organization and the Centers for Disease Control and Prevention. Includes bibliographical references.

Strauss, James, and Ellen Strauss. *Viruses and Human Disease.* New York: Elsevier, 2001. An undergraduate text that examines virology from a human disease perspective.

ECG or EKG. *See* Electrocardiography (ECG or EKG).

Eclampsia. *See* Preeclampsia and eclampsia.

Ectopic pregnancy
Disease/disorder

Also known as: Tubal pregnancy

Anatomy or system affected: Reproductive system

Specialties and related fields: Embryology, gynecology

Definition: The implantation of an embryo outside the uterine endometrium, most commonly in the Fallopian tube.

Causes and Symptoms

Although ectopic pregnancies can occur without any known cause, several factors increase a woman's risk. Studies have shown an increase in ectopic pregnancies in women with previous pelvic inflammatory disease (PID). An increase in such pregnancies is also seen in women who were using intrauterine devices (IUDs), especially those containing progesterone, at the time of conception and women who had tubal ligations and other surgeries of the Fallopian tubes. Endometriosis, multiple induced abortions, and pelvic adhesions also may increase a woman's chance of ectopic pregnancy. In general, women whose Fallopian tubes are damaged for any reason have a higher risk. The risk is heightened

---

Information on Ectopic pregnancy

Causes: Unknown; factors may include previous pelvic inflammatory disease, IUD use, tubal ligation, endometriosis, multiple abortions, pelvic adhesions

Symptoms: Similar to those of early pregnancy, followed by spotting, cramping, abdominal pain (especially on one side); if Fallopian tube ruptures, bleeding and severe pain

Duration: Acute

Treatments: Only in early cases, methotrexate to end pregnancy; usually surgical removal of embryo and Fallopian tube

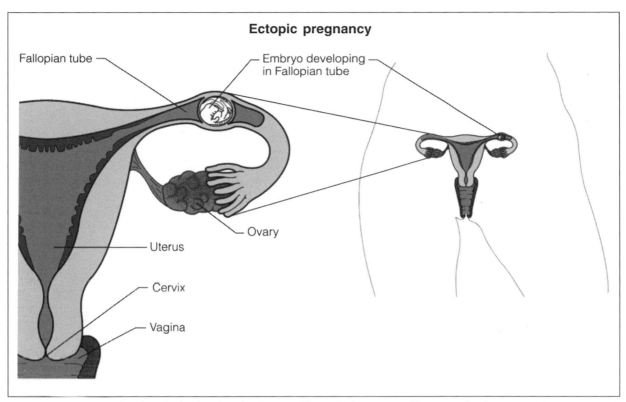

Ectopic pregnancy

Fallopian tube

Embryo developing
in Fallopian tube

Ovary

Uterus

Cervix

Vagina

Ectopic pregnancy results when the fertilized egg implants itself outside the uterus and begins to develop; surgical intervention is usually required.

because damage slows the progress of the developing embryo through the tube, allowing the embryo to be mature enough to implant itself before reaching the uterus. Another factor that may increase the chances of ectopic pregnancy is smoking. Nicotine slows the movement of cilia in the Fallopian tubes, thus slowing the progress of the embryo.

The symptoms of an early ectopic pregnancy are similar to those of any early pregnancy, except that spotting, cramping, and pain, especially on only one side of the abdomen, may occur as the embryo grows. Hormone levels mimic early pregnancy but usually do not rise as high as in a normal intrauterine implantation. If the tube ruptures, then bleeding and severe pain may occur.

TREATMENT AND THERAPY

If a tubal ectopic pregnancy is diagnosed early enough, methotrexate, a chemical that attacks quickly growing cells, may be administered. The drug causes the death of the embryo and flushes the material from the tube. Surgical removal is the most common treatment. The Fallopian tube may be split to remove the embryo, or all or part of the tube may be removed. Methotrexate may be administered to remove any remaining tissues from the pregnancy. Since there is no known way to implant the removed embryo in the uterus, surgical removal also results in the death of the embryo.

—*Richard W. Cheney, Jr., Ph.D.*

See also Conception; Contraception; Genital disorders, female; Miscarriage; Obstetrics; Pregnancy and gestation.

FOR FURTHER INFORMATION:

Carson, Sandra Ann, ed. *Ectopic Pregnancy*. Philadelphia: Lippincott-Raven, 1999.

Hey, Valerie, et al., eds. *Hidden Loss: Miscarriage and Ectopic Pregnancy*. 2d ed. London: Women's Press, 1997.

Leach, Richard E., and Steven J. Ory, eds. *Management of Ectopic Pregnancy*. Malden, Mass.: Blackwell Science, 2000.

Stabile, Isabel. *Ectopic Pregnancy: Diagnosis and Management*. New York: Cambridge University Press, 1996.

ECZEMA

DISEASE/DISORDER
ALSO KNOWN AS: Dermatitis
ANATOMY OR SYSTEM AFFECTED: Skin
SPECIALTIES AND RELATED FIELDS: Dermatology, pediatrics
DEFINITION: An inflammation of the skin.

CAUSES AND SYMPTOMS

The term "eczema" refers to a noncontagious inflammation of the skin. Several types of eczema exist, resulting in a range of symptoms that vary in appearance, duration, and severity. The common characteristic, however, is red, dry, and itchy skin. Other symptoms may include scaling, thickening, or cracking of the skin, leading to infections and severe discomfort.

Atopic dermatitis, the most common form of eczema, is characterized by itchy and cracked skin of the cheeks, arms, and legs. The onset of this chronic type of eczema occurs most often during infancy or childhood, although symptoms may continue into adulthood. The cause of atopic dermatitis is thought to be a hereditary predisposition to skin sensitivities to various environmental factors. These factors include irritants such as soaps, detergents, and rough clothes; allergens such as certain foods, pollen, or animal dander; and changes in

---

INFORMATION ON ECZEMA

CAUSES: Genetic sensitivity to irritants (soaps, detergents, rough clothes), allergens (certain foods, pollen, animal dander), and climate or temperature changes
SYMPTOMS: Red, dry, and itchy skin; scaling, thickening, or cracking of skin
DURATION: Often chronic
TREATMENTS: Minimal exposure to irritants, drugs (corticosteroid creams and ointments, antihistamines, antibiotics); in severe cases, oral corticosteroids or phototherapy

---

climate or temperature. Other forms of eczema, such as contact dermatitis, have similar environmental causes. Seborrheic eczema, nummular eczema, and dishydrotic eczema may result from a combination of several possible causes. Emotional factors, such as stress or frustration, may aggravate the symptoms.

The diagnosis of eczema requires a careful and detailed observation of symptoms. Family and personal medical histories are often useful to determine the presence of allergies or exposure to allergens or irritants. Dermatologists may also use skin biopsies or blood tests to determine a tendency toward elevated allergic or immune response.

TREATMENT AND THERAPY

The treatment of eczema involves minimizing exposure to possible causes while at the same time managing symptoms to maintain a high quality of life. Identifying known allergens and irritants specific to the individual is an important first step. Lifestyle changes aimed at avoiding exposure to these possible causes can lower the frequency and duration of symptoms dramatically. Proper skin care to avoid excessive drying of the skin, including the use of moisturizers or creams and minimizing exposure to water, may also help reduce skin irritation. Avoiding scratching of existing irritations and eliminating sources of emotional stress are other ways that patients can lessen the severity of their symptoms. Dermatologists may prescribe additional treatments, such as corticosteroid creams and ointments, antihistamines, or antibiotics. In more severe cases, systemic corticosteroid treatments or phototherapy, the use of ultraviolet (UV) light, may be tried.

The approval of a new type of treatment for eczema called topical immunomodulators has changed the way

Common Sites of Eczema

eczema is treated in recent years. This new class of drug counteracts the inflammation of the skin without interfering in the body's normal immune response. This treatment has been successful in preventing and even eliminating symptoms of eczema.

—*Paul J. Frisch*

See also Allergies; Dermatitis; Dermatology; Dermatology, pediatric; Itching; Rashes; Skin; Skin disorders; Wiskott-Aldrich syndrome.

FOR FURTHER INFORMATION:

National Eczema Society. http://www.eczema.org/.

Rakel, Robert E., and Edward T. Bope, eds. *Conn's Current Therapy 2003*. Philadelphia: W. B. Saunders, 2003.

Turkington, Carol A., and Jeffrey S. Dover. *Skin Deep: An A-Z of Skin Disorders, Treatments, and Health*. Updated ed. New York: Checkmark Books, 1998.

Westcott, Patsy. *Eczema: Recipes and Advice to Provide Relief*. New York: Welcome Rain, 2000.

EDEMA

DISEASE/DISORDER

ANATOMY OR SYSTEM AFFECTED: Blood vessels, circulatory system, liver, lungs, lymphatic system, respiratory system, skin

SPECIALTIES AND RELATED FIELDS: Internal medicine, nephrology, pulmonary medicine

DEFINITION: Accumulation of fluid in body tissues that may indicate a variety of diseases, including cardiovascular, kidney, liver, and medication problems.

KEY TERMS:

extracellular fluid: the fluid outside cells; includes the fluid within the vascular system and the lymphatic system and the fluid surrounding individual cells

hydrostatic pressure: the physical pressure on a fluid, such as blood; it tends to push fluids across membranes toward areas of lower pressure

interstitial fluid: the fluid between the vascular system and cells; nutrients from the vascular compartment must diffuse across the interstitial compartment to enter the cells

intracellular fluid: the fluid within cells

intravascular fluid: the fluid carried within the blood vessels; it is in a constant state of motion because of the pumping action of the heart

osmotic pressure: the ability of a concentrated fluid on one side of a membrane to draw water away from a less concentrated fluid on the other side

PROCESS AND EFFECTS

Edema is not a disease, but a condition that may be caused by a number of diseases. It signals a breakdown in the body's fluid-regulating mechanisms. The body's water can be envisioned as divided into three compartments: the intracellular compartment, the interstitial compartment, and the vascular compartment. The intracellular compartment consists of the fluid contained within the individual cells. The vascular compartment consists of all the water that is contained within the heart, the arteries, the capillaries, and the veins. The last compartment, and in many ways the most important for a discussion of edema, is called the interstitial compartment. This compartment includes all the water not contained in either the cells or the blood vessels. The interstitial compartment contains all the fluids between the intracellular compartment and the vascular compartment and the fluid in the lymphatic system. The sizes of these compartments are approximately as follows: intracellular fluid at 66 percent, interstitial fluid at 25 percent, and the vascular fluid at only 8 percent of the total body water.

When the interstitial compartment becomes overloaded with fluid, edema develops. To understand the physiology of edema formation, it may be helpful to follow a molecule of water as it travels through the various compartments, beginning when the molecule enters the aorta soon after leaving the heart. The blood has just been ejected from the heart under high pressure, and it speedily begins its trip through the body. It passes from the great vessel, the aorta, into smaller and smaller arteries that divide and spread throughout the body. At each branching, the pressure and speed of the water

---

INFORMATION ON EDEMA

CAUSES: Wide ranging; includes disease, heart failure, deep vein thrombosis, inadequate blood levels of albumin

SYMPTOMS: Varies; may include accumulated fluid, shortness of breath, pain and tenderness, impacted mobility

DURATION: Acute to chronic

TREATMENTS: Dependent on cause; may include frequent elevation of feet to heart level, support stockings, avoidance of prolonged standing or sitting, dietary changes, medications (*e.g.*, diuretics)

molecule decrease. Finally, the molecule enters a capillary, a vessel so small that red blood cells must flow in a single file. The wall of this vessel is composed only of the membrane of a single capillary cell. There are small passages between adjacent capillary cells leading to the interstitial compartment, but they are normally closed.

The hydrostatic pressure on the water molecule is much lower than when it was racing through the aorta, but it is still higher than the surrounding interstitial compartment. At the arterial end of the capillary, the blood pressure is sufficient to overcome the barrier of the capillary cell's membrane. A fair number of water and other molecules are pushed through the membrane into the interstitial compartment.

In the interstitial compartment, the water molecule is essentially under no pressure, and it floats amid glucose molecules, oxygen molecules, and many other compounds. Glucose and oxygen molecules enter the cells, and when the water molecule is close to a glucose molecule it is taken inside a cell with that molecule. The water molecule is eventually expelled by the cell, which has produced extra water from the metabolic process.

Back in the interstitial compartment, the molecule floats with a very subtle flow toward the venous end of the capillary. This occurs because, as the arterial end of the capillary pushes out water molecules, it loses hydrostatic pressure, eventually equaling the pressure of the interstitial compartment. Once the pressure equalizes, another phenomenon that has been thus far overshadowed by the hydrostatic pressure takes over—osmotic pressure. Osmotic pressure is the force exercised by a concentrated fluid that is separated by a membrane from a less concentrated fluid. It draws water molecules across the membrane from the less concentrated side. The more concentrated the fluid, the greater is the drawing power. The ratio of nonwater molecules to water molecules determines concentration.

The fluid that stays within the capillary remains more concentrated than the interstitial fluid for two reasons. First, the plasma proteins in the vascular compartment are too large to be forced across the capillary membrane; albumin is one such protein. These proteins stay within the vascular compartment and maintain a relatively concentrated state, compared to the interstitial compartment. At the same time, the concentration of the fluid in the interstitial compartment is being lowered constantly by the cellular compartment's actions. Cells remove molecules of substances such as glucose

to metabolize, and afterward they release water—a byproduct of the metabolic process. Both processes conspire to lower the total concentration of the interstitial compartment. The net result of this process is that water molecules return to the capillaries at the venous end because of osmotic pressure.

The water molecule is caught by this force and is returned to the vascular compartment. Back in the capillary, the molecule's journey is not yet complete. Now in a tiny vein, it moves along with blood. On the venous side of the circulatory system, the process of branching is reversed, and small veins join to form increasingly larger ones. The water molecule rides along in these progressively larger veins. The pressure surrounding the molecule is still low, but it is now higher than the pressure at the venous end of the capillary. One may wonder how this is possible if the venous pressure at the beginning of the venous system is essentially zero, and there is only one pump, the heart, in the body. As the molecule flows through the various veins, it occasionally passes one-way valves that allow blood to flow only toward the heart. The action of these valves, combined with muscular contractions from activities such as walking or tapping the foot, force blood toward the

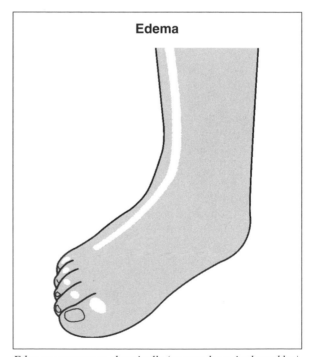

Edema

Edema may appear chronically (as seen here, in the ankles), with characteristic swelling and stretched, shiny skin; it can be a symptom of many diseases.

heart. Without these valves, it would be impossible for the venous blood to flow against gravity and return to the heart; the blood would simply sit at the lowest point in the body. Fortunately, these valves and contractions move the molecule against gravity, returning it to the heart to begin a new cycle.

In certain disease states, there is marked capillary dilation and excessive capillary permeability, and excessive amounts of fluid are allowed to leave the intravascular compartment. The fluid accumulates in the interstitial space. When capillary permeability is increased, plasma proteins also tend to leave the vascular space, reducing the intravascular compartment's osmotic pressure while increasing the interstitial compartment's osmotic pressure. As a result, the rate of return of fluid from the interstitial compartment to the vascular compartment is lowered, thus increasing the interstitial fluid levels.

Another route of return of interstitial fluid to the circulation is via the lymphatic system. The lymphatic system is similar to the venous system, but it carries no red blood cells. It runs through the lymph nodes, carrying some of the interstitial fluid that has not been able to return to the vascular compartment at the capillary level. If lymphatic vessels become obstructed, water in the interstitial compartment accumulates, and edema may result.

CAUSES AND SYMPTOMS

Heart failure is a major cause of edema. When the right ventricle of the heart fails, it cannot cope with all the venous blood returning to the heart. As a consequence, the veins become distended, the interstitial compartment is overloaded, and edema occurs. If the patient with heart failure is mostly upright, the edema collects in the legs; if the patient has been lying in bed for some time, the edema tends to accumulate in the lower back. Other clinical signs of right heart failure include distended neck veins, an enlarged and tender liver, and a "galloping" sound on listening to the heart with a stethoscope.

When the left ventricle of the heart fails, the congestion affects the pulmonary veins instead of the neck and leg veins. Fluid accumulates in the same fashion within the interstitial compartment of the lungs; this condition is termed pulmonary edema. Patients develop shortness of breath with minimal activity, upon lying down, and periodically through the night. They may need to sleep on several pillows to minimize this symptom. This condition can usually be diagnosed by listening to the lungs and heart through a stethoscope and by taking an X ray of the chest.

Deep vein thrombosis is another common cause of edema of the lower limbs. When a thrombus (a blood clot inside a blood vessel) develops in a large vein of the legs, the patient usually complains of pain and tenderness of the affected leg. There is usually redness and edema as well. If the thrombus affects a small vein, it may not be noticed. The diagnosis can be made by several specialized tests, such as ultrasound testing and/or impedance plethysmography. Other tests may be needed to make the diagnosis, such as injecting radiographic dye in a vein in the foot and then taking X rays to determine whether the flow in the veins has been obstructed, or using radioactive agents that bind to the clot. Risks for developing venous thrombosis include immobility (even for relatively short periods of time such as a long car or plane ride), injury, a personal or family history of venous thrombosis, the use of birth control pills, and certain types of cancer. Elderly patients are at particular risk because of relative immobility and an increased frequency of minor trauma to the legs.

When repeated or large thrombi develop, the veins deep inside the thigh (the deep venous system) become blocked, and blood flow shifts toward the superficial veins. The deep veins are surrounded by muscular tissue, and venous flow is assisted by muscular contractions of the leg (the muscular pump), but the superficial veins are surrounded only by skin and subcutaneous tissue and cannot take advantage of the muscular pump. As a consequence, the superficial veins become distended and visible as varicose veins.

When vein blockage occurs, the valves inside become damaged. Hydrostatic pressure of the venous system below the blockage then rises. The venous end of the capillary is normally where the osmotic pressure of the vascular compartment pulls water from the interstitial compartment back into the vascular compartment. In a situation of increased hydrostatic pressure, however, this process is slowed or stopped. As a result, fluid accumulates in the interstitial space, leading to the formation of edema.

A dangerous complication of deep vein thrombosis occurs when part of a thrombus breaks off, enters the circulation, and reaches the lung; this is called a pulmonary embolus. It blocks the flow of blood to the lung, impairing oxygenation. Small emboli may have little or no effect on the patient, while larger emboli may cause severe shortness of breath, chest pain, or even death.

Another potential cause of edema is the presence of a mass in the pelvis or abdomen compressing the large veins passing through the area and interfering with the venous return from the lower limbs to the heart. The resulting venous congestion leads to edema of the lower limbs. The edema may affect either one or both legs, depending on the size and location of the mass. This diagnosis can usually be established by a thorough clinical examination, including rectal and vaginal examinations and X-ray studies.

Postural (or gravitational) edema of the lower limbs is the most common type of edema affecting older people; it is more pronounced toward the end of the day. It can be differentiated from the edema resulting from heart failure by the lack of signs associated with heart failure and by the presence of diseases restricting the patients' degree of mobility. These diseases include Parkinson's disease, osteoarthritis, strokes, and muscle weakness. Postural edema of the lower limbs results from a combination of factors, the most important being diminished mobility. If a person stands or sits for prolonged periods of time without moving, the muscular pump becomes ineffective. Venous compression also plays an important role in the development of this type of edema. It will occur when the veins in the thigh are compressed between the weight of the body and the surface on which the patient sits, or when the edge of a reclining chair compresses the veins in the calves. Other factors that aggravate postural edema include varicose veins, venous thrombi, heart failure, some types of medication, and low blood albumin levels.

Albumin is formed in the liver from dietary protein. It is essential to maintaining adequate osmotic pressure inside the blood vessels and ensuring the return of fluid from the interstitial space to the vascular compartment. When edema is caused by inadequate blood levels of albumin, it tends to be quite extensive. The patient's entire body and even face are often affected. There are several reasons that the liver may be unable to produce the necessary amount of albumin, including malnutrition, liver impairment, the aging process, and excessive protein loss.

In cases of malnutrition, the liver does not receive a sufficient quantity of raw material from the diet to produce albumin; this occurs when the patient does not ingest enough protein. Healthy adults need at least 0.5 gram of protein for each pound of their body weight. Two groups of people are particularly susceptible to becoming malnourished: the poor and the elderly. Infants and children of poor families who cannot afford to pre-

pare nutritious meals often suffer from malnutrition. The elderly, especially men living on their own, are also vulnerable, regardless of their income.

A liver damaged by excessive and prolonged consumption of alcohol, diseases, or the intake of some type of medication or other chemical toxins will be unable to manufacture albumin at the rate necessary to maintain a normal concentration in the blood. Clinically, the patient shows other evidence of liver impairment in addition to edema. For example, fluid may also accumulate in the abdominal cavity, a condition known as ascites. The diagnosis of liver damage is made by clinical examination and supporting laboratory investigations. The livers of older people, even in the absence of disease, are often less efficient at producing albumin.

The albumin also can be deficient if an excessive amount of albumin is lost from the body. This condition may occur in certain types of diseases affecting the kidneys or the gastrointestinal tract. An excessive amount of protein also may be lost if a patient has large, oozing pressure ulcers, extensive burns, or chronic lung conditions that produce large amounts of sputum.

Patients with strokes and paralysis sometimes develop edema of the paralyzed limb. The mechanism of edema formation in these patients is not entirely understood. It probably results from a combination of an impairment of the nerves controlling the dilation, and a constriction of the blood vessels in the affected limb, along with postural and gravitational factors.

Severe allergic states, toxic states, or local inflammation are associated with increased capillary permeability that results in edema. The amount of fluid flowing out to the capillaries far exceeds the amount that can be returned to the capillaries at the venous end. A number of medications, including steroids, estrogens, some arthritis medications, a few blood pressure medications, and certain antibiotics, can induce edema by promoting the retention of fluid. Salt intake tends to cause retention of fluid as well. Obstruction of the lymphatic system often leads to accumulation of fluid in the interstitial compartment. Obstruction can occur in certain types of cancer, after radiation treatment, and in certain parasitic infestations.

TREATMENT AND THERAPY

The management of edema depends on the specific reason for its presence. To determine the cause of edema, a thorough history, including current medications, dietary habits, and activity level, is of prime importance.

Performing a detailed physical examination is also a vital step. It is frequently necessary to obtain laboratory, ultrasound, and/or X-ray studies before a final diagnosis is made. Once a treatable cause is found, then therapy aimed at the cause should be instituted.

If no treatable, specific disease is responsible for the edema, conservative treatment aimed at reducing the edema to manageable levels without inducing side effects should be initiated. Frequent elevation of the feet to the level of the heart, support stockings, and an avoidance of prolonged standing or sitting are the first steps. If support stockings are ineffective or are too uncomfortable, then custom-made, fitted stockings are available. A low-salt diet is important in the management of edema because a high salt intake worsens the fluid retention. If all these measures fail, then diuretics in small doses may be useful.

Diuretics work by increasing the amount of urine produced. Urine is made of fluids removed from the vascular compartment by the kidneys. The vascular compartment then replenishes itself by drawing water from the interstitial compartment. This reduction in the amount of interstitial fluid improves the edema. There are various types of diuretics, which differ in their potency, duration of action, and side effects. Potential side effects include dizziness, fatigue, sodium and potassium deficiency, excessively low blood pressure, dehydration, sexual dysfunction, the worsening of a diabetic's blood sugar control, increased uric acid levels, and increased blood cholesterol levels. Although diuretics are a convenient and effective means of treating simple edema, it is important to keep in mind that the cure should not be worse than the disease. When the potential side effects of diuretic therapy are compared to the almost total lack of complications of conservative treatment, one can see that mild edema which is not secondary to significant disease is best managed conservatively. Edema caused by more serious diseases, however, calls for more intensive measures.

PERSPECTIVE AND PROSPECTS

The prevalence of edema could decrease as people become more health-conscious and medical progress is made. Nutritious diets, avoidance of excessive salt, and an increased awareness of the dangers of excessive alcohol intake and of the benefits of regular physical exercise all contribute to decreasing the incidence of edema. Improved methods for the early detection, prevention, and management of diseases that may ultimately result in edema could also significantly reduce the scope of the problem. It is also expected that safer and more convenient methods of treating edema will become available.

—*Ronald C. Hamdy, M.D., Mark R. Doman, M.D., and Katherine Hoffman Doman*

See also Arteriosclerosis; Circulation; Elephantiasis; Embolism; Heart; Heart disease; Heart failure; Kidney disorders; Kidneys; Kwashiorkor; Liver; Liver disorders; Lungs; Malnutrition; Nutrition; Phlebitis; Pulmonary diseases; Pulmonary medicine; Pulmonary medicine, pediatric; Respiration; Thrombosis and thrombus; Varicose vein removal; Varicose veins; Vascular medicine; Vascular system; Venous insufficiency.

FOR FURTHER INFORMATION:

Andreoli, Thomas, et al., eds. *Cecil Essentials of Medicine.* 5th ed. Philadelphia: W. B. Saunders, 2001. A good introductory text to internal medicine that can also be easily understood by nonscientists.

Guyton, Arthur C. *Human Physiology and Mechanisms of Disease.* 6th ed. Philadelphia: W. B. Saunders, 1997. The standard reference text in human physiology. A background in basic physiology is helpful in understanding this work.

Marieb, Elaine N. *Human Anatomy and Physiology.* 6th ed. Redwood City, Calif.: Benjamin/Cummings, 2003. Details the inter-relationships of body organ systems, homeostasis, and how structure and function complement one another.

Michaelson, Cydney, ed. *Congestive Heart Failure.* St. Louis: C. V. Mosby, 1983. An excellent basic, yet thorough, treatise on the subject of heart failure. The authors discuss the circulatory system in states of both health and disease, low-salt diets, and the drug treatment for heart failure.

EDUCATION, MEDICAL
HEALTH CARE SYSTEM

DEFINITION: In the United States, the educational process that leads to obtaining and maintaining a state license to practice medicine, a process which generally involves obtaining two academic degrees and one or more medical certifications; the entire medical education takes a minimum of eleven years beyond high school.

KEY TERMS:

continuing medical education (CME): medical lectures given by hospitals, medical societies, specialists, and conferences that, in the United States, must be approved to meet the requirements for CME credits

generalist: a medical practitioner who belongs to one of the three largest specialties of medicine—family medicine, internal medicine, and pediatrics; sometimes, practitioners of obstetrics/gynecology (OB/GYN) and general surgery are considered to be generalists

internship: the first year of supervised, postgraduate training after receiving a Doctor of Medicine (M.D.) or Doctor of Osteopathy (D.O.) degree, which allows individuals to practice clinical medicine with a limited license; for M.D.'s, this is called year one of residency, and for D.O.'s this is called year one of internship

residency: a course of postgraduate medical education undertaken after receiving an M.D. or D.O. degree and leading to certification in a generalist or specialist branch of medicine

specialist: referring to specialties of medicine not categorized as generalist

STRUCTURE AND CURRICULUM

During the course of the twentieth century, the medical education system in the United States developed from a one-year or two-year program to the present requirement of eleven or more years of formal education and training after completion of secondary school.

College or university. A person who wishes to be licensed as a physician by one of the fifty states usually begins by completing a bachelor's degree at an accredited college or university. This is, by far, the norm, although it is not an absolute requirement. Some colleges and universities offer a premedical undergraduate program that emphasizes biology, chemistry, and other courses in scientific disciplines. In the past, medical schools preferred graduates of these premedical programs over those with liberal arts or science degrees. Today, many medical schools seek more well rounded students who have degrees in liberal arts disciplines. This change has been made in response to societal pressures to graduate more physicians who have a humanistic approach to medical practice. An effort has also been made to provide educational opportunities for members of disadvantaged and minority groups. Therefore, any person with a good grade-point average may consider applying to medical school regardless of the type or the nature of the bachelor-level education.

Preparation. The first choice that an individual must make when considering a career as a physician is, "What type of medical school do I wish to attend?" In the United States, two medical degrees are granted: Doctor of Medicine (M.D.) and Doctor of Osteopathy (D.O.). M.D.'s are occasionally referred to as allopathic physicians to distinguish them from osteopathic physicians. Historically, allopathic education stressed the importance of disease in causing illness. Laboratory tests and the prescription of medications are generally used in diagnosis and treatment. Osteopathic education historically looked to the musculoskeletal system with respect to health and illness. This distinction is largely a historic remnant. The curricula of both M.D. and D.O. schools are nearly identical. Both types of physicians train in the same residencies, and both receive the same license to practice medicine and surgery.

Medical school (preclinical). The first two years of medical school are generally devoted to the study of academic medicine. This period is known as preclinical education. These years stress the need to master material from basic sciences and to understand the scientific method of research. Courses such as anatomy, biochemistry, histology, immunology, microbiology, neurology, pathology, and physiology are taught. Achievement is marked by success in test taking through memorization, the analysis of detailed information, and the integration of new material. Actual contact with practicing physicians and their patients is not stressed. As a result, this phase is sometimes criticized for teaching medical knowledge that is separated from medical practice. Some medical schools are adjusting the curriculum in the preclinical years to reduce this dichotomy. At the end of the second year, students must pass the first component of the examination to obtain licensure.

Medical school (clinical). The second two years of medical education stress the clinical knowledge needed to become a physician. Classroom education is concerned with physical diagnosis, the identification of diseases, treatments, and associated procedures and techniques. Medical schools require students to observe physicians practicing medicine with patients in both hospital and office settings. Opportunities are available for students to spend time away from their medical school learning about various specialties. The standard curriculum requires all students to study internal medicine, surgery, pediatrics, obstetrics and gynecology, and psychiatry. Other specialties are studied on an elective basis. For example, a medical student may spend a month observing family practice physicians working in hospitals and their offices and receive a grade for that month. In this manner, students gain some experience by direct exposure to several medical specialties. At the end of the fourth year, students must

IN THE NEWS: AMA ENDORSES EIGHTY-HOUR RESIDENT WORKWEEK

For the first time in the history of U.S. medical education, mandated guidelines for the number of hours all medical residents are allowed to work went into effect July 1, 2003. The American Medical Association (AMA) endorsed limits placed on resident duty hours, which apply to all 7,800 accredited training programs.

The limits stemmed from fears of patient safety while in the care of sleep-deprived residents. A landmark case in the late 1980's implicated the training of residents as part of the problem that led to the death of an eighteen-year-old patient in New York. Following an investigation, the Bell Commission Report provided recommendations for changes in residents' hours that eventually became mandated in New York state law.

Over the years, various professional groups and organizations have voiced concern over the number of hours worked during residency. Several studies suggested that sleep deprivation had negative consequences on residents' performance and health and that many hours were spent in activities of little or no educational merit.

In 2001, consumer advocacy group Public Citizen, the Committee of Interns and Residents, and the American Medical Student Association jointly petitioned the Occupational Safety and Health Administration (OSHA) to federally regulate residents' hours. The petition cited the health and well-being of residents as the primary concern. The following year, both the Accreditation Council on Graduate Medical Education (ACGME) and the AMA set duty hour limits. The ACGME will monitor all accredited programs and enforce violations by probation or loss of accreditation. As a result, OSHA denied the petition for federal regulation.

The ACGME guidelines mandate that residents are not allowed to work more than eighty hours per week when averaged over a four-week period, unless approved to increase up to 10 percent more; they must have one day off out of seven, averaged over four weeks; they cannot be on call, on average, more than every third night; and they are limited to twenty-four hours on call, with up to six additional hours for transfer of care and educational activities.

The guidelines aim to improve the education and well-being of residents, enhance patient care, and provide a system for monitoring compliance. Many medical education professionals hope that these limits will prevent federal action, but others fear a negative impact on physician training. The AMA is conducting a ten-year survey to evaluate the impact of these changes.

—*Karen Lindell, M.S., R.D.*

pass the second component of the examination to obtain licensure.

Internship. In the past, many generalist physicians, after one year of internship, entered private practice. Today, the year of internship is completed under close medical supervision. This prepares a new physician for more independent practice. All new physicians complete their first year of internship in a residency program before receiving a full medical license in the second year of residency. Physicians who receive their medical education outside the United States must pass the same test as American medical students before being eligible to complete residency training. Some internships are spent rotating through the areas of medicine, surgery, pediatrics, and obstetrics before entering specialized training in areas such as radiology, dermatology, and some surgical specialties. During the first year of residency, a physician has a limited license to practice medicine. Upon completion of the internship or first-year residency and successful passage of the third portion of the standard licensure examination, a physician is granted a full license to practice medicine and surgery.

Residency. The three generalist areas in which resident physicians learn clinical medicine, also known as primary care specialties, are family medicine, internal medicine, and pediatrics. Family medicine treats the whole family throughout life, internal medicine treats adults, and pediatrics treats children and teenagers. The end of childhood and the beginning of adulthood are not clearly defined, and there is some overlap. Most pediatricians will treat patients up to the age of twenty-two, when they typically complete college. The lowest age for patients of internists is usually sixteen. The many specialist areas of medicine are concerned with specific organ systems, disease processes, or prevention. For example, a psychiatrist has a residency in the area of mental illness, while an emergency room (ER) physician has a residency in the practice of medicine in the ER.

Residency education is the time when a physician who has been graduated from medical school first becomes responsible for patient care, under both direct and indirect supervision. Residency teaches and evaluates the skill of a new physician in applying the knowledge gained in medical school to clinical practice. Residency programs are usually three to five years in length. After each year, the resident is given more independence of practice and more responsibility to supervise newer physicians. Upon completion of a residency program, a physician becomes eligible for certification by one of the generalist or specialist boards of medicine. Most boards require one or two years of independent practice before allowing candidates to seek board certification. A physician must take and pass yet another examination concerning knowledge related to the specialty area for which certification is desired. Many board certifications must be renewed periodically (every five to seven years) as a condition of retaining board-certified status.

Second residency (subspecialization). Some physicians choose to complete additional training in their medical specialties. This subspecialty medical education is usually called a fellowship. For example, a general surgeon may complete a multiyear residency in cardiac surgery, or a psychiatrist may complete a subspecialty residency in children's mental illness. Some highly subspecialized physicians need seven to ten years after medical school to complete their subspecialty training. An example of this level of specialization is forensic pathology, which requires residency training in pathology and fellowships in forensic and chemical pathology. Pediatric neurosurgery is another example.

Continuing medical education. All states require that physicians complete a certain number of continuing medical education (CME) credits in order to maintain their medical licensure. One hundred fifty CME credits over three years is a common requirement. Some specialties also require national examinations for recertification in the specialty. For physicians in the United States, medical education is an exercise in lifelong learning.

THE REQUIREMENTS FOR FULLY LICENSED PHYSICIANS

Place or Event	Degree or Program	Years
College or University	B.A. or B.S.	4
Medical School	Preclinical	2
Medical School	Clinical	2
Graduation	D.O. or M.D.	-
Internship or Residency	D.O. or M.D. Limited License	1
Residency (1st)	Generalist or Specialist	2-5
Residency (2d/3d)	Subspecialist (Optional)	0-5
Continuing Education	CME (150 credits)	every 3
	TOTAL	11-19+

ISSUES AND PHILOSOPHIES

American medical education is undergoing one of the greatest challenges in its history. Medical schools are being asked to teach physicians how to be effective and efficient caregivers to all persons. The corporate system of medical care demands medical care that is effective, cost-conscious or economically efficient, and delivered in a positive and caring manner. Health maintenance organizations (HMOs), preferred provider organizations (PPOs), and other organizational alliances of physicians expect the medical educational system to teach these values and skills.

The national government adds one more criterion: Physicians must be able to do the above for all citizens. In a pluralistic and democratic society, a physician must acknowledge various social, ethnic, cultural, and regional needs. Medical educators must train socially conscious physicians. Physicians must be available to practice in either rural or

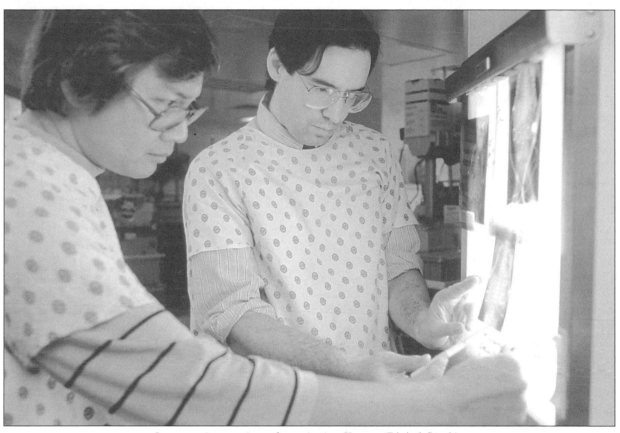

Interns gain experience by reviewing X rays. (Digital Stock)

inner-city areas. They must be able to treat various populations, such as African Americans and Native Americans, for their specific needs. Physicians are being asked to be cognizant of and caring toward all Americans.

The medical philosophy that allows for an increase of psychological skills and social awareness in medical education is called the biopsychosocial model. As the label indicates, it conceptualizes a medical education system which teaches physicians solid medical knowledge ("bio"), an improved ability to relate to patients ("psycho"), and an awareness of different social systems and cultural attitudes as they affect medical care ("social"). The biopsychosocial model of care is a proposed revision of what the medical education system should teach physicians. It may be the medical school curriculum of the future.

PERSPECTIVE AND PROSPECTS

The history of American medical education can be understood as falling into five periods of development. Each period stressed a certain philosophy and direction

unique to its times. The current philosophy of medical education has aspects of all five periods, affecting how and what physicians are taught.

The British period (1750-1815). American medical education was established on the British model. The emphasis in British medical education was on developing a physician's medical knowledge through direct observation of patient care in clinical settings. There were few formal centers for medical training. They functioned to instruct teaching physicians and to transmit new medical knowledge. In America, there were only six medical schools. Most medical education was clinical and taught by older physicians to younger physicians in office settings. There were no formal educational requirements. Most physicians could read and write, possessing the equivalent of only two or three years of formal education.

The French period (1815-1865). French physicians, who developed the skills of classification, influenced American medical education through methods of diagnosis and the use of hospitals. In the United States, many hospitals were built, and there was a significant expansion in the number of medical schools. Large groups of patients were admitted to hospitals and grouped on wards by diagnosis. The hospital-office model of medical education began to develop.

The German period (1865-1915). Laboratory methods and germ theory were introduced into medical education from Germany. Some medical schools began to educate physicians in the laboratory approach to medicine. Office practice was less important in medical education. The period of formal education was still relatively brief, often less than two years in total length. At the end of the German period, many medical schools that were not teaching laboratory methods were closed.

The American period (1915-1965). American medical education embraced a scientific approach, first detailed by Abraham Flexner in *Medical Education in the United States and Canada*, published in 1910 in a report on reforming American medical education. Physician-scientists were to be educated by quality medical schools to provide clinical medicine according to the scientific method. This model was successfully introduced into American medical education. It was considered the norm until the concerns of corporate interests and government interests became vital.

The corporate period (1965-   ). Medicare and Medicaid programs were created and supported by the national government in order to provide quality medical care to all Americans. Corporate interests require that medical education be effective in controlling health costs to industry. Many of the current challenges facing medical education revolve around teaching physicians the two concerns of access and cost-effectiveness.

In the early 1990's, the Council on Graduate Medical Education (COGME) suggested that certain humanistic and corporate medical education goals be reached by the year 2000. At least 50 percent of residency graduates should enter practice as generalist physicians. The number of underrepresented minority students should be doubled. Shortages of physicians in rural and urban areas should be eliminated. The purpose of these goals was to avoid a severe physician shortage for some populations, areas of specialty, and geographic centers. With a system of managed medical care in place, COGME projected a shortage of 35,000 generalist physicians and a surplus of 115,000 specialist physicians by the year 2000. COGME released a report in 1999 that noted the rate of growth in the physician supply had moderated slightly but still was likely to lead to a surplus of physicians, and that the number of generalist physicians was increasing.

In 1990, fewer than one-third of all American physicians practiced primary care. It appears that in the future, the trend toward specialization will be reversed. Those who plan, those who pay, and those who organize the various systems to deliver medical care in the United States no longer believe that so many specialty-trained physicians will be needed. Yet, the demand by Americans for specialized health care services has not diminished. A clash between recipients and providers appears to be inevitable. The next decades in American medicine are likely to be turbulent, as various stakeholders struggle to redefine the American system of health care.

There is an acknowledged maldistribution of physicians. Most prefer to practice in suburban and medical center settings, leaving significant numbers of Americans without easy access to adequate health care. Many planners also believe that the promised efficiency of managed care will result in a decreased need for physicians. In the mid-1990's, state legislatures began to reduce the amounts of support for medical education, effectively forcing medical schools to reduce the number of physicians that they graduate. The final outcomes of these policy changes are unclear. The results of this trend, however, will be felt by American society for decades.

—Gerald T. Terlep, Ph.D.; updated by
L. Fleming Fallon, Jr., M.D., Ph.D., M.P.H.

See also American Medical Association (AMA); Ethics; Hippocratic oath; Nursing; Osteopathic medicine; *specific specialties.*

FOR FURTHER INFORMATION:

Birenbaum, Aaron. *Wounded Profession: American Medicine Enters the Age of Managed Care.* Westport, Conn.: Greenwood Press, 2002. Traces the evolution of health care in the United States during the 1990's and examines the rising costs, consumer backlash, and new legislation.

Brown, Stanford J. *Getting Into Medical School.* 9th ed. Hauppauge, N.Y.: Barron's, 2001. Advice on recommended undergraduate courses, taking the Medical College Admission Test, applying to medical school, getting through the personal interview, and alternatives for students who have been rejected. Directory of American medical schools included.

Ludmerer, Kenneth M. *Time to Heal: American Medical Education from the Turn of the Century to the*

Managed Care Era. New York: Oxford University Press, 2000. Ludmerer looks at the future of medicine in America and reveals some very disturbing trends in managed care, education, and research funding. Contains a wealth of factual details and insightful questions.

Rivo, Marc L., et al. "Defining the Generalist Physician's Training." *Journal of the American Medical Association* 271 (May 18, 1994): 1499-1504. Rivo writes a clear, fact-filled article on major current issues in medical education. The article is accessible to the general reader. It also contains charts and references for further research.

Starr, Paul. "The Framework of Health Care Reform." *New England Journal of Medicine* 330, no. 15 (April 14, 1994): 1086-1088. This article reviews several proposals for health care reform. The author has provided commentary on the American health care system for many years.

Zabala, John A., et al. *Medical School Admissions: The Insider's Guide.* Nashville: Mustang, 1999. Written by medical students for medical students, gives practical advice on admission tasks such as the preparation of an effective application, improving scores on the MCAT, and writing a compelling personal essay.

EEG. *See* ELECTROENCEPHALOGRAPHY (EEG).

ELECTRICAL SHOCK
DISEASE/DISORDER
ANATOMY OR SYSTEM AFFECTED: Heart, nervous system, skin

SPECIALTIES AND RELATED FIELDS: Critical care, emergency medicine, neurology

DEFINITION: The physical effect of an electrical current entering the body and the resulting damage.

CAUSES AND SYMPTOMS
Electric shock ranges from a harmless jolt of static electricity to a power line's lethal discharge. The severity of the shock depends on the current flowing through the body, and the current is determined by the skin's electrical resistance. Dry skin has a very high resistance; thus 110 volts produces a small, harmless current. The resistance for perspiring hands, however, is lower by a factor of 100, resulting in potentially fatal currents. Currents traveling between bodily extremities are particularly dangerous because of their proximity to the heart.

> **INFORMATION ON ELECTRICAL SHOCK**
>
> **CAUSES:** Electrical current entering the body
> **SYMPTOMS:** Unconsciousness, moderate to severe pain, ventricular fibrillation, burning or charring of skin
> **DURATION:** Acute
> **TREATMENTS:** Resuscitation, emergency care

Electric shock causes injury or death in one of three ways: paralysis of the breathing center in the brain, paralysis of the heart, or ventricular fibrillation (extremely rapid and uncontrolled twitching of the heart muscle).

The threshold of feeling (the minimum current detectable) ranges from 0.5 to 1.0 milliamperes. Currents up to 5.0 milliamperes, the maximum harmless current, are not hazardous, unless they trigger an accident by involuntary reaction. Currents in this range create a tingling sensation. The minimum current that causes muscular paralysis occurs between 10 and 15 milliamperes. Currents of this magnitude cause a painful jolt. Above 18 milliamperes, the current contracts chest muscles, and breathing ceases. Unconsciousness and death follow within minutes unless the current is interrupted and respiration resumed. A short exposure to currents of 50 milliamperes causes severe pain, possible fainting, and complete exhaustion, while currents in the 100- to 300-milliampere range produce ventricular fibrillation, which is fatal unless quickly corrected. During ventricular fibrillation, the heart stops its rhythmic pumping and flutters uselessly. Since blood stops flowing, the victim dies from oxygen deprivation in the brain in a matter of minutes. This is the most common cause of death for victims of electric shock.

Relatively high currents (above 300 milliamperes) may produce ventricular paralysis, deep burns in the body's tissue, or irreversible damage to the central nervous system. Victims are more likely to survive a large but brief current, even through smaller, sustained currents are usually lethal. Burning or charring of the skin at the point of contact may be a contributing factor to the delayed death that often follows severe electric shock. Very high voltage discharges of short duration, such as a lightning strike, tend to disrupt the body's nervous impulses, but victims may survive. On the other hand, any electric current large enough to raise body temperature significantly produces immediate death.

Treatment and Therapy

Before medical treatment can be applied, the current must be stopped or the shock victim must be separated from the current source without being touched. Nonconducting materials such as dry, heavy blankets or pieces of wood can be used for this purpose. If the victim is not breathing, artificial respiration immediately applied provides adequate short-term life support, though the victim may become stiff or rigid in reaction to the shock. Victims of electric shock may suffer from severe burns and permanent aftereffects, including eye cataracts, angina, or disorders of the nervous system.

Electric shock can usually be prevented by strictly adhering to safety guidelines and using commonsense precautions. Careful inspection of appliances and tools, compliance with manufacturers' safety standards, and the avoidance of unnecessary risks greatly reduce the chance of an electric shock. Electrical appliances or tools should never be used when standing in water or on damp ground, and dry gloves, shoes, and floors provide considerable protection against dangerous shocks from 110-volt circuits.

Electrical safety is also provided by isolation, guarding, insulation, grounding, and ground fault interrupters. Isolation means that high-voltage wires strung overhead are not within reach, while guarding provides a barrier around high voltage devices, such as those found in television sets.

Old wire insulation may become brittle with age and develop small cracks. Defective wires are hazardous and should be replaced immediately. Most modern power tools are double-insulated; the motor is insulated from the plastic insulating frame. These devices do not require grounding, as no exposed metal parts become electrically live if the wire insulation fails.

In a home, grounding is accomplished by a third wire in outlets, connected through a grounding circuit to a water pipe. If an appliance plug has a third prong, it will ground the frame to the grounding circuit. In the event of a short circuit, the grounding circuit provides a low resistance path, resulting in a current surge which trips the circuit breaker.

In some instances the current may be inadequate to trip a circuit breaker (which usually requires 15 or 20 amperes), but current in excess of 10 milliamperes could still be lethal to humans. A ground-fault interrupter ensures nearly complete protection by detecting leakage currents as small as 5 milliamperes and breaking the circuit. This relatively inexpensive device operates very rapidly and provides an extremely high degree of safety against electrocution in the household. Many localities now have codes which require the installation of ground-fault interrupters in bathrooms, kitchens, and other areas where water is used.

—*George R. Plitnik, Ph.D.*

See also Burns and scalds; Critical care; Critical care, pediatric; Emergency medicine; Resuscitation; Shock; Unconsciousness.

For Further Information:

Atkinson, William. "Electric Injuries Can Be Worse than They Seem." *Electric World* 214, no. 1 (January/February, 2000): 33-36. Whether an electrical shock initially seems serious or mild, it is always a cause for concern. Aspects of electrical shock injuries are explored.

Bridges, J. E., et al., eds. *International Symposium on Electrical Shock Safety Criteria.* New York: Pergamon Press, 1985. The summary of a symposium covering the physiological effects of shock, bioelectrical conditions, and safety measures.

Hewitt, Paul G. *Conceptual Physics.* 8th ed. Reading, Mass.: Addison-Wesley, 1998. Comprehensive coverage of physics for the layperson, which includes detailed discussions of the laws of electricity and electrical devices.

Hogan, David E., and Jonathan L. Burstein. *Disaster Medicine.* Philadelphia: Lippincott Williams & Wilkins, 2002. Examines a wide range of relevant topics including natural, industrial, transportation and conflict-related disasters; and infectious diseases, winter storms, fires and mass burns.

Liu, Lynda. "Pullout Emergency Guide: Electric Shock." *Parents* 75, no. 1 (January, 2000): 65-66. A pull-out emergency guide for the prevention and treatment of electrical shock in children. Household hazards and electricity dos and don'ts are among the tips offered.

U.S. Department of Labor. Occupational Safety and Health Administration. *Controlling Electrical Hazards.* Rev. ed. Washington, D.C.: Government Printing Office, 1997. A report which identifies common electrical hazards and discusses their prevention.

Electrocardiography (ECG or EKG)

Procedure

Anatomy or system affected: Chest, circulatory system, heart

SPECIALTIES AND RELATED FIELDS: Biotechnology, cardiology, critical care, emergency medicine, exercise physiology, preventive medicine

DEFINITION: A noninvasive procedure that provides insight into the rate, rhythm, and general health of the heart.

KEY TERMS:

ECG waves: the repeated deflections of an electrocardiogram; one complete wave consists of a P wave, followed by a QRS complex, and then a T wave and represents one complete cardiac cycle, or heartbeat

electrocardiogram (ECG or EKG): a record of the waves produced by the rhythmically changing electrical conduction within the heart; often recorded by a strip chart recorder

INDICATIONS AND PROCEDURES

Electrocardiography is a useful medical diagnostic and evaluative procedure that reveals much information about the function or malfunction of a person's heart. ECG is a noninvasive, easy-to-use, and economical tool that is an essential part of diagnosing chest pain. It serves an important role in both cardiology and emergency medicine. ECG is also commonly used in preventive medicine to monitor heart health. For this purpose, ECG is frequently used in a format known as a stress test. Athletes often have ECG analysis performed as a part of their training and cardiovascular conditioning.

In a stress test, a person is studied for regularity of rhythm, rate, and unimpeded flow of electrical conduction within the heart. ECG recordings are first made while the person is at rest, then during light exercise, and, finally, if healthy enough, during rigorous exercise. Such exercise causes the heart to work harder and allows a physician to determine whether a person has a heart that beats with a regular, repetitive rhythm and at an appropriate pace for the level of rest or exercise. The stress of exercise can also help in assessing whether the heart muscle masses contract in the proper sequence: atrial contraction followed by ventricular contraction. An irregularity of electrical conduction, poor muscle contraction, dead regions of heart tissue (from a recent or old heart attack), and other maladies can be revealed.

In order to obtain an electrocardiogram, small metallic contact points are taped to the patient's skin via an electrically conductive adhesive or gel. The electric impulses travel across the skin to these contact points; from there, leads (plastic-coated wires) are attached to the recording device so that a complete circuit is made.

Either a monitor screen or a strip chart recorder traces the electrical impulses. The waves are plotted in units of millivolts (on the y-axis) versus time in units of seconds (on the x-axis).

A twelve-lead ECG has replaced the original four-lead type. A twelve-lead ECG allows the physician to explore the performance of the heart from twelve different orientations, or angles, so that much more of the heart mass can be evaluated. The leads (also called electrodes) are placed on the body as follows: one on the right leg, which serves as the ground electrode; one on each of the other extremities; and six on the precordium, which is the area around the sternum and on the left chest wall (over the heart). The leads are explored in different combinations.

USES AND COMPLICATIONS

Healthy people, including athletes or certain members of the armed services, may take stress tests in order to have their health and cardiovascular conditioning monitored during training. Some professionals are required to take stress tests on a regular basis, such as commercial airline pilots and astronauts. In addition, people who have a family history of cardiovascular disease, or who are concerned about their heart health for other reasons, may have a stress test performed to find early warning signs and allow intervention before a crisis occurs. Finally, it should be noted that some insurance companies require stress tests of their applicants in order to determine insurability before issuing or rejecting a policy.

Treatment for chest pain is highly dependent on the electrical patterns seen on the ECG. Drugs may be administered or withheld depending on the shape or duration reported for the P wave, QRS complex, and T-wave patterns. Left-sided versus right-sided heart disease can be discerned from the traces; infarction (heart attack) can be distinguished from angina. Although the waves in the electrocardiogram for an infarcted or anginal heart are abnormal, the patterns become abnormal in a predictable, and therefore diagnostic, manner.

Diagnostic patterns can also be seen for arrhythmias (unusual and abnormal beating patterns), such as ectopic foci, in which some part of the heart other than the sinoatrial (S-A) node (the natural pacemaker) is abnormally in control of determining when the heart contracts, or heart block, whereby electrical conduction is interrupted.

ECG is routinely used to keep close tabs on heart patients and in the postsurgery monitoring of patients who have had open heart or thoracic surgery. Certain

Electrocardiography

The electrical activity of the heart can be measured with an electrocardiograph (ECG or EKG) machine; characteristic patterns can be used to diagnose arrhythmias (irregular heartbeats). The patient may also be asked to walk on a treadmill while the heart is monitored in order to gauge its function during exercise.

kinds of neonatal or infant malformations or malfunctions may also be evaluated with ECG.

Because ECG is a superficial and noninvasive technique, there are no real risks associated with having this procedure performed.

Perspective and Prospects

Electrocardiography was once a wet, messy, and awkward procedure to perform: A patient dangled one arm in a huge jar filled with a conducting salt solution and placed the left leg in another saline-filled container. Changing the leads to include other limbs required the patient to take a good amount of soaking. Although it was a clumsy procedure, the basic premise of ECG remains unchanged: The heart exhibits regular patterns of electrical activity that can be useful diagnostically.

Recent advances in electrocardiography have involved the use of multiple electrode systems along with computers and recorders that allow rapid and simultaneous multiple-lead input and output. In addition, modern electronic instrumentation allows continuous ECG monitoring so that patients in intensive care units, coronary care units, or emergency rooms can be assessed on a second-by-second basis when seconds count. Undoubtedly, the ECG systems available today, coupled with thoughtful and informed interpretation by medical doctors and emergency medical technicians (EMTs), are responsible for saving many lives.

—*Mary C. Fields, M.D.*

See also Angina; Arrhythmias; Biofeedback; Cardiology; Cardiology, pediatric; Cardiopulmonary resuscitation (CPR); Critical care; Critical care, pediatric; Emergency medicine; Emergency medicine, pediatric; Exercise physiology; Heart; Heart attack; Paramedics; Stress; Stress reduction.

For Further Information:

Conover, Mary Boudreau. *Understanding Electrocardiography.* 8th ed. St. Louis: C. V. Mosby, 2002. This standard text is divided into four sections: introduction to the 12-lead electrocardiogram, arrhythmia recognition, abnormal 12-lead electrocardiograms, and special diagnostic and therapeutic procedures.

Phibbs, Brendan. *The Human Heart: A Complete Text on Function and Disease*. 5th ed. St. Louis: G. W. Manning, 1992. Designed for the general reader, this resource discusses cardiology. Includes bibliographical references and an index.

Rawlings, Charles A. *Electrocardiography*. Reprint. Redmond, Wash.: SpaceLabs, 1993. Discusses electrocardiography as a tool to measure the health of the heart. Includes bibliographical references and an index.

Surawicz, Borys, et al. *Electrocardiography in Clinical Practice*. 5th ed. Philadelphia: W. B. Saunders, 2001. Explores the values and limitations of the electrocardiogram and covers such topics as pericarditis and cardiac surgery, atrial and atrioventricular rhythms, ventricular arrhythmias, and effects of drugs on the ECG.

Thaler, Malcom S. *The Only EKG Book You'll Ever Need*. 4th ed. Philadelphia: Lippincott Williams & Wilkins, 2002. Many EKG texts delve heavily into the physics and myocardial electrophysiology associated with EKGs and overwhelm and confuse the early learner. This book avoids lengthy discussions of theory and uses wide spacing, open pages, simple text, and diagrams to allow for speedier mastery of the basics.

Wellens, Hein J. J., and Mary Boudreau Conover. *The ECG in Emergency Decision Making*. Philadelphia: W. B. Saunders, 1992. This resource offers guidance for the professional regarding the diagnosis of heart disease in an emergency setting.

Wiederhold, Richard. *Electrocardiography: The Monitoring and Diagnostic Leads*. Philadelphia: W. B. Saunders, 1999. This textbook is intended to be a primary or introductory text to the field of electrocardiography (ECG) for students in the health care professions or clinicians who are not cardiologists.

ELECTROCAUTERIZATION

PROCEDURE

ANATOMY OR SYSTEM AFFECTED: Blood vessels, cells, circulatory system, joints, ligaments, muscles, skin, uterus

SPECIALTIES AND RELATED FIELDS: Cardiology, critical care, dermatology, emergency medicine, family practice, general surgery, gynecology, internal medicine, vascular medicine

DEFINITION: The surgical control of bleeding from small blood vessels or the removal of unwanted tissue using a controlled electric current.

INDICATIONS AND PROCEDURES

Electrocauterization is a procedure used in many surgical operations. As a surgeon's scalpel penetrates layers of skin and tissue, numerous tiny blood vessels are cut open. To stop the associated bleeding, an assisting surgeon can seal these vessels immediately using an electrical instrument to burn just enough of the tissue to produce a tiny scar. Electrocauterization is also used to destroy unwanted tissue, such as skin lesions.

Prior to any surgery involving electrocautery, local anesthesia is applied by injection. Electrocauterization is carried out with a small needle probe that is heated with an electrical current. Enough current is applied to heat the probe to temperatures at which blood will coagulate. To prevent electrical shock, a grounding pad is placed on the patient and a small electrode is attached to the skin near the surgery site to direct any excess current away from the body. Depending on the surgery site and the size and shape of unwanted tissue, the cautery pattern may be circular, dotted, or linear. In some applications, a temperature sensor near the electrical probe allows a microprocessor-based control unit to regulate the delivered electrical power as a function of tissue temperature.

USES AND COMPLICATIONS

Electrocauterization is commonly used to destroy unwanted tissue. It has been applied to remove growths in the nasal passage, noncancerous polyps in the colon, canker sores, and lesions on or around the skin, muscles, ligaments, blood vessels, joints, and bones. It is used to stop bleeding during surgery and also when biopsies are performed. It has been used in women to remove abnormal tissue from the cervix and to stop abnormal bleeding from the uterus that is not caused by menstruation.

The healing time after electrocauterization procedures is usually two to three weeks. After electrocautery, a patient may experience pain, swelling, redness, drainage, bleeding, bruising, scarring, or itching at or around the surgery site. Headache, muscle aches, dizziness, fever, tiredness, and a general ill feeling may also occur following electrocauterization. The most serious complication can be the onset of infection. Antibiotics are typically administered if this occurs. Acetaminophen is used to diminish pain.

Excessive electrocautery can produce superficial to deep burns, which can be treated with cold packs. Electrocauterization of the cervix may lead to the misinterpretation of future Pap smear tests. When electrocauterization is performed multiple times to stop the occurrence of frequent nosebleeds, scar tissue can build up in the nose, leading to increased nosebleeds because of the lack of elasticity of scar tissue.

—Alvin K. Benson, Ph.D.

See also Biopsy; Canker sores; Cervical procedures; Colon and rectal polyp removal; Cryotherapy and cryosurgery; Dermatology; Dermatopathology; Genital disorders, female; Healing; Laser use in surgery; Nosebleeds; Skin; Skin disorders; Skin lesion removal; Surgery, general; Surgical procedures; Tumor removal; Tumors.

FOR FURTHER INFORMATION:

Bland, Kirby I., ed. *The Practice of General Surgery.* Philadelphia: W. B. Saunders, 2002.

Chasnoff, Ira J., and Jeffrey W. Ellis. *Family Medical and Health Guide.* Updated ed. Skokie, Ill.: Publications International, 1993.

Morreale, Barbara, David L. Roseman, and Albert K. Straus. *Inside General Surgery: An Illustrated Guide.* New Brunswick, N.J.: Johnson & Johnson, 1991.

ELECTROENCEPHALOGRAPHY (EEG)
PROCEDURE

ANATOMY OR SYSTEM AFFECTED: Brain, head, nervous system, psychic-emotional system

SPECIALTIES AND RELATED FIELDS: Biotechnology, critical care, emergency medicine, neurology, pathology, psychiatry, psychology, speech pathology

DEFINITION: The tracing of the electrical potentials produced by brain cells on a graphic chart, as detected by electrodes placed on the scalp.

KEY TERMS:

brain stem: the medulla oblongata, pons, and mesencephalon portions of the brain, which perform motor, sensory, and reflex functions and contain the corticospinal and reticulospinal tracts

cerebrum: the largest and uppermost section of the brain, which integrates memory, speech, writing, and emotional responses

epilepsy: uncontrollable excessive activity in either all or part of the central nervous system

lesion: a visible local tissue abnormality such as a wound, sore, rash, or boil which can be benign, cancerous, gross, occult, or primary

neurologic: dealing with the nervous system and its disorders

seizure: a sudden, violent, and involuntary contraction of a group of muscles; may be paroxysmal and episodic

INDICATIONS AND PROCEDURES

Clinical electroencephalography (EEG) uses from eight to sixteen pairs of electrodes called derivations. The "international 10-20" system of electrode placement provides coverage of the scalp at standard locations denoted by the letters F (frontal), C (central), P (parietal), T (temporal), and O (occipital). Subscripts of odd for left-sided placement, even for right-sided placements and z for midline placement further define electrode location. During the procedure, the patient remains quiet, with eyes closed, and refrains from talking or moving. In some circumstances, however, prescribed activities such as hyperventilation may be requested. An EEG test is used to diagnose seizure disorders, brain-stem disorders, focal lesions, and impaired consciousness.

Electrical potentials caused by normal brain activity have atypical amplitudes of 30 to 100 millivolts and irregular, wavelike variations in time. The main generators of the EEG are probably postsynaptic potentials, with the largest contribution arising from pyramidal cells in the third cortical layer. The ongoing rhythms on an EEG background recording are classified according to the frequencies that they produce as delta (less than 3.5 hertz), theta (4.0 to 7.5 hertz), alpha (8.0 to 13.0 hertz), and beta (greater than 13.5 hertz). In awake but relaxed normal adults, the background consists primarily of alpha activity in occipital and parietal areas and beta activity in central and frontal areas. Variations in this activity can occur as a function of behavioral state and aging. Alpha waves disappear during sleep and are replaced by synchronous beta waves of higher frequency but lower voltage. Theta waves can occur during emotional stress, particularly during extreme disappointment and frustration. Delta waves occur in deep sleep and infancy and with serious organic brain disease.

USES AND COMPLICATIONS

During neurosurgery, electrodes can be applied directly to the surface of the brain (intracranial EEG) or placed within brain tissue (depth EEG) to detect lesions or tumors. Electrical activity of the cerebrum is detected through the skull in the same way that the electrical activity originating in the heart is detected by an electrocardiogram (ECG or EKG) through the chest wall. The amplitude of the EEG, however, is much smaller than that of the ECG because the EEG is generated by cells that are not synchronously activated and are not geometrically aligned, whereas the ECG is generated by cells that are synchronously activated and aligned. Variations in brain wave activity correlate with neurological conditions such as epilepsy, abnormal psychopathological states, and level of consciousness such as during different stages of sleep.

The two general categories of EEG abnormalities are alterations in background activity and paroxysmal activity. An EEG background with global abnormalities indicates diffuse brain dysfunction associated with developmental delay, metabolic disturbances, infections, and degenerative diseases. EEG background abnormalities are generally not specific enough to establish a diagnosis—for example, the "burst-suppression" pattern may indicate severe anoxic brain injury as well as a coma induced by barbiturates. Some disorders do have characteristic EEG features: An excess of beta activity suggests intoxication, whereas triphasic slow waves are typical of metabolic encephalopathies, particularly as a result of hepatic or renal dysfunction. Psychiatric illness is generally not associated with prominent EEG changes. Therefore, a normal EEG helps to distinguish psychogenic unresponsiveness from neurologic disease. EEG silence is an adjunctive test in the determination of brain death, but it is not a definitive one because it may be produced by reversible conditions such as hypothermia. Focal or lateralized EEG abnormalities in the background imply similarly localized disturbances in brain function and thus suggest the presence of lesions.

Paroxysmal EEG activity consisting of spikes and sharp waves reflects the pathologic synchronization of neurons. The location and character of paroxysmal activity in epileptic patients help clarify the disorder, guide rational anticonvulsant therapy, and assist in determining a prognosis. The diagnostic value of an EEG is often enhanced by activation procedures, such as hyperventilation, photic (light) stimulation, and prolonged ambulatory monitoring, or by using special recording sites, such as nasopharyngeal leads, anterior temporal leads, and surgically placed subdural and depth electrodes. During a seizure, paroxysmal EEG activity replaces normal background activity and becomes continuous and rhythmic. In partial seizures, paroxysmal activity begins in one brain region and spreads to uninvolved regions.

PERSPECTIVE AND PROSPECTS

One of the most important uses of EEGs has been to diagnose certain types of epilepsy and to pinpoint the area in the brain causing the disturbance. Epilepsy is characterized by uncontrollable excessive activity in either all or part of the central nervous system and is classified into three types: grand mal epilepsy, petit mal epilepsy, and focal epilepsy. Additionally, EEGs are often used to localize tumors or other space-occupying lesions in the brain. Such abnormalities may be so large as to cause a complete or partial block in electrical activity in a certain portion of the cerebral cortex, resulting in reduced voltage. More frequently, however, a tumor compresses the surrounding nervous tissue and thereby causes abnormal electrical excitation in these areas.

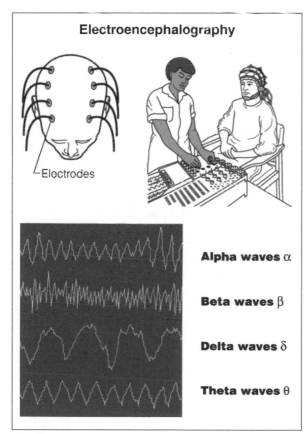

Electroencephalography

Electrodes

Alpha waves α

Beta waves β

Delta waves δ

Theta waves θ

The electrical activity of the brain can be measured with an electroencephalograph (EEG) machine; characteristic patterns can be used to diagnose some brain disorders and to determine levels of consciousness.

Some researchers predict new uses of EEG technology in the future, although many of these applications appear dubious. Attempts to interpret thought patterns so that an EEG could serve as a lie detector or measurement of intellectual ability, for example, have proven unsuccessful.

—*Daniel G. Graetzer, Ph.D.*

See also Brain; Brain disorders; Critical care; Critical care, pediatric; Emergency medicine; Epilepsy; Headaches; Neurology; Neurology, pediatric; Neurosurgery; Positron emission tomography (PET) scanning; Seizures; Tumor removal; Tumors.

FOR FURTHER INFORMATION:

Daube, Jasper R., ed. *Clinical Neurophysiology.* New York: Oxford University Press, 2002. Covers the basics of clinical neurophysiology, considers the assessment of disease by anatomical system, and explains how clinical neurophysiologic techniques are used in the clinical assessment of diseases of the nervous system. Electroencephalography is covered extensively.

Ebersole, John S., and Timothy A. Pedley, eds. *Current Practice of Clinical Electroencephalography.* 3d ed. Philadelphia: Lippincott, Williams and Wilkins, 2002. The thoroughly revised and greatly expanded third edition of this classic work covers the full range of applications of EEG and evoked potentials in current clinical practice. The most advanced instrumentation and techniques and their use in evaluating various disorders are discussed by more than twenty of the foremost authorities in the field.

Evans, J. R., and A. Abarbanel, eds. *Introduction to Quantitative EEG and Neurofeedback.* San Diego, Calif.: Academic Press, 1999. The stated purpose of this text is to provide "an overview of the basics of QEEG and neurofeedback in one source."

Hayakawa, Fumio, et al. "Determination of Timing of Brain Injury in Preterm Infants with Periventricular Leukomalacia with Serial Neonatal Electroencephalography." *Pediatrics* 104, no. 5 (November, 1999): 1077-1081. The authors determine the timing of brain injury in infants with periventricular leukomalacia with serial encephalography recordings during the neonatal period.

Powledge, Tabitha M. "Unlocking the Secrets of the Brain: Part II." *Bioscience* 47, no. 7 (July/August, 1997): 403-408. In the second article in a two-part series, Powledge discusses positron emission tomography (PET) scanning, electroencephalography, magnetoencephalography, and other imaging techniques that help provide an understanding of the brain.

Ricker, Joseph H., and Ross D. Zafonte. "Functional Neuroimaging and Quantitative Electroencephalography in Adult Traumatic Head Injury: Clinical Applications and Interpretive Cautions." *The Journal of Head Trauma Rehabilitation* 15, no. 2 (April, 2000): 859. This article provides an overview of the use of procedures such as positron emission tomography, single photon emission computed tomography, and quantitative electroencephalography in adults.

ELECTROLYTES. *See* FLUIDS AND ELECTROLYTES.

ELEPHANTIASIS

DISEASE/DISORDER

ALSO KNOWN AS: Bancroft's filariasis

ANATOMY OR SYSTEM AFFECTED: Lymphatic system

SPECIALTIES AND RELATED FIELDS: Environmental health, epidemiology, public health

DEFINITION: A grossly disfiguring disease caused by a roundworm parasite; it is the advanced stage of the disease Bancroft's filariasis, contracted through roundworms.

KEY TERMS:

acute disease: a disease in which symptoms develop rapidly and which runs its course quickly

chronic disease: a disease that develops more slowly than an acute disease and persists for a long time

host: any organism on or in which another organism (called a parasite) lives, usually for the purpose of nourishment or protection

inflammation: a response of the body to tissue damage caused by injury or infection and characterized by redness, pain, heat, and swelling

lymph nodes: globular structures located along the routes of the lymphatic vessels that filter microorganisms from the lymph

lymphatic system: a body system consisting of lymphatic vessels and lymph nodes that transports lymph through body tissues and organs; closely associated with the cardiovascular system

lymphatic vessels: vessels that form a system for returning lymph to the bloodstream

parasite: an organism that lives on or within another organism, called the host, from which it derives sustenance or protection at the host's expense

CAUSES AND SYMPTOMS

Elephantiasis is found worldwide, mostly in the tropics and subtropics. Most cases of elephantiasis are a result of infection with a parasitic worm called *Wuchereria bancrofti* (*W. bancrofti*). *W. bancrofti* belongs to a group of worms called filaria, or roundworms, and infection with a filarial worm is called filariasis. Filariasis caused by *W. bancrofti* is the most common and widespread type of human filarial infection and is often called Bancroft's filariasis. Elephantiasis is the advanced, chronic stage of Bancroft's filariasis, and only a small percentage of persons with Bancroft's filariasis will develop elephantiasis. During Bancroft's filariasis, adult forms of *W. bancrofti* live inside the human lymphatic system, and it is the person's reaction to the presence of the worm that causes the symptoms of the disease. The worm's life cycle is important in understanding how the disease is transmitted from one person to another, how the symptoms develop, and how to prevent and reduce the incidence of the disease.

The adult worms live in human lymphatic vessels and lymph nodes and measure about four centimeters in length for the male and nine centimeters in length for the female. Both are threadlike and about 0.3 millimeter in diameter. After mating, the female releases large numbers of embryos or microfilariae (microscopic roundworms), which are more than one hundred times smaller in length and ten times thinner than their parents. They make their way from the lymphatic system into the bloodstream, where they can circulate for two years or longer. Interestingly, most strains of microfilariae (all except those found in the South Pacific Islands) exhibit a nocturnal periodicity, in which they appear in the peripheral blood system (the outer blood vessels, such as those in the arms, legs, and skin) only at night, mostly between the hours of 10 P.M. and 2 A.M., and the remainder of the time they spend in the blood vessels of the lungs and other internal organs. This nighttime cycling into the peripheral blood is somehow related to the patient's sleeping habits, and although it is unknown exactly how or why the microfilariae do this, it is necessary for the survival of the worms. The microfilariae must develop through at least three different stages (called the first, second, and third larval stages) before they are ready to mature into adults; these stages take place not within humans, but within certain types of mosquitoes, which bite at night. Thus, the microfilariae appear in the peripheral blood just in time for the mosquitoes to bite an infected human and

extract them so that they can continue their life cycle. It is important to note, therefore, that both humans and the proper type of mosquito are needed to keep a filariasis infection going in a particular area.

Female night-feeding mosquitoes of the genera *Culex*, *Aedes*, and *Anopheles* serve as intermediate hosts for *Wuchereria bancrofti*. The mosquitoes bite an infected person and ingest microfilariae from the peripheral blood. The microfilariae pass into the intestines of the mosquito, invade the intestinal wall, and within a day find their way to the thoracic muscles (the muscles in the middle part of the mosquito's body). There they develop from first-stage to third-stage larvae in about two weeks, and the new third-stage larvae move from the thoracic muscles to the head and mouth of the mosquito. Only the third-stage larvae are able to infect humans successfully, and the third stage can mature only inside humans. When the mosquito takes a blood meal, infective larvae make their way through the proboscis (the tubular sucking organ with which a mosquito bites a person) and enter the skin through the puncture wound. After they enter the skin, the larvae move by an unknown route to the lymphatic system, where they develop into adult worms. It takes about one year or longer for the larvae to grow into adults, mate, and produce more microfilariae.

A person contracts Bancroft's filariasis by being bitten by an infected mosquito. Various forms of the disease can occur, depending on the person's immune response and the number of times the person is bitten. The period of time from when a person is first infected with larvae to the time microfilariae appear in the blood can be between one and two years. Even after this time some persons, especially young people, show no symptoms at all, yet they may have numerous microfilariae in their blood. This period of being a carrier of microfilariae without showing any signs of disease may last several years, and such carriers act as reservoirs for infecting the mosquito population.

In those patients showing symptoms from the infection, there are two stages of the disease: acute and chronic. In acute disease, the most common symptoms are a recurrent fever and lymphangitis and/or lymphadenitis in the arms, legs, or genitals. These symptoms are caused by an inflammatory response to the adult worms trapped inside the lymphatic system. Lymphangitis, an inflammation of the lymph vessels, is characterized by a hard, cordlike swelling or a red superficial streak that is tender and painful. Lymphadenitis is characterized by swollen and painful lymph nodes. The attacks of fever and lymphangitis or lymphadenitis recur at irregular intervals and may last from three weeks up to three months. The attacks usually become less frequent as the disease becomes more chronic. In the absence of reinfection, there is usually a steady improvement in the victim, each relapse being milder. Thus, without specific therapy, this condition is self-limiting and presumably will not become chronic in those acquiring the infection during a brief visit to an area where the disease is endemic.

The most obvious symptoms caused as a result of *W. bancrofti* infection, such as elephantiasis, are noted in the chronic stage. Chronic disease occurs only after years of repeated infection with the worms. It is seen only in areas where the disease is endemic and only occurs in a small percentage of the infected population. The symptoms are the result of an accumulation of damage caused by inflammatory reactions to the adult worms. The inflammation causes tissue death and a buildup of scar tissue that eventually results in the blockage of the lymphatic vessels in which the worms live. One of the functions of lymphatic vessels is to carry excess fluid away from tissues and bring it back to the blood, where it enters the circulation again as the fluid portion of the blood. If the lymphatic vessels are blocked, the excess fluid stays in the tissues, and swelling occurs. When this swelling is extensive, grotesque enlargement of that part of the body occurs. Elephantiasis is characterized by gross enlargement of a body part caused by the accumulation of fluid and connective tissue. It most frequently affects the legs, but may also occur in the arms, breasts, scrotum, vulva, or any other body part. The disease starts with the slight enlargement of one leg or arm (or other body part). The limb increases in size with recurrent attacks of fever. Gradually, the affected part swells, and the swelling, which is soft at first, becomes hard following the growth of

connective tissue in the area. In addition, the skin over the swollen area changes so that it becomes coarse and thickened, looking almost like elephant hide. The elephant-like skin, along with the enlarged body parts, gave the disease the name "elephantiasis."

TREATMENT AND THERAPY

One way in which doctors can tell whether a person has Bancroft's filariasis is by taking a sample of peripheral blood between 10 P.M. and 2 A.M. and looking at the blood under a microscope to try to find microfilariae. Sometimes, the ability to find microfilariae is enhanced by filtering the blood to concentrate the possible microfilariae in a smaller volume of liquid. Many persons infected with *W. bancrofti* have no detectable microfilariae in their blood, so other methods are available. In the absence of microfilariae, a diagnosis can be made on the basis of a history of exposure, symptoms

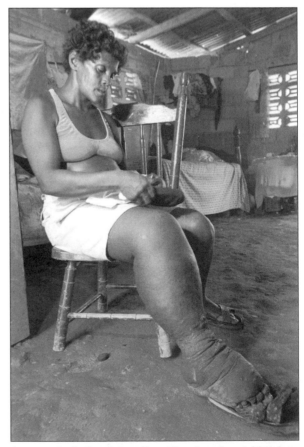

A woman in the Dominican Republic whose leg and foot have become crippled with elephantiasis, which affects many people in developing countries. (AP/Wide World Photos)

of the disease, positive antibody or skin tests, or the presence of worms in a sample of lymph tissue. It is important to note that occasionally a few other filarial worms and at least one bacteria can also cause elephantiasis; therefore, if symptoms of elephantiasis are observed, it is important to discover the correct cause so that the proper treatment can be given. Since chronic infection occurs after prolonged residence in areas where the disease occurs, patients with acute disease should be removed from those areas. They also should be reassured that elephantiasis is a rare complication that is limited to persons who have had constant exposure to infected mosquitoes for years.

The best way to avoid contracting filariasis when traveling to an affected area is to avoid being bitten by mosquitoes. Insect repellent, mosquito netting, and other methods are helpful in this regard. No drugs or vaccines are available to prevent infection once a person is bitten.

A problem in the treatment of all parasitic diseases is finding a drug that will kill the parasite without harming the human host. The drug diethylcarbamazine (DEC) is the drug of choice in treating Bancroft's filariasis. Its advantages are that it can be taken orally, patients have a relatively high tolerance to the drug, and it has relatively rapid, beneficial clinical effects. Generally, in the treatment of acute disease, excellent results are obtained when the proper dosage of the drug is given. There are only two relatively mild side effects of DEC. The first is nausea or vomiting. This symptom depends on the amount of the drug given; therefore, lower doses help alleviate this side effect. The second is fever and dizziness, the severity of which depends on the number of microfilariae a person has in his or her blood; the more microfilariae, the more severe the reaction. It is important to warn patients ahead of time about the fever reaction and encourage them to continue taking their doses anyway. The fever reaction is a sign that the patient is being cured, but the cure will not completely work if the patient does not finish the whole regimen of drug doses. Other drugs have been used in the treatment of filariasis (suramin, metrifonate, levamisole) but are generally less effective or more toxic than DEC. Additional treatment measures include bed rest and supportive measures, such as using hot and cold compresses to reduce swelling. The administration of antibiotics for patients with secondary bacterial infections and painkillers as well as anti-inflammatory agents during the painful, acute stage is helpful. Sometimes, swollen limbs can be wrapped in pressure bandages to force the lymph from them. If the distortion is not too great, this method is successful. It should also be noted that, although drugs such as DEC might be effective in killing *W. bancrofti*, the chronic lesions resulting from the infection are mostly incurable. Signs of chronic filariasis, such as elephantiasis of the limbs or the scrotum, are usually unaffected or only incompletely cured by medication, and it sometimes becomes necessary to apply surgical or other symptomatic treatments to relieve the suffering of the patients. Chronic obstruction in less advanced stages is sometimes improved by surgery. The surgical removal of an elephantoid breast, vulva, or scrotum is sometimes necessary.

Theoretically, it should be possible first to control and eventually to eliminate Bancroft's filariasis. Conditions that are highly favorable for continued propagation of the infection include a pool of microfilariae carriers in the human population and the right species of mosquitoes breeding near human habitations. Thus, control can be effected by treating all microfilariae carriers in an affected area and eliminating the necessary mosquitoes. Microfilariae carriers can be effectively treated with DEC. The decision usually is between giving mass drug treatment to the entire population in an affected area or only treating those persons who are microfilariae positive. Usually, if the infection is at a high rate and very widespread in an area, it is best to treat the entire population, since it would be very time consuming, difficult, and expensive to find all the microfilariae carriers. In other areas that are smaller or in which the pockets of infection are well defined, it is better to identify all the microfilariae-positive persons and treat only those persons until they are cured. The second control measure is to eliminate the mosquito population. It is important to note that eliminating the mosquitoes alone will not control the disease, especially in tropical areas, since the breeding period and season in which the disease can be transmitted is so extensive. In some temperate areas, where Bancroft's filariasis used to be endemic, measures that removed the mosquitoes alone aided in the elimination of the disease from that area, since in temperate areas the breeding period and thus the season for transmission is so short. In tropical areas, both DEC therapy and mosquito control must be applied in order to control the disease. The mosquito population can be controlled in four ways. First, general sanitation measures can be carried out in order to reduce the areas where the mosquitoes are breeding; for example, draining swamps. Second, insecticides can be used to kill the adult mosquitoes. Third, larvacides can be applied to sources of water where mosquitoes breed in order to kill the mosquito larvae. Finally, natural mosquito predators, such as certain species of fish, can be introduced into waters where mosquitoes breed to eat the mosquito larvae. Numerous problems stand in the way of eradication, such as poor sanitation, persons who do not cooperate with medical intervention, mosquitoes that become resistant to all known insecticides, increasing technology that yields increasing water supplies and therefore places for mosquitoes to breed, large populations, ignorance of the cause of the disease, and lack of medicine and a way of distributing that medicine.

Perspective and Prospects

Dramatic symptoms of elephantiasis, especially the enormous swelling of legs or scrotum, were recorded in much of the ancient medical literature of India, Persia, and the Far East. The embryonic form of microfilariae was first discovered and described by a Frenchman in Paris in 1863. The organism was named for O. Wucherer, who also discovered microfilariae in 1866, and Joseph Bancroft, who discovered the adult worm in 1876. Two important facts about *W. bancrofti*—namely, its development in mosquitoes and the nocturnal periodicity of the microfilariae—were discovered by Patrick Manson between 1877 and 1879. This was the first example of a disease being transmitted by a mosquito, and its discovery earned for Manson the title of Father of Tropical Medicine. These and most of the other essential facts of the disease were discovered before the end of the nineteenth century. Progress in the epidemiology and control of filariasis came after World War II. In 1947, DEC was shown to kill filariae in animals, and this result was followed by the successful use of DEC in the treatment of humans. The first promising results in the control of Bancroft's filariasis by mass administration of DEC were reported in 1957 on a small island in the South Pacific. Through subsequent studies, it has become clear that effective control of the infection can be achieved if sufficient dosages of DEC are administered to infected populations.

Filariasis is a serious health hazard and public health problem in many tropical countries. Infection with *Wuchereria bancrofti* has been recorded in nearly all countries or territories in the tropical and subtropical zones of the world. The infection occurs primarily in coastal areas and islands that experience long periods of high humidity and heat. Infections have also been noted from some temperate zone districts, such as mainland Japan, central China, and some European countries. There is more Bancroft's filariasis now than there was a hundred years ago, principally because of increases in population in affected areas and in increased resistance of mosquitoes to insecticides. In 1947, it was estimated that 189 million people were infected with *W. bancrofti*. More recently, the World Health Organization estimated that 250 million people are infected and 400 million are at risk.

Bancroft's filariasis was introduced into and became endemic to Charleston, South Carolina, until 1920. It disappeared in the United States before World War II, presumably because of a reduction of mosquitoes resulting from improved sanitation. Servicemen in the Pacific in World War II were concerned about contracting elephantiasis; although several thousand showed signs of acute filariasis, only twenty had microfilariae in their blood, and no one developed elephantiasis. In the United States today, the infection is most frequently seen in immigrants, military veterans, and missionaries. It is important for physicians to be aware of this and other tropical diseases so that they can treat the occasional patient who is suffering from one of them, since most of these diseases are more successfully treated in the early stages of the disease.

—*Vicki J. Isola, Ph.D.*

See also Arthropod-borne diseases; Bites and stings; Edema; Inflammation; Lymphadenopathy and lymphoma; Lymphatic system; Parasitic diseases; Roundworms; Tropical medicine; Worms; Zoonoses.

For Further Information:

Beaver, Paul C., and Rodney C. Jung. *Animal Agents and Vectors of Human Disease.* 5th ed. Philadelphia: Lea & Febiger, 1985. Discusses all major parasitic diseases. Chapter 12, "Filariae," which describes those diseases caused by filarial worms, contains helpful photographs and diagrams.

Biddle, Wayne. *Field Guide to Germs.* 2d ed. New York: Anchor Books, 2002. This comprehensive book is easily accessible to the nonspecialist and includes a discussion of nearly every virus, bacterium, and fungus known to cause human and nonhuman animal disease. The history of the microbe and the treatment of diseases are included.

Frank, Steven A. *Immunology and Evolution of Infectious Disease.* Princeton, N.J.: Princeton University Press, 2002. Blends research from molecular biology, immunology, pathogen biology, and population dynamics to discuss how and why parasites vary to escape recognition by the immune system, vaccine design, and the control of epidemics.

Ransford, Oliver. *"Bid the Sickness Cease."* London: John Murray, 1983. Discusses the effect of disease on the development of Africa. Chapter 6, "The Father of Tropical Medicine," describes how Patrick Manson made the original discoveries of the cause of elephantiasis.

Roberts, Larry S., and John Janovy, Jr., eds. *Gerald D. Schmidt and Larry S. Roberts' Foundations of Parasitology.* Rev. 6th ed. Boston: McGraw-Hill, 2000. Gives a good general description of all parasitic diseases, their causes, effects, and treatments. Deals specifically with diseases caused by filariae, including *Wuchereria bancrofti.*

Salyers, Abigail, and Dixie D. Whitt. *Bacterial Pathogenesis: A Molecular Approach.* Washington, D.C.: ASM Press, 2000. Examines the molecular mechanism involved in bacterial-host interactions that can produce infectious disease. Introductory chapters discuss host-parasite relationships.

Zinsser, Hans. *Zinsser Microbiology.* Edited by Wolfgang K. Joklik et al. 20th ed. Norwalk, Conn.: Appleton and Lange, 1992. The information presented in this textbook is thorough, logical, and supplemented by interesting diagrams, photographs, and charts. Contains a thorough description of Bancroft's filariasis.

EMBOLISM

DISEASE/DISORDER

ANATOMY OR SYSTEM AFFECTED: Blood vessels, brain, circulatory system, lungs, lymphatic system

SPECIALTIES AND RELATED FIELDS: Cardiology, internal medicine, neurology, vascular medicine

DEFINITION: A mass of undissolved matter traveling in the blood or lymphatic current.

CAUSES AND SYMPTOMS

An embolism is a mass of undissolved matter traveling in the vascular or lymphatic system. Although an embolism can be solid, liquid, or gaseous, the majority of emboli are solid. Likewise, emboli may consist of air bubbles, bits of tissue, globules of fat, tumor cells, or many other materials. The majority of emboli, however, are blood clots (thrombi) that originate in one portion of the body, then break loose and travel, eventually lodging in another part of the body. Where the traveling blood clot lodges will determine what kind of damage is done.

INFORMATION ON EMBOLISM

CAUSES: Blood clot, air bubble, tissue, fat globules, tumor cells, or other material lodging in part of the body

SYMPTOMS: If in the lung, shortness of breath and chest pain; if in the heart, symptoms of heart attack; if in the brain, symptoms of stroke; if in the leg, pain, cold, numbness

DURATION: Acute

TREATMENTS: Depends on system affected; may include blood-thinners (heparin), thrombolytic drugs, bypass surgery

---

If the thrombus starts in the veins of the legs, it may break loose, travel up the veins of the leg and abdomen, pass through the right side of the heart, and lodge in the arteries in the lungs. This condition, called a pulmonary embolism, is often fatal. If the embolism is small, it may cause only shortness of breath and chest pain. If it is even smaller, the embolism may produce no symptoms at all.

If a blood clot forms in the chambers of the heart, breaks loose, and eventually lodges in an artery in the brain, then the patient will experience a stroke. If a clot breaks loose and lodges in an artery in the leg, then the patient will experience pain, coldness, or numbness in that leg. A blood clot that lodges in the coronary arteries, the arteries that feed the heart muscle, may cause a heart attack.

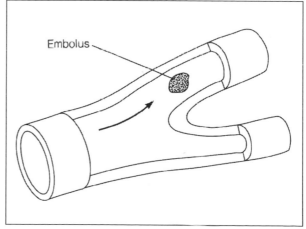

Embolus

An embolus is any material that is flowing in the bloodstream that obstructs a blood vessel; it may, for example, be a piece of a fatty plaque that has broken off an arterial wall.

TREATMENT AND THERAPY

Treatment will vary depending on what system has been affected by the embolus. If the clot lodges in the lungs, then the patient will likely be placed on a blood-thinning drug such as heparin. In severe cases, thrombolytic drugs, which dissolve clots, may be used. If the clot lodges in a coronary artery, then open-heart surgery may be performed to bypass the occluded artery. If the clot lodges in the leg, a surgeon may remove the clot from the artery. This procedure is possible only when the clot is discovered early, when it has not yet formed a strong attachment to the vessel wall. Another approach to this problem may be to bypass the occluded artery using an artificial artery or a graft.

PERSPECTIVE AND PROSPECTS

The prevention and treatment of emboli are constantly improving. Venous thrombosis, the most common cause of pulmonary emboli, is becoming easier to diagnose thanks to major advances in ultrasound imaging. Also, magnetic resonance imaging (MRI) is being used to make the identification of emboli in the lungs more accurate and safer. Imaging procedures of the chambers of the heart, a common spot where emboli form, are improving as well, making prevention easier.

—Steven R. Talbot, R.V.T.

See also Arteriosclerosis; Blood and blood disorders; Cholesterol; Circulation; Heart; Heart attack; Lungs; Phlebitis; Pulmonary diseases; Pulmonary medicine; Pulmonary medicine, pediatric; Respiration; Strokes; Thrombolytic therapy and TPA; Thrombosis and thrombus; Varicose vein removal; Varicose veins; Vascular medicine; Vascular system.

FOR FURTHER INFORMATION:

Bick, Roger L. *Disorders of Thrombosis and Hemostasis: Clinical and Laboratory Practice.* 3d ed. Philadelphia: Lippincott Williams and Wilkins, 2002.

Guinness, Alma E., ed. *ABC's of the Human Body: A Family Answer Book.* Pleasantville, N.Y.: Reader's Digest, 1987.

Verstrate, M., Valentin Fuster, and Eric Topol. *Cardiovascular Thrombosis: Thrombocardiology and Thromboneurology.* 2d ed. Philadelphia: Lippincott-Raven, 1998.

Virchow, Rudolf L. K. *Thrombosis and Emboli.* Translated by Axel C. Matzdorff and William R. Bell. Canton, Mass.: Science History, 1998.

EMBRYOLOGY

SPECIALTY

ANATOMY OR SYSTEM AFFECTED: All

SPECIALTIES AND RELATED FIELDS: Genetics, neonatology, obstetrics, perinatology

DEFINITION: The study of prenatal development from conception until the moment of birth.

KEY TERMS:

blastocyst: a small, hollow ball of cells which typifies one of the early embryonic stages in humans

cleavage: the process by which the fertilized egg undergoes a series of rapid cell divisions, which results in the formation of a blastocyst

congenital malformation: any anatomical defect present at birth

embryo: the developing human from conception until the end of the eighth week

fetus: the developing human from the end of the eighth week until the moment of birth

neural tube: the embryonic structure that gives rise to the central nervous system

teratogens: substances that induce congenital malformations when embryonic tissues and organs are exposed to them

zygote: the fertilized egg; the first cell of a new organism

SCIENCE AND PROFESSION

The study of human embryology is the study of human prenatal development. The three stages of development are cleavage (the first week), embryonic development (the second through eighth weeks), and fetal development (the ninth through thirty-eighth weeks).

After an egg is fertilized by sperm in the uterine, or Fallopian, tube, the resulting zygote begins to divide rapidly. This period of rapid cell division is known as cleavage. By the third day, the zygote has divided into a solid ball containing twelve to sixteen cells. The small ball of cells resembles a mulberry and is called the morula, which is Latin for "mulberry." The morula moves from the uterine tube into the uterus.

The morula develops a central cavity as spaces begin to form between the inner cells. At this stage, the developing human is called a blastocyst. The ring of cells on the outer edge of the hollow ball is called the trophoblast and will form a placenta, while the cluster of cells within becomes the inner cell mass and will form the embryo. By the end of the first week, the surface of the inner cell mass has flattened to form an embryonic disc, and the blastocyst has attached to the lining of the uterus and begun to embed itself.

During the second week of development, the trophoblast makes connections with the uterus to form the placenta. Blood vessels from the embryo link it to the placenta through the umbilical cord, through which the embryo receives food and oxygen and releases wastes. Two sacs develop around the embryo: the fluid-filled amniotic sac that surrounds and cushions the embryo and the yolk sac that hangs beneath to provide nourishment. Finally, a large chorionic sac develops around the embryo and the two smaller sacs.

During the third week, the cells of the embryo are arranged in three layers. The outer layer of cells is called the ectoderm, the middle layer is the mesoderm, and the inner layer is the endoderm. The ectoderm gives rise to the epidermis (outer layer) of the skin and to the nervous system; the mesoderm gives rise to blood, bone, cartilage, and muscle; and the endoderm gives rise to body linings and glands.

Other significant events of the third week are the development of the primitive streak and notochord. The primitive streak is a thickened line of cells on the embryonic disk indicating the future embryonic axis. Development of the primitive streak stimulates the formation of a supporting rod of tissue beneath it called the notochord. The presence of the notochord triggers the ectoderm in the primitive streak above it to thicken, and the thickened area will give rise to the brain and spinal cord. Later, when vertebrae and muscles develop around the neural tissue, the notochord will disappear.

The important event of the fourth week is the formation of the neural tube. After the thickened neural plate tissue has formed, an upward folding forms a groove, finally closing to form a neural tube. Closure begins at the head end and proceeds backward. The neural tube then sinks beneath surrounding ectodermal surface cells, which will become the skin covering the embryo.

Blocks of mesoderm cells line up along either side of the notochord and neural tube. These blocks are called somites, and eventually forty-two to forty-four pairs will form. They give rise to muscle, to the skeleton and cartilage of the head and trunk, and to the inner layer of skin. At the same time, embryonic blood vessels develop on the yolk sac. Because the human embryo is provided little yolk, there is need for early development of a circulatory system.

The heart is formed and begins to beat in the fourth week, though it is not yet connected to many blood vessels. During the fourth through eighth weeks, all the organ systems develop, and the embryo is especially vulnerable to teratogens (environmental agents that interfere with normal development). A noticeable change in shape is seen during the fourth week because the rapidly increasing number of cells causes a folding under at the edges of the embryonic disk. The flattened disk takes on a cylindrical shape, and the folding process causes curvature of the embryo and it comes to lie on its side in a C-shaped position.

The beginnings of arms and legs are first seen in the fourth week and are called limb buds, appearing first as small bumps. The lower end of the embryo resembles a tail, and the swollen cranial part of the neural tube constricts to form three early sections of the brain. The eyes and ears begin to develop from the early brain tissue.

During the fifth through eighth weeks, the head enlarges as a result of rapid brain development. The head makes up almost half the embryo, and facial features begin to appear. Sexual differences exist but are difficult to detect. Nerves and muscles have developed enough to allow movement. By the end of the eighth week the limb buds have grown and differentiated into appendages with paddle-shaped hands and feet and short, webbed digits. The tail disappears, and the embryo begins to demonstrate human characteristics. By convention, the embryo is now called a fetus.

The fetal stage of development is the period between the ninth and thirty-eighth weeks, until birth. Organs formed during the embryonic stage grow and differentiate during the fetal stage. The body has the largest growth spurt between the ninth and twentieth weeks, but the greatest weight gain occurs during the last weeks of pregnancy.

In the third month, the difference between the sexes becomes apparent, urine begins to form and is excreted into the amniotic fluid, and the fetus can blink its eyelids. The fetus nearly doubles in length during the fourth month, and the head no longer appears to be so disproportionately large. Ossification of the skeleton begins, and by the end of the fourth month, ovaries are differentiated in the female fetus and already contain many cells destined to become eggs.

During the fifth month, fetal movements are felt by the mother, and the heartbeat can be heard with a stethoscope. Movements until this time usually go unnoticed. The average length of time that elapses between the first movement felt by the mother and delivery is twenty-one weeks.

During the sixth month, weight is gained by the fetus, but it is not until the seventh month that a baby

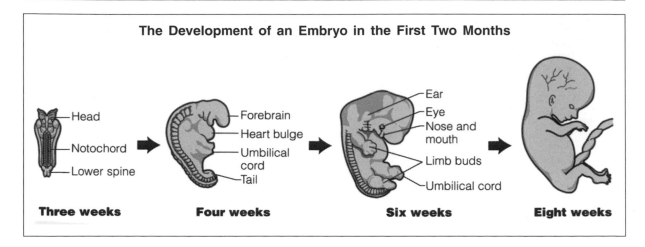

The Development of an Embryo in the First Two Months

Head
Notochord
Lower spine

Three weeks

Forebrain
Heart bulge
Umbilical cord
Tail

Four weeks

Ear
Eye
Nose and mouth
Limb buds
Umbilical cord

Six weeks

Eight weeks

usually can survive premature birth, when the body systems are mature enough to function. During the eighth month, the eyes develop the ability to control the amount of light that enters them. Fat accumulates under the skin and fills in wrinkles. The skin becomes pink and smooth, and the arms and legs may become chubby. In the male fetus, the testes descend into the scrotal sac. Growth slows as birth approaches. The usual gestation length is 266 days, or thirty-eight weeks after fertilization.

DIAGNOSTIC AND TREATMENT TECHNIQUES

Knowledge of normal embryonic development is very important both in helping women provide optimal prenatal care for their children and in promoting scientific research for improved prenatal treatment, better understanding of malignant growths, and insight into the aging process.

Environmental stress to the embryo during the fourth through eighth weeks can cause abnormal development and result in congenital malformation, which may be defined as any anatomical defect present at birth. Environmental agents that cause malformations are known as teratogens. Malformations may develop from genetic or environmental factors, but most often they are caused by a combination of the two. Some of the common teratogens are viral infections, drug use, a poor diet, smoking, alcohol consumption, and irradiation.

The genetic makeup of some individuals makes them particularly sensitive to certain agents, while others are resistant. The abnormalities may be immediately apparent at birth or hidden within the body and discovered later. Embryos with severe structural abnormalities often do not survive, and such abnormalities represent an important cause of miscarriages.

Genetic birth defects are passed on from one generation to another and result from a gene mutation at some time in the past. Mutations are caused by accidental rearrangement of deoxyribonucleic acid (DNA), the material of which genes are made, and range in severity from mild to life-threatening. They may cause such conditions as extra fingers and toes, cataracts, dwarfism, albinism, and cystic fibrosis. Gene mutations on a sex chromosome are described as sex-linked and are usually passed from mother to son; these include hemophilia, hydrocephalus (an excessive amount of cerebrospinal fluid), color blindness, and a form of baldness.

Abnormalities in the embryo may result because of unequal distribution of chromosomes in the formation of eggs or sperm. This imbalance can cause a variety of problems in development, such as Down syndrome and abnormal sexual development because of variable numbers of sex chromosomes. The normal human cell contains twenty-three chromosomes, twenty-two pairs of which are nonsex chromosomes, or autosomes. The last pair consists of the two sex chromosomes. Females normally have two X chromosomes, and males have an X and a Y chromosome.

When females have only one X, a set of conditions known as Turner syndrome results. The embryo will develop as a normal female, though ovaries will not fully form and there may be congenital heart defects. Because the single X chromosome does not cause enough estrogen to be produced, sexual maturity will not occur. If a male embryo should receive only the Y chromosome, it cannot survive. Sometimes a male will receive two (or more) X chromosomes along with a Y chromosome (XXY), producing Klinefelter syndrome. The appearance of the child is normal, but at puberty the breasts may enlarge and the testes will not mature, causing sterility. Males receiving two Y chromosomes (XYY) develop normally, but they may be quite tall and find controlling their impulses to be difficult.

Viral infections in the mother during the embryonic stages can cause problems in organ formation by disturbing normal cell division, fetal vascularization, and the development of the immune system. The organs most vulnerable to infection will be those undergoing rapid cell division and growth at the time of infection. For example, the lens of the eye is forming during the sixth week of development, and infection at this time could cause the formation of cataracts.

While most microorganisms cannot pass through the placenta to reach the embryo or fetus, those that can are capable of causing major problems in the embryonic development. Rubella, the virus that causes German measles, often causes birth defects in children should infection occur shortly before or during the first three months of pregnancy. The developing ears, eyes, and heart are especially susceptible to damage during this time. When a rubella infection occurs during the first five weeks of pregnancy, interference with organ development is most pronounced. After the fifth week, the risks of infection are not as great, but central nervous system impairment may occur as late as the seventh month.

The most common source of fetal infection may be the cytomegalovirus (CMV), a form of herpes which causes abortion during the first three months of pregnancy. If infection occurs later, the liver and brain are especially vulnerable and impairment in vision, hearing, and mental ability may result. Evidence has also suggested that the immune system of the fetus is adversely affected.

Other viruses may affect fetal development as well. When herpes simplex infects the fetus several weeks before birth, blindness or mental retardation may result. *Toxoplasma gondii*, a parasite of animals often kept as pets, may adversely affect eye and brain development without the mother having known that she had the infection. Syphilis infection in the mother leads to death or serious fetal abnormalities unless it is treated before the sixteenth week of pregnancy; if it is untreated, the fetus may possess hearing impairment, hydrocephalus, facial abnormalities, and mental retardation. Women infected with acquired immunodeficiency syndrome (AIDS) may transmit the virus to their infants before or during birth.

Certain chemicals can cross the placenta and produce malformation of developing tissues and organs.

During an embryo's first twenty-five days, damage to the primitive streak can cause malformation in bone, blood, and muscle. While bones and teeth are being formed, they may be adversely affected by antibiotics such as tetracycline.

At one time, thalidomide was widely used as an antinauseant in Great Britain and Germany and to some extent in the United States. Large numbers of congenital abnormalities began to appear in newborns, and the drug was withdrawn from the market after two years. Thalidomide caused failure of normal limb development and was especially damaging during the third to seventh weeks.

Exposure to other chemicals causes central nervous system disorders when the neural tube fails to close. When the anterior end of the tube does not close, development of the brain and spinal cord will be absent or incomplete and anencephaly results. Babies can live no more than a few days with this condition because the higher control centers of the brain are missing. If the posterior end of the tube fails to close, one or more vertebrae will not develop completely, exposing the spinal cord; this condition is called spina bifida. This condition varies in severity with the amount of neural tissue that remains exposed, because exposed tissue degenerates.

It has been long believed that neural tube disorders accompanied maternal depletion of folic acid, one of the B vitamins, and research has substantiated that relationship. Anencephaly and spina bifida rarely occur in the infants of women taking folic acid supplements. One of the harmful effects of alcohol and anticonvulsants is their depletion of the body's natural folic acid. A decrease in the mother's folic acid levels in the first through third months of pregnancy can cause abortion or growth deformities.

Maternal smoking is strongly implicated in low infant birth weights and higher fetal and infant mortality rates. Cigarette smoke may cause cardiac abnormalities, cleft lip and palate, and a missing brain. Nicotine decreases blood flow to the uterus and interferes with normal development, allowing less oxygen to reach the embryo.

Alcohol use may be the number-one cause of birth defects. Exposure of the fetus to alcohol in the blood results in fetal alcohol syndrome. Symptoms may include growth deficiencies, an abnormally small head, facial malformation, and damage to the heart and the nervous and reproductive systems. Behavioral disorders such as hyperactivity, attention deficit, and inability to relate to others may accompany fetal alcohol syndrome.

Radiation treatments given to pregnant women may cause cell death, chromosomal injury, and growth retardation in the developing embryo. The effect is proportional to the dosage of radiation. Malformations may be visible at birth, or a condition such as leukemia may develop later. Abnormalities caused by radiation include cleft palate, an abnormally small head, mental retardation, and spina bifida. Diagnostic X rays are not believed to emit enough radiation to cause abnormalities in embryonic development, but precautions should be taken.

Oxygen deficiency to the embryo or fetus occurs when mothers use cocaine. Maternal blood pressure fluctuates with the use of this drug, and the embryonic brain is deprived of oxygen, resulting in vision problems, lack of coordination, and mental retardation. Too little oxygen to the fetus may also cause death from lung collapse soon after birth.

Obvious physical malformations resulting from embryonic exposure to drugs have been recognized for a number of years, but recent investigators have found there are more subtle levels of effect that may show up later as behavioral problems. Physical abnormalities have been easily documented, but more attention is needed regarding the behavioral effects caused by teratogens.

PERSPECTIVE AND PROSPECTS

The first recorded observations of a developing embryo were performed on a chick by Hippocrates in the fifth century B.C.E. In the fourth century B.C.E., Aristotle wondered whether a preformed human unfolded in the embryo and enlarged with time, or whether a very simple embryonic structure gradually became more and more complex. This question was debated for nearly two thousand years until the early nineteenth century, when microscopic studies of chick embryos were carefully conducted and described.

Understanding human embryology is foundational for recognizing the relationships that exist between the body systems and congenital malformations in newborns. This field of study takes on new importance in the light of advances of modern technology, which have made prenatal diagnosis and treatment a reality.

The study of embryology is also making contributions toward finding the causes of malignant growth. Malignancy is a breakdown in the mechanisms for normal growth and differentiation first seen in the early embryo. Questions about uninhibited malignant growth may be answered by studying embryonic tissues and organs.

The study of old age is another area in which embryological research is valuable. Understanding the clock mechanisms of embryonic cells has led to greater understanding of the "winding down" of cells in old age. It is also important that researchers discover how environmental conditions modify rates of growth and affect the cell's clock. The degree to which the human life span can be expanded remains one of the most challenging questions in the area of aging.

In addition to the health benefits that may be derived from embryological research, this field is an important source of insight into some of the moral and ethical dilemmas facing humankind. Artificial insemination, contraception, and abortion regulations are some of the problems that will require close collaboration between ethicists and scientists, especially embryologists.

—*Katherine H. Houp, Ph.D.*

See also Abortion; Amniocentesis; Assisted reproductive technologies; Birth defects; Brain disorders; Cerebral palsy; Cesarean section; Chorionic villus sampling; Cloning; Conception; Down syndrome; Fetal alcohol syndrome; Fetal surgery; Gamete intrafallopian transfer (GIFT); Genetic counseling; Genetic diseases; Genetics and inheritance; Growth; Gynecology; In vitro fertilization; Miscarriage; Multiple births; Neonatology; Obstetrics; Perinatology; Placenta; Pregnancy and gestation; Premature birth; Reproductive system; Rh factor; Rubella; Sexual differentiation; Spina bifida; Stillbirth; Toxoplasmosis; Ultrasonography.

FOR FURTHER INFORMATION:

Mader, Sylvia S. *Inquiry into Life.* 10th ed. Dubuque, Iowa: W. C. Brown, 2002. An introductory-level college text designed to cover the entire range of biological topics. Gives a clear description of typical early developmental stages of all vertebrates and offers a section on human embryology and fetal development, adulthood, and aging.

Marieb, Elaine N. *Essentials of Human Anatomy and Physiology.* 6th ed. Redwood City, Calif.: Benjamin/Cummings, 2003. This introductory anatomy and physiology textbook, easily accessible to those with little science background, is richly illustrated with diagrams and photographs, which help to illuminate body systems and processes.

Moore, Keith L., and T. V. N. Persaud. *The Developing*

Human. 7th ed. Philadelphia: W. B. Saunders, 2003. An outstanding textbook on human embryonic development, with specific information about the causes of congenital malformations and common defects occurring in each of the body's systems. This widely used textbook gives a clear and careful description of normal human development during the entire prenatal period.

Riley, Edward P., and Charles V. Vorhees, eds. *Handbook of Behavioral Teratology.* New York: Plenum Press, 1986. An informative compilation of learning in the field of behavioral teratology. Covers historical context, general principles, and specific drugs and environmental agents that act as behavioral teratogens. Effects are listed for each agent that has been studied.

Tortora, Gerard J., and Sandra R. Grabowski. *Principles of Anatomy and Physiology.* 10th ed. New York: John Wiley & Sons, 2003. An intermediate-level college text widely used in fields of allied health. Chapters include overview of human prenatal development from fertilization through birth. Written in a very readable fashion; has excellent color diagrams and photographs on every page.

Tsiaras, Alexander, and Barry Werth. *From Conception to Birth: A Life Unfolds.* New York: Doubleday, 2002. Using state-of-the-art medical imaging technology, traces the development of a human life from conception through birth in spectacular, highly detailed photographs.

EMERGENCY MEDICINE
SPECIALTY
ANATOMY OR SYSTEM AFFECTED: All

SPECIALTIES AND RELATED FIELDS: Cardiology, critical care, gastroenterology, geriatrics and gerontology, neurology, nursing, obstetrics, pediatrics, pharmacology, psychiatry, public health, pulmonary medicine, radiology, sports medicine, toxicology

DEFINITION: The care of patients who are experiencing immediate health crises, a field defined by twenty-four-hour availability, the management of multiple patients simultaneously, and the need for broad-based skills and interventions.

KEY TERMS:

diagnostic: relating to the determination of the nature of a disease

emergency medical services: the complete chain of human and physical resources that provides patient care in cases of sudden illness or injury

heuristics: methods used to aid and guide in the discovery of a disease process when incomplete knowledge exists

paramedic: a person trained and certified to provide prehospital emergency medical care

pathologic: pertaining to the study of disease and the development of abnormal conditions

pathophysiology: an alteration in function as seen in disease

patient assessment: the systematic gathering of information in order to determine the nature of a patient's illness

triage: the medical screening of patients to determine their relative priority for treatment

SCIENCE AND PROFESSION

The field of emergency medicine is defined as care to acutely ill and injured patients, both in the prehospital setting and in the emergency room. It is practiced as patient-demanded and continuously accessible care and is defined by the location of its practice rather than by an anatomical concern. Emergency medicine encompasses all medical specialties and physical systems. The commitment to rapid, prudent intervention under stressful and often chaotic conditions is of paramount importance to the critically ill patient. This branch of medicine is characterized by its complexity of problems, its twenty-four-hour availability to a variety of patients, and its effective and broad-based understanding of disease and injury. These features are used to orchestrate the response of multiple hands with the ultimate goal of referring the patient to ongoing care.

The hourglass is an appropriate symbol of the nature of this medical division. It not only portrays the importance of time and the need for quick intervention, but its shape—wide at either end and narrowing in the middle—is an appropriate visualization of the pattern of emergency medical treatment. A large number of patients converge on a single area, the emergency room, where they are diagnosed, treated, and eventually released to other appropriate care, diverging on a wide range of follow-up options.

Unique to the field of emergency medicine is the importance of rapid definition and comprehension of the pathophysiology of the critically ill patient. Emergency care physicians must have a unique understanding of the practice of medicine, the nature of disease and injury, availing themselves of a host of clinical skills needed for the treatment of the variety of physical and psychological problems that require treatment. Emergency rooms are a melting pot of problems; most are medical, many are not. All of them reflect some person's perception of an emergency. Success in the emergency medical field often depends on the ability of personnel to use not only their medical knowledge but their knowledge of people as well.

Most often those seeking the assistance of emergency medical providers are people suffering from pain of illness or trauma; however, any patient may seek treatment at the emergency room. Often loneliness, disability, or homelessness serves as the motivation to seek treatment. Regardless of what brought the patient, the emergency physician strives to recognize and deal with the patient's "emergency," remembering that not all patients are as ill as they might think and that not all are as well as they might appear. Physicians of this specialty sift through a multitude of information. It is necessary to know the patient's pertinent medical history and the history of the present illness or complaint before appropriate and effective treatment can be prescribed. Patients rarely follow a preconceived plan. Emergency medicine works best, therefore, when its practitioners follow heuristics—that is, incomplete guides that lead to greater knowledge, a holistic approach.

Emergency medicine is primarily a hospital-based specialty; however, it also involves extensive prehospital responsibilities. Many times, patients seeking emergency care are first the responsibility of police, fire, or ambulance personnel. In these situations, the role of emergency medicine must be viewed under the wider context of the emergency medical system. This system—beginning with the first aid administered by bystanders leading to initial treatment and transportation by trained certified emergency medical technicians, paramedics, or flight nurses and culminating with care at an emergency room or a highly equipped trauma center—forms a uniquely structured unit. The emergency medical system is designed to provide rapid quality intervention regardless of prehospital conditions. The emergency medical physician is best viewed as a central part of a team whose knowledge and understanding of the whole allow the best possible care to patients undergoing health crises.

Emergency physicians are charged with the responsibility of providing the highest standard of care in the hospital setting. They ensure that both staff members and equipment are maintained at their utmost level of quality. Trends, breakthroughs, and recent advances are monitored via journals and other medical publica-

tions. Training of personnel must keep pace with medical advancement. Developing an overall program depends as much on its planning as its dissemination. The emergency physician often plays the role of teacher, actively influencing the overall quality of the program through education and skills development. Thus, the exercise of emergency medicine is truly a team effort, with all members acting in accordance with their training and level of competence in order to minimize further injury or discomfort.

In practice, emergency medicine encompasses any person or structure involved in the immediate decision making and/or actions necessary to prevent death or further disability of a patient in the midst of a health crisis. It represents a chain of human and physical resources brought together for the purpose of providing total patient care. In this respect, everyone has a part to play in the deliverance of emergency care. The bottom line of emergency medicine is the welfare of the patient. Thus, it is most appropriate to view the practice of emergency medicine in the context of the entire emergency medical system.

The components of the emergency medical system include recognition of the emergency, initiation of emergency medical response, treatment at the scene, transport by members of an emergency medical team to the appropriate facility, treatment in the emergency room or trauma center, and release of the patient. These components are only as strong as the weakest link.

DIAGNOSTIC AND TREATMENT TECHNIQUES

Recognition of an emergency is the first step in emergency care. Often this step is complicated by the patient's own denial and ignorance of basic symptoms. "Emergency" is in part defined by the patient's ability to identify, accept, and respond to a given situation. Regardless of the nature of the illness or injury, the sooner an emergency is defined the sooner care can be provided. The typical heart attack victim, for example, waits an average of three hours after experiencing symptoms before seeking help. In such cases, treatment by bystanders who have been trained in first aid and cardiopulmonary resuscitation (CPR) has proven effective.

In the United States, the response of emergency medical personnel has been aided by the implementation of the 911 emergency system. While not all communities have this capability, its use is increasing. It has been documented that patients who receive treatment at an appropriate facility within sixty minutes of the onset of a life-threatening emergency are more likely to survive. This "golden hour" is precious time.

Operating under protocols developed and approved by the emergency medical director and emergency medical councils of a given locale, emergency medical technicians (EMTs) and paramedics are trained and authorized to deliver care to the patient in need at the scene. EMTs and paramedics are charged with the initial assessment of the patient's condition, immediate stabilization prior to transport, and deliverance of care as far as his or her training allows, and the transport of the patient.

Unique to the field of emergency medicine is the special relationship of the paramedic with the doctor. Many people in need of emergency care are first treated outside the hospital. In these cases, emergency caregivers on the scene act as the eyes, ears, and hands of the physician. Through the EMT or paramedic, using telecommunications, an emergency doctor can speed the process of diagnosis. Signs and symptoms relayed through these trained professionals enable a doctor to make an accurate assessment of the patient's condition and to request a variety of treatments for a patient whom they cannot see or touch. Linked by telephone or radio, the medic and doctor can capitalize on the golden hour with the initiation of quality care.

Paramedics operate under the medical license of a medical command physician who has met all criteria set forth by the Department of Health and has been approved to provide medical directives to prehospital and interhospital providers. Protocols are the recognized practices that are within the training of the EMT and paramedic. They serve as standard procedures for prehospital treatment. While it is recognized that situations will arise which call for deviation from particular aspects of a given protocol, they are the standards under which the doctor and emergency personnel on the scene operate.

Treatment at the scene is followed by transport with advanced life support by members of the emergency medical system in 85 percent of all emergency cases. This requires much-needed equipment for the further

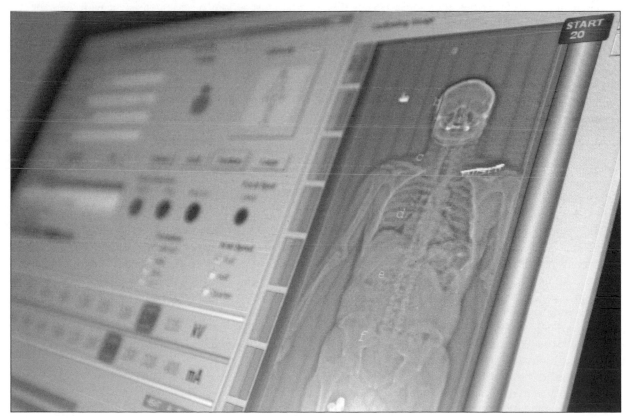

A monitor displays an image from Statscan, a low-dose, digital X-ray system that can provide a full-body scan in thirteen seconds without movement required from the patient. Such technology could prove lifesaving in emergency rooms. (AP/Wide World Photos)

treatment of patients. Deficiencies in the vehicle, equipment, or training of medical personnel can seriously endanger a patient. Thus, government agencies have been designated to grant permission for ambulance services and hospitals to engage in the practice of emergency medicine. This licensure process is designed to demand a level of competency for health care providers and ensure the public's protection.

Since only about 5 percent of all emergency department admissions constitute life-threatening situations, not all facilities stand at the same level of readiness for a given emergency. Transportation to the appropriate facility, therefore, requires a matching of patient's need to the hospital's capabilities. Hospitals are categorized according to their ability to render emergency intensive care, as well as to provide needed support services on a patient-demand basis. In general, they are viewed as emergency facilities and trauma facilities where trauma centers are designed to provide twenty-four-hour, comprehensive emergency intensive care, including operating rooms and intensive care nurses.

When the patient reaches the emergency facility, during the first five to fifteen minutes of care, many important decisions are made by the physician on duty. The process continues to overlap with needed diagnostic tests and consultations in an effort to provide quality care directed at the source of the illness or injury. The patient's immediate needs are cared for by emergency department staff until the patient is moved to a site of continued care or released to his or her own care.

Questions correctly phrased and sharply directed are effective tools for the rapid diagnosis needed in emergency medicine. The key to this field is the ability to triage, stabilize, prioritize, treat, and refer.

Triage is the system used for categorizing and sorting patients according to the severity of their problems. Emergency practitioners seek to ascertain the nature of the patient's problem and consider any life-threatening consequences of the present condition. This stage of triage allows for immediate care to the more seriously endangered person, relegating the more stable, less seriously ill or wounded patients to a waiting period. The emergency room, in other words, does not operate on a first come, first served basis.

Secondary to triage is stabilization. This term refers to any immediate treatment or intervening steps taken to alleviate conditions that would result in greater pain or defect and/or lead to irreversible or fatal consequences. Primary stabilization steps include ensuring an unobstructed airway and providing adequate ventilation and cardiovascular function.

Once patients have been stabilized, all illnesses must be looked at on the scale of their hierarchical importance. Life-threatening diseases or injuries are treated before more moderate or minor conditions. This system of prioritization can be illustrated from patient to patient: A heart attack victim, for example, is treated prior to the patient with an ankle sprain. It can also be applied for multiple conditions within the same patient. The heart attack victim with a sprained ankle receives treatment first for the life-threatening cardiovascular incident.

Treatment of the critically ill patient often poses a series of further questions. What is the primary disorder? Is there more than one active pathologic process present? How does the patient appear? Is the patient's presentation consistent with the initial diagnosis? Is a hospital stay warranted? What consultations are needed to diagnose and treat this patient?

The emergency physician's approach is to consider the most serious disease consistent with the patient's presentation and chief complaint. By rule of thumb, thinking the worst and hoping for the best is often the psychological stance of the emergency care provider. Only when more severe conditions have been ruled out are more minor processes considered. Often too, this broad view of patient assessment allows for multiple diagnosis. Through continued probing, alternate and additional conditions are often uncovered. It is not unlikely that the patient who seeks treatment for a head injury after a fall is diagnosed with a more serious condition which caused the fall. Focusing only on the immediate condition would endanger the patient. Success in this medical field therefore demands broad-based medical knowledge and diagnostic tools.

Emergency medicine is not practiced in a vacuum. Its very nature necessitates its interfacing with a variety of medical specialties. The emergency room is often only the first step in patient recovery. Initial diagnosis and stabilization must be coupled with plans for ongoing treatment and evaluation. Consultations and referrals play important roles in the overall care of a patient.

Perspective and Prospects

Historians are unable to document specific systems for emergency patients before the 1790's. The need to provide care to the battlefield wounded is seen as the first implementation of emergency response. Early wartime treatment did not, however, include prehospital treatment. Clara Barton is credited with providing the first professional-level prehospital emergency care for the wounded as part of the American Red Cross. Ambulance services began in major cities of the United States at the beginning of the twentieth century, but it was not until 1960 that the National Academy of Sciences' National Research Council actually studied the problem of emergency care.

Emergency medicine as a specialty is relatively new. Not until 1975, when the House of Delegates of the American Medical Association defined the emergency physician, did the medical community even recognize this branch of medicine. In 1981, the American College of Emergency Physicians added further recognition through the development of the definition of emergency medicine. Since then, growth and changes have enabled this field to develop as a major specialty, evolving to accept greater responsibility in both education and practice.

The development of emergency medicine and the increasing number of health care providers in this field have been dramatic. In 1990, there were a total of 23,000 emergency physicians, 85,000 emergency nurses, and 521,734 emergency technicians. These health care providers delivered care to the nearly 87 million emergency department patients seen that year.

Emergency medicine developed at a time when both the general public and the medical community recognized the need for quality accessible care in the emergency situation. It has grown to include a gamut of services provided by a community. In addition to responding to the acutely ill or injured, emergency medicine has grown to accept responsibilities of education, administration, and advocacy.

Included in the role of today's emergency medical providers is the administration of the entire emergency medical system within a community. This system includes the development of public education programs such as CPR instruction, poison control education, and the introduction of the 911 system. Emergency management systems and coordinators are now part of every state and local government. Disaster planning for both natural and human-made accidents also comes under the heading of emergency medicine.

Research, too, plays an important role in emergency medicine. The desire to identify, understand, and disseminate scientific rationale for basic resuscitative interventions, as well as the need to improve preventive medical techniques, are often driving forces in scientific research.

Finally, emergency medicine plays a key role in many of society's problems. Homelessness, drug use and abuse, acquired immunodeficiency syndrome (AIDS), and rising health costs have all contributed to the increase in the number of patients seen in the emergency room. In response, those administering emergency medical care have tried to communicate such problems to the general public and legislative bodies, as well as educate them regarding preventive measures. Being on the front line of medicine brings a special obligation to improve laws and services to ensure public safety and well-being.

—Mary Beth McGranaghan

See also Abdominal disorders; Altitude sickness; Amputation; Aneurysms; Antibiotics; Appendectomy; Appendicitis; Asphyxiation; Biological and chemical weapons; Bites and stings; Bleeding; Botulism; Burns and scalds; Cardiology; Cardiology, pediatric; Cardiopulmonary resuscitation (CPR); Catheterization; Cesarean section; Choking; Coma; Concussion; Critical care; Critical care, pediatric; Electrical shock; Electrocardiography (ECG or EKG); Electroencephalography (EEG); Emergency medicine, pediatric; Fracture and dislocation; Fracture repair; Frostbite; Grafts and grafting; Head and neck disorders; Heart attack; Heat exhaustion and heat stroke; Hospitals; Hyperthermia and hypothermia; Intoxication; Laceration repair; Meningitis; Nursing; Obstetrics; Paramedics; Peritonitis; Pneumonia; Poisoning; Radiation sickness; Resuscitation; Reye's syndrome; Salmonella infection; Shock; Snakebites; Spinal cord disorders; Splenectomy; Sports medicine; Staphylococcal infections; Streptococcal infections; Strokes; Thrombolytic therapy and TPA; Tracheostomy; Transfusion; Unconsciousness; Veterinary medicine; Wounds.

FOR FURTHER INFORMATION:

Bledsoe, Bryan E., Robert S. Porter, and Bruce R. Shade. *Brady Paramedic Emergency Care*. 3d ed. Upper Saddle River, N.J.: Brady Prentice Hall Education, Career & Technology, 1997. A comprehensive guide to the practice of emergency medicine as it applies to and is practiced by the paramedic. A solid overview of the basics of prehospital care. This text focuses on advanced life support practices.

Caroline, Nancy L. *Emergency Care in the Streets*. 5th ed. Boston: Little, Brown, 1995. This text provides a sophisticated understanding of the fundamental concepts of advanced life support and the underlying physiology. A focused approach written by a physician who has spent many hours in the field as a prehospital care provider. Includes new chapters on AIDS and other communicable diseases.

Grant, Harvey D., et al. *Brady Emergency Care.* 8th ed. Englewood Cliffs, N.J.: Brady Prentice Hall Education, Career, & Technology, 1998. This simple text has been acclaimed for its comprehensive, accurate, and up-to-the-minute treatment of emergency care. Easy to read, this book provides the contemporary standards on CPR from the American Heart Association and a full treatment on many emergency medical protocols for prehospital treatment.

Hamilton, Glenn C., ed. *Emergency Medicine: An Approach to Clinical Problem-Solving.* 2d ed. New York: W. B. Saunders, 2003. Addressed to students of medicine, this text provides a detailed, well-written script for the clinical setting. Facilitates the reader's understanding of the emergency scene. Actual medical cases are integrated into the chapters in order to reinforce concepts.

Marovchick, Vincent J., and Peter T. Pons. *Emergency Medicine Secrets.* 3d ed. New York: Elsevier, 2002. Details all aspects of emergency medicine in a question-and-answer format. Topics include nontraumatic illness, hematology/oncology, infectious disease, environmental emergencies, neonatal and childhood disorders, toxicologic emergencies, emergency medicine administration and risk management, and disaster management.

Rosen, Peter, ed. *Emergency Medicine: Concepts and Clinical Practice.* 2 vols. 5th ed. St. Louis: C. V. Mosby, 2002. A logical and straightforward presentation of current standards of emergency medicine. Intended to be a reference in busy emergency rooms. The writing is clear and to the point.

Tintinalli, Judith E., ed. *Emergency Medicine: A Comprehensive Study Guide.* 5th ed. New York: McGraw-Hill, 2000. This bible of emergency medicine provides a basic understanding of the field. Describes in detail key diagnostic techniques and treatments.

Emergency medicine, pediatric
Specialty

Anatomy or system affected: All
Specialties and related fields: Critical care
Definition: The decision making and actions necessary to prevent death or any further disability in children with life-threatening injuries, illnesses, and other health crises.

Key terms:
abc's: the basics of survival—*a* is for airway obstruction/choking, *b* is for breathing/respiratory distress, and *c* is for circulatory collapse/shock
pediatric emergency specialists: emergency physicians who focus their practices on emergency care for children, including research and teaching pediatric emergency medicine
triage: the process of choosing who will receive medical treatment first because of dire illness or injury

Science and Profession

The physician who specializes in pediatric emergency medicine has been trained to diagnose and treat patients in order to prevent death or any further disability for children in health crises. They are also skilled at health promotion and injury prevention efforts. For some young patients, emergency departments are increasingly the only source of routine medical care. Pediatric emergency physicians represent the front line of medicine.

Emergency medicine emphasizes the anticipation and recognition of a life-threatening process, rather than seeking a definitive diagnosis. The emergencies that these physicians treat are often the type parents hope never to see. The perceptions and complaints of the patients or the people who bring them to the emergency department or pediatric trauma center define the emergencies themselves. Most children treated in an emergency department will be seen in a general hospital whose staff is unlikely to include pediatric specialists. Each year, about one-third of the children who visit the emergency department are there because of an injury. Two-thirds of the visits are the result of illnesses such as debilitating asthma or life-threatening meningitis. Services are available twenty-four hours a day, seven days a week, 365 days a year in the hospital and in the field. They are provided by a network of health specialists, nurses, paramedics, emergency medical technicians, police officers, firefighters, and others dedicated to offering emergency medical services to children and adults.

Pediatric emergency specialists are needed because children are not little adults. The differences between children and adults are so great that they exist in virtually every organ system, body part, physiological process, and disease syndrome. For example, children's lungs are smaller and more fragile than those of adults, so that they require gentler thrusts during cardiopulmonary resuscitation (CPR). Children have faster heart and respiration rates than do adults, so that what may look like normal adult rates may be a sign of serious trouble in a child. Children require different and special equipment, different-sized instruments, different doses of different medicines, and different approaches to the psychological support and remedial care given to the ill or injured patient.

Physicians and other health care providers who lack pediatric emergency medical training and experience may find it difficult to recognize children who are critically ill and require the most urgent care. For example, infants may not develop a fever to signal infection. In children, respiratory arrest or shock signals the risk of cardiopulmonary arrest, rather than the arrhythmias that typically precede cardiac arrest in adults.

DIAGNOSTIC AND TREATMENT TECHNIQUES

A good medical outcome depends on the prompt identification and treatment of serious illness or injury in children. Emergency services personnel use a system called triage to decide whether patients are at risk for severe illness or imminent death, whether they have less urgent but still serious medical problems, or whether they have routine problems. Health care professionals use a system called the *abc*'s. Children who are choking (*a* for airway obstruction), in respiratory distress (*b* for breathing), or in shock (*c* for circulatory collapse) are treated immediately. The sickest patients always come first.

Doctors often make the most important decisions about a patient within the first five to fifteen minutes of care. The physician first determines whether the patient is in need of treatment and confirms or rules out the presence of catastrophic disease as quickly as possible. The doctor then stabilizes the patient's vital signs to reduce the risk of worsening symptoms or death. Next, the physician acts to relieve the most acute symptoms. The patient may then be hospitalized or discharged with directions about what to do next.

PERSPECTIVE AND PROSPECTS

Physicians have been treating pediatric emergencies for centuries. Only more recently, however, was there much recognition among the medical community or the public that pediatric emergency care requires unique training, equipment, and procedures.

Emergency medicine as a discipline in the United States dates to 1968, when the American College of Emergency Physicians was formed. During the 1970's, pediatricians and pediatric surgeons recognized that children's emergency care needs were not receiving adequate attention. The American Medical Association (AMA) and the American Board of Medical Specialties recognized emergency medicine as the twenty-third medical specialty in 1979. In the early 1980's, growing numbers of pediatric specialists and professional societies began to participate in the development of emergency medical systems. In 1993, a committee of the Institute of Medicine published a major study on the state of emergency care for children. The committee focused on standardizing the emergency care system so that the quality of emergency care would be consistent from state to state and community to community. It encouraged the creation of a nationwide 911 emergency response system and the establishment of minimum standards of care.

The tools, technologies, treatments, and problem-solving methods used by pediatric emergency physicians have been advancing rapidly. These specialists have gotten better at coping with the gamut of children's emergencies, including the medical and behavioral crises of newborns, infants, toddlers, young children, and adolescents. Emergency physicians have been and continue to be responsible for the development of new treatment techniques and the widespread availability of specialized pediatric equipment.

—Fred Buchstein

See also Allergies; Asthma; Biological and chemical weapons; Bites and stings; Bleeding; Burns and scalds; Cardiology, pediatric; Cardiopulmonary resuscitation (CPR); Cardiovascular system; Choking; Critical care, pediatric; Dizziness and fainting; Electrical shock; Fever; Food poisoning; Fracture and dislocation; Frostbite; Heat exhaustion and heat stroke; Meningitis; Physical examination; Pneumonia; Poisoning; Poisonous plants; Pulmonary medicine, pediatric; Rabies; Respiration; Respiratory distress syndrome; Seizures; Snakebites; Suicide.

FOR FURTHER INFORMATION:

Durch, Jane S., and Kathleen N. Lohr, eds. *Emergency Medical Services for Children*. Washington, D.C.: National Academy Press, 1993. This report of an Institute of Medicine study examines the nature and extent of acute illness and injury among children, reviews the origins and organization of emergency medical services (EMS) systems, describes the current state of effective care, and addresses data and standards needed for surveillance and evaluation of services and outcomes.

Hamilton, Glenn C., Arthur B. Sanders, Gary R. Strange, and Alexander T. Trott. *Emergency Medicine: An Approach to Clinical Problem-Solving.* 2d ed. Philadelphia: W. B. Saunders, 2003. A comprehensive textbook, in concise format, for residents and medical students.

Lynn, Stephan G., with Pamela Weintraub. *Medical Emergency! The St. Luke's-Roosevelt Hospital Center of Emergency Medicine.* New York: Hearst Books, 1996. This most helpful, informative, and well-arranged book tells how to be personally prepared for emergencies by having basic records and documents in wallet or purse and others in known places for easy location. It clarifies emergency tests and treatments and explains how family members and friends can act as emergency patient advocates.

Rogers, Janice Steiner. *Manual of Pediatric Emergency Nursing.* St. Louis: Mosby, 1998. A portable handbook summarizing most of the conditions seen in a pediatric emergency department. Includes the essential points and priorities for diagnosis, management, and follow-up care, as well as indications for hospitalization.

Strange, Gary R. *Pediatric Emergency Medicine: A Comprehensive Study Guide.* New York: McGraw-Hill, 2002. A handbook for a range of emergency situations encountered in pediatric care.

EMOTIONS: BIOMEDICAL CAUSES AND EFFECTS

BIOLOGY

ANATOMY OR SYSTEM AFFECTED: Brain, endocrine system, gastrointestinal system, immune system, muscles, musculoskeletal system, nerves, nervous system, psychic-emotional system

SPECIALTIES AND RELATED FIELDS: Neurology, psychiatry, psychology

DEFINITION: Agitations of the passions or sensibilities and the accompanying physiological changes.

KEY TERMS:

autonomic nervous system: the division of the nervous system that regulates involuntary action; comprises the sympathetic and parasympathetic systems

bipolar disorder: a syndrome characterized by alternating periods of mania and depression; also called manic-depressive disorder

Kluver-Bucy syndrome: a series of symptoms first observed in monkeys following temporal lobe removal, such as psychic blindness, abnormal oral tendencies, and changes in sexuality

loss-of-control syndrome: a pattern of behavior characterized by violent and emotional outbursts, occasionally associated with temporal lobe seizures

major depressive syndrome: a syndrome characterized by profound sadness and loss of pleasure in normal activities

sympathetic nervous system: the division of the autonomic nervous system concerned primarily with preparing the individual to expend energy

STRUCTURE AND FUNCTIONS

A central characteristic of being human is the ability to feel and express a wide range of emotions. Just what happens in the human brain and body to generate these feelings, however, is unclear. Over the years, it has been demonstrated that activity in the sympathetic nervous system is important in the expression and experience of emotional states, although the role of various regions of the brain in emotion has proved to be more elusive.

No consensus exists on how many different emotions humans are capable of experiencing, as so much depends on definitions and the type of evidence admitted. Most theorists agree, however, that emotions have a significant impact on human behavior. The term "emotion" usually means some subjectively felt effect. In addition, at least three other factors can be considered part of emotion: physiological arousal (increased heart rate, sweating palms), expressive changes of the muscles of the face and body (smiles, frowns), and behavior (striking with a fist, cringing).

The best-studied physical responses characteristic of emotional states are those produced by the sympathetic nervous system, which controls many different internal organs of the body, as well as the salivary and sweat glands. Several of the responses produced by this system occur in emotional states. These responses are recorded in an attempt to study, measure, and evaluate emotion. The most commonly used responses include changes in heart rate, blood pressure, dilation of the pupils, and sweat gland activity. Physiological arousal in emotion also includes changes in the secretion of some hormones such as adrenaline, testosterone, and cortisol, measured from their presence in such body fluids as urine, saliva, and blood plasma.

The nervous system provides for rapid communication in the body, as it is concerned with events that occur on the order of milliseconds. Its structural and functional unit is the neuron, or nerve cell. Neurons have certain distinctive regions. The dendrites, or bushy protrusions, are the part specialized in receiving excitation, whether from an external stimulus or from another cell. The axon, or elongated part of the cell, takes care of distributing excitation away from the dendrite zone. Axons can be very long and form bundles that make up nerves.

The entire nervous system is a functional unit, and an impulse arising in any receptor can be transmitted to every effector in the body. Synapses are the functional junctions where connections between neurons form. In this region, one cell comes into contact, or near contact, with another cell, thus influencing it. Nerve impulses are propagated electrochemical reactions. The neural message must jump from the axon of one neuron to the dendrite of another for transmission to occur. The most common way of achieving this is through a chemical transmitter substance, also called a neurotransmitter. Chemical transmission at a synapse involves two steps. The first is the release of the specific chemical or neurotransmitter on the arrival of a nerve impulse. The chemical is released from its storage place in the tip of the axon into the narrow space between adjacent neurons. Once this has taken place, the specific transmitter substance is attached to a specific molecular site in the dendrite of the other neuron. This attachment produces a change in the properties of its cell membrane so that a new nerve impulse is set up, and the transmission continues.

The rapidly acting neurotransmitters include norepinephrine, epinephrine, dopamine, serotonin, acetylcholine, gamma aminobutyric acid (GABA), glycine, glutamate, and probably aspartate and adenosine triphosphate (ATP). The action of these neurotransmitters depends on the chemistry of the receptor to which they bind, and there are several types of receptor for each neurotransmitter. Receptors for neurotransmitters are important targets for toxins and drugs. For example, psychoactive drugs exert their effects at synapses, mostly by binding to specific receptors, but also by interfering with the degradation or removal of the transmitter from the synaptic cleft so that it lingers longer in the system.

From research on people with spinal cord injuries, it was found that while emotions may not be caused by feedback from sympathetic activity, this activity does play an important role in reinforcing emotional feelings, making them more intense and longer lasting.

Many different regions of the brain participate in emotions. The neocortex is responsible for dealing with symbolic manipulation, and bodily responses to emotion involve circuits located in lower brain regions such as the hypothalamus. Hormonal changes bring the endocrine system into play.

Dramatic changes in personality and emotional expression often occur following damage to various areas of the brain, such as weakening of emotional control with an injury to the frontal lobes. There is controversy, however, regarding where in the brain emotion is actually experienced. Research has pointed to certain parts of the brain below the cerebral cortex, such as the hypothalamus and the amygdala, as possible key participants. Two syndromes corroborate this finding. In loss-of-control syndrome, emotional outbursts are caused by abnormal electrical discharges in the region of the temporal lobe and amygdala. These spontaneous discharges are characteristic of epilepsy and are thought to result from congenital defects, high fever, brain infection, or trauma. Epilepsy can be controlled with drugs that inhibit the electrical discharges, since uncontrolled discharges result in epileptic seizures. Violent behavior and periods of intense emotion are common prior to an epileptic attack, although in some cases the sensations that take place before the seizure are interpreted by the individual as ecstasy of the highest order. Kluver-Bucy syndrome refers to a series of symptoms first observed in monkeys following temporal lobe removal: psychic blindness, abnormal oral tendencies, changes in sexuality, tameness (a significant lack of emotion), and hypermetamorphosis (a tendency to examine and react to virtually everything in the environment). Some or all the symptoms described have been seen in human patients following strokes, brain injury, brain infections, and other traumas, although the presence of all five in a single individual is very rare. Subsequent research has suggested that changes in emotionality and sexuality are probably caused by damage to the amygdala, while psychic blindness is more likely attributable to the removal of the neocortex of the temporal lobe.

Besides the temporal lobe and the amygdala, portions of the limbic system such as the septal area and the hypothalamus are involved in emotional responses. The pleasure centers of the brain are found in the limbic system (which includes the septal area, amygdala, cingulate cortex, and hippocampus), the hypothalamus, and the brain stem. Brain regions can be classified as positive, negative, or neutral with respect to whether animals will work to turn on or turn off electrical stimulation of these particular areas. Virtually all the cerebral neurocortex and cerebellum is neutral, much of the limbic system and hypothalamus is positive, and some regions of the brain stem and hippocampus are negative. In some cases, electrical stimulation of positive sites mimics the effects of a naturally rewarding event so well that animals prefer the electrical stimulation to the actual experience.

Some research has indicated possible differences between the brain hemispheres in the understanding and expression of emotion. Such data come from the examination of neurological patients having brain damage confined to either side of the brain. Those patients with damage to the left hemisphere are more likely to suffer catastrophic reaction, characterized by intense fear, depressions, and a generally negative outlook on life. The ones with damage on the right side show an attitude of indifference or even unusual cheerfulness. One possible interpretation is that the observed emotions are a result of dominance by the healthy hemisphere, suggesting that the right side is responsible for negative emotional states such as fear, anger, and depression and that the left side produces more positive emotional states. Another possible explanation can reverse this conclusion, simply by stating that the damaged hemisphere becomes dominant in these cases. Identifying emotions with one side of the brain or the other, however, ignores some important data. For example, some patients with frontal lobe damage in either hemisphere will display changes in personality and emotional reactions.

The relationship between behavioral and physiological response processes has long provided an important focus for both laboratory and clinical studies of emotion. For example, research concerned with shyness in children is aimed at investigating the role of sympathetic arousal in emotion. It has been shown that children who are inhibited and quiet when placed in an unfamiliar social situation show larger sympathetic responses than more relaxed, spontaneous children.

Emotions are also the focus of research in the detection of deception, especially as it relates to criminal investigations. A polygraph is a device used to measure involuntary body responses such as changes in respiration, heart rate, and blood pressure in relation to various kinds of questions. It can determine whether the individual is trying to be deceptive. The use of a polygraph is based on two main assumptions: first, that physiological responses during emotional arousal are involuntary, and second, that only individuals with guilty knowledge will display emotional arousal to certain questions asked by the tester. There are three types of questions: irrelevant questions, such as "What is your name?"; control questions, which deal with issues similar to those under consideration but not directly relevant; and relevant questions. The questions are asked in an unpredictable order, sometimes more than once. It is assumed that the person is being deceptive if the polygraph shows more arousal to relevant questions than to control ones. In a controlled laboratory setting, the polygraph is 80 to 90 percent effective in identifying guilty individuals and 90 to 95 percent effective in identifying innocent individuals. It is a process filled with interpretive problems that have to be solved.

Almost every drug found to be effective in altering affective states in humans has also been found to exert effects upon catecholamines (such as norepinephrine and epinephrine) in the brain. These effects would suggest that catecholamines are involved in the mediation of affective states and in the action of the drugs that affect them. Drugs that are associated with depressive phenomena in humans normally cause the loss of catecholamines, while drugs that elevate the mood (antidepressants) have the opposite effect by blocking the mechanisms that destroy the compounds.

DISORDERS AND DISEASES

Mood disorders fall into one of two categories: major depressive disorder and bipolar disorder. Major depressive syndrome is characterized by profound sadness and loss of pleasure in normal activities. Bipolar (manic-depressive) disorder is characterized by alternating periods of mania and depression.

Major depressive syndrome can often be treated without drugs. In many cases, however, drugs accelerate the recovery process. Three main families of antidepressant drugs are the tricyclics, the monoamine oxidase inhibitors (MAOIs), and the selective serotonin reuptake inhibitors (SSRIs). One of the major tricyclic drugs is imipramine (Tofranil or Janimine), an example of an MAOI is isocarboxazid (Marplan), and the most commonly prescribed SSRI is fluoxetine (Prozac). All these drugs help lift depression by increasing the availability of monoamine neurotransmitters at synapses in critical circuits in the brain. Monoamine neurotransmitters include norepinephrine, epinephrine, dopamine, and serotonin. Tricyclic compounds increase the time that the neurotransmitter is available in the synapse, and thus the duration of neurotransmitter action. MAOIs inhibit the action of the enzyme that normally degrades monoamines. SSRIs inhibit serotonin, thus making more of it available to brain cells. Although these are the most common antidepressant drugs, not all of them belong to these families, and not all act by these mechanisms.

Antidepressants, like any other drugs, can have bothersome side effects that may include constipation, urinary retention, blurred vision, and weight gain. More severe side effects include abnormalities in heart function and blood pressure. SSRIs have fewer and more easily tolerated side effects. Antidepressants may be provided to the patient in one-week doses at a time, since a fatal dose is only ten to fifteen times the daily dose.

Electroconvulsive therapy (formerly called shock therapy) is another treatment for severe depression. It is a controversial therapy used as a last resort for severe cases, normally for patients who do not respond to other methods and who are at extreme risk for suicide. The process involves administration of a brief electric current through the head, enough to produce an electrical pattern resembling a grand mal epileptic seizure. Patients are given sedatives so that they are not aware of the current or convulsions. This treatment works for about 70 percent of the patients. Possible side effects include headaches and loss of memory for events just before the shock; sometimes this memory comes back, and sometimes it does not.

Bipolar mood disorder is much less common than major depressive syndrome. The main method of treatment is to administer lithium salts, although their mechanism of action is not known.

Anxiety disorders are the most common emotional disorders, as up to 8 percent of the population experiences them. Included in this group is panic disorder. A panic attack includes shortness of breath, dizziness, acceleration of heart rate, and sweating. It can take place by anticipation of something or for no reason at all. Although attacks last only a few minutes, they are very disturbing. These symptoms involve activation of the sympathetic division of the nervous system. Other anxiety disorders are phobias (chronic fears of certain situations) and obsessive-compulsive disorder. The benzodiazepines are drugs that are effective in the treatment of panic disorder. They include alprazolam (Xanax), chlordiazepoxide (Librium), and diazepam (Valium). These drugs enhance the inhibitory effect of GABA, a major inhibitory neurotransmitter, at synapses throughout the brain. Obsessive-compulsive disorder is characterized by stereotyped rituals or compulsions that develop in an attempt to deal with the anxiety produced by

obsessions (such as the fear of germs). It has been successfully treated with some of the tricyclic drugs, such as clomipramine.

PERSPECTIVE AND PROSPECTS

The word "passion" was frequently used by early philosophers to connote roughly what is now referred to as emotion: the phenomena of anger, fear, love, jealousy, and so on. In the fourth century B.C.E., Aristotle made a distinction between experiences that involve concurrent activity of both soul and body (such as appetites and passions) and those that involve activity of the soul alone (thinking). In the thirteenth century, Saint Thomas Aquinas was more explicit in affirming this belief in such a distinction, placing his argument within the context of Christian theology. In the seventeenth century, René Descartes directed his attention specifically to the passions. He reiterated that every passion experienced by the soul has its physical counterpart, and he emphasized the role of environmental stimulation in the generation of a passion and proposed a mechanism by which the environment created the passions. Descartes also established conceptual distinctions among passion (of the soul), bodily commotion (activity of the visceral organs), and action (motion of the somatic musculature) and indicated close correspondence among the three.

About two centuries passed without significant development in theoretical ideas about emotion. Interest was renewed, however, as a result of the publication of Charles Darwin's *The Expression of Emotions in Man and Animals* (1872), in which he drew attention to emotional behavior as the biologically significant aspect of emotion and pointed out the causal role of stimulus events or situations in producing behavior.

The American philosopher and psychologist William James proposed the first explicit psychological theory of emotion in 1884. He claimed that emotions are the result, not the cause, of bodily arousal. According to James, bodily arousal is produced by the action of the sympathetic system. These reactions he believed to be reflexive responses to emotion-provoking situations. The emotion would then be produced by feedback from nerves bringing input from various internal organs (the heart and stomach) and blood vessels affected by the sympathetic system. This theory triggered the serious experimental study of emotion. Danish physiologist Carl Lange independently published a similar theory in 1885, and as a result, the theory is known as the James-Lange theory of emotion. Although it was frequently criticized, this theory dominated the field of emotion research for more than fifty years.

In 1915, Walter Cannon provided convincing experimental evidence of endocrine and autonomic participation in emotional response patterns. In 1927, he conducted a dramatic experiment by removing the sympathetic nervous system of a few cats. All the nerve connections between sympathetic neurons and internal organs and blood vessels were eliminated. According to the James-Lange theory, the cats should feel no emotions. They still displayed clear-cut emotional behaviors, however, and Cannon proposed that external stimuli caused emotion by simultaneously activating neural circuits in the neocortex and triggering responses in the sympathetic nervous system. Most modern theories are more closely aligned with Cannon's work than with the James-Lange hypothesis.

In 1962, Stanley Schachter and Jerome Singer followed up on Gregorio Maranon's 1924 experiment on the role of bodily responses in emotion. They proposed that people need to attribute their feelings to some emotional state and that the complete emotional experience is a joint product of cognition and feedback from sympathetic arousal. The role of sympathetic activity in emotion is still an active topic of research.

Various experiments have sought to discover the functions of certain regions of the brain, as they relate to emotional responses. In 1939, psychologist Heinrich Kluver and neurosurgeon Paul Bucy were interested in identifying the regions of the brain where drugs produce hallucinations. They speculated that the temporal lobe might be involved since brief hallucinations precede temporal lobe epileptic attacks. Both temporal lobes of monkeys were removed, and a constellation of dramatic behavioral changes was observed, proving their theory. In 1954, James Olds and Peter Milner published a report that rats would press a lever for the sole reward of passing electrical current into certain regions of their brains. This phenomenon is known as self-stimulation, and it led to the discovery of the pleasure centers of the brain. Fearlike responses have been elicited from electrical stimulation of three regions of a cat's brain: the tectum, the thalamus, and portions of the hippocampus. Such sites are called negatively reinforcing regions.

As additional information is accumulated, the complexity of the human brain becomes increasingly evident. Emotion is no exception. The biochemical aspects of emotional states have been studied extensively, and considerable information has been acquired, largely in terms of the biochemical changes that accompany and feed back into the central emotional state. Yet there are still many areas to be explored, including complete elucidation of the mechanism of action of some drugs and thus better treatment options for certain disorders.

—Maria Pacheco, Ph.D.

See also Addiction; Aging; Alcoholism; Antidepressants; Anxiety; Asperger's syndrome; Autism; Bipolar disorder; Bonding; Brain; Brain disorders; Death and dying; Depression; Developmental stages; Endocrinology; Endocrinology, pediatric; Epilepsy; Grief and guilt; Hormones; Hypochondriasis; Light therapy; Midlife crisis; Nervous system; Nightmares; Obsessive-compulsive disorder; Panic attacks; Paranoia; Phobias; Postpartum depression; Post-traumatic stress disorder; Psychiatric disorders; Psychiatry; Psychiatry, child and adolescent; Psychiatry, geriatric; Psychoanalysis; Psychosis; Psychosomatic disorders; Puberty and adolescence; Schizophrenia; Seasonal affective disorder; Separation anxiety; Sexual dysfunction; Shock therapy; Sibling rivalry; Stress; Thumb sucking; Toilet training.

FOR FURTHER INFORMATION:

Cooper, J. R., F. E. Bloom, and R. H. Roth. *The Biochemical Basis of Neuropharmacology.* 8th ed. New York: Oxford University Press, 2003. A fine treatise on the drugs that affect the nervous system, such as psychotropic drugs that affect mood and behavior, sedatives, and other drugs that affect the autonomic nervous system.

Heilman, K. M., and Paul Satz, eds. *Neuropsychology of Human Emotion.* New York: Guilford Press, 1983. This book contains chapters by different authors on right-hemisphere involvement in emotion, the emotional changes associated with epilepsy, and other neurological and psychiatric diseases.

Henry, Helen L., and Anthony W. Norman, eds. *Encyclopedia of Hormones.* 3 vols. San Diego, Calif.: Academic Press, 2003. A comprehensive overview of the role of hormones, the major physiological systems in which they operate, and the biological consequences of an excess or deficiency of a particular hormone.

Kimble, D. P. *Biological Psychology.* 2d ed. Fort Worth, Tex.: Harcourt Brace Jovanovich, 1992. An excellent textbook which provides good suggestions for further readings of the various topics presented. A well-written, easy-to-read presentation of the topic of emotion and its causes.

Rosenzweig, Mark A., Arnold L. Leiman, and S. Marc Breedlove. *Biological Psychology: An Introduction to Behavioral, Cognitive, and Clinical Neuroscience.* 3d ed. Sunderland, Mass.: Sinauer Associates, 2002. This new edition examines each major topic in psychobiology from the perspectives of the description, evolution, and development of behavior as well as biological mechanisms underlying it.

EMPHYSEMA
DISEASE/DISORDER

ANATOMY OR SYSTEM AFFECTED: Chest, lungs, respiratory system

SPECIALTIES AND RELATED FIELDS: Internal medicine, pulmonary medicine

DEFINITION: A disease of the lung characterized by enlargement of the small bronchioles or lung alveoli, the destruction of alveoli, decreased elastic recoil of these structures, and the trapping of air in the lungs, resulting in shortness of breath, reduced oxygen to the body, and a variety of serious and eventually fatal complications.

KEY TERMS:

alveoli: tiny, delicate, balloonlike air sacs composed of blood vessels that are supported by connecting tissue and enclosed in a very thin membrane; these sacs are found at the ends of the bronchioles

bronchioles: small branches of the bronchi, which are extensions of the trachea (the central duct that conducts air from the environment to the pulmonary system)

bullous emphysema: localized areas of emphysema within the lung substance

centrilobular (centriacinar) emphysema: a type of emphysema that destroys single alveoli, entering directly into the walls of terminal and respiratory bronchioles

diffusion: the passage of oxygen into the bloodstream from the alveoli and the return or exchange of carbon dioxide across the membrane between the blood vessels and the alveoli

panlobular (panacinar) emphysema: a type of emphysema that involves weakening and enlargement of the air sacs, which are clustered at the end of respiratory bronchioles

perfusion: the flow of blood through the lungs or other vessels in the body

ventilation: the transport of air from the mouth through the bronchial tree to the air sacs and back through the nose or mouth to the outside; ventilation includes both inspiration (breathing in) and expiration (breathing out)

CAUSES AND SYMPTOMS

Emphysema is a lung disease in which damage to these organs causes shortness of breath and can lead to heart or respiratory failure. A discussion of the structure and function of the normal lung can illuminate the nature and effects of this damage.

Gases, smoke, germs, allergens, and environmental pollutants pass from the nose and mouth into a large duct called the trachea. The trachea branches into smaller ducts, the bronchi and bronchioles (small branches of the bronchi), which lead to tiny air sacs called alveoli. The respiratory system is like a tree: The trachea is the trunk, the bronchi and bronchioles are similar to the branches, and the alveoli are similar to the leaves. The blood vessels of the alveoli carry red blood cells, which pick up oxygen and transport it to the rest of the body. The cellular waste product, carbon dioxide, is released to the alveoli from the bloodstream and then exhaled. The alveoli are supported by a framework of delicate elastic fibers and give the lung a very distensible quality and the ability to "snap back," or recoil.

The lungs and bronchial tubes are surrounded by the chest wall, composed of bone and muscle and functioning like a bellows. The lung is elastic and passively increases in size to fill the chest space during inspiration and decreases in size during expiration. As the lung (including the alveoli) enlarges, air from the environment flows in to fill this space. During exhalation, the muscles relax, the elasticity of the lung returns it to a normal size, and the air is pushed out. Air must pass through the bronchial tree to the alveoli before oxygen can get into the bloodstream and carbon dioxide can get out, because it is the alveoli that are in contact with blood vessels. The bronchial tree has two kinds of special lining cells. The first type can secrete mucus as a sticky protection against injury and irritation. The second type of cell is covered with fine, hairlike structures called cilia. These cells are supported by smooth muscle cells and elastic and collagen fibers. The cilia wave in the direction of the mouth and act as a defense system by physically removing germs and irritating substances. The cilia are covered with mucus, which helps to trap irritants and germs.

INFORMATION ON EMPHYSEMA

CAUSES: Long-term exposure to dry air, smoke, or other environmental toxins; infection; allergies
SYMPTOMS: Shortness of breath, labored breathing, discolored skin, wheezing, difficulty coughing and talking
DURATION: Chronic
TREATMENTS: Eliminating causes of irritation, cleaning out airways via nebulizers and intermittent positive pressure breathing machine, medications (theophylline, antibiotics, steroids)

When alveoli are exposed to irritants such as cigarette smoke, they produce a defensive cell called an alveolar macrophage. These cells engulf irritants and bacteria and call for white blood cells, which aid in the defense against foreign bodies, to come into the lungs. The lung tissue also becomes a target for the enzymes or chemical substances produced by the alveolar macrophages and leukocytes (white blood cells). In a healthy body, natural defense systems inhibit the enzymes released by the alveolar macrophages and leukocytes, but it seems that this inhibiting function is impaired in smokers. In some cases, an individual may inherit a deficiency in an enzyme inhibitor. The enzymes vigorously attack the elastin and collagen of the lungs, the lung loses its elastic recoil, and air is trapped.

Emphysema, and a related disease, bronchitis, often work in concert. They are often lumped under the term "chronic obstructive pulmonary disease." Chronic bronchitis weakens and narrows the bronchi. Often, bronchial walls collapse, choking off the vital flow of air. Air is also trapped within the bronchial walls. Weakened by enzymes, the walls of the alveoli rupture and blood vessels die. Lung tissue is replaced with scar tissue, leaving areas of destroyed alveoli that appear as "holes" on an X ray. Small areas of destroyed alveoli are called blebs, and larger ones are called bullae.

As emphysema progresses, a patient has a set of large, overexpanded lungs with a weakened and partially plugged bronchial tree subject to airway collapse and air trapping with blebs and bullae. Breathing, especially exhalation, becomes a slow and difficult process. The patient often develops a "barrel chest" and is known, in medical circles, as a "blue bloater." The sci-entific world calls the mismatching of breathing to blood distribution a ventilation-to-perfusion imbalance; that is, when air arrives in the alveolus, there are no blood vessels there to transport their vital gaseous cargo to the cells (as a result of enzymatic damage). A person with chronic obstructive pulmonary disease has a bronchial tree with a narrow, defective trunk and sparse leaves.

The loss of elasticity of the lung and alveoli is a critical problem in the emphysemic patient. About one-half of the lungs' elastic recoil force comes from surface tension. The other half comes from the elastic nature of certain fibers throughout the lungs' structure. Emphysema weakens both of these forces because it destroys the elastic fibers and interferes with the surface tension. Fluid, a saline solution, bathes all the body's cells and surfaces. In the lung, this fluid contains surfactant, a substance that interferes with water's tendency to form a spherical drop with a pull into its center (and ultimate collapse). The tissue that gives shape to the lungs is composed of specialized fibers which contain a protein called elastin. These elastic fibers are also found in the alveolar walls and in the elastic connective tissue of the airways and air sacs. The amount of elastin in lung tissue determines its behavior. Healthy lungs maintain a proper balance between destruction of elastin and renewal. (Other parts of the body, such as bones, do this as well.) If too little elastin is destroyed, the lungs have difficulty expanding. If too much is destroyed, the lungs overexpand and cannot recoil properly.

The process of elastin destruction and renewal involves complex regulation. Specialized lung cells produce new elastin protein. Others produce elastase, an enzyme that destroys elastin. The liver plays a role in the production of a special enzyme known as alpha-1-antitrypsin, which controls the amount of elastase so that too much elastin is not digested. In emphysema, these regulatory systems fail: Too much elastin is destroyed because elastase is no longer controlled, apparently because alpha-1-antitrypsin production has been reduced to a trickle.

The loss of elastin (and thus elastic recoil) means that the lungs expand beyond the normal range during inspiration and cannot resume their resting size during expiration. Thus, alveoli overinflate and rupture. This further reduces elasticity because the loss of each alveolus further impairs the surface tension contribution to the lungs' ability to recoil. Thus, a state of hyperinflation is assumed in the emphysemic patient. This leads to stretched and narrowed alveolar capillaries, loss of elastic tissue, and dissolution of alveolar walls. The lungs increase in size, the thoracic (chest) cage assumes the inspiratory position, and the diaphragm becomes low and flat instead of convex. The patient becomes short of breath with any type of exertion. As the disease worsens, the patient's skin takes on a cyanotic color, as a result of poor oxygenation and perfusion. Wheezing is often present, and coughing is difficult and tiring. In the worst cases, even talking is enough ex-ertion to produce a spasmodic cough. The hyperinflated chest causes inspiration to become a major effort, and the entire chest cage lifts up, resulting in considerable strain. The head moves with each inspiration while the chest remains relatively fixed.

Emphysema may be diagnosed by the early symptom of dyspnea (shortness of breath) on exertion. In advanced cases, the distended chest, depressed diaphragm, increased blood carbon dioxide content, and severe dyspnea clearly point to the disease.

TREATMENT AND THERAPY

The initial step in treating emphysema is to open the airways by eliminating the causes of irritation: smoke, dry air, infection, and allergies. The second treatment is to clean out the airways. There are several techniques and medicines for loosening airway mucus and expelling it. In most chronic obstructive lung diseases, including emphysema, the mucus becomes thick and purulent; coughing up mucus of this type is difficult. In addition, in emphysema the natural cleansing action of the cilia and lung elasticity are impaired. Thus, treatment is aimed at the patient consciously taking over the function of cleaning out the lungs. Coughing is nature's way of bringing up mucus (phlegm), and the emphysemic patient is urged to cough. Since the mucus is thick, one needs to do whatever is necessary to thin it out and to lubricate the airways so that the mucus slips up easily with coughing. The cough must come from deep within the chest in order to be "productive" (to raise mucus).

Emphysema

Pleura
Rib
Enlarged alveoli
Intrapleural space
Mucus
Thickened mucosa
Bronchospasm
Lung

Air in

Trapped air in alveoli
Collapsed bronchiole

Air out

In emphysema, the body releases enzymes in response to inhaling irritants in the air, such as cigarette smoke; these enzymes reduce the lung's elasticity, compromising the bronchioles' ability to expand and contract normally. Air becomes trapped in the alveoli upon inhalation (top) and cannot escape upon exhalation (bottom). Over time, breathing becomes extremely difficult.

Moisture is helpful in loosening up thick mucus; hence, drinking large amounts of fluid is encouraged. Adding a humidifier or a vaporizer to a home is often helpful to the emphysemic patient. There are also machines known as nebulizers and intermittent positive pressure breathing (IPPB) machines that can help to add moisture to the airway of the patient with emphysema. Nebulizers are more effective in getting moisture beyond the throat and major airways than cold vaporizers. Nebulizers, which get their name from the Latin word for cloud or mist, create a mist that is a profusion of tiny droplets that keep themselves apart, even as they bump into one another. Nebulizers release only the smallest droplets—those which can penetrate far down into air passages, where thick mucus is likely to be. (Atomizers produce small droplets as well, but they also spray large droplets.) IPPBs have a special kind of valve that opens when one begins to breathe and allows the air to move into the lungs under mild pressure. As soon as the patient has come to the end of the inhalation, the valve closes and allows the patient to exhale freely.

When phlegm cannot be brought up by breathing mist, a technique called postural drainage is often combined with chest wall percussion or vibration. The idea is to move one's body to a position such that airways are perpendicular to the floor, or at least tilted down, so that gravity can help pull the mucus toward the larger airways, from which the phlegm can be coughed up. Percussion, or clapping the chest, is another way to loosen the mucus in the airways so that it can be coughed up.

A number of medications are useful in the treatment of emphysema. The bronchodilator drugs are xanthines, such as theophylline (Theo-Dur), that relieve bronchospasms, reduce wheezing and dyspnea, and improve respiratory muscle function. Theophylline is a drug that is similar chemically to caffeine. Whereas caffeine stimulates the skeletal muscles and the central nervous system, however, theophylline is potent as a cardiac stimulant and a smooth muscle relaxer. It has also been learned that theophylline stimulates mucociliary clearance of the airways, strengthens the diaphragm, and suppresses edema. Theophylline holds two benefits for the chronic obstructive pulmonary diseased patient: It helps get rid of mucus, and it strengthens the diaphragm, the main respiratory muscle. Common side effects are nausea, stomach pain, vomiting, insomnia, rapid heartbeat, loss of appetite, and restlessness. Another category of bronchodilator are the beta adrenergic stimulants such as metaproterenol (Alupent). Their side effects include nervousness, headache, nausea, and muscle cramps.

The antibiotics sometimes prescribed for emphysemic patients are used to combat bacterial infection. Common antibiotics include tetracycline, penicillin, cephalosporin, erythromycin, and sulfa drugs. Their side effects include a burning sensation in the stomach, vomiting, diarrhea, increased sensitivity to sunlight, rashes, itching, hives, fever, and weakness.

The steroid hormones, such as prednisone, decrease swelling, inflammation, and bronchospasms; they also relieve wheezing. Side effects include blurred vision, frequent urination, thirst, black stools, bone pain, mood changes, weight gain, swelling of the feet, muscle weakness, hoarseness, and a sore mouth.

Other drugs given for emphysema include digitalis, cardiac glycosides, diuretics, mast cell inhibitors, expectorants, and parasympatholytics. Digitalis and car-diac glycosides, such as digoxin, improve the strength of heart contractions and treat disturbances in heart rhythm. Side effects are loss of appetite, abdominal pain, nausea, slow uneven pulse, blurred vision, diarrhea, mood changes, and weakness. Diuretics, such as furosemide (Lasix), are often given to prevent excessive fluid retention. Such drugs cause loss of hearing, skin rashes, hives, bleeding, bruising, jaundice, an irregular or fast heartbeat, muscle cramps, lightheadedness, dizziness, and weakness. Mast cell inhibitors are a unique category of drugs that inhibit the release of body chemicals that cause wheezing and bronchospasm; however, they also cause weakness, nosebleeds, and nasal congestion. Expectorants, such as Robitussin, are used to thin secretions and have no known side effects. The parasympatholytics are a type of bronchodilator drug that inhibits the nerves that cause bronchospasm. They are apparently free from the many side effects associated with other bronchodilator drugs.

The emphysemic patient should avoid both excessive heat and excessive cold. If body temperature rises above normal, the heart works faster, as do the lungs. Excessive cold stresses the body to maintain its normal temperature. Smog, air pollution, dusts, powders, and hairspray should be avoided. Finally, a healthy diet consisting of foods high in calcium, vitamins, complex carbohydrates, proteins, and fiber is advised for the patient with lung disease.

A healthy core diet is high in complex carbohydrates; is low in sugars, fats, and cholesterol; and has adequate protein for moderate stress. It should be high in fiber and contain approximately 1,000 milligrams of calcium, 15,000 milligrams of vitamin A, and 250 milligrams of vitamin C. Snack foods can include skim milk, fruit, popcorn, and fresh salads. The respiratory distress of the emphysemic patient uses vast amounts of energy, and the patient should eat several small meals a day so as not to distend the stomach and limit movement of the diaphragm. Liquids are important in keeping airways clear. Good nutrition is helpful in maintaining strength and improving the quality of life for the patient with lung disease.

Perspective and Prospects

Chronic bronchitis and emphysema are responsible for at least fifty thousand deaths a year in the United States alone. An increase in air pollution and cigarette consumption are apparent causes for this rise. In males over forty, chronic obstructive pulmonary disease

(COPD) is second to heart disease as a cause of disability. With more females and young people smoking, the incidence of lung disease is likely to increase. Aside from death, a disease such as emphysema can cause long years of disability, joblessness, loss of income, depression, hospitalization, and an inability to perform normal activities.

Smoking is, by far, the single most important risk factor for emphysema. In the United States especially, social acceptance of women smokers began after World War II and has increased the number of women being diagnosed with COPD. Socioeconomic status also influences smoking habits. In many countries in Europe, the mortality rate from lung disease for the lowest socioeconomic class has been six times higher than for the highest. In the United States, the COPD mortality rate among unskilled and semiskilled laborers is twice as high as among professionals. Families with lower incomes usually live in small, often overcrowded apartments; such overcrowding makes respiratory infections more frequent. Often, family members of the COPD patient also smoke, increasing the surrounding air pollution.

In the United States, COPD causes 3 percent of all deaths. In some cases, it causes another 100,000 Americans to be too weak to survive other, unrelated medical conditions. Therefore, an annual figure of 150,000 deaths from COPD-related diseases is more realistic. The expanding COPD population is a growing market for pharmaceutical firms. For example, greater amounts of bronchodilator medications will be needed; hence, pharmaceutical firms are anxious to find longer-acting and more effective drugs for these patients to buy.

A number of economic pressures are likely to move COPD treatment from the hospital to the home. When effectively carried out by a well-trained health team, home care can lower medical costs. The COPD patient who finds a knowledgeable doctor and who begins a comprehensive rehabilitation program is the one who can look forward to a life that is more productive and more comfortable.

—*Jane A. Slezak, Ph.D.*

See also Chronic obstructive pulmonary disease (COPD); Cyanosis; Environmental diseases; Lungs; Oxygen therapy; Pulmonary diseases; Pulmonary medicine; Pulmonary medicine, pediatric; Respiration.

FOR FURTHER INFORMATION:

American Lung Association. http://www.lungusa.org/ asthma/. Includes in-depth information and recent research findings, a guide to local events and programs, and a section to share personal stories, among other features.

Bates, David V. *Respiratory Function in Disease*. 3d ed. Philadelphia: W. B. Saunders, 1989. Summarizes the effects of disease on pulmonary function. Also discussed are some of the more sophisticated pulmonary function tests. Exercise testing, obesity, and the effects of drugs are other topics reviewed in this work.

Decker, Caroline D. "Room to Breathe." *Saturday Evening Post* 266, no. 6 (November/December, 1994): 48-49. This article on emphysema discusses lung surgery. Illustrated with photographs.

Haas, François, and Sheila Sperber Haas. *The Chronic Bronchitis and Emphysema Handbook*. Rev. ed. New York: John Wiley & Sons, 2000. Helps patients with COPD learn to lead full and productive lives. Provides information pertinent to their disease and describes the treatments and medications available to them in order to improve their quality of life.

Hedrick, Hannah L., and Austin K. Kutscher, eds. *The Quiet Killer: Emphysema/Chronic Obstructive Pulmonary Disease*. Lanham, Md.: Scarecrow Press, 2002. Clinicians, researchers, and health educators combine their expertise in twenty-five chapters that discuss such topics as managing dyspnea, traveling with mechanical ventilation, encouraging patients to quit smoking, self-help groups, and hospice care.

Matthews, Dawn D. *Lung Disorders Sourcebook: Basic Consumer Health Information About Emphysema, Pneumonia and Other Lung Disorders*. Detroit: Omnigraphics, 2002. A comprehensive overview of lung anatomy, physiology, and dysfunctions taken from government agencies, the American Academy of Family Physicians, the American Lung Association, and the Mayo Foundation. Discusses thirty-five lung disorders in depth.

National Emphysema Foundation. http://www.emphysemafoundation.org/. Site offers tips on exercises, inhaler uses, and other helpful items for those with emphysema.

West, John B., and Karen Bartell. *Pulmonary Pathophysiology: The Essentials*. 6th ed. Philadelphia: Lippincott, Williams and Wilkins, 2003. Examines lungs afflicted with obstructive, restrictive, vascular, and environmental diseases.

Wolff, Ronald K. "Effects of Airborne Pollutants on Mucociliary Clearance." *Environmental Health Perspectives* 66 (April, 1986): 223-237. The role of mucociliary clearance as a lung defense mechanism is described in this article. The abnormal elimination of bronchial mucus is considered a possible factor in the pathogenesis of COPD. The role of certain pollutants, which pose a challenge to the mucociliary system, is detailed.

Encephalitis
Disease/disorder
Anatomy or system affected: Brain, nervous system

Specialties and related fields: Neurology, virology

Definition: A family of diseases resulting from viral infection or complications from another disease; inflammation of the brain resulting in a variety of usually serious symptoms and sometimes death.

Key terms:

athetosis: involuntary writhing movements of limbs and/or body, face, and tongue

dementia: loss of mental ability as a result of brain deterioration

diabetes insipidus: production of copious amounts of urine

hemiplegia: paralysis of one side of the body

nuchal: having to do with the nape of the neck

pleocytosis: an increase in the number of white blood cells in the cerebrospinal fluid

postencephalitic symptoms: symptoms commencing immediately after or years after an attack of encephalitis lethargica as a direct or indirect consequence of the infection

viremia: invasion of cells by viruses

Causes and Symptoms
Encephalitis, a noncontagious disease, is an inflammation of the brain. It most often results from viral infection, but it may also arise as a complication of measles, chickenpox, herpes simplex virus 1, or several other diseases. A nonviral form, encephalitis lethargica (sometimes referred to as "sleeping sickness") is implicated in parkinsonism. Between one thousand and five thousand cases are reported annually to the Centers for Disease Control in Atlanta, Georgia; the highest incidence is in the summer and early fall months, and worldwide, most cases are reported in the tropics. The disease affects the sexes equally, and no age group is unaffected.

The viruses that cause most cases of encephalitis are called arboviruses, animal viruses carried by arthropods and transmitted to vertebrate hosts. In a vertebrate, one of these viruses undergoes viremia, then multiplies in an arthropod when it feeds on the vertebrate host. The arthropod then passes the virus to another vertebrate, also while feeding. Arthropods implicated in passing on the virus to humans are mosquitoes, and rarely, ticks. Mosquitoes (and ticks) pick up the virus as they feed on an infected host. There are several variables, however, that determine whether the virus will be passed on to the next host. First, each different virus has a "preferred" arthropod carrier. Second, the concentration of the virus in the vertebrate host is crucial; more than 100,000 infectious doses per millimeter may be required for infection. Third, the incubation period for replication of the virus in the arthropod must be met; four days to two weeks generally must pass before the carrier can infect a vertebrate, but the virus may remain infective for several weeks after that. The incubation period is often influenced by environmental temperature; high temperature often accelerates incubation times and frequently results in epidemics.

Symptoms of encephalitis develop one to two weeks after the bite of the mosquito and may come on gradually or quite suddenly and forcefully. Acute viral infection of the central nervous system varies from disease to disease because each virus may affect different parts of the nervous system and/or nerve cells. For example, if the meninges (outer covering of the brain and cord) are infected, symptoms may include headache, fever, stiff neck, and pleocytosis. If the fundamental tissues of the brain (parenchymal cells) are involved, loss of consciousness, seizures, focal neurological deficits, and an increased pressure within the brain (such is the case with encephalitis) may also occur. In addition to all other symptoms, if the hypothalamic-pituitary region becomes involved, sudden increases or decreases in body temperature may occur, and diabetes insipidus may result from a lack of antidiuretic hormone secretion. Swelling of the brain may lead to coma and is often followed by cardiac and respiratory arrest. In these cases, the disease may be deemed fatal. If the spinal cord becomes infected, symptoms manifested include paralysis of bowel and bladder.

The three most common symptoms of the acute state (with sudden, forceful onset) are headache, disturbances of sleep rhythm, and visual abnormalities (blurred vision or double vision). Headaches, though common, are not often severe but may accompany vomiting and other body aches. Sleep disturbances generally include lethargy during the day and insomnia at night. More severe cases suffer fever and delirium. Other common symptoms might include drowsiness, stupor, and eye muscle weakness. Because of the infrequency with which encephalitis strikes and the complete change in symptoms in the latter half of the twentieth century, the acute stage may never be observed. Still, in a study of two thousand cases, 38 percent of the patients died, all during the acute phase. These deaths occurred during the first month, most frequently on the fourteenth day. Those most likely to succumb were children under one year of age and adults over the age of seventy. Young adults between the ages of twenty and thirty were most likely to survive. Complete recovery, however, occurred in only about one-fourth of the cases. The remainder of the survivors suffered some degree of dementia.

Symptoms of the chronic stage include sleep disturbances (lethargy and/or insomnia), some dementia, depression, irritability, and anxiety in adults. Children often experience such behavior disorders as stealing, animal cruelty, and other criminal mischief. Respiratory disorders are common in chronic cases, but visual disturbances persist in only a few cases. Since the epidemic during and after World War I that brought so much attention to the disease, the symptoms have undergone remarkable changes. With the epidemic form, the symptoms came on suddenly and with force. Years later, the onset became less terrifying but the chronic stage was often more severe. The most noted symptom in current cases is not during the course of the disease but later. Such is the case with those suffering post-encephalitic parkinsonism. The long-range effects may be delayed as long as forty years before onset. Other lingering aftereffects may be deterioration of mental faculties. In children who have contracted the disease, behavioral disorders may result.

Very infrequently, encephalitis has been implicated in epilepsy. This link would be likely only if the disease caused lesions in the brain. Injuries to or inflammation of a child's nervous system may be the basis for hyperactivity in as many of 80 percent of those children suffering from hyperactivity. Although there are many ways these events can happen, it is not unreasonable to expect that some children who have recovered from encephalitis will experience hyperactivity. In fact, their hyperactivity may be the only real neurological aftermath of the disease.

The encephalitis that was prevalent during World War I was usually accompanied by sleep lasting days or even weeks. (Sometimes called "sleeping sickness" or "sleepy sickness," this type of encephalitis is not to be confused with African sleeping sickness, which is caused by the parasite trypanosoma, borne by the tsetse fly.) Its scientific name is encephalitis lethargica, and it is sometimes referred to as von Economo's disease. This sleep results from lesions in the midbrain as well as the hypothalamic and subthalamic regions of the brain. The lesions also induce continual drowsiness as well as motor deficiencies. Encephalitis lethargica is a type of coma, but the patient can be easily roused with stimulation although he or she lies inert, making no sound. The patient's eyes can follow movement or watch the observer carefully. Rarely, encephalitis lethargica may produce symptoms suggestive of chorea (characterized by involuntary movements).

Postinfection encephalitis may occur during, or as a result of, infectious diseases such as influenza or measles. It may also appear after vaccination against rabies, smallpox, or measles. Postinfection encephalitis does not occur as frequently as the other types, but neither is it affected by the sufferer's age. Because children are most often vaccinated, however, they are more susceptible to postinfection encephalitis.

In the United States, five types of encephalitis are commonly recognized. St. Louis encephalitis is geographically the most widespread as well as the most common type of arbovirus-induced encephalitis. It is found primarily in the South and Midwest and mostly victimizes the elderly. Affected areas of the nervous system include the basal ganglia, brainstem, and white matter of the brain and occasionally the spinal cord. The usual symptoms are fever, reduced heart rate, drowsiness, stupor, nuchal rigidity, athetoses and tremors of the hands, and sometimes seizures. Unusual symptoms may include urinary dysfunction (painful urination and pus in the urine), uncoordinated muscular movements, diabetes insipidus as a result of a lack of antidiuretic hormone, and oculomotor paralysis. Even so, recovery rates are considered to be good for St. Louis encephalitis.

Eastern equine encephalitis is very rare, but the most deadly, with 20 to 40 percent mortality. It is mostly found all along the East Coast where there are horses and pheasants. Eastern equine encephalitis produces numerous large lesions in the brain and is accompanied by high fever, drowsiness, cyanosis (lack of oxygen because of respiratory distress), twitching, seizures, and nuchal rigidity. Not only are mortality rates high, but there is likelihood of severe disabilities including speech difficulties, paralyses, and mental retardation as well.

California encephalitis, sometimes called Western encephalitis, is also rare. Found west of the Mississippi, it is not often fatal or serious. It comes on strong with headache, fever, vomiting, confusion, stupor with perhaps coma, seizures, and respiratory failure. The respiratory failure may cause death in 5 percent of the cases. Aftereffects are rare but might include parkinsonism or learning difficulties. A fourth type of encephalitis found in the United States is LaCrosse, which occurs in the north-central states and West Virginia. Its victims are most often young children.

West Nile virus is a mosquito-borne flavivirus causing severe human meningoencephalitis. West Nile virus was first recognized in Uganda in 1937 and is commonly identified in humans, birds, horses, and other vertebrates in Africa, West Asia, and the Middle East. Prior to 1999, the virus had never been documented in the Americas. During the summer of 1999, an outbreak of West Nile virus occurred in the New York metropolitan area infecting humans, horses, cats, dogs, bats, chipmunks, raccoons, and sixty types of birds, most commonly crows. In 1999, sixty-two cases of severe disease in humans were reported, resulting in seven deaths. In 2003, the virus was documented in forty-seven U.S. states and throughout Canada, with more than 6,000 cases and 145 deaths reported that year. The origin of the Western Hemisphere outbreak of West Nile virus is not known, but the virus is genetically related to strains found in a similar outbreak in Israel during the late 1990's.

The vector between continents is suspected to have been migrating birds, shipborne mosquitoes, or an infected human international traveler. The virus is spread most commonly by the bite of an infected mosquito. Mosquitoes become infected when they feed on infected birds. The virus has been identified in eight varieties of North American mosquitoes, including the bird-loving *Culex pipiens* and the *Aedes vexans*, which prefers to feed on mammals, especially humans, and has a habitat range from the Arctic to Mexico. The fact that *Culex* mosquitos can survive through winter in an adult stage and that annually migrating infected birds will likely transmit the virus to mosquitoes in new areas makes permanent establishment and widespread transmission of West Nile virus in the Western Hemisphere likely. Most people who are infected with West Nile virus will not have any type of illness. It is estimated that 20 percent of the people who become infected will develop West Nile fever. Human symptoms of West Nile virus include fever, head and body aches, skin rash, swollen lymph glands, stupor, disorientation, coma, tremors, convulsions, and paralysis. At its most serious, the virus causes permanent neurological damage. Death occurs in 15 percent of cases.

Encephalitis may occur sporadically as a result of other viral infections such as herpes simplex virus 1, measles (it rarely follows German measles), mumps, rabies, and even during the course of human immunodeficiency virus (HIV) infection. The most common form of fatal sporadic encephalitis is caused by herpes simplex virus 1. It accounts for 5 to 10 percent of the total number of encephalitis cases in the United States each year. If untreated, it is fatal in as many as 70 percent of the cases. Herpes simplex-induced encephalitis produces fever, headache, seizures, and coma and is sometimes preceded by a span of bizarre behavior. These personality changes are likely the result of lesions in the temporal lobes and may include terror and hallucinations. The patient may suffer some paralysis, particularly of the face and arm. Deep coma with respiratory arrest may occur. Of those surviving herpes-induced encephalitis, about half continue to suffer major motor and sensory deficits, speech problems, and frequently, an amnestic syndrome (Korsakoff's psychosis). Two antiviral agents are used to combat the disease with moderate success: acyclovir (often the drug of choice) and adenosine arabinoside. Acyclovir is active only in the cells invaded by the herpes simplex virus and inhibits deoxyribonucleic acid (DNA) replication (effectively halting cell division and numerical growth). HIV-infected patients often experience herpes simplex virus 1, which means that acquired immunodeficiency syndrome (AIDS) patients with this herpes virus may develop encephalitis.

Occasionally, a child under two years of age apparently fights off a bout of measles, only to succumb to a slow invasion of encephalitis that may be fatal. The encephalitis may appear before the rash, with the rash, or after the rash. It may not make an appearance until the child is between ages four and eighteen. In these rare cases (one in every 200,000 cases), known as subacute sclerosing panencephalitis (SSPE), the initial symptoms may be mild. The child may experience poor concentration at first; then symptoms might progress through stages of erratic jerking of the limbs, blindness, severe mental retardation, and then death. There may be a sudden onset with symptoms of fever, lethargy, delirium, catatonia, or excitement. Seizures are common, and mortality rates are high. SSPE results when the measles virus persists in the brain, killing some nerve cells and destroying the myelin sheath surrounding others. SSPE is rare because of the widespread use of antimeasles vaccines.

Another disease of the nervous system that most frequently affects children is acute toxic encephalitis. The difference occurs in the changes it induces in the nervous system. There is not only brain cell degeneration but also edema of the brain and small hemorrhages. Acute toxic encephalitis may also occur in children suffering from burns because of the toxemic effects that burns have on nerve cells.

Several theories have been proposed to answer why other diseases lead to encephalitis. One of these is that the central nervous system reacts to the virus that caused the original disease. Another theory suggests that there may be poisonous substances that develop during the course of the original disease that induce encephalitis. The least popular theory is that enzymes already in the patient or enzymes produced by the original disease are activated. These enzymes destroy the myelin around the nerve cells. Still others believe that postinfection encephalitis is an autoimmune disease. Because of the rarity of postinfection encephalitis, it may be years before the answer is found.

TREATMENT AND THERAPY

Generally, in order to diagnose a patient with encephalitis (which is often indistinguishable from viral meningitis), a physician must review the patient's medical history in the light of the presence or absence of an epidemic, as well as the presence of signs and symptoms. If they indeed are indicative of the possibility, a lumbar puncture and examination of spinal fluid are performed. The amount of pressure the fluid exerts is checked; if pleocytosis and an elevated protein level are found, they too, indicate the likelihood of encephalitis. In some cases, the blood is found to contain increased numbers of neutralizing antibodies. Because the onset of fever, the aches and pains, and other symptoms characterize many infections and diseases as well as encephalitis, specific diagnosis can be made only by isolating the virus or sometimes through a blood workup. Because it is extremely difficult to isolate the virus in the blood, successful diagnosis may be made when two specific antibodies increase in the blood. Although sometimes misdiagnosed as poliomyelitis or multiple sclerosis, encephalitis can be distinguished from these diseases by the sleep disturbances it causes and by the visual disturbances that it may induce. It is unlikely to cause paralysis and only infrequently results in convulsions, unlike the other diseases. Encephalitis is also occasionally misdiagnosed as meningitis but differs from it in that the spinal fluid does not contain an excess of cells as in meningitis. An electroencephalogram (EEG) can be useful because it might show the appropriate disturbance of cerebral activity.

At one time, as many as seventy-five methods of treatment for encephalitis were reported. Yet none of these actually influences how the disease progresses. The only thing that can be treated, therefore, is the symptoms. Placement in intensive care as early as possible is desirable because of the rapid progression of the illness. Relieving the headache and reducing the fever so the sufferer can be as comfortable as possible would likely be the first course taken. Seizures can be treated with anticonvulsant drugs such as phenytoin. Intracranial pressure should be monitored, and if the pressure does rise, nasotracheal intubation (a tube placed in the nose) with hyperventilation from a ventilator might aid in decreasing pressure. During convalescence, speech and physical therapy may be necessary. The length of convalescence depends on how severe the illness has been, but it may take several months for recovery. The prognosis for those with viral encephalitis depends on the causative agent.

In order to control the spread of the mosquito-borne encephalitis virus, a thorough knowledge and understanding of the mosquito population is necessary. Breeding sites must be located, and the distribution and density of the adult mosquito population must be determined, especially those in areas near human populations. This information can be used to contain the mosquito population by using larvivorous fish or chemical insecticides. If one is in an area that is experiencing an outbreak, the best prevention is to remain indoors after dark, thereby avoiding the time that mosquitoes are feeding. If one must go out, one should spray exposed areas with insect repellent and/or wear long sleeves and pants of tightly woven material. The use of window screens, residual insecticide application on and around screen doors, and mosquito netting over cribs offers other ways to retard the number of mosquitoes that can enter the house or to prevent mosquito bites.

PERSPECTIVE AND PROSPECTS

A look at history reveals numerous cases and minor epidemics of encephalitis. In 1580, Europe was inundated with a fever-causing lethargic disease resulting in parkinsonism and other long-lasting neurological effects. Other serious epidemics occurred in London between 1672 and 1673 and again between 1673 and 1675. The most common (and highly unusual) symptom of this epidemic was hiccuping. Epidemics also occurred in the German city of Tübingen from 1712 to 1713, in France and Germany in the latter half of the eighteenth century, and in Italy following a deadly influenza outbreak in 1889 and 1890. None of these epidemics, however, was nearly as widespread as the pandemic that began in the winter of 1916-1917. This major outbreak began in the European city of Vienna, and within three years it had spread worldwide. It seemed each case was different; no two patients experienced the same signs and symptoms the same way. Because of such variations, diagnosis such as epidemic delirium, epidemic schizophrenia, epidemic parkinsonism, rabies, and polio were erroneously made. Seemingly, thousands of new diseases were instantly pervading the globe. It was Constantin von Economo who, through his pathological studies on the brain tissues of many of those who died, not only found a unique pattern of damage but also isolated the virus common to all. Von Economo named this "new" disease encephalitis lethargica.

As this epidemic seized the world, more than five million people were either killed or severely affected. It lasted ten years, leaving as suddenly as it had come. Of those who died, one-third succumbed during the acute stages of the sleeping sickness (in such a deep comatose state as to preclude arousal, or in such a state of sleeplessness as to invalidate sedation). Even those who survived the coma/wakefulness attacks were so affected that they failed to recover to their predisease

alertness. Many were simply conscious, unaware, speechless, motionless, and without energy, motivation, appetite, or desire. They knew what was occurring around them but were totally apathetic to the events, showing no behavior at all.

Sixty years after the epidemic of World War I, many survivors were still alive. Some had active lives despite parkinsonism, tics, and other problems. They were the lucky few; most postencephalitic patients suffered gross debilitating neurological damage, never to function independently again. Many of the survivors were bedridden and robbed of movement, speech, and perhaps memory. Most of them were banished to asylums, nursing homes, or other "special" places where they were untreated and forgotten.

—Iona C. Baldridge;
updated by Randall L. Milstein, Ph.D.

See also Arthropod-borne diseases; Bites and stings; Brain; Brain disorders; Dementias; Hemiplegia; Nervous system; Neurology; Neurology, pediatric; Parasitic diseases; Sleeping sickness; Viral infections; West Nile virus.

FOR FURTHER INFORMATION:

Aminoff, Michael J., ed. *Neurology and General Medicine.* 3d ed. New York: Churchill Livingstone, 2001. This compilation by numerous contributors relates neurological disorders that may occur as a result of or in conjunction with general medical disorders. The intended audience is medical professionals.

Booss, John, Margaret Esiri, and Margaret M. Esin, eds. *Viral Encephalitis in Humans.* Washington, D.C.: ASM Press, 2003. Details the causes, symptoms, diagnosis, and treatment of the disease.

Dana.org. http://www.dana.org/. A nonprofit organization of neuroscientists, which was formed to provide information about the personal and public benefits of brain research. The Web site is research oriented and gives excellent information and links on current brain studies, new diagnosis and treatment technology, and brain-related news stories.

Donaghy, Michael. *Brain's Diseases of the Nervous System.* 11th ed. Oxford, England: Oxford University Press, 2001. A lengthy, complex volume written to educate and inform medical professionals on all aspects of neurological dysfunctions. Its completeness provides a wide range of material, but it is intended for diagnostic usage.

Goddard, Jerome. *Physician's Guide to Arthropods of Medical Importance.* 4th ed. Boca Raton, Fla.: CRC Press, 2002. Nontechnical description of a wide variety of arthropods and conditions related to their stings or bites. Topics include the signs and symptoms of arthropod-borne diseases.

Johnson, Richard T. *Viral Infections of the Nervous System.* 2d ed. New York: Raven Press, 1998. A readable volume, with a clinical audience in mind; punctuated with pictures and tables. Emphasizes the biology of nervous system infections, and references to laboratory diagnoses, prevention, and therapy are also included.

Parker, James N., and Philip M. Parker, eds. *The Official Patient's Sourcebook on Rasmussen's Encephalitis.* San Diego, Calif.: Icon Health, 2002. Draws from public, academic, government, and peer-reviewed research to provide a wide-ranging handbook for patients with encephalitis.

Sacks, Oliver. *Awakenings.* New York: Summit Books, 1987. An insightful and intriguing look into twenty case histories of patients suffering from postencephalitic symptoms. Traces the history of the first drug treatment of these patients and their reentry into "life."

Service, M. W., ed. *Encyclopedia of Arthropod-Transmitted Infections.* New York: Oxford University Press, 2001. Offers basic information related to the transmission, symptoms, treatment, and control of infections transmitted by biting midges, ticks, lice, and related organisms.

Sompayrac, Lauren. *How Pathogenic Viruses Work.* 5th ed. Sudbury, Mass.: Jones and Bartlett, 2002. Engaging exploration of the basics of virology. The author uses twelve of the most common viral infections to demonstrate how viruses "devise" various solutions to stay alive.

Strauss, James, and Ellen Strauss. *Viruses and Human Disease.* New York: Elsevier, 2001. An undergraduate text that examines virology from a human disease perspective.

ENDARTERECTOMY

PROCEDURE

ANATOMY OR SYSTEM AFFECTED: Blood vessels, circulatory system, neck

SPECIALTIES AND RELATED FIELDS: General surgery, vascular medicine

DEFINITION: A surgical procedure used to remove plaque from the lining of the carotid arteries in the neck.

INDICATIONS AND PROCEDURES

The internal carotid artery lies in the side of the neck, slightly in front of and beneath the sternocleidomastoid muscle. A skin incision is made anterior to this muscle. The branches of the carotid artery, adjacent blood vessels, and nerves are freed and inspected. A clamp is applied to the common carotid artery. Two additional clamps are applied to the external and internal carotid arteries to prevent bleeding and to prevent emboli from migrating to the brain during the procedure.

A lengthwise incision is made in the internal carotid artery from a point about 3.8 centimeters (1.5 inches) above the beginning of the vessel into the common carotid artery, about 2.5 centimeters (1 inch) below the beginning of the vessel. The edges of the artery are retracted, and the interior is exposed. The plaque can usually be scraped off the walls of the artery. The internal lining of the artery is carefully closed, and any tears are sutured. The carotid artery is then sewed together with fine suture material. If the underlying disease has been extensive or if the lining of the artery was damaged, a

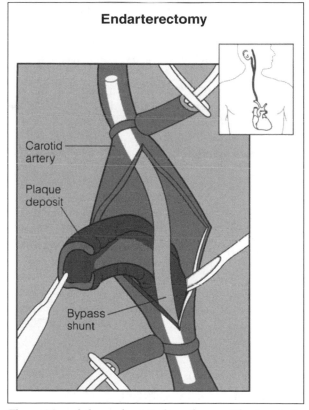

Endarterectomy

Carotid artery

Plaque deposit

Bypass shunt

The excision of plaque deposits from the carotid artery in the neck is called endarterectomy; the inset shows the location of the carotid artery.

portion of the saphenous vein in the patient's leg is used to repair the arterial wall.

Restoring blood flow is crucial; it is important to avoid both leaks in the artery and the formation of emboli. The clamp on the external carotid artery is briefly released, and a small amount of blood is allowed to flow back into the repaired area to check for leaks under low pressure. This clamp is reapplied. The clamp on the common carotid artery is removed to check for leaks under high pressure. The clamp to the external carotid artery is removed next. Blood is allowed to flow, flushing any emboli from the operative site and away from the brain. If all is well, the clamp on the internal carotid artery is removed.

The structures that were pulled away from the carotid artery are released and briefly inspected to ensure that no damage has been done. The edges of the skin are then brought together and closed with sutures. The patient returns in about a week for a checkup and removal of the sutures.

USES AND COMPLICATIONS

Endarterectomy is used to restore adequate blood flow to the brain, thus preventing periods of ischemia that can result in loss of consciousness. Complications include emboli, which cause strokes by blocking important blood vessels.

Endarterectomy is successful in most patients and restores more normal circulation. It has decreased the incidence of strokes in younger patients.

—*L. Fleming Fallon, Jr., M.D., Ph.D., M.P.H.*

See also Angioplasty; Arteriosclerosis; Bypass surgery; Circulation; Embolism; Strokes; Vascular medicine; Vascular system.

FOR FURTHER INFORMATION:

Ancowitz, Arthur. *Strokes and Their Prevention: How to Avoid High Blood Pressure and Hardening of the Arteries.* New York: Van Nostrand Reinhold, 1975.

Browse, Norman L., and A. O. Mansfield. *Carotid Endarterectomy: A Practical Guide.* Boston: Butterworth Heinemann, 2000.

Loftus, Christopher M., and Timothy F. Kresowik. *Carotid Artery Surgery.* New York: Thieme, 2000.

Rutherford, Robert B., ed. *Vascular Surgery.* 5th ed. Philadelphia: W. B. Saunders, 2000.

Wissler, R. W., and J. C. Geer, eds. *The Pathology of Atherosclerosis.* Baltimore: Williams & Wilkins, 1982.

ENDOCARDITIS
DISEASE/DISORDER

ANATOMY OR SYSTEM AFFECTED: Circulatory system, heart

SPECIALTIES AND RELATED FIELDS: Bacteriology, cardiology, internal medicine, vascular medicine

DEFINITION: Inflammatory lesions of the endocardium, the lining of the heart.

CAUSES AND SYMPTOMS

The lesions of endocarditis may be noninfective, as in rheumatic fever, or infective. The latter are characterized by direct invasion of the endocardium by microorganisms, most often bacteria. Bacterial endocarditis may occur on normal or previously damaged heart valves and also on artificial (prosthetic) heart valves. Rarely, endocarditis may occur on the wall (mural surface) of the heart or at the site of an abnormal hole between the pumping chambers of the heart, called a ventricular septal defect.

In areas of turbulent blood flow, platelet-fibrin deposition can occur, providing a nidus for subsequent bacterial colonization. Transient bacteremia may accompany infection elsewhere in the body or some medical and dental procedures, and these circulating bacteria can adhere to the endocardium, especially at platelet-fibrin deposition sites, and produce endocarditis. Intravenous drug abusers using unsterile equipment and drugs often inject bacteria along with the drugs, which can result in endocarditis. The lesions produced by these depositions plus bacteria are called vegetations. Clinical symptoms and signs usually begin about two weeks later.

Bacterial endocarditis usually involves either the mitral or the aortic heart valve. In intravenous drug abusers, the tricuspid heart valve is more commonly affected because it is the first valve to be reached by the endocardium-damaging drugs and contaminating bacteria. The pulmonic valve is only rarely the site of endocarditis. Occasionally, more than one heart valve

---

INFORMATION ON ENDOCARDITIS

CAUSES: Bacterial infection
SYMPTOMS: Fever, malaise, fatigue, dyspnea, chest pain, heart murmurs
DURATION: Temporary
TREATMENTS: Antibiotics

is infected; this occurs most often in intravenous drug abusers or patients with multiple prosthetic heart valves.

Gram-positive cocci are the most common cause of bacterial endocarditis. Different species predominate in various conditions or situations: *Streptococcus viridans* in native valves, *Staphylococcus aureus* in the valves of intravenous drug abusers, and *Staphylococcus epidermidis* in prosthetic heart valves. Gram-negative bacilli are found in association with prosthetic heart valves or intravenous drug addiction.

The clinical manifestations of endocarditis are varied and often nonspecific. Early symptoms are similar to those encountered in most infections: fever, malaise, and fatigue. As the disease progresses, more cardiovascular and renal-related symptoms may appear: dyspnea, chest pain, and stroke. Fever and heart murmurs are found in most patients. Enlargement of the spleen, skin lesions, and evidence of emboli are commonly present.

The key to the diagnosis of bacterial endocarditis is to suspect the presence of the illness and obtain blood cultures. Febrile patients who have a heart murmur, cardiac failure, a prosthetic heart valve, history of intravenous drug abuse, preexisting valvular disease, stroke (especially in young adults), multiple pulmonary emboli, sudden arterial occlusion, unexplained prolonged fever, or multiple positive blood cultures are likely to have endocarditis. The hallmark of bacterial endocarditis is continuous bacteremia; thus, nearly all blood cultures will be positive. Other nonspecific blood tests, such as an erythrocyte sedimentation rate, or specific blood tests, such as tests for teichoic acid antibodies, may be helpful in establishing a diagnosis.

TREATMENT AND THERAPY

Endocarditis may be prevented by administering prophylactic antibiotics to patients with preexisting heart abnormalities that predispose them to endocarditis when they are likely to have transient bacteremia. An example would be a patient with an artificial heart valve scheduled to have a dental cleaning.

Endocarditis is one of the few infections that is nearly always fatal if mistreated. Antibacterial therapy with agents capable of killing the offending bacteria, along with supportive medical care and cardiac surgery when indicated, cures most patients.

PERSPECTIVE AND PROSPECTS

The first demonstration of bacteria in vegetations associated with endocarditis was by Emmanuel Winge of

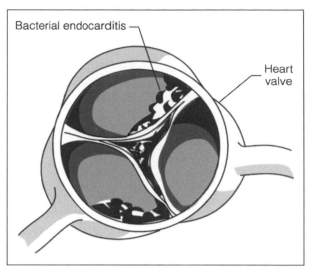

Bacterial endocarditis of a heart valve occurs when bacteria invade and cause inflammatory lesions; untreated, the condition is usually fatal.

Oslo, Norway, in 1869. Fifty years later, a fresh section was cut from the preserved heart valve described by Winge, and staining by modern methods revealed a chain of streptococci verifying his discovery. It was not until 1943, when Leo Loewe successfully treated seven cases of bacterial endocarditis with penicillin, that the era of modern therapy of this serious illness began.

Endocarditis accounts for approximately one case in every 1,000 hospital admissions in the United States. The incidence remained fairly constant between the 1960's and the 1990's, but the type of patient has changed: Heroin addicts, the elderly, and patients with prosthetic heart valves constitute an increasing percentage of endocarditis cases.

—*H. Bradford Hawley, M.D.*

See also Bacterial infections; Cardiology; Cardiology, pediatric; Circulation; Heart; Heart disease; Heart valve replacement; Mitral valve prolapse; Rheumatic fever; Vascular medicine; Vascular system.

FOR FURTHER INFORMATION:

American Heart Association. http://www.american heart.org/. A group dedicated to reducing disability and death from cardiovascular diseases and stroke. Offers thorough information on a wide range of cardiovascular diseases, referrals to emergency cardiovascular care classes, and research statistics and articles.

Crawford, Michael, ed. *Diagnosis and Treatment in Cardiology.* New York: McGraw-Hill, 2002. Discusses advances in cardiac diagnostics, treatments, and prognostic indicators and includes extensive information on prevention techniques.

Eagle, Kim A., and Ragavendra R. Baliga. *Practical Cardiology: Evaluation and Treatment of Common Cardiovascular Disorders*. Philadelphia: Lippincott Williams & Wilkins, 2003. Details advances in cardiac medicine.

Giessel, Barton E., Clint J. Koenig, Robert L. Blake, Jr. "Information from Your Family Doctor: Bacterial Endocarditis, A Heart at Risk." *American Family Physician* 61, no. 6 (March 15, 2000): 1705. This patient handout sheet contains information about bacterial endocarditis, an infection of the valves and inner lining of the heart. It includes information on prevention, complications, and treatment.

Kaye, Donald, ed. *Infective Endocarditis*. 2d ed. New York: Raven Press, 1992. An excellent text covering all the features of endocarditis in the modern era.

Magilligan, Donald J., Jr., and Edward L. Quinn, eds. *Endocarditis: Medical and Surgical Management*. New York: Marcel Dekker, 1986. Discusses the treatment of endocarditis and its complications.

Muirhead, Greg. "Targeting Therapy for Infective Endocarditis." *Patient Care* 33, no. 16 (October 15, 1999): 127-149. The diagnosis of infective endocarditis remains difficult, as does the treatment of this uncommon but potentially deadly disease. Discussed here are the better diagnostic criteria, developed in recent years, which allow for more effective therapy.

ENDOCRINE DISORDERS
DISEASE/DISORDER

ANATOMY OR SYSTEM AFFECTED: Endocrine system, glands

SPECIALTIES AND RELATED FIELDS: Endocrinology

DEFINITION: Breakdowns in the normal functioning of the endocrine system, which controls the metabolic processes of the body.

KEY TERMS:

cyclic AMP: a chemical that acts as a second messenger to bring about a response by the cell to the presence of some hormones at their receptors

endocrine: a secretion into the bloodstream rather than by way of a duct, such as hormones

feedback: the mechanism whereby a hormone inhibits its own production; often involves the inhibition of the hypothalamus and tropic hormones

hypothalamohypophysial: relating to the hypothalamus and the hypophysis (pituitary gland)

target cell or organ: a cell or organ possessing the specific hormone receptors needed to respond to a given hormone

tropic: hormones that feed a particular physiological state

tropin: hormones that cause a "turning toward" a particular physiological state

PROCESS AND EFFECTS

In order to understand endocrine disorders, it is necessary to review briefly the location of the principal endocrine glands, the hormones secreted, and the normal functions of the hormones. The hormones are released into the bloodstream and are carried throughout the body, where they affect target cells or organs that have receptors for the given hormone.

The pituitary gland, or hypophysis, is sometimes called the master gland because of its widespread influences on many other endocrine glands and the body as a whole. It is located in the midline on the lower part of the brain just above the posterior part of the roof of the mouth. The pituitary has three lobes: the posterior lobe, the intermediate lobe, and the anterior lobe.

The posterior lobe does not synthesize hormones, but it does have nerve fibers coming into it from the hypothalamus of the brain. The ends of these axons release two hormones that are synthesized in the hypothalamus, oxytocin and antidiuretic hormone (ADH). Oxytocin causes the contraction of the smooth muscles of the uterus during childbirth and the contraction of tissues in the mammary glands to release milk during nursing. ADH causes the kidneys to reabsorb water and thereby reduce the volume of urine to normal levels when necessary.

The intermediate lobe of the pituitary secretes melanocyte-stimulating hormone (MSH), a hormone with an uncertain role in humans but known to cause the darkening of melanocytes in animals. Sometimes, the intermediate lobe is considered to be a part of the anterior lobe.

The anterior lobe of the pituitary is under the control of releasing hormones produced by the hypothalamus and carried to the anterior lobe by special blood vessels. In response to these releasing hormones, some stimulatory and some inhibitory, the anterior lobe produces thyroid-stimulating hormone (TSH), adrenocorticotropic hormone (ACTH), follicle-stimulating hormone (FSH), luteinizing hormone (LH), prolactin, and somatotropin or growth hormone (GH). TSH stimulates the thyroid to produce thyroxine, ACTH stimulates the adrenal cortex to produce some of its hormones, FSH stimulates the growth of the cells surrounding eggs in the ovary and causes the ovary to produce estrogen, LH induces ovulation (the release of an egg from the ovary) and stimulates the secretion of progesterone by the ovary, prolactin is essential for milk production and various metabolic functions, and GH is needed for normal growth.

The pineal gland, or epiphysis, is a neuroendocrine gland attached to the roof of the diencephalon in the brain. It produces melatonin, which is released into the bloodstream during the night and has important functions related to an individual's biological clock.

The thyroid gland is located below the larynx in the front of the throat. It produces the hormones thyroxine (T_3) and triiodothyronine (T_4), which are essential for maintaining a normal level of metabolism and heat production, as well as enabling normal development of the brain in young children. C cells in the thyroid produce calcitonin, which is involved in blood calcium regulation. This is also true for parathyroid hormone, a product of the nearby parathyroid glands. The thymus, located under the breast bone or sternum, produces the hormone thymosin that stimulates the immune system. Even the heart is an endocrine gland: It produces atrial natriuretic factor, which stimulates sodium excretion by the kidneys. The pancreas, located near the stomach and small intestine, produces digestive enzymes that pass to the duodenum, but also it produces insulin and glucagon in special cells called pancreatic islets. Insulin causes blood sugar (glucose) to be taken up from the blood into the tissues of the body, and glucagon causes stored starch (glycogen) to be broken down in the liver and thereby increases blood glucose levels.

The pair of adrenal glands, located on the kidneys, are made up of two components: first, a cortex that produces glucocorticoids, mineralocorticoids, and sex steroids or androgens; and second, a medulla, or inner part, that secretes adrenaline and noradrenaline. The gonads, testes or ovaries, are located in the pelvic region and produce several hormones, including the estrogen and progesterone that are essential for reproduction in females and the testosterone that is essential for reproduction in males. The kidneys and digestive tract also produce hormones that regulate red blood cell formation and the functioning of the digestive tract, respectively.

COMPLICATIONS AND DISORDERS

A wide variety of endocrine disorders can be treated successfully. In fact, the ability to restore normal endocrine function with replacement therapy has long been one of the techniques for showing the existence of hypothesized hormones.

The posterior pituitary releases both oxytocin and ADH. Chemicals similar to oxytocin are sometimes given to induce contractions in pregnant women so that birth will occur at a predetermined time. The other hormone released from the posterior pituitary, ADH, normally causes the reabsorption of water within the tubules of the kidney. A deficiency of ADH leads to diabetes insipidus, a condition in which many liters of water a day are excreted by the urinary system; this necessitates that the patient drink huge quantities of water simply to stay alive. A synthetic form of ADH, desmopressin acetate, can be given in the form of a nasal spray that diffuses into the bloodstream and thus restores the reabsorption of water by the kidneys.

The anterior lobe of the pituitary produces six known hormones. The production of these hormones is stimulated and/or inhibited by special releasing hormones secreted by the hypothalamus and carried to the anterior lobe by the hypothalamohypophysial portal system of blood vessels. Thus, the source of some anterior pituitary disorders can reside in the hypothalamus. Tumors of anterior pituitary cells can result in the overproduction of a hormone, or if the tumor is destructive, the underproduction of a hormone. Radiation or surgery can be used to destroy tumors and thereby restore normal pituitary functioning.

Anterior pituitary hormones can be the basis of a variety of disorders. As with other hormones, there may be below-normal production of the hormone (hyposecretion) or overproduction of the hormone (hypersecretion). Because the pituitary hormones are often supportive of hormone secretion by the target organ or tissue, hyposecretion or hypersecretion of the tropic or

Glands of the Endocrine System

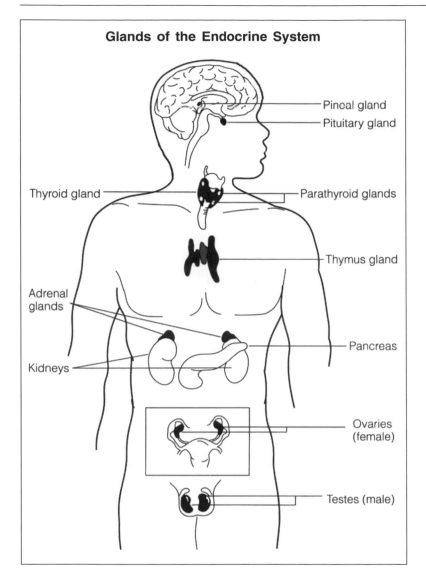

duce thyroxine causes high blood levels of TSH and an abnormal growth of the thyroid that results in a greatly enlarged thyroid, called a goiter. The addition of iodine to salt has eliminated the incidence of goiter in developed countries. Even with an adequate supply of iodine in the diet, however, hypothyroidism can still develop from other sources. The usual treatment is to ingest a dose of thyroxine daily.

Other examples of anterior pituitary disorders include those involving changes in GH secretion. Undersecretion of GH can lead to short stature or even dwarfism, in which an individual has normal body proportions but is smaller than normal. Now it is possible to obtain human GH from bacteria genetically engineered to produce it. Replacement GH can be given during the normal growth years to enhance growth. A tumor sometimes develops in the pituitary cells that produce GH, and this can cause abnormally increased growth or gigantism. If the tumor develops during the adult years, only a few areas of abnormal growth can occur, such as in the facial bones and the bones of the hands and feet. This condition is called acromegaly. Abraham Lincoln is thought to have had abnormal levels of GH that caused

supportive hormone leads to a similar change in the production of hormones by the target organ or tissue.

For example, hyperthyroidism, or Graves' disease, can be caused by excessive secretion of TSH by the pituitary, leading to hypersecretion of thyroxine, or by nodules within the thyroid that produce excessive thyroxine. In the diagnosis process, blood levels of both TSH and thyroxine are usually measured to determine the specific cause of the disorder. Similarly, hypothyroidism can be induced by deficits at several levels. The lack of iodine in the diet can prevent the production of thyroxine, which requires iodide as part of its molecular composition. The production of thyroxine usually has a negative feedback effect on the hypothalamus and pituitary, reducing TSH production. The failure to pro-

gigantism in his youth and then acromegaly in his later years. Acromegaly can be treated by radiation or surgery of the anterior pituitary.

Pineal gland tumors have been associated with precocious puberty, in which children become sexually developed in early childhood. It is thought that melatonin normally inhibits sexual development during this period. The pineal gland is influenced by changes in the daily photo-period, so that the highest levels of melatonin appear in the blood during the night, especially during the long nights of winter. Seasonal affective disorder (SAD), a mental depression that occurs during the late fall and winter, has been linked to seasonally high melatonin levels. Daily exposure to bright lights to mimic summer has been used to treat SAD. The pineal gland and melatonin are also being studied with regard to jet lag and disorders associated with shift work. The pineal gland thus seems to be involved in the functioning of the body's biological clock.

The pancreatic islets, also called the islets of Langerhans, produce insulin and glucagon. Diabetes mellitus is caused by insufficient insulin production (type 1 or juvenile-onset diabetes) or by the lack of functional insulin receptors on body cells (type 2 or maturity-onset diabetes). Type 1 diabetes can be treated with insulin injections, an implanted insulin pump, or even a transplant of fetal pancreatic tissue. Type 2 diabetes is treated with diet and weight loss. Weight loss induces an increase in insulin receptors. In addition to the symptoms of high blood sugar levels in the diabetic, long-term damage to the kidneys, blood vessels to the retina, and blood vessels in the legs and feet are important concerns.

The adrenal cortex produces glucocorticoids, mineralocorticoids, and androgens, any of which can be the basis of hyposecretion or hypersecretion. Addison's disease is caused by hyposecretion, whereas Cushing's syndrome is caused by hypersecretion or more-than-sufficient replacement therapy. Similar to those of the thyroid, the adrenal cortex secretions have a negative feedback on the hypothalamus and the anterior pituitary. Addison's disease is characterized by low blood pressure and a poor physiological response to stress. The high levels of ACTH—high because of inadequate feedback of corticoids on the hypothalamus and anterior pituitary—cause a bronzing of the skin because ACTH is similar in its molecular composition to MSH. During an adrenal crisis, exogenous adrenal corticoids are essential to avoid death. Corticoids can be given to prevent inflammation, but their overuse can lead to adrenal cortex suppression by the negative feedback mechanism. The abuse of androgens by athletes wanting to build up their muscles can also result in adrenal suppression, sterility, and damage to the heart. Tumors of androgen-producing cells in women can cause beard growth, increased muscle development, and other changes associated with sex hormones.

Perspective and Prospects

The early history of endocrinology noted that boys who were castrated failed to undergo the changes associated with puberty. A. A. Berthold in 1849 described the effects of castration in cockerels. The birds failed to develop large combs and waddles and failed to show male behavior. He noted that these effects could be reversed if testes were transplanted back into the cockerels. W. M. Bayliss and E. H. Starling in 1902 first introduced the term "hormone" to refer to secretin. They found that secretin is produced by the small intestine in response to acid in the chyme and that secretin causes the pancreas to release digestive enzymes into the small intestine. Most important, F. G. Banting and G. H. Best in 1922 reported their extraction of insulin from the pancreas of dogs and their success in alleviating diabetes in dogs by means of injections of the insulin. Fredrick Sanger in 1953 established the amino acid sequence for insulin and later won a Nobel Prize for this achievement.

Another Nobel Prize was awarded to Earl W. Sutherland, Jr., in 1971 for his demonstration in 1962 of the role of cyclic AMP as a second messenger in the sequence involved in the stimulation of cells by many hormones. Andrew V. Schally and Roger C. L. Guillemin in 1977 received a Nobel Prize for their work in isolating and determining the structures of hypothalamic regulatory peptides.

More recent achievements in endocrinological research have centered on the identification of receptors that bind with the hormone when the hormone stimulates a cell and on the genetic engineering of bacteria to produce hormones such as human growth hormone. The use of fetal tissues in endocrinological research and therapy—the host usually does not reject fetal implants—continues to be an area for future research.

—John T. Burns, Ph.D.

See also Addison's disease; Adrenalectomy; Amenorrhea; Corticosteroids; Cushing's syndrome; Diabetes mellitus; Dwarfism; Dysmenorrhea; Endocrinology; Endocrinology, pediatric; Endometriosis; Fructosemia; Gigantism; Glands; Goiter; Growth; Hashimoto's thyroiditis; Hormone replacement therapy (HRT); Hormones; Hyperparathyroidism and hypoparathyroidism; Hypoglycemia; Infertility in females; Infertility in males; Insulin resistance syndrome; Liver; Menopause; Menorrhagia; Ovarian cysts; Pancreas; Pancreatitis; Parathyroidectomy; Pregnancy and gestation; Prostate gland; Prostate gland removal; Puberty and adolescence; Steroids; Testicular surgery; Thyroid disorders; Thyroid gland; Thyroidectomy.

For Further Information:

Griffin, James E., and Sergio R. Ojeda, eds. *Textbook of Endocrine Physiology.* 4th ed. New York: Oxford University Press, 2000. A detailed account of normal and abnormal functioning of the endocrine system written by specialists. Intended for first year medical students.

Hadley, Mac E. *Endocrinology*. 5th ed. Englewood Cliffs, N.J.: Prentice Hall, 2000. A college-level text covering the endocrine system, primarily in humans and mammals. Recommended for a technical but understandable coverage of the field.

Henry, Helen L., and Anthony W. Norman, eds. *Encyclopedia of Hormones*. 3 vols. San Diego, Calif.: Academic Press, 2003. A comprehensive overview of the role of hormones, the major physiological systems in which they operate, and the biological consequences of an excess or deficiency of a particular hormone.

Martini, Frederic. *Fundamentals of Anatomy and Physiology*. 5th ed. Englewood Cliffs, N.J.: Prentice Hall, 2001. A good place to start for a solid overview of the anatomy and physiology of the endocrine system before considering the details of disease states.

Scanlon, Valerie, et al. *Essentials of Anatomy and Physiology*. 4th ed. Philadelphia: F. A. Davis, 2002. A text designed around three themes: the relationship between physiology and anatomy, the interrelations among the organ systems, and the relationship of each organ system to homeostasis.

Shaw, Michael, ed. *Everything You Need to Know About Diseases*. Springhouse, Pa.: Springhouse Press, 1996. This well-illustrated consumer reference, compiled by more than one hundred doctors and medical experts, describes five hundred illnesses and conditions, their causes, symptoms, diagnosis, treatment, and prevention. Of particular interest is chapter 12, "Hormone and Gland Disorders."

Wilson, Jean D. *Wilson's Textbook of Endocrinology*. 10th ed. New York: Elsevier, 2003. Text that covers the spectrum of information related to the endocrine system, including thyroid disorders, diabetes, endocrinology and aging, female reproduction and fertility control, sexual function and dysfunction, kidney stones, and endocrine hypertension.

ENDOCRINOLOGY
SPECIALTY

ANATOMY OR SYSTEM AFFECTED: Brain, endocrine system, glands, immune system, nervous system, pancreas, psychic-emotional system, reproductive system, uterus

SPECIALTIES AND RELATED FIELDS: Biochemistry, genetics, gynecology, immunology

DEFINITION: The science dealing with how the internal secretions from ductless glands in the body act both in normal physiology and in disease states.

KEY TERMS:

adrenal gland: an endocrine gland situated immediately above the upper pole of each kidney; it consists of an inner part or medulla, which produces epinephrine and norepinephrine, and an outer part or cortex, which produces steroid hormones

endocrine pancreas: specialized secretory tissue dispersed within the pancreas called islets of Langerhans, which are responsible for the secretion of glucagon and insulin

hypothalamus: the region of the brain called the diencephalon, forming the floor of the third ventricle, including neighboring associated nuclei

metabolism: the process of tissue change, which may be synthetic (anabolic) or degradative (catabolic)

parathyroid gland: one of four small endocrine glands situated underneath the thyroid gland, whose main product is parathyroid hormone, which is responsible for the regulation of serum calcium levels

pituitary gland: a small (0.5-gram), two-lobed endocrine gland that is attached by a stalk to the brain at the level of the hypothalamus

thyroid gland: a 20-gram endocrine gland that sits in front of the trachea and consists of two lateral lobes connected in the middle by an isthmus

SCIENCE AND PROFESSION

The rates of metabolic pathways in the body are controlled mainly by the endocrine system, in conjunction with the nervous system. These two systems are integrated in the neuroendocrine system, which controls the secretion of hormones by the endocrine glands. The study of endocrinology deals with the normal physiology and pathophysiology of endocrine glands. The endocrine glands that are typically the main focus of clinical endocrinologists are the hypothalamus, pituitary gland, thyroid, parathyroid, adrenal glands, endocrine pancreas, ovaries, and testes. The endocrine system regulates virtually all activities of the body, including growth and development, homeostasis, energy production, and reproduction.

The hypothalamus is a highly specialized endocrine organ that sits at the base of the brain and that functions as the master gland of the endocrine system. It is the main integrator for the endocrine and nervous systems. The hypothalamus produces a number of chemical mediators which have direct control over the pituitary gland. These chemicals are made in the cells of the hypothalamus and reach the pituitary gland, which sits just below it, by a special hypophyseoportal blood system. In adult humans, the pituitary is divided into two lobes: the anterior lobe (adenohypophysis) and the posterior lobe (neural lobe).

Vasopressin and oxytocin are the two main hormones that are made in the hypothalamus but stored in the posterior lobe of the pituitary for release when needed. Vasopressin (also known as antidiuretic hormone, or ADH) is a hormone that maintains a normal water concentration in the blood and is a regulator of circulating blood volume. Oxytocin is a hormone that is involved in lactation and obstetrical labor.

The hypothalamic-pituitary-thyroid axis is important in the control of basal metabolic rate. There are a number of releasing hormones secreted from the hypothalamus that control the release of anterior pituitary hormones, which then cause the release of hormone at the end organ. Most of these hormones have the chemical structures of peptides. Thyrotropin-releasing hormone (TRH) was the first hypothalamic releasing hormone that was synthesized and used clinically. TRH, secreted in nanogram quantities, is a cyclic tripeptide that causes release of thyrotropin-stimulating hormone (TSH) from the thyrotropic cells of the anterior pituitary gland. The release of TSH is in microgram quantities and leads to an increase in thyroid hormone release by the thyroid gland. The amount of thyroid hormone synthesized is on the order of milligrams. Therefore, the secretion of minute amounts of the TRH allows for the production of thyroid hormone that is a millionfold greater than the amount of TRH itself. This is an example of an amplifying cascade, a system by which the central nervous system can control all metabolic processes with the secretion of very small amounts of hypothalamic releasing hormones. This intricate system possesses controls to stop the production of too much hormone as well. Such negative feedback is an important concept in endocrinology. In the case of the thyroid, an increased amount of thyroid hormone produced by the thyroid gland will cause the pituitary and hypothalamus to decrease the amounts that they produce of TSH and TRH, respectively. Many hormones are subject to the laws of negative feedback control. TRH also causes potent release of the anterior pituitary hormone called prolactin. Thyroid hormone is important in determining basal metabolism and is needed for proper development in the newborn child. The thyroid gland produces

both thyroxine (T_4, also called tetraiodothyronine) and triiodothyronine (T_3), both of which it synthesizes from iodine and the amino acid tyrosine.

The hypothalamic-pituitary-adrenal axis is critical in the reaction to stress, both physical and emotional. Corticotropin-releasing hormone (CRH) is a polypeptide, consisting of forty-one amino acids, that causes the production of the proopiomelanocortin molecule by the corticotropic cells of the anterior pituitary. The proopiomelanocortin molecule is cleaved by proteolytic enzymes to yield adrenocorticotropic hormone (ACTH, also called corticotropin), melanocyte-stimulating hormone, and lipotropin. It is ACTH made by the anterior pituitary which then stimulates the adrenal cortex to produce steroid hormones. The main stress hormone produced by the adrenal cortex in response to ACTH is the glucocorticoid cortisol. ACTH also has some control over the production of the mineralocorticoid aldosterone and the androgens dehydroepiandrosterone and testosterone. These steroids are synthesized from cholesterol. The production of cortisol (also known as hydrocortisone) is subject to negative feedback by CRH and ACTH.

The hypothalamic-pituitary-gonadal axis is involved in the control of reproduction. Gonadotropin-releasing hormone (GnRH), also known as luteinizing hormone-releasing hormone (LHRH), is produced by the hypothalamus and stimulates the release of luteinizing hormone (LH) and follicle-stimulating hormone (FSH) from the gonadotrophic cells of the anterior pituitary. LH and FSH have different effects in men and women. In men, LH controls the production and secretion of testosterone by the Leydig's cells of the testes. The release of LH is regulated by negative feedback from testosterone. FSH along with testosterone acts on the Sertoli cells of the seminiferous tubule of the testis at the time of puberty to start sperm production. In women, LH controls ovulation by the ovary and also the development of the corpus luteum, which produces progesterone. Progesterone is a steroid hormone that is critically important for the maintenance of pregnancy. FSH in women stimulates the development and maturation of a primary follicle and oocyte. The ovarian follicle in the nonpregnant woman is the main site of production of estradiol. Estradiol is the principal estrogen made in the reproductive years by the ovary and is responsible for the development of female secondary sexual characteristics.

Growth hormone-releasing hormone (GHRH) is a polypeptide with forty-four amino acids that stimulates the release of growth hormone (GH) from the somatotrophic cells of the anterior pituitary. The regulation of GH secretion is under dual control. While GHRH positively releases GH, somatostatin (a polypeptide with fourteen amino acids, also released from the hypothalamus) inhibits the release of GH. Somatostatin has a wide variety of functions, including the suppression of insulin, glucagon, and gastrointestinal hormones. GH released from the pituitary circulates in the bloodstream and stimulates the production of somatomedins by the liver. Several somatomedins are produced, all of which have a profound effect on growth, with the most important one in humans being somatomedin C, also called insulin-like growth factor I (IGF I). Molecular biological techniques have shown that many cells outside the liver also produce IGF I; in these cells, IGF I acts in autocrine or paracrine ways to cause the growth of the cells or to affect neighboring cells.

Prolactin is a peptide hormone that is secreted by the lactotrophs of the anterior pituitary. It is involved in the differentiation of the mammary gland cells and initiates the production of milk proteins and other constituents. Prolactin may also have other functions, as a stress hormone or growth hormone. Prolactin is under tonic negative control. The inhibition of prolactin release is caused by dopamine, which is produced by the hypothalamus. Thus, while dopamine is normally considered to be a neurotransmitter, in the case of prolactin release it acts as an inhibitory hormone. Serotonin, also classically thought of as a neurotransmitter, may cause the stimulation of prolactin release from the anterior pituitary.

DIAGNOSTIC AND TREATMENT TECHNIQUES

One of the most common medical problems seen by specialists in the field of endocrinology is a patient with type I diabetes mellitus, sometimes also called juvenile-onset or insulin-dependent diabetes mellitus. "Insulin-dependent" is probably more appropriate, as not all patients with type I diabetes mellitus develop the disease in childhood. Type I diabetes is an autoimmune disease in which antibodies to different parts of the pancreatic beta cell, the cell that normally produces insulin, are produced. Some of these antibodies are cytotoxic; that is, they actually destroy the pancreatic beta cell. The most striking characteristic of patients with type I diabetes is that they produce very little insulin. The symptoms of type I diabetes include increased thirst, increased urination, blurring of vision, and weight loss. A doctor would confirm the diagnosis by running blood tests for glucose and insulin. The glucose level would be high, and the insulin level would be low. The treatment includes controlled diet, exercise, insulin therapy, and self-monitoring of blood glucose. With proper control of blood glucose, patients with type I diabetes can lead normal, productive lives.

Graves' disease is another autoimmune disease that is commonly seen by endocrinologists. Graves' disease is caused by the production of thyroid-stimulating immunoglobulin antibodies that bind to and activate TSH receptors. As a result, the thyroid gland produces too much thyroid hormone and the thyroid gland enlarges in size. The antibodies also commonly affect the eyes, causing a characteristic bulging. The clinical symptoms of hyperthyroidism include increased heart rate, anxiety, heat sensitivity, sleeplessness, diarrhea, and abdominal pain. Patients often lose considerable weight, despite having a great appetite and eating large amounts of food. Sometimes, the diagnosis is missed, leading to an extensive evaluation for a variety of other diseases. Often, a family history of thyroid disease or other endocrine disease can be found.

The usual method of screening for Graves' disease is with a simple blood test for thyroid function, which includes testing for T_4, T_3, and TSH. In patients with Graves' disease, both T_4 and T_3 will be elevated, and TSH will be very low. If the blood test reveals this pattern, the next usual step is to proceed to a radioactive iodine uptake and scan test, which involves giving a very small amount of radioactive iodine by mouth and having the patient return twenty-four hours later for a scan. The thyroid gland normally accumulates iodine and thus will accumulate the radioactive iodine as well. The radioactive iodine emits a gamma-ray energy that can be picked up by a solid-crystal scintillation counter placed over the thyroid gland. With this device, one can determine the percentage of iodine uptake and also obtain a picture of the thyroid gland. The normal radioactive iodine uptake is about 10 to 30 percent of the dose, depending somewhat on the amount of total body iodine, which is derived from the diet. Patients with Graves' disease will have high radioactive iodine uptakes.

Those who suffer from Graves' disease can be treated by three different means, depending on the circumstances. The first treatment that is often tried is antithyroid drugs, either propylthiouracil or methimazole. These drugs belong to the class of sulfonamides and inhibit the production of new thyroid hormone by blocking the attachment of iodine to the amino acid tyrosine. Another mode of therapy is the use of radioactive iodine. A dose of radioactive iodine (on the order of 5 to 10 millicuries) is used to destroy part of the thyroid gland. The gamma-ray energy emitted from the iodine molecule that has traveled to the thyroid gland is enough to kill some thyroid cells. An alternative way to destroy the thyroid gland is to remove it surgically (thyroidectomy). Endocrinologists rarely send patients for surgery, as the other therapies are often effective. The goal of all treatments is to bring the level of thyroid hormone into the normal range, as well as to shrink the thyroid gland. After treatment, the patient's level of thyroid hormone sometimes falls to levels that are below normal. The symptoms of hypothyroidism are the opposite of hyperthyroidism and include fatigue, weight gain, cold sensitivity, constipation, and dry skin. If this happens, the patient is treated with thyroid hormone replacement. The dose is adjusted for each individual to produce normal levels of T_4, T_3, and TSH.

A less common but important endocrine disorder is the existence of a pituitary tumor that secretes prolactin, called a prolactinoma. Prolactinomas are diagnosed earlier in women than in men, as women with the disorder often complain of a lack of menstrual periods and spontaneous milk production from the breasts, known as galactorrhea. These tumors, which can be quite small, are called microadenomas because they are less than 10 millimeters in size. They can affect men as well, causing decreased sex drive and impotence. Macroadenomas are tumors greater than 10 millimeters in size. When the tumors increase in size, they can cause symptoms such as headache and decreased vision. It is important to note that most microadenomas never progress to macroadenomas. Vision loss and/or decreased eye movement can be seen with a macroadenoma and are reason for immediate treatment.

Doctors screen patients for a prolactinoma by running a blood test for prolactin. There are other reasons for mild elevations in prolactin levels, including the use of certain psychiatric drugs such as phenothiazines or the antihypertensive drugs reserpine and methyldopa, primary hypothyroidism, cirrhosis, and chronic renal failure. If a pituitary tumor is suspected, then other biochemical tests of pituitary function are conducted to determine if the rest of the gland is functioning normally. At that time, imaging tests are often done to get a picture of the hypothalamic-pituitary area; this can be done with either computed tomography (CT) scanning or magnetic resonance imaging (MRI). Patients with macroadenomas will require treatment. In patients with little neurological involvement, medical therapy may be initiated. Bromocriptine, a semisynthetic ergot alkaloid which is an inhibitor of prolactin secretion, may be used. It has been shown that patients treated with this drug have reduction in tumor size. Patients can be maintained on the drug indefinitely because prolactin levels return to pretreatment levels when the drug is stopped. If there is severe neurologic involvement, with loss of vision and other eye problems, immediate surgery may be indicated. There is a very high incidence of tumor recurrence after surgery, requiring medical and/or radiation therapy.

PERSPECTIVE AND PROSPECTS

The field of endocrinology is a continuously evolving one. Advances in biomedical technology, including molecular biology and cell biology, have made it a demanding job for the clinician to keep up with all the breakthroughs in the field. The challenge for endocrinology will be to apply many of these new technologies to novel treatments for patients with endocrine diseases.

An example of the progression of the field of endocrinology can be seen in the history of pituitary diseases. The start of pituitary endocrinology is ascribed to Pierre Marie, the French neurologist who in 1886 first described pituitary enlargement in a patient with acromegaly (enlargement of the skull, jaw, hands, and feet) and linked the disease to a pituitary abnormality. During the first half of the twentieth century, many of the hypothalamic and pituitary hormones were isolated and characterized. The field of endocrinology was revolutionized by the development of the radioimmunoassay, which allows sensitive and specific measurements of hormones. The radioimmunoassay replaced bioassay techniques, which were laborious, time-consuming, and not always precise. This technique has allowed for rapid measurement of hormones and improved screening for endocrine diseases involving hormone deficiency or hormone excess.

The development of new hormone assays has been complemented by the development of noninvasive imaging techniques. Before the advent of CT scanning in the late 1970's, it was an ordeal to diagnose a pituitary tumor. Pneumoencephalography was often performed, which involved injecting air into the fluid-containing structures of the brain, with associated risk and discomfort to the patient. In the 1980's, with new generations of high-resolution CT scanners that were more sensitive than early scanners, smaller pituitary lesions could be detected and diagnosed. That decade also ushered in the use of MRI to diagnose disorders of the hypothalamic-pituitary unit. MRI has allowed doctors to evaluate the hypothalamus, pituitary, and nearby structures very precisely; it has become the method of choice for evaluating patients with pituitary disease. MRI can easily visualize the optic chiasm in the forebrain and the vascular structures surrounding the pituitary.

In patients who require surgery, advances have helped decrease mortality rates. Harvey Cushing pioneered the transsphenoidal technique in 1927 but abandoned it in favor of the transfrontal approach. This involves reaching the pituitary tumor by retracting the frontal lobes to visualize the pituitary gland sitting underneath. The modern era of transsphenoidal pituitary surgery was developed by Gérard Guiot and Jules Hardy in the late 1960's. Transsphenoidal surgery done with an operating microscope to visualize the pituitary contents allows for selective removal of the tumor, leaving the normal pituitary gland intact. The advantage of this approach from below, instead of from above, includes minimal movement of the brain and less blood loss. This technique requires a neurosurgeon with much skill and experience. There are also new drug treatments for patients with pituitary diseases, such as bromocriptine for use in patients with prolactinomas and octreotide (a somatostatin analogue) to lower growth hormone levels in patients with acromegaly.

—*RoseMarie Pasmantier, M.D.*

See also Addison's disease; Adrenalectomy; Chronobiology; Corticosteroids; Cushing's syndrome; Diabetes mellitus; Dwarfism; Endocrine disorders; Endocrinology, pediatric; Enzymes; Fructosemia; Gestational diabetes; Gigantism; Glands; Goiter; Growth; Gynecology; Hair loss and baldness; Hashimoto's thyroiditis; Hormone replacement therapy (HRT); Hormones; Hot flashes; Hyperparathyroidism and hypoparathyroidism; Hypoglycemia; Hysterectomy; Melatonin; Menopause; Menstruation; Obesity; Paget's disease; Pancreas; Pancreatitis; Parathyroidectomy; Pharmacology; Pharmacy; Prostate gland; Prostate gland removal; Puberty and adolescence; Sex change surgery; Sexual differentiation; Steroids; Thyroid disorders; Thyroid gland; Thyroidectomy; Weight loss and gain.

FOR FURTHER INFORMATION:

Braverman, Lewis E., and Robert D. Utiger, eds. *Werner and Ingbar's The Thyroid: A Fundamental and Clinical Text.* 8th ed. Philadelphia: J. B. Lippincott, 2000. An exhaustive textbook on all aspects of the thyroid, including history, anatomy, biology, pathology, basic and clinical research, and the thyroid in development and pregnancy.

Brooks, S. J., and Robert S. Bar. *Early Diagnosis and Treatment of Endocrine Disorders.* Totowa, N.J.: Humana Press, 2003. Reviews the early signs and symptoms of common endocrine diseases, surveys the clinical testing needed for a diagnosis, and presents recommendations for therapy.

Davidson, Mayer B. *Diabetes Mellitus.* 4th ed. Philadelphia: W. B. Saunders, 1998. A very good, practical approach to the overall management of the endocrine patient with diabetes mellitus.

Imura, Hiroo, ed. *The Pituitary Gland.* 2d ed. New York: Raven Press, 1994. Good discussion of the master gland, the hypothalamic-pituitary unit.

Lebovitz, Harold E., ed. *Therapy of Diabetes Mellitus and Related Disorders.* 3d ed. Alexandria, Va.: American Diabetes Association, 1998. A comprehensive treatise on the treatment of various aspects of diabetes mellitus. The different chapters are written by experts in the field.

Speroff, Leon, Robert H. Glass, and Nathan G. Kase, eds. *Clinical Gynecologic Endocrinology and Infertility.* 6th ed. Baltimore: Williams & Wilkins, 1999. An excellent textbook which brings together all aspects of endocrinology in women from embryology to old age. Good discussion of the problems seen in infertile couples.

Wilson, Jean D. *Wilson's Textbook of Endocrinology.* 10th ed. New York: Elsevier, 2003. Text that covers the spectrum of information related to the endocrine system, including thyroid disorders, diabetes, endocrinology and aging, female reproduction and fertility control, sexual function and dysfunction, kidney stones, and endocrine hypertension.

ENDOCRINOLOGY, PEDIATRIC
SPECIALTY

ANATOMY OR SYSTEM AFFECTED: Brain, endocrine system, glands, immune system, nervous system, pancreas, psychic-emotional system

SPECIALTIES AND RELATED FIELDS: Biochemistry, genetics, immunology, neonatology, pediatrics

DEFINITION: The study of the normal and abnormal function of the endocrine (ductless) glands in children and adolescents.

KEY TERMS:

hormone: a chemical molecule produced in either the hypothalamus or one of the endocrine glands that is secreted and travels (usually via the bloodstream) to a target organ or to specific receptor cells, causing a specific response

hypothalamus: a very small portion of the base of the brain, immediately adjacent to the pituitary gland

insulin: a hormone that is essential in regulating blood glucose, as well as in assimilating carbohydrates for growth and energy

pancreas: a large gland near the stomach which has both exocrine and endocrine functions and which produces insulin

pituitary gland: a very small gland at the base of the brain that is referred to as the master gland; with the hypothalamus, it regulates most of the endocrine systems

thyroid: a gland in the anterior neck which regulates the level of the body's metabolism and which is instrumental in normal physical and mental growth

SCIENCE AND PROFESSION

Pediatric endocrinology is a major subspecialty, limited to children and adolescents, which involves the study of normal as well as abnormal functions of the endocrine system, which comprises the glands of internal or ductless secretions. These practitioners, referred to as endocrinologists or pediatric endocrinologists, are doctors of medicine or osteopathy who have completed three years of pediatric residency training and an additional two to three years of fellowship training in endocrinology.

Endocrinology is one of the most interesting and challenging fields in pediatrics because it requires a blend of basic science and technology in the clinical setting. Some of the diagnoses are very difficult, yet they are almost always completely logical. Endocrinology is tightly related to other areas of pediatrics, such as adolescent medicine, genetics, growth, development, nutrition, and metabolism. These relationships make this field even more complex and intellectually stimulating.

Pediatric endocrinology and adult endocrinology are relatively young fields, probably beginning with the discovery in 1888 that "myxedema" (hypothyroidism) could be improved by feeding the patient thyroid extract. Both fields deal with the major endocrine glands and their disorders, such as diabetes mellitus or hypothyroidism, but there are several key differences, most related to growth (both physical and mental), potential, and genetics. Some major areas of specific emphasis in pediatric endocrinology include diabetes mellitus (which presents very differently in children), disorders of growth, disorders of sexual maturation and differentiation, genetic disorders, and adolescent medicine.

DIAGNOSTIC AND TREATMENT TECHNIQUES

In pediatric endocrinology, as in all medical fields, history taking and physical examination are the starting points and usually the most useful tools for diagnosis. Endocrinology is a specialty that is particularly aided by science. Blood and urine chemistries, hormone assays, chromosomal analyses, X rays, computed tomography (CT) scans, magnetic resonance imaging (MRI), and a host of other sophisticated tests have advanced diagnosis and treatment and have made this specialty one of the favorites for physicians who like science. Virtually all the known hormones can be assayed accurately and quickly.

Since insulin was first available for injection in 1922, there have been amazing advances in treatment. Many of the treatments in endocrinology involve hormone therapy. In 1985, recombinant growth hormone was synthesized for the first time. This development has allowed endocrinologists to treat not only pituitary dwarfism but also other kinds of growth deficiencies, such as Turner syndrome.

Turner syndrome is a relatively common chromosomal abnormality affecting females and resulting in short stature and lack of sexual development. While these girls will never become fertile, the combination of growth hormone for stature and other hormonal therapy for the development of secondary sexual characteristics enables them to have a normal female body. Studies have shown that normal body image and the presence of menstruation is essential for the self-esteem of these patients.

Diabetes mellitus is the most common significant endocrine disorder in both adults and children. What was commonly referred to as juvenile diabetes years ago is now called diabetes mellitus, type I. Unlike type II, which usually presents insidiously in middle-aged and older adults, type I presents rapidly, and the patient will need daily injectable insulin treatments. Diabetes in children is complex to manage not only because of the insulin treatment but also because of the patients' growth, metabolism, fluctuating activity levels, and the physiologic and psychological changes that occur, especially in adolescence.

Now small portable and quite accurate glucometers allow patients to measure blood glucose (sugar) at home, making diabetes management much simpler.

Tighter control of blood glucose will decrease or delay the onset of long-term complications of the disease, such as blindness, heart disease, and kidney disease. In the United States, newborn screening, which is now performed in all fifty states, has virtually eliminated cretinism, which tragically resulted when congenital hypothyroidism was not diagnosed until later in childhood. These children were irreversibly mentally retarded.

Enhanced techniques in pediatric surgery and neurosurgery, greatly aided by scans, play a role in the treatment of some endocrine disorders. Very small tumors and masses can be identified and often removed successfully. Often, endocrinologists and oncologists work together in concert with the surgeon.

Although this subspecialty is one of the most scientific and laboratory-based in pediatrics, it is also a field where emotional support, counseling, and often mental health care is given. Children do not like being "different," and body image is very important in children and particularly in teenagers. Even when a child appears absolutely normal, the frustration of ongoing monitoring and treatment is resented and can result in rebellion, especially in children with diabetes. Often, a team approach is needed, which involves professionals, teachers, family, and peers.

PERSPECTIVE AND PROSPECTS

The future promises ever-advancing and dramatic tools for the diagnosis and treatment of endocrine disorders, as well as for their prevention. On the immediate horizon, an implantible glucose pump, which can serve as a substitute pancreas, can change the lives of diabetic patients dramatically. A method for rapidly analyzing blood glucose using the surface of the skin has been developed. In addition, genetic engineering may revolutionize the approaches to treating many of these diseases.

—*C. Mervyn Rasmussen, M.D.*

See also Addison's disease; Adrenalectomy; Chronobiology; Corticosteroids; Diabetes mellitus; Dwarfism; Endocrine disorders; Endocrinology; Enzymes; Fructosemia; Gigantism; Glands; Growth; Gynecology; Hormone replacement therapy (HRT); Hormones; Hyperparathyroidism and hypoparathyroidism; Hypoglycemia; Melatonin; Menstruation; Obesity; Pancreas; Pancreatitis; Parathyroidectomy; Pediatrics; Pharmacology; Pharmacy; Puberty and adolescence; Steroids; Thyroid disorders; Thyroid gland; Thyroidectomy; Weight loss and gain.

FOR FURTHER INFORMATION:

Brooks, S. J., and Robert S. Bar. *Early Diagnosis and Treatment of Endocrine Disorders*. Totowa, N.J.: Humana Press, 2003. Reviews the early signs and symptoms of common endocrine diseases, surveys the clinical testing needed for a diagnosis, and presents recommendations for therapy.

Handwerger, Stuart. *Molecular and Cellular Pediatric Endocrinology*. Totowa, N.J.: Humana Press, 1999. The chapters in this book reflect the genetic and molecular bases of many of the fundamental problems of differentiation and growth in a manner appropriate for a pediatrics textbook.

Little, Marjorie. *Diabetes*. New York: Chelsea House, 1991. A clearly written overview directed toward a nonspecialized audience. Includes a fourteen-page chapter on type I (juvenile) diabetes.

Sperling, Mark A., ed. *Pediatric Endocrinology*. 2d ed. Philadelphia: W. B. Saunders, 2002. Discusses endocrine diseases in infancy and childhood. Includes a bibliography and an index.

Wales, Jerry, and Jan Maarten Wit. *Pediatric Endocrinology and Growth*. Philadelphia: W. B. Saunders, 2003. An illustrated text that outlines specific endocrine problems, from growth disorders to glucose homeostasis, early or late sexual development, abnormal genitalia, goiter, failure to thrive, and obesity.

Wilson, Jean D. *Wilson's Textbook of Endocrinology*. 10th ed. New York: Elsevier, 2003. Text that covers the spectrum of information related to the endocrine system, including thyroid disorders, diabetes, endocrinology and aging, female reproduction and fertility control, sexual function and dysfunction, kidney stones, and endocrine hypertension.

ENDODONTIC DISEASE
DISEASE/DISORDER

ANATOMY OR SYSTEM AFFECTED: Mouth, teeth
SPECIALTIES AND RELATED FIELDS: Dentistry
DEFINITION: Disease of the dental pulp and sometimes also the soft tissues and bone around the tip of the root.

CAUSES AND SYMPTOMS

The most common cause of endodontic disease is infection of the dental pulp by the bacteria that cause tooth decay. The pulp is composed of connective tissue, nerves, blood vessels, and tooth regenerative cells. It fills the root canal, a narrow channel in the center of the

INFORMATION ON ENDODONTIC DISEASE

CAUSES: Bacterial infection of dental pulp
SYMPTOMS: Gum inflammation and pain, which is severe if abscess forms
DURATION: Chronic if untreated
TREATMENTS: Root canal treatment

tooth root, which is embedded in the jawbone. Teeth usually contain one to four root canals. Decay-causing bacteria reach the pulp after dissolving their way through the two, hard outer layers of the tooth—the enamel and dentin. Bacteria may also reach the pulp through a crack or facture in a tooth and through tooth wear or abrasion. Many kinds of bacteria can infect the pulp.

Pulp infected by bacteria becomes inflamed and has no place to swell because it is surrounded by dentin, which is rigid. Pain may result. Eventually, the entire pulp may become infected and die. If not treated, the infection can spread to the soft tissue and bone surrounding the tip of the root and form an abscess, which often produces severe pain.

TREATMENT AND THERAPY

To treat damaged or dead pulp tissue and preserve the tooth, endodontic therapy, or root canal treatment, is required. Endodontists specialize in this procedure. One or two visits are usually required. A small hole is made in the top (crown) of the infected tooth, and all the pulp tissue is removed. Then an inert material, usually a piece of rubberlike gum called gutta percha, is inserted in place of the pulp and secured in place with a sealer or cement. A tooth that has had root canal treatment is commonly considered to be dead, but the fibers of the periodontal ligament that hold the tooth in the jawbone are still alive. Following this procedure, additional dental treatments are necessary to preserve the weakened tooth.

PERSPECTIVE AND PROSPECTS

Historically, the only remedy for endodontic disease was tooth extraction. Since the mid-twentieth century, endodontic research has yielded treatments that preserve infected teeth. Furthermore, there has been an increased appreciation of the role of dental hygiene in preventing tooth decay and the endodontic infections that can result from it. Research on the causes and prevention of endodontic disease, and treatments for it, is being conducted at dental schools and at the National Institute of Dental and Cranio-Facial Research.

—Jane F. Hill, Ph.D.

See also Cavities; Dental diseases; Dentistry; Gingivitis; Gum disease; Periodontal surgery; Periodontitis; Root canal treatment; Teeth; Tooth extraction; Toothache.

FOR FURTHER INFORMATION:

Beers, Mark, ed. *The Merck Manual of Medical Information.* 2d ed. Rahway, N.J.: Merck Research Laboratories, 2003.

Christensen, Gordon J. *A Consumer's Guide to Dentistry.* 2d ed. St. Louis: Mosby, 2002.

Smith, Rebecca W., and the Columbia University School of Dental and Oral Surgery. *The Columbia University School of Dental and Oral Surgery's Guide to Family Dental Care.* New York: W. W. Norton, 1997.

ENDOMETRIAL BIOPSY

PROCEDURE

ANATOMY OR SYSTEM AFFECTED: Genitals, reproductive system, uterus
SPECIALTIES AND RELATED FIELDS: General surgery, gynecology
DEFINITION: A procedure designed to obtain a sample of the uterine lining (endometrium) for diagnostic analysis.

INDICATIONS AND PROCEDURES

Endometrial biopsy is a diagnostic procedure used to assess such medical disorders as female infertility and abnormal vaginal bleeding. It is an outpatient procedure performed with local anesthesia, and it takes only thirty seconds. A small plastic cylinder is placed into the uterus through the cervix. A suction device or metal scraping instrument in the cylinder removes a small sample of the endometrium. The sample is sent to a laboratory for microscopic analysis.

USES AND COMPLICATIONS

If infertility testing reveals no obvious physical problems or abnormalities in sperm number and viability of a couple, further procedures are conducted, including an endometrial biopsy. The quality of the uterine lining is distinctly different while under the influence of estrogen, just prior to ovulation, as compared to its quality while progesterone is being produced after ovulation. Endometrial tissue analysis can reveal if the woman is not ovulating or is producing inadequate progesterone to support a pregnancy after ovulation. This procedure can be performed between a week after ovulation to the first day of the woman's menstrual period.

If the cause of infertility is a lack of ovulation, a variety of drug and hormone therapies are available to induce ovulation. Inadequacies in maintaining the uterine lining after ovulation may be treated with natural progesterone or other medications.

Bleeding between menstrual periods or a heavy increase in menstrual flow may be indicative of a host of conditions. In some cases, an endometrial biopsy may be performed to analyze the uterine lining for abnormal cell growth that may be indicative of cancer or such conditions as uterine polyps and fibroids. Surgical removal of abnormal growths and/or cancer therapies are initiated when appropriate.

Possible complications of endometrial biopsy include minor cramping and spotting after the procedure. Some physicians believe that there may be a small risk to a newly implanted embryo and advise the use of birth control during the several weeks prior to the biopsy.

—*Karen E. Kalumuck, Ph.D.*

See also Biopsy; Cancer; Cervical, ovarian, and uterine cancers; Cervical procedures; Genital disorders, female; Gynecology; Infertility in females; Oncology; Reproductive system.

FOR FURTHER INFORMATION:

Boston Women's Health Book Collective. *Our Bodies, Ourselves for the New Century.* New York: Simon & Schuster, 1998.

Cunningham, F. Gary. *Williams Obstetrics.* 21st ed. Stamford, Conn.: Appleton-Century-Crofts, 2001.

Dechnery, William. *Current Obstetric and Gynecological Diagnosis and Treatment.* 7th ed. Norwalk, Conn.: Appleton and Lange, 1991.

Henderson, Lorraine, and Ros Wood. *Explaining Endometriosis.* 2d ed. St. Leonards, Australia: Allen and Unwin, 2001.

Novak, Emil, and Jonathan S. Berek, eds. *Novak's Gynecology.* 13th ed. Philadelphia: Lippincott Williams & Wilkins, 2002.

Phillips, Robert H., and Glenda Motta. *Coping with Endometriosis: A Practical Guide to Understanding, Treating, and Living with Chronic Endometriosis.* New York: Putnam, 2000.

ENDOMETRIOSIS
DISEASE/DISORDER

ANATOMY OR SYSTEM AFFECTED: Reproductive system, uterus

SPECIALTIES AND RELATED FIELDS: Gynecology

DEFINITION: Growth of cells of the uterine lining at sites outside the uterus, causing severe pain and infertility.

KEY TERMS:

cervix: an oval-shaped organ that separates the uterus and the vagina

dysmenorrhea: painful menstruation

dyspareunia: painful sexual intercourse

endometrium: the tissue that lines the uterus, builds up, and sheds at the end of each menstrual cycle; when it grows outside the uterus, endometriosis occurs

Fallopian tubes: two tubes extending from the ovaries to the uterus; during ovulation, an egg travels down one of these tubes to the uterus

hysterectomy: surgery that removes part or all of the uterus

implant: an abnormal endometrial growth outside the uterus

laparoscopy: a surgical procedure in which a small incision made near the navel is used to view the uterus and other abdominal organs with a lighted tube called a laparoscope

laparotomy: a surgical procedure, often exploratory in nature, carried out through the abdominal wall; it may be used to correct endometriosis

laser: a concentrated, high-energy light beam often used to destroy abnormal tissue

oophorectomy (or *ovariectomy*): removal of the ovaries, which is often necessary in cases of severe endometriosis

prostaglandins: fatlike hormones that control the contraction and relaxation of the uterus and other smooth muscle tissue

CAUSES AND SYMPTOMS

Endometriosis, the presence of endometrial tissue outside its normal location as the lining of the uterus, is a disabling disease in women that causes severe pain and in many cases infertility. The classic symptoms of endometriosis are very painful menstruation (dysmenorrhea), painful intercourse (dyspareunia), and infertility. Some other common endometriosis symptoms include nausea, vomiting, diarrhea, and fatigue.

It has been estimated that endometriosis affects between five million and twenty-five million American women. Often, it is incorrectly stereotyped as being a disease of upwardly mobile, professional women. According to many experts, the incidence of endometriosis worldwide and across most racial groups is probably very similar. They propose that the reported occurrence rate difference for some racial groups, such as a lower incidence in African Americans, has been a socioeconomic phenomenon attributable to the social class of women who seek medical treatment for the symptoms of endometriosis and to the highly stratified responses of many health care professionals who have dealt with the disease.

The symptoms of endometriosis arise from abnormalities in the effects of the menstrual cycle on the endometrial tissue lining the uterus. The endometrium normally thickens and becomes swollen with blood (engorged) during the cycle, a process controlled by female hormones called estrogens and progestins. This engorgement is designed to prepare the uterus for conception by optimizing conditions for implantation in the endometrium of a fertilized egg, which enters the uterus via one of the Fallopian tubes leading from the ovaries.

By the middle of the menstrual cycle, the endometrial lining is normally about ten times thicker than that at its beginning. If the egg that is released into the uterus is not fertilized, pregnancy does not occur and decreases in production of the female sex hormones result in the breakdown of the endometrium. Endometrial tissue mixed with blood leaves the uterus as the menstrual flow and a new menstrual cycle begins. This series of uterine changes occurs repeatedly, as a monthly cycle, from puberty (which usually occurs between the ages of twelve and fourteen) to the menopause (which usually occurs between the ages of forty-five and fifty-five).

In women who develop endometriosis, some endometrial tissue begins to grow ectopically (in an abnormal position) at sites outside the uterus. The ectopic endometrial growths may be found attached to the ovaries, the Fallopian tubes, the urinary bladder, the rectum, other abdominal organs, and even the lungs. Regardless of body location, these implants behave as if they were still in the uterus, thickening and bleeding each month as the menstrual cycle proceeds. Like the endometrium at its normal uterine site, the ectopic tissue responds to the hormones that circulate through the body in the blood. Its inappropriate position in the body prevents this ectopic endometrial tissue from leaving the body as menstrual flow; as a result, some implants grow to be quite large.

INFORMATION ON ENDOMETRIOSIS

CAUSES: Unknown
SYMPTOMS: Painful menstrual periods, discomfort during sexual intercourse, localized pain, infertility
DURATION: Chronic
TREATMENTS: Chemotherapy, surgery

In many cases, the endometrial growths that form between two organs become fibrous bands called adhesions. The fibrous nature of adhesions is attributable to the alternating swelling and breakdown of the ectopic tissue, which yields fibrous scar tissue. The alterations in size of living portions of the adhesions and other endometrial implants during the monthly menstrual cycle cause many afflicted women considerable pain. Because the body location of implants varies, the site of the pain may be almost anywhere, such as the back, the chest, the rectum, or the abdomen. For example, dyspareunia occurs when adhesions hold a uterus tightly to the abdominal wall, making its movement during intercourse painful.

The presence of endometriosis is usually confirmed by laparoscopy, viewed as being the most reliable method for its diagnosis. Laparoscopy is carried out after a physician makes an initial diagnosis of probable endometriosis from a combined study including an examination of the patient's medical history and careful exploration of the patient's physical problems over a period of at least six months. During prelaparoscopy treatment, the patient is very often maintained on pain medication and other therapeutic drugs that will produce symptomatic relief.

For laparoscopy, the patient is anesthetized with a general anesthetic, a small incision is made near the navel, and a flexible lighted tube—a laparoscope—is inserted into this incision. The laparoscope, equipped with fiber optics, enables the examining physician to search the patient's abdominal organs for endometrial implants. Visibility of the abdominal organs in laparoscopic examination can be enhanced by pumping harmless carbon dioxide gas into the abdomen, causing it to distend. Women who undergo laparoscopy usually require a day of postoperative bed rest, followed by seven to ten days of curtailed physical activity. After a laparoscopic diagnosis of endometriosis is made, a variety of surgical and therapeutic drug treatments can be employed to manage the disease.

About 40 percent of all women who have endometriosis are infertile; contemporary wisdom evaluates this relationship as one of cause and effect, which should make this disease the second most common cause of fertility problems. The actual basis for this infertility is not always clear, but it is often the result of damage to the ovaries and Fallopian tubes, scar tissue produced by implants on these and other abdominal organs, and hormone imbalances.

Because the incidence of infertility accompanying endometriosis increases with the severity of the disease, all potentially afflicted women are encouraged to seek early diagnosis. Many experts advise all women with abnormal menstrual cycles, dysmenorrhea, severe menstrual bleeding, abnormal vaginal bleeding, and repeated dyspareunia to seek the advice of a physician trained in identifying and dealing with endometriosis. Because the disease can begin to present symptoms at any age, teenagers are also encouraged to seek medical attention if they experience any of these symptoms.

John Sampson coined the term "endometriosis" in the 1920's. Sampson's theory for its causation, still widely accepted, is termed retrograde menstruation. Also called menstrual backup, this theory proposes that the backing up of some menstrual flow into the Fallopian tubes, and then into the abdominal cavity, forms the endometrial implants. Evidence supporting this theory, according to many physicians, is the fact that such backup is common. Others point out, however, that the backup is often found in women who do not have the disease. A surgical experiment was performed on female monkeys to test this theory. Their uteri were turned upside down so that the menstrual flow would spill into the abdominal cavity. Sixty percent of the animals developed endometriosis postoperatively—an inconclusive result.

Complicating the issue is the fact that implants are also found in tissues (such as in the lung) that cannot be reached by menstrual backup. It has been theorized that the presence of these implants results from the entry of endometrial cells into the lymphatic system, which returns body fluid to the blood and protects the body from many other diseases. This transplantation theory is supported by the occurrence of endometriosis in various portions of the lymphatic system and in tissues that could not otherwise become sites of endometriosis.

A third theory explaining the growth of implants is the iatrogenic, or nosocomial, transmission of endometrial tissue. These terms both indicate an accidental creation of the disease through the actions of physicians. Such implant formation is viewed as occurring most often after cesarean delivery of a baby when passage through the birth canal would otherwise be fatal to mother and/or child. Another proposed cause is episiot-

---

IN THE NEWS: LINK BETWEEN ENDOMETRIOSIS AND OTHER DISEASES

In the October, 2002, issue of *Human Reproduction*, the Endometriosis Association and the National Institutes of Health (NIH) announced the results of a study involving 3,680 women who were members of the Endometriosis Association and who had been diagnosed with endometriosis. The study suggested that women with endometriosis are significantly more likely than other women to contract a number of serious autoimmune diseases including lupus, Sjögren's syndrome, rheumatoid arthritis, and multiple sclerosis.

Although a study conducted in 1980 established a link between endometriosis and immune dysfunctions, the new study sought to identify specific diseases for which women with endometriosis are at higher risk. In addition to the connection between endometriosis and autoimmune diseases, researchers found that the women in the study were more than one hundred times more likely than women in the general population to suffer from chronic fatigue syndrome; twice as likely to suffer from fibromyalgia (recurrent pain in the muscles, tendons, and ligaments), and seven times as likely to suffer from hypothyroidism (which can also be an autoimmune disorder). Researchers also found that the women studied reported higher rates of allergies and asthma than women in the general population.

Researchers warn that the study may not be representative of all patients with endometriosis, both because members of the Endometriosis Association are most probably those patients suffering pain from their condition and because the survey was completed predominantly by white, educated women. Even so, this new information provides more light on an enigmatic disease and should help health care professionals treat patients.

—*Cassandra Kircher, Ph.D.*

omy—widening of the birth canal by an incision between the anus and vagina—to ease births.

Any surgical procedure that allows the spread of endometrial tissue can be implicated, including surgical procedures carried out to correct existing endometriosis, because of the ease with which endometrial tissue implants itself anywhere in the body. Abnormal endometrial tissue growth, called adenomyosis, can also occur in the uterus and is viewed as a separate disease entity.

Other theories regarding the genesis of endometriosis include an immunologic theory, which proposes that women who develop endometriosis are lacking in antibodies that normally cause the destruction of endometrial tissue at sites where it does not belong, and a hormonal theory, which suggests the existence of large imbalances in hormones such as the prostaglandins that serve as the body's messengers in controlling biological processes. Several of these theories—retrograde menstruation, the transplantation theory, and iatrogenic transmission—all have support, but none has been proved unequivocally. Future evidence will identify whether one cause is dominant, whether they all interact to produce the disease, or whether endometriosis is actually a group of diseases that simply resemble one another in the eyes of contemporary medical science.

TREATMENT AND THERAPY

Laparoscopic examination most often identifies endometriosis as chocolate-colored lumps (chocolate cysts) ranging from the size of a pinhead to several inches across or as filmy coverings over parts of abdominal organs and ligaments. Once a diagnosis of the disease is confirmed by laparoscopy, endometriosis is treated by chemotherapy, surgery, or a combination of both methods. The only permanent contemporary cure for endometriosis, however, is the onset of the biological menopause at the end of a woman's childbearing years. As long as menstruation continues, implant development is likely to recur, regardless of its cause. Nevertheless, a temporary cure of endometriosis is better than no cure at all.

The chemotherapy that many physicians use to treat mild cases of endometriosis (and for prelaparoscopy periods) is analgesic painkillers, including aspirin, acetaminophen, and ibuprofen. The analgesics inhibit the body's production of prostaglandins, and the symptoms of the disease are merely covered up. Therefore, analgesics are of quite limited value except during a prelaparoscopy diagnostic period or with mild cases

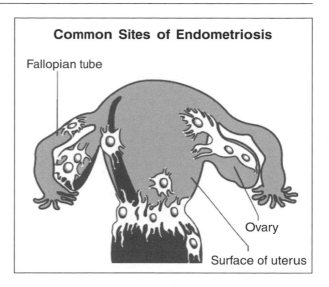

Common Sites of Endometriosis

Fallopian tube

Ovary

Surface of uterus

of endometriosis. In addition, the long-term administration of aspirin will often produce gastrointestinal bleeding, and excess use of acetaminophen can lead to severe liver damage. In some cases of very severe endometriosis pain, narcotic painkillers are given, such as codeine, Percodan (oxycodone and aspirin), or morphine. Narcotics are addicting and should be avoided unless absolutely necessary.

More effective for long-term management of the disease is hormone therapy. Such therapy is designed to prevent the monthly occurrence of menstruation—that is, to freeze the body in a sort of chemical menopause. The hormone types used, made by pharmaceutical companies, are chemical cousins of female hormones (estrogens and progestins), male hormones (androgens), and a brain hormone that controls ovulation (gonadotropin-releasing hormone, or GnRH). Appropriate hormone therapy is often useful for years, although each hormone class produces disadvantageous side effects in many patients.

The use of estrogens stops ovulation and menstruation, freeing many women with endometriosis from painful symptoms. Numerous estrogen preparations have been prescribed, including the birth control pills that contain them. Drawbacks of estrogen use can include weight gain, nausea, breast soreness, depression, blood-clotting abnormalities, and elevated risk of vaginal cancer. In addition, estrogen administration may cause endometrial implants to enlarge.

The use of progestins arose from the discovery that pregnancy—which is maintained by high levels of a natural progestin called progesterone—reversed the symptoms of many suffering from endometriosis. This realization led to the utilization of synthetic progestins to cause prolonged false pregnancy. The rationale is that all endometrial implants will die off and be reabsorbed during the prolonged absence of menstruation. The method works in most patients, and pain-free periods of up to five years are often observed. In some cases, however, side effects include nausea, depression, insomnia, and a very slow resumption of normal menstruation (such as lags of up to a year) when the therapy is stopped. In addition, progestins are ineffective in treating large implants; in fact, their use in such cases can lead to severe complications.

In the 1970's, studies showing the potential for heart attacks, high blood pressure, and strokes in patients receiving long-term female hormone therapy led to a search for more advantageous hormone medications. An alternative developed was the synthetic male hormone danazol (Danocrine), which is very effective. One of its advantages over female hormones is the ability to shrink large implants and restore fertility to those patients whose problems arise from nonfunctional ovaries or Fallopian tubes. Danazol has become the drug of choice for treating millions of endometriosis sufferers. Problems associated with danazol use, however, can include weight gain, masculinization (decreased bust size, facial hair growth, and deepened voice), fatigue, depression, and baldness. Those women contemplating danazol use should be aware that it can also complicate pregnancy.

Because of the side effects of these hormones, other chemotherapy was sought. Another valuable drug that has become available is GnRH, which suppresses the function of the ovaries in a fashion equivalent to surgical oophorectomy (removal of the ovaries). This hormone produces none of the side effects of the sex hormones, such as weight gain, depression, or masculinization, but some evidence indicates that it may lead to osteoporosis.

Thus, despite the fact that hormone therapy may relieve or reduce pain for years, contemporary chemotherapy is flawed by many undesirable side effects. Perhaps more serious, however, is the high recurrence rate of endometriosis that is observed after the therapy is stopped. Consequently, it appears that the best treatment of endometriosis combines chemotherapy with surgery.

The extent of the surgery carried out to combat endometriosis is variable and depends on the observations made during laparoscopy. In cases of relatively mild endometriosis, conservative laparotomy surgery removes endometriosis implants, adhesions, and lesions.

This type of procedure attempts to relieve endometriosis pain, to minimize the chances of postoperative recurrence of the disease, and to allow the patient to have children. Even in the most severe cases of this type, the uterus, an ovary, and its associated Fallopian tube are retained. Such surgery will often include removal of the appendix, whether diseased or not, because it is very likely to develop implants. The surgical techniques performed are the conventional excision of diseased tissue or the use of lasers to vaporize it. Many physicians prefer lasers because it is believed that they decrease the chances of recurrent endometriosis resulting from retained implant tissue or iatrogenic causes.

In more serious cases, hysterectomy is carried out. All visible implants, adhesions, and lesions are removed from the abdominal organs, as in conservative surgery. In addition, the uterus and cervix are taken out, but one or both ovaries are retained. This allows female hormone production to continue normally until the menopause. Uterine removal makes it impossible to have children, however, and may lead to profound psychological problems that require psychiatric help. Women planning to elect for hysterectomy to treat endometriosis should be aware of such potential difficulties. In many cases of conservative surgery or hysterectomy, danazol is used, both preoperatively and postoperatively, to minimize implant size.

The most extensive surgery carried out on the women afflicted with endometriosis is radical hysterectomy, also called definitive surgery, in which the ovaries and/or the vagina are also removed. The resultant symptoms are menopausal and may include vaginal bleeding atrophy (when the vagina is retained), increased risk of heart disease, and the development of osteoporosis. To counter the occurrence of these symptoms, replacement therapy with female hormones is suggested. Paradoxically, this hormone therapy can lead to the return of endometriosis by stimulating the growth of residual implant tissue.

PERSPECTIVE AND PROSPECTS

Modern treatment of endometriosis is viewed by many physicians as beginning in the 1950's. A landmark development in this field was the accurate diagnosis of endometriosis via the laparoscope, which was invented in Europe and introduced into the United States in the 1960's. Medical science has progressed greatly since that time. Physicians and researchers have recognized the wide occurrence of the disease and accepted its symptoms as valid; realized that hysterectomy will not necessarily put an end to the disease; utilized chemotherapeutic tools, including hormones and painkillers, as treatments and as adjuncts to surgery; developed laser surgery and other techniques that decrease the occurrence of formerly ignored iatrogenic endometriosis; and understood that the disease can ravage teenagers as well and that these young women should be examined as early as possible.

As pointed out by Niels H. Lauersen and Constance DeSwaan in *The Endometriosis Answer Book* (1988), more research than ever is "exploring the intricacies of the disease." Moreover, the efforts and information base of the proactive American Endometriosis Association, founded in 1980, have been very valuable. As a result, a potentially or presently afflicted woman is much more aware of the problems associated with the disease. In addition, she has a source for obtaining objective information on topics including state-of-the-art treatment, physician and hospital choice, and both physical and psychological outcomes of treatment.

Many potentially viable avenues for better endometriosis diagnosis and treatment have become the objects of intense investigation. These include the use of ultrasonography and radiology techniques for the predictive, nonsurgical examination of the course of growth or the chemotherapeutic destruction of implants; the design of new drugs to be utilized in the battle against endometriosis; endeavors aimed at the development of diagnostic tests for the disease that will stop it before symptoms develop; and the design of dietary treatments to soften its effects.

Regrettably, because of the insidious nature of endometriosis—which has the ability to strike almost anywhere in the body—some confusion about the disease still exists. New drugs, surgical techniques, and other aids are expected to be helpful in clarifying many of these issues. Particular value is being placed on the study of the immunologic aspects of endometriosis. Scientists hope to explain why the disease strikes some women and not others, to uncover its etiologic basis, and to solve the widespread problems of iatrogenic implant formation and other types of endometriosis recurrence.

—*Sanford S. Singer, Ph.D.*

See also Amenorrhea; Cervical, ovarian, and uterine cancers; Childbirth complications; Dysmenorrhea; Endometrial biopsy; Genital disorders, female; Gynecology; Hysterectomy; Infertility in females; Menorrhagia; Menstruation; Pregnancy and gestation; Reproductive system.

FOR FURTHER INFORMATION:

Endometriosis.org. http://www.endometriosis.org/. A Web site that offers FAQs about the disease, research articles, case histories, information about local support groups, diagnosis and treatment information, and a glossary.

Henderson, Lorraine, and Ros Wood. *Explaining Endometriosis*. 2d ed. St. Leonards, Australia: Allen and Unwin, 2001. Details possible causes, diagnosis, surgeries, and current treatment options for endometriosis.

Novak, Emil, and Jonathan S. Berek, eds. *Novak's Gynecology*. 13th ed. Philadelphia: Lippincott Williams & Wilkins, 2002. A standard text covering all aspects of gynecology with an emphasis on diagnosis and treatment. Topics include biology and physiology, family planning, sexuality, evaluation of pelvic infections, early pregnancy loss, benign breast disease, benign gynecologic conditions, malignant diseases of the reproductive tract, and breast cancer.

Phillips, Robert H., and Glenda Motta. *Coping with Endometriosis: A Practical Guide to Understanding, Treating, and Living with Chronic Endometriosis*. New York: Putnam, 2000. Educates the reader on current research and addresses the psychological and emotional concerns brought on by a diagnosis.

Shaw, Michael, ed. *Everything You Need to Know About Diseases*. Springhouse, Pa.: Springhouse Press, 1996. This well-illustrated consumer reference, compiled by more than one hundred doctors and medical experts, describes five hundred illnesses and conditions, their causes, symptoms, diagnosis, treatment, and prevention. Of particular interest is chapter 9, "Gynecologic Disorders."

Sherwood, Lauralee. *Human Physiology: From Cells to Systems*. 4th ed. Belmont, Calif.: Wadsworth, 2001. This college text contains much useful biological information. Included are details about the menstrual cycle, hormones, the endometrium, and many helpful definitions. Clearly written, the book is a mine of information for interested readers.

2000 Physician's Desk Reference. Montvale, N.J.: Medical Economics, 2000. This atlas of prescription drugs includes the drugs used against endometriosis, the companies that produce them, their useful dose ranges, their effects on metabolism and toxicology, and their contraindications.

Weinstein, Kate. *Living with Endometriosis*. Reading, Mass.: Addison-Wesley, 1987. The main divisions of this handy book are medical aspects, treatments and outcomes, emotional problems, and pain and psychiatric problems. Highlights include the complete description of the female reproductive system and menstruation, the glossary, and appendices on organizations, literature, and pain management centers.

Weschler, Toni. *Taking Charge of Your Fertility*. Rev. ed. New York: HarperCollins, 2001. Explores common health issues of women and their role in preventing pregnancy.

ENDOSCOPY

PROCEDURE

ANATOMY OR SYSTEM AFFECTED: Abdomen, anus, bladder, gastrointestinal system, intestines, joints, knees, lungs, stomach, urinary system

SPECIALTIES AND RELATED FIELDS: Gastroenterology, gynecology, obstetrics, orthopedics, proctology, pulmonary medicine, urology

DEFINITION: The use of a flexible tube to look into body structures in order to inspect and sometimes correct pathologies.

KEY TERMS:

biopsy: the collection and study of body tissue, often to determine whether it is cancerous

fiber optics: the transmission of light through thin, flexible tubes

pathology: a disease condition; also the study of diseases

INDICATIONS AND PROCEDURES

Early endoscopes were simply rigid hollow tubes with a light source. They were inserted into body orifices, such as the anus or the mouth, to allow the physician to look directly at processes within. Modern instruments are more sophisticated. They use fiber optics in flexible cables to penetrate deep into body structures. For example, one form of colonoscope can be threaded though the entire lower intestine, allowing the physician to search for pathologies all the way from the anus to the cecum of the colon (large intestine).

There are eight basic types of endoscope: gastroscope, colonoscope, bronchoscope, cystoscope, laparoscope, colposcope, arthroscope, and amnioscope. Their primary uses are diagnostic; however, they can be fitted with special instruments to perform many different tasks, including taking bits of tissue for biopsy and carrying out surgical procedures.

USES AND COMPLICATIONS

The gastroscope and its variants are used to inspect structures of the gastrointestinal system. The name of one class of procedure gives an idea of how sophisticated the gastroscope has become: esophagogastroduodenoscopy. As the term implies, this technique can be used to investigate the esophagus (the tube leading to the stomach), the stomach itself, and the intestines all the way into the duodenum (the first link of the small intestine). Further, in a procedure called endoscopic retrograde cholangiopancreatography, the endoscope can be used to investigate processes in the gallbladder, the cystic duct, the common hepatic duct, and the common bile duct. By far the most common use of the gastroscope is in the diagnosis and management of esophageal and stomach problems. The gastroscope is used to confirm the suspicion of stomach ulcers and other gastroesophageal conditions and to monitor therapy.

The colonoscope and its variants are critical in the diagnosis of diseases in the lower intestine and in some aspects of therapy. The long, flexible fiber-optic tube can be threaded through the anus and rectum into the S-shaped sigmoid colon (flexible fiber-optic sigmoidoscopy). The tube can be made to rise up the descending colon, across the transverse colon, and down the ascending colon to the cecum. With the colonoscope, the physician can discover abnormalities such as polyps, diverticula, and blockages and the presence of cancer, Crohn's disease, ulcerative colitis, and many other diseases. The physician can also use the colonoscope to remove polyps; this is the major therapeutic use of colonoscopy.

Like most other forms of endoscopy, bronchoscopy is used for both diagnosis and treatment. The bronchoscope allows direct visualization of the trachea (the tube leading from the throat to the lungs) and the bronchi (the two main airducts leading into the lungs). It will show certain forms of lung cancer, various infectious states, and other pathologies. The bronchoscope can also be used to remove foreign objects, excise local tumors, remove mucus plugs, and improve bronchial drainage.

The cystoscope is used for visual inspection of the urethra and bladder. The bladder stores urine; the urethra is the tube through which it is eliminated. Cystoscopy discovers many of the conditions that can afflict these organs: obstruction, infection, cancer, and other disorders.

The laparoscope is used to look into the abdominal cavity for evidence of a wide variety of conditions. It can inspect the liver, help evaluate liver disease, and take tissue samples for biopsy. Laparoscopy can confirm the diagnosis of ectopic pregnancy (a condition in which a fetus develops outside the womb, usually in one of the Fallopian tubes). It can confirm the presence or absence of abdominal cancers and diagnose disease conditions in the gallbladder, spleen, peritoneum (the membrane that surrounds the abdomen), and the diaphragm, as well as give some views of the small and large intestine. In an important, relatively new development, the laparoscope is being used to remove gallbladders (cholecystectomy). This procedure is far less traumatic than the old surgery, often permitting release of the patient a day or two after the operation rather than requiring weeks of recuperation.

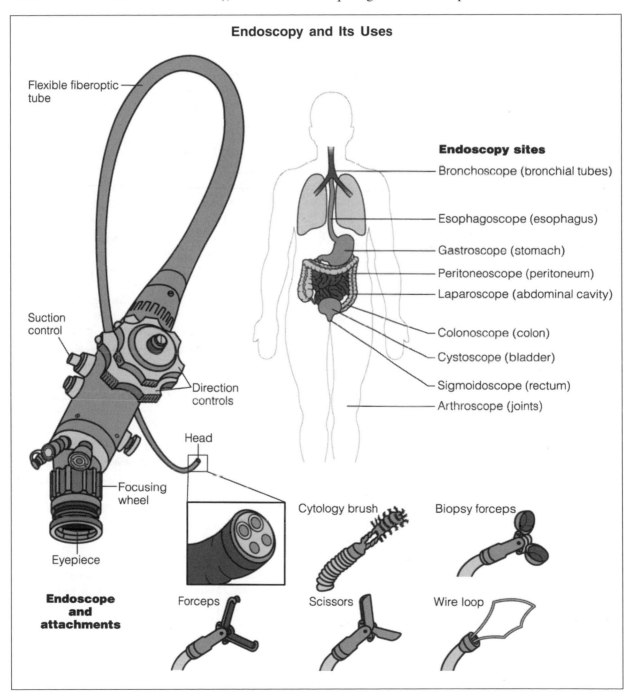

Endoscopy and Its Uses

Flexible fiberoptic tube

Suction control

Direction controls

Head

Focusing wheel

Eyepiece

Endoscope and attachments

Forceps

Cytology brush

Scissors

Biopsy forceps

Wire loop

Endoscopy sites

Bronchoscope (bronchial tubes)

Esophagoscope (esophagus)

Gastroscope (stomach)

Peritoneoscope (peritoneum)

Laparoscope (abdominal cavity)

Colonoscope (colon)

Cystoscope (bladder)

Sigmoidoscope (rectum)

Arthroscope (joints)

The colposcope is used to inspect vaginal tissue and adjacent organs. Common reasons for colposcopy include abnormal bleeding and suspicion of tumors.

Arthroscopy, the investigation of joint structures by endoscopy, is now the most common invasive technique used on patients with arthritis or joint damage. In addition to viewing the area, the arthroscope can be fitted with various instruments to perform surgical procedures.

The term "amnioscope" comes from the amnion, the membrane that surrounds a fetus. This type of endoscope is used to enter the uterus and inspect the growing fetus in the search for any visible abnormalities.

Endoscopy is one of the most useful and most-used techniques for diagnosis because it permits the investigation of many internal body organs without surgery. It is extraordinarily safe in the hands of experienced practitioners and is relatively free of pain and discomfort. In addition, specialized endoscopes are assuming greater roles in therapy. Many procedures that once involved major surgery can now be conducted through the endoscope, saving the patient pain, trauma, and expense.

PERSPECTIVE AND PROSPECTS

Endoscopes have become highly sophisticated instruments with enormous range throughout the body and enormous potential. Colonoscopy, for example, promises to revolutionize the treatment of cancerous and precancerous polyps by helping physicians attain a clearer understanding of the polyp-to-cancer progression. The laparoscope has revolutionized gallbladder removal, as the arthroscope has revolutionized joint surgery. The gastroscope gives the physician new security and control in the management of gastrointestinal conditions, and the bronchoscope facilitates many lung procedures.

Similarly throughout the entire range of endoscopy, new opportunities are opening and leading to significant improvements in therapy, and these improvements will continue. Electronic and video techniques are being introduced into endoscopy, and this new technology promises to widen the applications and therapeutic range of endoscopy still further.

—*C. Richard Falcon*

See also Abdominal disorders; Arthritis; Arthroscopy; Biopsy; Cholecystectomy; Colon and rectal polyp removal; Colon cancer; Colonoscopy and sigmoidoscopy; Cystoscopy; Gallbladder diseases; Gastrointestinal disorders; Invasive tests; Laparoscopy; Pulmonary diseases; Stone removal; Stones.

FOR FURTHER INFORMATION:

Classen, Meinhard, and C. J. Lightdale. *Gastroenterological Endoscopy*. New York: Thieme Medical, 2002. Text that examines such topics as the impact of endoscopy, its history of use, diagnostic procedures and techniques, therapeutic procedures, descriptions of diseases involving the upper and lower intestine, endoscopic features of infectious diseases of the GI tract, and pediatric endoscopy.

Emory, Theresa S., Herschel A. Carpenter, Christopher J. Gostout, and Leslie H. Sobin. *Atlas of Gastrointestinal Endoscopy and Endoscopic Biopsies*. Washington, D.C.: Armed Forces Institute of Pathology, 2000. This resource is divided into four major sections that correspond to the major endoscopic divisions of the gastrointestinal tract. Each section begins with an overview of the endoscopic examination and the histology.

Horton, Edward, et al., eds. *The Marshall Cavendish Illustrated Encyclopedia of Family Health*. 24 vols. London: Marshall Cavendish, 1986. The surgical listing covers a wide range of topics from anesthesia and aseptic techniques to surgical tools and sutures.

Larson, David E., ed. *Mayo Clinic Family Health Book*. 3d ed. New York: William Morrow, 2003. Perhaps the best general medical text for the layperson, this book covers the entire medical field. While the information is derived from a wide variety of highly technical sources, the articles are written to be easily understood by a general audience.

ENEMAS
PROCEDURE

ANATOMY OR SYSTEM AFFECTED: Abdomen, anus, gastrointestinal system, intestines

SPECIALTIES AND RELATED FIELDS: Gastroenterology

DEFINITION: A procedure to assist the body in evacuating fecal material from the bowel.

INDICATIONS AND PROCEDURES

Enemas are used primarily for two purposes: cleansing and retention. Many solutions have been used to promote cleansing. The most commonly used is made up of mild soapsuds and tap water. Commercially prepared solutions containing premeasured mild soap and water are also available.

To receive an enema, the patient should lie on the left side of the body with the upper thigh drawn up to the abdomen. The solution should be slightly above body temperature. The source of the enema fluid should be 30 to 45 centimeters (12 to 18 inches) above the anus. All air should be removed from the tubing that connects the enema reservoir and the tip. The tip is warmed in the hands, lubricated with a commercial preparation or a bit of soapy water, and gently inserted into the anus with a combination of soft pressure and a twisting motion. The tip should not be inserted more than 10 centimeters (4 inches) into the rectum. The solution is allowed to flow slowly into the rectum to prevent cramping.

A towel may be held gently against the rectum to prevent leakage. If cramping does occur, the flow should be interrupted by pinching the tubing. For an adult, approximately 1 liter (1 quart) of solution is probably sufficient; the patient should hold the solution for two to three minutes. The enema tube is tightly clamped and slowly withdrawn; a towel is again held against the anus to catch any leakage. A readily available bedpan or toilet stool is used while the patient evacuates the bowel. Depending on the need for the enema, the procedure may be repeated.

The procedure for administering a retention enema is similar except that the solution is instilled very slowly to promote retention. Lubricants or medicines are administered in this fashion. The patient holds the instilled solution as long as possible before evacuating the bowel.

USES AND COMPLICATIONS

Cleansing enemas are used to promote bowel evacuation by softening fecal material and stimulating the movement by bowel walls (peristalsis). Retention enemas are used to lubricate or soothe the mucosal lining of the rectum, to apply medication to the bowel wall or for absorption by the colon, and to soften feces.

There is no physiological need to have a bowel movement every day; normality is defined as from three to ten per week. Enemas should not be used routinely for cleansing because the bowel quickly becomes dependent on them. This problem is especially common among older individuals.

—*L. Fleming Fallon, Jr., M.D., Ph.D., M.P.H.*

See also Colon and rectal polyp removal; Colon and rectal surgery; Colon cancer; Colonoscopy and sigmoidoscopy; Gastroenterology; Gastrointestinal system; Hemorrhoid banding and removal; Hemorrhoids; Internal medicine; Intestines; Peristalsis; Proctology; Surgery, general.

FOR FURTHER INFORMATION:

Heuman, Douglas M., A. Scott Mills, and Hunter H. McGuire, Jr. *Gastroenterology*. Philadelphia: W. B. Saunders, 1997.

Mitsuoka, Tomotari. *Intestinal Bacteria and Health*. Translated by Syoko Watanabe. Tokyo: Harcourt Brace Jovanovich, 1978.

Peikin, Steven R. *Gastrointestinal Health*. Rev. ed. New York: HarperCollins, 1999.

ENTEROCOLITIS
DISEASE/DISORDER

ALSO KNOWN AS: Acute infectious diarrhea

ANATOMY OR SYSTEM AFFECTED: Gastrointestinal system, intestines

SPECIALTIES AND RELATED FIELDS: Family practice, gastroenterology, pediatrics

DEFINITION: Inflammation of the small and large intestines, which may be caused by a severe bacterial infection.

CAUSES AND SYMPTOMS

Enterocolitis is characterized by copious and sometimes bloody diarrhea, abdominal pain, vomiting, and dehydration. A high fever usually exists in young children. Cultures of the stool and blood can establish the exact organism involved.

Campylobacter enterocolitis, resulting from infection with *Campylobacter* bacteria, is the most common bacterial cause of diarrhea. It is endemic in developing countries, and epidemics are seen in Western countries in daycare centers. Salmonella enterocolitis is an infec-

---

INFORMATION ON ENTEROCOLITIS

CAUSES: Bacterial infection; unknown for necrotizing enterocolitis

SYMPTOMS: For bacterial infection, copious and sometimes bloody diarrhea, abdominal pain, vomiting, dehydration, high fever in young children; for necrotizing enterocolitis, poor feeding, abdominal distention or tenderness, decreased bowel sounds, apnea, lethargy, shock, cardiovascular collapse

DURATION: Acute

TREATMENTS: For bacterial infection, intravenous fluids and antibiotics; for necrotizing enterocolitis, surgery (intestinal resection)

tion in the lining of the small intestine caused by *Salmonella* bacteria acquired through the ingestion of contaminated food or water or exposure to reptiles. This type of enterocolitis can range from mild to severe and lasts from one to two weeks.

A different type of enterocolitis is necrotizing enterocolitis (NEC), the most common gastrointestinal medical emergency occurring in newborns. It is more prevalent in premature infants. NEC may begin with poor feeding, abdominal distention or tenderness, and decreased bowel sounds. If it becomes systemic, then symptoms can include apnea, lethargy, shock, and cardiovascular collapse. Outbreaks of NEC seem to follow an epidemic pattern, suggesting an infectious disease, but a specific causative organism has not been identified. Research suggests that several factors may be involved.

TREATMENT AND THERAPY

The treatment of bacterial enterocolitis involves intravenous fluids and antibiotics. In underdeveloped countries, where medical care is poor, enterocolitis is responsible for more than 60 percent of all deaths in children under age five.

Infants with NEC cannot take food by mouth and often must be fed through a central venous catheter. Those with severe disease may require surgical intervention such as intestinal resection. The mortality rate for NEC approaches 50 percent in infants weighing less than 1,500 grams.

—*Connie Rizzo, M.D.;
updated by Tracy Irons-Georges*
See also Antibiotics; Bacterial infections; Dehydration; Diarrhea and dysentery; Fever; Gastroenterology, pediatric; Gastrointestinal system; Intestinal disorders; Intestines; Nausea and vomiting; Salmonella infection.

FOR FURTHER INFORMATION:

Gilchrist, Brian F., ed. *Necrotizing Enterocolitis*. Georgetown, Tex.: Eurekah.Com, 2000.

Janowitz, Henry D. *Your Gut Feelings: A Complete Guide to Living Better with Intestinal Problems*. Rev. and updated ed. New York: Oxford University Press, 1994.

Stoll, Barbara J., and Robert M. Kliegman, eds. *Necrotizing Enterocolitis*. Philadelphia: W. B. Saunders, 1994.

Thompson, W. Grant. *Gut Reactions: Understanding Symptoms of the Digestive Tract*. New York: Plenum Press, 1989.

ENURESIS. *See* BED-WETTING.

ENVIRONMENTAL DISEASES
DISEASE/DISORDER
ANATOMY OR SYSTEM AFFECTED: All
SPECIALTIES AND RELATED FIELDS: Environmental health, epidemiology, occupational health, public health, toxicology
DEFINITION: A wide variety of conditions and diseases resulting from largely human-mediated hazards in both the natural and artificial (for example, home and workplace) environments; an area of special concern given rapid environmental degradation during the twentieth century.
KEY TERMS:
emphysema: the overinflation of bronchial tubes and alveoli with air, resulting in reduced lung function
environment: the biological, physical, cultural, and mental factors that influence health; anything external to an individual
food chain: a sequence—plant, herbivore, primary carnivore, and secondary and tertiary carnivore—in which each level depends on the stored energy from the lower level and often concentrates contaminants in the process
mutagen: a substance or event that effects a permanent, inheritable change in the genetic makeup of an organism
organic compound or waste: a chemical compound based on carbon, with or without hydrogen and other elements—in the context of environmental disease, usually a manufactured product
risk factor: a factor that increases the chances of an effect
teratogen: a substance or event that causes malformation in a developing fetus

CAUSES AND SYMPTOMS

Environmental health explores the influence of external factors on human health and disease. Technically, almost any condition except those of purely genetic origin could be considered as environmentally caused or having an environmental component, but the term "environmental disease" is usually applied to the effects of human alterations in the physical environment and excludes transmissible disease caused by pathogenic organisms, except in cases where human alteration of the environment is an important factor in epidemiology. Health hazards generally classed as environmental include air and water (including groundwater) pollution, toxic wastes, lead, asbestos, pesticides and herbicides, ionizing and nonionizing radiation, noise, and light.

In the United States, the Clean Air Act of 1970 established maximum levels for sulfur and nitrogen dioxide, particulates, hydrocarbons, ozone, and carbon monoxide—the most common air pollutants of concern in urban environments. Even with increasingly stringent controls on emissions from automobiles and industry, air quality in urban areas frequently does not meet minimum standards. Carbon monoxide lowers the oxygen-carrying capacity of the blood, nitrogen and sulfur dioxide react with water to form acids which damage lung tissue, ozone damages tissue directly, and particulates may accumulate in the lungs. The result is decreased lung capacity and function. Cigarette smoking increases susceptibility to other forms of lung damage.

Indoor air quality poses additional concerns. Emphasis on energy efficiency in building design decreases air exchange. Carpets and furniture release organic compounds, and cleaning solvents leave a volatile residue. Formaldehyde from foam stuffing and insulation in-

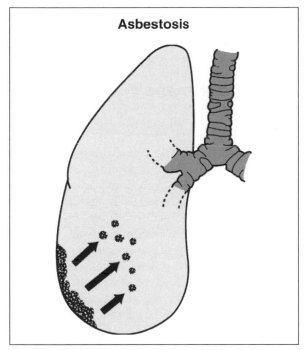

Asbestosis

Asbestosis—the progressive destruction of respiratory tissues via inhalation of dust-sized asbestos fibers that attach to the walls of the lung and then spread outward—is often the result of prolonged exposure to asbestos-containing materials (in shipyards, office buildings, manufacturing plants); it is one of a wide variety of environmental diseases.

hibits liver function and is a suspected carcinogen. Breathing in an enclosed space decreases atmospheric oxygen and increases carbon dioxide. In some areas, radioactive radon gas released by the soil becomes concentrated in buildings. A ventilation system which draws its air from a polluted outdoor environment, such as a loading dock, will fail to perform its function. Secondhand cigarette smoke poses the same hazards of emphysema and lung cancer to people chronically exposed to it in an enclosed environment as to the smokers themselves. The phenomenon known as "sick building syndrome," in which large numbers of people in one building complain of respiratory illness, headaches, and impaired concentration, results from a combination of these factors.

Lead additives in gasoline were once a significant source of atmospheric lead, but they are being phased out; unfortunately, they leave a permanent residue in soils of high-traffic areas. Levels of 20 micrograms per deciliter of lead in the blood inhibit hemoglobin production, slow the transmission of nerve impulses, and are suspected of causing cognitive impairment in children; higher levels cause anemia, weakness, stomach pains, and nervous system impairment. Even levels below 5 micrograms may be hazardous to children. Because of lead in the paint and plumbing in old houses and soil contamination, blood lead levels high enough to cause developmental impairment in children occur frequently in older parts of cities; low-income residents are most likely to be at risk. Mercury, another metallic neurotoxin, is introduced into water in small amounts through industrial effluent but becomes concentrated in the food chain, where it poses a hazard to people who eat large quantities of fish. Any waterborne pollutant that is not rapidly degraded has the potential for being concentrated in the food chain. Shellfish, which filter nutrients from seawater, can concentrate toxins. The most notorious cause of shellfish poisoning is a naturally occurring neurotoxic alga, but polychlorinated biphenyls (PCBs) and pesticides have also been implicated. Some metals, including lead, arsenic, and mercury, remain toxic indefinitely and are exceedingly difficult to remove from an environment into which they have been introduced.

Inhalation of asbestos fibers carries a high risk of developing lung cancer after an interval of twenty or thirty years, a connection first established among shipyard workers. Between 1940 and 1970, asbestos was used extensively in public buildings as insulation. It is estimated that three to five million workers in the

United States were exposed to unacceptably high levels of airborne fibers during this period, and millions of people continue to be exposed when building materials deteriorate. Asbestos abatement adds considerably to the cost of renovating old public buildings.

Urban drinking water in industrialized countries is monitored for hazardous contaminants; there is some question as to whether chlorine and fluoride, added for legitimate health reasons, are completely without negative effects. Well water in irrigated agricultural areas may have high levels of nitrates, which decrease blood oxygen and have been implicated in miscarriages and birth defects.

Organic chemical compounds make up 60 percent of the hazardous wastes generated by industry. This category includes PCBs (including dioxin), chlorofluorocarbons, phthalate esters, chlorinated benzenes, chloromethanes, solvents (such as benzene and carbon tetrachloride), plasticizers, fire retardants, pesticides, and herbicides. Many are acutely toxic—dioxin is one of the most potent toxins known—and require elaborate precautions to prevent worker exposure or accidental contamination of foodstuffs. PCBs, which are used in a wide variety of manufacturing processes, have been shown to cause cancer and reproductive disorders in laboratory animals and have been linked to these conditions in humans. The herbicide 2,4,5-T, the defoliant Agent Orange used during the Vietnam War, is the subject of continuing claims against the manufacturer and the Veterans Administration by soldiers who later developed neurological symptoms, immune disorders, or cancer, or who had children with birth defects.

The burial of toxic by-products of manufacturing processes in landfills has created an ongoing environmental health crisis as containers rupture and chemicals leach into the sur-rounding soil. Underground fuel storage tanks pose a similar problem. Toxins leached from a waste dump eventually enter streams and become disseminated or, if volatile, enter the atmosphere. Residents of the infamous Love Canal site in New York State were

IN THE NEWS: AGENT ORANGE LINKED TO LEUKEMIA

Agent Orange and other herbicides were used extensively during the Vietnam War to defoliate jungle canopies in South and North Vietnam, parts of Cambodia, and Laos. The purpose of defoliation was to reveal enemy troop concentrations, jungle camps and refuge areas, and resupply roads. Defoliation was also employed to rid areas of vegetation in preparation for the establishment of a U.S. military base.

Following the end of the war, increased incidence of cancers among veterans and birth defects in the children of veterans prompted concerns about possible links between exposure to Agent Orange and the health of Vietnam veterans. In 1978, the Department of Veterans Affairs (VA) established the Agent Orange Registry Examination to identify Vietnam veterans exposed to Agent Orange during their tour of duty. The Agent Orange Act of 1991 formally recognized the possible relationship between exposure to Agent Orange and susceptibility to cancers and other diseases among Vietnam veterans. The act also established disability compensation for affected personnel and initiated research to evaluate the correlation between herbicide exposure and incidence of disease; these tasks were entrusted to the Institute of Medicine (IOM), a branch of the privately operated organization called the National Academics of Science (NAM).

The initial report of the IOM stated that there was insufficient or inadequate evidence to link Agent Orange exposure to subsequent occurrence of leukemia in exposed military and support personnel. Following this report, however, the VA requested a separate evaluation of the incidence of chronic lymphocytic leukemia (CLL), which is similar to non-Hodgkin's lymphoma, a disease that had already been associated with exposure to Agent Orange.

Results of the new investigation, presented in the 2002 report of *Veterans and Agent Orange*, documented evidence of an association between the incidence of CLL in Vietnam veterans and exposure to 2,4-D, 2,4,5-T (or its contaminant TCDD), picloram, and/or cacodylic acid. This finding is critical for Vietnam veterans who currently have CLL because it will allow them to receive health care benefits. The results will also promote a proactive approach to the continued investigation and evaluation of Agent Orange exposure and the incidence of CLL in Vietnam veterans.

—Dwight G. Smith

made ill by fumes from contaminated soil and ground-water.

High energy from X-ray sources and radioactive materials is termed "ionizing" because such radiation can cause chemical changes in molecules, including genetic material. Chronic exposure to ionizing radiation poses a high risk of cancer, inheritable mutations, and fetal malformation. Exposure may be occupational, as with workers in the nuclear power industry or hospital radiology laboratories. Some radioactive by-products of nuclear weapons testing and reactor accidents (such as strontium 90 or carbon 14) are exceptionally hazardous because they are structurally incorporated into living tissue and become concentrated in the food chain. The by-products of the nuclear reactor accident in Chernobyl, Ukraine, in 1987 were disseminated across international boundaries and will continue to endanger the health of millions of people in Belarus, Ukraine, and Eastern Europe. Whether widespread atmospheric testing of nuclear weapons in the 1950's caused radiation damage in the population at large is unknown; military personnel involved in the testing and inhabitants of the regions near test sites report increased rates of suspected radiation-induced illness.

Hazards of nonionizing radiation (visible, ultraviolet, infrared, or microwave) are less well established. Intense visible light can damage vision. Artificial lighting is known to disrupt reproductive cycles in plants and invertebrates and could have subtle effects on human biology. That the level of microwave radiation to which the public at large is inadvertently exposed is well below levels known to produce adverse effects is not completely reassuring. Ultraviolet light, principally from sunlight, is a factor in skin cancer, which is increasing both because of the popularity of sunbathing and because ozone depletion increases ultraviolet exposure.

A category of severe lung disease affects workers in environments with a high concentration of particulate matter in the air: black lung disease, from coal dust in coal mines; silicosis, from fine rock powder in mines; and byssinosis, from textile fibers in spinning and weaving mills. The result of long-term breathing of particulates is obstruction and emphysema, which may be fatal.

Electromagnetic fields produced by power lines and electrical devices are an area of increasing controversy as electricity becomes more ubiquitous. One study found a higher-than-average rate of childhood leukemia near high-tension power lines; other studies have failed to confirm this finding. Women who work con-stantly at video display terminals have somewhat higher miscarriage rates than other office workers.

Exposure to industrial solvents has been a significant source of workplace illness. Among the most dangerous solvents are benzene, used in a variety of processes and produced as a by-product in the coking industry; vinyl chloride, used in plastics manufacture; and formaldehyde. All these chemicals are carcinogenic.

Repetitive motion injuries are an increasing occupational hazard. Any body part subject to constant, selective hard use, especially where tasks and workstations are poorly designed, may develop problems. The most common compensation claims arise from damage to the spinal column from lifting heavy objects and damage to nerves in the hand and forearm from repetitive, rapid hand movements (such as carpal tunnel syndrome).

SOCIETAL INTERVENTION

In order to improve environmental health, health professionals and regulatory agencies must anticipate and minimize future hazards, identify existing health problems that may have an environmental component and attempt to determine whether a connection exists, and redress the mistakes of the past. It is notoriously difficult to prove that an illness has an environmental cause. Suspicion arises when epidemiological statistics on reportable illnesses show that some condition known to be influenced by environmental factors—such as cancer, endocrine disorders, reproductive disorders, or immunodeficiency—occurs at an unusually high frequency in some subset of the population, occurs in a restricted geographical area, or is increasing throughout the general population. Even then, the cause may not be environmental; the acquired immunodeficiency syndrome (AIDS) epidemic was thought by some to be an environmental effect until the causative organism was identified.

The time interval between exposure and illness can be as long as twenty or thirty years, during which the exposed population may have dispersed and may no longer be readily identifiable. Subtle effects such as mild immunosuppression or cognitive impairment may escape detection or be dismissed as psychosomatic. Multiple environmental, behavioral, and even genetic factors are often involved, confounding efforts to pinpoint a cause. In the United States and Western Europe, high rates of exposure to pollutants are correlated with poverty and thus with higher-than-normal rates of malnutrition, alcohol and drug abuse, and inadequate access to health care. Tobacco smoking is a common confounding behavioral factor in environmental diagnosis. Where liability is involved, there are powerful financial incentives on the side of disproving the environmental or occupational linkage.

When a new technology or chemical is introduced, regulations in most countries require an assessment of health impact, which includes experimentation with animal models and risk assessment to determine the probable impact on the human population. Animal experimentation is most effective at demonstrating short-term and acute effects of toxic materials, but it is poor at demonstrating effects of long-term, low-level exposure. Risk assessment must take into consideration unusually susceptible individuals (pregnant women, for example), deliberate or accidental overexposure, and synergistic effects. In the realm of environmental legislation, risk assessment is also influenced by psychology; people are more willing to accept familiar risks over which they have personal control.

Perspective and Prospects

Concern for occupational health began with the Industrial Revolution in the early nineteenth century, and found some of its earliest expression in the recognition that some industrial jobs were inappropriate for children. Although many occupations in preindustrial societies carried a high risk of trauma, only a few involved chronic exposure to toxic substances. The combined effects of heavy physical labor and malnutrition are not infrequently seen in skeletons from archaeological excavations, but injury caused by repetitive motion under assembly-line conditions is a modern phenomenon.

Concerns about the effects of pollution and toxic wastes on the general population are of even more recent origin. Sanitarians in the first half of the twentieth century directed their attention toward reducing transmissible disease through the prevention of water and food supply contamination and the control of insect vectors. Several factors increased public awareness of environmental health problems in the United States and led to creation of agencies and legislation to address the problem, beginning in 1970: Urban-industrial air pollution contributed to hundreds of deaths from respiratory disease in Pennsylvania (1948) and London (1952); there was much publicity surrounding the dangers of pesticides to wildlife in the 1960's; a variety of health problems, including increased cancer risk, were found at Love Canal, a housing development in New York State built on a toxic waste dump; and it was dem-

onstrated that urban lead levels were high enough to impair psychomotor development in children.

The increase in the proportion of morbidity and mortality attributable to environmental factors in the late twentieth century was the result not only of the exponential increase in energy use and the output of complex synthetic chemicals but also of changing demographics. Effects of low-level exposure to toxins may take decades to produce disease and may never become apparent in populations with a low life expectancy. In developing countries, where environmental protection is rudimentary and life expectancies are increasing rapidly, the adverse health effects of environmental degradation are particularly visible.

In the United States, specific legislation addresses compensation for miners, asbestos workers, and other specific victims of exposure to hazardous materials. On a worldwide basis, monitoring of hazardous substances is a prime concern of the World Health Organization. As incidents such as the accidental release of cyanide from a fertilizer plant in Bhopal, India, indicate, provisions for industrial safety and for separating residential and industrial areas in the developing world are unsatisfactory. The former Soviet Union represents what in many ways is a worst-case scenario combining rapid, concentrated industrialization with poor environmental controls. Some of the earliest signs that the Communist regime was weakening came from the environmental movement in its agitation for better protection for human and natural resources. Safeguarding environmental health and addressing existing hazards and environmentally caused illnesses requires a major expenditure of funds and effort, which is likely to continue growing as the delayed effects of industrial practices introduced since World War II continue to become apparent.

—*Martha Sherwood-Pike, Ph.D.*

See also Allergies; Asthma; Bronchitis; Cancer; Carpal tunnel syndrome; Chronic obstructive pulmonary disease (COPD); *E. coli* infection; Emphysema; Environmental health; Epidemiology; Food poisoning; Gulf War syndrome; Lead poisoning; Lung cancer; Malignant melanoma removal; Multiple chemical sensitivity syndrome; Occupational health; Poisoning; Pulmonary diseases; Radiation sickness; Respiration; Skin cancer; Skin lesion removal; Toxicology.

For Further Information:

Baron-Faust, Rita. *The Autoimmune Connection.* New York: McGraw-Hill, 2003. Examines myriad health issues in women and investigates their possible environmental triggers, among other causes.

Carson, Rachel. *Silent Spring*. 40th anniversary ed. New York: Houghton Mifflin, 2002. A classic book first published in 1962 that alerted a large audience to the health risks associated with pesticide use.

Cooper, M. G., ed. *Risk: Man-Made Hazards to Man*. Oxford, England: Clarendon Press, 1985. A book about how people perceive and assess risks, factors that affect environmental legislation. In addition to a discussion of statistics and the effects of publicity, this British publication adopts a conservative view that hazards are often overstated.

Davis, Derva Lee. *When Smoke Ran Like Water: Tales of Environmental Deception and the Battle Against Pollution*. New York: Basic Books, 2002. Written by an epidemiologist and nominated for the 2002 National Book Award in nonfiction, this work explores the impact of air pollution on public health by examining historical air pollution crises in London, Los Angeles, and Donora, Pennsylvania, among other locales.

Goldstein, Inge F., and Martin Goldstein. *How Much Risk? A Guide to Understanding Environmental Health Hazards*. New York: Oxford University Press, 2001. A critical analysis of environmental health hazards and their threat to the public. Includes discussions of radiation from nuclear testing, radon in the home, the connection between electromagnetic fields and cancer, environmental factors and asthma, and pesticides and breast cancer.

Greenberg, Michael R., ed. *Public Health and the Environment: The United States Experience*. New York: Guilford Press, 1987. This text explores modern environmental problems from the point of view of public health. Part 1, a survey of the contribution of the environment to disease, includes sections on worker health and lifestyle as a factor in chronic disease.

Journal of Environmental Health, 1963-   . This journal published by the National Environmental Health Association offers articles on a wide variety of environmental and occupational health issues. The journal also acts as a forum for concerns of environmental health professionals and sanitarians.

Martens, Pim Josef, and Anthony J. McMichael, eds. *Environmental Change, Climate and Health: Issues and Research Methods*. Cambridge, Mass.: Cambridge University Press, 2002. Text that explores the health effects of global environmental change.

Morgan, Monroe T. *Environmental Health*. 3d ed. New York: Wadsworth, 2002. Examines the links between environmental sciences and human population, focusing on the practices that support human life as well as the need to control factors that are harmful to human life.

Rom, William N., ed. *Environmental and Occupational Medicine*. 2d ed. Boston: Little, Brown, 1992. The emphasis in this textbook is on industrial occupational safety, with approximately a third of the work devoted to the diagnosis and pathology of occupational lung diseases, including byssinosis and black lung disease. The effects of acute and chronic exposure to heavy metals, solvents, and other toxic substances are organized by agent.

Steenland, Kyle, and David A. Savits. *Topics in Environmental Epidemiology*. New York: Oxford University Press, 1997. A comprehensive survey of the epidemiology of common environmental exposures, this volume covers diet, water, particulates in outdoor air, nitrogen dioxide, ozone, environmental tobacco smoke, radon in homes, electromagnetic fields, and lead.

ENVIRONMENTAL HEALTH
SPECIALTY

ANATOMY OR SYSTEM AFFECTED: All

SPECIALTIES AND RELATED FIELDS: Epidemiology, occupational health, preventive medicine, psychology, public health, pulmonary medicine, toxicology

DEFINITION: The control of all factors in the physical environment that exercise, or may exercise, a deleterious effect on human physical development, health, and survival.

KEY TERMS:

community: a group of people living in the same locality

hygiene: the science of health and the prevention of disease

pollutant: a noxious substance that contaminates the environment

remediation: correcting an evil, fault, or error

sanitation: the application of measures designed to protect public health

SCIENCE AND PROFESSION

The environment is the sum of all external influences and conditions affecting the life and development of an organism. For humans, a healthy environment means that the surroundings in which humans live, work, and play meet some predetermined quality standard. The field of environmental health encompasses the air that humans breathe, the water that they drink, the food that they consume, and the shelter that they inhabit. The definition also includes the identification of pollutants, waste materials, and other environmental factors that adversely affect life and health. The study of environmental health encompasses the fields of environmental engineering and sanitation, public health engineering, and sanitary engineering. The majority of professionals working in the field of environmental health are trained as civil engineers, environmental engineers, geologists, toxicologists, or preventive medicine specialists. Many are also qualified in subspecialties such as hydrogeology, epidemiology, public sanitation, and occupational health.

Environmental health deals with the control of factors in the physical environment that cause (or may cause) a negative effect on the health and survival of communities. Consideration is given to the physical, economic, and social impact of the controlling measures. These measures include controlling, modifying, or adapting the physical, chemical, and biological factors of the environment in the interest of human health, comfort, and social well-being. Environmental health is concerned not only with simple survival and the prevention of disease and poisoning but also with the maintenance of an environment that is suited to efficient human performance and that preserves human comfort and enjoyment.

DIAGNOSTIC AND TREATMENT TECHNIQUES

The field of environmental health covers an extremely broad area of human living space. For practical purposes, those involved in the profession of environmental health concern themselves with the impact of humans on the environment and the impact of the environment on humans, balancing their appraisals and allocations of available resources. The scope of environmental health research and community environmental health planning usually involves the following topics: water supplies, water pollution and wastewater treatment, solid waste disposal, pest control, soil pollution, food hygiene, air pollution, radiation control, noise control, transportation control, safe housing, land use planning, public recreation, abuse of controlled substances, resource conservation, postdisaster sanitation, accident prevention, medical facilities, and occupational health, particularly the control of physical, chemical, and biological hazards.

The implementation of effective environmental health strategies must take place within the context of comprehensive regional or area-wide community planning. Planning considerations for a community's environmental health are based on individual community aspirations and goals, priorities, local resources, and the availability of outside resources required to meet projected health standards. The planning and implementation of environmental health activities directly involve engineers, sanitarians, medical specialists, planners, architects, geologists, biologists, chemists, geophysicists, technicians, naturalists, and related personnel. The natural and physical scientists provide research necessary for communities to locate and use available resources responsibly, and they also identify potential and existing health hazards. The engineering specialties provide know-how to communities concerning the design, installation, and operation of equipment. When a problem is identified or an emergency occurs, it is often the engineering professionals who direct remediation efforts. Medical specialists, with scientific backup, determine dangers to a community's physical health; if health problems arise, they concern themselves with curing disease. The implementation of any environmental health strategy is clearly a team effort.

PERSPECTIVE AND PROSPECTS

The concept of environmental health in modern society is considerably expanded from that of the past. Activities in the field of environmental health were once controlled only because they were known to be disease-related. The present concept of environmental health aims to provide a high quality of living.

The field of environmental health concerns itself with the control of physical factors affecting the health of humans and is different from the prevention and control of individual illness and the preservation of human health. Most environmental health problems are the direct result of human activities and interactions with natural resources. Human manipulation of natural resources causes changes to the environment. These changes can be local or global, anticipated or unanticipated. At the present time, humans are living in a polluted environment, the result of centuries of lack of concern for and appreciation of the ecologic consequences of human activities. The cumulative effects of human actions on the environment have risen steeply and continuously, while human response to mounting problems of environmental quality has been sporadic and targeted toward high-profile or emergency problems. As a result, environmental programs have been developed to preserve wildlife, maintain clean groundwater supplies, manage resources, combat communicable disease, increase agricultural production, and ensure healthy and sanitary living conditions for human populations.

As a direct reflection of the public's concern about environmental degradation, environmental health has become a rapidly growing specialty in the fields of engineering, medicine, environmental science, geology, and resource management. As public awareness of the devastating effects of pollution and resource depletion grows, the demand for qualified environmental health professionals and administrators increases. Whether these sought-after professionals are asked to offer stopgap measures for environmental problems that have already progressed to dangerous, possibly unresolvable levels or whether they are employed to foster a new, more holistic approach to the natural world will depend on the environmental conscience of modern civilization.

—*Randall L. Milstein, Ph.D.*

See also Allergies; Arthropod-borne diseases; Asthma; Bacteriology; Biological and chemical weapons; Cholera; Chronic obstructive pulmonary disease (COPD); Environmental diseases; Environmental health; Epidemiology; Food poisoning; Frostbite; Gulf war syndrome; Heat exhaustion and heat stroke; Hyperthermia and hypothermia; Immune system; Immunization and vaccination; Immunology; Interstitial pulmonary fibrosis (IPF); Lead poisoning; Legionnaires' disease; Lice, mites, and ticks; Lung cancer; Lungs; Lyme disease; Malaria; Microbiology; Nasopharyngeal disorders; Occupational health; Parasitic diseases; Plague; Poisoning; Poisonous plants; Preventive medicine; Pulmonary diseases; Pulmonary medicine; Pulmonary medicine, pediatric; Salmonella infection; Skin cancer; Snakebites; Stress; Stress reduction; Toxicology; Tropical medicine.

FOR FURTHER INFORMATION:

Environmental Defense. http://www.environmental defense.org.

Higgins, Thomas. *Hazardous Waste Minimization Handbook.* Chelsea, Mich.: Lewis, 1989.

Moeller, D. W. *Environmental Health.* Rev. ed. Cambridge, Mass.: Harvard University Press, 1997.

Morgan, Monroe T. *Environmental Health.* 3d ed. New York: Wadsworth, 2002.

Philp, Richard B. *Ecosystems and Human Health: Toxicology and Environmental Hazards.* 2d ed. Boca Raton, Fla.: CRC Press, 2001.

Raven, Peter H., and Linda R. Berg. *Environment.* 4th ed. Fort Worth, Tex.: Harcourt Brace College, 2004.

Steger, Will, and Jon Bowermaster. *Saving the Earth: A Citizen's Guide to Environmental Action.* New York: Alfred A. Knopf, 1990.

Yassi, Annalee, et al. *Basic Environmental Health.* New York: Oxford University Press, 2001.

ENZYME THERAPY

TREATMENT

ALSO KNOWN AS: Enzyme replacement therapy

ANATOMY OR SYSTEM AFFECTED: All

SPECIALTIES AND RELATED FIELDS: Alternative medicine, biochemistry, genetics

DEFINITION: The use of enzymes as drugs to treat specific medical problems.

INDICATIONS AND PROCEDURES

Enzymes are large, complex protein molecules that catalyze chemical reactions in living organisms. The phrase "enzyme therapy" is sometimes used to refer to enzyme preparations given as dietary supplements, often as digestive aids. Such treatment is of questionable value because enzymes, like all proteins, are degraded in the stomach. Legitimate enzyme therapy is an innovative procedure based on emerging technology. Enzymes used to treat various medical conditions are delivered intravenously.

Enzyme therapy is used to dissolve clots in stroke and cardiac patients. Enzymes such as streptokinase, plasmin, and human tissue plasminogen activator (TPA) are able to dissolve clots when injected into the bloodstream.

Some types of adult leukemia can be treated by injection of the enzyme asparaginase, which destroys asparagine. Tumors in these patients require asparagine, and the asparaginase removes it from the blood, thus inhibiting the ability of these tumors to grow.

Enzyme therapy can also be used to treat certain inherited diseases. One of these is Fabry's disease. These patients are deficient in an enzyme called alpha-galactosidase A. Without this enzyme, harmful levels of a substance called ceremide trehexoside accumulate in the heart, brain, and kidneys. If left untreated, patients usually die in their forties or fifties after a lifetime of pain. On the other hand, patients injected with alpha-galactosidase A once every two weeks lead nearly normal lives.

Gaucher's disease is another severe inherited disease characterized by a deficiency in an enzyme that normally prevents the buildup of a chemical to injurious levels. It can be treated by injections of the enzyme glucocerebrosidase.

USES AND COMPLICATIONS

The use of enzymes to treat clotting problems and genetic diseases started in the early 1990's; thus, the long-term effects are unknown. Enzyme therapy does not cure genetic disease, so the therapy must be lifelong.

Some people are encouraged to swallow enzyme preparations to aid digestion. For example, the enzyme papain is promoted as a digestive aid. Although papain is very effective at breaking down proteins in the laboratory or as a meat tenderizer in the kitchen, it does not function well in the stomach. Papain is most effective at a nearly neutral pH of 6.2, whereas the stomach is highly acidic with a pH of about 2.0. On the other hand, papain is active in the more neutral esophagus. Although normally little or no food is found in the esophagus, papain has the potential to damage the esophageal lining, especially in people with esophageal disorders.

—*Lorraine Lica, Ph.D.*

See also Blood and blood disorders; Digestion; Enzymes; Fatty acid oxidation disorder; Fructosemia; Galactosemia; Gaucher's disease; Genetic diseases; Glycogen storage diseases; Heart attack; Leukemia; Metabolism; Mucopolysaccharidosis (MPS); Niemann-Pick disease; Oncology; Pharmacology; Strokes; Tay-Sachs disease; Thrombolytic therapy and TPA; Thrombosis and thrombus; Tumors.

FOR FURTHER INFORMATION:

Devlin, Thomas M., ed. *Textbook of Biochemistry: With Clinical Correlations.* 5th ed. New York: Wiley-Liss, 2002.

Rimoin, David L., et al., eds. *Emery and Rimoin's Principles and Practice of Medical Genetics.* 4th ed. New York: Churchill Livingstone, 2002.

Scriver, Charles R., et al., eds. *The Metabolic and Molecular Bases of Inherited Disease.* 8th ed. New York: McGraw-Hill, 2001.

ENZYMES
BIOLOGY

ANATOMY OR SYSTEM INVOLVED: Cells, immune system
SPECIALTIES AND RELATED FIELDS: Biochemistry, cytology, endocrinology, genetics, pharmacology
DEFINITION: Large molecules, produced by cells, that catalyze chemical reactions inside living organisms.

KEY TERMS:

active site: the part of an enzyme where the substrate is bound; this is the site where the reaction occurs
activity: a measure of the ability of an enzyme to catalyze its reaction
amino acid: the fundamental building blocks of proteins; there are twenty amino acids, each with a different chemistry
catalysis: increasing the speed of a chemical reaction
molecule: a collection of atoms bonded together; normally neutral because it has an equal number of protons and electrons
mutation: a substitution of one amino acid for another in the amino acid sequence of a protein
protein: large molecules made up of amino acids connected by peptide bonds; the sequence of amino acids in a protein determines its three-dimensional structure
substrates: reactants that enzymes convert into products; every enzyme is specific for one specific substrate

STRUCTURE AND FUNCTIONS

Enzymes are remarkable molecules because they increase rates of biochemical reactions. Each enzyme within a cell selectively speeds up, or catalyzes, one particular reaction or type of reaction. The vast majority of enzymes belong to the class of large molecules known as proteins. Proteins are built by combining amino acids. There are twenty amino acids, which can be divided into three classes: hydrophobic, charged, and polar. Hydrophobic amino acids behave chemically like oils, avoiding contact with water. Charged amino acids are ionic, containing one extra or one less electron than do neutral molecules. Polar amino acids are attracted to water and other polar amino acids. Each of these three classes of amino acids has a distinct chemistry. The specific order of the amino acid sequence defines the structure and function of every protein. Inside cells, enzymes catalyze reactions so that they occur millions of times faster than they would without the presence of these proteins. Each cell in the body produces many different enzymes. Different sets of enzymes are found in different tissues, reflecting the specialized function of each particular enzyme. Thousands of different enzymes are at work in the body; many have yet to be discovered.

Protein enzymes work by bringing the reactants in a chemical reaction together in the most favorable geometrical arrangement, so that bonds can be easily broken and reformed. This is possible because different enzymes have different three-dimensional shapes. It is the shape of the enzyme that determines its chemistry. Each enzyme combines with a specific substrate, or reactant, and catalyzes its characteristic reaction. When the reaction is over, the substrate has been converted into products. The enzyme remains unchanged, ready to catalyze another reaction with the next substrate molecule it encounters.

Enzymes play a significant role in treating diseases. Because enzymes have specific functions, a particular enzyme that has the required function to treat the disorder can be administered. Modern methods of genetic engineering allow the production of desired enzymes. Scientists can use bacteria as factories to produce large amounts of enzyme from an organism by copying the gene from the organism of interest into bacterial cells. The bacteria are then grown in culture, producing the enzyme of interest as they grow. This procedure is a much safer method than the old procedure of isolating enzyme from animal tissues, because the enzymes produced are free of viruses and other contaminants present in animal tissues. Proteins produced by genetic engineering techniques are called recombinant proteins.

Sometimes enzymes can be used as drugs for the treatment of specific diseases. Streptokinase is an enzyme mixture that is useful in clearing blood clots that occur in the heart and the lower extremities. Another useful enzyme for dissolving blood clots that occur as a result of heart attacks is human tissue plasminogen activator (TPA). Recombinant TPA is produced by genetic engineering techniques, using bacteria cultures to produce large quantities of human TPA. The administration of TPA within an hour of the formation of a blood clot in a coronary artery dramatically increases survival rates of heart attack victims. Some types of adult leukemia are treated by intravenous administration of the asparaginase enzyme. Tumor cells require the molecule asparagine to grow, and they scavenge it from the bloodstream. Asparaginase drastically reduces the amount of asparagine in the blood, thus slowing the growth of the tumor. Because most enzymes do not last long in blood, huge amounts of enzymes are required for therapeutic effects. In classic hemophilia, the factor VIII enzyme is missing or is genetically mutated so that it has a very low activity. This enzyme is essential for inducing the formation of blood clots. In the past, it was a laborious task to collect a concentrated blood plasma sample containing factor VIII, which was administered to hemophiliacs to stop hemorrhages.

This treatment carried the risk of infecting the patient with viruses that cause acquired immunodeficiency syndrome (AIDS), hepatitis, and other diseases. Purified recombinant factor VIII is now available. Because the recombinant human factor VIII is produced by bacteria, it cannot be infected with the viruses that cause hepatitis and AIDS.

A classic enzyme inhibitor used as a drug is penicillin. Penicillin was discovered in 1928 by Alexander Fleming, after he noticed that bacterial growth was prevented by a contaminating mold known as *Penicillium*. Ten years later, Howard Florey and Ernst Chain performed the key experiments that led to the isolation, characterization, and clinical use of this wonder drug antibiotic. In 1957, Joshua Lederberg showed that penicillin interferes with the synthesis of the cell walls of bacteria. In 1965, James Park and Jack Strominger independently discovered that penicillin blocks the last step in cell wall synthesis. The last step is the cross-linking of different strands of the wall and is catalyzed by the enzyme glycopeptide transpeptidase. The shape of penicillin resembles that of the normal substrate of glycopeptide transpeptidase, so that penicillin binds to the active site of the transpeptidase enzyme. Once bound to the active site, penicillin forms a permanent bond with one of the amino acid residues. This chemical reaction permanently inhibits the glycopeptide transpeptidase enzyme, thus preventing the transpeptidase from cross-linking the bacterial wall.

Several anticancer drugs work by blocking the synthesis of deoxythymidylate (dTMP), as an abundant supply of dTMP is required for rapid cell division to be sustained. Drugs that inhibit the enzymes thymidylate synthase and dihydrofolate reductase are very effective agents in cancer chemotherapy. Thymidylate synthase, which makes dTMP from deoxyuridylate, is irreversibly inhibited by the drug fluorouracil. This drug is converted into fluorodeoxyuridylate (F-dUMP), which chemically reacts with thymidylate synthase so that the enzyme can no longer function in its normal role of making dTMP from deoxyuridylate. The synthesis of dTMP can also be blocked by drugs that inhibit the enzyme dihydrofolate reductase. The normal substrate for dihydrofolate reductase is the molecule dihydrofolate. Drugs such as aminopterin and methotrexate bind to the active site of the reductase enzyme, inhibiting rapid cell growth. Methotrexate is very effective at inhibiting rapidly growing tumors such as acute leukemia and choriocarcinoma. Unfortunately methotrexate kills all rapidly dividing cells, including stem cells in

The Function of Some Enzymes

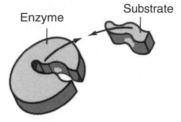

Enzyme

Substrate

An enzyme combines with a substrate that has molecules of a complementary shape.

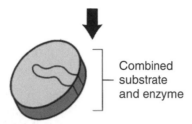

Combined substrate and enzyme

The interaction between the enzyme and substrate causes a chemical change in the substrate, splitting it in two.

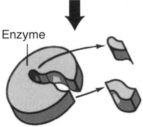

Enzyme

The enzyme is unchanged and can repeat the process with another substrate molecule.

bone marrow, epithelial cells of the intestinal tract, and hair follicles, which explains the many toxic side effects of this drug. Computer-aided drug design has been applied to the dihydrofolate reductase enzyme, with encouraging results.

The activity of an enzyme is a measure of how efficiently a particular enzyme catalyzes its reaction. A loss in activity corresponds to a decrease in catalytic efficiency, and an increase in activity corresponds to an increase in catalytic efficiency. Many drugs increase enzyme activity (enzyme induction), and many decrease enzyme activity (enzyme inhibition). Both enzyme induction and enzyme inhibition result from the interaction of the drug with the enzyme, altering the surface of the enzyme where the substrate normally is bound during catalysis. In enzyme induction, the surface is altered such that the substrate is bound tighter than usual, while in enzyme inhibition, the surface is altered so that the substrate cannot bind to the enzyme. The structures of many enzyme inhibitors are similar to the structures of substrates. Inhibitors bind at active sites of enzymes. Drugs that are enzyme inhibitors are very powerful medical tools, as they bind to the enzyme and are not easily removed.

Universities, government agencies, and pharmaceutical companies are continually seeking to develop drugs that specifically bind and inhibit enzymes responsible for disease. Much effort is spent trying to design drugs in a rational manner, using the most powerful tools of chemistry. Techniques such as X-ray crystallography, nuclear magnetic resonance (NMR) spectroscopy, and computational chemistry allow researchers to determine the shapes of enzymes, their substrates, and their inhibitors. These efforts allow the research team to design drugs that bind more specifically to the target enzyme, thus increasing the effectiveness and lowering the toxicity of the drug.

Disorders and Diseases

Defects in enzymes, known as mutations, can cause disease. A protein molecule is mutated when one or more of the original amino acids in the protein is replaced by a different amino acid. For example, if an enzyme consists of one hundred amino acids, and amino acid number 35 is changed from one kind of amino acid to a different kind, the protein is now a mutant. A mutated enzyme has a slightly altered shape compared to the original enzyme. If the change in shape causes the enzyme to perform its chemistry more slowly than the original enzyme, then the cell and tissue have an impaired function. In particular, if an amino acid is changed from one of the three classes (hydrophobic, charged, or polar) to a different class, then the mutation is more likely to cause a change in the structure and function of the enzyme. Not all mutations are harmful, but a single mutation in a key region of an enzyme can be fatal to a living organism.

Many diseases are diagnosed by measuring enzyme concentrations and activities in the body. Enzyme concentration refers to the amount of enzyme present, while enzyme activity refers to the ability of the enzyme to perform its chemistry. Enzyme concentrations and activities can be measured in blood or in tissue. Disease of tissues and organs can cause cellular damage, so that enzymes that are normally not present in significant quantities in blood are raised to very high levels as they flow from the damaged tissue into the blood plasma. Detection of particular enzymes in blood plasma indicates a diseased organ. The higher the concentration of enzyme in the blood, the more extensive the damage to that tissue or organ. The detection of these enzymes in the blood is a diagnostic tool, indicating a particular disorder. Genetic diseases caused by a mutation in an enzyme can be detected by laboratory tests that measure enzyme activity or enzyme shape.

Disease diagnosis is often made by measuring the concentration or activity of enzymes. Isozymes are enzymes that catalyze the same reaction but have slightly different structures. Most isozymes are enzymes consisting of two or more subunits, with different combinations of the subunits differentiating the isozymes. Isozymes of the enzymes lactate dehydrogenase, creatine kinase, and alkaline phosphatase are used for clinical applications. Monitoring of the isozyme concentrations and activities of lactate dehydrogenase and creatine kinase in the blood shows whether a patient has suffered a heart attack. Creatine kinase consists of two subunits. The two possible subunits are M, which stands for muscle type, and B, which stands for brain type. There are three possible isozymes: MM, BB, and MB. The MM isozyme consists of two M subunits and is the only isozyme found in skeletal muscle, the BB isozyme consists of two B subunits and is the only isozyme found in the brain, and the MB isozyme consists of one M and one B subunit and is found only in the heart. Lactate dehydrogenase consists of four subunits, made from five combinations of two subunits. The two subunits are the heart subunit, designated by H, and the muscle subunit, designated by M. The HHHH and HHHM isozymes are found in the heart and in red blood cells, the HHMM isozyme is found in the brain and kidney, and the MMMM isozyme is found in the liver and skeletal muscle. After a heart attack, the cellular breakup of heart tissue releases the MB isozyme of creatine kinase into the bloodstream within six to eighteen hours. Release of lactate dehydrogenase into the blood is slower than that of creatine kinase, occurring one to two days after the appearance of creatine kinase. In a healthy person, the activity of the HHHM isozyme of lactate dehydrogenase is higher than that of the HHHH isozyme. In heart attack victims, however, the activity of the HHHH isozyme becomes greater than that of the HHHM isozyme between twelve and twenty-four hours after the attack. Measurement of increased concentration of the MB isozyme a short while after a suspected heart attack, followed by the switch in lactate

dehydrogenase activity between the HHHH and HHHM isozymes, indicates that a heart attack occurred. Secondary complications of a heart attack can also be followed with isozyme measurements. For example, increased activity of the MMMM isozyme of lactate dehydrogenase is an indication of liver congestion.

Certain medical conditions can be screened by using immobilized enzymes as reagents in desktop clinical analyzers. For example, screening tests for cholesterol and triglycerides can be completed in a few minutes using 0.01 milliliter of blood plasma. The enzymes cholesterol oxidase and lipase are immobilized, or fixed in place, in a detection kit. If cholesterol is present, cholesterol oxidase breaks off hydrogen peroxide from the cholesterol. The enzyme peroxidase and a colorless dye are included in the detection kit, and peroxidase catalyzes the reaction of the colorless dye and hydrogen peroxide to form a colored dye that can be easily measured from the amount of light reflected from the solution. The enzyme lipase allows the accurate determination of triglycerides in blood.

A mutation in a protein that acts as a natural inhibitor of an enzyme can cause disease. For example, emphysema is a destructive lung disease in which the alveolar walls of the lungs are destroyed by an enzyme known as elastase. A person with emphysema breathes much harder to exchange the same volume of air because the alveoli, or air pockets, have become much less efficient. Normally, the elastase enzyme is prevented from destroying lung tissue by the protein antitrypsin. Antitrypsin is made in the liver and flows to the lungs, where it binds to the active site of elastase and prevents it from digesting lung tissue. Emphysema can occur when the negatively charged amino acid at position 53 of the amino acid sequence of antitrypsin is replaced with a positively charged amino acid. This mutation changes the chemical nature of antitrypsin such that the mutant antitrypsin is released from the liver at a much slower rate. The level of this mutant antitrypsin in the lungs is 15 percent of the normal level. The net result of this one amino acid mutation in the antitrypsin protein is that most of the elastase enzyme is free to destroy lung tissue. Cigarette smoking dramatically increases the incidence of emphysema in people who have the mutant antitrypsin. Cigarette smoke reacts with the hydrophobic amino acid at position 358 of antitrypsin, adding one oxygen atom at this position in the amino acid sequence. The addition of this one extra oxygen atom at this critical place in antitrypsin changes the chemical nature of the hydrophobic amino acid so that the antitrypsin no longer can bind to elastase. Because only 15 percent of the mutant antitrypsin gets from the liver to the lungs in the first place, cigarette smoking puts people with this particular mutation at grave risk for developing emphysema.

PERSPECTIVE AND PROSPECTS

Enzymatic reactions have been used by humankind since prehistoric times. It has been known for more than six thousand years that fermentation processes transform grapes into wine, but it was not until the nineteenth century that it was understood that the conversion of grape sugar to alcohol is a process catalyzed by enzymes found in yeast. In the 1700's, Antoine Lavoisier showed that a solution of sugar could be fermented if provided with the sediment of a previous fermentation and that the sugar was converted to alcohol and carbon dioxide in this process. At this time, it was thought that there was a vital force responsible for the workings of a living cell. This notion of a vital force slowed the development of the discipline of biochemistry considerably, as many good scientists struggled to understand the fermentation process. In 1828, Friedrich Wöhler synthesized urea in a test tube, providing strong evidence against the concept of a vital force. In 1833, Anselme Payen and Jean Persoz discovered the first enzyme, diastase (now known as amylase), which converted starch into sugar. The next year, Johann Eberle showed that the presence of a stomach is not required for gastric digestion to take place. In 1836, Theodor Schwann made the very important discovery that the active ingredient in digestion, which he called pepsin, could be extracted from the stomach wall.

The next year, Jöns Jakob Berzelius developed the idea of catalysis, making the point that both living and inorganic systems had catalysts. In the late 1850's, Louis Pasteur confirmed and extended the earlier experiments of Schwann. Despite his brilliant experimental abilities, however, Pasteur was handicapped in his research by his belief that fermentation could happen only within a living organism. In 1860, Marcelin Berthelot showed that a living being was not the ferment, but produced the ferment, in sharp contrast to Pasteur's vitalist ideas. Pasteur's response to this work was that Berthelot and he meant different things by the use of the word "ferment." Moritz Traube, a German wine merchant, realized that chemical processes and living bodies were mostly based on ferment actions, and he published these ideas in 1858 and again in 1878. In 1878, Friedrich Kühne proposed that to remove the discrepancy over the meaning of the word "ferment," the word "enzyme" should be used, as it means "in yeast." It was not until 1897 that Eduard Buchner showed that living cells are not essential for fermentation to occur, as he extracted from yeast a cell-free juice containing the entire fermentation system.

From 1894 to 1898, Emil Fischer used synthetic organic chemistry for the preparation of substrates of known structure and configuration. He showed that enzymes have a very high degree of specificity for their own particular substrate and developed the famous "lock-and-key" hypothesis. This theory, which has been only slightly modified, states that the shape of a substrate and the enzyme's active site must be complementary for catalysis to occur. Purification of enzymes remained a difficult problem, and it was not until 1926 that James Summer crystallized the first enzyme, jack bean urease. The sequence of protein enzymes could be determined experimentally after 1952, when Frederick Sanger developed his methods for amino acid sequencing. In 1965, David Phillips produced the first three-dimensional picture of an enzyme, determining the shape of lysozyme. The advent of genetic engineering techniques in the 1970's revolutionized the field of enzyme research and the use of enzymes in medical applications by enabling the production of copious amounts of recombinant proteins.

—*George C. Shields, Ph.D.*

See also Antibiotics; Bacteriology; Blood and blood disorders; Blood testing; Cholesterol; Digestion; Emphysema; Enzyme therapy; Fatty acid oxidation disorders; Food biochemistry; Fructosemia; Gaucher's disease; Genetic diseases; Genetic engineering; Genetics and inheritance; Glycogen storage diseases; Glycolysis; Hemophilia; Laboratory tests; Leukemia; Maple syrup urine disease (MSUD); Metabolism; Mucopolysaccharidosis (MPS); Mutation; Niemann-Pick disease; Oncology; Pharmacology; Pulmonary medicine; Screening; Tay-Sachs disease; Thrombolytic therapy and TPA.

FOR FURTHER INFORMATION:

Campbell, Neil A. *Biology: Concepts and Connections*. 6th ed. San Francisco: Benjamin/Cummings, 2002. This classic introductory textbook provides an excellent discussion of essential biological structures and mechanisms. Its extensive and detailed illustrations help to make even difficult concepts accessible to the nonspecialist. Of particular interest is the chapter on enzymes, titled "An Introduction to Metabolism."

Copeland, Robert Allen. *Enzymes: A Practical Introduction to Structure, Mechanism, and Data Analysis.* 2d ed. New York: Wiley, 2000. An introductory text that examines the structural complexities of proteins and enzymes and the mechanisms by which enzymes perform their catalytic functions.

Fruton, Joseph S. *Molecules and Life.* New York: Wiley-Interscience, 1972. Fruton, a Yale biochemist, has filled his book with historical essays on the interplay of chemistry and biology. The first part of the book, "From Ferments to Enzymes," is an interesting account of how science progressed from the known results of fermentation to the chemical knowledge that enzymes were the molecules responsible for this and all other biochemical processes.

Kornberg, Arthur. *For the Love of Enzymes.* Cambridge, Mass.: Harvard University Press, 1989. Both an autobiography of a great biochemist and a history of the study of enzymes. Arthur Kornberg won a Nobel Prize for the laboratory synthesis of deoxyribonucleic acid (DNA). An excellent scientific biography.

Liska, Ken. *Drugs and the Human Body with Implications for Society.* Englewood Cliffs, N.J.: Prentice Hall, 2003. An easy-to-read book about the effects of drugs on the human body. A good overview of how drugs interact with various molecules in the body, including many cases in which enzymes are drug targets.

Palmer, Trevor. *Understanding Enzymes.* 4th ed. London: Prentice Hall, 1995. A standard text on enzymes and how they function. Includes a bibliography and an index.

Richard B. Silverman. *Organic Chemistry of Enzyme-Catalyzed Reactions.* Rev. ed. New York: Elsevier, 2002. A text that examines the general mechanisms used by enzymes and stresses that enzymology is simply a biological application of physical organic chemistry.

Voet, Donald, and Judith G. Voet. *Biochemistry.* Rev. ed. New York: Wiley, 2002. A text that approaches biochemistry via organic chemistry reactions.

EPIDEMIOLOGY

SPECIALTY

ANATOMY OR SYSTEM AFFECTED: All

SPECIALTIES AND RELATED FIELDS: Environmental health, microbiology, pathology, public health

DEFINITION: The scientific study of the distribution of disease in human populations, as well as its causes and effects.

KEY TERMS:

endemic disease: a disease which is usually present in a population and whose frequency does not fluctuate greatly

epidemic: a marked increase in the frequency of a disease in a population, compared to historical experience

infectivity: the ability of an organism to enter and reproduce within a host

pathogenicity: the ability of an organism to cause disease

virulence: a measure of the severity of disease

SCIENCE AND PROFESSION

While etiology studies the causes of disease in individuals, epidemiology studies the causes and effects of disease in populations. Historically, epidemics of contagious disease have been one of the most important causes of human mortality and have played a profound role in influencing human history; the emergence of acquired immunodeficiency syndrome (AIDS) and the resurgence of other epidemic diseases have demonstrated the continuing importance of epidemiology to medical science.

An epidemic is characterized by a large increase in the frequency of a disease within a population. Until relatively recently, the term was used primarily for outbreaks of contagious diseases caused by infectious agents, but current epidemiology also concerns itself with environmentally caused diseases, such as radiation-induced cancers, and with mental and behavioral problems, such as drug use. Outbreaks of diseases in plants and animals are also loosely termed epidemics but are more properly termed epiphytotics and epizootics, respectively.

The defining characteristic of an epidemic is not the absolute frequency of the disease or its severity, but the abrupt increase in its frequency. In contrast, an endemic disease is one whose frequency within a population does not vary markedly with time. An epidemic may be local in scope and limited in its effects; an endemic disease may be widespread and an important source of mortality within a population. The extreme case is a pandemic, an epidemic which transcends national boundaries and affects huge numbers of individuals on a worldwide basis. The most notorious pandemics in recorded history were the bubonic plague that swept Eurasia in the fourteenth century, killing an estimated one-third of the population of Europe, and the influenza epidemic of 1918-1919, which killed approximately 20 million people worldwide. The AIDS epidemic, not recognized in the United States and Europe as a major public health threat until the early 1980's, has reached pandemic status; because of its predominantly sexual mode of transmission and relatively low infectivity, however, the number of infected individuals is far lower than would be the case for a disease transmitted by casual contact.

Epidemics have played an important role in human life since the dawn of recorded history. Studies of animal populations and of primitive hunting communities, however, suggest that epidemics are more a burden of civilization than a part of the human condition, because effective spread of disease between humans requires high population densities. A virulent, easily transmitted pathogen simply cannot be sustained in a self-contained group of a few dozen or hundred individuals who have few contacts with the world at large. Even with the advent of agriculture and settled life, the inhabitants of the Americas, Australia, and Oceania enjoyed relative freedom from epidemic diseases before the coming of Europeans. Although human pathogens are derived from animal pathogens—many of them, presumably, through long coevolution with humans and their hominid ancestors, others through mutations in more recent times—the most common animal reservoirs of human disease are those animals most closely related to humans. Thus Africa and tropical Asia, home to the great apes and humankind's immediate ancestors, have always harbored the greatest diversity of human pathogens, while Australia and isolated Pacific islands had very few.

The devastating effect of the introduction of Eurasian and African diseases, chiefly of an epidemic nature, into Australia, Oceania, and the Americas eclipses even the great plague pandemic of the 1300's in its historical impact. The decimation of native populations in these areas under European influence must be ascribed first to disease and second to impoverishment and social dislocation, with direct military action as a poor, insignificant third. In the period between 1770 and 1870, the native population of Hawaii declined by 90 percent, and the native population of Tasmania became extinct. As much as 50 percent of Mexico's estimated pre-Columbian population of 25 million may have perished of smallpox and other epidemic diseases during and immediately after the Spanish Conquest; a hundred years later, the population had declined by 90 percent. In contrast, European colonial activity in West Africa and Southeast Asia did not result in precipitous native population decline.

Surveying a wide variety of historical evidence, William McNeill concluded that the historical experience of Mexico and Hawaii represented the usual result of the confluence of disease pools and the introduction of a virulent pathogen into a previously unexposed population: destruction of 30 percent to 50 percent of the population in a few years, followed by more gradual decline until the remaining human population becomes genetically resistant, the pathogen disappears because of a lack of hosts, or the human population becomes extinct. Parallels to the Amerindian experience can be found in Japan, where diseases (principally the plague) introduced from China killed half the population in the eighth century; in medieval Europe; and perhaps in late antiquity, according to McNeill's hypothesis that the depopulation of the Roman Empire between 150 and 400 was caused by measles and smallpox introduced from the Orient.

The nature and severity of an epidemic of infectious disease are influenced by the nature of the pathogen and by the physical and social makeup of the affected population. Characteristics of the pathogen include transmissibility (the ease with which a pathogen is passed from one host to another), infectivity (its ability to grow and multiply in that host), pathogenicity (its ability to produce clinical disease), and virulence (the severity of the disease produced). The worst epidemic diseases, such as smallpox, are highly transmissible, infective, pathogenic, and virulent. Chickenpox is highly transmissible and infective but not very virulent. Diseases that are not highly transmissible, such as leprosy, or are selectively pathogenic, such as tuberculosis, are more likely to be endemic than epidemic.

Each infectious disease has characteristic modes of transmission that must be understood for the purpose of disease prevention. Respiratory diseases transmitted as airborne particles—smallpox, influenza, measles, pneumonic plague—spread rapidly and are difficult to control through sanitation and quarantine. Diseases spread through fecal contamination of water and food—cholera, hepatitis, typhoid, poliomyelitis—are more easily avoided and, in industrialized countries, tend to occur in localized outbreaks with identifiable sources. Blood-borne diseases transmitted by biting arthropods—malaria, yellow fever, typhus, bubonic plague—can erupt in devastating epidemics when both host and vector populations are high. Localized outbreaks of arthropod-transmitted diseases that have natural animal reservoirs (including yellow fever, St. Louis encephalitis, bubonic plague, murine typhus, and

Lyme disease) occur throughout the world, but human-to-human chains of transmission are most likely to occur in Third World countries beset by social upheaval. The spread of sexually transmitted diseases is also aided by war and social dislocation. The transmission of blood-borne viral diseases through contaminated hypodermic needles became significant in the latter part of the twentieth century.

Human resistance to disease is a function of genetic makeup, age, and general health. The impact of a measles epidemic illustrates these relationships. Europeans, through many generations of epidemics that killed the most susceptible individuals, inherit an immune system which is effective at fighting this virus. Disease resistance decreases with increasing age. Although no specific treatment for measles existed until a vaccine was developed in the 1960's, mortality rates in the United States declined dramatically between 1850 and 1950 as a result of improved nutrition and housing and better nursing care. The mortality rate of untreated measles among American children in the 1950's was one in two hundred or three hundred, among poor European slum dwellers in the nineteenth century was one in twenty or thirty, and among Amerindians and Polynesians, who were both impoverished and lacking genetic resistance, was one in two or three.

Diseases caused by behavioral and environmental factors can also be viewed as occurring in epidemics. A major explanation for the increased prominence of noninfectious diseases as causes of mortality and morbidity has been an increasing life span; the cumulative effects of environmental toxins and unhealthy behavior exhibit themselves only as an individual ages. The age-specific frequency of Alzheimer's disease in the United States remained relatively constant in the twentieth century, but because of increasing longevity, the frequency increased dramatically.

Both longevity and changes in behavior contributed to the increase in mortality from lung cancer in industrialized countries in the twentieth century. The various lines of investigation linking this epidemic to tobacco smoking are a good example of epidemiological research. Recent increases in the incidence of skin cancer seem to be linked partly to the popularity of sunbathing and partly to increases in ultraviolet radiation caused by pollution.

Localized clusters of disease and mortality often point to a single environmental hazard. The long-term adverse effects of lead, asbestos, and herbicides have been identified and characterized based on observa-tions of groups of peoples with high levels of exposure to these substances.

DIAGNOSTIC AND TREATMENT TECHNIQUES

Epidemiologists may be actively involved in the diagnosis and collection of field data, or they may rely on data submitted by physicians, hospitals, and public health workers. The data generated by the study of epidemiology are used for a variety of purposes: to suggest hypotheses and avenues of research in the case of a condition whose cause or causes (etiology) are unknown, to assist health care workers in diagnosis and treatment, to encourage private and public agencies to adopt policies to slow the spread of disease, and to influence public and private policy so as to reduce underlying social and environmental causes of disease.

Cultural practices that have their root in informal epidemiological observation and serve to accomplish one of the four aims outlined above can be found throughout history. For example, not eating pork is a way of preventing the transmission of trichinosis. Mongols, who avoided trapping marmots in the belief that they were the reincarnations of deceased ancestors, were less likely to contract bubonic plague than the Chinese, who had no such cultural taboo. Scientific epidemiology, which relies on a correct understanding of the causes of disease, dates from the mid-nineteenth century. The classic pioneering study is that of John Snow, who conducted a thorough investigation of cholera cases during an epidemic in London in 1854. By mapping the distribution of cases, he was able to link them to specific contaminated water sources. He recommended the boiling of drinking water, strict hygiene in the tending of infected patients, and better sanitation in food preparation; the result was real progress in reducing the severity of that and subsequent epidemics. It is interesting to note that the understanding of the etiology of certain major plant diseases (wheat stem rust, bunt, potato blight) and the epidemiological recommendations for their control antedate corresponding developments in human diseases by a half century.

The discoveries by Robert Koch, Louis Pasteur, and others linking specific microorganisms to human disease ushered in an era when the most effective method for improving human health was the prevention of infection, principally through epidemiological public health measures. Sewage treatment, water purification, and the inspection of food preparation facilities reduced the incidence of cholera, typhoid, and hepatitis; draining and channeling stagnant water to control mosquitoes made malaria and yellow fever rare diseases in the United States and southern Europe. The pesticide DDT (although subsequently condemned because of the serious environmental problems that it caused) performed a laudable service to human health in the aftermath of World War II, killing the vectors of louse-borne typhus and other diseases.

In the field of nontransmissible disease, the early twentieth century saw great progress in the understanding of nutritional deficiencies. Pellagra (a niacin deficiency) and scurvy (a vitamin C deficiency) may still occur in epidemics among institutionalized persons, but they are treated with simple dietary methods.

Today, the World Health Organization of the United Nations coordinates epidemiological efforts between nations and within poorer countries that do not have the resources to address their internal epidemiological problems. Most countries have a central agency which monitors the occurrence of disease within the country; states, provinces, and other political divisions also have epidemiological public health agencies. In countries with a national health service, the activities of primary care physicians and clinics are closely coordinated with public health administration.

Statistics are the raw material of epidemiological investigation. Death certificates record both the primary and contributing causes of death, the age and sex of the deceased, and the place of death. Census figures give a picture of the community in which epidemiological events occur, such as its racial and socioeconomic composition, age structure, and population density. Physicians and hospitals are required to notify the public health authorities of the occurrence of certain "reportable" diseases, such as AIDS, syphilis, and tuberculosis. Hospital admission records will reflect increases in conditions requiring hospitalization, while school and workplace attendance figures reflect outbreaks of milder communicable diseases.

Some outbreaks are routine and predictable, and the measures for controlling them are well established. When influenza cases increase, public health authorities identify the strain responsible and take steps to immunize those individuals who are most at risk for severe disease. Identifying the source of contaminated food or water is critical to controlling outbreaks of hepatitis A and typhoid in industrialized countries. When war or natural disaster disrupts the normal infrastructure of modern life, it is considered prudent to inoculate the affected population against a variety of infectious diseases.

The history of the discovery of Lyme disease illustrates how epidemiology works. Physician and hospital records indicated a clustering of cases diagnosed as juvenile arthritis near Lyme, Connecticut. By comparing the cases and observing their common characteristics, epidemiologists deduced that an arthropod-transmitted organism normally found on wild animals was probably responsible. Armed with this information, they surveyed microorganisms found in biting arthropods and were able to establish that the same spirochete was found in wild deer, deer ticks, and patients exhibiting symptoms of juvenile arthritis. This organism, and the chronic disease that it causes, proved to be widespread, although not particularly common among humans. Knowing the etiology of the disease enabled physicians to diagnose the condition correctly and to treat it.

Environmentally and behaviorally caused diseases are less amenable to control by health professionals alone, and consequently can prove much more intractable. This is particularly true when there are powerful economic factors working at cross purposes to disease control measures. The epidemiologist can demonstrate that the increase in lung cancer in the twentieth century paralleled an increase in tobacco consumption and that smokers account for most cases of lung cancer. The biomedical investigator studying etiology can show that tobacco derivatives cause cancer in laboratory animals and may ultimately be able to explain how this is brought about at the molecular level. Physicians can advise patients not to smoke, and psychologists can devise therapies to help people quit smoking. None of these efforts, however, will achieve definitive success as long as there are powerful forces encouraging people to smoke and undermining the efforts of the health professionals. The difficulty is compounded, as with any addictive drug, by the active participation of the very people who are the victims of the epidemic in perpetuating the conditions that favor it.

PERSPECTIVE AND PROSPECTS

Tremendous progress was made in controlling epidemic disease over the course of the twentieth century, so much so that there was a period when epidemics of life-threatening contagious diseases were viewed as past history in industrialized countries and there was optimism that the same result could be achieved in the Third World as well. The gradual elimination of smallpox was viewed as a model. A worldwide scourge until vaccination was discovered in the eighteenth century, smallpox had become rare in Europe and the United

States by the end of the nineteenth century. In the 1960's, when the World Health Organization embarked on a worldwide campaign to eliminate smallpox, it was endemic only in parts of Africa and India. Since 1980, no new cases have been reported worldwide. Poliomyelitis, the subject of a massive worldwide inoculation campaign, was declared to be absent from the Western Hemisphere in 1989. With diseases for which an effective vaccine is available, it is possible at relatively low cost to inoculate a high proportion of the population, breaking the chain of infection. Water purification and the destruction of insect vectors are also effective in reducing disease incidence.

Yet the worldwide epidemic of AIDS and the resurgence of malaria, tuberculosis, and cholera as epidemic diseases in the late twentieth century are ample evidence that the epidemiological battle against disease is far from won, and that medical science's current arsenal of weapons against infectious disease has serious inadequacies. The factors favoring an increase in epidemics of transmissible disease in the last decades of the twentieth century included an increase in the speed and frequency of international travel, the emergence of drug-resistant strains of a wide variety of pathogens, and a high level of political and social instability in developing nations. Some scientists believe that increasing exploitation of tropical rain forests is responsible for bringing humans into contact with the diseases of nonhuman primates, which then have the potential to spread throughout the world. Such is probably the case with AIDS, whose spread from a center of origin in tropical Africa was aided by the fact that infected individuals can carry and transmit the virus for years without exhibiting clinical symptoms of disease. Most methods of preventing and treating viral illnesses in humans rely on bolstering the normal human immune response, so a virus which undermines this response poses a difficult challenge to medical science.

AIDS is only one notable example of dozens of tropical diseases that have the potential for causing lethal worldwide epidemics. Commenting on Ebola virus, a virulent pathogen responsible for a 1976 epidemic in Zaire in which 90 percent of the victims died, a prominent virologist confessed to being afraid and noted that "fortunately, Ebola does not have a significant respiratory component, or the world would be a far different place today. There would be a lot fewer of us." A related virus, lethal to monkeys and infective but nonvirulent in humans, swept a primate quarantine facility in Mary-

land, and another member of this virus group caused a localized lethal epidemic among monkeys and laboratory workers in Marburg, Germany. Many other lethal transmissible viruses have been identified.

AIDS, the widespread use of immunosuppressant drugs, and the aging of the population have created significant numbers of individuals who have weakened immune systems and are susceptible to infection by animal pathogens. It is worth noting that the worst pandemic in recorded human history, the fourteenth century bubonic plague epidemic, occurred when an animal pathogen became established in a human population and then mutated from a moderately transmissible, arthropod-borne disease to a highly transmissible, airborne infection. The likelihood that animal pathogens will spread to humans and that they will be disseminated internationally is increasing, and the chances of a mutation toward increased transmissibility or virulence increases with the number of infected individuals. The potential for a worldwide pandemic capable of overwhelming the efforts of modern medical science certainly exists, although its probability cannot be estimated.

—*Martha Sherwood-Pike, Ph.D.*

See also Acquired immunodeficiency syndrome (AIDS); Anthrax; Arthropod-borne diseases; Bacterial infections; Bacteriology; Biological and chemical weapons; Biostatistics; Centers for Disease Control and Prevention (CDC); Childhood infectious diseases; Cholera; Creutzfeldt-Jakob disease (CJD); Disease; *E. coli* infection; Ebola virus; Elephantiasis; Environmental diseases; Environmental health; Food poisoning; Forensic pathology; Hanta virus; Hepatitis; Influenza; Laboratory tests; Legionnaires' disease; Leprosy; Lice, mites, and ticks; Malaria; Measles; Microbiology; National Institutes of Health; Necrotizing fasciitis; Noroviruses; Occupational health; Parasitic diseases; Pathology; Plague; Poisoning; Poliomyelitis; Prion diseases; Pulmonary diseases; Rabies; Salmonella infection; Severe acute respiratory syndrome (SARS); Sexually transmitted diseases (STDs); Stress; Tropical medicine; Veterinary medicine; Viral infections; World Health Organization; Yellow fever; Zoonoses.

FOR FURTHER INFORMATION:

Alcamo, I. Edward. *Microbes and Society: An Introduction to Microbiology.* Sudbury, Mass.: Jones and Bartlett, 2002. A nonscientific text for the liberal arts student that explores the importance of microbes to human life and their role in food production and agriculture, in biotechnology and industry, in ecology and the environment, and in disease and bioterrorism.

Bhopal, Raj S. *Concepts of Epidemiology: An Integrated Introduction to the Ideas, Theories, Principles, and Methods of Epidemiology.* New York: Oxford University Press, 2002. Discusses the language, principles, and methods underlying the science of epidemiology and examines its applications to policy making, health service planning, and health promotion.

Gerstman, B. Burt. *Epidemiology Kept Simple: An Introduction to Classic and Modern Epidemiology.* 2d ed. New York: Wiley, 2003. Accessible, introductory text on the subject. Includes practical exercises, case studies, and real-world applications.

Giesecke, Johan. *Modern Infectious Disease Epidemiology.* 2d ed. London: Hodder Arnold, 2001. Divided into two sections, the first covers the tools and principles of epidemiology from an infectious disease perspective. The second covers the role of contact pattern from an assessment angle, exploring such topics as infectivity, incubation periods, sero-epidemiology, and immunity.

Goldsmid, John. *The Deadly Legacy: Australian History and Transmissible Disease.* Kensington, New South Wales, Australia: New South Wales University Press, 1988. This book discusses the disease history of Aborigines and settlers, as well as the history of government efforts to control epidemics from the early nineteenth century to the late twentieth century, with good coverage of the control measures in effect in 1988.

Preston, Richard. "A Reporter at Large: Crisis in the Hot Zone." *The New Yorker* 68 (October 26, 1992): 58. Focusing on how U.S. government epidemiologists controlled an outbreak of deadly Ebola virus in a primate quarantine facility in Maryland, this article gives a good overview of the various "new" human diseases that have surfaced, including AIDS, and the worldwide threat that they pose.

Ranger, Terence, and Paul Slack, eds. *Epidemics and Ideas: Essays on the Historical Perception of Pestilence.* Cambridge, England: Cambridge University Press, 1997. A collection of papers describing the interplay among perceptions of the etiology of disease, social and religious attitudes, and politics in epidemics from classical antiquity to the present.

Timmreck, Thomas C. *An Introduction to Epidemiology.* 3d ed. Boston: Jones and Bartlett, 2002. A book in the Jones and Bartlett series in health sciences. Discusses epidemiological methods. Includes a bibliography and an index.

EPIGLOTTITIS

DISEASE/DISORDER

ALSO KNOWN AS: Supraglottitis

ANATOMY OR SYSTEM AFFECTED: Respiratory system, throat

SPECIALTIES AND RELATED FIELDS: Bacteriology, emergency medicine, family practice, internal medicine, pediatrics

DEFINITION: An acute, life-threatening inflammation of the epiglottis.

CAUSES AND SYMPTOMS

Epiglottitis is an acute, severe infection that commonly affects children between ages two and six. It is most commonly caused by the bacterium *Haemophilus influenzae*, but it can also be caused by other bacteria such as *Staphylococcus aureus* or *Streptococcus pneumoniae*, fungi such as *Candida albicans*, and viruses.

Epiglottitis presents classically with a fever and sore throat in a young child, who progresses rapidly within a few hours to an inability to eat and drooling, with signs of respiratory obstruction such as stridor. The epiglottis is a thin flap of cartilage at the back of the tongue that closes the respiratory tract while swallowing. When it is inflamed, considerable swelling and consequent respiratory obstruction result. Drooling occurs as the child is unable to swallow his or her own saliva. This is an emergency situation, as the respiratory distress can progress rapidly and become life-threatening within minutes.

It is strongly advised that the mouth and larynx not be examined using a tongue depressor, as this could

---

INFORMATION ON EPIGLOTTITIS

CAUSES: Usually bacterial infection; sometimes fungal or viral infection

SYMPTOMS: Sore throat, fever, inability to eat, drooling, stridor

DURATION: Acute

TREATMENTS: Hospitalization, humidified oxygen, antibiotics, intravenous fluids, corticosteroids, emergency tracheostomy if needed

precipitate a spasm of the epiglottis and exacerbate respiratory distress. Epiglottitis is diagnosed by a clinician through laryngoscopy, with efforts made to secure the airway first. Neck X rays reveal a characteristic "thumbprint" sign caused by an enlarged epiglottis. A blood culture may reveal the causative organism, and an elevated white blood cell count may be observed.

TREATMENT AND THERAPY

In most cases of epiglottitis, hospitalization is required, and the patient is usually admitted to the intensive care unit (ICU). The foremost concern is to secure and maintain an airway as soon as possible. Humidified oxygen, which has been moistened to help the patient breathe better, is administered. An emergency tracheostomy or needle cricothyrotomy may be needed to secure the airway. Antibiotics, intravenous fluids, and corticosteroids may also be administered to decrease the swelling. With proper and prompt treatment, the prognosis is very good.

PERSPECTIVE AND PROSPECTS

Epiglottitis, which was first described in 1848, is an acute inflammation of the epiglottis that should be distinguished from laryngotracheobronchitis or croup. Also, children ingesting hot liquids may present with similar symptoms. The disease must be managed efficiently and in a clinical setting only. Since the causative agent of the disease is infectious, family members must also be screened and treated for the disease. The aggressive immunization of children against *Haemophilus influenzae B* by the *Hib* vaccine has resulted in a significant decrease in the incidence of epiglottitis.

—*Venkat Raghavan Tirumala, M.D., M.H.A.*

See also Antibiotics; Bacterial infections; Childhood infectious diseases; Choking; Otorhinolaryngology; Pulmonary medicine, pediatric; Respiration; Sore throat.

FOR FURTHER INFORMATION:

Braunwald, Eugene, et al., eds. *Harrison's Principles of Internal Medicine*. 15th ed. New York: McGraw-Hill, 2001.

Rakel, Robert E., ed. *Textbook of Family Practice*. 6th ed. Philadelphia: W. B. Saunders, 2002.

Tapley, Donald F., et al., eds. *The Columbia University College of Physicians and Surgeons Complete Home Medical Guide*. 3d rev. ed. New York: Crown, 1995.

EPILEPSY
DISEASE/DISORDER
ANATOMY OR SYSTEM AFFECTED: Brain, head, nerves, nervous system
SPECIALTIES AND RELATED FIELDS: Neurology
DEFINITION: A serious neurologic disease characterized by seizures, which may involve convulsions and loss of consciousness.
KEY TERMS:
anticonvulsant: a therapeutic drug that prevents or diminishes convulsions
aura: a sensory symptom or group of such symptoms that precedes a grand mal seizure
clonic phase: the portion of an epileptic seizure that is characterized by convulsions
electroencephalogram (EEG): a graphic recording of the electrical activity of the brain, as recorded by an electroencephalograph
grand mal: a type of epileptic seizure characterized by severe convulsions, body stiffening, and loss of consciousness during which victims fall down; also called tonic-clonic seizure
idiopathic disease: a disease of unknown origin
petit mal: a mild type of epileptic seizure characterized by a very short lapse of consciousness, usually without convulsions; the epileptic does not fall down
seizure: a sudden convulsive attack of epilepsy that can involve loss of consciousness and falling down
seizure discharges: characteristic brain waves seen in the EEGs of epileptics; their strength and frequency depend upon whether a seizure is occurring and its type
status epilepticus: a rare, life-threatening condition in which many sequential seizures occur without recovery between them
tonic-clonic seizure: another term for a grand mal seizure
tonic phase: the portion of an epileptic seizure characterized by loss of consciousness and body stiffness

CAUSES AND SYMPTOMS

Epilepsy is characterized by seizures, commonly called fits, which may involve convulsions and the loss of consciousness. It was called the "falling disease" or "sacred disease" in antiquity and was mentioned in 2080 B.C.E. in the laws of the famous Babylonian king Hamurabi. Epilepsy is a serious neurologic disease that usually appears between the ages of two and fourteen. It does not affect intelligence, as shown by the fact that the range of intelligence quotients (IQs) for epileptics is quite similar to that of the general population. In addition, many suspected epileptics have achieved fame, such as Alexander the Great, Julius Caesar, Russian novelist Fyodor Dostoevski, and Dutch artist Vincent van Gogh.

In 400 B.C.E., Hippocrates of Cos proposed that epilepsy arose from physical problems in the brain. This origin of the disease is now known to be unequivocally true. Despite many centuries of exhaustive study and effort, however, only a small percentage (20 percent) of cases of epilepsy caused by brain injuries, brain tumors, and other diseases are curable. This type of epilepsy is called symptomatic epilepsy. In contrast, 80 percent of epileptics can be treated to control the occurrence of seizures but cannot be cured of the disease, which is therefore a lifelong affliction. In these cases, the basis of the epilepsy is not known, although the suspected cause is genetically programmed brain damage that still evades discovery. Most epilepsy is, therefore, an idiopathic disease (one of unknown origin), and such epileptics are thus said to suffer from idiopathic epilepsy.

A common denominator in idiopathic epilepsy, and also in symptomatic epilepsy, is that it is evidenced by unusual electrical discharges, brain waves, seen in the electroencephalograms (EEGs) of epileptics. These brain waves are called seizure discharges. They vary in both their strength and their frequency, depending on whether an epileptic is having a seizure and what type of seizure is occurring. Seizure discharges are almost always present and recognizable in the EEGs of epileptics, even during sleep.

There are four types of common epileptic seizures. Two of these are partial (local) seizures called focal motor and temporal lobe seizures, respectively. The others, grand mal and petit mal, are generalized and may involve the entire body. A focal motor seizure is characterized by rhythmic jerking of the facial muscles, an arm, or a leg. As with other epileptic seizures, it is caused by abnormal electrical discharges in the portion of the brain that controls normal movement in the body part that is affected. This abnormal electrical activity is always seen as seizure discharges in the EEG of the affected part of the brain.

In contrast, temporal lobe seizures, again characterized by seizure discharges in a distinct portion of the cerebrum of the brain, are characterized by sensory hallucinations and other types of consciousness alteration, a meaningless physical action, or even a babble of some incomprehensible language. Thus, for example, tem-

---

INFORMATION ON EPILEPSY

CAUSES: Brain injury, brain tumors, disease, possible genetic factors
SYMPTOMS: Seizures, loss of consciousness
DURATION: Typically chronic
TREATMENTS: Surgery to remove tumor or causative brain tissue abnormality, anticonvulsant drugs

---

poral lobe seizures may explain some cases of people "speaking in tongues" in religious experiences or in the days of the Delphic oracles of ancient Greece.

The term "grand mal" refers to the most severe type of epileptic seizure. Also called tonic-clonic seizures, grand mal attacks are characterized by very severe EEG seizure discharges throughout the entire brain. A grand mal seizure is usually preceded by sensory symptoms called an aura (probably related to temporal lobe seizures), which warn an epileptic of an impending attack. The aura is quickly followed by the grand mal seizure itself, which involves the loss of consciousness, localized or widespread jerking and convulsions, and severe body stiffness.

Epileptics suffering a grand mal seizure usually fall to the ground, may foam at the mouth, and often bite their tongues or the inside of their cheeks unless something is placed in the mouth before they lose consciousness. In a few cases, the victim will lose bladder or bowel control. In untreated epileptics, grand mal seizures can occur weekly. Most of these attacks last for only a minute or two, followed quickly by full recovery after a brief sense of disorientation and feelings of severe exhaustion. In some cases, however, grand mal seizures may last for up to five minutes and lead to temporary amnesia or to other mental deficits of a longer duration. In rare cases, the life-threatening condition of status epilepticus occurs, in which many sequential tonic-clonic seizures occur over several hours without recovery between them.

The fourth type of epileptic seizure is petit mal, which is often called generalized nonconvulsive seizure or, more simply, absence. A petit mal seizure consists of a brief period of loss of consciousness (ten to forty seconds) without the epileptic falling down. The epileptic usually appears to be daydreaming (absent) and shows no other symptoms. Often a victim of a petit mal seizure is not even aware that the event has occurred. In some cases, a petit mal seizure is accompanied by mild jerking of hands, head, or facial features and/or rapid blinking of the eyes. Petit mal attacks can be quite dangerous if they occur while an epileptic is driving a motor vehicle.

Diagnosing epilepsy usually requires a patient history, a careful physical examination, blood tests, and a neurologic examination. The patient history is most valuable when it includes eyewitness accounts of the symptoms, the frequency of occurrence, and the usual duration range of the seizures observed. In addition, documentation of any preceding severe trauma, infection, or episodes of addictive drug exposure provides useful information that will often differentiate between idiopathic and symptomatic epilepsy.

Evidence of trauma is quite important, as head injuries that caused unconsciousness are often the basis for later symptomatic epilepsy. Similarly, infectious diseases of the brain, including meningitis and encephalitis, can cause this type of epilepsy. Finally, excessive use of alcohol or other psychoactive drugs can also be a causative agent for symptomatic epilepsy.

Blood tests for serum glucose and calcium, electroencephalography, and computed tomography (CT) scanning are also useful diagnostic tools. The EEG will nearly always show seizure discharges in epileptics, and the location of the discharges in the brain may localize problem areas associated with the disease. CT scanning is most useful for identifying tumors and other serious brain damage that may cause symptomatic epilepsy. When all tests are negative except for abnormal EEGs, the epilepsy is considered idiopathic.

It is thought that the generation of epileptic symptoms occurs because of a malfunction in nerve impulse transport in some of the billions of nerve cells (neurons) that make up the brain and link it to the body organs that it innervates. This nerve impulse transport is an electrochemical process caused by the ability of the neurons to retain substances (including potassium) and to excrete substances (including sodium). This ability generates the weak electrical current that makes up a nerve impulse and that is registered by electroencephalography.

A nerve impulse leaves a given neuron via an outgoing extension (or axon), passes across a tiny synaptic gap that separates the axon from the next neuron in line, and enters an incoming extension (or dendrite) of that cell. The process is repeated until the impulse is transmitted to its site of action. The cell bodies of neurons make up the gray matter of the brain, and axons and dendrites (white matter) may be viewed as connecting wires.

Passage across synaptic gaps between neurons is mediated by chemicals called neurotransmitters, and it is now believed that epilepsy results when unknown materials cause abnormal electrical impulses by altering neurotransmitter production rates and/or the ability of sodium, potassium, and related substances to enter or leave neurons. The various nervous impulse abnormalities that cause epilepsy can be shown to occur in the portions of the gray matter of the cerebrum that control high-brain functions. For example, the frontal lobe—which controls speech, body movement, and eye movements—is associated with temporal lobe seizures.

TREATMENT AND THERAPY

Idiopathic epilepsy is viewed as the expression of a large group of different diseases, all of which present themselves clinically as seizures. This is extrapolated from the various types of symptomatic epilepsy observed, which have causes that include faulty biochemical processes (such as inappropriate calcium levels), brain tumors or severe brain injury, infectious diseases (such as encephalitis), and the chronic overuse of ad-

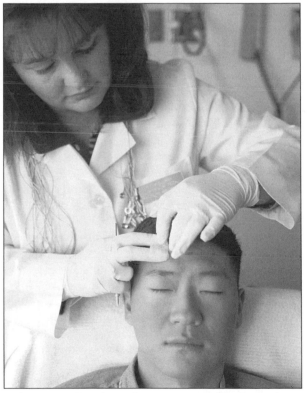

A doctor attaches electrodes to a patient's head in order to monitor his epilepsy. (PhotoDisc)

dictive drugs. As to why idiopathic epilepsy causes are not identifiable, the general biomedical wisdom states that present technology is too imprecise to detect its causes.

Symptomatic epilepsy is treated with medication and either by the extirpation of the tumor or other causative brain tissue abnormality that was engendered by trauma or disease or by the correction of the metabolic disorder involved. The more common, incurable idiopathic disease is usually treated entirely with medication that relieves symptoms. This treatment is essential because without it most epileptics cannot attend school successfully, maintain continued employment, or drive a motor vehicle safely.

A large number of anticonvulsant drugs are presently available for epilepsy management. It must, however, be made clear that no one therapeutic drug will control all types of seizures. In addition, some patients require several such drugs for effective therapy, and the natural history of a given case of epilepsy may often require periodic changes from drug to drug as the disease evolves. Furthermore, every therapeutic antiepilepsy drug has dangerous side effects that may occur when it is present in the body above certain levels or after it is used beyond some given time period. Therefore, each epileptic patient must be monitored at frequent intervals to ascertain that no dangerous physical symptoms are developing and that the drug levels in the body (monitored by the measurement of drug content in blood samples) are within a tolerable range.

More than twenty antiepilepsy drugs are widely used. Phenytoin (Dilantin) is very effective for grand mal seizures. Because of its slow metabolism, phenytoin can be administered relatively infrequently, but this slow metabolism also requires seven to ten days before its anticonvulsant effects occur. Side effects include cosmetically unpleasant hair overgrowth, swelling of the gums, and skin rash. These symptoms are particularly common in epileptic children. More serious are central nervous effects including ataxia (unsteadiness in walking), drowsiness, anemia, and marked thyroid deficiency. Most such symptoms are reversed by decreasing the drug doses or by discontinuing it. Phenytoin is often given together with other antiepilepsy drugs to produce optimum seizure prevention. In those cases, great care must be taken to prevent dangerous synergistic drug effects from occurring. High phenytoin doses also produce blood levels of the drug that are very close to toxic 25 micrograms per milliliter values.

Carbamazepine (Tegretol) is another frequently used antiepileptic drug. Chemically related to the drugs used as antidepressants, it is useful against both psychomotor epilepsy and grand mal seizures. Common carbamazepine side effects are ataxia, drowsiness, and double vision. A more dangerous, and fortunately less common, side effect is the inability of bone marrow to produce blood cells. Again, very serious and unexpected complications occur in mixed-drug therapy that includes carbamazepine, and at high doses toxic blood levels of the drug may be exceeded.

Phenobarbital, a sedative hypnotic also used as a tranquilizer by nonepileptics, is a standby for treating epilepsy. It too can have serious side effects, including a lowered attention span, hyperactivity, and learning difficulties. In addition, when given with phenytoin, phenobarbital will speed up the excretion of that drug, lowering its effective levels.

Four major lessons can be learned from these three drugs. First, individual antiepilepsy drugs have many different side effects. Second, there are concrete reasons that epileptics taking therapeutic drugs must be monitored carefully for physical symptoms. Third, at high antiepileptic drug doses, the blood levels attained may closely approximate and even exceed toxic values. Fourth, drug interactions in mixed-drug therapy can be counterproductive.

About 20 percent of idiopathic epileptics do not achieve adequate seizure control after prolonged and varied drug therapy. Another option for some—but not all—such people is brain surgery. This type of brain surgery is usually elected after two conditions are met. First, often-repeated EEGs must show that most or all of the portion of the brain in which the seizures develop is very localized. Second, these affected areas must be in a brain region that the patient can lose without significant mental loss (often in the prefrontal or temporal cerebral lobes). When such surgery is carried out, it is reported that 50 to 75 percent of the patients who are treated and given chronic, postoperative antiepilepsy drugs become able to achieve seizure control.

The most frequent antiepilepsy surgery is temporal lobectomy. The brain has two temporal lobes, one of which is dominant in the control of language, memory, and thought expression. A temporal lobectomy is carried out by removing the nondominant temporal lobe, when it is the site of epilepsy. About 6 percent of temporal lobectomies lead to a partial loss of temporal lobe functions, which may include impaired vision, movement, memory, and speech.

Another common type of antiepilepsy surgery is called corpus callosotomy. This procedure involves partially disconnecting the two cerebral hemispheres by severing some of the nerves in the corpus callosum that links them. This surgery is performed when an epileptic has frequent, uncontrollable grand mal attacks that cause many dangerous falls. The procedure usually results in reduced numbers of seizures and decreases in their severity.

Physicians now believe that many cases of epilepsy may be prevented by methods aimed at avoiding head injury (especially in children) and the use of techniques such as amniocentesis to identify potential epileptics and treat them before birth. Furthermore, the prophylactic administration of antiepilepsy drugs to nonepileptic people who are afflicted with encephalitis and other diseases known to produce epilepsy is viewed as wise.

PERSPECTIVE AND PROSPECTS

A great number of advances have occurred in the treatment of epilepsy via therapeutic drugs and surgical techniques. With the exception of symptomatic epilepsy, drug therapy has been the method of choice because it is less drastic than surgery, easier to manage, and rarely has the potential for irreversible damage to patients that can be caused by the removal of a portion of the brain. The main antiepileptic drugs are phenytoin, carbamazepine, and phenobarbital, but a tremendous variety of other chemical therapies has been investigated and utilized successfully.

Such treatments include high doses of vitamins, injections of muscle relaxants, and changes in diet. The variety is unsurprising, considering the vast number of disease issues that can cause seizures. For example, the rare genetic disease phenylketonuria (PKU) can cause epilepsy. Phenylketonuric epilepsy is often treated by use of a ketogenic diet rich in fats; the clear value of this treatment is unexplained. Readers are encouraged to investigate the many epilepsy treatments that have not been noted. Such an examination may be quite valuable because there are about a million epileptics in the United States alone, and some estimates indicate that four of every thousand humans are likely to develop some epileptic symptoms during their lifetime.

Modern surgical treatment of epilepsy reportedly began in 1828, with the efforts of Benjamin Dudley, who removed epilepsy-causing blood clots and skull fragments from five patients, who all survived despite primitive and nonsterile operating rooms. The next landmark in such surgery was the removal of a brain tumor by the German physician R. J. Godlee, in 1884, without the benefit of X rays or EEG techniques, which did not then exist.

By the 1950's EEGs were used to locate epileptic brain foci, and physicians such as the Canadians Wilder Penfield and Herbert Jasper pioneered its use to locate brain regions to remove for epilepsy remission without damaging vital functions. After considerable evolution over the course of forty years, antiepilepsy surgery by the 1990's had become widespread, commonplace, and relatively safe.

Nevertheless, because of the imperfections of all available methodologies, 5 to 8 percent of epileptics cannot achieve seizure control by any method or method combination, and even the "well-managed" epilepsy treatment regimen has its flaws. There is still much to be learned about curing epilepsy. It is hoped that the efforts of ongoing biomedical research, both in basic science and in clinical settings, will eliminate epilepsy through the development of new therapeutic drugs and sophisticated advances in surgery and other nondrug methods.

—*Sanford S. Singer, Ph.D.*

See also Auras; Brain; Brain disorders; Computed tomography (CT) scanning; Electroencephalography (EEG); Nervous system; Neurology; Neurology, pediatric; Neurosurgery; Phenylketonuria (PKU); Seizures; Unconsciousness.

FOR FURTHER INFORMATION:

Berkow, Robert, and Andrew J. Fletcher, eds. *The Merck Manual of Diagnosis and Therapy.* 17th ed. Rahway, N.J.: Merck Sharp & Dohme Research Laboratories, 1999. Contains a compendium of data on the characteristics, etiology, diagnosis, and treatment of adult epilepsy. Also discusses seizure disorders of children and newborns. Designed for physicians, the material is also useful to less specialized readers.

Bloom, Floyd E., et al., eds. *The Dana Guide to Brain Health.* New York: Simon & Schuster, 2003. An easy-to-understand health guide to the brain from neuroscience, neurology, and psychiatry perspectives. More than seventy psychiatric and neurological disorders, their diagnoses, and their treatments are covered.

Devinsky, Orrin. *Epilepsy: Patient and Family Guide.* 2d ed. Philadelphia: F. A. Davis, 2001. An excellent lay guide to the medical and social topics relevant to epilepsy. Topics include diagnosis and treatment, epilepsy in children and adults, legal and financial issues, and research resources.

Epilepsy Foundation. http://www.epilepsyfoundation .org/. A national organization dedicated to education, research, and advocacy. Web site offers information on careers and employment, parent support groups and children's programs, and online "Interest Groups," among many other features.

Freeman, John M., et al. *Seizures and Epilepsy in Childhood: A Guide*. 3d ed. Baltimore: Johns Hopkins University Press, 2002. Designed for parents, an overall guide to the symptoms, diagnosis and treatment of children with epilepsy. Third edition includes new chapters on alternative therapies and medicines, routine health care, insurance issues, and research resources.

Gumnit, Robert J., ed. *Living Well with Epilepsy*. New York: Demos, 1990. Designed to give people with epilepsy the outlook necessary to live successfully with the disease. Among the topics covered are causes and treatment, high-quality care, medical and surgical options, the problems of epileptic children, sexuality and pregnancy, the workplace, rights, and resources.

Hopkins, Anthony. *Epilepsy: The Facts*. 2d ed. New York: Oxford University Press, 1996. The author wishes to eliminate misunderstanding about epilepsy and educate people about it. This is done nicely by clear coverage of topics including explanation of epilepsy, seizure types and causes, epilepsy treatment methods, and information on living with the disease.

Nolte, John. *Human Brain: An Introduction to Its Functional Anatomy*. 5th ed. New York: Elsevier, 2001. Text covering major concepts and structure-function relationships in the human neurological system.

Weaver, Donald F. *Epilepsy and Seizures: Everything You Need to Know*. Toronto, Ont.: Firefly Books, 2001. A lay guide covering research advances, history of the disease, different types, the mechanisms, diagnosis and treatment, and special situations, such as epilepsy in pregnant women, children, and the elderly.

EPISIOTOMY

PROCEDURE

ANATOMY OR SYSTEM AFFECTED: Anus, genitals, reproductive system

SPECIALTIES AND RELATED FIELDS: Gynecology, obstetrics

DEFINITION: A surgical cut made in the pelvic floor to enlarge the vagina for the facilitation of childbirth.

INDICATIONS AND PROCEDURES

An episiotomy is performed to enlarge the vaginal opening and ease the delivery of a baby during childbirth. While not a routine procedure, some circumstances which indicate the need for an episiotomy include rapid delivery, breech delivery, and presentation of the baby with face to the front of the birth canal, all of which prevent the perineum (the area between the vagina and the anus) from stretching rapidly enough to prevent tearing. Scarring from vaginal surgeries also limits the ability of the vagina to expand.

During the procedure, a local anesthetic is injected into the perineum. The obstetrician uses straight-bladed blunt scissors to snip the tissue between the vagina and anus, avoiding the anal sphincter muscle. After delivery, the incision is carefully stitched together, along with any minor tears in the birth canal.

USES AND COMPLICATIONS

The birth canal has very limited space to accommodate an infant, and situations such as feet-first or face-forward presentation can lead to compression of the umbilical cord and interruption of the oxygen supply to the baby, or even to potential crushing of the infant. An episiotomy can facilitate a rapid delivery in these circumstances, thereby preventing serious injury to the infant. Failure of the perineum to stretch sufficiently to accommodate the child can result in severe, irregular tears of the vagina and even of the anal sphincter muscles. Ragged tears are very difficult to repair surgically and are much more prone to infection. Tearing of the anal sphincter could lead to permanent incontinence. The easily repaired incisions of episiotomy eliminate these potential difficulties.

Healing of the incisions is rapid and straightforward, but the area may itch and be somewhat painful for a few weeks. Painkilling drugs may be prescribed, and ice packs can be used to alleviate pain. Women who do not desire episiotomies and have controlled, problem-free deliveries may try to stretch the perineum gradually by massaging it with warm oil during the delivery.

—Karen E. Kalumuck, Ph.D.

See also Childbirth; Childbirth complications; Incontinence; Obstetrics.

FOR FURTHER INFORMATION:

Carlson, Karen J., Stephanie A. Eisenstat, and Terra Ziporyn. *The Harvard Guide to Women's Health.* Cambridge, Mass.: Harvard University Press, 1996.

Cunningham, F. Gary, et al., eds. *Williams Obstetrics.* 21st ed. Stamford, Conn.: Appleton and Lange, 2001.

Goldberg, Roger P. *Ever Since I Had My Baby: Understanding, Treating, and Preventing the Most Common Physical After-Effects of Pregnancy and Childbirth.* New York: Crown, 2003.

Gonik, Bernard, and Renee A. Bobrowski. *Medical Complications in Labor and Delivery.* Cambridge, Mass.: Blackwell Scientific, 1996.

Reynolds, Karina, Christoph Lees, and Grainne McCarten. *Pregnancy and Birth: Your Questions Answered.* Rev. ed. New York: DK, 2002.

Sears, William, and Martha Sears. *The Birth Book.* Boston: Little, Brown, 1994.

Simkin, Penny, Janet Whalley, and Ann Keppler. *Pregnancy, Childbirth, and the Newborn: A Complete Guide for Expectant Parents.* Rev. ed. New York: Simon & Schuster, 2001.

Stoppard, Miriam. *Conception, Pregnancy, and Birth.* Rev. ed. London: Dorling Kindersley, 2000.

Warhus, Susan. *Countdown to Baby: Answers to the One Hundred Most Asked Questions About Pregnancy and Childbirth.* Omaha, Nebr.: Addicus Books, 2003.

EPSTEIN-BARR VIRUS. *See* CHRONIC FATIGUE SYNDROME; MONONUCLEOSIS.

ESTROGEN REPLACEMENT THERAPY. *See* HORMONE REPLACEMENT THERAPY (HRT).

ETHICS

ALSO KNOWN AS: Bioethics, medical ethics

DEFINITION: Ethics is a code of conduct based on established moral principles. Medical ethics is the study of the conduct of professionals in the field of medicine.

KEY TERMS:

autonomy: independence and self-reliance, especially referring to decision making

beneficence: doing good

informed consent: the dialogue between physician and patient prior to an invasive procedure

justice: the rationing of scarce resources according to a prearranged plan

nonmaleficence: avoiding evil

paternalism: acting in the manner of a father to his children

PRINCIPLES

Ethics deals with a code of conduct based on established moral principles. When applied to a particular professional field, abstract theories as well as concrete principles are considered. Often the consequences of a particular course of action dictate its rightness or wrongness. Bioethics is the study of ethics by professionals in the fields of medicine, law, philosophy, or theology. Some also refer to this area as applied ethics. The term "bioethics" is often used interchangeably with "medical ethics," but purists would define medical ethics as the study of conduct by professionals in the field of medicine. Codes of ethics promulgated by professional groups or associations define obligations governing members of a given profession.

Initial questions concerning medical ethics entail purpose, to whom a duty is owed (legal or moral) and how far that duty extends. Does it extend solely to patients, or does it extend to their families or to society as a whole? For example, public health obligations to society involve a duty to prevent disease, maintain the health of the populace, and oversee the delivery of health care.

In the 1972 article "Models for Ethical Practice in a Revolutionary Age," Robert M. Veatch proposed four models for ethical medicine. The first is the engineering model, in which the physician becomes an applied scientist interested in treating disease rather than caring for a patient. The Nazi physicians during World War II acting as so-called scientists and technicians are examples of the engineering model taken to its extreme. The second is the priestly model, in which the physician assumes a paternalistic role of moral dominance, treating the patient as a child. The main principle of this model is the traditional one of *primum non nocere*, or "first do no harm." It neglects principles of patient autonomy, dignity, and freedom. The third is the collegial model, in which physician and patient are colleagues cooperating in pursuing a common goal, such as preserving health, curing illness, or easing pain. This model requires mutual trust and confidence, demanding a continued dialogue between the parties. The fourth is the contractual model, in which the relationship between health care provider and patient is analogous to a legal contract, with rights and obligations on both sides. The contractual model can be modified to provide for shared decision making and cooperation between physician and patient and tailored to the particular physician-patient relationship involved, resulting in a collegial association.

Autonomy and informed consent. Since the Nuremberg trials, which presented horrible accounts of medical experimentation in Nazi concentration camps, the issue of consent has been one of primary importance. These basic concepts recognize an individual's uniqueness and inherent decision-making ability without coercion or undue influence from others. Respect for privacy and freedom are fundamental to human dignity. Even when people present difficult problems, such as being unconscious or in a coma, they must continue to be respected. Rational decision making by patients or their surrogates must be followed, and those with specialized knowledge or expertise are not authorized to impose their will on another person or limit that person's freedom.

Informed consent seeks to encourage open communication between patient and health care provider, to protect patients and research subjects from harm, and to encourage health care providers to act responsibly vis-à-vis patients and subjects, ultimately preserving autonomy and rational decision making. Especially applicable in invasive procedures, such as those involving surgery or treatments with serious risks, informed consent requires the presence of certain conditions, including a patient's competency or decision-making capacity, in order to understand the relative consequences of a proposed course of treatment and its effect on a patient's life and health. (Absent informed consent, an invasive procedure would constitute a legal cause of action in battery, or a harmful or offensive touching). The health care provider must inform patients of alternative courses of action, if any, and the fact that patients have the option to refuse treatment, even if that alternative is contrary to the recommendation of the physician. The information conveyed to the patient must include the diagnosis, nature of the proposed treatment, known risks and consequences (excluding those that are too remote or improbable to bear significantly on the ultimate decision whether to proceed on a course of treatment, as well as those that are so well known that they are obvious to everyone), benefits from the proposed treatment, alternatives, prognosis without treatment, economic cost, and how the treatment plan will impact the patient's lifestyle. The patient should also be made aware that once given, an informed consent can be withdrawn. Hospital consent forms do not provide this type of information.

The information conveyed must be material and important to this patient, not a fictional reasonable and prudent person. A factor is material if it could change the decision of that patient. Inherent problems include speculation into the factors that would have a dramatic impact on the patient's life, requiring a dialogue between patient and health care provider. It is also important to recognize the role of the physician's time constraints as well as the patient's overall stress level while the information is being conveyed, including possible information overload. Not only must the information be conveyed adequately, but it must also be assimilated and understood. The ability of an individual to process information raises substantial issues about understanding. Comprehension is not always easily ascertainable. Sometimes a person's ability to make decisions is affected by problems of nonacceptance of information, even if it was comprehended. A patient may voluntarily waive informed consent, so that the patient asks not to be informed, thereby relieving the physician of the obligation to obtain informed consent and ultimately delegating decision-making authority to the physician.

Medical emergencies constitute exceptions to the informed consent requirement, provided that four conditions are met: The patient, whose wishes are unknown because no advance directive or living will exists, is incapable of giving consent because of the emergency; no surrogate is available; the medical condition poses a danger to the patient's life or seriously impairs the patient's health; and immediate treatment is required to avert the danger to life or health. This exception is justified on the grounds that consent can be assumed in cases in which a reasonable person would consent if informed. If the patient is not in imminent danger, or if consent can be obtained at a later time, the emergency exception does not apply. The second exception is the therapeutic privilege in which health care providers are justified in legitimately withholding information from a patient when they reasonably believe that disclosure will have an adverse effect on the patient's condition or health, as in the case of a depressed, emotionally drained, or unstable patient. Again, the decision is subjective, referring to this patient, decided on a case-by-case basis. The privilege does not apply if the health care provider withholds information based on the belief that the patient will refuse consent if told all the facts. In that instance, withholding information amounts to misrepresentation or deception.

Another ethical dilemma involving intentional deception or incomplete disclosure concerns the therapeutic use of placebos. One defense is that deception is moral when it is used for the patient's welfare.

Paternalism. From the Latin word *pater*, meaning "father," paternalism refers to controlling others as a father acts in his relationship with his children. In medical ethics, paternalism involves overriding one's own wishes in order to act to benefit or avert harm to the patient. Intervention by a health care provider to prevent competent patients from harming themselves is called strong paternalism. Strong paternalism is generally rejected by ethicists because of the view that health care providers do not know all the factors influencing the life of another person and therefore lack the competence to decide what is best for another person. Weak paternalism exists when the health care provider overrules the wishes of an incompetent or questionably competent patient. It is sometimes justified in nonemergencies without informed consent to relieve serious pain and suffering. Another example of weak paternalism is the temporary use of restraints, justified on the grounds that confused and disoriented patients are otherwise likely to injure themselves. When restraints are necessary, the surrogate is generally asked to give consent, recognizing that restraints, albeit temporary, constitute a limitation of one's liberty.

Beneficence and nonmaleficence. The principles of beneficence (doing good) and nonmaleficence (avoiding evil) are both expressed in the Hippocratic oath: "I will use treatment to help the sick according to my ability and judgment, but I will never use it to injure or wrong them." Each principle has a bearing on the other, and each is limited by the other. The obligations in beneficence are also limited by obligations to avoid evil. One may perform an act that risks evil if the following conditions are present (the principle of double effects): The action is good or morally indifferent; the agent intends a good effect; the evil effect is not the means to achieving good; and proportionality exists between good and evil. The principle of proportionality states that provided that an action does not go directly against the dignity of the individual, there must be a proportionate good to justify risking evil consequences. Items to be considered are the possible existence of an alternative means with less evil or no evil, the level of good intended and the level of evil risked, and the certitude or probability of good or evil. The latter is called the wedge principle, referring to the fact that putting the tip of a wedge into a crack in a log and striking the wedge will split the log and destroy it; by analogy, in defending a given position, even a small concession can de-

stroy that position. The last element is the causal influence of the agent, recognizing that most effects result from many causes and that a particular agent is seldom the sole cause. For example, as noted by Thomas M. Garrett and colleagues in *Health Care Ethics: Principles and Problems* (2001), lung cancer can be triggered not only by smoking but also by conditions in the workplace, the environment, and heredity.

Obligations are imposed on the patient that demand the use of ordinary but not extraordinary means of preserving and restoring health. In other words, the patient should use means that produce more good than harm and evaluate the effects on the self, family, and society, including pain, cost, and health benefits to life, its meaning and quality. The health care provider's obligation demands that the benefits outweigh the burdens on the patient. An overarching obligation to society exists to provide health care information and leadership to ensure the equitable distribution of scarce medical resources accomplished in ways that allow the goals of health care to be achieved. Finally, the surrogate's obligation depends on whether the wishes of the once-competent patient are known or can be ascertained. If so, the surrogate should decide accordingly (the substituted judgment principle). Overruling the person's wishes would constitute a denial of the patient's autonomy. If the person has never been competent or has never expressed his or her wishes, the surrogate should act in the best interests of the patient alone, disregarding the interests of family, society, and the surrogate. Another approach requires the surrogate to choose what the patient would have chosen if and when competent after having considered all relevant information and the interests of others.

Certain conditions justify the decision to omit treatment, such as pointless or futile treatment, especially with regard to the dead or those who are dying, and situations in which the burdens of treatment outweigh the benefits. It should be noted that no bright line exists here because these cases are not decided easily. Ethicists as well as those in the medical professions debating these issues have not reached a clear-cut solution that applies in every case.

Justice. Also called distributive justice, justice establishes principles for the distribution of scarce resources in circumstances where demand outstrips supply and rationing must occur. Needs are to be considered in terms of overall needs and the dignity of members of society. Aside from the biological and physiological elements, the social context of health and disease may influence a given problem and its severity. Individual prejudices and presuppositions may enlarge the nature and scope of the disease, creating a demand for health care that makes it even more difficult to distribute scarce resources for all members of society. Principles of fair distribution in society often supersede and become paramount to the concerns of the individual. Questions about who shall receive what share of society's scarce resources generate controversies about a national health policy, unequal distributions of advantages to the disadvantaged, and the rationing of health care.

Similar problems recur with regard to access to and distribution of health insurance, medical equipment, and artificial organs. The lack of insurance as well as the problem of underinsurance constitutes a huge economic barrier to health care access in the United States. In *Principles of Biomedical Ethics* (2001), Tom L. Beauchamp and James F. Childress point out that the acquired immunodeficiency syndrome (AIDS) crisis has presented dramatic instances of the problems of insurability and underwriting practices, in which insurers often appeal to actuarial fairness in defending their decisions while neglecting social justice. Proposals to alleviate the unfairness to those below the poverty line have been based on charity, compassion, and benevolence toward the sick rather than on claims of justice. The ongoing debate over the entitlement to a minimum of health care in the United States involves not only government entitlement programs but also complex social, political, economic, and cultural beliefs.

Decisions concerning the allocation of funds will dictate the type of health care that can be provided and for which problems. Numerous resources, supplies, and space in intensive care units (ICUs) have been allocated for specific patients or classes of patients. A life-threatening illness complicates this decision. In the United States, health care has often been allocated by one's ability to pay rather than by other criteria; rationing has at times been based on ranking a list of services or a patient's age.

Confidentiality and privacy. In the United States, the medical profession has always strived to maintain the confidentiality of physician-patient communications, as well as the privacy of a patient's medical records. While admirable, these values have not been absolute, and no uniformity exists among the fifty states regarding access to one's medical records. As technology improved, with computers and fax machines transmitting health care data to distant locations and medical records themselves existing in electronic form, no laws had been created to protect medical records adequately. In the late twentieth and early twenty-first centuries, the administrations of Bill Clinton and George W. Bush sought to enact legislation that would bridge the privacy gaps and create uniform standards, at the same time eliminating discrimination in employment and insurance coverage based on one's genetic predisposition. The Health Insurance Portability and Accountability Act (HIPAA) became law in 1997.

APPLICATION OF ETHICAL PRINCIPLES

Advances in medical technology have expanded the scope of what medicine can accomplish. As capabilities grow and become more sophisticated, medical ethics also seeks to resolve age-old dilemmas and to evaluate the use of new technologies. Certain ethical dilemmas have garnered sharp disagreement. Chief among these is the issue of death and dying, which brings into controversy two theories about the nature of health care. The "curing" approach is based on traditional medical ethical principles that date back to Hippocrates and include the principles of beneficence, nonmaleficence, and justice. The "caring" approach focuses on patient autonomy, proper bedside manners by health care providers, the preparation of advance directives, and the hospice movement.

The "curing" approach to medical ethics equates medicine with healing. The sanctity of life is important because it is a gift from God and must be sustained to the extent reasonably possible. All ordinary measures must be taken to preserve life. This tradition holds that only God can decide the time of death, and even in the face of suffering, the health care provider must not take measures to shorten life. Physicians are the primary decision makers and in the best position to recommend and advise the patient and to direct the treatment plan. The model is paternalistic.

In the "caring" approach, the health care provider's role is to minimize pain, to present alternatives and the relative consequences of various options, and ultimately to proceed according to the patient's determination. The "caring" approach is subjective, as each case is decided individually. The quality of life rather than the sanctity of life becomes the guiding principle.

Issues regarding futility of treatment arise, as well as the recognition that prolonging life does not always benefit patients. Physicians are not obligated to provide futile treatment, which may violate the physician's duty not to harm patients because such treatments are often burdensome and invasive, exacerbating the patient's pain and discomfort. Patients cannot ethically compel health care workers to provide treatment that violates the worker's own personal beliefs or the standards of the profession. Other issues in this area deal with physician-assisted suicide and whether to provide or withhold lifesaving treatments.

The transplantation of vital organs—notably the heart, liver, and kidney—raises difficult ethical questions. As organ transplantation has become routine at many medical centers, its success has opened a Pandora's box of ethical questions involving the allocation of scarce donor organs. One example is whether the sickest person on the waiting list for an organ should be the recipient, or whether it should go to someone more robust who may live longer. Another is whether live donors should be compensated for donating an organ, just as blood donors are compensated. Many countries outside the United States and the United Kingdom condone the sale of organs; the 1984 National Organ Transplant Act makes selling organs illegal in the United States. Ethicists are debating animal-to-human organ transplants to alleviate the scarcity of human donor organs for transplantation.

Assisted reproduction in the form of in vitro fertilization (IVF), egg freezing, and sperm banking is largely an unregulated industry. Couples seeking help must make complex ethical decisions dealing with the preselection of embryos based on genetic traits through screening of a single cell. Other decisions deal with how many eggs should be fertilized and whether the remainder should be disposed of or frozen. The rights of the participants and the children created through assisted reproduction remain undefined. State laws vary widely regarding whether a child conceived by IVF or donor eggs or sperm has the right to know the identity of the biological parents.

The identification of human embryonic stem cells has been widely acknowledged as extremely valuable because it will assist scientists in understanding basic mechanisms of embryo development and gene regulation. It also holds the promise of allowing the development of techniques for manipulating, growing, and cloning stem cells to create designer cells and tissues. Stem cells are created in the first days of pregnancy. Scientists hope to direct stem cells to grow into replacement organs and tissues to treat a wide variety of diseases. Embryos are valued in research for their ability to produce stem cells, which can be harvested to grow a variety of tissues for use in transplantation to treat seri-

ous illnesses such as cancer, heart disease, and diabetes. In so doing, however, researchers must destroy days-old embryos, a procedure condemned by the Catholic Church, some antiabortion activists, and some women's rights organizations. Other research points to similar promise using stem cells harvested from adults, so that no embryos are destroyed.

PERSPECTIVE AND PROSPECTS

Medical ethics in Western culture has its roots in ancient Greek and Roman medicine, the Greek physician Hippocrates and the Roman physician Galen. In ancient Greece, as in most early societies, healing wounds and treating disease first appeared as folk practice and religious ritual. The earliest statement about ethics appears in a clinical and epidemiological book entitled *Epidemics I*, attributed to Hippocrates. It is in this work that the admonition "to help and not to harm" first appeared. The book itself deals with prognosis rather than treatment, which is the approach taken by Hippocrates. Galen asserted that any worthwhile doctor must know philosophy, including the logical, the physical, and the ethical, and be skilled at reasoning about the problems presented to him, understanding the nature and function of the body within the physical world.

From the fourth to the fourteenth centuries, medicine became firmly established in the universities and in the public life of the emerging nations of Europe. During this time, the Roman Catholic Church had a strong influence on Western civilization. Medicine was deeply touched by the doctrine and discipline of the Church, and its theological influence shaped the ethics of medicine. The early Church endorsed the use of human medicine and encouraged care of the sick as a work of charity. One of the greatest physicians during this period was the Jewish Talmudic scholar Maimonides, whose writings sometimes dealt with ethical questions in medicine.

The duty to comfort the sick and dying was a moral imperative in Christianity and Judaism. As the bubonic plague swept across Europe over the following several centuries, Protestant leader Martin Luther urged doctors and ministers to fulfill the obligation of Christian charity by faithful service, but John Calvin argued that physicians and ministers could depart if the preservation of their lives was in the common interest.

The ethical debates surrounding the plague moved medical ethics ahead. As noted by Albert R. Jonsen in *A Short History of Medical Ethics* (2000), the question became, "Under what circumstances does a person who has medical skills have a special obligation to serve the community?" When syphilis emerged in epidemic proportions at the end of the fifteenth century, a similar question regarding service to the sick at the cost of danger to oneself resurfaced, and members of the medical profession struggled with the link between medical necessity and moral correctness. Not until the nineteenth century did a consensus appear, mandating that the physician should take personal risks to serve the needy without appraising the morality of a patient's behavior.

—*Marcia J. Weiss, J.D.*

See also Abortion; Aging: Extended care; Animal rights vs. research; Assisted reproductive technologies; Cloning; Contraception; Euthanasia; Fetal tissue transplantation; Genetic engineering; Hippocratic oath; In vitro fertilization; Law and medicine; Malpractice; Medicare; Resuscitation; Screening; Stem cells; Suicide; Terminally ill: Extended care; Transplantation; Xenotransplantation.

FOR FURTHER INFORMATION:

Beauchamp, Tom L., and James F. Childress. *Principles of Biomedical Ethics.* 5th ed. New York: Oxford University Press, 2001. Regarded as one of the basic texts of bioethics. An excellent source for a detailed discussion of fundamental principles.

Beauchamp, Tom L., and LeRoy Walters, eds. *Contemporary Issues in Bioethics.* 6th ed. Belmont, Calif.: Wadsworth, 2003. A compilation of scholarly articles and major legal cases in bioethics.

Garrett, Thomas M., Harold W. Baillie, and Rosellen M. Garrett. *Health Care Ethics: Principles and Problems.* 4th ed. Englewood Cliffs, N.J.: Prentice-Hall, 2001. A basic and succinct text outlining the principles and problems of health care ethics.

Jonsen, Albert R. *A Short History of Medical Ethics.* New York: Oxford University Press, 2000. A concise and comprehensive chronicle of the history of ethics and medicine.

Pence, Gregory E. *Re-creating Medicine: Ethical Issues at the Frontiers of Medicine.* Lanham, Md.: Rowman & Littlefield, 2000. A subjective and skeptical (not balanced) discussion of the major bioethical issues at the beginning of the twenty-first century, such as organ donation, reproduction and its progeny, genetics, and other controversial subjects.

Torr, James D., ed. *Medical Ethics.* San Diego, Calif.: Greenhaven Press, 2000. Part of the Current Controversies series, this book presents reprints of articles illustrating both sides of controversial and contested issues in medical ethics.

Veatch, Robert M. "Models for Ethical Practice in a Revolutionary Age." *Hastings Center Report* 2, no. 3 (June, 1972): 5-7. A major figure in the bioethics movement, Veatch outlines four ethical medical models.

EUTHANASIA

ETHICS

DEFINITION: The intentional termination of a life, which may be active (resulting from specific actions causing death) or passive (resulting from the refusal or withdrawal of life-sustaining treatment), voluntary (with the patient's consent) or involuntary (on behalf of infants or others who are incapable of making this decision, such as comatose patients).

KEY TERMS:

active euthanasia: administration of a drug or some other means that directly causes death; the motivation is to relieve patient suffering

durable power of attorney: designation of a person who will have legal authority to make health care decisions if the patient becomes incapable of making decisions for himself or herself

living will: a legal document in which the patient states a preference regarding life-prolonging treatment in the event that he or she cannot choose

nonvoluntary euthanasia: a decision to terminate life made by another when the patient is incapable of making a decision for himself or herself

passive euthanasia: ending life by refusing or withdrawing life-sustaining medical treatment

voluntary euthanasia: a patient's consent to a decision which results in the shortening of his or her life

THE CONTROVERSY SURROUNDING EUTHANASIA

In the past, the role of the doctor was clear: The physician should minimize suffering and save lives whenever possible. In the present, it is possible for these two goals to be at odds. Saving lives in some situations seems to prolong the misery of the patient. In other cases, procedures or treatments may only marginally postpone the time of death. Advances in medical technology enable many to live who would have died just a few years ago, and massive amounts of money are spent each year on medical research with the goal of prolonging life. Experts in U.S. population trends indicate that by the year 2030, those over the age of sixty-five will comprise about 20 percent of the country's total population. These people will probably be healthy and alert well into their eighties; however, in the last years of their lives they will probably require significant medical care, putting financial stress on the health care system.

The complex issues surrounding death, suffering, and economics create an insistency for answers to difficult ethical questions. Does all life have value? Should one fight against death even when suffering is intense? Should suffering be lessened if the time of death is brought nearer? Should a patient be given the right to refuse medical treatment if the result is death? Should others be allowed to make this decision for the patient? Should other factors such as the financial or emotional burden on the family be part of the decision-making process? Once a decision has been made to terminate suffering by death, is there any ethical difference between discontinuing medical treatment and giving a lethal dosage of painkilling medication? Should laws be put into place that offer guidelines in these situations, or should each case be decided on an individual basis? And who should decide? There is a wide range of opinion and much uncertainty involving euthanasia and what constitutes a "good" death.

Euthanasia comes from a Greek word that can be translated as "good death" and is defined in several ways, depending on the philosophical stance of the one giving the definition. Tom Beauchamp, in his book *Health and Human Values* (1983), defines euthanasia as

putting to death or failing to prevent death in cases of terminal illness or injury; the motive is to relieve comatoseness, physical suffering, anxiety or a serious sense of burdensomeness to self and others. In euthanasia at least one other person causes or helps to cause the death of one who desires death or, in the case of an incompetent person, makes a substituted decision, either to cause death directly or to withdraw something that sustains life.

Most patients who express a wish to die more quickly are terminally ill; however, euthanasia is sometimes considered as a solution for nonterminal patients as well. An example of the latter would be seriously deformed or retarded infants whose futures are judged to have a poor "quality of life" and who would be a serious burden on their families and society.

When discussing the ethical implications of euthanasia, the types of cases have been divided into various classes. A distinction is made between voluntary and nonvoluntary euthanasia. In voluntary euthanasia, the patient consents to a specific course of medical action in which death is hastened. Nonvoluntary euthanasia would occur in cases in which the patient is not able to make decisions about his or her death because of an inability to communicate or a lack of mental facility. Each of these classes has advocates and antagonists. Some believe that voluntary euthanasia should always be allowed, but others would limit voluntary euthanasia to only those patients who have a terminal illness. Some, although agreeing in principle that voluntary euthanasia in terminal situations is ethically permissible, nevertheless oppose euthanasia of any type because of the possibility of abuses. With nonvoluntary euthanasia, the main ethical issues deal with when such an action should be performed and who should make the decision. If a person is in an irreversible coma, most agree that that person's physical life could be ended; however, arguments based on "quality of life" can easily become widened to include persons with physical or mental disabilities. Infants with severe deformities can sometimes be saved but not fully cured with medical technology, and some individuals would advocate nonvoluntary euthanasia in these cases because of the suffering of the infants' caregivers. Some believe that family members or those who stand to gain from the decision should not be allowed to make the decision. Others point out that the family is the most likely to know what the wishes of the patient would have been. Most believe that the medical care personnel, although knowledgeable, should not have the power to decide, and many are reluctant to institute rigid laws. The possibility of misappropriated self-interest from each of these parties magnifies the difficulty of arriving at well-defined criteria.

The second type of classification is between passive and active euthanasia. Passive euthanasia occurs when sustaining medical treatment is refused or withdrawn and death is allowed to take its course. Active euthanasia involves the administration of a drug or some other means that directly causes death. Once again, there are many opinions surrounding these two types. One position is that there is no difference between active and passive euthanasia because in each the end is premeditated death with the motive of prevention of suffering. In fact, some argue that active euthanasia is more compassionate than letting death occur naturally, which may involve suffering. In opposition, others believe that there is a fundamental difference between active and passive euthanasia. A person may have the right to die, but not the right to be killed. Passive euthanasia, they argue, is merely allowing a death which is inevitable to occur. Active euthanasia, if voluntary, is equated with suicide because a human being seizes control of death; if nonvoluntary, it is considered murder.

Passive euthanasia, although generally more publicly acceptable than active euthanasia, has become a topic of controversy as the types of medical treatment that can be withdrawn are debated. A distinction is sometimes made between ordinary and extraordinary means. Defining these terms is difficult, since what may be extraordinary for one patient is not for another, depending on other medical conditions that the patient may have. In addition, what is considered an extraordinary technique today may be judged ordinary in the future. Another way to assess whether passive euthanasia should be allowed in a particular situation is to weigh the benefits against the burdens for the patient. Although most agree that there are cases in which high-tech equipment such as respirators can be withdrawn, there is a question about whether administration of food and water should ever be discontinued. Here the line between passive and active euthanasia is blurred.

Religious and Legal Implications

Decisions about death concern everyone because everyone will die. Eventually, each individual will be the patient who is making the decisions or for whom the decisions are being made. In the meantime, one may be called upon to make decisions for others. Even those not directly involved in the hard cases are affected, as taxpayers and subscribers to medical insurance, by the decisions made on the behalf of others. In a difficult moral issue such as this, individuals look to different institutions for guidelines. Two sources of guidance are the church and the law.

In 1971, the Roman Catholic church issued a statement entitled *Ethical and Religious Directives for Catholic Health Facilities*. Included in this directive was the statement, "[I]t is not euthanasia to give a dying person sedatives and analgesics for alleviation of pain, when such a measure is judged necessary, even though they may deprive the patient of the use of reason or shorten his life." This thinking was reaffirmed by a 1980 statement from the Vatican which considers suffering and expense for the family legitimate reasons to withdraw medical treatment when death is imminent. Bishops from The Netherlands, in a letter to a government commission, state "[B]odily deterioration alone does not have to be unworthy of a man. History shows how many people, beaten, tortured and broken in body,

sometimes even grew in personality in spite of it. Dying becomes unworthy of a man, if family and friends begin to look upon the dying person as a burden, withdraw themselves from him. . . ." When speaking of passive euthanasia, the bishops state, "We see no reason to call this euthanasia. Such a person after all dies of his own illness. His death is neither intended nor caused, only nothing is done anymore to postpone it." Christians from Protestant churches may reflect a wider spectrum of positions. Joseph Fletcher, an Episcopal priest, defines a person as one having the ability to think and reason. If a patient does not meet these criteria, according to Fletcher, his or her life may be ended out of compassion for the person he or she once was. The United Church of Christ illustrates this view in its policy statement: "When illness takes away those abilities we associate with full personhood . . . we may well feel that the mere continuance of the body by machine or drugs is a violation of their person. . . . We do not believe simply the continuance of mere physical existence is either morally defensible or socially desirable or is God's will."

These varied positions generally are derived from differing emphases on two truths concerning the nature of God and the role of suffering in the life of the believer. First is the belief that God is the giver of life and that human beings should not usurp God's authority in matters of life and death. Second, alleviation of suffering is of critical importance to God, since it is not loving one's neighbor to allow him or her to suffer. Those who give more weight to the first statement believe as well that God's will allows for suffering and that the suffering can be used for a good purpose in the life of the believer. Those who emphasize the second principle insist that a loving God would not prolong the suffering of people needlessly and that one should not desperately fight to prolong a life which God has willed to die.

C. Everett Koop, former surgeon general of the United States, differentiates between the positive role of a physician in providing a patient "all the life to which he or she is entitled" and the negative role of "prolonging the act of dying." Koop has opposed euthanasia in any form, cautioning against the possibility of sliding down a slippery slope toward making choices about death that reflect the caregivers' "quality of life" more than the patient's.

Dr. Jack Kevorkian, a Michigan physician, became the most well known advocate of assisted suicide in the United States. From 1990 to 1997, Kevorkian assisted at least sixty-six people in terminating their lives. According to Kevorkian's lawyer, many other assisted suicides have not been publicized. Kevorkian believes that physician-assisted suicide is a matter of individual choice and should be seen as a rational way to end tremendous pain and suffering. Most of the patients assisted by him spent many years suffering from extremely painful and debilitating diseases, such as multiple sclerosis, bone cancer, and brain cancer.

The American Medical Association (AMA) has criticized this view, calling it a violation of professional ethics. When faced with pain and suffering, the AMA asserts that it is a doctor's responsibility to provide adequate "comfort" care, not death. In the AMA's view, Kevorkian served as "a reckless instrument of death." Three trials in Michigan for assisting in suicide resulted in acquittals for Kevorkian before another trial delivered a guilty verdict on the charge of second-degree murder in March, 1999.

During the course of reevaluating the issues involved in terminating a life, the law has been in a state of flux. The decisions that are made by the courts act on the legal precedents of an individual's right to determine what is done to his or her own body and society's position against suicide. The balancing of these two premises has been handled legally by allowing refusal of treatment (passive euthanasia) but disallowing the use of poison or some other method that would cause death (active euthanasia). The latter is labeled suicide, and anyone who assists in such an act can be found guilty of assisting a suicide, or of murder. Following the Karen Ann Quinlan case in 1976, in which the family of a comatose woman secured permission to withdraw life-sustaining treatment, the courts routinely allowed family members to make decisions regarding life-sustaining treatment if the patient could not do so. The area of greatest legal controversy involves the withdrawal of food and water. Some courts have charged doctors with murder for the withdrawal of basic life support measures such as food and water. Others have ruled that invasive procedures to provide food and water (intravenously, for example) are similar to other medical procedures and may be discontinued if the benefit to the patient's quality of life is negligible.

In 1994, 51 percent of the voters in Oregon passed the world's first "death with dignity" law. It allowed physician-assisted suicide. Doctors could begin prescribing fatal overdoses of drugs to terminally ill patients. The vote was reaffirmed in 1997 by 60 percent of the state's voters, despite opposition from the Roman Catholic Church, the AMA, and various anti-abortion and right-to-life groups. The 9th United States Circuit Court of Appeals in San Francisco then lifted a lower court order blocking implementation of the law. Since 1999, several states, including Hawaii, Vermont, New Hampshire, Maine, and North Carolina, have witnessed attempts to legalize physician-assisted suicide but the cases have either been withdrawn or defeated by voters or in state legislature.

Doctors in Oregon became free to prescribe fatal doses of barbiturates to patients with less than six months to live. Physicians were required to file forms with the Oregon Health Division before prescribing the overdose. Then, there would be a fifteen-day waiting period between the request for suicide assistance and the approval of the prescription. Opponents of the Oregon law charged that it perverted the practice of medicine and forced many suffering people to "choose" an early death to save themselves from expensive medical care or pain that could be manageable if physicians were aware of new methods of pain control. The National Right to Life Committee indicated that it would continue to fight implementation of the law in federal courts.

Although the laws vary from state to state, most states allow residents to make their wishes known regarding terminal health care either by writing a living will or by choosing a durable power of attorney. A living will is a document in which one can state that some medical treatments should not be used in the event that one becomes incapacitated to the point where one cannot choose. Living wills allow the patient to decide in advance and protect health care providers from lawsuits. Which treatment options can be terminated and when this action can be put into effect may be limited in some states. Most states have a specific format that should be followed when drawing up a living will and require that the document be signed in the presence of two witnesses. Often, qualifying additions can be made by the individual that specify whether food and water may be withdrawn and whether the living will should go into effect only when death is imminent or also when a person has an incurable illness but death is not imminent. A copy of the living will should be given to the patient's physician and become a part of the patient's medical records. The preparation or execution of a living will cannot affect a person's life insurance coverage or the payment of benefits. Since the medical circumstances of one's life may change and a person's ethical stance may also change, a patient may change the living will at any time by signing a written statement.

A second way in which a person can control what kind of decisions will be made regarding his or her death is to choose a decision maker in advance. This person assumes a durable power of attorney and is legally allowed to act on the patient's behalf, making medical treatment decisions. One advantage of a durable power of attorney over a living will is that the patient can choose someone who shares similar ethical and religious values. Since it is difficult to foresee every medical situation that could arise, there is more security with a durable power of attorney in knowing that the person will have similar values and will therefore probably make the same judgments as the patient. Usually a primary agent and a secondary agent are designated in the event that the primary agent is unavailable. This is especially important if the primary agent is a spouse or a close relative who could, for example, be involved in an accident at the same time as the patient.

PERSPECTIVE AND PROSPECTS

Although large numbers of court decision, articles, and books suggest that the issues involved in euthanasia are recent products of medical technology, these questions are not new. Euthanasia was widely practiced in Western classical culture. The Greeks did not believe that all humans had the right to live, and in Athens, infants with disabilities were often killed. Although in general they did not condone suicide, Pythagoras, Plato, and Aristotle believed that a person could choose to die earlier in the face of an incurable disease and that others could help that person to die. Seneca, the Roman Stoic philosopher, was an avid proponent of euthanasia, stating:

> Against all the injuries of life, I have the refuge of death. If I can choose between a death of torture and one that is simple and easy, why should I not select the latter? As I choose the ship in which I sail and the house which I shall inhabit, so I will choose the death by which I leave life.

The famous Hippocratic oath for physicians acted in opposition to the prevailing cultural bias in favor of euthanasia. Contained in this oath is the statement, "I will never give a deadly drug to anybody if asked for it . . . or make a suggestion to this effect." Interestingly, the AMA has reaffirmed this position in a policy statement:

> . . . the intentional termination of the life of one human being by another—"mercy killing"—is contrary to that for which the medical profession stands and is contrary to the policy of the American Medical Association.

Jewish and Christian theology has traditionally opposed any form of euthanasia or suicide, avowing that since God is the author of life and death, life is sacred. Therefore, a man rebels against God if he prematurely shortens his life, because he violates the Sixth Commandment, "Thou shalt not kill." Suffering was viewed not as an evil to be avoided at all costs but as a condition to be accepted. The Apostle Paul served as an example for early Christians. In 2 Corinthians, he prayed for physical healing, yet when it did not come, he accepted his weakness as a way to increase his dependence on God. This position was affirmed by Saint Augustine in his work *De Civitate Dei* (413-426; *The City of God*) when he condemned suicide as a "detestable and damnable wickedness" which was worse than murder because it left no room for repentance. These strong indictments from the Church against suicide and euthanasia were largely responsible for changing the Greco-Roman attitudes toward the value of human life. They were accepted as society's position until the advent of technologies that made it possible to extend life beyond what would have been the point of death a few years ago.

Although these issues have been debated among both physicians and philosophers for centuries, there is a heightened need for thoughtful discussion and resolution today. Clearly, the decisions surrounding the issue of euthanasia are very complicated. The choice is not simply between commitments to "sanctity of life" or "quality of life" viewpoints. No consensus has yet been reached across the spectrum of society, and instead a variety of alternatives are supported by groups of individuals. A clear understanding of all positions in the debate is the best preparation for making personal decisions at the time of death.

—Katherine B. Frederich, Ph.D.;
updated by Leslie V. Tischauser, Ph.D.

See also Aging: Extended care; Critical care; Critical care, pediatric; Death and dying; Ethics; Hippocratic oath; Law and medicine; Pain management; Psychiatry; Psychiatry, geriatric; Suicide; Terminally ill: Extended care.

FOR FURTHER INFORMATION:

Corr, Charles A., Clyde M. Nabe, and Donna M. Corr. *Death and Dying, Life and Living.* 4th ed. Belmont, Calif.: Wadsworth, 2002. This book provides perspective on common issues associated with death and dying for family members and others affected by life-threatening circumstances.

Dowbiggin, Ian Robert. *Merciful End: The Euthanasia Movement in Modern America*. New York: Oxford University Press, 2003. Blends social history, medical knowledge, and political analysis to trace the evolution of euthanasia and its perception in the United States throughout the twentieth century.

Gorovitz, Samuel. *Drawing the Line*. Reprint. New York: Oxford University Press, 1993. This book reflects on the author's seven-week sabbatical-in-residence at Beth Israel Hospital. Gorovitz presents numerous insights drawn from conversations with patients and medical personnel.

Harron, Frank, John Burnside, and Tom Beauchamp. *Health and Human Values*. New Haven, Conn.: Yale University Press, 1983. Using a case-study approach, the authors consider the different types of euthanasia and report on policy statements from interested social groups.

Leone, Daniel A. *The Ethics of Euthanasia*. San Diego, Calif.: Greenhaven Press, 1999. This volume includes ten essays on the ethics and morality of euthanasia, potential abuse, distinctions between active and passive euthanasia, and whether euthanasia is consistent with Christian belief.

Magnusson, Roger, and Peter H. Ballis. *Angels of Death: Exploring the Euthanasia Underground*. New Haven, Conn.: Yale University Press, 2002. Explores the existence of a euthanasia underground in Australia and the United States using firsthand accounts of health professionals who have been involved in assisted death.

Rebman, Renee C. *Euthanasia and the Right to Die: Pro/Con Issues*. Berkeley Heights, N.J.: Enslow, 2002. Part of the "Hot Pro/Con Issues" series for young adults, offers a balanced perspective on a range of issues surrounding euthanasia.

Spring, Beth, and Ed Larson. *Euthanasia*. Portland, Oreg.: Multnomah Press, 1988. This book considers the spiritual, medical, and legal issues in terminal health care, citing numerous perspectives from the religious community. Contains two chapters detailing practical guidelines for writing living wills and durable powers of attorney.

Torr, James D. *Euthanasia*. San Diego, Calif.: Greenhaven Press, 1999. Designed for students in grades nine through twelve, this volume brings together essays by authorities in diverse vocations. The four chapters explore whether euthanasia is ethical, if it should be legalized, if legalization would lead to in-voluntary killing, and under what circumstances, if any, doctors should assist in suicide.

Wennberg, Robert N. *Terminal Choices*. Grand Rapids, Mich.: Wm. B. Eerdmans, 1989. The author presents a helpful history of the euthanasia debate and also discusses possible moral distinctions between treatment refusal and treatment withdrawal.

EWING'S SARCOMA
DISEASE/DISORDER

ALSO KNOWN AS: Bone cancer

ANATOMY OR SYSTEM AFFECTED: Bones, musculoskeletal system

SPECIALTIES AND RELATED FIELDS: Oncology, orthopedics, pediatrics, radiology

DEFINITION: A rare bone cancer involving any part of the skeleton but found commonly in the long bones (60 percent), the pelvis (18 percent), and the ribs (15 percent) of children and young adults.

CAUSES AND SYMPTOMS

The specific cause of Ewing's sarcoma is unknown, but it may be associated with recurrent trauma, metal implants, congenital anomalies, unrelated tumors, or exposure to ionizing radiation. Approximately 90 percent of patients are between five and twenty-five years of age; rarely are patients younger than five or older than forty.

The initial symptom is pain, discontinuous at first and then intense, in the long bones, vertebra, or pelvis. Swelling may follow. Neurological signs involving the nerve roots or spinal cord depression are characteristic of nearly one-half of patients with involvement of the axial skeleton. Weight loss may occur, with remittent fever and mild anemia.

INFORMATION ON EWING'S SARCOMA

CAUSES: Unknown; possibly related to recurrent trauma, metal implants, congenital anomalies, unrelated tumors, exposure to ionizing radiation

SYMPTOMS: Pain in long bones, vertebra, or pelvis; swelling; neurological disorders; weight loss; fever; mild anemia

DURATION: Long-term

TREATMENTS: Surgery, chemotherapy, radiation

The phases of Ewing's sarcoma are based on degree of metastasis: the local phase (a nonmetastatic tumor), the regional phase (lymph node involvement), and the distant phase (involvement of the lungs, bones, and sometimes the central nervous system).

TREATMENT AND THERAPY

Patients are of two types, those with localized tumors and those with metastasized tumors. Depending on where the tumor is located, the treatment of Ewing's sarcoma is complex in all stages of disease and requires a multidisciplinary perspective. It is best treated when diagnosed early. Obtaining a bone biopsy is recommended in nearly all cases.

Surgery may be used to remove a tumor, followed by chemotherapy administered to kill any remaining cancer cells. Radiation may be prescribed to kill cancer cells and shrink tumors.

PERSPECTIVE AND PROSPECTS

Ewing's sarcoma is one of the most malignant of all tumors. It may be localized or metastasize to the lungs and other bones. The primary tumor can be controlled by irradiation, but the prognosis is poor. Often, amputation is not justifiable. Recent developments in multiagent chemotherapy, however, are encouraging. Long-term survival of patients with Ewing's sarcoma is 50 to 70 percent or more with localized disease; the rate drops to less than 30 percent for metastatic disease.

—*John Alan Ross, Ph.D.*

See also Cancer; Bone cancer; Bone disorders; Bones and the skeleton; Orthopedics, pediatric.

FOR FURTHER INFORMATION:

Cady, Blake, ed. *Cancer Manual.* 7th ed. Boston: American Cancer Society, 1986.

Children's Cancer Web. http://www.cancerindex.org/ccw/.

Dollinger, Malin, Ernest H. Rosenbaum, and Greg Cable. *Everyone's Guide to Cancer Therapy.* 4th rev. ed. Kansas City, Mo.: Andrews & McMeel, 2002.

Dorfman, Howard D., and Bogdan Czerniak. *Bone Tumors.* St. Louis: Mosby, 1998.

Grealy, Lucy. *Autobiography of a Face.* New York: HarperCollins, 2003.

Holleb, Arthur I., ed. *The American Cancer Society Cancer Book: Prevention, Detection, Diagnosis, Treatment, Rehabilitation, Cure.* Garden City, N.Y.: Doubleday, 1986.

Janes-Hodder, Honna, and Nancy Keene. *Childhood Cancer: A Parent's Guide to Solid Tumor Cancers.* 2d ed. Cambridge, Mass.: O'Reilly and Associates, 2002.

Morra, Marion, and Eve Potts. *Choices: Realistic Alternatives in Cancer Treatment.* New York: Avon Books, 1987.

Murphy, G., L. Morris, and D. Lange. *Informed Decisions: The Complete Book of Cancer Diagnosis, Treatment, and Recovery.* New York: Viking, 1997.

EXERCISE PHYSIOLOGY

SPECIALTY

ANATOMY OR SYSTEM AFFECTED: Circulatory system, heart, joints, knees, lungs, muscles, musculoskeletal system, respiratory system, tendons

SPECIALTIES AND RELATED FIELDS: Cardiology, family practice, nutrition, physical therapy, preventive medicine, sports medicine

DEFINITION: The science that studies the effects on the body of various intensities and types of physical activity, including cellular metabolism, cardiovascular responses, respiratory responses, neural and hormonal adaptations, and muscular adaptations to exercise.

KEY TERMS:

adenosine triphosphate (ATP): a high-energy compound found in the cell which provides energy for all bodily functions

aerobic: metabolism involving the breakdown of energy substrates using oxygen

anaerobic: metabolism involving the breakdown of energy substrates without using oxygen

atherosclerosis: hardening and thickening of the walls of the arteries caused by a buildup of fatty deposits

electrocardiogram (ECG): a graphic record of electrical currents of the heart

glycogen: the form that glucose takes when it is stored in the muscles and liver

heart rate: the number of times the heart contracts, or beats, per minute

maximal oxygen uptake: the maximum rate of oxygen consumption during exercise

metabolic equivalent (MET): a unit used to estimate the metabolic cost of physical activity; 1 MET is equal to 3.5 milliliters of oxygen consumed per kilogram of body weight per minute

SCIENCE AND PROFESSION

The primary focus of research in the field of exercise physiology is to gain a better understanding of the quantity and type of exercise needed for health maintenance and rehabilitation. A major goal of professionals in exercise physiology is to find ways to incorporate appropriate levels of physical activity into the lifestyles of all individuals.

Physiology is the science of physical and chemical factors and processes involved in the function of living organisms. The study of exercise physiology examines these factors and processes as they relate to physical exertion. The physical responses that occur are specific to the intensity, duration, and type of exercise performed.

Low or moderate exercise intensity relies on oxygen to release energy for work. This process is often referred to as aerobic exercise. In the muscles, carbohydrates and fats are broken down to produce adenosine triphosphate (ATP), the basic molecule used for energy. Aerobic exercise can be sustained for several minutes to several hours.

Higher-intensity exercise is predominantly fueled anaerobically (in the absence of oxygen) and can be sustained for up to two minutes only. Muscle glycogen is broken down without oxygen to produce ATP. Anaerobic metabolism is much less efficient at producing ATP than is aerobic metabolism.

During anaerobic metabolism, a by-product called lactic acid begins to accumulate in the blood as blood lactate. The point at which this accumulation begins is called the anaerobic threshold (AT), or the onset of blood lactate accumulation (OBLA). Blood lactate can cause muscle soreness and stiffness, but it also can be used as fuel during aerobic metabolism.

A third and less often used energy system is the creatine phosphate (ATP-CP) system. Utilizing the very limited supply of ATP that is stored in the muscles, phosphate molecules are exchanged between ATP and CP to provide energy. This system provides only enough fuel for a few seconds of maximum effort.

The type of muscle fiber recruited to perform a specific type of exercise is also dependent on exercise intensity. Skeletal muscle is composed of "slow-twitch" and two types of "fast-twitch" muscle fibers. Slow-twitch fibers are more suited to using oxygen than are fast-twitch fibers, and they are recruited primarily for aerobic exercise. One type of fast-twitch fiber also functions during aerobic activity. The second type of fast-twitch fiber serves to facilitate anaerobic, or high-intensity, exercise.

Exercise mode is also a factor in the physiological responses to exercise. Dynamic exercise (alternating muscular contraction and relaxation through a range of motion) using many large muscles requires more oxygen than does activity utilizing smaller and fewer muscles. The greater the oxygen requirement of the physical activity, the greater the cardiorespiratory benefits.

Many bodily adaptations occur over a training period of six to eight weeks, and other benefits are gradually manifested over several months. The positive adaptations include reduced resting and working heart rates. As the heart becomes stronger, there is a subsequent increase in stroke volume (the volume of blood the heart pumps with each beat), which allows the heart to beat less frequently while maintaining the same cardiac output (the volume of the blood pumped from the heart each minute). Another beneficial adaptation is increased metabolic efficiency. This is partially facilitated by an increase in the number of mitochondria (the organelles responsible for ATP production) in the muscle cells.

One of the most recognized representations of aerobic fitness is the maximum volume of oxygen (VO_{2max}) an individual can use during exercise. VO_{2max} is improved through habitual, relatively high-intensity aerobic activity. After three to six months of regular training, levels of high-density lipoproteins (HDLs) in the blood increase. HDL molecules remove cholesterol (a fatty substance) from the tissues to aid in protecting the heart from atherosclerosis.

Various internal and external factors influence the metabolic processes that take place during and after exercise. Internally, nutrition, degree of hydration, body composition, flexibility, sex, and age are some of the variables that play a role in the physiological responses. Other internal variables include medical conditions such as heart disease, diabetes, and hypertension (high blood pressure). Externally, environmental conditions such as temperature, humidity, and altitude alter how the exercising body functions.

Various modes of exercise testing and data collection are used to study the physiological responses of the body to exercise. Treadmills and cycle ergometers (instruments used to measure work and power output) are among the most common methods of evaluating maximum oxygen consumption. During these tests, special equipment and computers analyze expired air, heart rate is monitored with an electrocardiograph (ECG), and blood pressure is taken using a sphygmomanometer. Blood samples and muscle fiber samples can also be extracted to aid in identifying the fuel system and type of muscle fibers being used. Other data sometimes collected, such as skin temperatures and body core temperatures, can provide pertinent information.

Metabolic equivalent units, or METs, are often used to translate a person's capability into workloads on various pieces of exercise equipment or into everyday tasks. For every 3.5 milliliters of oxygen consumed per kilogram of body weight per minute, the subject is said to be performing at a workload of one MET. One MET is approximately equivalent to 1.5 kilocalories per minute, or the amount of energy expended per kilogram of body weight in one minute when a person is at rest.

Another factor greatly affecting the physical response to exercise is body composition. The three major structural components of the body are muscle, bone, and fat. Body composition can be evaluated using a combination of anthropometric measurements. These measurements include body weight, standard height, measurements of circumferences at various locations using a tape measure, measurements of skeletal diameters using a sliding metric stick, and measurements of skinfold thicknesses using calipers.

Body fat can be estimated using several methods, the most accurate of which is based on a calculation of body density. This method is called hydrostatic weighing, which involves weighing the subject under water while taking into account the residual volume of air in the lungs. The principle underlying this measurement of body density is based on the fact that fat is less dense than water and will float, whereas bone and muscle, which are denser than water, will sink. One biochemical technique often used to determine levels of body fat is based on the relatively constant level of potassium 40 naturally existing in lean body mass. Another method utilizes ultrasound waves to measure the thickness of fat layers. X rays and computed tomography (CT) scanning can be used to provide images from which fat and bone can be measured. Bioelectrical impedance (BIA) is a method of estimating body composition based on the resistance imposed on a low voltage electrical current sent through the body. The most widely used and easily assessable method, however, involves measurement of skinfolds at various sites on the body using calipers. In all cases, mathematical formulas have been devised to interpret the collected data and provide the best estimate of an individual's body composition.

Other tests have been developed to determine muscular strength, muscular endurance, and flexibility. Muscular strength is often measured by performance of one maximal effort produced by a selected muscle group. Muscular endurance of a muscle or muscle group is often demonstrated by the length of time or number of repetitions a particular, submaximal workload or skill can be performed.

Two major types of flexibility have been identified. One type consists of the flexibility through the range of motion of a muscle group or joint. This is called static flexibility. It can be measured using a metric stick or a protractor-type instrument called a goniometer. Dynamic flexibility is the other major identified type of flexibility. It is the torque of or resistance to movement. Methods to measure dynamic flexibility have not been developed.

Overlapping the science of exercise physiology are the studies of biomechanics or kinesiology (sciences dealing with human movement) and nutrition. Only through an understanding of efficient body mechanics and proper nutrition can the physiological responses of the body to exercise be identified correctly.

Diagnostic and Treatment Techniques

Exercise prescription is the primary focus in the application of exercise physiology. General health maintenance, cardiac rehabilitation, and competitive athletics are three major areas of exercise prescription.

Before making recommendations for an exercise program, an exercise physiologist must evaluate the physical limitations of the exerciser. In a normal, health maintenance setting—often called a "wellness" program—a health-related questionnaire can reveal relevant information. Such a questionnaire should include questions about family medical history and the subject's history of heart trouble or chest pain, bone or joint problems, and high blood pressure. The presence of any of these problems suggests the need for a physician's consent prior to exercising. After the individual has been deemed eligible to participate, an assessment of the level of physical fitness should be performed. Determining or estimating VO_{2max}, muscular strength, muscular endurance, flexibility, and body composition is usually included in this assessment. It is then possible to design a program best suited to the needs of the individual.

For the healthy adult participant, the American College of Sports Medicine (ACSM), a widely recognized authoritative body on exercise prescription, recommends three to five sessions of aerobic exercise weekly. Each session should include a five- to ten-minute warm-up period, twenty to sixty minutes of aerobic exercise at a predetermined exercise intensity, and a five- to ten-minute cool-down period.

In order to recommend an appropriate aerobic exercise intensity, the exercise physiologist must determine

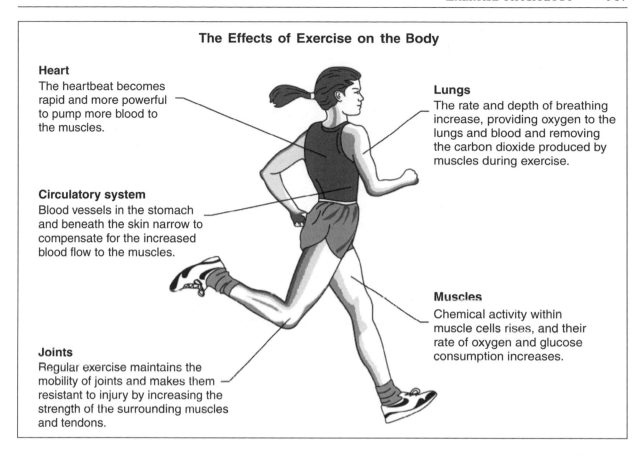

The Effects of Exercise on the Body

Heart
The heartbeat becomes rapid and more powerful to pump more blood to the muscles.

Lungs
The rate and depth of breathing increase, providing oxygen to the lungs and blood and removing the carbon dioxide produced by muscles during exercise.

Circulatory system
Blood vessels in the stomach and beneath the skin narrow to compensate for the increased blood flow to the muscles.

Muscles
Chemical activity within muscle cells rises, and their rate of oxygen and glucose consumption increases.

Joints
Regular exercise maintains the mobility of joints and makes them resistant to injury by increasing the strength of the surrounding muscles and tendons.

an individual's maximum heart rate. The best way to obtain this maximum heart rate is to administer a maximal exercise test. Such a test can be supervised by an exercise physiologist or an exercise test technician; it is advisable, especially for the older participant, that a cardiologist also be in attendance. An ECG is monitored for irregularities as the subject walks, runs, cycles, or performs some dynamic exercise to exhaustion or until the onset of irregular symptoms or discomfort.

Exercise prescription using heart rate as a measure can be achieved by various methods. A direct correlation exists between exercise intensity, in terms of oxygen consumption, and heart rate. From data collected during a maximal exercise test, a target heart rate range of 40 percent to 85 percent of functional capacity can be calculated. Another method used to determine an appropriate heart rate range is based on the difference between an individual's resting heart rate and maximum heart rate, called the heart rate reserve (HRR). Values representing 60 percent and 80 percent of the heart rate reserve are calculated and added to the resting heart rate, yielding the individual's target heart rate range. A third method involves calculating 70 percent and 85

percent of the maximum heart rate. Although this method is less accurate than the other two methods, it is the simplest way to estimate a target heart rate range.

Intensity of exercise can also be prescribed using METs. This method relies on the predetermined metabolic equivalents required to perform activities at various intensities. Activity levels reflecting 40 percent to 85 percent of functional capacity can be calculated.

The rating of perceived exertion (RPE) is another method of prescribing exercise intensity. Verbal responses by the participant describing how an exercise feels at various intensities are assigned to a numerical scale, which is then correlated to heart rate. Through practice, the participant can correlate heart rate with the RPE, reducing the necessity of frequent pulse monitoring in the healthy individual.

Adequate physical fitness can be defined as the ability to perform daily tasks with enough reserve for emergency situations. All aspects of health-related fitness direct attention toward this goal. Aerobic exercise often provides some conditioning for muscular endurance, but muscular strength and flexibility need to be addressed separately.

The ACSM recommends resistance training using the "overload principle," which involves placing habitual stress on a system, causing it to adapt and respond. For this training, it is suggested that eight to twelve repetitions of eight to ten strengthening exercises of the major muscle groups be performed a minimum of two days per week.

Flexibility of connective tissue and muscle tissue is essential to maximize physical performance and to limit musculoskeletal injuries. At least one stretching exercise for each major muscle group should be executed three to four times per week while the muscles are warm. Three methods of stretching that have been designed to improve flexibility are ballistic stretching, static stretching, and proprioceptive neuromuscular facilitation (PNF). Ballistic stretching incorporates a bouncing motion and is generally prescribed only in sports that replicate this type of movement. During a static stretch, the muscles and connective tissue are passively stretched to their maximum lengths. PNF involves a contract-relax sequence of the muscle.

In addition to exercise prescription for cardiorespiratory fitness, muscular fitness, and flexibility, it is appropriate for the exercise physiologist to make recommendations concerning body composition. Exercise is an effective tool in fat loss. Dietary caloric restriction without exercise results in a greater loss of muscle mass along with fat loss than if exercise is part of a weight loss program.

For persons with special health concerns, such as diabetes mellitus or high blood pressure, the exercise physiologist works with the participant's physician. The physician is responsible for prescribing necessary medications and often decides which modes of exercise are contraindicated (those that should be avoided).

A second application, cardiac rehabilitation, takes exercise prescription a step further. Participation of the heart patient is more individualized than in wellness programs. The condition of the circulatory system, pulmonary system, and joints are only a few of the special concerns. Secondary conditions such as obesity, diabetes, and hypertension must also be considered. The responsibilities of cardiac rehabilitation specialists include monitoring blood sugar in diabetic patients and blood pressure in all patients, especially those with hypertension. Many drugs affect heart rate or blood pressure, and most of these participants are taking more than one type of medication. Patients with heart damage caused by a heart attack may display atypical heart rhythms, which can be seen on an ECG monitor. Furthermore, the stage of recovery of the postsurgical pa-

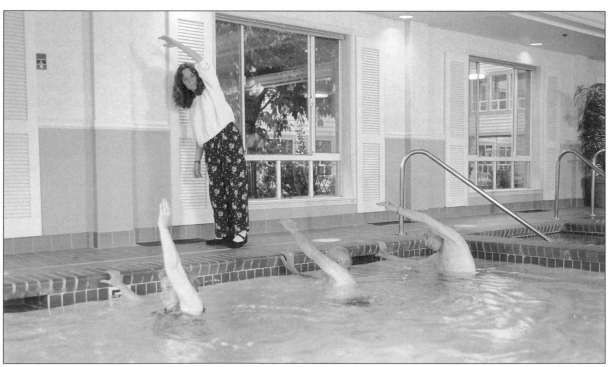

Elderly individuals may find low-impact exercise, such as swimming, to be a safer and easier way to stay fit. (PhotoDisc)

tient is a major factor in recommending the type, frequency, intensity, and duration of exercise.

Patient education is also important. Lifestyle is usually the main factor in the development of heart disease. Cardiac patients often have never participated in a regular exercise program. Frequently, they are smokers, are overweight, and have poor eating habits. Helping them to identify and correct destructive health-related behaviors is the focus of education for the heart patient.

A third application of the study of exercise physiology involves dealing with the competitive athlete. In this case, findings from the most recent research are constantly applied to yield the best athletic performance possible. A delicate balance of aerobic training, anaerobic training, strength training, endurance training, and flexibility exercises are combined with the optimum percentage of body fat, proper nutrition, and adequate sleep. The program that is designed must enhance the athletic qualities that are most beneficial to the sport in which the athlete participates.

The competitive athlete usually pushes beyond the boundaries of general exercise prescription in terms of intensity, duration, and frequency of exercise performance. As a result, the athlete risks suffering more injuries than the individual who exercises for health benefits. If the athlete sustains an injury, the exercise physiologist may work in conjunction with an athletic trainer or sports physician to return the athlete to competition as soon as possible.

PERSPECTIVE AND PROSPECTS

The modern study of exercise physiology developed out of an interest in physical fitness. In the United States, and possibly much of the world, that interest was primarily driven by a desire to prepare soldiers for war adequately.

In the United States, the concern for development and maintenance of physical fitness was well established by the end of the twentieth century. As early as 1819, Stanford and Harvard universities offered professional physical education programs. At least one textbook on the physiology of exercise was published by that time.

Much of the pioneer work in this field, however, was done in Europe. Nobel Prize-winning European research on muscular exercise, oxygen utilization as it relates to the upper limits of physical performance, and production of lactic acid during glucose metabolism dates back to the 1920's.

In the early 1950's, poor performance by children in the United States on a minimal muscular fitness test helped lead to the formation of what is now known as the President's Council on Physical Fitness and Sport. Concurrently, a significant number of deaths of middle-aged American males were found to be caused by poor health habits associated with coronary artery disease. A need for more research in the areas of health and physical activity was recognized by the mid-1960's. The subsequent research was facilitated by the existence of fifty-eight exercise physiology research laboratories in colleges and universities throughout the country.

Organizations such as the American Physiological Society (APS), the American Alliance of Health, Physical Education, and Recreation (AAHPER), and the American College of Sports Medicine (ACSM) were established by the mid-1950's. In an effort to ensure that well-trained professionals were involved in cardiac rehabilitation programs, the ACSM developed a certification program in 1975. Certifications for fitness personnel were added later.

A better understanding of fundamental physiological mechanisms should stem from increasingly more sophisticated testing equipment, allowing practitioners to be more effective in measuring physical fitness and in prescribing exercise programs. Health maintenance has become a priority as the number of adults over the age of fifty continues to increase. Advances in medical techniques also increase the survival rate of victims of heart attacks, creating a need for more cardiac rehabilitation programs and practitioners. Health care professionals and the general population need to be made more aware of the benefits of exercise in the maintenance of good health and in the rehabilitation of individuals with medical problems.

—Kathleen O'Boyle

See also Biofeedback; Bones and the skeleton; Cardiac rehabilitation; Cardiology; Electrocardiography (ECG or EKG); Glycolysis; Heart; Kinesiology; Lungs; Metabolism; Muscle sprains, spasms, and disorders; Muscles; Nutrition; Orthopedics; Orthopedics, pediatric; Oxygen therapy; Physical rehabilitation; Physiology; Preventive medicine; Pulmonary medicine; Respiration; Sports medicine; Steroid abuse; Tendinitis; Vascular system.

FOR FURTHER INFORMATION:

American College of Sports Medicine. *ACSM's Guidelines for Exercise Testing and Prescription.* 6th ed. Philadelphia: Lippincott Williams & Wilkins, 2000. This manual provides guidelines for professionals working in preventive exercise programs or in cardiac rehabilitation. The recommendations are based on the most up-to-date research available at the time of publication.

_____. *Resource Manual for Guidelines for Exercise Testing and Prescription.* 4th ed. Baltimore: Williams & Wilkins, 2001. Based on the objective of providing safe and effective exercise programs for all individuals, this publication provides an excellent overview of many of the topics of concern to the exercise physiologist. Specific recommendations regarding stress testing and exercise prescription are included in the text.

Beim, Gloria, and Ruth Winter. *The Female Athlete's Body Book: How to Prevent and Treat Sports Injuries in Women and Girls.* New York: McGraw-Hill, 2003. Organized by sport, covers common injuries and how to prevent and treat them and guidelines for off-season training, among other topics.

Brooks, George A., and Thomas D. Fahey. *Fundamentals of Human Performance.* New York: Macmillan, 1987. This textbook was written for students of physical education, nursing, nutrition, and physical therapy who need a practical introduction to exercise physiology. The theoretical basis and practical application of physical activity are explained through a discussion of metabolic phenomena.

McArdle, William, Frank I. Katch, and Victor L. Katch. *Exercise Physiology: Energy, Nutrition, and Human Performance.* 5th ed. Philadelphia: Lippincott Williams & Wilkins, 2001. A wide-ranging text on exercise and the human body, covering topics such as nutrition, energy transfer, exercise training, systems of energy delivery and utilization, enhancement of energy capacity, the effect of environmental stress, and the effect of exercise on successful aging and disease prevention.

Plowman, Sharon A., and Denise L. Smith. *Exercise Physiology for Health, Fitness, and Performance.* San Francisco: Benjamin/Cummings, 2002. Discusses the basics of exercise physiology as well as special topics such as the impact of altitude on exercise training, pollution and exercise, and children and the cardiovascular risk factors of physical activity.

Powers, Scott K., and Edward T. Howley. *Exercise Physiology: Theory and Application to Fitness and Performance.* New York: McGraw-Hill, 2000. The upper-level undergraduate or beginning graduate student will find detailed information concerning exercise physiology in this useful textbook. Designed for students who are serious about the study of exercise science.

EXTENDED CARE FOR THE AGING. *See* **AGING: EXTENDED CARE.**

EXTENDED CARE FOR THE TERMINALLY ILL. *See* **TERMINALLY ILL: EXTENDED CARE.**

EXTREMITIES. *See* **FEET; FOOT DISORDERS; LOWER EXTREMITIES; UPPER EXTREMITIES.**

EYE DISORDERS. *See* **BLINDNESS; CATARACTS; EYES; GLAUCOMA; TRACHOMA; VISUAL DISORDERS.**

EYE SURGERY
PROCEDURE

ANATOMY OR SYSTEM AFFECTED: Eyes
SPECIALTIES AND RELATED FIELDS: General surgery, geriatrics, ophthalmology, optometry
DEFINITION: Surgical removals from or repairs to the eye.
KEY TERMS:

canal of Schlemm: a tiny vein at the angle of the anterior eye chamber that drains aqueous humor into the bloodstream

choroid: the vascular, intermediate coat furnishing nourishment to parts of the eyeball

cornea: the clear, transparent portion of the eye's outer coat, forming the covering of the aqueous chamber

iris: a colored circular membrane suspended behind the cornea and in front of the lens, regulating the amount of light entering the eye by changing the size of the pupil

lens: the transparent biconvex body of the eye

retina: the innermost coat of the eye, formed from sensitive nerve elements and connected with the optic nerve

sclera: the white part of the eye; with the cornea, it forms the eye's external protective coat

trabeculae: the portion of the eye in front of the canal of Schlemm and within the angle created by the iris and cornea

INDICATIONS AND PROCEDURES

Compared to surgery performed on internal organs and any number of outpatient procedures, eye surgery can fill patients with added fears, often concerned with great suffering and the possibility of permanent sight loss. Surgery to an internal organ is usually perceived as happening in a remote location in an unseen portion of the body, and most patients have little idea of the organ's function. Often, if an internal growth or organ is removed, the body continues to function quite well. Most patients have some knowledge of the eye, unlike most internal organs, and thus are more likely to develop anxiety about even common surgical procedures involving it. Patients know what eyes are and what they are used for and that they are extremely sensitive and painful to touch. A grain of sand or a hair touching the eye is painful, so the thought of contacting the eye with a needle or making an incision in it with a scalpel or laser can be almost unimaginable. Patients with ocular problems requiring surgery fear damage to the eye and know all too well the consequences of removal. In most instances, the general public has little to no knowledge or understanding of the function and mechanics of eye surgery. Common eye surgeries include, but are not limited to, cataract surgery, corneal transplantation, vision correction, pterygium removal, retinal detactment repair, and tear duct surgery.

A cataract is an opacity on the eye's lens. A cataract may be minimal in size and low in density, so that light transmission is not appreciably affected, or it may be large and opaque so that light cannot gain entry into the interior eye. When the cataract is pronounced, the interior of the patient's eye cannot be seen with clarity, and the patient cannot see out clearly. Over time, the lens takes on a yellowish hue and begins to lose transparency. As the lens thus becomes "cloudy," the patient needs brighter and brighter lights for visual clarity. If the lens becomes completely opaque, then the patient is functionally blind. A cataract is removed when it endangers the health of the eye or interferes with a patient's ability to function. Conditions such as contrast sensitivity, glare, pupillary constriction, and ambient light may significantly affect a patient's functionality.

The objective of cataract surgery is to remove the crystalline lens of the eye that has become cloudy. Modern surgical procedures involve removing the lens, either intact or in pieces after shattering it with high-frequency sound. The surgery is usually performed under an operating microscope because magnification is necessary. Many methods are used for cataract surgery, including an extracapsular procedure, an intracapsular procedure, and phacoemulsification. Most surgeons perform cataract surgery in freestanding surgical centers on an outpatient basis.

In extracapsular surgery, an incision is made at the superior limbus and a small opening is made into the anterior chamber. A viscoelastic substance is introduced and then a small, bent needle, or cystotome, is introduced. An incision is made into the anterior capsule in a circular, triangular, or D-shaped fashion. The wound is enlarged to a diameter of 10 to 11 millimeters, allowing removal of the cataractous nucleus.

The most common cataract surgical procedure is phacoemulsification, or small-incision cataract surgery. A stair-stepped incision of between 1.5 and 4.0 millimeters is made in the front of the eye. A cystotome is inserted to cut the anterior capsule of the lens. An emulsifier and aspirator is inserted to remove the collapsed lens. The missing lens is then replaced by an artificial substitute that is folded and inserted through the incision and rotated into place. The wound is sealed with a single suture or no suture at all. This procedure has become favored because it causes less tissue destruction, less wound reaction, and less astigmatism, and patients can resume normal activities immediately after surgery. Vision is then fine-tuned with glasses or contact lenses, if needed.

Another common eye surgery is corneal transplantation. The cornea is the clear portion in the front part of that eye. When injured, degenerated, or infected, the cornea can become cloudy and vision disrupted. Corneal surgery restores lost vision by replacing a portion of the cornea with a clear window taken from a donor eye. Usually, the donor cornea is taken from a recently deceased person. However, not everyone with corneal disease can be helped by corneal transplantation.

The cornea was one of the first structures of the body to be transplanted. Because the cornea is devoid of blood vessels, it is one of the few tissues in the human body that may be transplanted from one human to another with a high degree of success. The absence of blood vessels in the donor cornea reduces immune system reactions.

Two types of corneal transplants are performed: partial penetration, in which a half thickness of the cornea is transplanted, and penetrating transplantation, which involves the full thickness of the cornea. In partial penetration, the anterior of the eye is not entered; only the outer half or two-thirds of the cornea is transplanted. Union is made by several sutures around the periphery of the donor tissue. Depending on the extent of the disease, the donor tissue may be 6 to 10 millimeters in diameter. In a penetrating transplantation, surgery involves entering the anterior chamber of the eye, inserting the donor cornea, and establishing a tight fit with a continuous suture.

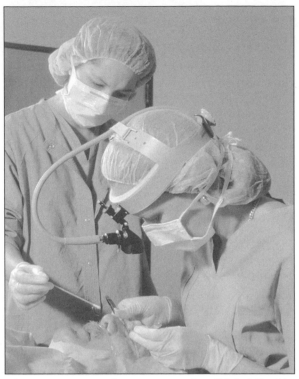

An eye surgeon performs an operation. (Digital Stock)

Glaucoma is an ocular disease affecting roughly 2 percent of the population over forty. The major characteristic of the condition is a sustained increase in intraocular pressure so great that the fibrous scleral coat cannot expand significantly and the eye cannot withstand the increasing pressures against surrounding soft tissue without damage to its structure and vision impairment. The results of this pressure increase include excavation of the optic disc, hardness of the eyeball, reduced vision, the appearance of colored halos around lights, visual field defects, and headaches. Surgical procedures are performed to relieve this pressure. Although many types of surgical procedures are performed to treat glaucoma, they are all basically fistulizing surgeries, attempting to create an opening between the anterior chamber and the subconjunctival space or between the surgically prepared layers of the sclera.

Glaucoma surgery involves a small incision made either directly through the cornea at the upper limbus or under a flap of conjunctival tissue. The iris is grasped with small forceps and pulled out of the eye, and a small portion of the trabecular meshwork is partially removed, allowing the aqueous fluid to filter out of the anterior chamber. The cornea is then sutured and the

eye bandaged. The most popular procedure of this type is trabeculectomy. As a whole, glaucoma surgeries are performed less often today because of the success of nonsurgical treatments and management with drug therapies. A major consequence of some glaucoma surgery is the development of cataracts. For this reason, early surgery is advocated, especially if factors place patients at high risk.

A common early stage nonincisive procedure in treating glaucoma is laser trabeculoplasty. This procedure involves lasing the middle to anterior portion of the trabecular meshwork with eighty to one hundred equally spaced burns. The argon laser reopens blocked drainage channels and reduces fluid pressure in the eye. More than 90 percent of patients experience successful outcomes from this treatment. Surgery is performed only if patients continue to lose the visual field.

A pterygium is a fibrovascular membrane that extends from the medial aspect of the bulbar conjunctiva and invades the cornea. It is a progressive growth related to overexposure to ultraviolet (UV) light. In time, it can make its way to the central portion of the cornea and interfere with vision. Pterygia are most common in southern climates, where people have greater exposure to UV light. In northern regions, people who work outdoors, especially in open fields or on open water, are most prone to developing a pterygium growth.

The purpose of removing a pterygium is to excise the membrane before it can interfere with vision. The operation requires incision into the cornea as well as the conjunctiva, then removal of the pterygium tissue or its transplantation to another position to redirect its growth.

In a normal eye, the retina lays against the choroidal layer, from which it receives part of its blood supply and nourishment. The retina is loosely attached to the choroid, but when it becomes separated from the choroid, it flaps and hangs within the eye's vitreous fluid. Retinal detachment does not allow adequate nutrients to reach the retina and thus causes poor function, and it eventually leads to vision loss. Retinal detachment may be caused by injury, myopia, or previous eye surgeries. Often, a tear or hole permits fluid to collect under the retina, causing the detachment.

Retinal detachment surgery corrects the loose retina by bringing it back to the choroid or by pushing the choroid up to the retina. To bring the retina back into place, scleral punctures are made to drain fluids that lay between the retina and the choroid. When the retina returns to lay against the choroid, either electrocoagulation or cryotherapy with a cold probe against the sclera unites the retina to the choroid. Then the retina and choroid are brought together with a silicone buckling band to exert inward pressure. If the retina is not attached at this point, then air, special gases, or oil is injected into the vitreous fluid to push the retina back against the choroid.

Surgery involving corrective procedures to tear ducts is common, especially in older patients. A blockage in the nasolacrimal passage may result in a condition called epiphora, in which the tear ducts water constantly. Such a blockage of the tear canal may result from some form of obstruction. These obstructions are cleared by a surgical procedure called dacryocystorhinostomy. In this procedure, a large incision of 8 to 10 millimeters is made in the wall of the nose, and a union is created between the mucosal lining of the nose and the lacrimal sac. In this way, the lacrimal sac opens directly into the nose. The operation is usually successful in curing the tearing and infection problems arising from stagnation in the blocked tear duct.

Elective refractive eye surgery for the purpose of vision correction began in the Soviet Union in the 1970's and gained popularity in the United States in the 1990's with the use of lasers. It is performed for the relief of myopia, hypermyopia, and astigmatism, with the goal of eliminating the need for either eyeglasses or contact lenses. It is also used to correct refractive errors caused by cataract surgery and corneal transplantation.

Two of the most common refractive surgeries are radial keratotomy (RK) and photorefractive keratectomy (PRK), also known as excimer laser surgery. Myopic patients suffer from a cornea that is either too convex or has an axial length that is too long, causing light to converge at a focal point anterior to the retina. In refractive surgery, corneal reshaping is the important concept. The surgical goal is to flatten the center of the cornea so that light will focus more posteriorly.

RK reshapes the cornea by radial incisions made with a diamond knife. This process weakens the cornea, so normal intraocular pressure pushes the center of the cornea outward, flattening the central cornea. PRK uses a laser to remove the superficial layers of the central cornea, about 50 to 100 microns of tissue, to achieve a similar reshaping of the cornea.

USES AND COMPLICATIONS

The introduction of lasers to eye surgery has proved both beneficial and controversial, depending on its use. An excimer laser can remove any opacifications of the superficial layers of the cornea while retaining the health and clarity of deeper corneal layers. The laser can be used to remove injury-related and surgical corneal scars and to treat astigmatism that may follow implant cataract surgery. The excimer laser also enables surgeons to treat diseases such as fungal ulcers and to smoothe out pterygium irregularities.

Patients interested in pursuing elective refractive surgeries, however, should be aware of the inherent risks of the procedures and that some ophthalmologists are hesitant to use these procedures to correct nearsightedness. The leading cause of skepticism is a reluctance to operate on an essentially healthy eye, thus putting it at risk. These operative procedures have been developed to correct only refractive vision errors. Refractive surgery does not treat glaucoma, cataracts, or other disorders that affect or damage vision.

PERSPECTIVE AND PROSPECTS

As experience and long-term results from the use of laser energy as a surgical tool increase, other forms of therapy will be investigated. Noninvasive glaucoma procedures and laser disruptions of vitreous opacities and retinal traction bands are already being performed. Ablation procedures to control late-stage glaucoma and techniques to emulsify and remove cataract lenses with lasers in a noninvasive procedure have undergone positive trials.

Today, lasers share space in many clinics and operating rooms along with traditional surgical techniques. Laser technology is providing new types of therapy and is treating more challenging forms of eye disease.

—*Randall L. Milstein, Ph.D.*

See also Blindness; Blurred vision; Cataract surgery; Cataracts; Corneal transplantation; Eyes; Glaucoma; Laser use in surgery; Myopia; Ophthalmology; Optometry; Sense organs; Surgery, general; Visual disorders.

FOR FURTHER INFORMATION:

Bartlett, Jimmy D., and Siret D. Jaanus, eds. *Clinical Ocular Pharmacology.* 4th ed. Boston: Butterworth-Heinemann, 2001. A well-illustrated and descriptive account of diseases of the eye, as well as surgical and pharmacological treatments. Though aimed at medical professionals, the book is a valuable reference for any interested reader.

Eden, John. *Physician's Guide to Cataracts, Glaucoma, and Other Eye Problems.* Yonkers, N.Y.: Consumer Reports Books, 1992. A book about eye problems and surgeries aimed at the general reader. The explanations and descriptions are easy to read and follow. The book contains no illustrations.

Johnson, Gordon J., et al., eds. *The Epidemiology of Eye Disease*. 2d ed. London: Edward Arnold, 2003. A university-level text concerning eye disease. Very descriptive and richly illustrated with color images. The book is well referenced and provides researchers and interested readers with timely data sources.

Newell, F. W. *Ophthalmology: Principles and Concepts*. 8th ed. St. Louis: Mosby, 1996. A medical textbook of general ophthalmology. Written for the medical professional, it describes diagnostic and operational techniques for disorders of the eye.

Stein, Harold A., Bernard J. Slatt, and Raymond M. Stein. *The Ophthalmic Assistant: A Guide for Ophthalmic Medical Personnel*. 7th ed. St. Louis: Mosby, 2000. A teaching text for ophthalmic surgical assistants. Very descriptive and well illustrated, with overviews of diseases, disorders, and infections, as well as most surgical procedures. Though written for students training in the field, the text is well referenced to the appendix and glossary.

Vaughan, Daniel, Taylor Asbury, and Paul Riordan-Eva. *General Ophthalmology*. 15th ed. Stamford, Conn.: Appleton & Lange, 1999. An in-depth medical text on the general practice and science of ophthalmology. It is very technical and not for the general reader, though rich in information and illustrations.

Eyes

Anatomy

Anatomy or system affected: Nervous system

Specialties and related fields: Ophthalmology, optometry

Definition: The body structures that receive and transform information about objects into neural impulses that can be translated by the brain into visual images.

Key terms:

accommodation: adjustments of the crystalline lens that are necessary for clear vision at various distances

cornea: the transparent structure forming the anterior part of the fibrous tunic of the eye; light must pass through this structure to reach the retina

crystalline lens: the transparent focusing mechanism of the eye; it is a biconvex structure situated between the posterior chamber and the vitreous body of the eye

diopter: a unit of power of a lens equal to the reciprocal of the focal length of the lens in meters

iris: the circular pigmented membrane behind the cornea, perforated by the pupil; the most anterior portion of the vascular tunic of the eye

photoreceptor: a light-responsive nerve cell or receptor which is located in the retina of the eye

pupil: the opening at the center of the iris through which light passes

retina: the innermost of the three tunics of the eyeball, which is situated around the vitreous body and is continuous posteriorly with the optic nerve; it contains the photoreceptors

sclera: the tough outer coat or fibrous tunic of the eyeball, which covers the posterior five-sixths of its surface and is continuous anteriorly with the cornea

visual acuity: clarity or clearness in vision

Structure and Functions

The eye captures pictures from the environment and transforms them into neural impulses that are processed by the brain into visual images. The retina, with its light-sensitive cells, acts as a camera to "put the picture on film," while neural processing in the brain "develops the film" and forms a visual image that is meaningful and informative for the individual.

The human eye originates during development, that is, while the individual is being formed as an embryo in the uterus. Eye formation begins during the end of the third week of development when outgrowths of brain neural tissue, called the optic vesicles, form at the sides of the forebrain region. The optic vesicle induces overlying embryonic tissue to thicken in one region, forming a primitive lens structure called the lens placode. The lens placode, in turn, induces the optic vesicles to form a cuplike structure, the optic cup, while the brain's connection of the vesicles narrows into a slender stalk that forms the optic nerve. The inner part of the optic cup forms the neural or sensory retina, with its photoreceptors, while the outer part of the optic cup develops into the layers of tissues, or tunics, that make up the wall of the eyeball. The lens placode further condenses and solidifies by forming lens fibers that become transparent. The function of the lens will eventually be to focus light onto the retina. The major structures of the eye—the retina, lens, and eyeball coats—are initially formed by the fifth month of fetal development. During the remainder of the prenatal period, eye structures continue to enlarge, mature, and form increasingly complex neural networks with the visual processing regions of the brain.

At birth, an infant's eyes are about two-thirds the size of adult eyes. Until after their first month of life, most newborns lack complete retinal development, especially in the area that is responsible for visual acuity. As a result, infants cannot focus their eyes properly and typically have a vacant stare during their first weeks of life. Most of the subsequent eye growth occurs rapidly during the remainder of the first year of life. From the second year of life until puberty, the rate of eye growth progressively slows. After puberty, eye growth is negligible.

The adult human eye weighs approximately 7.5 grams and measures approximately 24.5 millimeters in its anterior-to-posterior diameter. All movement of the eyeball, or globe, is accomplished by six voluntary muscles attached anteriorly by ligaments to the outer coat of the globe and posteriorly to a tendinous ring located behind the globe. One voluntary muscle elevates the upper lid.

Three concentric tunics form the globe itself. The outermost fibrous tunic consists of two portions. In the small, anterior portion, the tunic fibrils are arranged in a regular pattern, forming the transparent cornea. Posteriorly, the tunic fibrils are irregularly spaced, forming the opaque, white sclera. The innermost tunic, or nervous tunic, consists of two parts: the pars optica, or retina, containing photoreceptor cells, and the pars ceca lining the iris and ciliary body. Tucked between the outer and inner tunics lies the vascular tunic, consisting of the pigmented iris, which gives the eye its distinctive color; the ciliary body, which forms the aqueous humor to provide nourishment for the anterior structures of the globe; and the highly vascular choroid, which provides nourishment for the retina and also acts as a cooling system by regulating blood flow to the chemically active retina. In the center of the circular, pigmented iris lies the pupil, which is a small opening into the posterior parts of the eyeball.

The cavity that contains the globe, circumscribed by the concentric tunics, is filled with a clear, jellylike substance called the vitreous body. This substance is anteriorly bounded in the vitreous cavity by the transparent crystalline lens that lies just posterior to the pupil. The crystalline lens is elastic in structure, allowing for variations in thickness that change the focusing power of the eye.

The eye can refract, or bend, light rays because of the curved surfaces of two transparent structures, the cornea and the crystalline lens, through which light rays must pass to reach the retina. Any curved surface, or lens, will refract light rays to a greater or lesser degree depending on the steepness or flatness of the surface curve. The steeper the curve, the greater the refracting power. If a curved surface refracts light rays to an intersection point one meter away from the refracting lens, this lens is defined as having 1 diopter of power. The human eye has approximately 59 diopters of power in its constituent parts, including the cornea and crystalline lens.

Light rays emitted from a distant point of light enter the eye in a basically parallel pattern and are bent to intersect perfectly at the retina, forming an image of the distant point of light. If the point of light is near the eye, the rays that are emitted are divergent in pattern. These divergent rays must also be refracted to meet at a point on the retina, but these rays require more bending hence, a steeper curved surface is needed. By a process called accommodation, the human eye automatically adjusts the thickness of the crystalline lens, forming a steeper curve on its surface and thereby creating a perfect image on the retina. Variations from the normal in either the length of an eyeball or the curves of the cornea and crystalline lens will result in a refractive error or blurred image on the retina.

The major task of the eye is to focus environmental light rays on the photoreceptor cells, the rods and cones of the retina. These photoreceptors absorb the light energy, transforming it into electrical signals that are carried to the visual center of the brain. Cones are specialized for color or daylight vision and have greater visual discrimination or acuity than the rods, which are specialized for black-and-white or nighttime vision.

The fovea is a pin-sized depression in the center of the retina that contains only cone cells in high concentrations. This makes the fovea the point of the most distinct vision, or greatest visual acuity. When the eye focuses on an object, the object's image falls on the retina in the area of the fovea. Immediately surrounding the fovea is a larger area called the macula lutea that contains a relatively high concentration of cones. Macula lutea acuity, while not as great as in the fovea, is much greater than in the retina's periphery, which contains fewer cones. The concentration of cones is greatest in the fovea and declines toward the periphery of the retina. Conversely, the concentration of the rods is greater at the more peripheral areas of the retina than in the macula luteal area. The retina of each eye contains about 100 million rod cells and about 300 million cone cells.

The optic nerve carries impulses from the photoreceptors to the brain. This nerve exits the retina in a central location called the blind spot. No image can be detected in this area because it contains neither rods nor cones. Normally, an individual is not aware of the retinal blind spot because the brain's neural processing compensates for the missing information when some portion of a peripheral image falls across this part of the retina.

On a cellular level, rod and cone photoreceptors consist of three parts: an outer segment that detects the light stimulus, an inner segment that provides the metabolic energy for the cell, and a synaptic terminal that transmits the visual signal to the next nerve cell in the visual pathway leading to the brain. The outer segment is rod-shaped in the rods and cone-shaped in the cones (hence their names). This segment is made of a stack of flattened membranes containing photopigment molecules that undergo chemical changes when activated by light.

The rod photopigment, called rhodopsin, cannot discriminate between various colors of light. Thus rods provide vision only in shades of gray by detecting different intensities of light. Rhodopsin is a purple pigment (a combination of blue and red colors), and it transmits light in the blue and red regions of the visual spectrum while absorbing energy from the green region of the spectrum. The light that is absorbed best by a photopigment is called its absorption maximum. Thus at night, when rods are used for vision, a green car is seen far more easily than a red car, because red light is poorly absorbed by rhodopsin. Only absorbed light produces the photochemical reaction that results in vision.

When rhodopsin absorbs light, the photopigment dissociates or separates into two parts: retinene, which is derived from vitamin A, and opsin, a protein. This separation of retinene from opsin, called the bleaching reaction, causes the production of nerve impulses in the photoreceptors. In the presence of bright light, practically all the rhodopsin undergoes the bleaching reaction and the person is in a light-adapted state. When a light-adapted person initially enters a darkened room, vision is poor since the light sensitivity of the rod photoreceptors is very low. After some time in the dark, however, a gradual increase in light sensitivity, called dark adaptation, occurs as increased amounts of retinene and opsin are recombined by the rods to form rhodopsin. The increased level of rhodopsin occurs after a few minutes in the dark and reaches a maximum sensitivity in about twenty minutes.

Each kind of cone—red, green, and blue—is distinguished by its unique photopigment, which responds to a particular wavelength or color of light. Combinations of cone colors provide the basis for color vision. While each type of cone is most sensitive to the particular wavelength of light indicated by its color—red, green, or blue—cones can respond to other colors with varying degrees. One's perception of color rests on the differential response of each cone type to a particular wavelength of light. The extent that each cone type is activated is coded and sent in separate parallel pathways to the brain. A color vision center in the brain combines and processes these parallel inputs to create the perception of color. Color is thus a concept in the mind of the viewer.

The intricacies of the human visual system require various methods to assess eye structure and function. Visual acuity is a measure of central cone function. Clinically, the most common method for testing visual acuity is by the use of a Snellen chart, consisting of a white background with black letters. All symbols on the chart create, or subtend, a visual angle at the approximate center of the eye. The smaller the symbol, the smaller the angle and the more difficult cone recognition becomes. At the standard distance of twenty feet, the smallest letters on the Snellen chart subtend an angle of five minutes of arc at the eye's center. The larger letters on the chart are calibrated such that each consecutively larger letter subtends a multiple unit of five minutes of arc. If the eye can detect the smallest letters on the chart, the patient is said to have normal (20/20) vision. The numerator of the clinical fraction designates the test distance of twenty feet. The denominator varies with the patient's visual function, identifying the distance at which the smallest letter recognized by the patient subtends an angle of five minutes of arc. For example, if the smallest letter recognized is fifty minutes of arc in size, the fraction used to record this visual acuity is 20/200 because the letter with fifty minutes of arc is ten times bigger than the smallest letters on the chart. Therefore, the distance needed for this letter to create five minutes of arc at the eye is ten times farther than the normal twenty feet. In this example, the patient is said to have a refractive error.

DISORDERS AND DISEASES

Commonly existing refractive errors are astigmatism, myopia, hyperopia, and presbyopia. Presbyopia is an anomaly that occurs with aging when the crystalline lens loses its ability to accommodate. Causes include

The Anatomy of the Human Eye

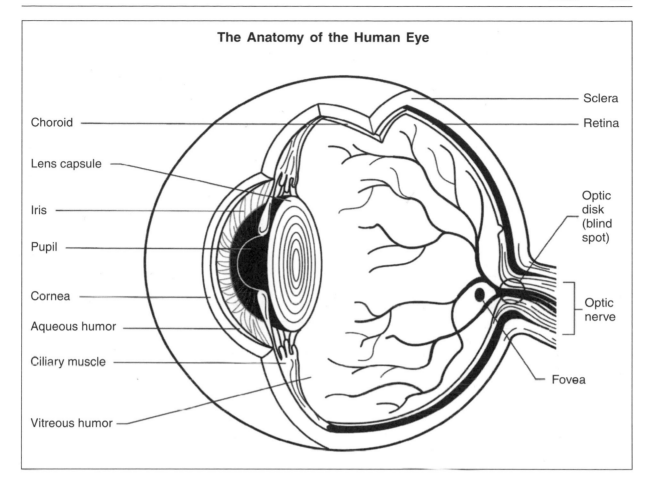

Choroid

Lens capsule

Iris

Pupil

Cornea

Aqueous humor

Ciliary muscle

Vitreous humor

Sclera

Retina

Optic disk (blind spot)

Optic nerve

Fovea

thickening of the lens and changes in the attachment fibers that anchor the lens. Because of these alterations, the lens is not able to change its shape and the eye remains focused at a specific distance. To compensate for this problem, bifocal spectacles are normally prescribed, with the upper region of the lens focused for distant vision and the lower lens focused for near vision. Hyperopia, also called farsightedness, results when an eyeball is too short. Because light rays are not bent sufficiently by the lens system, the image is focused not on the retina but behind the retina. To compensate for this problem, spectacles with convex lenses are prescribed, which bring the focus point back on the retina. Conversely, myopia, or nearsightedness, results from an abnormally long eyeball. In this case, the lens system focuses in front of the retina. This abnormal vision can be corrected by spectacles with a concave lens. Astigmatism results from a refractive error of the lens system, usually caused by an irregular shape in the cornea or less frequently by an irregular shape in the lens. The consequence of this anomaly is that some light rays

are focused in front of the retina and some behind the retina, creating a blurred image. To correct the focusing error, a special irregular spectacle must be made to correct the abnormal irregularity of the eye's lens system.

An examiner can assess the amount of refractive error based on a patient's verbal choice as to which of a given series of lenses sharpens the retinal image of the letters on the Snellen chart. Refractive error can also be determined when a patient is not capable of response. A retinoscope is often used to shine a light through the pupil onto the retina. An image of the light is reflected back out to the examiner who, in turn, can assess refractive error by the movement and shape of the image.

Visual field testing is a measure of the integrity of the neural pathways to the vision center in the brain. To test visual fields clinically, the patient focuses on a central target. While continuing to focus centrally, test targets are serially brought into the patient's peripheral vision, or visual field. The smaller and dimmer the test target, the more sensitive the test. The simplest visual field test technique is by confrontation. The patient and examiner sit facing each other one meter apart. If both patient and examiner cover their right eyes, the patient's left visual field is being tested. Since the patient's left visual field is congruent to the examiner's left visual field, the examiner can detect visual field defects when the patient is not responsive to a test target brought into view from the side. Lesions to some portion of the visual pathway to the brain will result in a scotoma, or blind area, in the corresponding visual field.

A biomicroscope, or slitlamp microscope, is commonly used to assess external eye structures, including the eyelids, lashes, conjunctiva, cornea, sclera, and one internal structure, the crystalline lens. The white part of the eye, or sclera, is covered with a thin, transparent covering called the conjunctiva. Infections and tumors often invade this external structure. Though the normally transparent crystalline lens is essentially free of infections and tumors, it can become cloudy or opaque and develop a cataract. Causes for cataract formation are multiple, the most common being the aging process; less frequently, trauma to the lens or a secondary symptom of systemic disease can result in cataracts. When the cataract is so dense that it obstructs vision, the crystalline lens is surgically removed and replaced with an artificial, plastic lens.

To view internal eye structures, the pupil is dilated to allow more light to be introduced into the interior and posterior regions of the eyeball. Two commonly used instruments are the handheld ophthalmoscope and the head-mounted indirect ophthalmoscope. Diseases of the retina include retinal tears, detachments, artery or vein occlusions, degenerations, and retinopathies secondary to systemic disease.

Glaucoma is an eye disease characterized by raised pressure inside the eye. Normal eye pressure is stabilized by the balance between the production and removal of the aqueous humor, the solution that bathes the internal, anterior structures of the eye. Abnormal pressures are often associated with defects in the visual, or optic, nerve and in the visual field. Approximately 300 people per 100,000 are affected by glaucoma. Clinically, intraocular pressure is assessed by numerous methods in a process called tonometry.

Abnormalities of the eye muscles constitute a significant portion of visual problems. Binocular vision and good depth perception are present when both eyes are aligned properly toward an object. A weakness in any of the six rotatory eye muscles will result in a tendency for that eye to deviate away from the object, resulting in an obvious or latent eye turn called strabismus. Associated signs are eye fatigue, abnormal head postures, and double vision. To alleviate objectionable double vision, a patient often suppresses the retinal image at the brain level, resulting in functional amblyopia (often called lazy eye), in which visual acuity is deficient.

Color blindness, a trait that occurs more frequently in men than in women, is caused by a hereditary lack of one or more types of cones. For example, if the green-sensitive cones are not functioning, the colors in the visual spectral range from green to red can stimulate only red-sensitive cones. This person can perceive only one color in this range, since the ratio of stimulation of the green-red cones is constant for the colors in this range. Thus this individual is considered to be green-red color-blind and will have difficulty distinguishing green from red.

PERSPECTIVE AND PROSPECTS

Early physicians recognized the importance of good eyesight, but because of limited understanding they had minimal means to treat major eye disorders. During the Middle Ages, surgeons performed eye operations, including ones for cataracts in which the lens was pushed down and out of the way with a needle inserted into the eyeball. In the 1700's, this operation was improved when cataract lenses were extracted from the eye. In the early 1600's, Johannes Kepler described how light was focused by the lens of the eye on the retina, thus providing insight into why spectacles are valuable in cases of poor eyesight. In 1801, Thomas Young published a foundational text entitled *On the Mechanics of the Eye*. Hermann von Helmholtz in the 1800's invented the first ophthalmoscope, which allowed inspection of the interior structures of the eye. Young and Helmholtz also developed theories to explain the phenomenon of color vision. From the invention of the ophthalmoscope, the range of clinical observation was extended to the inside of the eyeball, allowing the diagnosis of eye disorders. The modern understanding of eyesight and vision is increasing with contributions from ongoing research.

Ophthalmology is the study of the structure, function, and diseases of the eye. An ophthalmologist is a physician who specializes in the diagnosis and treatment of eye disorders and diseases with surgery, drugs, and corrective lenses. An optometrist is a specialist with a doctorate in optometry who is trained to examine and test the eyes and treats defects in vision by prescribing corrective lenses. An optician is a technician who fits, adjusts, and dispenses corrective lenses that are based on the prescription of an ophthalmologist or optometrist.

Vision care personnel are vital to industry, public health, recreation, highway safety, education, and the community. Since 85 percent of learning is visual-based, good vision is extremely important in education, work, and play. Good vision enhances the production and morale of workers, and athletic performance is improved when vision problems are corrected. Vision care specialists work to promote the prevention of eye injuries and diseases while supporting practices that enhance good health and vision. Vision therapy may be used to correct many disorders of the eye such as amblyopia, reduced visual perception, reading disorders, poor eye coordination, and reduced visual acuity.

—*Elva B. Miller, O.D., and Roman J. Miller, Ph.D.*

See also Albinos; Astigmatism; Blindness; Cataract surgery; Cataracts; Chlamydia; Color blindness; Conjunctivitis; Corneal transplantation; Diabetes mellitus; Dyslexia; Eye surgery; Face lift and blepharoplasty; Glaucoma; Gonorrhea; Jaundice; Laser use in surgery; Macular degeneration; Microscopy, slitlamp; Myopia; Ophthalmology; Optometry; Optometry, pediatric; Pigmentation; Ptosis; Sense organs; Sjögren's syndrome; Strabismus; Styes; Systems and organs; Trachoma; Transplantation; Visual disorders.

FOR FURTHER INFORMATION:

Buettner, Helmut, ed. *Mayo Clinic on Vision and Eye Health: Practical Answers on Glaucoma, Cataracts, Macular Degeneration, and Other Conditions.* Rochester, Minn.: Mayo Foundation for Medical Education and Research, 2002. A helpful handbook on all the medical, social, and emotional facets of vision impairment.

Guyton, Arthur C. *Human Physiology and Mechanisms of Disease.* 6th ed. Philadelphia: W. B. Saunders, 1997. Guyton is a nationally recognized authority on medical physiology, having written and edited numerous college-level and medical school textbooks on the subject. His writing style is understandable to the nonmedical specialist and student. This college-level text contains two chapters on the eye: The first deals with the optics of vision and the function of the retina; the second emphasizes the neurophysiology of vision.

Larson, David E., ed. *Mayo Clinic Family Health Book.* 3d ed. New York: HarperResource, 2003. Perhaps the best general medical text for the layperson, this book covers the entire medical field. While the information is derived from a wide variety of highly technical sources, the articles are written to be easily understood by a general audience.

National Eye Research Foundation. http://www.nerf.org. Site provides consumers and professionals with access to developing technology for treating impaired vision.

Prevent Blindness America. http://www.preventblindness.org/. Founded in 1908, this group is dedicated to fighting blindness and saving sight. Their efforts are focused on promoting a continuum of vision care, public and professional education, certified vision screening training, and community and patient service programs and research.

Tortora, Gerard J., and Sandra R. Grabowski. *Principles of Anatomy and Physiology.* 10th ed. New York: John Wiley & Sons, 2003. An outstanding textbook of human anatomy and physiology, contains a well-written chapter on the special senses, emphasizing eyesight and vision.

Vaughan, Daniel, Taylor Asbury, and Paul Riordan-Eva, eds. *General Ophthalmology.* 16th ed. New York: McGraw-Hill, 2003. This well-illustrated textbook is an excellent reference for the serious student who desires more in-depth information on any aspect of the eye or its diseases.

FACE LIFT AND BLEPHAROPLASTY
PROCEDURE

ANATOMY OR SYSTEM AFFECTED: Eyes, skin
SPECIALTIES AND RELATED FIELDS: General surgery, plastic surgery
DEFINITION: Techniques used to remove unwanted wrinkles and other indicators of aging from the face.

INDICATIONS AND PROCEDURES

Aging may create serious problems among individuals for whom success in their occupations depends on appearance. Premature wrinkling of skin on the face and eyelids or premature looseness of these tissues can create an insurmountable psychological barrier. In these situations, cosmetic surgery such as face lift (rhytidectomy) and/or blepharoplasty (the removal of excess tissue around the eyelids) is indicated.

Surgical face lifting involves making an incision at the hairline and extending it downward in front of the ear toward the angle of the jaw; the length of the incision is dependent on the amount of skin sagging that is present. The skin is gently separated from the underlying fascia and is pulled back and tightened until the desired degree of wrinkle elimination is achieved. Excess skin at the posterior (back) margins is removed. The edges are carefully brought together and secured with fine sutures or adhesive closures. The patient returns to the plastic surgeon in seven to ten days for follow-up evaluation.

Blepharoplasty refers to the surgical alteration of the eyelids. The surgery is similar to that described for a total face lift. An incision is made along the lower margin of the eyebrow. Skin is separated from the fascia.

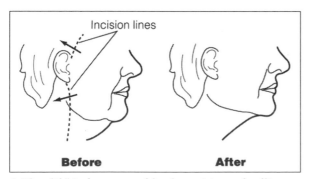

A *"face lift" is the term used for the excision and pulling upward of sagging skin on the face. This cosmetic procedure can smooth wrinkles and provide a more attractive profile, but there are drawbacks: The patient's appearance may be changed too dramatically, and the procedure must be repeated periodically to maintain the desired results.*

Sometimes, small amounts of fat are also removed. The skin of the upper eyelid is tightened. After excess tissue is removed, the free edges are attached with fine sutures. Cosmetic alteration of the lower eyelid can also be accomplished surgically. The incision is made along a natural crease in the skin just below the lower eyelid. The skin above the incision is separated from its underlying fascia. Some fat may be removed. Typically, excess skin is removed before the edges are reattached, again using very fine sutures. The patient returns to the plastic surgeon in approximately one week for removal of the sutures. Chemical peeling or dermabrasion are additional techniques that can be used to remove fine wrinkles and lines in skin.

USES AND COMPLICATIONS

A face lift is a form of cosmetic surgery and is usually undertaken for aesthetic reasons. Short-term problems include bruising and swelling. Possible long-term complications include infection, scarring, and insufficient removal of unwanted wrinkles. Proper techniques can reduce the first two problems. Realistic expectations can minimize disappointment.

Because of the eyelid's good blood circulation blepharoplasty performed under sterile conditions seldom results in serious infection. However, the procedure can result in a number of other complications: continued bleeding that requires reopening the eyelid wound and either the cauterization of the bleeding vessel or evacuation of a clot; the edges of the eyelid skin closure may separate, requiring either support tape or sutures; eyelid asymmetry whereby the eyelids look fine individually but do not match as a pair; and finally, either insufficient or excessive skin removal.

PERSPECTIVE AND PROSPECTS

At birth, human skin contains relatively large amounts of a molecule called collagen. Collagen provides strength to the skin; this is technically called turgor. The function of collagen is similar to the fibers in fiberglass or steel reinforcement in concrete: strength. Living on Earth, people are constantly subjected to the effects of gravity and ultraviolet radiation, which over time cause slight damage to the collagen in skin. The turgor is slowly lost. Without sufficient collagen, the skin starts to sag under the influence of gravity. Excessive exposure to the sun accelerates this process. The use of tanning beds in salons can increase the amount of harmful ultraviolet radiation, which also accelerates the aging process. With sufficient time and

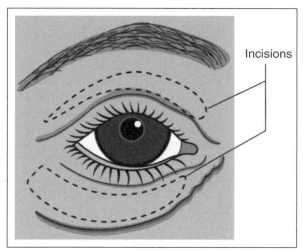

Blepharoplasty is the removal of excess, baggy skin around the eyes.

exposure, the typical appearance of skin in old age is seen.

There is no way to stop the human body from aging; accepting this inevitable reality can reduce both stress and anxiety. Cosmetic surgical procedures such as blepharoplasty and face lifts are temporary and enable an individual to maintain only an approximation of youthfulness. Over time, the skin will continue to change, necessitating repeat procedures. Each time the procedure is repeated, the result is diminished in comparison to an earlier procedure. Cosmetic surgery can thus only retard the appearance of aging rather than re-create youth.

—*L. Fleming Fallon, Jr., M.D., Ph.D., M.P.H.*
See also Aging; Botox; Plastic surgery; Skin; Skin disorders.

FOR FURTHER INFORMATION:
Bosniak, Stephen L., and Marian Cantisano Zilkha. *Cosmetic Blepharoplasty and Facial Rejuvenation.* 2d ed. Baltimore: Lippincott Williams & Wilkins, 1999.

Grabb, William C., and James Walter Smith. *Grabb and Smith's Plastic Surgery.* 5th ed. Philadelphia: Lippincott-Raven, 1997.

Henry, Kimberly A. *The Face-Lift Sourcebook.* Los Angeles: Lowell House, 2000.

Lewis, Wendy. *The Beauty Battle: The Insider's Guide to Wrinkle Rescue and Cosmetic Perfection from Head to Toe.* Berkeley, Calif.: Laurel Glen Books, 2003.

Loftus, Jean. *The Smart Woman's Guide to Plastic Surgery.* New York: McGraw-Hill, 2000.

Marfuggi, Richard A. *Plastic Surgery: What You Need to Know Before, During, and After.* New York: Berkeley, 1998.

Narrins, Rhoda, and Paul Jarrod Frank. *Turn Back the Clock Without Losing Time: Everything You Need to Know About Simple Cosmetic Procedures.* New York: Crown, 2002.

Turkington, Carol. *Encyclopedia of Skin and Skin Disorders.* New York: Facts On File, 2002.

Wyer, E. Bingo. *The Unofficial Guide to Cosmetic Surgery.* New York: Simon & Schuster/Macmillan, 1999.

FACIAL PALSY. *See* BELL'S PALSY.

FACTITIOUS DISORDERS
DISEASE/DISORDER
ANATOMY OR SYSTEM AFFECTED: Psychic-emotional system, most bodily systems

SPECIALTIES AND RELATED FIELDS: Family practice, internal medicine, psychiatry, psychology

DEFINITION: Psychophysiological disorders in which individuals intentionally produce their symptoms in order to play the role of patient.

CAUSES AND SYMPTOMS

Although factitious disorders cover a wide array of physical symptoms and are believed to be closely related to a subset of psychophysiological disorders (somatoform disorders), they are unique in all of medicine for two reasons. The first distinguishing factor is that whatever the physical disease for which treatment is sought and regardless of how serious, the patients who seek its treatment have deliberately and intentionally produced the condition. They may have done so in one of three ways, or in any combination of these three ways. First, patients fabricate, invent, lie about, and make up symptoms that they do not have; for example, they claim to have fever and night sweats or severe back pain that they actually do not have. Second, patients have the actual symptoms that they describe, but they intentionally caused them; for example, they might inject human saliva into their own skin to produce an abscess or ingest a known allergic food to cause the predictable reaction. Third, someone with a known condition such as pancreatitis has a pain episode but exaggerates its severity, or someone else with a history of migraines claims his or her headache to be yet another migraine when it is not.

The second element that makes these disorders unique (and at the same time both fascinating to study and frustrating to treat) is that the sole motivation for causing or claiming the symptoms is for these patients to become and remain patients, to assume the sick role wherein little can be expected from them. These patients are not malingerers, individuals who consciously use actual or feigned symptoms for some other gain (such as claiming a fever so one does not have to go to work or school, or insisting that one's post-traumatic stress is worse than it is to enhance the judgment in a lawsuit). In fact, it is the absence of any discernible external benefit that makes these disorders so intriguing.

Technically, psychiatrists and psychologists understand factitious disorders as having three subtypes. In the first, patients claim to have predominantly psychological symptoms such as memory loss, depression, contemplation of suicide, the hearing of voices, or false memory of childhood molestation. Characteristically, the symptoms worsen whenever the patients know themselves to be under observation. In the second, patients have predominantly physical symptoms that at least superficially suggest some general medical condition. In a more extreme form called Münchausen syndrome, individuals will have spent much of their lives getting admitted to medical facilities and, once there, remaining as long as possible. While common complaints include vomiting, dizziness, blacking out, generalized rashes, and bleeding, the symptoms can involve any organ and seem limited only to the individuals' medical knowledge and experience with the medical system. The third subtype combines both psychological and physical complaints in such a way that neither predominates.

Regardless of subtype, factitious disorders are difficult to diagnose. Usually, the diagnosis is considered when the course of treating either a medical or a mental illness becomes atypical and protracted. Often, the person with a factitious disorder will present in a way which seems odd to the experienced clinician. The person may have an unusually extensive history of traveling, much familiarity with medical procedures and terminology, a complex medical and surgical history, few visitors during the hospitalization, behavioral disruptions and disturbances while hospitalized, exacerbation of symptoms while under observation, and/or fluctuating illness with new symptoms and complications arising as the workup proceeds. When present, these traits along with others make suspicion of factitious disorders reasonable.

No one knows how many people suffer with facti-

tious disorders, but the condition is generally regarded as uncommon. It is certainly rarely reported, but this in part may be attributable to the difficulties in determining the diagnosis. While brief episodes of the condition occur, most people who claim a factitious disorder have it chronically, and they usually move on to another physician or facility when they are confronted with the true nature of their illness. It is therefore likely that some individuals are reported more than once by different hospitals and providers.

There is little certainty about what causes factitious disorders. This is true in large measure because those who know the most about the subject—patients with the disorder—are notoriously unreliable in providing information about their psychological state and often seem only dimly aware of what they are doing to themselves. It may be that they are generally incapable of putting their feelings into words. They are unaware of having inner feelings and may not know, for example, that they are sad or angry. It is possible that they experience emotions more physically, behaviorally, and concretely than do most others.

Another view suggests that people learn to distinguish their primitive emotional states through the responsivity of their primary caretaker. A normal, healthy, average mother responds appropriately to her infant's differing affective states, thereby helping the infant, as he or she develops, to distinguish, define, and eventually name what he or she is feeling. When a primary caretaker is, for any of several reasons, incapable of responding in consistently appropriate ways, the infant's emotional awareness remains undifferentiated and the child experiences confusion and emotional chaos.

It is possible, too, that factitious disorder patients are motivated to assume what sociology defines as a sick role wherein people are required to acknowledge that they are ill and are required to relinquish adult responsibilities as they place themselves in the hands of designated caretakers.

TREATMENT AND THERAPY

Internists, family practitioners, and surgeons are the specialists most likely to encounter patients with factitious disorder, although psychiatrists and psychologists are often consulted in the management of these patients. These patients pose a special challenge because in a real sense they do not wish to become well even as they present themselves for treatment. They are not ill in the usual sense, and their indirect communication and manipulation often make them frustrating to treat using standard goals and expectations.

Sometimes mental and medical specialists' joint, supportive confrontation of these patients results in a disappearance of the troubling and troublesome behavior. During these confrontations, the health professionals are acknowledging that such extreme behavior evidences extreme distress in these patients, and as such is its own reason for psychotherapeutic intervention. These patients are not psychologically minded, however; they also have trouble forming relationships that foster genuine self-disclosure, and they rarely accept the recommendation for psychotherapeutic treatment. Because they believe that their problems are physical, not psychological, they often become irate at the suggestion that their problems are not what they believe them to be.

—*Paul Moglia, Ph.D.*

See also Hypochondriasis; Münchausen syndrome by proxy; Psychiatric disorders; Psychiatry; Psychiatry, child and adolescent; Psychiatry, geriatric; Psychoanalysis; Psychosomatic disorders.

FOR FURTHER INFORMATION:

American Psychiatric Association. *Diagnostic and Statistical Manual of Mental Disorders: DSM-IV-TR.* Rev. 4th ed. Washington, D.C.: Author, 2000. This reference book lists the clinical criteria for psychiatric disorders, including mood disorders.

Feldman, Marc D., and Charles V. Ford. *Patient or Pretender? Inside the Strange World of Factitious Disorders.* New York: John Wiley & Sons, 1994. Recounting fascinating case histories, psychiatrists Feldman and Ford examine the minds of people whose craving for attention leads them to fake illnesses, sometimes to the point of death.

Phillips, Katherine A. *Somatoform and Factitious Disorders.* Washington, D.C.: American Psychiatric Association, 2001. A comprehensive examination of such topics as epidemiology, etiology/pathology, and treatment modalities for somatoform and factitious disorders.

Viederman, M. "Somatoform and Factitious Disorders." In *The Personality Disorders and Neuroses,* edited by Arnold M. Cooper, Allen J. Frances, and Michael H. Sacks. New York: Basic Books, 1986. A chapter in a reference work on personality and neurotic disorders. Includes bibliographical references and an index.

FAILURE TO THRIVE

DISEASE/DISORDER

ALSO KNOWN AS: Growth impairment, stunting, wasting

ANATOMY OR SYSTEM AFFECTED: Bones, brain, endocrine system, psychic-emotional system

SPECIALTIES AND RELATED FIELDS: Endocrinology, family practice, gastroenterology, genetics, neonatology, pediatrics, psychiatry, psychology

DEFINITION: A disorder of early childhood growth that includes disturbances in psychosocial skills and development.

CAUSES AND SYMPTOMS

Failure to thrive may be organic or inorganic; in many children, the etiology is multifactorial. The onset of growth problems may be prenatal as a result of maternal substance abuse, most notably alcohol use, or of maternal infection, particularly with rubella, cytomegalovirus (CMV), or toxoplasmosis. Small size in infants secondary to prematurity resolves by two to three years of age unless there are complications.

Many children with failure to thrive are both stunted (linear growth-affected) and wasted (weight-affected). Assessing which of the two conditions predominates can be done using the body mass index (BMI), which is calculated by dividing weight in kilograms by height in meters squared. A low BMI is a sign of malnutrition. Children with environmental failure to thrive fall into this category.

A child who is small but has an appropriate BMI has short stature rather than failure to thrive. The two leading causes of short stature are familial short stature and constitutional delay.

TREATMENT AND THERAPY

The main focus of the medical intervention with failure to thrive is to ensure a nurturing environment and

---

INFORMATION ON FAILURE TO THRIVE

CAUSES: Maternal substance abuse or infection during prenatal phase, familial short stature, constitutional delay

SYMPTOMS: Stunted growth, weight impairment

DURATION: Two to three years

TREATMENTS: Nurturing environment, nutritional intervention, family counseling

adequate nutrition. Nutritional intervention can be achieved in many ways, such as by securing adequate access to food for the family and offering concentrated formulas, nutritional supplementation, and calorie-dense food, depending on the age of the child. Developmental intervention should also be provided if delay is detected. Likewise, family counseling, especially focusing on parenting skills, may be indicated.

PERSPECTIVE AND PROSPECTS

The term "failure to thrive" originated in 1933; it replaced the term "cease to thrive," which appeared in 1899. Initially, the condition was reported in institutionalized children, including those in orphanages. In the 1940's, it was recognized as a condition that could also affect children living at home with their biological or adoptive parents.

Although the list of conditions that can cause growth impairment in children is quite extensive, a systematic approach using history and both physical and psychosocial assessment will provide clues to the diagnosis. Intervention ensures an adequate outcome, with improved prospects for physical growth and brain development.

—*Carol D. Berkowitz, M.D.*

See also Bonding; Cognitive development; Cytomegalovirus (CMV); Fetal alcohol syndrome; Growth; Malnutrition; Neonatology; Nutrition; Pediatrics; Rubella; Toxoplasmosis; Weight loss and gain.

FOR FURTHER INFORMATION:

Berk, Laura E. *Child Development*. 6th ed. Boston: Allyn and Bacon, 2003.

Garrow, J. S., and W. P. T. James, eds. *Human Nutrition and Dietetics*. 10th ed. New York: Churchill Livingstone, 2000.

Kreutler, Patricia A., and Dorice M. Czajka-Narins. *Nutrition in Perspective*. 2d ed. Englewood Cliffs, N.J.: Prentice Hall, 1987.

Nathanson, Laura Walther. *The Portable Pediatrician: A Practicing Pediatrician's Guide to Your Child's Growth, Development, Health, and Behavior from Birth to Age Five*. 2d ed. New York: HarperCollins, 2002.

Shore, Rima. *Rethinking the Brain: New Insights into Early Development*. New York: Families and Work Institute, 1997.

Whitney, Eleanor Noss, and Sharon Rady Rolfes. *Understanding Nutrition*. 9th ed. St. Paul, Minn.: West, 2002.

Winick, Myron, Brian L. G. Morgan, Jaime Rozovski, and Robin Marks-Kaufman, eds. *The Columbia Encyclopedia of Nutrition*. New York: G. P. Putnam's Sons, 1988.

FAINTING. *See* DIZZINESS AND FAINTING.

FAMILY PRACTICE

SPECIALTY

ANATOMY OR SYSTEM AFFECTED: All

SPECIALTIES AND RELATED FIELDS: Geriatrics and gerontology, internal medicine, obstetrics, osteopathic medicine, pediatrics, preventive medicine, psychiatry, psychology

DEFINITION: The specialty concerned with the primary health maintenance and medical care of an undifferentiated patient population, in the context of family and community.

KEY TERMS:

ambulatory care: health care provided outside the hospital, usually in a clinic or office and sometimes in the patient's home

biopsychosocial model: a model that examines the effects of illness on all spheres in which the patient functions—the biological sphere, the psychological sphere, and the social sphere

general practice: a primary care field with care provided by physicians who usually have completed less than three years of residency training; the organization from which family practice evolved

generalism: a medical and political movement concerned with primary care, often associated with the medical specialties of family practice, general internal medicine, general pediatrics, and sometimes obstetrics and gynecology

health maintenance: the practice of anticipating, finding, preventing, and/or dealing with potential or established medical problems at the earliest possible stage to minimize adverse effects on the patient

internship: a synonym for the first year of residency training

patient advocacy: the representation of the patient's interest in medical diagnosis and treatment decisions, in which the physician acts as an information source and counselor for the patient

primary care: first-line or entry-level care; the health care that most people receive for most illnesses

residency training: medical training provided in a specialty after graduation from medical school; similar to an apprenticeship and designed to mimic real-life practice as closely as possible

specialist: any physician who practices in a specialty other than the generalist areas of family practice, general internal medicine, general pediatrics, and obstetrics and gynecology

undifferentiated patient population: patients seen by family physicians regardless of age, sex, or type of problem

SCIENCE AND PROFESSION

Family practice is the direct descendant of general practice. For many years, most physicians were general practitioners. In the mid- to late twentieth century, however, the explosion of medical knowledge led to the specialization of medicine. For example, increased knowledge of the function and diseases of the heart seemed to demand creation of the specialty of cardiology. The model of the country doctor or jack-of-all-trades physician taking care of a wide range of medical problems seemed doomed to sink in the sea of subspecialization in medicine. The general practitioner, the venerable physician who hung out his or her shingle after medical school and one or more years of internship or residency training, appeared to be headed for extinction. Indeed, in their then-existent forms, the general practitioner and general practice would not have survived. Several forces came into play which did result in the passing of general practice but which also changed general practice into family practice.

The primary force pushing for general practice to survive and improve was the desire of the general public to retain the family doctor. The services that these physicians rendered and the relationships developed between physician and patients were held in high esteem. Through such voices as the Citizen Commission on Graduate Medical Education appointed by the American Medical Association (AMA), the public requested the rescue of the family doctor.

Other major players in the movement to revive and reshape general practice included the AMA itself and the American Academy of General Practice. On February 8, 1969, approval was granted for the creation of family practice as medicine's twentieth official specialty. The American Academy of General Practice became the American Academy of Family Physicians (AAFP), and a certifying board, the American Board of Family Practice (ABFP), was established. After these steps were completed, three-year training programs (residencies) in family practice were established in medical universities and larger community hospitals to provide the necessary training for family physicians.

Family physicians are trained to provide comprehensive ongoing medical care and health maintenance for their patients. Those people who choose to become family physicians tend to value relationships over technology and service over high financial rewards. Many family physicians find themselves providing service to underserved populations and in mission work both inside and outside the United States. Family physicians often become advocates, providing counseling and advice to patients who are trying to sort out medical treatment options. They generally enjoy close relationships with their patients, who often hold them in high esteem.

Following graduation from medical school, students interested in a career in family practice begin a three-year residency in the specialty. During the residency, these physicians train in actual practice settings under the supervision of faculty physicians. Family practice residency training consists of three years of rotations with other medical specialties, such as internal medicine, pediatrics, surgery, and psychiatry. The unifying thread in family practice residency training is the continuity clinic. Throughout their training, the residents see their own patients several days a week under the supervision of family practice faculty physicians. Every effort is made to make this training as close as possible to experiences in the real world. Family practice residents will deliver their patients' babies, hospitalize their patients, and deal with the emotional issues of death and dying, chronic illness, and disability.

Family practice residents receive intensive training in behavioral and psychosocial issues, as well as "bedside manner" training. Scientific research has shown that many patients who seek care from family physicians have problems that require the physician to be a good listener and a skilled counselor. Family practice residency training emphasizes these skills. It also emphasizes the functioning (or malfunctioning) of the family as a system and the effect of major changes (such as the birth of a child or retirement) on the health and functioning of the family members.

The length of training (three years versus one year) and the emphasis on psychosocial and family systems training are two of the major differences in the training of a family physician and the training of a general practitioner. Moreover, family physicians spend up to 30 percent of their training time outside the hospital in a clinic. Family practice was the first medical specialty to emphasize this type of training, and family physicians spend more time in ambulatory (clinic) training than virtually any other specialist.

Following the successful completion of a residency program, a family physician may take a competency examination devised and administered by the American Board of Family Practice. Passing this examination allows the physician to assume the title of Diplomate of the American Board of Family Practice and makes him or her eligible to join the American Academy of Family Physicians, the advocacy and educational organization of family practice.

If family physicians wish to retain their diplomate status, they must take at least fifty hours per year of medical education. After a family physician fulfills all educational and other requirements of the American Board of Family Practice, that physician must then retake the certifying examination every seven years or the certification will lapse. This periodic retesting is required by the American Board of Family Practice to make sure that family physicians keep up their medical education and maintain their knowledge level and clinical skills. Family practice was the first specialty to require periodic reexamination of its physicians. In fact, since family practice has mandated reexaminations, many other medical specialty organizations now require periodic reexamination of their members or are considering such a move. Many former general practitioners who did not have a chance to do a three-year family practice residency took the American Board of Family Practice certifying examination and became diplomates based on their years of practice experience and successful completion of the certifying examination. This option was closed to general practitioners in 1988.

Currently, the American Academy of Family Physicians requires new active physician members to be residency-trained in family practice. Diplomate status reflects only an educational effort by the physician and does not directly affect medical licensure. Medical licensure is based on a different testing mechanism, and license requirements vary from state to state. There are more than fifty thousand family physicians providing health care in the United States, the District of Columbia, the Virgin Islands, Guam, and Puerto Rico. Family practice residency programs are approximately four hundred in number and usually have about seven thousand residents in training.

DIAGNOSTIC AND TREATMENT TECHNIQUES
Service to patients is the primary concern of family practice and all those who practice, teach, administer,

or foster the specialty. Of all the family physicians in practice, more than 93 percent are involved in direct patient care. While family physicians by no means constitute a majority of physicians, they are among the busiest when measured in terms of ambulatory patient visits. Family physicians see 30 percent of all ambulatory patients in the United States, which is more than the number of ambulatory visits to the next two specialty groups combined. Because of their training, family physicians can successfully care for more than 85 percent of all patient problems they encounter. Consultation with other specialty physicians is sought for the problems that are outside the scope of the family physician's knowledge or abilities. This level of consultation is not unique to family physicians, as other specialty physicians find it necessary to seek consultation for 10 to 15 percent of their patients as well.

Family physicians can be found in all areas of the United States and in virtually all types of practice situations, providing a wide range of medical services. Family physicians can successfully practice in metropolitan areas or rural communities of one thousand people (or less), and they can be found teaching or doing research in medical colleges. Because of their training and the fact that they see a truly undifferentiated patient population, family physicians deliver a wide range of medical services. Besides seeing many patients in their offices, family physicians care for patients in nursing homes, make house calls, and admit patients to the hospital. Within the hospital, many family physicians care for patients in intensive care and other special care units and assist in surgery when their patients have operations. A small number perform extensive surgical procedures in the hospital setting. A sizable minority of family physicians take care of pregnant women and deliver their children; some of these physicians also perform cesarean sections. Because family physicians see anyone that walks through the door, it is not unheard of for a family physician to deliver a child in the morning, see the siblings in the office in the afternoon, and make a house call to the grandparents in the evening.

The thing that makes family physicians different from other physicians is their attention to the physician-patient relationship. The family physician has first contact with the patient and is in a position to bond with the patient. The family physician evaluates the patient's complete health needs and provides personal care in one or more areas of medicine. Such care is not limited to any particular type of problem, be it biological, behavioral, or social, and the patients seen are not screened according to age, sex, or illness. The family physician utilizes knowledge of the patient's functioning in the family and community and maintains continuity of care for the patient in a hospital, clinic, or nursing home or in the patient's own home. Thus, in family practice, the patient-physician relationship is initiated, established, and nurtured for both sexes, for all ages, and across time for many types of problems.

Because of their training, family physicians are highly sought-after care providers. Small rural communities, insurance companies, and government agencies at all levels actively seek family physicians to care for patients in a wide variety of settings. In this respect, family practice is the most versatile medical specialty. Family physicians are able to practice and live in communities that are too small to support any other types of physician. In the early 1990's, 28.4 percent of family physicians were practicing in towns with a population of ten thousand or less. As a result, family physicians, along with general pediatricians, are the lowest paid of all physicians.

While the vast majority of family physicians find themselves providing care for patients, there is a minority of family physicians who serve in other, equally important roles. Roughly 3.5 percent of family physicians serve as administrators and educators. They can be found working in state, federal, and local governments; in the insurance industry; and in residency programs and medical schools. Family physicians in residency programs provide instruction and role modeling for family practice residents in community-based and university-based residency programs. Family physicians in medical colleges design, implement, administer, and evaluate educational programs for medical students during the four years of medical school. The Society of Teachers of Family Medicine (STFM) is the organization that supports family physicians in their teaching role. A major problem facing the United States, particularly acute for family physician faculty, is the shortage of family physicians. In 1993, it was estimated that, if every medical school graduate went into family practice, there would be just enough family physicians by the year 2003. In reality, only about 10 to 13 percent of U.S. medical students choose family practice, which is barely enough to keep up with the loss of family physicians through death and retirement. This problem can be addressed through a variety of initiatives by family physicians, government entities, foundations, and the medical insurance industry.

One problem facing the specialty of family practice is the very small percentage who are dedicated to re-search: only 0.3 percent of all family physicians. There is a large need for research in family practice to determine the natural course of illnesses, how best to treat them, and the effects of illness on the functioning of the family unit. The need for research in the ambulatory setting is especially acute because, while most medical research is done in the hospital setting, most medical care in the United States is provided in clinics and offices. This problem will not be easily solved because of the service focus of family practice training and the small number of family physicians dedicated to research.

The organizations representing family physicians are also concerned about providing service to the American people. The American Academy of Family Physicians has worked since its founding to increase the numbers and improve the quality of family physicians, and it proposed a plan to improve health care access for those Americans who are underserved because of financial or other barriers. Another organization of family physicians is Doctors Oughta Care (DOC). DOC is a medical activist organization that works against the number-one and number-two killers in American society: tobacco and alcohol. DOC takes a tongue-in-cheek approach and ridicules the tobacco and alcohol industries. Its members were in large part responsible for bringing a lawsuit against the tobacco industry alleging that it actively markets cigarettes to children.

PERSPECTIVE AND PROSPECTS

Family practice developed as a medical specialty because of the demands of the citizens of the United States; it is the only medical specialty with that claim. The ancestor of family practice was general practice, and there is a direct link from the family physician to the general practitioner. Family practice has grown and evolved into the specialty best suited to provide for the primary health care needs of most patients. Because of their broad scope of practice, cost-effective methods, and versatility, family physicians are found in virtually every type of medical and administrative setting. Family physicians provide a large portion of all ambulatory health care in the United States, and in some settings they are the sole providers of health care. General practice has been around as long as there have been physicians—Hippocrates was a general practitioner—but family practice has a definite point of origin. It was created from general practice on February 8, 1969.

The present role of the family physician is and will continue to be to seek to improve the health of the people of the United States at all levels. Major problems exist for family practice, including attrition as older family physicians retire or die, lack of medical student interest in family practice as a career choice, and the lack of a solid cadre of researchers to advance medical knowledge in family practice. The major strengths supporting family practice are its service ethic, attention to the physician-patient relationship, and cost-effectiveness.

After their near demise as a recognizable group in the mid-twentieth century, family physicians have a number of reasons to expect that they will have expanded opportunities to provide for the health care needs of their patients in the future. As the United States, for example, examines its system of health care, which is the most costly and the least effective of any health care system in the developed world, many medical and political leaders look to generalism, and particularly family practice, to provide answers. Research has shown that, for many medical problems, family physicians can provide outcomes very similar to those provided by specialists. When one couples that fact with the versatility and cost-effectiveness of generalist physicians, it can be argued that to save health care dollars the nation must reverse the 30 percent to 70 percent ratio of generalist to specialist physicians. A ratio of 50 percent to 50 percent generalist to specialist physicians has been proposed at many levels in medicine and government.

Those who champion family practice can be heartened by several developments. First, it is hoped that changes in legislation will soon enhance payment for family physicians for the services they provide. Also, family physicians have formed alliances with medical specialties and other organizations concerned with the promotion of generalism. Finally, the field's solid organizational structure, which is highly regarded and very effective in its areas of operation, has made tremendous strides in promoting and nurturing family practice.

There has been a growing acceptance of family practice since its inception. Building on its long history of enjoying the respect and admiration of patients, family practice is finding itself more and more popular. Government agencies and medical insurance companies look to family physicians to meet their needs, and family practice is now found in most U.S. medical schools. For these and other reasons, it appears that the United States may be coming full circle back to the days of the country doctor.

—Paul M. Paulman, M.D.

See also Allergies; Anemia; Athlete's foot; Bacterial infections; Bronchitis; Chickenpox; Childhood infectious diseases; Cholesterol; Common cold; Constipation; Coughing; Cytomegalovirus (CMV); Death and dying; Diarrhea and dysentery; Digestion; Dizziness and fainting; Domestic violence; Exercise physiology; Fatigue; Fever; Fungal infections; Geriatrics and gerontology; Grief and guilt; Halitosis; Headaches; Healing; Heartburn; Hypercholesterolemia; Hyperlipidemia; Hypertension; Hypoglycemia; Indigestion; Infection; Inflammation; Influenza; Laryngitis; Measles; Mononucleosis; Mumps; Muscle sprains, spasms, and disorders; Nutrition; Obesity; Osteopathic medicine; Pain; Pediatrics; Pharmacology; Pharmacy; Physical examination; Pneumonia; Poisonous plants; Preventive medicine; Psychology; Puberty and adolescence; Rashes; Rheumatic fever; Rubella; Scabies; Scarlet fever; Sciatica; Shingles; Shock; Sinusitis; Sore throat; Strep throat; Stress; Tetanus; Tonsillitis; Toxicology; Ulcers; Viral infections; Vitamins and minerals; Whooping cough; Wounds.

FOR FURTHER INFORMATION:

American Academy of Family Physicians. *Facts About Family Practice 1998*. Kansas City, Mo.: Author, 1998. This reference guide provides a list of facts about family practice physicians. Included in this publication are statistics about the location of family physicians and the scope of their practice.

American Academy of Family Physicians' Membership Directory, 1973-   . Available from the American Academy of Family Physicians, this annual publication provides a state-by-state, city-by-city listing of family physicians by name.

Behrman, Richard E., et al. *Nelson Textbook of Pediatrics*. 17th ed. New York: Elsevier, 2003. Text covering all medical and surgical disorders in children with authoritative information on genetics, endocrinology, aetiology, epidemiology, pathology, pathophysiology, clinical manifestations, diagnosis, prevention, treatment, and prognosis.

Rakel, Robert E. *Essentials of Family Practice*. 2d ed. Philadelphia: W. B. Saunders, 1998. This book outlines the core content essentials for family practice training.

Scherger, Joseph E., et al. "Responses to Questions by Medical Students About Family Practice." *The Journal of Family Practice* 26, no. 2 (1988): 169-176. Although aimed at medical students, this popular medical article provides good background information about the scope and socioeconomic aspects of family practice.

Sloane, Phillip D., et al. *Essentials of Family Medicine.* 4th ed. Philadelphia: Lippincott Williams & Wilkins, 2002. A basic introductory reference text to family medicine with three sections: "Principles of Family Medicine," "Preventive Care," and "Common Problems."

FATIGUE
DISEASE/DISORDER
ANATOMY OR SYSTEM AFFECTED: All

SPECIALTIES AND RELATED FIELDS: Family practice, geriatrics and gerontology, internal medicine, psychiatry

DEFINITION: A general symptom of tiredness, malaise, depression, and sometimes anxiety associated with many diseases and disorders; in some cases, no specific cause can be found.

KEY TERMS:

physical deconditioning: a condition that results when a person who has previously been exercising (has become conditioned) stops exercising

psychogenic fatigue: fatigue caused by mental factors, such as anxiety, and not attributable to any physical cause

sleep apnea: cessation of breathing during sleep, which may result from either an inhibition of the respiratory center (central apnea) or an obstruction to the flow of air (obstructive apnea)

sleep disorders: conditions resulting in sleep interruption, interfering with the restorative functions of sleep

syndrome: a collection of complaints (symptoms) and signs (abnormal findings on clinical examination) which do not match any specific disease

CAUSES AND SYMPTOMS

Almost all people suffer from fatigue at some point in their lives. It is a nonspecific complaint including tiredness, lack of energy, listlessness, or malaise. Patients often confuse fatigue with weakness, breathlessness, or dizziness, which indicate the existence of other physical disorders. Rest or a change in the daily routine ordinarily alleviates fatigue in healthy individuals. Though normally short in duration, fatigue occasionally lasts for weeks, months, or even years in some individuals. In such cases, it limits the amount of physical and mental activity in which the person can participate.

Long-term fatigue can have serious consequences. Often, patients begin to withdraw from their normal activities. They may withdraw from society in general and may gradually become more apathetic and depressed. As a result of this progression, a patient's physical and mental capabilities may begin to deteriorate. Fatigue may be aggravated further by a reduced appetite and inadequate nutritional intake. Ultimately, these symptoms lead to malnutrition and multiple vitamin deficiencies, which intensify the fatigue state and trigger a vicious circle.

This fatigue cycle ends with a person who lacks interest and energy. Such patients may lose interest in daily events and social contacts. In later stages of fatigue, they may neglect themselves and lose track of their goals in life. The will to live and fight decreases, making them prime targets for accidents and repeated infections. They may also become potential candidates for suicide.

Physical and/or mental overactivity commonly cause recent-onset fatigue. Management of such fatigue is simple: Adequate physical and/or mental relaxation typically relieve it. Fortunately, many persistent fatigue states can be easily diagnosed and successfully treated. In some cases, however, fatigue does not respond to simple measures.

Fatigue can stem from depression. Depressed individuals often reflect boredom and a lack of interest, and frequently express uncertainty and/or anxiety about the future. These people usually appear "down." They may walk slowly with their head down, slump their shoulders, and sigh frequently. They often take unusually long to respond to questions or requests. They also show little motivation. Depressed individuals typically relate feelings of dejection, sadness, worthlessness, or helplessness. Often, they complain of feeling tired when they wake up in the morning, and no amount of sleep or rest improves their condition. In fact, they feel weary all day and frequently complain of feeling weak. They often have poor appetites and sometimes lose weight. Once these patients are questioned by a physician, however, it may become apparent that their state of fatigue actually fluctuates. At times they feel exhausted, while at other times (sometimes only minutes later) they feel refreshed and full of energy.

Other manifestations of depression include sleep disorders (particularly early morning waking), reduced appetite, altered bowel habits, and difficulty concentrating. Depressed individuals sometimes fail to recognize their condition. They may channel their depres-

INFORMATION ON FATIGUE

CAUSES: Disease, depression, sleep disorders, physical and/or mental overactivity, excessive intake of stimulants, medications

SYMPTOMS: Tiredness, malaise, depression, anxiety, withdrawal

DURATION: Typically short-term but can be chronic

TREATMENTS: Rest and relaxation, medications, counseling

sion into physical complaints such as abdominal pain, headaches, joint pain, or vaguely defined aches and pains. In older people, depression sometimes manifests itself as impaired memory.

Anxiety, another major cause of fatigue, interferes with the patient's ability to achieve adequate mental and physical rest. Anxious individuals often appear scared, worried, or fearful. They frequently report multiple physical complaints, including neck muscle tension, headaches, palpitations, difficulty in breathing, chest tightness, intestinal cramping, and trouble falling asleep. In some cases, both depression and anxiety may be present simultaneously.

Medications also constitute a major cause of fatigue. All drugs—prescription, over-the-counter, or recreational—can cause fatigue. Sleeping medications, antidepressants, antianxiety medications, muscle relaxants, allergy medications, cold medications, and certain blood pressure medications can lead to problems with fatigue.

An excessive intake of stimulants, paradoxically, sometimes leads to easy fatigability. Stimulants can interfere with proper sleeping habits and relaxation. Common culprits include caffeine and medications (such as some diet pills and nasal decongestants) that can be purchased without a prescription. So-called recreational drugs can also contribute to chronic fatigue. Depending on their tendencies, they function to cause fatigue in much the same way as the prescription and over-the-counter drugs already discussed. Cocaine and amphetamines, for example, act as stimulants. Narcotics such as heroin and barbiturates (downers) possess strong sedative qualities. Alcohol consumption in an attempt to escape loneliness, depression, or boredom may further exacerbate a sense of fatigue. Alcohol produces fatigue in two ways. It has sedative qualities, and it also intensifies the sedative effects of other medications, if taken with them.

Other drugs that may induce fatigue include diuretics and those that lower blood pressure. These medications increase the excretions of many substances through the kidneys. If inappropriately given or regulated, these drugs may alter the blood concentration of other medications taken concurrently.

Painkillers can lead to fatigue in a different way. In some individuals, they irritate the lining of the stomach and cause it to bleed. Such bleeding usually occurs in small amounts and goes unnoticed by the patient. This slight blood loss can gradually lead to anemia and fatigue.

Medications are particularly likely to cause fatigue in elderly individuals. With many drugs, their elimination from the body through metabolism or excretion may decrease with age. This often leads to higher drug concentrations in the blood than intended, resulting in a state of constant sedation and lethargy. Also, elderly individuals' brains may be more sensitive to sedation than those of younger individuals. Finally, the elderly tend to take more medication for more illnesses than younger adults. The additive side effects of multiple medicines can add to fatigue problems.

Sleep deprivation or frequent sleep interruptions lead to fatigue. A change in environment can induce sleep disorders, especially if accompanied by unfamiliar noises, excessive lighting, uncomfortable temperatures, or an excessive degree of humidity or dryness. Total sleep time may be adequate under such conditions, but quality of sleep is usually poor. Nightmares can also interrupt sleep, and if numerous and recurring, they also cause fatigue.

Some sleep interruptions are not so readily apparent. In sleep apnea, a specific and increasingly diagnosed sleep disorder, the patient temporarily stops breathing while sleeping. This results in reduced oxygen levels and increased carbon dioxide levels in the blood. When a critical level is reached, the patient awakens briefly, takes a few deep breaths, and then falls asleep again. Many episodes of sleep apnea may occur during the night, making the sleep interrupted and less refreshing than it should be. The next day, the patient often feels tired and fatigued but may not recognize the source of the problem. Obstructive sleep apnea normally develops in grossly overweight patients or in those with large tonsils or adenoids. Patients with obstructive sleep apnea usually snore while sleeping, and typically they are unaware of their snoring and/or sleep disturbance.

A number of diseases can lead to easy fatigability. In most illnesses, rest relieves fatigue and individuals awake refreshed after a nap or a good night's sleep. Unfortunately, they also tire quickly. Unlike psychogenic fatigue or fatigue induced by drugs, disease-related fatigue is not usually the patient's main symptom. Other symptoms and signs frequently reveal the underlying diagnosis. Individuals who suffer from severe malnutrition, anemia, endocrine system malfunction, chronic infections, tuberculosis, Lyme disease, bacterial endocarditis (a bacterial infection of the valves of the heart), chronic sinusitis, mononucleosis, hepatitis, parasitic infections, and fungal infections may all experience chronic fatigue.

In early stages of acquired immunodeficiency syndrome (AIDS), fatigue may be the only symptom. Persons at high risk for contracting the human immunodeficiency virus (HIV)—those with multiple sexual partners, homosexual men, those with a history of blood transfusion, or intravenous drug users—who complain of persistent fatigue should be tested for HIV infection.

Abnormalities of mineral or electrolyte concentrations—potassium, sodium, chloride, and calcium are the most important of these—may also cause fatigue. Such abnormalities may result from medications (diuretics are frequently responsible), diarrhea, vomiting, dietary fads, and endocrine or bone disorders.

Some less common medical causes of chronic fatigue include dysfunction of specific organs such as kidney failure or liver failure. Allergies can also produce chronic fatigue. Cancer can cause fatigue, but other symptoms usually surface and lead to a diagnosis before the patient begins to notice chronic weariness.

TREATMENT AND THERAPY

When an individual's fatigue persists in spite of adequate rest, medical help becomes necessary in order to determine the cause. Common diseases known to be associated with fatigue should be considered. Initially, the physician makes detailed inquiries about the severity of the fatigue and how long ago it started. Other important questions include whether it is progressive, whether there are any factors that make it worse or relieve it, or whether it is worse during specific times of the day. An examination of the patient's psychological state may also be necessary.

The physician should ask about the presence of any symptoms that occur along with the general sense of fatigue. For example, breathlessness may indicate a cardiovascular or respiratory disease. Abdominal pain might arouse the suspicion of a gastrointestinal disease.

Weakness may point to a neuromuscular collagen disease. Excessive thirst and increased urine output may suggest diabetes mellitus, and weight loss may accompany metabolic or endocrine abnormalities, chronic infections, or cancer.

Whether they have been prescribed by a physician or purchased over-the-counter, the medications taken regularly by a patient should be reviewed. The doctor should also inquire about alcohol and tobacco use and dietary fads. A thorough physical examination may be required. During an examination, the doctor sometimes uncovers physical signs of fatigue-inducing diseases. Blood tests and other laboratory investigations may also be needed, especially because a physical examination does not always reveal the cause.

Often, however, despite an extensive workup, no specific cause for the persistent fatigue appears. At this stage, the diagnosis of chronic fatigue syndrome should be considered. In order to fit this diagnosis, patients must have several of the symptoms associated with this syndrome. They must have complained of fatigue for at least six months, and the fatigue should be of such an extent that it interferes with normal daily activities. Since many of the symptoms associated with chronic fatigue syndrome overlap with other disorders, these other fatigue-inducing conditions must be considered and ruled out.

In order to fit the diagnosis of chronic fatigue syndrome, patients must have at least six of the classic symptoms. These include a mild fever and/or sore throat, painful lymph nodes in the neck or axilla, unexplained generalized weakness, and muscle pain or discomfort. Patients may describe marked fatigue lasting for more than twenty-four hours that is induced by levels of exercise that would have been easily tolerated before the onset of fatigue. They may suffer from generalized headaches of a type, severity, or pattern that is different from headaches experienced before the onset of chronic fatigue. Patients may also have joint pain without swelling or redness and/or neuropsychologic complaints such as a bad memory and excessive irritability. Confusion, difficulty in thinking, inability to concentrate, depression, and sleep disturbances are also on the list of associated symptoms.

No one knows the exact cause of chronic fatigue syndrome. Researchers continue to study the disease and come up with hypotheses, though none have proven entirely satisfactory. One theory argues that since patients with chronic fatigue syndrome appear to have a reduced aerobic work capacity, defects in the muscles may cause the condition. This, however, constitutes only one of many theories concerning the syndrome and its origin.

Many patients with chronic fatigue syndrome relate that they suffered from an infectious illness immediately preceding the onset of fatigue. This pattern causes some scientists to suspect a viral origin. Typically, the illness that precedes the patient's problems with fatigue is not severe, and resembles other upper respiratory tract infections experienced previously. The implicated viruses include the Epstein-Barr virus, Coxsackie B virus, herpes simplex virus, cytomegalovirus, human herpesvirus 6, and the measles virus. It should be mentioned, however, that some patients with long-term fatigue do not have a history of a triggering infectious disease before the onset of fatigue.

Patients with chronic fatigue syndrome sometimes have a number of immune system abnormalities. Laboratory evidence exists of immune dysfunction in many patients with this syndrome, and there have been reports of improvement when immunoglobulin (antibody) therapy was given. The significance of immunological abnormalities in chronic fatigue syndrome, however, remains uncertain. Most of these abnormalities do not occur in all patients with this syndrome. Furthermore, the degree of immunologic abnormality does not always correspond with the severity of the symptoms.

Some researchers believe that the acute infectious disease that often precedes the onset of chronic fatigue syndrome forces the patient to become physically inactive. This inactivity leads to physical deconditioning, and the progression ends in chronic fatigue syndrome. Experiments in which patients with chronic fatigue syndrome were given exercise testing, however, do not support this theory completely. In the case of physical deconditioning, the heart rates of patients with chronic fatigue syndrome should have risen more rapidly with exercise than those without the syndrome. The exact opposite was found. The data were not determined consistent with the suggestion that physical deconditioning causes chronic fatigue syndrome.

A high prevalence of unrecognized psychiatric disorders exists in patients with chronic fatigue, especially depression. Depression affects about half of chronic fatigue syndrome patients and precedes other symptoms in about half of them as well. Yet a critical question remains unanswered concerning chronic fatigue syndrome: Are patients with this syndrome fatigued because they have a primary mood disorder, or has the mood disorder developed as a secondary component of the chronic fatigue syndrome?

No completely satisfactory treatment exists for chronic fatigue syndrome, since the cause remains a mystery. A group of researchers using intravenous immunoglobulin therapy met with varying degrees of success, but other investigators could not reproduce these results. Other therapeutic trials used high doses of medications such as acyclovir, liver extract, folic acid, and cyanocobalamine. A mixture of evening primrose oil and fish oil was also administered with some degree of success. Claims have also been made that patients administered magnesium sulfate improved to a larger extent than those receiving a placebo. Other therapeutic options include cognitive behavioral therapy, programs of gradually increasing physical activity, analgesics, nonsteroidal anti-inflammatory drugs (NSAIDs), and antidepressants. Finally, a number of self-help groups exist for chronic fatigue sufferers.

The prognosis and natural history of chronic fatigue syndrome are still poorly defined. Chronic fatigue syndrome does not kill patients, but it does significantly decrease the quality of life for sufferers. For the physician, management of this syndrome remains challenging. In addition to correcting any physical abnormalities present, the physician should attempt to find an activity that interests the patient and encourage him or her to become involved in it.

PERSPECTIVE AND PROSPECTS

Fatigue is generally considered a normal bodily response, protecting the individual from excessive physical and/or mental activity. After all, the normal levels of performance for individuals who do not rest usually decline. In the case of overactivity, fatigue should be viewed as a positive warning sign. Using relaxation and rest (mental and/or physical), the individual can often alleviate weariness and optimize performance.

In some cases, however, fatigue does not derive from physical or mental overactivity, nor does it respond adequately to relaxation and rest. In these instances, it interferes with an individual's ability to cope with everyday life and enjoy usual activities. The patient begins referring to fatigue as the reason for not participating in normal physical, mental, and social activities.

Unfortunately, physicians, health care professionals, society, and even the patients themselves dismiss fatigue as a trivial complaint. As a result, sufferers seek medical help only after the condition becomes advanced. This dangerous, negative attitude can delay the correct diagnosis of the underlying pathology and threaten the patient's chances for a quick recovery.

The diagnosis and management of chronic fatigue syndrome prove challenging for both physician and patient. It is important to note that chronic fatigue syndrome often stems from nonmedical causes. While the possibility of a serious medical illness should be addressed, illness-related fatigue usually occurs along with other, more prominent symptoms. The causes of chronic fatigue syndrome are numerous and can take time to define. Patients need to answer all questions related to their complaints as thoroughly and accurately as possible, so that their physicians can reach accurate diagnoses using the minimum number of tests. Extensive testing for rare medical causes of fatigue can become extraordinarily expensive and uncomfortable, so doctors select the tests that they are ordering cautiously. They must balance the benefit, the cost, and the risk of each test to the patient. Such decisions should be based on their own experience and on the available data.

Open communication between the patient and doctor is of paramount importance. It ensures a correct diagnosis, followed by the most effective treatment. Follow-up visits and reassurance may be the best therapy in many cases. Professional counselors can offer assistance with fatigue-inducing psychological disorders. Examination of sleep and relaxation habits can reveal potential problems, and steps can be taken to ensure adequate rest.

Persistent fatigue should not be regarded lightly, and serious attempts should be made to determine its underlying causes. In this respect, it may be appropriate to recall one of Hippocrates' aphorisms, "Unprovoked fatigue means disease."

—*Ronald C. Hamdy, M.D., Mark R. Doman, M.D., and Katherine Hoffman Doman*

See also Aging; Anemia; Anxiety; Apnea; Chronic fatigue syndrome; Depression; Dizziness and fainting; Fibromyalgia; Malnutrition; Multiple chemical sensitivity syndrome; Narcolepsy; Sleep disorders; Sleeping sickness; Stress; Stress reduction.

FOR FURTHER INFORMATION:

Archer, James, Jr. *Managing Anxiety and Stress*. 2d ed. Muncie, Ind.: Excellerated Development, 1991. Anxiety is a common cause of persistent fatigue. This text examines the nature of anxiety. Contains several methods to combat anxiety and stress, ranging from management skills, personal relations, nutrition, and exercise to meditation and relaxation techniques.

DePaulo, J. Raymond, Jr., and Leslie Ann Horvitz. *Understanding Depression: What We Know and What You Can Do About It*. New York: Wiley, 2003. A leading expert on depression examines the disease's nature, causes, effects, and treatments.

Feiden, Karyn. *Hope and Help for Chronic Fatigue Syndrome: The Official CFS-CFIDS Network*. New York: Prentice Hall, 1990. A complete review of chronic fatigue syndrome, presenting the many aspects of this disease. The history of this syndrome, symptomatology, theories of causation, and experimental therapies are addressed.

Goroll, Allan H., Lawrence A. May, and Albert G. Mulley, Jr., eds. *Primary Care Medicine*. Rev. 4th ed. Philadelphia: J. B. Lippincott, 2000. The essential text for the medical office practice of adult medicine. It is problem-oriented and easily read even by individuals without medical training. The section on the causes of fatigue is one of the best available.

Patarca-Montero, Roberto. *Chronic Fatigue Syndrome and the Body's Immune Defense System*. New York: Haworth Medical Press, 2002. Patarca-Montero, a leading immunologist, examines the connections between the disease and immunology, reviews how therapeutic tools such as herbal medicine, vaccines, and cell therapy are being used in CFS research, and discusses the connection between CFS and fibromyalgia, Gulf War syndrome, sick building syndrome, and multiple chemical sensitivity.

Talley, Joseph. *Family Practitioner's Guide to Treating Depressive Illness*. Chicago: Precept Press, 1987. Depression is probably the most common cause of persistent fatigue. This well-written text examines the multiple facets of depression. It also reviews the various therapies available, different philosophies of depressive treatments, and the use of psychotherapy.

Wilson, James L. *Adrenal Fatigue: The Twenty-First Century Stress Syndrome*. Petaluma, Calif.: Smart, 2001. The author, a clinician for more than two decades, helps readers assess their condition and symptoms and determine causes, and suggests treatment of the condition through lifestyle and dietary modification.

Zgourides, George D., and Christie Zgourides. *Stop Feeling Tired: Ten Mind-Body Steps to Fight Fatigue and Feel Your Best*. Oakland, Calif.: New Harbinger, 2003. A self-help book that stresses holistic tools for eliminating tension and improving quality of life.

Explores relaxation methods adapted from both Western and Eastern disciplines, such as cognitive-behavioral strategies, simple meditation, visualization, and energy-balancing techniques.

FATTY ACID OXIDATION DISORDERS
DISEASE/DISORDER

ANATOMY OR SYSTEM AFFECTED: Heart, liver, muscles

SPECIALTIES AND RELATED FIELDS: Biochemistry, biotechnology, nutrition, pediatrics, perinatology

DEFINITION: Inherited metabolic defects that prevent the breakdown of fatty acids in the liver, muscles, and heart.

INFORMATION ON FATTY ACID OXIDATION DISORDERS

CAUSES: Genetic enzyme deficiency

SYMPTOMS: Only under fasting conditions (overnight or when exacerbated by infection or fever), vomiting, coma, and sometimes death; some disorders largely asymptomatic

DURATION: Chronic with acute episodes

TREATMENTS: Minimizing of fasting (snacking before sleep), intravenous glucose for acute episodes

---

CAUSES AND SYMPTOMS

Fatty acid oxidation disorders are inherited defects in the enzymes that break down fatty acids to generate metabolic energy. Defects in at least eleven of the twenty enzymes involved with this process have been identified and can be diagnosed by enzymatic analysis of a tissue biopsy. Some generate unique profiles of metabolites in the blood or urine that can be used for diagnosis. These disorders are inherited as autosomal recessive traits, and, in many cases, the causative deoxyribonucleic acid (DNA) mutations have been determined. Fatty acid oxidation disorders can affect the liver, which breaks down fatty acids for its own needs and, by converting them to ketone bodies, for energy generation in other body tissues; they can also affect muscles and the heart, which use fatty acids as a source of energy.

Symptoms appear only under fasting conditions, either overnight or when exacerbated by infection or fever. Under these conditions, as glycogen stores are depleted, the body depends increasingly on fatty acids for energy. If fatty acids cannot be broken down completely, an energy deficit and the accumulation of deleterious intermediates lead to vomiting, coma, and, in severe cases, death. The levels of blood glucose are low because the energy needed for its synthesis is lacking. The first episode may occur in the first two years of life; such an episode can be fatal and may be mistakenly attributed to sudden infant death syndrome (SIDS). Some fatty acid oxidation disorders, however, are largely asymptomatic.

TREATMENT AND THERAPY

The general treatment for fatty acid oxidation disorders is to minimize fasting, as by snacking before sleep, and, in acute episodes, to administer intravenous glucose. This treatment restores depleted blood glucose and reduces the demand for fatty acid oxidation. Some defects also benefit from a low intake of dietary fat. Fasting or low carbohydrate diets, for weight loss or other reasons, are contraindicated for individuals with these disorders.

One of these diseases is attributable to the defective cellular uptake of carnitine, which is needed to transport fatty acids into mitochondria, where they are oxidized; this type can be treated with supplemental carnitine. In acute episodes with some other disorders, treatment with carnitine has proven beneficial in increasing the urinary excretion of deleterious intermediates.

PERSPECTIVE AND PROSPECTS

The first observation of a defect in fatty acid oxidation was made in 1972. Although not reported until 1982, one such disorder, medium-chain acyl-coenzyme A dehydrogenase (MCAD) deficiency, is among the most common inborn errors of metabolism, with a frequency of 1 in 9,000 live births. Each disorder of fatty acid oxidation is a candidate for enzyme replacement therapy or gene replacement therapy, although these remain experimental treatments.

—*James L. Robinson, Ph.D.*

See also Enzyme therapy; Enzymes; Food biochemistry; Glycogen storage diseases; Metabolism.

FOR FURTHER INFORMATION:

Devlin, Thomas M., ed. *Textbook of Biochemistry with Clinical Correlations.* 5th ed. New York: Wiley-Liss, 2002.

Hay, William W., Jr., et al., eds. *Current Pediatric Diagnosis and Treatment.* 16th ed. New York: McGraw-Hill, 2003.

Roe, C. R., and J. Ding. "Mitochondrial Fatty Acid Oxidation Disorders." In *The Metabolic and Molecular Bases of Inherited Disease*, edited by Charles R. Scriver et al. 8th ed. New York: McGraw-Hill, 2001.

Feet

Anatomy

Anatomy or system involved: Bones, musculoskeletal system

Specialties and related fields: Orthopedics, podiatry

Definition: The lowest extremities, composed of a complex system of muscles and bones, that act as levers to propel the body and that must support the weight of the body in standing, walking, or running.

Key terms:

distal: referring to a particular body part that is farther from the point of attachment or farther from the trunk than another part

extension: movement that increases the angle between the bones, causing them to move further apart; straightening or extension of the ankle occurs when the toes point away from the shin

flexion: a bending movement that decreases the angle of the joint and brings two bones closer together; flexion of the ankle pulls the foot closer to the shin

hallucis: a term referring to the big toe; the flexor hallucis longus is a muscle which flexes the big toe

inferior: situated below another part; the ankle bones are inferior to the bones of the lower leg

lateral: toward the side with respect to the body's imaginary midline; away from the midline of the body, a limb, or any understood point of reference

medial: closer to an imaginary midline dividing the body into equal right and left halves than another part

plantar: having to do with the sole of the foot (for example, a plantar wart)

podiatry: the branch of medicine that deals with the study, examination, diagnosis, treatment, and prevention of diseases and malfunctions of the foot

proximal: referring to a particular body part that is closer to a point of attachment than another part

superior: above another part or closer to the head; the ankle bones are superior to the bones of the feet

Structure and Functions

The anatomy of the foot is very similar to that of the hand; however, the foot is adapted to perform very different functions. The human hand has the ability to perform fine movements such as grasping and writing, while the foot is involved mainly in support and movement. Therefore, the bones and muscles of the foot tend to be heavier and function without the same dexterity as the hand.

The twenty-six bones of the foot include the tarsals, metatarsals, and phalanges. The proximal portion of the foot next to the ankle is composed of seven tarsal bones: the calcaneus, talus, navicular, cuboid, medial cuneiform, intermediate cuneiform, and lateral cuneiform. The bones are rather irregular in shape and form gliding joints; these joints allow only a limited movement when compared to other joints in the body. The calcaneus forms the large heel bone, which serves as a major attachment for the muscles that are located in the back of the lower leg. Just above the calcaneus is another large foot bone called the talus. The talus rests between the tibia and the fibula, the two lower leg bones. Interestingly, the talus is the single bone that receives the entire weight of the body when an individual is standing; it must then transmit this weight to the rest of the foot below. The cuboid and the three cuneiform bones meet the proximal end of the long foot bones, the metatarsals.

The five separate metatarsal bones are relatively long and thin when compared to the tarsal bones. Anatomists distinguish between the five metatarsals by number. If one begins numbering from the medial (or inside) part of the foot, that metatarsal is number one and the lateral (or outside) metatarsal is number five. The distal portion of each metatarsal articulates (meets) with the toe bones, or phalanges.

Humans have toes that are very similar to their fingers. In fact, the numbers and names of the toe and finger bones, phalanges, are identical. The major differences lie in the fact that the finger phalanges are longer than the phalanges that make up toes. Hinge joints are located between each phalanx and allow for flexion and extension movements only. Human toes (or fingers) are made up of fourteen different phalanges. Each toe (or finger) has three phalanges except for the big toe (or thumb), which has only two. The toes are named in a similar way as the metatarsals; that is, the big toe is number one and the little toe is number five. The three phalanges that make up each toe (except for the big toe) are named according to location. The phalanx meeting the metatarsal is referred to as the proximal phalanx. The bone at the tip of the toe is the distal phalanx, and the one in between is the middle phalanx. Since the big toe only has two phalanges, they are called proximal and distal phalanges.

Although it seems that there is only a single arch in each foot, podiatrists and anatomists identify three arches: the medial and lateral longitudinal arches and the transverse, or metatarsal, arch. The medial longitudinal arch, as the name implies, is located on the medial surface of the foot and follows the long axis from the calcaneus to the big toe. Likewise, the lateral longitudinal arch is on the lateral surface and runs from the heel to the little toe. The transverse, or metatarsal, arch crosses the width of the foot near the proximal end of the metatarsals. The bones are only one factor that maintains arches in the feet and prevents them from flattening under the weight of the body. Ligaments (which connect bones), muscles, and tendons (which attach muscles to bones) are primarily responsible for the support of the arches. The arches function to distribute body weight between the calcaneus and the distal end of the metatarsals (the balls of the feet). They also are flexible enough to absorb some of the shock to the feet from walking, running, and jumping.

While the feet seem to be composed of only bones, tendons, and ligaments, the movements of the toes and feet require an extensive system of muscles. Most of the larger muscles that act on the foot and toes are actually located in the lower leg. Anatomists divide these muscles into separate compartments: anterior, posterior, and lateral.

The muscles of the anterior compartment move the foot upward (dorsiflex) and extend the toes. These muscles include the tibialis anterior, extensor digitorum longus, extensor hallucis longus, and peroneus tertius. The tibialis anterior is attached to the top of the first metatarsal and pulls the medial part of the foot upward and slightly lateral. All the toes except the big toe are pulled up (extended) by the extensor digitorum longus. The extensor hallucis longus moves only the big toe upward, while the peroneus tertius is attached to the fifth metatarsal and moves the foot upward.

The muscles of the lateral compartment act to move the foot in a lateral or outward direction. The peroneus longus and peroneus brevis are attached to the first and fifth metatarsal, respectively. Using these attachments, the muscles can pull the foot laterally.

The muscles of the posterior compartment are the largest group and act to flex the foot and toes. All these muscles share a common tendon, the calcaneus (or Achilles) tendon. As the name suggests, this large tendon attaches to the calcaneus bone. The larger, more superficial muscles include the gastrocnemius, soleus, and plantaris; these powerful muscles are commonly called the calf muscles. Also in the posterior compartment are four smaller muscles located beneath the calf muscles: the popliteus (located directly behind the knee joint), flexor hallucis longus, flexor digitorum longus, and tibialis posterior. The popliteus rotates the lower leg medially. The flexor hallucis longus flexes the big toe. The remaining toes are flexed by the flexor digitorum longus, while the tibialis posterior acts opposite the tibialis anterior to flex the foot.

Within the foot itself are some muscles known as the intrinsic foot muscles. All but one of these muscles are located on the bottom surface of the foot. This one muscle extends all the toes except the little toe. The remaining intrinsic muscles are on the plantar (bottom) surface and serve to flex the toes.

The major vessels that provide blood to the foot include branches from the anterior tibial artery. This relatively large artery is located along the anterior surface of the lower leg and branches into the dorsalis pedis artery, which serves the ankle and upper part of the foot. Physicians often check for a pulse in this foot artery to provide information about circulation to the foot and circulation in general, as this is the point farthest from the heart. The bottom parts of the feet are supplied with blood by branches of the peroneal artery. At the ankle, this artery branches into plantar arteries, which supply the structures on the sole of the foot. The human toes receive most of their blood from branches of the plantar arteries called the digital arteries.

DISORDERS AND DISEASES

Even though the anatomy of the foot is resistant to the tremendous amount of force that the body places on it, it can be injured. Force injuries to the foot commonly result in fractures or breaks of the metatarsals and pha-

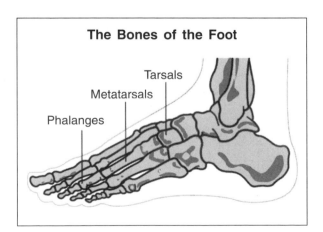

The Bones of the Foot

Tarsals

Metatarsals

Phalanges

langes. Occasionally, the calcaneus may fracture from a fall on a hard surface. More commonly, patients complain of painful heel syndrome.

Because the shock-absorbing pads of tissue on the heel become thinner with age, repeated pressure on the heel can cause pain. Prolonged standing, walking, or running can add to the pressure, as can being overweight. One cause of pain is plantar fasciitis, an inflammation of the tough band of connective tissue on the sole. The inflammation occurs when the muscles located on the back of the lower leg that are attached to the connective tissue at the calcaneus pull under stress. This may even be associated with small fractures. X rays may show small spurs of bone near the site of stress; however, these spurs are not believed to be the cause of pain.

Deformities of the foot at birth are fairly common and include clubfoot, flat foot, and clawfoot. The cause of these anomalies is abnormal development. The foot of the fetus normally goes through stages where it is turned outward and inward but gradually assumes a normal position by about the seventh month of gestation. In the case of clubfoot, arrested development in the stage when the foot is turned inward causes the muscles, bones, and joints to develop in this abnormal anatomical position. At the time of birth, the deformity is readily observable and the foot immobile. Treatment includes splints, casting, and surgery. If treatment is begun at birth, the foot may look relatively normal after approximately one year.

Almost everyone is born with feet that are flat because the arches do not begin to develop until the ligaments and muscles function normally. In most people, the arches are fully formed by the age of six. In some individuals, however, the ligaments and muscles remain weak and the feet do not develop a normal arch. Flat feet can also develop in adult life, at which time they are called "fallen arches." Body weight moves along a precise path during walking or running, beginning with the heel touching the ground. Then, as the foot steps, the arch receives the forces pushing down on the foot. Because the bones, muscles, and ligaments form an arch in the foot, the arch can deform slightly and absorb some of the downward force. With further movement, the weight passes to the ball of the foot (the distal metatarsals). A fallen arch has lost this flexibility and shock-absorbing capability. The arch "falls" because of improper weight distribution along the foot, causing the arch to stretch excessively and to weaken with time. Without proper arch support, the foot begins to twist inward, or medially, causing the body weight to be trans-

mitted to the inside of the foot rather than in a straight line toward the toes. This problem often occurs in runners who have improperly fitted shoes or a poor running style (although anyone can suffer from fallen longitudinal arches, regardless of the individual's level of physical activity). As a runner increases distance and speed without correcting his or her shoes or running form, the force applied to the feet increases. Fallen arches appear to occur particularly in runners or joggers who exercise on hard surfaces without proper technique or arch support.

A number of disorders can affect the skin of the foot. Corns are small areas of thickened skin on a toe that are usually caused by tight-fitting shoes. People with high arches are affected most because the arch increases the pressure applied to the toes during walking. If the corn becomes painful, the easiest treatment is for the person to wear better-fitting shoes. If the pain persists, a clinician can pare down the growth with a scalpel.

Plantar warts appear on the skin of the sole and are caused by a papillomavirus. Because of pressure from the weight of the body, the plantar wart is often flattened and forced into the skin of the sole. The wart may disappear without treatment. If it persists, surgery or chemical therapy can be used to relieve the discomfort.

Athlete's foot is a common fungal infection which causes the foot to become itchy, sore, and cracked. It is usually treated with antifungal agents such as miconazole. Preventive measures including keeping the feet dry and disinfecting areas where the fungus may live, such as shower stalls.

Another common deformity is a bunion, which is a bursa (fluid-filled pad) overlying the joint at the base of the big toe. Normal structure of the first metatarsal, first phalange, and their joint is necessary to withstand the force applied to them in everyday activities. A bunion is caused by an abnormal outward projection of the joint and an inward projection of the big toe. Treatment involves correcting the position of the big toe and keeping it in a normal position. Sometimes surgery is necessary if the tissues become too swollen. In fact, some severe cases of bunions have required complete reconstruction of the toe. Unless treated, a bunion will get progressively worse.

Gout is a metabolic disorder, mainly found in men, which causes uric acid crystals to form in joints. Even though any joint can be affected, the big toe joint is likely the major site for gout because it is under chronic stress from walking. The joint is usually red, swollen, and very tender and painful. The first attack usually involves only one joint and lasts a few days. Some patients never experience another attack, but most have a second episode between six months and two years after the first. After the second attack, more joints may become involved. Treatment includes anti-inflammatory drugs and colchicine. These drugs help reduce the pain by decreasing the amount of inflammation around the joint. Physicians may also prescribe allopurinol to reduce the amount of uric acid that the body produces. Drugs are also available that increase the kidneys' ability to excrete uric acid; examples of these agents are probenecid and sulfinpyrazone.

PERSPECTIVE AND PROSPECTS

Even though the feet constitute a relatively small area of the body, ailments of the feet afflict more than half the world's population. For a long time, disorders of the foot were not taken as seriously as those found in other parts of the body. It is now known, however, that poor foot health can have serious effects. For example, in children a painful foot condition not properly diagnosed and treated can result in lost school days and decreased participation in other activities. More important, an uncorrected congenital abnormality, if neglected, could have irreversible consequences. For the elderly, foot problems hinder or prevent normal activities such as taking care of personal needs, exercising, and socializing. Anything that affects the feet affects that individual's overall health and well-being.

Because of the potentially devastating problems of improper foot care, a branch of medicine developed that specifically addresses problems of the feet. Physicians known as podiatrists practice a specialized branch of medicine called podiatry. It is the job of the podiatrist to assess the cause of the foot problem and the patient's general medical condition in determining the need for and the course of treatment. This assessment often calls for contact with the patient's primary care physician for access to the patient's medical records, as many diseases affect the whole body but present signs and symptoms in the feet. The podiatrist or other physician, such as an orthopedist, will evaluate a disorder through physical exams, laboratory tests, and anatomical tests to examine the internal structures; the latter may include X rays, computed tomography (CT) scans, or magnetic resonance imaging (MRI). The physician will then diagnose and begin treating the disorder using surgery, medical therapy, or physical therapy.

As more individuals become physically active throughout their lives, clinicians who practice sports medicine are paying closer attention to problems of the foot. Many people seek to improve their health by walking, jogging, and bicycling. All these activities have proven to be excellent for maintaining cardiovascular health, but all place additional stress on the foot. Physicians who counsel patients on physical fitness programs attempt to identify individuals who may be injury-prone. Failure to recognize an anatomical anomaly of the feet could lead to an injury or series of injuries that restrict certain activities or even cause permanent damage. Occasionally, individuals are too enthusiastic about their exercise program and experience overuse injuries involving the feet. Such injuries may cause a sudden cessation of the physical activity and may have a significant demoralizing effect on individuals who finally decide to take steps to improve their health and well-being.

People commonly neglect their feet and underemphasize the importance of the normal functional anatomy of the foot. Individuals who experience a foot injury, however, begin to appreciate the absolute importance of this rather complex but often overlooked structure.

—Matthew Berria, Ph.D.

See also Anatomy; Athlete's foot; Bones and the skeleton; Bunions; Cysts; Flat feet; Foot disorders; Frostbite; Ganglion removal; Gout; Hammertoe correction; Hammertoes; Heel spur removal; Lower extremities; Nail removal; Nails; Orthopedic surgery; Orthopedics; Orthopedics, pediatric; Podiatry; Sports medicine; Tendon repair; Warts.

FOR FURTHER INFORMATION:

Currey, John D. *Bones: Structures and Mechanics.* Princeton, N.J.: Princeton University Press, 2002. Very accessible overview of a range of information related to whole bones, bone tissue, and dentin and enamel. Topics include stiffness, strength, viscoelasticity, fatigue, fracture mechanics properties, buckling, impact fracture, and properties of cancellous bone.

Hales, Dianne. *An Invitation to Health.* 9th ed. Belmont, Calif.: Wadsworth Thomson Learning, 2000. This text should be read by anyone who wishes an overview of health topics. Chapter 7 deals with exercise and contains a section on the importance of wearing the correct shoes for a given activity.

Hole, John W., Jr. *Essentials of Human Anatomy and Physiology.* 8th ed. Dubuque, Iowa: Wm. C. Brown, 2002. The authors do an excellent job of describing the rather complex anatomy of the foot and lower leg. Several views of the internal and external anatomy of the foot are given.

Lippert, Frederick G., and Sigvard T. Hansen. *Foot and Ankle Disorders: Tricks of the Trade.* New York: Thieme, 2003. Details common foot disorders and their causes and treatment.

Mader, Sylvia S. *Human Biology.* 7th ed. Dubuque, Iowa: Wm. C. Brown, 2001. Provides an excellent overview of lower limb anatomy and physiology. It also addresses common medical terminology relating to foot movement.

Marieb, Elaine N. *Human Anatomy and Physiology.* 7th ed. Redwood City, Calif.: Benjamin/Cummings, 2003. This text discusses the functional significance of various anatomical structures, including the foot. Readers will enjoy the excellent pictures and diagrams of the foot and associated body parts.

Van De Graaff, Kent M., and Stuart I. Fox. *Concepts of Human Anatomy and Physiology.* 5th ed. Dubuque, Iowa: Wm. C. Brown, 2000. Van De Graaff has taught human anatomy for years, and anyone would appreciate the approach that he has taken in presenting human structures. Chapters 7, 9, and 10 cover the anatomy of the foot and some problems that can occur if the anatomy is abnormal. Chapter 10 includes the surface anatomy of the lower leg and foot.

Fetal alcohol syndrome
Disease/disorder

Anatomy or system affected: Brain, musculoskeletal system, nervous system, reproductive system

Specialties and related fields: Embryology, neonatology, obstetrics, perinatology, public health

Definition: Growth retardation and mental or physical abnormalities in a child resulting from alcohol consumption by the mother during pregnancy.

Fetal alcohol syndrome was first identified in the early 1970's. Whether consumed as beer, wine, or hard liquor, alcohol is a teratogen, a toxic substance that can cause abnormalities in unborn children. The damage ranges from subtle to severe, depending on the quantity consumed and the stage of pregnancy when the exposure occurs. A critical period is in early pregnancy, when a woman may not know that she is pregnant. Even one or two drinks a day by the mother may have an effect on her child.

> ## Information on
> ## Fetal Alcohol Syndrome
>
> **Causes:** Alcohol consumption by mother during pregnancy
> **Symptoms:** Growth retardation, certain facial anomalies, central nervous system impairment, clumsiness, behavioral problems, brief attention span, poor judgment, impaired memory, diminished capacity to learn from experience
> **Duration:** Chronic
> **Treatments:** None; preventive measures during pregnancy

There are three diagnostic criteria for fetal alcohol syndrome: growth retardation, certain facial anomalies, and central nervous system impairment. Growth retardation begins in utero, causing low birth weight. Babies with low birth weight are at risk for delayed growth and development and even death. Growth impairment affects not only the skeleton but also the brain and face. The resulting head and facial abnormalities are characterized by thin lips; small, wide-set eyes; a short, upturned nose; a receding chin; and low-set ears. Fetal alcohol syndrome children have intelligence quotients (IQs) well below the mean of the population because of impaired brain growth that results in irreversible mental retardation. Fetal alcohol syndrome is a leading cause of mental retardation. Abnormalities often originate during the first trimester, when bones and organs are forming. Major organ systems such as the heart, kidney, liver, and skeleton can be impaired.

Less specific problems that result from alcohol damage are clumsiness, behavioral problems, a brief attention span, poor judgment, impaired memory, and a diminished capacity to learn from experience. These symptoms are often labeled "fetal alcohol effects."

Alcohol enters the fetal bloodstream as soon as the mother has a drink. It not only can damage the brain but also may impair the function of the placenta, which is the organ interface between maternal and fetal circulation. The exact mechanism for this damage is not completely understood. The most probable cause is that alcohol creates a glucose or oxygen deficit for the fetus. Because it is not known what dose of alcohol is safe, the best preventive measure is to abstain from alcohol during pregnancy and even when planning a pregnancy.

—*Wendy L. Stuhldreher, Ph.D., R.D.*

See also Addiction; Alcoholism; Birth defects; Childbirth; Childbirth complications; Embryology; Genetic diseases; Neonatology; Obstetrics; Perinatology; Pregnancy and gestation.

For Further Information:

Abel, Ernest L., ed. *Fetal Alcohol Syndrome: From Mechanism to Prevention*. Boca Raton, Fla.: CRC Press, 1996.

Armstrong, Elizabeth M. *Conceiving Risk, Bearing Responsibility: Fetal Alcohol Syndrome and the Diagnosis of Moral Disorder*. Baltimore: Johns Hopkins University Press, 2003.

Hannigan, John H., et al., eds. *Alcohol and Alcoholism: Effects on Brain and Development*. Mahwah, N.J.: Lawrence Erlbaum, 1998.

Huebert, Kathryn M., and Cindy Raftis. *Fetal Alcohol Syndrome and Other Alcohol-Related Birth Defects*. Edmonton: Alberta Alcohol and Drug Abuse Commission, 1996.

National Organization of Fetal Alcohol Syndrome. http://www.nofas.org/main/index2.htm. A group committed to raising public awareness of FAS and to developing and implementing plans for prevention, intervention, education, and advocacy.

Spohr, Hans-Ludwig, and Hans-Christoph Steinhausen, eds. *Alcohol, Pregnancy, and the Developing Child*. New York: Cambridge University Press, 1996.

Stratton, Kathleen, Cynthia Howe, and Frederick Battaglia, eds. *Fetal Alcohol Syndrome: Diagnosis, Epidemiology, Prevention, and Treatment*. Washington, D.C.: National Academy Press, 1996.

Streissguth, Ann Pytkowicz. *Fetal Alcohol Syndrome: A Guide for Families and Communities*. Baltimore: Paul H. Brookes, 1997.

Fetal surgery

Procedure

Anatomy or system affected: Bladder, blood, brain, liver, lungs, respiratory system, urinary system

Specialties and related fields: Cardiology, ethics, genetics, neonatology, obstetrics, pediatrics, urology

Definition: Surgical intervention in utero, before birth, if the fetus has a life-threatening condition or congenital abnormality that can be alleviated.

Key terms:

amniocentesis: the drawing of amniotic fluid through the abdominal wall of a pregnant woman in the fifteenth or sixteenth week of pregnancy to test for fetal abnormalities, particularly Down syndrome

diaphragmatic hernia: a protrusion of the stomach into the diaphragm

hiatal hernia: a protrusion of the stomach into the opening normally occupied in the diaphragm by the esophagus

hydronephrosis: swelling (distension) of the kidney

hypotonic: the presence of a low osmotic pressure

in utero: the Latin term for "inside or within the womb"

neonatologist: a physician who specializes in treating newborn infants

osmotic pressure: the pressure between two solutions

teratoma: a tumor composed of tissue not normally found at that site

thorax: the bone and cartilage cage attached to the sternum; generally referred to as the rib cage

uropathy: any disease of the urinary tract

Indications and Procedures

As early as the 1960's, some unborn infants suffering from progressive anemia caused by antibodies that drew away their strength were saved by receiving blood transfusions in utero. These early procedures marked the beginnings of invasive medical intervention in dealing with fetal problems.

Not until the technical advances of the 1970's and beyond, however, was it possible to observe human fetuses in the uterus. With the development of ultrasound imaging, it became possible to examine in considerable detail the size, growth, and contour of fetuses. The use of ultrasound enabled physicians to assess with considerable accuracy the age of fetuses and to predict their probable date of birth.

Laparoscopes with diameters of less than 0.1 inch make it possible to examine the fetal stomach. The use of lasers and tiny instruments guided by computers has allowed methods of fetal surgery that were inconceivable at mid-twentieth century. These instruments greatly reduce blood loss in all types of surgery, including fetal surgery, and greatly improve the prognosis in such procedures. They are used to repair ruptured membranes in fetuses, to install shunts to relieve blockages, and, with the laser excision of placental vessels, to equalize osmotic pressure in twin-twin transfusion syndrome.

It has become possible for obstetricians to observe all significant fetal organs. Whereas physicians earlier could barely hear the beat of the fetal heart, they now can monitor all four of its chambers in the unborn to detect defects early, and, in some cases, to repair them surgically. Ultrasound enables physicians to observe fetal movement within the uterus and to monitor fetal breathing and swallowing.

Because physicians can now gather specific information about the fetus and its health, abnormalities and life-threatening physical problems can be detected several months prior to delivery. Whereas neonatologists have regularly encountered such problems as intestinal and urinary tract obstructions, heart defects, protrusions of the wall of the stomach into the thorax (diaphragmatic hernia) or into the esophageal region (hiatal hernia), swelling of the kidney (hydronephrosis), tumors (sacrococcygeal teratomas), hydrocephalus (water on the brain), and defects of the chromosomes shortly after the birth of a child, it is now possible to detect and, in some cases, to treat these defects surgically in utero.

In cases where fetal surgery appears to offer the most reasonable solution to a difficult problem, the mother may be sent to one of the few centers in the United States where this highly specialized and controversial form of surgery is performed regularly. With the development of sophisticated computer-operated instrumentation, surgeons geographically distant from their patients can perform highly specialized surgery on them. Eventually, such surgery will likely be performed without uprooting mothers.

The current success rate of fetal surgery is not encouraging, although some remarkable outcomes have occurred through its use. Fetal surgical procedures often result in miscarriages and sometimes in the death of both the mother and the fetus.

Two conditions that frequently require fetal surgery are obstructions in the urinary tract that, if untreated until birth, may lead to kidney failure, and hydrocephalus, in which cerebral swelling makes it difficult or impossible for brain fluids to circulate. Both conditions, which occur in 1 of every 5,000 to 10,000 births, require immediate attention to prevent long-term problems or death. Stents can overcome blockages. Instruments have been developed to drain fluid from the brain in instances of hydrocephalus.

When surgery is performed to allow fetal lungs to develop normally, the fetus, attached to the mother through the umbilical cord, exists in the most protective environment it is ever likely to know. If corrections are made in the uterus,

then the fetal lungs are in the safest possible environment for becoming stronger before they are forced to function on their own.

In cases of obstructive urinopathy (obstruction of the urinary tract), surgery may help injured kidneys to recover and develop. Hypotonic urine found in fetal samples indicates that normal kidney function might be restored and suggests that surgery may permit the affected kidneys to gain strength within the uterus. On the other hand, the presence of isotonic urine in fetal samples indicates kidneys that are too badly compromised to regain normal function. Treatments currently available offer no solution to this problem.

One of the more routine procedures connected with pregnancy is amniocentesis, testing for chromosomal abnormalities through the analysis of amniotic fluid drawn through the abdominal wall of the mother and of blood drawn from the umbilical cord. This procedure is not without risks to mothers and fetuses. It is commonly used, however, because the benefits derived from it are generally thought to outweigh the risks.

Nevertheless, amniocentesis remains a controversial procedure, and major ethical questions surround its use. If the test reveals a chromosomal abnormality, the

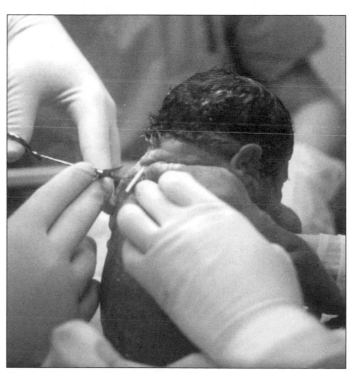

Shortly after birth, doctors examine the shunt that was inserted into a baby two months earlier in an effort to correct his hydrocephalus. (AP/Wide World Photos)

parents are left with the decision of whether to seek a therapeutic abortion to terminate the pregnancy, which in many jurisdictions would be considered a realistic option. With many such abnormalities, however, the fetus might be delivered alive and, although significantly handicapped, have a life expectancy of many years.

Fetal surgery is indicated when physicians are convinced that a fetus will not survive long enough to be delivered or when it appears certain that the newborn will be unable to survive long after its birth. For example, if it appears through ultrasound that a fetus suffers from a severe kind of congenital diaphragmatic hernia in which the liver is in the chest, then it is obvious that the development of the lungs will be seriously compromised without surgical intervention. Fetal surgery becomes a stopgap measure in such cases to lessen the severity of the problem so that the fetus can grow to term and be delivered, after which corrective surgery outside the uterus can be undertaken. This procedure involves substantial risk, however, because the liver can be destroyed in the process of trying to restore it to its normal position in utero.

Sometimes ultrasound reveals noncancerous sacrococcygeal tumors. Such tumors, if untreated, can become large enough in a fetus to put a strain on the heart sufficient to cause heart failure. This severely compromises the survival of the fetus. Guided by ultrasound imagery, surgeons can cut off the blood supply to such tumors and starve them before they do irreparable damage to the fetus. When this procedure is used, the destroyed tumor can be removed surgically after birth.

Another growing use of fetal surgery is in cases where spina bifida, usually identified through ultrasound around the sixteenth week of pregnancy, is present. This congenital defect involves a malformation in the vertebral arch, in which the neural tube connected to the brain and the spine is exposed. When this condition is diagnosed and treated early in the development of the fetus, considerable spinal cord function can be preserved. This makes postnatal treatment more effective than it would be were the condition not discovered until after delivery.

There are essentially two major forms of fetal surgery. The more drastic of these involves performing a cesarean section, after which the fetus is carefully removed from the uterus and treated. It is then returned to the uterus, which is closed with sutures. The umbilical cord is not cut, so that the fetus is still receiving oxygen and need not breathe on its own before its lungs have developed sufficiently. This procedure is indicated when some congenital defect, possibly a teratoma (tumor), blocks the airway. Clearing the fetal airway enables the baby to breathe independently upon delivery. The other form of fetal surgery is done without removing the fetus from the uterus and is made possible by the use of laparoscopes and other specialized instruments. This is the preferred method if a choice is offered.

USES AND COMPLICATIONS

As fetal surgery becomes more significant and more common in the treatment and elimination of many threatening prenatal conditions, numerous complications, both ethical and physical, necessarily arise. Any surgery involves risk, and in fetal surgery a dual risk exists: risk to the fetus and risk to the mother. Therefore, physicians who perform fetal surgery have simultaneously as patients both prospective mothers and fetuses. Because fetuses cannot speak for themselves or make their own decisions, fetal surgeons often find themselves in an ethical quagmire. Most physicians hestitate to recommend fetal surgery except in such extreme cases that fetal death or severe disability without such surgery seems inevitable.

Sometimes wrenching decisions must be made about whether to save the life of the mother or the life of the fetus. Questions also arise about whether to allow a fetus to come to term if it is obvious that it will suffer from birth defects that will either severely limit the length of its life or adversely compromise its quality of life, which in some cases may involve a normal life span. Many notable people who suffered from severe birth defects have made significant contributions to society and have led productive and rewarding lives.

One of the more significant uses of fetal surgery is in the treatment of twin-twin transfusion syndrome. In the United States, this syndrome occurs in about one thousand pregnancies each year. Twin-twin transfusion syndrome results in a pair of twins being of unequal size in the fetal state because of abnormal circulation of amniotic fluid between them within the placenta that they share. The larger of the two is surrounded by considerably more amniotic fluid than the smaller one. This disproportion can result in the death of one or both of the fetuses. Attempts can be made to equalize the amniotic fluid by inserting a hollow needle through the mother's abdomen and drawing out excess fluid, a procedure that can threaten the viability of one or both of the fetuses.

Another more sophisticated treatment of twin-twin transfusion syndrome involves inserting a fetoscope into the uterus and using heat from a laser to seal off the blood vessels between the fetuses. This treatment is directed toward separating the circulation between the twins, which accounts for the condition. Regardless of which treatment is employed, the mortality rate is currently quite high in such cases, and premature delivery is a virtual given in them. Without intervention, however, these fetuses inevitably die in the uterus.

One of the greatest complications of fetal surgery is premature delivery. Fetuses were once thought to be viable only in the seventh month and beyond. Now the means are available to make survival outside the uterus possible earlier than that, although extraordinary care, attention, and equipment are required for extended periods following the delivery of a baby short of seven months and hospitalization in the neonatal intensive care unit (NICU) may continue for many months following such a birth.

When fetal surgery is performed, the mother is routinely medicated with drugs that will both reduce her pain and substantially decrease the possibility of miscarriage or premature delivery. As the field grows and becomes increasingly sophisticated, many of the current problems that it poses will surely be overcome.

Perspective and Prospects

The development of highly specialized instruments, including fiber-optic telescopes and instruments specially designed to enter the uterus through minute incisions, has made possible the field of fetal surgery. Obstetrical surgeons can now correct life-threatening defects and malformations through the smallest, least invasive of openings while the fetus remains within the protection of the mother's body. This procedure, referred to as fetoscopic surgery, is the method preferred whenever it is possible because it reduces substantially the danger of bringing about premature labor at a time when the fetus cannot breathe on its own.

Because fetal surgery is in its infancy, relatively few surgeons specialize in it and the full range of its uses and promises has yet to be explored. The two major centers in the United States that have pioneered development in this field are the Children's Hospital in Philadelphia and the University of California Hospital in San Francisco.

Considerable research in fetal surgery is being conducted at both of these institutions and in laboratories and hospitals throughout the country. It is a matter of time before improved technology will exist to eradicate some of the major barriers to more extensive fetal sur-

gery. Surgery of all kinds is becoming less invasive, which reduces considerably the shock that it delivers to patients' bodies, including blood loss and recovery time. Noninvasive fetal surgery is particularly important to ensure the physical welfare of both the fetus and the mother.

—*R. Baird Shuman, Ph.D.*

See also Abortion; Amniocentesis; Birth defects; Brain disorders; Cesarean section; Chorionic villus sampling; Down syndrome; Embryology; Ethics; Genetic diseases; Genetics and inheritance; Hernia; Hernia repair; Hydrocephalus; Laparoscopy; Miscarriage; Multiple births; Neonatology; Obstetrics; Perinatology; Pregnancy and gestation; Premature birth; Spina bifida; Stillbirth; Ultrasonography; Umbilical cord.

For Further Information:

Barron, S. L., and D. F. Roberts, eds. *Issues in Fetal Medicine: Proceedings of the Twenty-ninth Annual Symposium of the Galton Institute, London, 1992.* New York: St. Martin's Press, 1995. Chapter 7, "Fetal Surgery," by Don K. Nakauyama, and chapter 8, "Fetal Therapy," by Martin J. Whittle, deal directly with matters relating to fetal surgery, clearly outlining the medical problems that it is generally directed toward treating. In chapter 1, "The Galton Lecture for 1992: The Changing Status of the Fetus," Barron also touches briefly on intravenous transfusion and limited exchange transfusion in utero.

Harrison, Michael, et al. *The Unborn Patient: The Art and Science of Fetal Therapy.* 3d ed. Philadelphia: W. B. Saunders, 2001. Deals with correcting hydrocephalus through fetal surgery that results in the reduction of fluid in the brain.

O'Neill, J. A., Jr. "The Fetus as a Patient." *Annals of Surgery* 213 (1991): 277-278. This brief editorial raises cogent ethical concerns surrounding fetal surgery.

Wise, Barbara, et al., eds. *Nursing Care of the General Pediatric Surgical Patient.* Gaithersburg, Md.: Aspen, 2000. Of particular relevance is chapter 9, "Fetal Surgery," by Lori J. Howell, Susan K. Von Nessen, and Kelli M. Burns, which explores the varieties of surgeries generally performed on fetuses.

Fetal tissue transplantation

Procedure

Anatomy or system affected: Blood, brain, nervous system, pancreas, spine

Specialties and related fields: Ethics, neurology

DEFINITION: The controversial use of tissue from aborted human fetuses to replace damaged tissue in patients with diseases in which the patient's own tissue has been destroyed (such as parkinsonism or diabetes mellitus).

KEY TERMS:

cannula: a narrow tube used in surgery to drain fluid or to deliver cell suspensions for a transplant

fetal: in humans, a term normally referring to the developmental period following eight weeks of gestation; in fetal tissue transplantation, refers to tissue from earlier developmental stages as well

in utero: a Latin term meaning "in the womb"

parkinsonism: a disease in which the dopamine-secreting cells of the midbrain degenerate, resulting in uncontrolled movement and rigidity

stereotaxic computed tomography: a method of imaging using a series of X rays that are compiled by a computer to give a three-dimensional image of internal structures

INDICATIONS AND PROCEDURES

Advances in technology sometimes catapult a society into ethical arenas that are not yet circumscribed by laws and clear moral boundaries. Fetal tissue transplantation is one of these advances. It is a technology that carries the hope of curing a diverse array of severe, often tragic, ailments but one that raises many difficult questions. Tissues from aborted fetuses have been shown in experimental trials to be an excellent source of replacement tissue for patients whose diseases have destroyed their own vital tissues. Parkinson's, Huntington's, and Alzheimer's diseases (in which regions of the brain deteriorate) or juvenile-onset diabetes mellitus (in which insulin-secreting cells of the pancreas degenerate) theoretically could be cured with suitable tissue replacement.

The two sources of tissue used in transplantations, donations from cadavers and from aborted fetuses, differ significantly in their suitability. Tissues from cadavers have the severe disadvantage of being immunologically rejected when grafted into anyone who is not an identical twin. The body's surveillance system that protects against infection is designed to attack and destroy any cells that carry molecular markers identifying them as foreign. Patients receiving tissue transplants from other individuals, therefore, will tolerate the tissue graft only if their immune systems are first suppressed with a battery of potent drugs, leaving the patient dangerously unarmed against infection. Fetal tissues, however, do not induce a full-scale immune response when transplanted. Fetal cells are said to be immunologically naïve since they have not yet acquired the cell surface molecular markers that are recognized by the immune system. When transplanted into a patient, they seem to be invisible to the patient's immune system and are tolerated without the use of immunosuppression.

Other properties add to the suitability of fetal tissue for transplantation. Because it is not yet fully differentiated, fetal tissue is said to be very plastic in its abilities to adapt to new locations. Moreover, once placed in a patient, it secretes factors that promote its own growth and those of the new blood vessels at the site. Tissue from an adult source does not have these properties and consequently is slow-growing and poorly vascularized. Though growth factors can be added along with the graft, adult tissue is less responsive to these hormones than is fetal tissue.

It is the source of fetal tissue that has fired such debate over its use for transplantation. Though there has been general acceptance of using tissue from spontaneous abortions or from ectopic pregnancies which, because of their location outside of the womb, endanger the life of the mother and must be terminated, these sources are not well suited to transplantation. Spontaneous abortions rarely produce viable tissue, since in most cases the fetus has died two to three weeks before it is expelled. In addition, there are usually major genetic defects in the aborted fetus. In ectopic pregnancies as well, more than 50 percent of the fetuses are genetically abnormal, and most resolve themselves in spontaneous abortion outside a clinic setting. These types of abortions are almost always accompanied by a sense of tragic loss felt by the parents. Many researchers find it unacceptable to request permission from these parents to transplant tissue from the lost fetus.

The alternative source of fetal tissue is elected abortions. One-and-a-half million of these abortions occur in the United States every year. The debate over the ethical correctness of elected abortions has left a cloud of confusion over the issue of using this tissue for transplantation.

When an abortion is performed in a clinic, the tissue is removed by suction through a narrow tube. Normally, the tissue would be thrown away. If it is to be used for transplantation, written permission must be obtained from the woman after the abortion is completed. No discussion of transplantation is to take place prior to the abortion, and no alteration in the abortion procedure, except to keep the tissue sterile during collection, is to be made. The donor may not be paid for the tissue, and both the donor and the recipient of the tissue must remain anonymous to each other.

Once collected, the tissue is searched through to locate suitable tissue for transplantation. Normally only a small block of tissue is used, about eight cubic millimeters (the size of a thin slice of pencil eraser). The tissue is screened for infectious diseases such as hepatitis B and human immunodeficiency virus (HIV). Tissue that is collected is washed a number of times in a sterile solution to ensure that there is no bacterial contamination, and then it is maintained in a sterile, buffered salt solution until it is used. In order to increase the amount of usable tissue, the tissue may be grown in culture on a nutritive medium under carefully controlled conditions of humidity (95 percent), temperature (37 degrees Celsius), and gas (5 percent carbon dioxide in air) to stimulate normal growing conditions. Preservation of the tissue for long-term storage has been made possible by the highly refined technique of freezing the tissue in liquid nitrogen. Fetal tissue has been kept for as long as ten months in this manner before being used successfully in a transplantation. The technique should provide methods of maintaining tissue indefinitely.

The actual transplantation of the tissue is usually relatively quick and noninvasive. Often the tissue is injected into the patient as a suspension of individual cells. This permits the use of a small-bore tube called a cannula to deliver the cells to the target organ, thereby avoiding large surgical incisions. Because of modern stereotaxic imaging equipment such as computed tomography (CT) scanning and ultrasound, the physician is able to determine with extreme precision exactly where the cells are to be delivered and can visualize the position of the needle as the cells are injected. In this way, an entire region of an organ can be seeded with fetal cells. Often the patient is under only a local anesthetic. This aspect of the surgery is especially important when fetal cells are being inserted into the brain, since the physicians can then monitor the patient's ability to speak and move, to ensure that no major damage to the brain is occurring. Usually, antibiotics are given on the day of the transplantation procedure and for two additional days to avoid infection. The procedure is not dangerous, recovery is quick, and patients often go home in less than three days.

Fetal tissue transplantation is still considered an experimental procedure, and further trials are needed to fine-tune the techniques. For example, the precise age of fetal tissue that would be most effective in various cases is uncertain, though it is generally agreed that tissue from a first-trimester fetus is optimal, and it is not known which patients would respond best to the therapy. Researchers are also uncertain about whether immunosuppressive drugs should be administered. In animal trials using rats and monkeys, fetal transplants even of human tissue have been well tolerated in the absence of immunosuppression. In humans as well, fetal tissue appears to be readily accepted, with no signs of rejection, and in one study, patients did better without immunosuppression. Some surgeons, however, unwilling to risk tissue rejection, routinely give the transplant patient immunosuppressive drugs, such as cyclosporine and prednisone.

Uses and Complications

The major focus for fetal tissue transplantation has been the treatment of patients with Parkinson's disease, and results have been encouraging. Parkinsonism is caused by a deterioration of dopamine-secreting regions of the brain, primarily in the putamen and caudate nucleus of the midbrain. There is an accompanying loss of motor control causing tremors, rigidity, and finally paralysis, which is eventually fatal. The drugs used to treat the disorder, dopamine precursors such as L-dopa, produce side effects that cause unrelenting and uncontrolled movement of the limbs, periods in which the patient is completely frozen, and hallucinations.

Patients with parkinsonism who have received fetal tissue transplants have shown remarkable improvement and diminished requirements for drug treatment. The first case in the United States to be treated was a man with a twenty-year history of parkinsonism symptoms. He had frequent freezing spells, could not walk without a cane, and suffered from chronic constipation. He also was unable to whistle, a beloved hobby of his. He was operated on by Dr. Curt R. Freed and his associates in 1988. Following the operation, initial improvement was slow, but within a year, he was walking without a cane, his speed of movement had considerably improved, and his constipation had resolved itself. He also had regained his ability to whistle. Even after four years, improvements continued. Such results have occurred with many parkinsonism patients receiving fetal tissue transplants.

Even better results have been obtained in patients with induced Parkinson-like symptoms. In 1982, some intravenous drug users developed Parkinson-like symptoms after using a homemade preparation of "synthetic heroin" that was contaminated with 1-methyl-4-

phenyl-1,2,5,6-tetrahydropyridine (MPTP). MPTP destroys dopamine-secreting cells of the substantia nigra, a region of the midbrain which communicates with the caudate nucleus and putamen. Though the region of the brain destroyed by the drug is slightly different from that of patients with parkinsonism, the manifestations of the destruction are the same. Some of these patients received fetal tissue transplants. Within a year after their operation, they were able to walk with a normal gait, resume chores, and be virtually free of their previously uncontrollable movements.

Because no patient with parkinsonism or with Parkinson-like symptoms has yet been cured by a fetal tissue transplant, some have considered the results of such experiments to be disappointing. The expectation of complete cures from a technique that is still in its early experimental phase, however, is overly optimistic. Many parkinsonism patients themselves are encouraged, and many have resumed driving and the other tasks of normal daily life.

That transplanted fetal brain tissue can replace damaged brain tissue to any extent has opened the doors of hope for many diseases. For example, Huntington's disease, a genetic disorder that destroys a different set of neurons but in the same region as that affected by parkinsonism, brings a slow death to those carrying the dominant trait. Its severe dementia and uncontrollable jerking and writhing that steadily progress have had no treatment and no cure. In animal studies in which fetal brain tissue was transplanted into rats with symptoms mimicking Huntington's disease, results have been encouraging enough to warrant human trials, and one human trial, reported by a surgeon in Mexico, has shown limited success. Researchers are hopeful, though less optimistic, that Alzheimer's disease, a form of dementia that is characterized by neuronal death within the brain, also may be treatable with fetal tissue transplants. Because the destruction is so widespread, however, it is difficult to determine where the transplants should be placed.

Type I insulin-dependent diabetes, often called juvenile-onset diabetes, also has been treated with fetal tissue transplants. More than a million people in the United States suffer from this disease caused by the destruction of pancreatic beta cells, the insulin-secreting cells that regulate sugar metabolism. Though the disease can be controlled with regular insulin shots, the long-term effects of diabetes can lead to blindness, premature aging, and renal and circulatory problems. After animal tests showed a complete reversal of the disease when fetal pancreatic tissue was transplanted into diabetic rats, human trials were initiated with great expectations. Though complete success has not been achieved, the sixteen diabetic patients who were given fetal pancreatic tissue transplants by Dr. Kevin Lafferty between 1987 and 1992 all showed significant drops in the amount of insulin needed to manage their disease. The transplanted tissue continued to pump out insulin.

An unusual variation of such procedures has been to transplant fetal tissue into fetuses diagnosed with severe metabolic diseases. It is more effective to treat the condition while the fetus is still in the womb than to wait until after birth, when damage from the disease may already be extensive. Fetuses with Hurler's syndrome and similar "storage" diseases have been treated in this way. Hurler's syndrome is a lethal condition in which tissues become clogged with stored mucopolysaccharides, long-chain sugars that the body is unable to break down because it lacks the appropriate enzyme. One of the fetuses to receive this treatment was the child of a couple who had lost two children to the disease. With the transplanted tissue, the child lived and by one year of age was producing therapeutic levels of the enzyme. It has been estimated that there are at least 155 other genetic disorders that could be similarly treated by fetal tissue transplants in utero.

The list of ailments that fetal tissue transplants may alleviate includes some of the major concerns of modern medicine. In addition to those already mentioned are sickle cell disease, thalassemias, metabolic disorders, immune deficiencies, myelin disorders, and spinal cord injuries. In interpreting the value of these applications, however, it is important to separate the politics of abortion from the medical issue of fetal tissue transplantation.

Perspective and Prospects

Though controversy surrounds the use of fetal tissue for transplantation, such controversy has not included all facets of fetal tissue research. Indeed, fetal cells were used in the 1950's to develop the Salk polio vaccine and later the vaccine against rubella (German measles). With the scourge of acquired immunodeficiency syndrome (AIDS), in the 1990's fetal cells were first used to help design treatments against the AIDS virus. Even the early attempts at fetal tissue transplantation occurred quietly. Reports date as far back as 1928, when Italian surgeons attempted unsuccessfully to cure a patient with diabetes using fetal pancreatic tissue, a procedure repeated, again unsuccessfully, in the United States in

1939. In 1959, American physicians tried to cure leukemia with fetal tissue transplants, but again without success. The first real indicator that such techniques might work came in 1968, when fetal liver cells were used to treat a patient with DiGeorge syndrome. The success of this procedure resulted in its becoming the accepted treatment for this usually fatal genetic disorder.

It was not until 1987 that ethical issues over fetal tissue transplants truly surfaced in the United States. Debate was precipitated when the director of the National Institutes of Health (NIH) submitted a request to the Department of Health and Human Services to transplant fetal tissue into patients with parkinsonism. Rather than receiving approval, the request was tabled, pending a thorough study of the issue by an NIH panel on fetal tissue transplantation. The panel made a detailed report on the ethical, legal, and scientific implications of fetal tissue transplantation, concluding that it was acceptable public policy. Despite the report, however, the Secretary of Health and Human Services instituted a ban against the use of government funds for transplanting fetal tissue derived from elected abortions. While in effect, the ban influenced private funding as well. Physicians who performed fetal tissue transplants, unable to obtain grant money, were forced to charge their patients—a bill that could reach as high as forty thousand dollars per transplant. President Bill Clinton's lifting of the ban in 1993, on his third day in office, paved the way for research advances, including isolating and propagating human stem cells. However, the opposition of Clinton's successor, George W. Bush, to the use of fetal tissue and stem cells for scientific purposes led to several legislative battles and cast some doubts on the future of this field.

The debates over fetal tissue transplantation are far from over. Though a strict set of guidelines are in place concerning the procurement of fetal tissue, ensuring that the needs never influence decisions concerning abortion, other issues have not been addressed. Some ask whether a fetal tissue bank should be established and, if so, whether it should be government-funded to avoid commercialization. As technology continues to create increasingly complicated ethical issues, society's responsibility increases, as does its need to be scientifically informed.

—*Mary S. Tyler, Ph.D.*

See also Abortion; Alzheimer's disease; Brain; Brain disorders; Diabetes mellitus; Ethics; Genetic diseases; Genetic engineering; Neurology; Pancreas; Parkinson's disease; Stem cells; Transplantation.

For Further Information:

Beardsley, Tim. "Aborting Research." *Scientific American* 267, no. 2 (August, 1992): 17-18. An excellent encapsulation of the debate over fetal tissue transplantation and the instances in which it has been used.

Beauchamp, Tom, and James F. Childress. *Principles of Biomedical Ethics*. 5th ed. New York: Oxford University Press, 2001. A classic text that introduces the field of ethics, its theories, and their application to biomedical issues and presents ten cases covering a wide range of issues in biomedical ethics, some of which have led to landmark decisions.

Begley, Sharon. "From Human Embryos, Hope for 'Spare Parts.'" *Newsweek*, November 16, 1998, 73. Researchers have teased out clumps of cells from human embryos and induced them to burst into a veritable cellular symphony, forming most of the 210 kinds of cells that constitute the human body. These colonies could revolutionize transplantation medicine.

"Fetal Cell Study Shows Promise for Parkinson's." *Los Angeles Times*, April 22, 1999, p. 29. The first federally funded trial to study the effectiveness of fetal cell transplants for Parkinson's disease has proved that it works for some patients, mainly those under the age of sixty.

Freed, Curt R., Robert Breeze, and Neil Rosenberg. "Transplantation of Human Fetal Dopamine Cells for Parkinson's Disease." *Archives of Neurology* 47, no. 5 (May 1, 1990): 505-512. A historically important paper describing the techniques used by Freed, an American doctor who has been a pioneer in the technique of fetal tissue transplantation. Though written for a medical audience, most of the paper is readily understandable to a lay audience.

Holland, Suzanne, et al. *The Human Embryonic Stem Cell Debate: Science, Ethics, and Public Policy*. Cambridge, Mass.: MIT Press, 2001. Tackles difficult questions such as the nature of human life, the limits of intervention into human cells and tissues, who should approve controversial research, and what constitutes human dignity, respect, and justice.

Lindvall, Olle, Patrik Brundin, and Håkan Widner. "Grafts of Fetal Dopamine Neurons Survive and Improve Motor Function in Parkinson's Disease." *Science* 247 (February 2, 1990): 574-577. A landmark reference describing the technique of a group of physicians led by Lindvall of Sweden. This and the paper by Freed's group encompass the extent of variation in the technique, and the degrees of success.

Marshak, Daniel R., et al., eds. *Stem Cell Biology.* Cold Springs Harbor, N.Y.: Cold Springs Harbor Press, 2002. An excellent, multidisciplinary examination of recent advances in the field and their impact on medicine and science.

Singer, Peter, H. Kuhse, S. Buckle, K. Dawson, and P. Kasimba, eds. *Embryo Experimentation.* Cambridge, England: Cambridge University Press, 1990. This text provides an excellent discussion of the moral questions raised by the use of fetal tissue for transplantation.

U.S. Congress. Senate. Committee on Labor and Human Resources. *Finding Medical Cures: The Promise of Fetal Tissue Transplantation Research.* 102d Congress, 1st session, 1992. Senate Report 1902. A surprisingly readable and gripping set of testimonies from physicians, interest groups, and citizens concerning the debate over the use of fetal tissue for transplantations.

Wade, Nicholas. "Primordial Cells Fuel Debate on Ethics." *The New York Times*, November 10, 1998, p. 1. Two groups of scientists, one led by James A. Thomson of the University of Wisconsin at Madison and the other led by John D. Gearhart of The Johns Hopkins University in Baltimore, have recently reported success in the attempt to grow primordial human cells outside the body.

FEVER

DISEASE/DISORDER

ANATOMY OR SYSTEM AFFECTED: All

SPECIALTIES AND RELATED FIELDS: Family practice, internal medicine, pediatrics, virology

DEFINITION: A symptom associated with a variety of diseases and disorders, characterized by body temperature above normal (98.6 degrees Fahrenheit, or 37 degrees centigrade or Celsius); considered very serious at 104 degrees Fahrenheit (40 degrees Celsius) and higher.

KEY TERMS:

antipyretic drugs: drugs that are employed to reduce fevers, such as sodium salicylate, indomethacin, acetophenetidin, and paracetamol

ectotherms: organisms that rely on external temperature conditions in order to maintain their internal temperature

endotherms: organisms that control the internal temperature of their bodies by the conversion of calories to heat

febrile response: an upward adjustment of the thermoregulatory set point

metabolic rate: a measurement of the Calories (kilocalories) that are converted into heat energy in order to maintain body temperature and/or for physical exertion

pyrogens: protein substances that appear at the outset of the process that leads to a fever reaction

thermoregulatory set point: the ultimate neural control that maintains the human internal body temperature at 37 degrees Celsius and can either raise or lower it

CAUSES AND SYMPTOMS

Although the symptoms that often accompany a fever are familiar to everyone—shivering, sweating, thirst, hot skin, and a flushed face—what causes fever and its function during illness are not fully clear even among medical specialists. Considerable literature exists on the differences between warm-blooded organisms (endotherms) and cold-blooded organisms (ectotherms) in what is called the normal state, when no symptoms of disease are present. Cold-blooded organisms depend on temperature conditions in their external environment to maintain various levels of temperature within their bodies. These fluctuations correspond to the various levels of activity that they need to sustain at given moments. Thus, reptiles, for example, may "recharge" themselves internally by moving into the warmth of the sun. Warm-blooded organisms, on the other hand, including all mammals, utilize energy released from the digestion of food to maintain a constant level of heat within their bodies. This level—a "normal" temperature—is approximately 37 degrees Celsius (98.6 degrees Fahrenheit) in humans. An internal body temperature which rises above this level is called a febrile temperature, or a fever.

If the temperature in the surrounding environment is low, warm-blooded organisms must raise their metabolic rate (a measurement, in Calories, of converted energy) accordingly to maintain a normal internal body temperature. In humans, this rate of energy expenditure is about 1,800 Calories per day. If insufficient food is taken in to supply the necessary potential energy for this metabolic conversion into heat, the body will draw on its storage resource—fat—to fulfill this vital need. The potentially fatal condition called hypothermia, in which the body is too fatigued to maintain metabolic

INFORMATION ON FEVER

CAUSES: Infection, various diseases
SYMPTOMS: Shivering, sweating, thirst, hot skin, flushed face
DURATION: Acute
TREATMENTS: Medication, comfort measures (*e.g.*, cool compress), rest

functions or has exhausted all of its stores of calories, occurs when the internal temperature falls below normal. Although cold-blooded animals must also protect themselves against the danger that their body heat may fall too low to sustain life functions, they can support adjustments in their own internal temperature down to about 20 degrees Celsius At the same time, metabolic expenditures, as measured in Calories, are very low in cold-blooded animals; for example, alligators must expend only 60 Calories per day to create the same amount of heat as 1,800 Calories per day in warm-blooded humans.

The question of internal temperature in warm-blooded animals is closely tied to management efficiency in the body. This function becomes critical when one considers abnormally high internal temperature, or fever. Generally speaking, all essential biochemical functions in the human body can be carried out at optimal levels of efficiency at the set point of 37 degrees Celsius. In the simplest of terms, any increase or decrease in temperature creates either more or less kinetic energy and has the potential to affect the chemistry of all body functions.

Endotherms are able to tolerate a certain range of involuntary change in their internal body temperature (brought about by disease or illness), but there is an upper limit of 45 degrees Celsius, which constitutes a high fever. If the self-regulating higher set point associated with fever goes beyond this point, destructive biochemical phenomena will occur in the body—in particular, a breaking down of protein molecules. If these phenomena are not checked, they can bring about death.

Modern scientific approaches to the internal body processes that lead to fever, like a medical discussion of the effects that occur once fever is operating in the body, are much more complicated. They revolve around the concept of a change in the set point monitored in the brain. When this change in the brain's normal (37 degree) thermostatic signal is called for, a process called phagocytosis begins, leading to a higher internal body heat level throughout the organism.

Phagocytosis, the ingestion of a solid substance (especially foreign material such as invading bacteria), involves the appearance in the host's system of large numbers of leukocyte cells. When these cells ingest the bacteria, small quantities of protein called leukocytic pyrogens are produced. According to most modern theories, these protein pyrogens trigger the biochemical reactions in the brain that alter the body's temperature set point. After this point, changes that occur throughout the system and raise the body's internal temperature depend on a component of the bacterial cell wall called endotoxin. By the end of the 1960's, researchers had drawn attention to at least twenty effects that activated endotoxins may have on the host organism. Key effects include enhancement of the production of new white blood cells (leukocytosis), enhancement of various forms of immunological resistance, reduction of serum iron levels, and lowering of blood pressure.

Most, if not all, of these effects brought about by endotoxins are accompanied by higher levels of heat throughout the body, the definition of fever. Closer biochemical examination of the source of the added heat yielded the suggestion, made by P. B. Beeson in 1948, that the host's endotoxin-affected cells begin to produce a distinct form of protein, now called endogenous pyrogens. Pyrogens are thought to induce the first stage of fever by interacting with cells in tissues very close to the brain, specifically in the brain stem itself. Laboratory experiments in the first half of the twentieth century allowed researchers to produce almost immediate fever reactions when they injected pyrogen protein material into rabbits. Studies of the induced febrile state in laboratory animals, and therefore presumably also in humans, linked fever to immunological (virus-resistant and bacteria-resistant) reactions, not necessarily in the initially affected tissues around the brain but in various places throughout the organism.

Although scientific research has produced many hypotheses concerning the origins of fever in the body, experts admit that the process is not well understood. Matthew J. Kluger, in *Fever: Its Biology, Evolution, and Function* (1979), claims that "the precise mechanism behind endogenous pyrogens' effect on the thermoregulatory set-point is unknown."

TREATMENT AND THERAPY

The febrile response has been noted in five of the seven extant classes of vertebrates on earth (Agnatha, such as lampreys, and Chondrichthyes, such as sharks, are excluded). Scientists have determined that its function as a reaction to bacterial infection can be traced back as far as 400 million years in primitive bony fishes. The question of whether the natural phenomenon of fever actually aids in combating disease in the body, however, has not been fully resolved.

In ancient and medieval times, it was believed that fever served to "cook" and separate out one of the four essential body "humors"—blood, phlegm, yellow bile, and black bile—that had become excessively dominant. Throughout the centuries, such beliefs even caused some physicians to try to induce higher internal body temperatures as a means of treating disease. Use of modern antipyretic drugs to reduce fever remained unthinkable until the nineteenth century.

It was the German physician Carl von Liebermeister who, by the end of the nineteenth century, set some of the guidelines that are still generally observed in deciding whether antipyretic drugs should or should not be used to reduce a naturally occurring fever during illness. Liebermeister insisted that the phenomenon of fever was not one of body temperature gone "out of control" but rather a sign that the organism was regulating its own temperature. He also demonstrated that part of the process leading to increased internal temperature could be seen in reactions that actually reduce heat loss at the body's surface, notably decreases in skin blood flow and evaporative cooling through perspiration. Liebermeister determined that one of the positive effects of higher temperatures inside the body was to im-

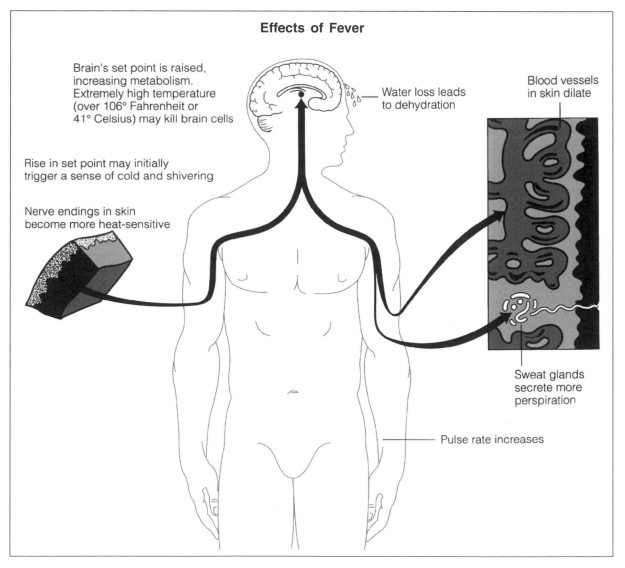

Effects of Fever

Brain's set point is raised, increasing metabolism. Extremely high temperature (over 106° Fahrenheit or 41° Celsius) may kill brain cells

Rise in set point may initially trigger a sense of cold and shivering

Nerve endings in skin become more heat-sensitive

Water loss leads to dehydration

Blood vessels in skin dilate

Sweat glands secrete more perspiration

Pulse rate increases

pede the growth of harmful microorganisms. At the same time, however, other side effects of fever during illness were deemed to be negative, such as loss of appetite and, in some cases, actual degeneration of key internal organs. Liebermeister's generation of physicians, therefore, tended to rely on antipyretic drugs only when high fevers persisted for long periods of time. Moderate fevers or even high fevers, if they did not continue too long, were deemed to contribute to the overall process of natural body resistance to disease.

In fact, a limited school of physicians followed the teaching of 1927 Nobel laureate Julius Wagner-Jauregg, who claimed that "fever therapy" methods should be adopted for the treatment of certain diseases. Wagner-Jauregg himself had pioneered this theory by inoculating victims of neurosyphilis with fever-producing malaria. Part of his argument in favor of this experimental therapy was that malaria, with its accompanying fever, was a treatable disease (through the use of quinine) and could be controlled at regular intervals during its "service" as a fighter against a disease that still had no known cure. Later use of fever therapy for treatment of other sexually transmitted diseases, specifically gonorrhea, proved to be moderately successful. When typhoid vaccine was used to induce fevers in some patients, however, side effects such as hypotension (low blood pressure) or cardiovascular shock introduced what some considered to be dangerous risk factors. Nevertheless, certain fields of medicine, especially those involved with eye diseases and related eye ailments, have proved that fever-inducing agents (specifically those contained in typhoid and typhoid-paratyphoid vaccines) also induce beneficial secretion of the anti-inflammatory hormone cortisol.

By the second half of the twentieth century, the medical use of antipyretic drugs, containing such components as salicylates and indomethacin, had become widespread. This phenomenon was not caused by any compelling reversal of earlier general assumptions that moderate levels of fever, being a natural body reaction, were not necessarily harmful to patients suffering from a wide variety of diseases. Rather, physicians may have opted to use such drugs as much for their pain-relieving qualities as for their fever-reducing characteristics. Although patients receiving such drug treatment notice a diminishing of severe pains or general aching, the cause of the disease has not been combated merely by the removal of such symptoms as fever and pain.

Modern medical science has tended to support further study of particular circumstances in which induced

fevers can actually produce disease-combating reactions. A newly emerging field by the late 1970's, for example, involved studying the benefits of higher temperatures in newborn infants fighting viral infections. Although specific circumstances and the nature of disease prevent a generalized conclusion in terms of the use of induced fevers as a form of treatment, researchers have shown that an elevated body temperature serves to increase the speed at which white blood cells, the body's natural enemies against disease, move to infected areas.

PERSPECTIVE AND PROSPECTS

Although doctors have been aware of the symptoms of fever since the beginnings of medical history, centuries passed before its importance as an indicator of disease was accepted. A certain degree of sophistication in the study of fevers became possible largely as a result of the development of the common thermometer, in a rudimentary form in the seventeenth century and then with greater technical accuracy in the eighteenth century. Systematic use of the thermometer in the eighteenth century enabled doctors to observe such phenomena as morning remission and evening peaking of fever intensity. Studies involving the recording of temperature in healthy individuals also yielded important discoveries. One such discovery was made in 1774, when use of the thermometer showed that, even in a room heated to the boiling point of water (100 degrees Celsius), healthy subjects maintained an internal body heat that was very close to the normal 37-degree level.

Medical reports as late as the end of the eighteenth century, however, indicate that even internationally recognized pioneers of science were still not close to understanding the causes of fever. The English doctor John Hunter, for example, declared himself opposed to the prevailing view that rising body heat came from the circulation of warmer blood throughout the body. Hunter suspected that the warmth was produced by an entirely different agent that was independent of the circulatory system. He never learned what that agent might be, however, and failed in defense of his theory that the source of added body heat was in the stomach. Even the famous French chemist Antoine-Laurent Lavoisier erred when he tried to explain fever in terms of some form of chemical "combustion" involving hydrogen and carbon. Lavoisier identified the lungs as the possible location for this spontaneous production of internal body heat.

Although these theories were identified as erroneous, the late eighteenth and early nineteenth centuries left one legacy that would develop into the twentieth century and is still practiced by physicians: systematic thermometry. In essence, thermometry involves the tracing of the upward or downward direction of fever during illness in order to judge the course of the disease and the effects brought about by different stages of treatment. In many diseases, for example, clinical records of the full course of previous cases can be studied by doctors responsible for treating an individual patient. With thermometry, the doctor is able to determine how far the body's struggle against a certain disease has progressed. If thermometry shows a marked departure from what clinical records have charted as the normal course of disease under certain forms of treatment, then the physician may look for signs of another disease.

—*Byron D. Cannon, Ph.D.*

See also Bacterial infections; Common cold; Heat exhaustion and heat stroke; Hyperthermia and hypothermia; Influenza; Reye's syndrome; Rheumatic fever; Scarlet fever; Typhoid fever and typhus; Viral infections; Yellow fever; *specific diseases.*

FOR FURTHER INFORMATION:

Bartfai, Tamas, Charles A. Dinarello, and Matthew J. Kluger. *Molecular Mechanisms of Fever.* Baltimore: Johns Hopkins University Press, 1999. The authors place major emphasis on recent advances using molecular tools such as cytokine knockout mice, cloned cytokines, descriptions of molecular pathways for signal transduction, and heat shock proteins.

Kemper, Kathi J. *The Holistic Pediatrician: A Pediatrician's Comprehensive Guide to Safe and Effective Therapies for the Twenty-five Most Common Ailments of Infants, Children, and Adolescents.* New York: HarperCollins, 2002. Integrates mainstream and alternative medicine to aid parents in dealing with the most common childhood health problems such as fever, diaper rash, ear infections, and allergies.

Kluger, Matthew J. *Fever: Its Biology, Evolution, and Function.* Princeton, N.J.: Princeton University Press, 1979. An accessible book-length study of the phenomenon of fever. Although some parts of the discussion are more technical in nature, the general level is comprehensible.

Larson, David E., ed. *Mayo Clinic Family Health Book.* 3d ed. New York: HarperResource, 2003. Perhaps the best general medical text for the layperson, this book covers the entire medical field. While the information is derived from a wide variety of highly technical sources, the articles are written to be easily understood by a general audience.

Mackowiak, Philip A., ed. *Fever: Basic Mechanisms and Management.* 2d ed. Philadelphia: Lippincott-Raven, 1997. This text explains the physiology behind fever and addresses ways to treat it. Includes a bibliography and an index.

Nathanson, Laura Walther. *The Portable Pediatrician: A Practicing Pediatrician's Guide to Your Child's Growth, Development, Health, and Behavior from Birth to Age Five.* 2d ed. New York: HarperCollins, 2002. An engaging, easy-to-read guide for parents to assess their child's development, medical symptoms, and behavioral problems.

FIBROCYSTIC BREAST DISEASE. *See* BREAST DISORDERS.

FIBROMYALGIA

DISEASE/DISORDER

ANATOMY OR SYSTEM AFFECTED: Brain, head, muscles, musculoskeletal system, nerves, nervous system, psychic-emotional system

SPECIALTIES AND RELATED FIELDS: Rheumatology

DEFINITION: A connective, soft tissue disease involving chronic, spontaneous, and widespread musculoskeletal pain, as well as recurrent fatigue and sleep disturbance.

KEY TERMS:

connective tissue: the supporting framework of the body, particularly tendons and ligaments

fibrositis: an earlier, less common term for fibromyalgia

flare-up: an episode of heightened pain and debilitation in fibromyalgia; sometimes flare-ups do not have an immediate, precipitating cause that is identifiable, while other times they are associated with humidity, cold, physical exertion, or psychological stress

functional somatic syndromes: a continuum or spectrum of disorders (such as chronic fatigue syndrome, Epstein-Barr virus, and primary headaches) characterized by complex interactions between symptoms and patients' personal stress

tender points: specific, precise, and localized areas of moderately to severely intense pain

CAUSES AND SYMPTOMS

The cause of fibromyalgia is unknown. Some researchers believe that an injury or trauma to the central nervous system causes the disorder. Other researchers believe that changes in muscle and connective tissue metabolism produce decreased blood flow, beginning a pathological cycle of weakness, fatigue, and decreased strength that eventually results in the full-blown syndrome. Still others believe that an as-yet-undiscovered virus or infectious agent attacks people who are naturally susceptible to the infection, who then develop the syndrome.

The most salient feature of fibromyalgia syndrome is pain. Described by sufferers as "having no boundaries," the pain is characteristically variable. The same sufferer experiences pain ranging from deep muscle aching to throbbing, stabbing, or shooting pains to a burning sensation that has been called "acid running through blood vessels." The pain frequently causes joint and muscle stiffness. Pain and stiffness may be worse in the morning and may be more intense in the joints and muscle groups that are used more often. Patients may have tender points, as in the knee, hips, spine, shoulders, and neck. There are typically eighteen potential tender points, and at least eleven must be painful for a diagnosis of fibromyalgia to be made.

Sufferers also experience fatigue and weakness, ranging from mild to debilitating. Patients liken the fatigue to having their arms and legs tied to concrete, and many feel that they are living in a kind of mental fog, unable to focus or concentrate. Between 40 and 70 percent of patients also have some variation of irritable bowel syndrome (IBS): frequent abdominal cramping, nausea, and chronic constipation or diarrhea. About half of all sufferers also experience concurrent migraine or tension headaches. The condition is often mental as well as physical, as sufferers may also suffer from major depressive disorder and anxiety.

Less common, but readily found, are a constellation of symptoms that, in order of prevalence, include jaw, face, and head pain, which is easily misdiagnosed as temporomandibular joint syndrome (TMJ); hypersensitivities to odors, bright lights, and even fibromyalgia medications; painful menstruation; memory problems; and muscle twitching. Weather (particularly exposure to cold), normal hormonal fluctuation, stress, anxiety, depression, and physical exertion can aggravate fibromyalgia and produce flare-ups.

TREATMENT AND THERAPY

Because the cause of fibromyalgia is unknown, only its symptoms can be addressed. The treatment plan must be individualized and flexible and is considered long-term management. Rigid, stereotyped approaches can be worse than no management at all.

Because difficulty sleeping and pain can be both contributors to and outcomes of fibromyalgia, traditional treatment approaches focus on improving quality of sleep and reducing pain. Physicians commonly prescribe medications that increase the neurotransmitters serotonin and norepinephrine, which modulate sleep, pain, and the immune system. Amitriptyline (Elavil), paroxetine (Paxil), doxepin (Sinequan), cyclobenzaprine (Flexeril), clonazepam (Klonopin), and similar medications may be prescribed in low doses; they benefit one-third to one-half of patients. Alone or in combination, these medicines improve sleep staging, elevate mood, and relax overtense, stiff, and spasm-prone muscle groups.

More comprehensive are approaches that use medications as part of a well-rounded treatment plan. Physical therapy, massage therapy, acupuncture, and behavioral health are other treatment options. Physical therapy and aerobic exercises such as swimming and walking reduce muscle tenderness and pain while improving muscle conditioning and fitness. Because of fibromyalgia sufferers' sensitivity to cold and frequent stiffness, applied heat and therapeutic massage can render short-term relief. Though acupuncture is less well studied, anecdotal accounts claim its effectiveness, making it a sought-after therapy. Psychological counseling, or psychotherapy, can be effective for patients who are overwrought, overstressed, often wrongly blamed for having fibromyalgia, and in need of lifestyle adjustments.

INFORMATION ON FIBROMYALGIA

CAUSES: Unknown; possibly injury or trauma to central nervous system, changes in muscle and connective tissue metabolism, or infectious agent

SYMPTOMS: Severe muscle pain; joint and muscle stiffness; tender points in knee, hips, spine, shoulders, and neck; fatigue; weakness; sometimes concurrent irritable bowel syndrome (IBS) and migraine or tension headaches

DURATION: Chronic with acute episodes

TREATMENTS: Alleviation of symptoms through medications, physical therapy, massage therapy, acupuncture, behavioral therapy

PERSPECTIVE AND PROSPECTS

Until the 1990's, fibromyalgia syndrome—or fibrositis, as it was then more often called—was not widely accepted by primary care specialists as a legitimate condition. Difficult to diagnose, it was often mistaken as chronic fatigue syndrome (itself a condition not widely recognized in primary care medicine), a sort of chronic pain syndrome, or some condition that was completely psychosomatic (that is, all in the patient's head). Fibromyalgia syndrome was often thought of as a "garbage can diagnosis": a little bit of everything, but not a real syndrome that could be treated. Sufferers had difficulty finding sympathetic medical help and were often at odds with family, friends, and co-workers who misattributed the causes of this connective, soft tissue disease whose existence could not be proven.

Advances in rheumatological research and the American College of Rheumatology's establishment of diagnostic criteria for fibromyalgia have made it a legitimate medical condition for which treatment can be sought. Previously, fibromyalgia patients often suffered from this painful, fatiguing condition and felt blamed for causing it—or worse, "making it up." Even today, the Fibromyalgia Network, a grass roots informational clearinghouse, underscores research that proves fibromyalgia syndrome is real.

Despite differing theories about the cause of fibromyalgia, ongoing research has produced some results that all investigators consider reliable. This syndrome seems to involve a relationship among the nervous system, the endocrine system, and sleep. When sleep electroencephalograms (EEGs) for patients known to have fibromyalgia are compared with those for nonpatient subjects, disturbances in the non-rapid eye movement (non-REM) stages become evident. There are five well-known and easily recognized stages of sleep: four non-REM stages and then a REM stage. Most people effortlessly progress through non-REM and REM stages. When they reach stage 4, a non-REM stage, they have reached sleep at its deepest. This is the stage during which tissue repair, antibody production, and possibly neurotransmitter regulation occur. Fibromyalgia EEGs show that these patients revert to stage 2 after stage 3, without having reached stage 4. Specialists refer to this sleep disorder as the alpha-EEG anomaly.

This EEG finding corresponds directly with fibromyalgia patients' anecdotal reports that they frequently do not feel rested or refreshed after a night's sleep. This result also contributes to an understanding of why sufferers are fatigued so often. The disturbance of non-REM sleep helps to produce the symptoms of insufficient sleep: Tiredness, reduced mental acuity, irritability, and autoimmune susceptibilities. The various stages of sleep also have corresponding hormonal activity, with different hormones and different levels released during each. Stages 3 and 4 are when growth hormones, including insulin growth factor (IGF), are primarily released. Fibromyalgia patients have low IGF levels.

A few other characteristic findings in these patients are not related to sleep. First, the neurotransmitter cerebrospinal fluid P (CSF P), also called substance P, is found in fibromyalgia patients at three times the normal level. Significantly, CSF P is associated with enhanced pain perception. Second, sufferers have low cortisol levels, suggesting that the hypopituitary-adrenal axis is adversely altered. Among much else, this axis mediates the fight-or-flight response and relaxation. Third, using an office procedure called tilt table testing, fibromyalgia symptoms can be provoked, accompanied by a rapid lowering of blood pressure in fibromyalgia patients but not in nonpatients. These findings all provide evidence that problems in the autonomic and endocrine systems cause fibromyalgia. What would set these problems into motion in the first place, however, is unknown, although many sufferers have experienced significant physical and/or psychological trauma before any syndrome-specific symptoms began.

—*Paul Moglia, Ph.D.*

See also Anxiety; Chronic fatigue syndrome; Depression; Fatigue; Headaches; Irritable bowel syndrome (IBS); Migraine headaches; Muscle sprains, spasms, and disorders; Muscles; Pain; Pain management; Sleep disorders; Stress; Stress reduction.

FOR FURTHER INFORMATION:

Fibromyalgia Network. http://www.fmnetnews.com.

Goldenberg, Don L. *Fibromyalgia: A Leading Expert's Guide to Understanding and Getting Relief from the Pain That Won't Go Away.* Berkeley, Calif.: Berkeley Publishing Group, 2001.

Pellegrino, Mark. *Inside Fibromyalgia.* Columbus, Ohio: Anadem, 2001.

Teitelbaum, Jacob. *From Fatigue to Fantastic.* New York: Avery, 2001.

Wallace, Daniel J., and Janice Brook Wallace. *All About Fibromyalgia.* New York: Oxford University Press, 2002.

FIFTH DISEASE
DISEASE/DISORDER
ALSO KNOWN AS: Erythema infectiosum
ANATOMY OR SYSTEM AFFECTED: Nose, skin, throat
SPECIALTIES AND RELATED FIELDS: Family practice, pediatrics
DEFINITION: An infectious disease of children characterized by an erythematous (reddish) rash and low-grade fever.

INFORMATION ON FIFTH DISEASE

CAUSES: Viral infection
SYMPTOMS: "Slapped cheek" rash, fever, sore throat, achiness, malaise
DURATION: Ten to fourteen days
TREATMENTS: Alleviation of symptoms through bed rest, administration of liquids

---

CAUSES AND SYMPTOMS

Fifth disease is caused by infection with the human parvovirus (HPV) B19. The disease is more prevalent during late winter or early spring. Fifth disease is most commonly observed in young children, with the peak attack rate between five and fourteen years of age. Adults may become infected, but they rarely show evidence of disease.

The virus is spread from person to person through nasal secretions or sneezing. Following an incubation period of several days, a rash develops on the face, which has the appearance of slapped cheeks. The bright red color fades as the rash spreads over the rest of the body. An erythematous, pimply eruption may also appear on the trunk or extremities. A mild fever, sore throat, and nasal stuffiness may also be apparent. The rash generally lasts from ten days to two weeks. Often, it will fade only to reappear a short time later. Sunlight may aggravate the skin during this period, also causing a reappearance of the rash.

The diagnosis of fifth disease is primarily clinical, based on the symptoms. Laboratory tests for the virus are generally not performed.

TREATMENT AND THERAPY

No antibiotic therapy is available for fifth disease. Since the disease is rarely serious, treatment is mainly symptomatic. Bed rest and the administration of liquids, as commonly used in treating mild illness in children, are generally sufficient. Isolation is unnecessary since transmission is unlikely following appearance of the rash.

PERSPECTIVE AND PROSPECTS

Fifth disease was first described during the late nineteenth century as the fifth in the series of erythematous illnesses often encountered by children; the others are measles, mumps, chickenpox, and rubella. HPV B19 was isolated in 1975 and shown to be the etiological agent of the disease in the mid-1980's.

The disease is common and generally benign. HPV B19 has been implicated, however, in certain forms of hemolytic anemias and arthritis in adults, and research continues on the virus.

—*Richard Adler, Ph.D.*

See also Childhood infectious diseases; Fever; Rashes; Sneezing; Sore throat; Viral infections.

FOR FURTHER INFORMATION:

Behrman, Richard E., ed. *Nelson Textbook of Pediatrics*. 17th ed. Philadelphia: W. B. Saunders, 2003.

Burg, Fredric D., ed. *Treatment of Infants, Children, and Adolescents*. Philadelphia: W. B. Saunders, 1990.

Kemper, Kathi J. *The Holistic Pediatrician: A Pediatrician's Comprehensive Guide to Safe and Effective Therapies for the Twenty-five Most Common Ailments of Infants, Children, and Adolescents*. New York: HarperCollins, 2002.

Robbins, Stanley L., Ramzi S. Cotran, and Vinay Kumar, eds. *Robbins' Pathologic Basis of Disease*. 6th ed. Philadelphia: W. B. Saunders, 1999.

Sompayrac, Lauren. *How Pathogenic Viruses Work*. 5th ed. Sudbury, Mass.: Jones and Bartlett, 2002.

FINGERNAIL REMOVAL. *See* NAIL REMOVAL.

FISTULA REPAIR
PROCEDURE
ANATOMY OR SYSTEM AFFECTED: Abdomen, anus, bladder, blood, gallbladder, gastrointestinal system, intestines, reproductive system, urinary system, uterus
SPECIALTIES AND RELATED FIELDS: Gastroenterology, general surgery, pediatrics, proctology
DEFINITION: The removal of any abnormal passage associated with body sites or tissues.
KEY TERMS:
anorectal: associated with the anal portion of the large intestine

arteriovenous: associated with arteries and/or veins

Crohn's disease: a chronic inflammation of the bowel, often as a result of an autoimmune disease

crypt: a pit or depression in the body

fistulectomy: the surgical elimination of a fistula

INDICATIONS AND PROCEDURES

A fistula represents any abnormal opening or passage between internal organs or between an internal organ and the surface of the body. Fistulas can occur nearly anywhere in the body, but they are most commonly associated with the anorectal portion of the anatomy. Some fistulas may result from congenital defects, while others may be created surgically in association with specific procedures. For example, an arteriovenous fistula may be created to allow the insertion of a cannula (tube) for hemodialysis.

Anorectal fistulas usually begin as an abscess within the anal region or internal crypt that then spreads to adjacent tissue or to the surface of the body. Pain, itching, or tenderness in the region is often the first sign of a problem. The discomfort may be aggravated by bowel movements. Since infection is common, the opening may become purulent (pus-producing).

Treatment of anorectal fistulas usually requires surgery. A crypt hook may be used if the site of the original crypt must be located, an observation which is often unnecessary. The crypt may also be observed through an anoscope, or as part of a proctoscopic examination. Often, digital examination of the anal canal may detect a nodule, representing the abscess itself.

Any abscess must first be drained and treated. If the fistula is small, it may heal itself. The surgical procedure, commonly referred to as a fistulectomy, is a relatively simple operation carried out under general anesthesia. The fistula must be reduced or removed. Surgical repair begins at the primary opening, and generally the entire tract is opened, both to allow for proper drainage of infectious material and to promote healing. If the surgery is carried out properly, the incision should heal relatively quickly.

Difficult labor in women may create a variety of fistulas. A vesicovaginal fistula, created between the urinary bladder and the vagina, may be indicated by the presence of urine in the vaginal tract. As with any opening to the surface of the body, infection may develop. Likewise, a rectovaginal fistula, between the rectum and vagina, was formerly a possible serious complication of difficult childbirth. As with any fistulas, such openings have to be opened, drained, and sutured for healing.

Fistula formation may also be internal, as in biliary fistulas between the gallbladder and intestine. Such connections can occur as a consequence of gallstones, ulcers, or tumor formation. Often, the major symptom may be an intestinal blockage resulting from the stone or tumor itself. Bile may leak from the gallbladder into the peritoneum or body cavities, resulting in infection. Therapy for such fistula formation first requires an analysis of the channel itself. If the fistula is external, contrast material may be injected into the site to analyze the tract. If the fistula is internal, the extent of the tract may require cholangiography, the injection of a radiopaque material to outline the bile duct. General surgery is required for the proper correction of any underlying problem.

USES AND COMPLICATIONS

Surgical repair of a fistula has a number of functions, in addition to the elimination of the fistula itself. The goal of repair is to support the healing process, while at the same time attempting to maintain the normal function (and appearance, when applicable) of the tissue.

The anal fistula represents one of the more common types. Frequently, it begins as an abscess or break in the

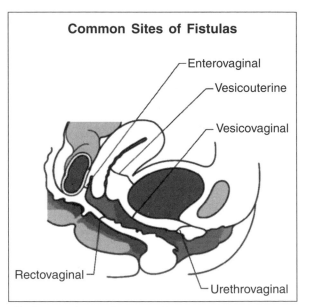

Common Sites of Fistulas

Enterovaginal

Vesicouterine

Vesicovaginal

Rectovaginal

Urethrovaginal

Fistulas are abnormal passages between organs or an organ and the outside of the body. They are more common in the rectal and genital regions of women, such as between the intestines and vagina (enterovaginal), the bladder and uterus (vesicouterine), the bladder and vagina (vesicovaginal), the urethra and vagina (urethrovaginal), and the rectum and vagina (rectovaginal).

anal or rectal wall. Not infrequently, the underlying cause may be inflammation of the colon as a result of ulcerative colitis or Crohn's disease, an autoimmune disease which can cause ulceration of the intestinal wall. The fistula itself may become chronically infected, resulting in pain and discomfort. Cancer development in the area of the fistula, while uncommon, has been known to occur.

The major complication of anorectal surgery to repair the fistula is delayed healing. If not completely drained or covered, the area may continue to become infected. If the fistula is deep, damage to muscles during surgical repair may result in incontinence. Assuming that the fistula does not recur and postoperative care is properly provided, however, the prognosis is generally excellent.

Surgical procedures can also be used in the intentional formation of a fistula. For example, a site must be prepared for insertion of a cannula to carry out hemodialysis, the removal of waste from the blood under conditions of renal insufficiency. Generally, such a fistula between an artery and a vein is prepared one to two months prior to insertion of the cannula. The fistula is created either by grafting a section of bovine carotid artery into the site or by using a graft prepared from synthetic material. Proper circulation through the fistula must be monitored to ensure that infection does not develop.

PERSPECTIVE AND PROSPECTS

The development and widespread use of antibiotics in the mid-twentieth century provided a means for the effective treatment of the major complication associated with fistula development: infection. Fistulas may result in abscess formation or may be secondary to problems elsewhere, as with Crohn's disease. Better treatment of those infections associated with fistula formation, such as tuberculosis, has reduced their incidence. Likewise, proper prenatal care has largely controlled fistula development secondary to difficult labor in women.

—*Richard Adler, Ph.D.*

See also Abscess drainage; Abscesses; Childbirth complications; Colon and rectal surgery; Crohn's disease; Gastroenterology; Gastroenterology, pediatric; Gastrointestinal disorders; Gastrointestinal system; Grafts and grafting; Gynecology; Infection; Proctology; Reproductive system; Stone removal; Stones; Tumor removal; Tumors; Ulcer surgery; Ulcers; Urinary system; Urology; Urology, pediatric.

FOR FURTHER INFORMATION:

Clayman, Charles, B., ed. *The American Medical Association Family Medical Guide.* New York: Random House, 1994. An excellent reference for the beginner. The scientific accuracy of the text is not compromised by its accessibility.

Peikin, Steven R. *Gastrointestinal Health.* Rev. ed. New York: HarperCollins, 1999. Examines a range of gastrointestinal ailments in depth, including diarrhea and colitis, and offers tips for managing them via diet, stress management, and drugs.

Saibil, Fred. *Crohn's Disease and Ulcerative Colitis: Everything You Need to Know.* Rev. ed. Toronto: Firefly Books, 2003. A leading expert on IBD, Saibil covers topics such as signs and symptoms, how the gastrointestinal system works normally and how IBD affects it, procedures and instruments used to diagnose IBD, effects of diet, children and IBD, and effects on sexual activity and child-bearing.

Tierney, Lawrence M., Jr., et al., eds. *Current Medical Diagnosis and Treatment 2004.* 43d ed. New York: McGraw-Hill, 2003. This text, updated yearly, is the point of reference for physicians and other health care practitioners. It incorporates each year's biomedical research discoveries that have immediate, relevant, and applicable use for the patient.

Way, Lawrence W., and Gerard M. Doherty, eds. *Current Surgical Diagnosis and Treatment.* 11th ed. New York: Lange Medical Books/McGraw Hill, 2003. A reference work on general surgery for physicians, this tome is nevertheless comprehensible to laypersons familiar with medical terminology. Presents succinct overviews of the stoma procedures and their potential complications and contains finely detailed illustrations.

FLAT FEET
DISEASE/DISORDER

ALSO KNOWN AS: Pes planus, talipes planus

ANATOMY OR SYSTEM AFFECTED: Feet, ligaments, muscles, musculoskeletal system

SPECIALTIES AND RELATED FIELDS: Orthopedics, podiatry

DEFINITION: A congenital or acquired flatness of the longitudinal arch of the foot.

CAUSES AND SYMPTOMS

Congenital flat feet are considered to be hereditary. Acquired flat feet can be caused by stretching of the arch ligaments and a weakness of the muscles found in the

INFORMATION ON FLAT FEET

CAUSES: Congenital weakness of muscles in arches, changes in shape of foot bones, short Achilles tendon, injury

SYMPTOMS: Delays in learning how to walk, pain, clumsiness in walking

DURATION: Typically short-term

TREATMENTS: Depends on severity; ranges from orthopedic shoes with arch supports, foot exercises, and rest to casts or surgery

arches; this produces flexible flat feet. Rigid flat feet are caused by changes in the shape of the foot bones or a short Achilles tendon. Other causes of flat feet include injury and a lack of muscle tone or weak foot muscles that cannot sustain the body's weight.

All infants appear to be flat-footed because of a pad of fat under each instep. Arch formation in the feet takes place once they begin walking. Flat feet are often detected by parents when an infant experiences delays in learning how to walk.

Flat feet usually are painless and do not contribute to changes in posture or the ability to walk. Adolescents and adults are occasionally prone to fallen arches, or temporary foot strain caused by an activity that overstretches the ligaments in the arch; this condition is accompanied by pain. Rigid flat feet caused by a short Achilles tendon and spastic flat feet caused by a deformity of the heel result in pain and clumsiness in walking.

TREATMENT AND THERAPY

Flexible, pain-free flat feet require no treatment. Special orthopedic shoes with arch supports do not change the shape of the feet over time, while foot exercises and prescribed changes in gait are hard to enforce in children.

In cases of fallen arches accompanied by fatigue or pain, however, rest, foot exercises, and the use of arch supports are recommended. If the Achilles tendon is too short or tight, it can be stretched by placing the foot in a cast. Severe cases of flat feet require surgery that removes excess bone or reconstructs the soft tissue of the foot.

—*Rose Secrest*

See also Arthritis; Bone disorders; Bones and the skeleton; Foot disorders; Lower extremities; Orthopedics; Orthopedics, pediatric; Podiatry.

FOR FURTHER INFORMATION:

Copeland, Glenn, and Stan Solomon. *The Foot Doctor.* Emmaus, Pa.: Rodale Press, 1986.

Currey, John D. *Bones: Structures and Mechanics.* Princeton, N.J.: Princeton University Press, 2002.

Lippert, Frederick G., and Sigvard T. Hansen. *Foot and Ankle Disorders: Tricks of the Trade.* New York: Thieme, 2003.

Lorimer, Donald L., ed. *Neal's Common Foot Disorders: Diagnosis and Management.* 6th ed. New York: Churchill Livingstone, 2001.

Van De Graaff, Kent M. *Human Anatomy.* 5th ed. Dubuque, Iowa: Wm. C. Brown, 2000.

FLUIDS AND ELECTROLYTES

BIOLOGY

ANATOMY OR SYSTEM AFFECTED: Blood, cells, respiratory system

SPECIALTIES AND RELATED FIELDS: Biochemistry, cytology, hematology, histology, pharmacology, pulmonary medicine, serology, urology

DEFINITION: Body fluids are intracellular or extracellular solutions of water and other substances, the concentrations of which must be regulated to achieve proper physiological functioning; electrolytes are chemicals that become electrically charged particles when they dissolve in water.

KEY TERMS:

adenosine triphosphate: a chemical that, when it reacts to lose a phosphate group, gives off free energy that is available for bodily processes

edema: the abnormal accumulation of fluid in tissues or cavities of the body

electrolyte: a chemical that, when it dissolves in water, dissociates to form positive and negative ions so that the resulting solution is an electrical conductor

homeostasis: the tendency of the body to maintain a beneficial balance among its parts

physiology: the study of the processes and mechanisms by which living organisms function

resorption: the process in which bones dissolve and return their components to the body fluids

semipermeable membrane: a barrier that allows some materials to pass but blocks others

solute: a material that has gone into solution and in so doing has changed its phase

STRUCTURE AND FUNCTIONS

Humans live in a wide variety of environmental conditions. Some days are hot and wet, others are cold and dry, and most are somewhere between. At the same time, as foods and liquid are taken in, the body is exposed to a variety of chemical substances over a wide range of concentrations. Amid these widely changing circumstances, the internal environment, to which the body's cells are exposed, remains essentially unchanged. This regulation of the internal environment, which is called homeostasis, is necessary for the correct functioning of the body. Essentially, all the organs and tissues of the body play roles in the homeostatic processes, and the main control mechanism operates through the movement of body fluids.

There are several different body fluids, but they are all solutions of solutes in water. The identity of the solutes and their concentrations differentiates one body fluid from another. Among the solutes, two categories exist. Some solutes dissociate into electrically charged particles when they dissolve and are thus called electrolytes. Others remain as neutral particles dissolved in the water and are nonelectrolytes. Both types of solutes play important roles in the correct physiological functioning of the body, but it is the electrolytes that draw the most attention. This is the case because the fluids and the electrolytes are interdependent and because imbalances of these factors are associated with a vast array of illnesses.

Although subject to some variation with age, gender, and physical condition, the body is composed of about 60 percent water by weight. For purposes of classification, this water is considered to be present in compartments. It is important to recognize that this terminology is conceptual only and does not refer to the existence of any real, separate, water-containing compartments in the body. Approximately 25 cubic decimeters of water are contained within the body's cells; this is the intracellular fluid. Most of the remaining fluid, about 12 cubic decimeters, is termed extracellular and exists in the regions exterior to cells. The extracellular fluid is further subdivided into the categories of interstitial fluid, which surrounds the cells; intravascular fluid, which is located within the blood vessels; and transcellular fluid, which includes the fluid found in the spinal column, the region of the lungs, the area surrounding the heart, the sinuses, and the eyes, along with sweat and digestive secretions. These subcategories are listed in order of the amount of fluid present. Of all these types, only the intravascular fluid is directly affected when a person drinks or eliminates fluid. Alterations in the other regions occur in response to that change, however, and there is a continual dynamic exchange of fluid among all compartments. The balance of conditions created by this exchange determines the state of health of the individual.

The solutes that are electrolytes generate positively charged ions called cations and negatively charged ions called anions. The amount of positive charge present in a solution is always equal to the amount of negative charge. The major cations present are hydrogen, sodium, potassium, calcium, and magnesium. The most important anions are chloride, hydrogen carbonate, hydrogen phosphate, sulfate, and those derived from organic acids such as acetic acid. Several other ions of both types are present at very low levels. The nonelectrolytes present include urea, creatinine, bilirubin, and glucose. All these solutes are involved with particular biological changes in the body, so their presence at the correct concentration is vital.

The fluid and its solutes move within the body by means of several transport mechanisms, some of which move solutes through the fluid and some of which move either water or the solutes from one side of a cell membrane to the other. The mechanisms available are diffusion, active transport, filtration, and osmosis. Diffusion is the movement of particles through a solution from a region in which the concentration of the particles is high to a region in which it is lower. The energy that drives this motion is thermal energy, and the transport rate is increased by increasing the temperature, which increases the concentration difference from point to point and is faster for smaller particles. Cell walls are a barrier to this type of transport unless the solute particles are small enough to pass through pores in the wall or are soluble in the cell wall itself. Active transport provides another means of moving solutes across cell walls. The energy for such movement is provided by a series of chemical reactions involving adenosine triphosphate. The movement of sodium out of and potassium into cells, as well as the transport of amino acids into cells, occurs in this manner. Filtration is a means by which both water and some solutes are transported through a porous membrane. The solutes transported are those that are small enough to pass through the pores in the membrane. The driving force for filtration is provided by a difference in pressure on the two sides of the membrane, and the motion occurs from the high-pressure side to the low-pressure side. The pressure in this case results from gravity and from the pumping action of the heart. Osmosis is a process by which water is moved across a semipermeable membrane as the result of the influence of a different type of pressure. When two solutions of different concentrations of solute particles are separated by a semipermeable membrane, an osmotic pressure develops that acts as the driving force to move water from the side of the membrane where the concentration of solute particles is lower to the side where the solute particle concentration is higher.

A solute's concentration in the body fluid has a great effect on the transport of materials and thus on the body's health. Concentrations in body fluids are expressed in several ways. Electrolyte concentration is often expressed in terms of milliequivalents of solute per cubic decimeter of solution. This is a measure of the amount of change, positive or negative, provided by that solute. A solution with twice the number of milliequivalents per cubic decimeter will have twice the concentration of change. This also measures the solute's combining power, because one milliequivalent of cations will chemically combine with one milliequivalent of anions. Osmolality, osmolarity, and tonicity refer to a solution's ability to provide an osmotic pressure. Osmolality and osmolarity are proportional to the number of particles of solute present in the solution. When solutions of different osmolalities or osmolarities are separated by a semipermeable membrane, there will be a flow of solvent across the membrane. Isotonic solutions have equal osmotic effects. Tonicity is a way of comparing the osmotic potential of solutions by referring to one as being hypotonic, isotonic, or hypertonic to the other.

DISORDERS AND DISEASES

There are two ways to approach thinking about the health role of body fluids and electrolytes. One is to consider one particular fluid component, such as sodium, that is out of balance and proceed to trace possible causes of the imbalance and appropriate treatment modes. It must be noted, however, that there are many possible illnesses that could cause any particular imbalance. The second approach is to consider a representative number of specific diseases and to look at their effect on the fluid and electrolyte balance and how such effects may be treated.

The first of these two approaches is adopted here because it highlights the fluids and electrolytes themselves rather than the diseases. Two imbalances will be considered as examples of the types of effects seen. First to be considered is the volume of fluid itself. Second, the balance of calcium will be given attention because of the connection of calcium deficiency with the bone brittleness that often occurs during aging.

Volume imbalance that is larger than the system's normal regulatory ability to control may occur in either the intracellular or extracellular fluid or both and may be in the direction of too little fluid (dehydration) or too much (overhydration). Both of these effects may result from a number of underlying illnesses, but each is, by itself, life-threatening and requires direct treatment. Often, this treatment precedes the diagnosis of the root cause.

The body apparently senses fluid volume imbalance with receptors near the heart, and several coping responses are triggered. Dehydration can be the result of vomiting, diarrhea, excessive perspiration, or blood loss. In such cases, the body's responses are in the direction of maintaining the flow of blood to vital organs. Vessels at the extremities are constricted, and those in the regions of the vital organs are dilated. Kidney function is greatly slowed, the reabsorption of sodium is increased, and the production of urine is markedly decreased, ensuring water retention. Centers in the hypothalamus respond and cause the individual to become thirsty. Thus, the body acts to protect its most important functions while at the same time stimulating actions from the individual that will bring additional fluid volume into the system. The manner in which the individual responds to being thirsty will determine other bodily changes. If plain water is used to quench the thirst, the extracellular fluid becomes less concentrated in electrolytes than is the intracellular fluid, causing an osmotic pressure imbalance that the body regulates by transporting more water into the cells, producing overhydration there and aggravating the original dehydration in the extracellular fluid. Notice that this means that drinking large amounts of water can, strange though it may seem, cause dehydration. If saltwater is ingested, the reverse occurs, with a resulting dehydration of the cells that in turn triggers extreme thirst but few cardiovascular problems. Proper volume replacement thus requires that the water brought into the system be of the same electrolyte concentration as the cellular fluids—that is, that they be isotonic. In that case, the osmotic pressure remains balanced and the fluid volumes in both of the major compartments can be built up.

Overhydration is a less common occurrence that is usually associated with cardiovascular disease, severe malnutrition and kidney disease, or surgical stress. When the heart is not able to act as an effective pump, a back pressure builds in the circulatory system that causes fluid to be filtered through the walls of the vessels and that results in the accumulation of fluid in the interstitial regions around the heart and lungs. A decrease in proteins in the bloodstream, resulting from either malnutrition or kidney malfunction, lowers the osmotic pressure in the blood and causes water retention in the interstitial spaces. Accumulation of excess fluid in the interstitial spaces is called edema. This same end condition also arises when the kidney excessively filters fluid from the bloodstream into the interstitial spaces. The treatment of overhydration takes the form of fluid intake restriction, restriction of dietary sodium, and the use of diuretic therapy to stimulate urine production.

Calcium, much of which comes from milk and milk products, is the fifth most abundant ion in the body and is involved with the formation of the mineral component of teeth and bones, the contraction of muscles, proper blood clotting, and the maintenance of cell wall permeability. Calcium is added to extracellular fluid as a result of the intestinal absorption of dietary calcium and bone resorption. It is lost from the extracellular fluid via secretion into the intestinal tract, urinary excretion, and deposition in bone. The maintenance of a proper calcium level mainly depends on processes occurring in the intestinal tract. Only a very small part of the body's total calcium is in fluids. Both hypocalcemia and hypercalcemia, the shortage and the overabundance of calcium in the fluids, may occur. Unlike the case of water shortage or excess, however, there are few direct visual consequences of a calcium imbalance; one must rely on laboratory testing of the fluid and on indirect physical assessment.

Hypocalcemia in the blood is associated with reduced intake, increased loss, or altered regulation, as in hypoparathyroidism. Bone, a living material, continually absorbs and desorbs calcium. The parathyroid gland secretes a hormone that regulates bone resorption and thus can raise the calcium level in the extracellular fluid at the expense of decreasing the amount of bone. Obviously, this cannot be a long-term mechanism to provide calcium. The same hormone also regulates the absorption of calcium from the intestines and the kidneys. Vitamin D is an essential, although indirect, factor in permitting the absorption of calcium from the intestine. A deficiency of this vitamin is a major cause of hypocalcemia. When the calcium level in the extracellular fluid falls below normal, the nervous system becomes increasingly excited. If the level continues to fall, the nerve fibers begin to discharge spontaneously, passing impulses to the peripheral skeletal muscles,

where they cause a contractive spasm. Often, this is first seen in a contracting of the fingers. Generalized muscular spasming can be lethal if the calcium imbalance is not corrected quickly. Immediate calcium deficiency is treated with the administration of either oral or intravenous calcium compounds, with vitamin D therapy, and with the inclusion of foods of high calcium content in the diet. In the longer term, treatment of the underlying illness is necessary.

The opposite imbalance, hypercalcemia, can occur as a result of an excessive intake of calcium supplements and vitamin D, in conjunction with a high-calcium diet. Calcium excess is also associated with some tumors and with kidney or glandular diseases. It has also been found to be caused by prolonged immobility, in which case the bones resorb because of the lack of bone stress. This later effect has been of major concern in the space program. Too high a level of calcium in the intercellular fluid causes a depression of the nervous system and a slowing of reflexes. Lack of appetite and constipation are also common results. At very high levels, calcium salts may precipitate in the blood system, an effect that can be rapidly lethal. Again, in the long term, the underlying cause of the imbalance must be corrected, but treatments do exist for more immediate alleviation. As long as the kidneys are functioning correctly, intravenous treatment with saline serves as a means of flushing out excess calcium. Calcium also can be bound to phosphate that is delivered intravenously, but there is a risk of causing soft tissue precipitation of the calcium phosphate compound. Dietary control is used, at times in concert with steroid therapy, to counter high calcium levels. If resorption is the cause of the excess, there are therapies, both chemical and physical, that are effective in increasing bone deposition.

PERSPECTIVE AND PROSPECTS

From the earliest times, those concerned with the treatment of illnesses have had their attention drawn to the fluids present in or exuded by the human body. The color, smell, and texture of fluids being given off by a sick or injured person provided clues to the nature of the illness or injury. Bleeding was commonly practiced as a means of venting the illness so that health could be restored. Lancing of ulcerative conditions was also practiced by early healers. These early attempts at understanding and of treatment have been greatly refined, and the search for better understanding and improved treatment modes continues.

This concern with fluids and electrolytes is easy to understand. The fluids and their components constitute both the external and the internal environment for all the body's tissues and cells. Any abnormality in the cells or tissues is reflected in a variation from normal conditions in the fluids. All major illnesses and many minor ones have associated with them a fluid and electrolyte disorder. Fluids are more readily accessible for study than are tissues from deep within the body; hence, a considerable effort has been directed at measuring fluid constituents and interpreting the findings. The testing of fluids has evolved from highly labor intensive measurements of a few components to highly automated testing procedures applied to dozens of components. The reliability and precision of the measurements continue to increase, and the scope of measurements continues to expand.

Not all that is to be known about fluids and electrolytes, however, depends on laboratory testing. Some knowledge can be collected from close observation of the patient. Although the resulting measurements are not precise, they are nevertheless important because they are much more immediately available. Physical symptoms that carry information about fluids and electrolytes include the following: sudden weight gain or loss; changes in abdominal girth; changes in either the intake or output of fluids; body temperature; depth of respiration; heart rate; blood pressure; skin moisture, color, and temperature; the skin's ability to relax to normal after being pinched; the swelling of tissue; the condition of the tongue; the appearance of visible veins; reflexive responses; apparent mental state; and thirst. Each of these observations, and more, is readily available to one who is monitoring the health of an individual.

As is the case with most testing and data-gathering situations, interpreting the test and observation results is the critical step. Any one measure, by itself, points to a vast array of possible illnesses. Only by considering the whole and recognizing the existence of patterns in the information can a health professional narrow the possibilities. It is this recognition of patterns that develops with education and experience, and it is this step that relies on judgment that makes medicine an art as well as a science.

—*Kenneth H. Brown, Ph.D.*

See also Acid-base chemistry; Blood and blood disorders; Cells; Circulation; Cytology; Edema; Fever; Hypertension; Lipids; Physiology; Vascular system; Weight loss and gain.

FOR FURTHER INFORMATION:

Campbell, Neil A. *Biology: Concepts and Connections.* 4th ed. Redwood City, Calif.: Benjamin/Cummings, 2002. This classic introductory textbook provides an excellent discussion of essential biological structures and mechanisms. Of particular interest are the five chapters comprising the unit titled "The Cell."

Chambers, Jeanette K., Marilyn J. Rantz, and Meridean Maas, eds. *Common Fluid and Electrolyte Disorders and Nursing Diagnoses: Implementation.* Philadelphia: W. B. Saunders, 1987. The first part of this two-part book contains twelve short chapters, each targeted to an aspect of the subject. The book is designed for nurses, and the material is presented on a very practical level.

Guyton, Arthur C. *Human Physiology and Mechanisms of Disease.* 6th ed. Philadelphia: W. B. Saunders, 1997. This college-level physiology text contains several chapters relevant to the appreciation of the importance of body fluids and electrolytes. Although written at an advanced level, the writing is well done, and the major points are clearly presented. The text allows the subject to be placed in context of the whole of human physiology.

Horne, Mima M., and Ursula Easterday Heitz. *Fluid, Electrolyte, and Acid-Base Balance: A Case Study Approach.* St. Louis: Mosby Year Book, 1991. This book, written for nursing students but readable by those with minimum science background, provides an excellent summary of the subject and places the material in the context of human health. Its particular strength is in relating fluids and electrolytes to specific illnesses and in discussing treatment modes.

Kee, Joyce L. *Fluids and Electrolytes with Clinical Applications: A Programmed Approach.* 6th ed. New York: John Wiley & Sons, 2000. This is a well-presented self-instruction text that begins with the basics and then refines the topic. The thrust is the connection of the assessment of fluid and electrolyte imbalance with an understanding of illness and treatment.

Lee, Carla A. Bouska, C. Ann Barrett, and Donna D. Ignatavicius, eds. *Fluids and Electrolytes: A Practical Approach.* Rev. 4th ed. Philadelphia: F. A. Davis, 1996. The authors have aimed for a pragmatic and simplified treatment of the subject matter that is related directly to the clinical situation. Following sections that summarize the principles, the book uses a case study approach to connect principles and practice.

Speakman, Elizabeth, and Norma Jean Weldy. *Body Fluids and Electrolytes*. 8th ed. New York: Elsevier, 2001. A classic text that details clinical conditions such as pH imbalance, electrolyte imbalance, and fluid overload or under load.

FLUORIDE TREATMENTS
PROCEDURE

ANATOMY OR SYSTEM AFFECTED: Gums, mouth, teeth

SPECIALTIES AND RELATED FIELDS: Bacteriology, biochemistry, dentistry, microbiology

DEFINITION: Treatment of the teeth with a fluoride-releasing substance to help the enamel resist tooth decay.

INDICATIONS AND PROCEDURES

Tooth decay involves the solubility of food during eating. Consumed carbohydrates are oxidized to organic acids, such as lactic acid, by the action of specific bacteria that adhere to the teeth. These acids dissolve tooth enamel, which mainly consists of a mineral called hydroxyapatite and is considered to be the hardest substance in the body. The protection of the enamel, and thus the inner part of the tooth, from decomposition can be achieved through fluoride treatments.

Fluoride treatment involves the ingestion of fluoride ions in drinking water, toothpaste, and other sources to change the nature and composition of hydroxyapatite by producing a new compound called fluorapatite. Because it is less basic than hydroxyapatite, fluorapatite forms a more resistant enamel. Because of its effectiveness in preventing cavities, fluoride is added in the form of sodium fluoride or sodium hexafluorosilicate to the public water supply of many municipalities in the United States in concentrations of about 1 milligram per milliliter, or 1 part per million.

USES AND COMPLICATIONS

As a result of this so-called fluoridation process, a drastic reduction in dental decay has been observed. In addition, more than 80 percent of all toothpastes and gels now sold in the United States contain fluoride, in the form of stannous fluoride, sodium monofluorophosphate, and/or sodium fluoride in concentrations of about 0.1 percent fluoride by weight.

The recommended annual or semiannual dental cleaning by a dentist or oral hygienist removes accumulated plaque and may include further application with a fluoride substance. Generally, only children and teen-

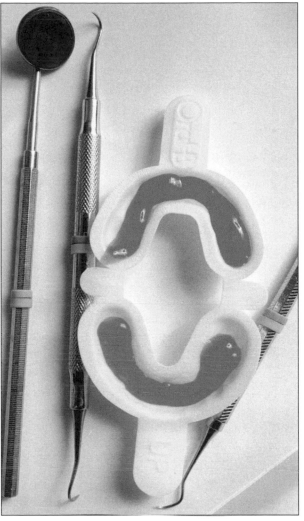

Children may be given fluoride treatments as a gel in a foam mouthpiece in order to protect against the formation of cavities. (AP/Wide World Photos)

agers receive such a fluoride treatment, although some adults may also have it.

It must be noted that fluoride ions are toxic in large quantities. As a result, when the fluoride concentration in water is about 2 to 3 parts per million, discoloration (mottling) or damage of the teeth may occur.

—*Soraya Ghayourmanesh, Ph.D.*

See also Cavities; Dental diseases; Dentistry; Dentistry, pediatric; Teeth; Wisdom teeth.

FOR FURTHER INFORMATION:

Ash, Major M., and Stanley J. Nelson. *Dental Anatomy, Physiology, and Occlusion*. 8th ed. New York: Elsevier, 2002.

Foster, Malcolm S. *Protecting Our Children's Teeth: A Guide to Quality Dental Care from Infancy Through Age Twelve.* New York: Insight Books, 1992.

Smith, Rebecca W. *The Columbia University School of Dental and Oral Surgery's Guide to Family Dental Care.* New York: W. W. Norton, 1997.

Woodall, Irene R., ed. *Comprehensive Dental Hygiene Care.* 4th ed. St. Louis: C. V. Mosby, 1993.

FLUOROSCOPY. *See* IMAGING AND RADIOLOGY.

FOOD AND DRUG ADMINISTRATION (FDA)

ORGANIZATION

ALSO KNOWN AS: Bureau of Chemistry (1906-1927); Food, Drug, and Insecticide Administration (1927-1931)

DEFINITION: An agency in the United States Department of Health and Human Services whose responsibilities include protecting citizens against harmful or falsely labeled foods, food additives, drugs, cosmetics, or medical devices.

KEY TERMS:

Generally Recognized as Safe (GRAS) list: food ingredients or chemicals designated by the FDA as harmless to human beings when used as intended

generic drugs: copycat versions of brand-name originals that are no longer protected by patents

orphan drug: a drug developed for a very rare disease (legally, drugs for two hundred thousand or fewer potential users)

thalidomide: a sedative and sleep-inducing drug that was found to produce phocomelia (a birth defect in which hands or feet are attached to the body by short, flipperlike stumps) in developing fetuses and newborns

STRUCTURE AND FUNCTION

The mission of the Food and Drug Administration (FDA) is to protect the nation's health. Consequently, the U.S. Congress empowered this agency to prevent the sale of harmful products. The FDA's specific duty is to enforce the numerous federal laws that have been passed to ensure that foods and drugs are pure and safe and that all such products are correctly labeled. With the multiplication of its responsibilities over time came a concomitant growth in the FDA's administrative, technical, and service staffs both in Washington, D.C., and in ten regions around the country. Officials in each region are responsible for enforcing the relevant laws in their jurisdictions, and they are helped in this by inspectors and scientists.

The activities of FDA personnel include research, inspection, and legal action. In FDA laboratories scientists verify manufacturers' claims of the safety and effectiveness of food additives, drugs, and cosmetics before they are put onto the market. In addition to studying the long-term effects of various products, FDA workers also study how foods are processed, preserved, packaged, and stored. Using their field staffs, FDA officials send their inspectors to monitor manufacturing facilities and assist industrial employees in setting up procedures to prevent violations of the law. The FDA also has the duty of enforcing laws against illegal sales of prescription drugs, and FDA employees periodically examine imports of foods, drugs, cosmetics, and therapeutic devices to make sure that they comply with federal laws.

Even though the FDA has the responsibility of protecting consumers from various lawbreakers, its enforcement of relevant laws is limited by the courts. In fact, the agency must have the cooperation of attorneys and judges to prosecute persons or firms, impose fines, or seize products. FDA inspectors collect evidence of violations, and administrators review this evidence before deciding which cases will be presented to the federal courts for action. As a federal agency, the FDA is restricted to products involved in interstate commerce.

Because of physicians' professional concerns with nutrition, prescription and nonprescription drugs, and medical technologies, they have a vested interest in the FDA and its activities. According to several studies, physicians are protective of their independence and the integrity of the doctor-patient relationship, and many doctors are wary of governmental involvement in how they practice medicine. On the other hand, critics have pointed out the dangers of the close relationship that has developed between doctors and drug companies.

The FDA supervises the development and marketing of all drugs sold in the United States. New drugs originate in pharmaceutical or chemical companies, government laboratories, medical schools, or universities. An inventor or discoverer of a new drug can be granted a patent for the drug itself or for how it is made or used. Patents give the developer exclusive rights to a drug for seventeen years. After a patent has expired, other companies may sell a generic version of the drug, usually at a much lower price. The FDA's approval of a generic drug is based on laboratory studies to guarantee that the copy has the safety and effectiveness of the original. Since the generic drug manufacturer who is first to market a new generic drug reaps huge financial rewards, great pressures exist on the FDA to facilitate this process.

In 1988 generic drugs became the focus of a congressional subcommittee. It discovered that three generic drug companies were receiving accelerated approval of their applications in exchange for payoffs to FDA employees. When this generic drug scandal was over, federal courts had convicted ten companies and forty-two people of corruption. This scandal also revealed a potentially corrupting collusion between FDA workers and pharmaceutical companies, since FDA employees often leave their government jobs for highly paid positions at the companies they had formerly regulated.

Controversies and Ethical Debates

As the federal agency charged with protecting the health of Americans, the FDA is often entangled in controversial and ethical issues. For example, it is responsible for the regulation of investigational new drugs (INDs)—drugs approved for testing but not for sale. For a drug to become an IND, it must first be given to animals, since a correlation often exists between a drug's adverse effect on animals and its similar effect on humans. The FDA's procedure for testing INDs includes three phases: In Phase I, small groups of healthy volunteers are given the IND to help researchers study its effectiveness, dosage, and metabolism; in Phase II, one to two hundred patients with the drug-targeted disease are monitored for the drug's safety, efficacy, and side effects; in Phase III, even larger numbers of patients take the drug to refine optimum dosages and, with the use of placebos, to make sure that the IND's effects are not due to chance or the developer's optimism.

In the 1970's, the FDA's handling of INDs came under attack. The General Accounting Office (GAO) studied ten of the more than six thousand drugs then classified as INDs, concluding that in eight cases the FDA failed to halt human tests after receiving indications that the new drugs were unsafe. Furthermore the GAO found that drug companies delayed reporting adverse drug effects to the FDA. Others pointed out that the FDA tested INDs singly, whereas some drugs have the potential of causing great harm when they interact with other drugs (the so-called synergistic effect). Some criticized the FDA for approving too many drugs too quickly, thereby increasing risks, while others blamed the FDA for increasing risks by approving too few drugs too slowly. Defenders of the FDA responded by saying that it is impossible to eliminate all risks from the use of medicines.

A specific example of what some see as the FDA's excessive regulation of foods and drugs is the controversy over dietary supplements. Initially the FDA tried to restrict the public's right to choose these supplements. Some scientists thought that the FDA's vitamin regulations were reasonable, but public discontent forced Congress to pass a law guaranteeing consumers freedom to choose nutritional supplements. In the 1970's, this debate centered on laetrile (also known as vitamin B_{17}), a substance found naturally in apricot pits. Many countries permitted the sale of laetrile as a supplement, but the FDA banned it, pointing out that it causes the release of cyanide in the body. Advocates believed that laetrile relieved the symptoms and slowed the growth of cancers, and some states legalized laetrile, challenging the FDA ban. However, in 1979, the Supreme Court ruled unanimously that the FDA had the power to ban the interstate sale and distribution of laetrile. This and such controversies as disputes over artificial hearts, cigarettes as "drug-delivery devices," and various acquired immunodeficiency syndrome (AIDS) drugs helped define the FDA's role in American society, just as similar controversies have throughout the history of the agency.

Perspective and Prospects

Most scholars trace the history of the FDA to the Pure Food and Drug Act of 1906. This law, like many that would follow it, originated from public outrage over tragedies caused by impure foods and drugs. More than a century ago, food producers commonly added water to milk and adulterated coffee with charcoal. They colored foods and drinks with harmful dyes, and they used such injurious preservatives as formaldehyde, sodium benzoate, and borax. Consumers had to choose drugs based on false or misleading labels. This intolerable situation inspired the crusade of Harvey Wiley, who, because of his attacks on adulterated or pernicious foods and drugs, became known as the "Father of the Pure Food and Drug Law." In his position as chief of the Bureau of Chemistry of the Department of Agriculture, Wiley gathered a group of idealistic young chemists, nicknamed the "Poison Squad," to study the physiological effects of various chemical additives in foods. Their studies aroused public concern over food additives, but "Wiley's Law" would never have become a reality were it not for Upton Sinclair, whose novel *The Jungle* (1906) dramatized unsanitary practices in the meatpacking industry, and for President Theodore Roosevelt, who, disgusted by scandals in the drug trade, prodded members of Congress to pass the law. The Food and Drug Act of 1906 prohibited the "manufacture, sale, or transportation of adulterated or misbranded or poisonous or deleterious foods, drugs, medicines, and liquors." The Bureau of Chemistry administered the new law, and Wiley and his successors developed an organization that won many victories for pure foods and drugs in the courts.

In 1928, Congress authorized the creation of the Food, Drug, and Insecticide Administration as the executor of the Pure Food and Drug Act. The Agricultural Appropriation Act of 1931 changed the agency's name to the Food and Drug Administration. When Franklin D. Roosevelt became president in 1933, he and his team of "New Dealers" tried to get through Congress a number of fiscal and social reforms, including an expansion of the FDA's mission, since companies were continuing to make dangerous medicines. Little was accomplished until 1937, when the Massengill Company shipped its Elixir Sulfanilamide to pharmacists. This drug, which was intended to cure infections, eventually caused the deaths of 107 people. Within months of this tragedy, Congress finally passed the Federal Food, Drug, and Cosmetic Act of 1938. This law required drug manufacturers to provide scientific proof, through tests on animals and humans, that all their new drugs were safe before they were put on the market.

To isolate the FDA from advocacy groups, it became part of the Federal Security Agency in 1940. World War II expanded the FDA's workload, especially with the discovery of new "wonder drugs" that had to be tested. After the war, the number, variety, and power of new drugs increased dramatically. With the FDA's emphasis on prescription drugs, new industries emerged and, because of high profits, these companies grew in size and influence. The profitability of the postwar food and drug industries brought both abuses and legislative remedies.

During the 1950's and 1960's the 1938 act was periodically amended, including the Humphrey-Durham Drug Prescription Act (1951), the Food Additives Amendment (1958), the Color Additives Amendment (1961), and the Kefauver-Harris Drug Amendment (1962). After the FDA became part of the Department of Health, Education, and Welfare in 1953, it used these new laws to concentrate control of powerful new drugs

in the hands of FDA officials and doctors. Some of these new laws gave the FDA responsibility for determining the safety of food ingredients, even those on the Generally Recognized as Safe (GRAS) list that had previously been used with no apparent ill effects. For example, sodium cyclamate, an additive used as an artificial sweetener, had originally been classified as GRAS but was later banned as being possibly carcinogenic. The Delaney Clause (1958) prohibited the use of substances in food if they caused cancer in laboratory animals. This law led to a controversial ban of another artificial sweetener, saccharin, a weak carcinogen (the Delaney Clause was replaced, in 1996, by a less stringent standard).

In the late 1950's, the thalidomide tragedy in Europe, during which thousands of deformed infants were born, helped to enhance public support for legislation strengthening the Food, Drug, and Cosmetic Act. Widespread use of thalidomide in America was prevented by Dr. Frances Kelsey, an FDA examiner, who used the pretext of insufficient information to turn down a company's repeated applications to market this drug in the United States. Congress responded to the thalidomide tragedy by passing the Kefauver-Harris Amendment in 1962. This law changed the ways in which drugs were created, tested, developed, prescribed, and sold. The burden was now on the companies sponsoring a new drug to show that it was safe and effective. The FDA also issued new regulations that made the drug review process extremely stringent; some said too stringent, because FDA officials, fearful of another thalidomide-like tragedy, delayed new drug approval by asking for study after study.

During the 1970's, 1980's, and 1990's, the Food, Drug, and Cosmetic Act of 1938 was constantly revised and amended. For example, an amendment in 1976 strengthened the FDA's authority to regulate medical devices, and in 1980 serious illnesses in babies caused Congress to pass an Infant Formula Act requiring strict controls over the nutritional content and safety of commercial baby foods. In 1982 seven deaths from cyanide poisoning later traced to Tylenol capsules caused the FDA to issue regulations requiring tamper-resistant packaging. The Orphan Drug Act of 1983 offered economic inducement to encourage pharmaceutical companies to develop drugs for rare diseases affecting small populations. However, the multiplication of regulations did not prevent the generic drug scandals of the late 1980's. In fact, for many critics, the FDA had become an inefficient agency, under constant attack from congressional subcommittees, newspaper reporters, public interest groups, and industry executives.

In the 1990's, the FDA struggled to retrieve its credibility and authority by becoming once again the guardian of the nation's health. In 1992, the Prescription Drug User Fee Act required $100,000 for each new drug application, rising to $233,000 per application in five years. In return, the FDA hired six hundred new examiners to cut the review time for important new drugs. The FDA also improved standards of risk assessment for food additives, drugs, and medical devices, and it increased inspections of food and drug factories. By the end of the twentieth century, the FDA was an agency trying to keep up with the revolutionary advances in the chemical, biological, and medical sciences.

The beginning of the twenty-first century introduced an interesting era for the FDA. Because of a slowdown in the creation of innovative drugs and medical devices, the FDA rolled out new guidelines to help pharmaceutical companies better prove how a drug works in efforts to streamline the process of approval and get new treatments to the consumer market faster. Noting that drug companies went from sending a high of sixty never-before-seen drugs in 1995 for FDA approval down to just seventeen in 2002, the agency decided to make their requirements for approval more clear so that companies could do better research faster and be more willing to take chances on truly novel treatments instead of safer "copycat" medications. Some of these requirements included helping companies avoid incomplete applications, developing special guidelines for brand-new technology so that companies can design the right studies from the beginning, and providing more training of FDA reviewers.

The terrorist attacks on the World Trade Center and the Pentagon in 2001 also introduced a change in the FDA's approval process. In order to help in the development of bioterrorism antidotes, the agency announced that it would approve certain drugs based only on animal studies if human drug testing would be impossible. The new approach to the evaluation process includes only those drugs that would treat or prevent the potentially lethal or disabling toxicity of chemical, biological, or nuclear substances.

—*Robert J. Paradowski, Ph.D.*

See also Animal rights vs. research; Antibiotics; Anti-inflammatory drugs; Clinical trials; Creutzfeldt-Jakob disease (CJD); Food biochemistry; Food poisoning; Iatrogenic disorders; Pharmacology; Pharmacy; Screening.

FOR FURTHER INFORMATION:

Burkholz, Herbert. *The FDA Follies.* New York: Basic-Books, 1994. Analyzes in lurid detail how the FDA failed in its mission to protect the health of Americans during the Reagan and Bush administrations.

Grabowski, Henry G., and John M. Vernon. *The Regulation of Pharmaceuticals.* Washington, D.C.: American Enterprise Institute for Public Policy Research, 1983. Argues that the FDA does not deal with new drugs neutrally, since the cost of rejecting a good drug is borne by manufacturers and patients while the cost of accepting a bad drug is borne by FDA officials.

Hilts, Philip J. *Protecting America's Health: The FDA, Business, and One Hundred Years of Regulation.* New York: Alfred Knopf, 2003. Provides a thorough history of the FDA and its battles with self-serving political and industrial interests.

Jackson, Charles O. *Food and Drug Legislation in the New Deal.* Princeton, N.J.: Princeton University Press, 1970. A political and historical analysis of the complex struggle leading to the Food, Drug, and Cosmetic Act of 1938.

Liska, Ken. *Drugs and the Human Body with Implications for Society.* Englewood Cliffs, N.J.: Prentice Hall, 2003. Examines the use of drugs in the North American culture by discussing such topics as what constitutes a drug and where drugs come from, drug metabolism, the different classifications of drugs, and federal laws that can be applied generally to many drug categories, including over-the-counter and prescription drugs.

Lucas, Scott. *The FDA.* Millbrae, Calif.: Celestial Arts, 1978. An analysis of the structure, purpose, practices, and abuses of the FDA, and how all these affect the general public.

Parrish, Richard. *Defining Drugs: How Government Became the Arbiter of Pharmaceutical Fact.* Somerset, N.J.: Transaction, 2003. Traces the development of drug regulation in the United States, explains the social construction of this system, and argues for a "therapeutic reformation."

Patrick, William. *The Food and Drug Administration.* New York: Chelsea House, 1988. Investigates the primary question facing the FDA: how much to regulate, and when?

Pisano, Douglas. *Essentials of Pharmacy Law.* Boca Raton, Fla.: CRC Press, 2002. A clear, user-friendly text that compiles and comments on selected federal laws and regulations pertaining to the general practice of pharmacy in the United States.

Temin, Peter. *Taking Your Medicine: Drug Regulation in the United States.* Cambridge, Mass.: Harvard University Press, 1980. Both a narrative of drug regulation and an analysis of the U.S. government's paternalistic assumption that neither consumers nor doctors can wisely choose drugs for themselves.

Young, James Harvey. *Pure Food: Securing the Federal Food and Drugs Act of 1906.* Princeton, N.J.: Princeton University Press, 1989. A historical study of how pure-food advocates, chemists, and politicians helped make the Pure Food and Drug Law into a reality.

FOOD BIOCHEMISTRY
BIOLOGY

ANATOMY OR SYSTEM AFFECTED: Cells, gastrointestinal system, pancreas, stomach

SPECIALTIES AND RELATED FIELDS: Biochemistry, cytology, gastroenterology, nutrition, pharmacology

DEFINITION: The breakdown of food by cells, a process in which nutrients are converted to energy and other components needed by the body.

KEY TERMS:

amino acids: the organic compounds that make up proteins; twenty are necessary for growth, nine of which must be obtained in the diet

Calorie: the basic unit of energy; the amount of heat needed to change the temperature of one liter of water from 14.5 degrees Celsius to 15.5 degrees Celsius

carbohydrates: a group of organic compounds that includes the sugars and the starches; one of three classes of nutrients and a basic source of energy

fats: a group of organic compounds, also called lipids, that store energy; one of three classes of nutrients

glycolysis: a metabolic pathway that converts the sugar glucose to pyruvate for energy without the use of oxygen

metabolism: the totality of a cell's biochemical processes; the process by which food molecules release their stored energy

minerals: inorganic compounds that are essential for human life; seventeen are required in the diet

proteins: organic compounds that are composed of amino acids and function as enzymes, speeding up metabolic reactions; one of three classes of nutrients

vitamins: organic compounds, essential for life but required in very minute quantities, that participate in biochemical reactions and help to release energy from the three classes of nutrients

STRUCTURE AND FUNCTIONS

Food biochemistry is concerned with the breakdown of food in the cell as a source of energy. Each cell is a factory that converts the nutrients of the food one eats to energy and other structural components of the body. The amount of energy that these nutrients supply is expressed in Calories (kilocalories). The number of Calories consumed will determine the energy balance of the individual and whether one loses or gains weight. The nutrients come in a variety of forms, but they can be divided into three major categories: carbohydrates, lipids (fats), and proteins. These nutrients are broken down by the cell metabolically to produce energy for cellular processes. Other components are used by the cell and the entire body for structure and transport. Each of these nutrients is essential to a well-balanced diet and good health. Two other components of a successful diet are vitamins and minerals.

Carbohydrates are molecules composed of carbon, hydrogen, and oxygen. They range from the simple sugars all the way to the complex carbohydrates. The simplest carbohydrates are the monosaccharides (one-sugar molecules), primarily glucose and fructose. The simple monosaccharides are usually joined to form disaccharides (two-sugar molecules), such as sucrose (glucose and fructose, or cane sugar), lactose (glucose and galactose, or milk sugar), and maltose (two glucoses, which is found in grains). The complex carbohydrates are the polysaccharides (multiple sugar molecules), which are composed of many monosaccharides, usually glucose. There are two main types: starch, which is found in plants such as potatoes, and glycogen, in which form humans store carbohydrate energy for the short term (up to twelve hours) in the liver.

The next major group of molecules is the lipids, which are made up of the solid fats and liquid oils. These molecules are primarily composed of carbon and hydrogen. They form three major groups: the triglycerides, phospholipids, and sterols. The triglycerides are composed of three fatty acids attached to a glycerol (a three-carbon molecule); this is the group that makes up the fats and oils. Fats, which are primarily of animal origin, are triglycerides that are solid at room temperature; such triglycerides are saturated, which means that there are no double bonds between their carbon molecules. Oils are liquid at room temperature, primarily of plant origin, and either monounsaturated or polyunsaturated (there are one or more double bonds between the carbon molecules in the chain). This group provides long-term energy in humans and is stored as adipose (fat) tissue. Each gram of fat stores approximately 9 Calories of energy per gram, which is about twice that of carbohydrates and proteins (4 Calories per gram). The adipose tissue also provides important insulation in maintaining body temperature. Phospholipids are similar to triglycerides in structure, but they have two fatty acids and a phosphate attached to the glycerol molecule. Phospholipids are the building blocks of the cell membranes that form the barrier between the inside and the outside of the cell. Sterols are considered lipids, but they have a completely different structure. This group includes cholesterol, vitamin D, estrogen, and testosterone. The sterols function in the structure of the cell membrane (as cholesterol does) or as hormones (as do testosterone and estrogen).

The last major group of molecules is that of the proteins, which are composed of carbon, hydrogen, oxygen, and nitrogen. Proteins are long chains of amino acids; each protein is composed of varying amounts of the twenty different amino acids. Proteins are used in the body as enzymes, substances that catalyze (generally, speed up) the biochemical reactions that take place in cells. They also function as transport molecules (such as hemoglobin, which transports oxygen) and provide structure (as does keratin, the protein in hair and nails). The human body can synthesize eleven of the twenty amino acids; the other nine are considered essential amino acids because they cannot be synthesized and are required in the diet.

Two other groups of essential compounds are necessary in the diet for the body's metabolism: vitamins and minerals. The vitamins are organic compounds (made up of carbon) that are required in only milligram or microgram quantities per day. The vitamins are classified into two groups: the water-soluble vitamins (the B vitamins and vitamin C) and the fat-soluble vitamins (vitamins A, D, E, and K). Vitamins are vital components of enzymes.

The minerals are inorganic nutrients that can be divided into two classes, depending on the amounts needed by the body. The major minerals are required in amounts greater than 100 milligrams per day; these minerals are calcium, phosphorus, magnesium, sodium, chloride, sulfur, and potassium. The trace elements, those needed in amounts of only a few milligrams per day, are iron, zinc, iodine, fluoride, copper, selenium, chromium, manganese, and molybdenum. Although they are required in small quantities, the minerals play an important role in the human body. Calcium is involved in bone and teeth formation and muscle contractions. Iron is found in hemoglobin and aids in the transportation of oxygen throughout the body. Potassium helps nerves send electrical impulses. Sodium and chloride maintain water balance in tissues and vascular fluid.

An adequate diet is one that supplies the body and cells with sources of energy and building blocks. The first priority of the diet is to supply the bulk nutrients—carbohydrates, fats, and proteins. An average young adult requires between 2,100 and 2,900 Calories per day, taking into account the amount of energy required for rest and work. Carbohydrates, fats, and proteins are taken in during a meal and digested—that is, broken into smaller components. Starch is broken down to glucose, and sucrose is broken down to fructose and glucose and absorbed by the bloodstream. Fats are broken down to triglycerides, and proteins are divided into their separate amino acids, to be absorbed by the bloodstream and transported throughout the body. Each cell then takes up essential nutrients for energy and to use as building parts of the cell.

Once the nutrients enter the cell, they are broken down into energy through a series of metabolic reactions. The first step in the metabolic process is called glycolysis. Glucose is broken down through a series of reactions to produce adenosine triphosphate (ATP), a molecule used to fuel other biochemical pathways in the cell. Glycolysis gives off a small amount of energy and does not require oxygen. This process can provide the energy for a short sprint; lactic acid buildup in the muscles will lead to fatigue, however, if there is insufficient oxygen.

Long-term energy requires oxygen. Aerobic respiration can metabolize not only the sugars produced by glycolysis but triglycerides and amino acids as well. The molecules enter what is called the Krebs cycle, an aerobic pathway that provides eighteen times more energy than glycolysis. The waste products of this pathway are carbon dioxide and water, which are exhaled.

DISORDERS AND DISEASES

Diet plays a major role in the metabolism of the cells. One major problem in diet is the overconsumption of Calories, which can lead to weight gain and eventual obesity. Obesity is defined as being 20 percent over one's ideal weight for one's body size. A number of problems are associated with obesity, such as high blood pressure, high levels of cholesterol, increased risk of cancer, heart disease, and early death.

At the other end of the scale is malnutrition. Carbohydrates are the preferred energy source in the form of either blood glucose or glycogen, which is found in the liver and muscles. This source gives a person approximately four to twelve hours of energy. Long-term storage of energy occurs as fat, which constitutes anywhere from 15 percent to 25 percent of body composition. During times of starvation, when the carbohydrate reserve is almost zero, fat will be mobilized for energy. Fat will also be used to make glucose for the blood because the brain requires glucose as its energy source. In extreme starvation, the body will begin to degrade the protein in muscles down to its constituent amino acids in order to produce energy.

Malnutrition can also occur if essential vitamins and minerals are excluded from the diet. Vitamin deficiencies affect the metabolism of the cell since these compounds are often required to aid the enzymes in producing energy. A number of medical problems are associated with vitamin deficiencies. A deficiency in thiamine will result in the metabolic disorder called beriberi. A loss of the thiamine found in wheat and rice can occur in the refinement process, making it more difficult to obtain enough of this vitamin from the diet. Alcoholics have an increased thiamine requirement, to help in the metabolism of alcohol, and usually have a low level of food consumption; thus, they are at risk for developing beriberi. Lack of vitamin A results in night blindness, and lack of vitamin D results in rickets, in which the bones are weakened as a result of poor calcium uptake.

One interesting feature about diet and the metabolic pathways concerns how different molecules are treated. Some people mistakenly believe that it is better to eat fruit sugar than other sugars. Fruit sugar, the simple sugar fructose, is chemically related to glucose. Because glucose and fructose are converted to each other during glycolysis, it does not matter which sugar is eaten. Far more important to proper nutrition is what accompanies the sugar. Table sugar provides only calories, while a piece of fruit contains both fruit sugar and vitamins, minerals, and fiber for a more complete diet.

Many errors in metabolism occur because genes do not carry the proper information. The result may be an enzyme that, although critical to a biochemical pathway, does not function properly or is missing altogether. One disorder of carbohydrate metabolism is called galactosemia. Mother's milk contains lactose, which is normally broken down into galactose and glucose. With galactosemia, the cells take in the galactose but are unable to convert it to glucose because of the lack of an enzyme. Thus, galactose levels build up in the blood, liver, and other organs, impairing their function. This condition can lead to death in an infant, but the effects of galactosemia are usually detected and the diet modified by use of a milk substitute.

Amino acid metabolism can also be defective, leading to the accumulation of toxic by-products. One of the best-known examples involves the amino acid phenylalanine. About one in ten thousand infants is born with a defective pathway, a disorder called phenylketonuria (PKU). If PKU is not discovered in time, by-products can accumulate, causing poor brain development and severe mental retardation. PKU must be diagnosed early in life, and a special, controlled diet must be given to the infant. Because phenylalanine is an essential amino acid, limited amounts are included in the diet for proper growth, but large amounts need to be excluded. The artificial sweetener aspartame (NutraSweet) poses a problem for those with PKU. Aspartame is composed of two amino acids, phenylalanine and aspartic acid. When aspartame is broken down during digestion, phenylalanine enters the bloodstream. Individuals with PKU should not ingest aspartame; there is a warning to that effect on products containing this chemical.

Other errors of metabolism are noted later in life. One example is lactose intolerance, in which lactose is cleaved by the enzyme lactase into glucose and galactose. The enzyme lactase, found in the digestive tract, is very active in suckling infants, but only Northern Europeans and members of some African tribes retain lactase activity into adulthood. Other groups, such as Asian, Arab, Jewish, Indian, and Mediterranean peoples, show little lactase activity as adults. These people cannot digest the lactose in milk products, which then cannot be absorbed in the intestinal tract. A buildup of lactose can lead to diarrhea and colic. Usually in those parts of the world milk is not used by adults as food. In the United States, one can purchase milk that contains lactose which has been partially broken down into galactose and glucose. One can also purchase the lactase enzyme itself and add it to milk.

Another error of metabolism results in diabetes mellitus, which means "excessive excretion of sweet urine." A telltale sign of this condition is sugar, specifically glucose, in the urine. In normal people, blood glucose levels remain relatively stable. After a meal, when the blood glucose levels rise, the pancreas starts to secrete the hormone insulin. Insulin causes the cells to take in the extra blood glucose and convert it to glycogen or fat, thus storing the extra energy. In diabetics, there is little or no insulin production or release, or the target cells may have faulty receptors. As a result, the blood glucose level remains high. The excess glucose is then excreted in the urine, leading to the symptom of excess thirst. The body is forced to rely much more heavily on fats as an energy source, leading to high levels of circulating fats and cholesterol in the blood. These substances can be deposited in the blood vessels, causing high blood pressure and heart disease. Excess fats, in levels that exceed the body's ability to metabolize and burn them, may produce acetone, which gives the breath of diabetics a sweet odor. A buildup of acetone can lead to ketoacidosis, a pathologic condition in which the blood pH drops from 7.4 to 6.8. Complications arising from diabetes also include blindness, kidney disease, and nerve damage. Furthermore, resulting peripheral vascular disease, in which the body's extremities do not get enough blood, leads to tissue death and gangrene.

Perspective and Prospects

The study of food biochemistry has evolved over the years from a strictly biochemical approach to one in which diet and nutrition play a major role. An understanding of diet and nutrition required vital information about the metabolic processes occurring in the cell, supplied by the field of biochemistry.

This information started to become available in 1898 when Eduard Buchner discovered that the fermentation of glucose to alcohol and carbon dioxide could occur in a cell-free extract. The early 1900's led to the complete discovery of the glycolytic pathway and the enzymes that were involved in the process. In the 1930's, other pathways of metabolism were elucidated.

In conjunction with Buchner's discovery, British physician Archibald Garrod in 1909 hypothesized that genes control a person's appearance through enzymes that catalyze certain metabolic processes in the cell. Garrod thought that some inherited diseases resulted from a patient's inability to make a particular enzyme, and he called them "inborn errors of metabolism." One example he gave was a condition called alkaptonuria, in which the urine turns black upon exposure to the air.

Some of the earliest nutritional studies date back to the time of Aristotle, who knew that raw liver contained an ingredient that could cure night blindness. Christiaan Eijkman studied beriberi in the Dutch East Indies and traced the problem to diet. Sir Frederick Hopkins was an English biochemist who conducted pioneering work on vitamins and the essentiality of amino acids in the early 1900's. Hopkins realized that the type of protein is important in the diet as well as the quantity. Hopkins hypothesized that some trace substance in addition to proteins, fats, and carbohydrates may be required in the diet for growth; this substance was later identified as the vitamin. Hopkins was the first biochemist to explore diet and metabolic function.

Working with this broad base, scientists have made tremendous advances in the study of diet and nutrition based on the biochemistry of the cell. In 1943, the first recommended daily (or dietary) allowances (RDAs) were published. They provide standards for diet and good nutrition and are revised every five years as new information becomes available. The RDAs suggest the amounts of protein, fats, carbohydrates, vitamins, and minerals required for adequate nutrient uptake. The major uses of the RDAs are for schools and other institutions in planning menus, obtaining food supplies, and preparing food labels.

Since the 1970's, research has consistently associated nutritional factors with six of the ten leading causes of death in the United States: high blood pressure, heart disease, cancer, cardiovascular disease, chronic liver disease, and non-insulin-dependent diabetes mellitus. This research has led to improvements in the American diet.

—*Lonnie J. Guralnick, Ph.D.*

See also Antioxidants; Caffeine; Cholesterol; Cytology; Diabetes mellitus; Digestion; Enzymes; Fatty acid oxidation disorders; Glycogen storage diseases; Glycolysis; Lactose intolerance; Malnutrition; Metabolism; Nutrition; Phenylketonuria (PKU); Phytochemicals; Supplements; Vitamins and minerals.

For Further Information:

American Dietetic Association Complete Food and Nutrition Guide. 2d ed. New York: Wiley, 2002. Experts from the American Dietetic Association detail advances in nutrition research and provide authoritative answers to questions regarding food and nutrition.

Bonci, Leslie. *American Dietetic Association Guide to Better Digestion.* New York: Wiley, 2003. A user-friendly guide to help analyze one's eating habits, map out a dietary plan to manage and reduce the uncomfortable symptoms of digestive disorders, and find practical recommendations for implementing lifestyle changes.

Campbell, Neil A. *Biology: Concepts and Connections.* 4th ed. Redwood City, Calif.: Benjamin/Cummings, 2002. An introductory college textbook geared for the biology major but easily understood by the high school student. One chapter covers the process of digestion and nutritional requirements. References at the end of the chapter are provided for further reading. Contains useful tables and diagrams.

Clark, Nancy. *Sports Nutrition Guidebook: Eating to Fuel Your Active Lifestyle.* Rev. ed. Champaign, Ill.: Leisure Press, 1996. An easy-to-read book that covers the subject of nutrition for the sports-minded reader. Dispels a number of nutritional myths. Explores many applications of food biochemistry, and offers recipes and references in the appendix.

Lehninger, Albert L. "Human Nutrition." In *Principles of Biochemistry.* New York: Worth, 1982. A well-written chapter in an elementary biochemistry college textbook. Easy to read even for the beginner who has little understanding of biochemistry. References are included at the end of the chapter.

Margen, Sheldon. *Wellness Foods A to Z: An Indispensable Guide for Health-Conscious Food Lovers.* New York: Rebus, 2002. In encyclopedic format, offers a nutritional and market profile of the health benefits of myriad foods; a guide to food groups, vitamins and minerals, and herbs and spices; how to read food labels; and a cooking glossary.

Nasset, Edmund S. *Nutrition Handbook.* 3d ed. New York: Harper & Row, 1982. A small, easy-to-read book that describes the three classes of nutrients. Covers digestion and absorption, and discusses how the body utilizes nutrients and vitamins. A valuable glossary is provided at the end of the book.

Nieman, David C., Diane E. Butterworth, and Catherine N. Nieman. *Nutrition.* Dubuque, Iowa: Wm. C. Brown, 1990. A good textbook that links food biochemistry to health and nutrition. Chapters 5, 6, and 7 cover the basics on carbohydrates, lipids, and proteins. Easy to read, with an excellent chapter outline at the beginning of each chapter. Tables and diagrams are included.

Food poisoning
Disease/disorder

Anatomy or system affected: Gastrointestinal system, intestines, stomach

Specialties and related fields: Environmental health, epidemiology, gastroenterology, public health, toxicology

Definition: Food-borne illness caused by bacteria, viruses, or parasites consumed in food and resulting in acute gastrointestinal disturbance that may include diarrhea, nausea, vomiting, and abdominal discomfort.

Key terms:

contamination: infection of a food item by a pathogen

food-borne infection: disease caused by eating foods contaminated by infectious microorganisms, with onset occurring within twenty-four hours (for example, salmonellosis)

food-borne intoxication: disease caused by eating foods containing microorganisms that produce toxins, with onset occurring within six hours (for example, botulism)

microorganism: an organism which is too small to be seen with the naked eye

parasite: an organism which lives on another organism (the host) and causes harm to the host while it benefits

pathogen: a disease-causing organism

thermal death point: the lowest temperature that can destroy a food-borne organism

Causes and Symptoms

Often a person feeling the symptoms of nausea, vomiting, diarrhea, and abdominal discomfort assumes that he or she has contracted influenza. The presence of a true influenza virus, however, is uncommon. More likely, these symptoms are caused by eating food that contains undesirable bacteria, viruses, or parasites. This is called food-borne illness, or food poisoning. Most food-borne pathogens are colorless, odorless, and tasteless. Fortunately, there are recommendations based on scientific principles to help prevent food-borne illness.

Food poisoning is a worldwide problem. In developing countries, diarrhea is a factor in child malnutrition and is estimated to cause 3.5 million deaths per year. Despite advances in modern technology, food-borne illness is a major problem in developed countries as well. In the United States, an estimated 24 million cases of food-borne diarrheal disease occur each year, which means that about one out of ten people experience a food-associated illness in a given year.

Certain foods, particularly foods with a high protein and moisture content, provide an ideal environment for the multiplication of pathogens. The foods with high risk in the United States are raw shellfish (especially mollusks), underdone poultry, raw eggs, rare meats, raw milk, and cooked food that another person handled before it was packaged and chilled. In addition to those foods listed, some developing countries could add raw vegetables, raw fruits that cannot be peeled, foods from sidewalk vendors, and tap water or water from unknown sources. Most of the documented cases of food-borne illness are caused by only a few bacteria, viruses, and parasites.

Bacteria known as *Salmonella* are ingested by humans in contaminated foods such as beef, poultry, and eggs; they may also be transmitted by kitchen utensils and the hands of people who have handled infected food or utensils. Once the bacteria are inside the body, the incubation time is from eight to twenty-four hours. Since the bacteria multiply inside the body and attack the gastrointestinal tract, this disease is known as a true food infection. The main symptoms are diarrhea, abdominal cramps, and vomiting. The bacteria are killed by cooking foods to the well-done stage.

The major food-borne intoxication in the United States is caused by eating food contaminated with the toxin of *Staphylococcus* bacteria. Because the toxin or poison has already been produced in the food item that is ingested, the onset of symptoms is usually very rapid (between one-half hour and six hours). Improperly stored or cooked foods (particularly meats, tuna, and potato salad) are the main carriers of these bacteria. Since this toxin cannot be killed by reheating the food items to a high temperature, it is important that foods are properly stored.

Botulism is a rare food poisoning caused by the toxin of *Clostridium botulinum*. It is anaerobic, meaning that it multiplies in environments without oxygen, and is mainly found in improperly home-canned food items. Originally one of the sources of the disease was from eating sausages (the Latin word for which is *botulus*)—hence, the name "botulism." A very small amount of toxin, the size of a grain of salt, could kill hundreds of people within an hour. Danger signs include double vision and difficulty swallowing and breathing.

Though everyone is at risk for food-borne illness, certain groups of people develop more severe symptoms and are at a greater risk for serious illness and death. Higher-risk groups include pregnant women, very young children, the elderly, and immunocompromised individuals, such as patients with acquired immunodeficiency syndrome (AIDS) and cancer.

Bacteria known as *Listeria* were first documented in 1981 as being transmitted by food. Most people are at low risk of becoming ill after ingesting these bacteria; however, pregnant women are at high risk. *Listeria* infection is rare in the United States, but it does cause serious illness. It is associated with consumption of raw (unpasteurized) milk, nonreheated hot dogs, undercooked chicken, various soft cheeses (Mexican style, feta, Brie, Camembert, and blue-veined cheese), and food purchased from delicatessen counters. *Listeria* cause a short-term illness in pregnant women; however, this bacteria can cause stillbirths and spontaneous abortions. A parasite called *Toxoplasma gondii* is also of particular risk for pregnant women. For this reason, raw or very rare meat should not be eaten. (In addition, since cats may shed these parasites in their feces, it is recommended that pregnant women avoid cleaning cat litter boxes.)

As the protective antibodies from the mother are lost, infants become more susceptible to food poisoning. Botulism generally occurs by ingesting the toxin or poison; however, in infant botulism it is the spores that germinate and produce the toxin within the intestinal tract of the infant. Since honey and corn syrup have been found to contain spores, it is recommended that they not be fed to infants under one year of age, especially those under six months.

Determining whether a disease is caused by a food-borne organism is highly skilled work. The Centers for Disease Control (CDC) in Atlanta, Georgia, investigate diseases and their causes. It has been estimated that the true incidence of food-borne illness in the United States is ten to one hundred times greater than that reported to the CDC. The CDC report some of the more interesting cases and outbreaks in narrative form in the *Morbidity and Mortality Weekly Report*.

TREATMENT AND THERAPY

In cases of severe food poisoning marked by vomiting, diarrhea, or collapse—especially in cases of botulism and ingestion of poisonous plant material such as suspicious mushrooms—emergency medical attention should be sought immediately, and, if possible, specimens of the suspected food should be submitted for analysis. Identifying the source of the food is especially

---

INFORMATION ON FOOD POISONING

CAUSES: Bacteria, viruses, or parasites consumed in food

SYMPTOMS: Diarrhea, nausea, vomiting, fever, abdominal discomfort

DURATION: One to three days

TREATMENTS: Rest, avoidance of food, extra fluid intake

important if that source is a public venue such as a restaurant, because stemming a widespread outbreak of food poisoning may thereby be possible. In less severe cases of food poisoning, the victim should rest, eat nothing, but drink fluids that contain some salt and sugar; the person should begin to recover after several hours or one or two days and should see a doctor if not well after two or three days.

The best "treatment" for food poisoning is prevention. While there is ample information regarding the prevention of food poisoning, many outbreaks still occur as a result of carelessness in the kitchen. Good food safety is basically good common sense, yet it can make sense only when one has acquired some knowledge of how food-borne pathogens spread and how to apply food safety steps to prevent food-borne illness. Based on the research literature, as well as on the suggestions made by the World Health Organization (WHO) and other groups, the recommendations are to cook foods well, to prevent cross-contamination, and to keep hot foods hot and cold foods cold.

Cooking foods well means cooking them to a high enough temperature in the slowest-to-heat part and for a long enough time to destroy pathogens that have already gained access to foods. Cooking foods well is only a concern when they have become previously contaminated from other sources or are naturally contaminated. There are a number of possible sources of contamination of food products.

Coastal water may contaminate seafood. Filter-feeding marine animals (such as clams, scallops, oysters, cockles, and mussels) and some fish (such as anchovies, sardines, and herring) live by pumping in seawater and sifting out organisms that they need for food. Therefore, they have the ability to concentrate suspended material by many orders of magnitude. Shellfish grown in contaminated coastal waters are the most frequent carriers of a virus called hepatitis A.

Contaminated eggs can be another vehicle of food-borne illness. Contamination of eggs can occur from external as well as internal sources. If moist conditions are present and there is a crack in the shell, the fecal material of hens carrying the microorganism can penetrate the shell and membrane of the egg and can multiply. In the early 1990's, *Salmonella enteritidis* began to appear in the intact egg, particularly in the northeastern part of the United States. It is hypothesized that contamination occurs in the oviduct of the hen before the egg is laid. Food vehicles in which *Salmonella enteritidis* has been reported include sandwiches dipped in eggs and cooked, hollandaise sauce, eggs Benedict, commercial frozen pasta with raw egg and cheese stuffing, Caesar salad dressing, and blended food in which cross-contamination had occurred. Foods such as cookie or cake dough or homemade ice cream made with raw eggs are other possible vehicles of food-borne illness.

Milk, especially raw milk, can be contaminated. Sources of milk contaminants could be an unhealthy cow (such as from mastitis, a major infection of the mammary gland of the dairy cow) or unclean methods of milking, such as not cleaning the teats well before attaching them to the milker or unclean utensils (milking tanks). If milk is not cooled fast enough, contaminants can multiply.

Modern mechanized milking procedures have reduced but not eliminated food-borne pathogens. Post-pasteurization contamination may occur, especially if bulk tanks or equipment have not been properly cleaned and sanitized. In 1985 in Chicago, one of the largest salmonellosis outbreaks occurred, with the causal food being pasteurized milk. More than sixteen thousand people were infected, and ten died. A small connecting piece in the milk tank which allowed milk and microorganisms to collect was determined to be the source of the contamination. Bulk tanks should be properly maintained and piping should be inspected regularly for opportunities for raw milk to contaminate the pasteurized product.

Recommendations for cooking temperatures are based not only on the temperature required to kill food-borne pathogens but also on aesthetics and palatability. Generally, a margin of safety is built into the cooking temperature because of the possibility of nonuniform heating. Based on generally accepted temperature requirements, cooking red meat until 71 degrees Celsius (160 degrees Fahrenheit) will reach the thermal death point. Hamburger should be well cooked so that it is medium-brown inside. If pressed, it should feel firm and the juices that run out should be clear. Cooking poultry to the well-done stage is done for palatability. Tenderness is indicated when there is a flexible hip joint, and juices should run clear and not pink when the meat is pierced with a fork. Fish should be cooked until it loses its translucent appearance and flakes when pierced with a fork. Eggs should be thoroughly cooked until the yolk is thickened and the white is firm, not runny. Cooked or chilled foods that are served hot (that is, leftovers) should be reheated so that they come to a rolling boil.

Cross-contamination occurs when microorganisms are transmitted from humans, cutting boards, and utensils to food. Contamination between foods, especially from raw meat and poultry to fresh vegetables or other ready-to-eat foods, is a major problem.

One of the best ways to prevent cross-contamination is simply washing one's hands with soap and water. Twenty seconds is the minimum time span that should be spent washing one's hands. In order to prevent the spread of disease, it is also recommended that the hands be dried with a paper towel, which is then thrown away. Thoroughly washed hands can still be a source of bacteria, however, so one should use tongs and spoons when cooking to prevent contamination.

It is especially important to wash one's hands after certain activities, such as blowing the nose or sneezing, using the lavatory, diapering a baby, smoking, petting animals or pets, and before cooking or handling food.

Other sources of cross-contamination include utensils and cutting surfaces. If people use the same knife and cutting board to cut up raw chicken for a stir-fry and peaches for a fruit salad, they are putting themselves at great risk for food-borne illness. The bacteria on the cutting board and the knife could cross-contaminate the peaches. While the chicken will be cooked until it is well done, the peaches in the salad will not be. In this situation, one could cut the fruit first and then the chicken, and then wash and sanitize the knife and cutting board.

Cleaning and sanitizing is actually a two-step process. Cleaning involves using soap and water and a scrubber or dishcloth to remove the major debris from the surface. The second step, sanitizing, involves using a diluted chloride solution to kill bacteria and viruses.

Wooden cutting boards are the worst offenders in terms of causing cross-contamination. Since bacteria and viruses are small, they can adhere to and grow in the grooves of a wooden cutting board and spread to other foods when the cutting board is used again. Use of a plastic or acrylic cutting board prevents this problem.

The danger zone in which bacteria can multiply is a range of 4.4 degrees Celsius (40 degrees Fahrenheit) to 60 degrees Celsius (140 degrees Fahrenheit). Room temperature is generally right in the middle of this danger zone. The danger zone is critical because, even though they cannot be seen, bacteria are increasing in number. They can double and even quadruple in fifteen to thirty minutes. Consequently, perishable foods such as meats, poultry, fish, milk, cooked rice, leftover pizza, hard-cooked eggs, leftover refried beans, and potato salad should not be left in the danger zone for more than two hours. Keeping hot foods hot means keeping them at a temperature higher than 60 degrees Celsius.

Keeping cold foods cold means keeping them at a temperature lower than 4.4 degrees Celsius.

Other rules are helpful for preventing contamination. When shopping, the grocery store should be the last stop so that foods are not stored in a hot car. When meal time is over, leftovers should be placed in the refrigerator or freezer as soon as possible. When packing for a picnic, food items should be kept in an ice chest to keep them cold or brought slightly frozen. Much serious illness and death could be prevented if such food safety rules were followed.

PERSPECTIVE AND PROSPECTS

When the lifestyle of people changed from a hunting-and-gathering society to a more agrarian one, the need to preserve food from spoilage was necessary for survival. As early as 3000 B.C.E., salt was used as a meat preservative and the production of cheese had begun in the Near East. The production of wine and the preservation of fish by smoking also were introduced at that time. Even though throughout history people had tried many methods to preserve foods and keep them from spoiling, the relationship between illness and pathogens or toxins in food was not recognized and documented until 1857. It was then that the French chemist Louis Pasteur demonstrated that the microorganisms in raw milk caused spoilage.

Stories from the American Civil War (1860-1865) demonstrate the problems of institutional feeding of many people for long periods of time. Gastrointestinal diseases were rampant during that time period. During the first year of the war, of the people who had diarrhea and dysentery, the morbidity rate was 640 per 1,000 and increased to 995 per 1,000 in 1862. More men died of disease and illness than were killed in battle.

Food can be contaminated by disease-causing organisms at any step of the food-handling chain, from the farm to the table. An important role of government and industry is to ensure a safe food supply. In the United States, setting and monitoring of food safety standards are the responsibility of the Food and Drug Administration (FDA) under the auspices of the U.S. Department of Health and Human Services and the Food Safety and Inspection Service (FSIS) under the auspices of the U.S. Department of Agriculture (USDA). The FDA is responsible for the wholesomeness of all food sold in interstate commerce, except meat and poultry, while the USDA is responsible for the inspection of meat and poultry sold in interstate commerce and internationally. Some major food safety laws and policies that have guided the provision of safe food are the Federal Food and Drugs Act in 1906; the Federal Meat Inspection Act in 1906-1907; the Food, Drug, and Cosmetic Act in 1938; and the Poultry Products Inspection Act in 1957. The food supply in the United States has been credited as being among the safest in the world.

Historically, the diseases of tuberculosis, scarlet fever, strep throat, typhoid fever, and diphtheria have been associated with raw or unpasteurized milk. The reporting of food-borne illness was initiated in the 1920's by the U.S. Public Health Service (USPHS) when annual summaries of outbreaks of milk-borne disease were recorded and reported. Later, reports of waterborne and food-borne diseases were added.

The public attitude about what is hazardous in the food supply and that of the FDA have often differed. The public generally believes that the safety of additives and chemical contaminants in food is of a higher priority than that of the microbiological and nutritional hazards—the exact opposite of the FDA's priorities. (For example, in the mid-1980's, the story about Alar, a chemical used to slow the ripening of apples, represented a very emotional topic. There was particular concern about the risks that this chemical might pose to children who ate large amounts of apple products.) As more reliable information is available about both areas of concern, the situation regarding priorities is likely to change.

—Martha M. Henze, M.S., R.D.;
updated by Maria Pacheco, Ph.D.

See also Bacterial infections; Biological and chemical weapons; Botulism; Diarrhea and dysentery; *E. coli* infection; Gangrene; Gastroenterology; Gastroenterology, pediatric; Gastrointestinal disorders; Gastrointestinal system; Indigestion; Intestinal disorders; Intestines; Lead poisoning; Nausea and vomiting; Noroviruses; Parasitic diseases; Poisoning; Salmonella infection; Shigellosis; Trichinosis; Ulcers; Viral infections.

For Further Information:

Cliver, Dean O., ed. *Foodborne Diseases.* 2d ed. San Diego, Calif.: Academic Press, 2002. An exceptional college textbook providing chapters written by experts in the field. This important work provides not only background information but also in-depth reference information on the most common food-borne pathogens.

Food and Drug Administration Center for Food Safety and Applied Nutrition. http://vm.cfsan.fda.gov/list .html. Site provides information on food safety, nutrition, and wholesomeness, as well as the regulation of cosmetics safety.

Gaman, P. M. *The Science of Food: An Introduction to Food Science, Nutrition, and Microbiology.* 4th ed. New York: Pergamon Press, 1996. An easy-to-read book dealing with food composition and microbiology. Includes good bibliographical references and an index.

Hobbs, Betty C. *Food Poisoning and Food Hygiene.* London: Edward Arnold, 1993. A nontechnical handbook of the causes of food poisoning and other food-borne diseases for those in the fields of food microbiology and food hygiene. Emphasis is given to the main aspects of hygiene necessary for the production, preparation, sale, and service of safe and palatable food.

Jay, James Monroe. *Modern Food Microbiology.* 6th ed. New York: Van Nostrand Reinhold, 2000. This excellent textbook summarizes the current state of knowledge of the biology and epidemiology of the microorganisms that cause food-borne illness.

Leon, Warren, and Caroline Smith DeWaal. *Is Our Food Safe? A Consumer's Guide to Protecting Your Health and the Environment.* New York: Crown, 2002. Focuses on three themes—food safety and food-borne illnesses, environmental aspects of food choices, and sound diet and nutrition—and answers common questions about the safety of meat, dairy products, fish, fruits, and other foods that make up American diets.

Longree, Karla, and Gertrude Armbruster. *Quantity Food Sanitation.* 5th ed. New York: John Wiley & Sons, 1996. An excellent reference guide on food safety for quantity cooking in institutions such as hospitals and restaurants.

Marriot, Norman G. *Principles of Food Sanitation.* 4th ed. New York: Chapman and Hall, 1999. A reference work that provides students and food industry personnel with the information necessary to ensure hygienic practices in food production and specific directions for applying these fundamentals to attain hygienic conditions in various food processing and food preparation facilities.

Nestle, Marion. *Safe Food: Bacteria, Biotechnology, and Bioterrorism.* Berkeley: University of California Press, 2003. Argues that ensuring safe food involves politics, its connections with industry, government, and consumers, and issues of values, economics, and political power.

Ray, Bibek. *Fundamental Food Microbiology*. 2d ed. Boca Raton, Fla.: CRC Press, 2001. A comprehensive text on the basic principles of food microbiology. Includes bibliographical references and an index.

U.S. Department of Agriculture/Food and Drug Administration Foodborne Illness Education Information Center. http://www.nalusda.gov/fnic/foodborne/foodborn.htm. Site provides information on foodborne illnesses.

Wilson, Michael, Brian Henderson, and Rod McNab. *Bacterial Virulence Mechanisms*. New York: Cambridge University Press, 2002. Basing their discussion on research advances in microbiology, molecular biology, and cell biology, the authors describe the interactions that exist between bacteria and human cells both in health and during infection.

FOOT DISORDERS
DISEASE/DISORDER

ANATOMY OR SYSTEM AFFECTED: Bones, feet, muscles, musculoskeletal system

SPECIALTIES AND RELATED FIELDS: Orthopedics, podiatry

DEFINITION: Disorders involving the muscles, bones, nerves, or skin of the feet.

Because of the constant and heavy use of feet by humans as bipeds, they are prone to many problems. In spite of what is commonly believed, most cases of foot bone and joint abnormalities are developmental in origin instead of being caused by poorly fitting footwear.

Developmental, muscle, and bone disorders of the feet. Clubfoot, also called talipes, is one of the developmental, or congenital, disorders affecting the feet. It occurs in approximately 1 of every 1,000 live human births and is characterized by deformities such as the

---

> ### INFORMATION ON FOOT DISORDERS
>
> **CAUSES:** Congenital and developmental factors, improper footwear, muscle weakness, incorrect weight-bearing, short Achilles tendon, nerve disorders, dermatologic disorders
>
> **SYMPTOMS:** Pain, swelling, limping, numbness, tingling
>
> **DURATION:** Short-term or chronic
>
> **TREATMENTS:** Medication, ointments, surgery, orthopedic footwear

foot turning down and under, such that a child will walk on the top of his or her foot. Over time, tendon and ligament contraction reinforces the deformity; thus, either casting or surgery is needed for realignment.

Flat foot, or pes planus, is an abnormally flat arch in the foot, accompanied by a characteristic gait, both of which can occur in varying degrees. Muscle weakness, incorrect weight-bearing, a short Achilles tendon, and developmental defects may all contribute to this deformity. Flat foot may or may not produce a pathologic condition such as arthritis.

A bunion is the relocation of bone from the first metatarsal to the inner portion of the joint connecting it to the big toe. This prominence at the base of the big toe makes the soft tissue in the area subject to pressure from shoes, causing swelling and pain in the protective sac above the metatarsophalangeal joint in a condition called bursitis. Cortisone injections may relieve symptoms, but surgery is required in extreme cases to realign the first metatarsal. Flat foot usually accompanies bunions and is a factor in their development.

Muscular imbalances inherent in the foot are the reason for the curvature of the individual bones of the toes. Abnormally curved bones produce hammertoe, or claw

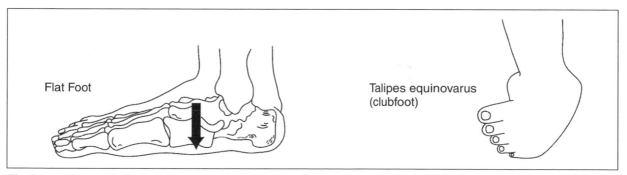

Flat feet, or abnormally flat arches, can arise from muscle weakness, improper walking, or developmental defects. Clubfoot is a congenital disorder that may require surgical realignment.

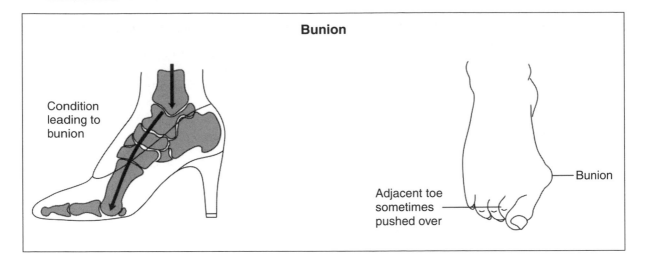

Bunion

Condition leading to bunion

Adjacent toe sometimes pushed over

Bunion

toe, which usually requires little treatment other than a padding of the shoes to avoid corn or callus development. Excessive muscle tension at the heel can produce bony growths called heel spurs or calcaneal exostoses. Inflammation may develop in a neighboring joint's bursa, causing a throbbing pain.

Apophysitis of the calcaneus or heel bone can occur in childhood while the heel is still in the process of fusing from two bones. Injury can result because the connecting, softer cartilage between the two bones has not yet been replaced with bone. This affliction usually disappears as a child grows.

Nerve and skin disorders of the feet. Factors including footwear, the structures of the foot itself, and harmful external forces acting on the foot may all contribute to the irritation and/or damage to the nerves of the foot. Morton's neuroma is the thickening of the nerve located between the metatarsals of the third and fourth toes, followed by the formation of a small benign tumor. Painful burning, numbness, or tingling sensations may be alleviated by wearing more comfortable footwear or by the surgical removal of the tumor. Tarsal tunnel syndrome occurs when a nerve traveling along the bottom of the foot through a channel called the tarsal canal becomes compressed and damaged. Cortisone injections into this canal can relieve pressure on the nerve, and surgery can be used to treat severe cases.

The skin of the foot is subject to much pressure and rubbing; thus, it responds by producing changes, termed dermatologic disorders, which themselves cause pain. A corn, or heloma, is a small, sharply defined, raised area of thickened skin containing much of the fibrous protein called keratin. Calluses are also composed of keratin but are flatter and do not possess the defined borders of corns. Both types of thickened keratinized skin are usually attributed to incorrect positioning of the underlying bone.

Warts, or verrucae, are actually skin tumors caused by the human papillomavirus. They occur most commonly on the sole of the foot, where they are named plantar warts. Warts can be transmitted from person to person, and the lymphatic communication between warts within an individual explains their ability to spread. Warts on the foot are invariably benign, however, and should not be treated with X-ray or radium therapy lest the surrounding areas undergo change themselves and eventually produce tumors.

Dermatitis venenata is often caused by chemicals used in the binding or dyeing of shoes. Angiokeratoma is a lesion on the bottom of the foot commonly mistaken for a wart. Fibroma is the name of the benign growth that may spread under the toenails as a result of insect bites in the vicinity or manifestations of other skin diseases.

Ingrown toenails, or onychocryptoses, occur when the free end of the toenail penetrates the surrounding soft tissue. Reasons for this painful disorder are commonly badly fitted footwear, nail disease, and foot or nail structural abnormalities.

Systemic diseases affecting the feet. Rheumatoid arthritis is a condition involving connective tissue, unknown in origin, in which the synovial membrane of joints proliferates while invading and even destroying cartilage and bone. Women acquire this disease three times more often than do men. Steroid hormones are sometimes applied to aid in the treatment of rheumatoid arthritis, but gold salt injection is the only therapy resulting in a permanent cure. The chances of a cure are greater when this disease occurs in children. The condition is then known as juvenile rheumatoid arthritis, or Still's disease.

Several normally fatal diseases may accompany rheumatoid arthritis. Systemic lupus erythematosus can be masked by the arthritic condition until inflammation spreads to small arteries of the body's organs. Polyarteritis nodosa also involves arteries throughout the body, and its true diagnosis may be prevented by the misleading arthritic condition. Scleroderma involves the thickening of the skin on the face, hands, and feet; depigmentation; loss of hair; and lesions. Sarcoidosis manifests itself in the hands and feet and causes microscopic lesions in the bone that eventually become visible by X-ray examination. Schoenlein-Henoch syndrome is an allergic reaction which can resemble the synovitis of rheumatic fever.

Rheumatic fever affects fibrous tissues in a widespread fashion involving the joints and later the heart. It is related to streptococcal infections and occurs as a migrating arthritis producing no lasting joint damage in the feet, but it can cause permanent damage to the cardiac valve. Osteoarthritis causes the degeneration of cartilage and the overgrowth of bone surfaces. The effects of this condition are limited to the joints, unlike rheumatoid arthritis, which can spread to nearby cartilage and bone. Staphylococci, streptococci, and coliform bacteria are the infective agents involved in pyogenic arthritis. In this condition, the organism is carried by the blood to the joint interior. Ulcers of the feet may be caused by a variety of conditions including diabetes mellitus, syphilis, anemia, and leprosy.

If there is sustained pain in the foot or ankle with no known cause such as injury, a continuously low leukocyte count, and negative laboratory tests for the presence of bacteria, then a viral infection is likely present. An elevated leukocyte count is often indicative of a bacterial infection.

—*Ryan C. Horst and Roman J. Miller, Ph.D.*

See also Athlete's foot; Birth defects; Bones and the skeleton; Bunions; Feet; Flat feet; Fracture and dislocation; Frostbite; Fungal infections; Ganglion removal; Gout; Hammertoe correction; Hammertoes; Heel spur removal; Lower extremities; Nail removal; Nails; Orthopedic surgery; Orthopedics; Orthopedics, pediatric; Podiatry; Tendon repair; Warts.

FOR FURTHER INFORMATION:

American Podiatric Medical Association. http://www .apma.org/foot.html.

Copeland, Glenn, and Stan Solomon. *The Foot Doctor.* Emmaus, Pa.: Rodale Press, 1986.

Lippert, Frederick G., and Sigvard T. Hansen. *Foot and Ankle Disorders: Tricks of the Trade.* New York: Thieme, 2003.

Lorimer, Donald L., ed. *Neal's Common Foot Disorders: Diagnosis and Management.* 6th ed. New York: Churchill Livingstone, 2001.

Van De Graaff, Kent M. *Human Anatomy.* 5th ed. Dubuque, Iowa: Wm. C. Brown, 2000.

FORENSIC PATHOLOGY

SPECIALTY

ANATOMY OR SYSTEM AFFECTED: All

SPECIALTIES AND RELATED FIELDS: Dentistry, epidemiology, hematology, histology, pathology, psychology, public health, pulmonary medicine, serology, toxicology

DEFINITION: A science that brings medical knowledge to bear in order to resolve legal issues, usually through the performance of an autopsy.

KEY TERMS:

anthropology: the study of human remains, especially skeletal ones

autopsy: the examination of a body to determine the cause and circumstances of death

forensic: having to do or in connection with the operation of the law, usually criminal law

histology: the microscopic study of plant and animal tissue

odontology: the study of teeth

pathology: the study of disease and the deviations from normalcy that it causes

psychiatry: the medical discipline concerned with mental, emotional, and behavioral disorders

serology: the study of body fluids

toxicology: the study of poisons and their effects

trace evidence: minute, often microscopic, signs or indications of an event or a presence

SCIENCE AND PROFESSION

Forensic medicine probably is best known to most people because of the work of forensic pathologists, principally for the autopsies that they perform as coroners and medical examiners. Other experts, however, also are key participants in the field. They include anthropologists, histologists, odontologists, psychiatrists, serologists, toxicologists, police officers, and specialists in trace evidence. Except for the forensic psychiatrist, who is called on to determine the sanity of an accused individual and thus that person's fitness to stand trial, the above-listed specialists generally do not become involved in the work of forensic medicine until a death has occurred that obviously is other than from natural causes.

In the United States, a forensic pathologist is a medical doctor who typically will spend three to four years preparing in that field after being graduated from medical school and two or so years beyond that before being certified by the American Society of Clinical Pathologists. Other forensic specialties generally require a four-year college degree as well as specialized training after that.

Forensic medicine is not a crowded field. Indeed, there is a shortage of trained and qualified people because most such jobs are in the public sector, where salaries are good but not as high as similar skills and knowledge will command in the private sector. Those who choose careers in forensic medicine, however, find the fascinating and exciting work, intellectual challenge, and personal satisfaction that private-sector jobs seldom offer.

DUTIES AND INVESTIGATIVE TECHNIQUES

As a general rule, the coroner, supported to a greater or lesser extent by one or more of the specialists listed above, will become involved in a death when a person dies of criminal or other violent means, by suicide, suddenly when in apparent good health, or in any suspicious or unusual manner. In such a case, the coroner typically is charged by law with determining the cause, mode, and manner of death, with each of those terms having a specific meaning. The physical cause of death is a purely medical determination. Legal considerations, on the other hand, are broader and more inclusive.

Both medical and legal aspects, however, are so interrelated that they cannot be separated. For example, to determine the physical cause of death, it would be sufficient to show a penetrating wound to the heart. To determine the mode of death, however, it would be necessary to establish whether the wound was caused by a bullet or a sharp instrument. An autopsy would reveal the mode of death. The next question is legal: What was the manner of death? In other words, how was the wound inflicted? Was it self-inflicted? If it was, was it intentional (suicide) or accidental? If it was inflicted by another person, was it an accident or was it homicide? Investigation of the scene where the injury was sustained, examination of the evidence found there, and

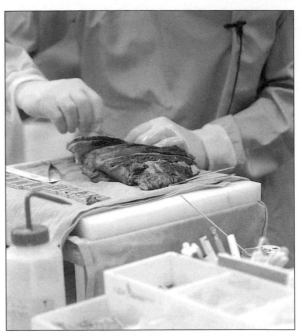

A pathologist studies a tissue sample. (PhotoDisc)

statements of witnesses would furnish information as to the circumstances of the incident.

The actual autopsy involves the dissection and examination of a dead body—surgery performed postmortem. It begins with what is called a gross examination—that is, a visual examination with the naked eye, first externally and then internally. For the internal examination, a Y-shaped incision is made beginning at each shoulder, running down to and meeting just below the sternum or breastbone and continuing as a single cut down to the lower portion of the abdomen just above the genital area. Rib cutters are used to expose the thoracic area. The internal organs are removed and examined. Fluids are drawn for laboratory tests, and tissue samples are taken for microscopic examination. Access to the brain is gained by using a small powersaw to remove the top part of the skull. The third portion of the autopsy involves the toxicological examination of body fluids, including blood, urine, and the vitreous humor of the eye. After examination, the body is restored, and the incisions are carefully sewn.

PERSPECTIVE AND PROSPECTS

Probably the first well-known person to be the subject of a postmortem examination was Julius Caesar. A physician named Antisius determined that of the twenty-three wounds that Caesar sustained, the one that perforated the thorax was the cause of death. The Justinian

Code of the sixth century required the opinion of a physician in certain circumstances and often is credited as the first recognition of the correlation of law and medicine in effecting legal justice. By the sixteenth century in England, investigations were being made by a representative of the king, who had the title of *Custos Placitorum Coronae* (guardian of the decrees of the crown), from which comes the word "coroner." It is believed that William Penn appointed the first coroner in the American colonies. In the nineteenth century, forensic medicine became established as a distinct specialty and has continued to mature into the advanced and sophisticated field that it is today.

The capabilities of and advances in forensic medicine traditionally are tied to those of science in general and applicable medical specialties. They set the pace for the development of forensic medicine. The future should prove no different. The advances in overall knowledge of deoxyribonucleic acid (DNA), the development of scanning electron microscopy, improvements in spectrographic analysis, and advances in computer graphics capabilities, for example, occurred outside the field of forensic medicine and subsequently were adopted by it.

—John M. Shaw;
updated by Karen E. Kalumuck, Ph.D.

See also Anatomy; Autopsy; Death and dying; DNA and RNA; Histology; Laboratory tests; Law and medicine; Pathology; Suicide; Toxicology.

FOR FURTHER INFORMATION:

Browning, Michael, and William R. Maples. *Dead Men Do Tell Tales: The Strange and Fascinating Cases of a Forensic Anthropologist*. New York: Main Street Books, 1995. From a skeleton, a skull, a mere fragment of burnt thighbone, Dr. Maples can deduce the age, gender, and ethnicity of a murder victim, the manner in which the person was dispatched, and, ultimately, the identity of the killer.

Camenson, Blythe, and Anita Hufft. *Opportunities in Forensic Science Careers*. New York: McGraw-Hill, 2001. Provides those seeking a career in forensics with information on training and education requirements and salary statistics, and lists professional and Internet resources.

Evans, Colin. *The Casebook of Forensic Detection: How Science Solved One Hundred of the World's Most Baffling Crimes*. New York: John Wiley & Sons, 1996. This book describes the development of forensics from the nineteenth century to the present. Cases are classified by fifteen forensic types then arranged chronologically.

Genge, N. E. *The Forensic Casebook: The Science of Crime Scene Investigation*. New York: Random House, 2002. Uses true crime stories and draws on interviews with police personnel and forensic scientists—including animal examiners, botanists, zoologists, firearms specialists, and autoposists—to provide an encyclopedic view of the underworkings of criminal investigation.

James, Stuart H., and Jon J. Nordby. *Forensic Science: An Introduction to Scientific and Investigative Techniques*. Boca Raton, Fla.: CRC Press, 2002. An introductory text that covers a range of topics, including trace evidence, forensic toxicology, DNA analysis, crime scene investigation, fingerprints, traumatic death, forensic anthropology, bloodstain patterns, and criminal profiling, among many others.

Joyce, Christopher, and Eric Stover. *Witnesses from the Grave: The Stories Bones Tell*. Boston: Little, Brown, 1991. Journalists Joyce and Stover explore the history and investigative methods of forensic anthropology, focusing on one of its foremost practitioners, Clyde Snow, who has participated in civil, criminal, and human rights investigations, and who was called upon in 1985 to identify the skeletal remains of Nazi doctor Josef Mengele.

Klawans, Harold L. *Trials of an Expert Witness: Tales of Clinical Neurology and the Law*. Boston: Little, Brown, 1998. This book is written by a physician who has learned the ropes of the court system and who entertains the reader with forensic medical tales. Although Dr. Klawans is a frequent medical expert witness for both sides of the versus, he does not hesitate to use the term "hired gun" for impartial medical experts and minces no words in describing the shortcomings of the tort system.

Miller, Hugh. *What the Corpse Revealed: Murder and the Science of Forensic Detection*. New York: St. Martin's Press, 1999. This resource examines a number of cases in which forensic medicine played a role in criminal investigations. Each chapter is devoted to a different case. Includes an index.

Ubelaker, Douglas H., and Henry Scammel. *Bones: A Forensic Detective's Casebook*. New York: M. Evans, 2000. Among the dozens of true stories in this volume are accounts of homicide, cannibalism, ritual sacrifice, and other horrific crimes, solved and unsolved, from Ubelaker's own personal casebooks and those of the Smithsonian.

FRACTURE AND DISLOCATION

DISEASE/DISORDER

ANATOMY OR SYSTEM AFFECTED: Arms, bones, hands, hips, joints, knees, legs, musculoskeletal system

SPECIALTIES AND RELATED FIELDS: Emergency medicine, orthopedics

DEFINITION: A fracture is a break in a bone, which may be partial or complete; a dislocation is the forceful separation of bones in a joint.

KEY TERMS:

anesthesia: a state characterized by loss of sensation, caused by or resulting from the pharmacological depression of normal nerve function

callus: a hard, bonelike substance made by osteocytes which is found in and around the ends of a fractured bone; it temporarily maintains bony alignment and is resorbed after complete healing or union of a fracture occurs

ecchymosis: a purplish patch on the skin caused by bleeding; the spots are easily visible to the naked eye

embolus: an obstruction or occlusion of a vessel (most commonly, an artery or vein) caused by a transported blood clot, vegetation, mass of bacteria, or other foreign material

epiphysis: the part of a long bone from which growth or elongation occurs

instability: excessive mobility of two or more bones caused by damage to ligaments, the joint capsule, or fracture of one or more bones

ischemia: a local anemia or area of diminished or insufficient blood supply due to mechanical obstruction, commonly narrowing of an artery

osteoblast: a bone-forming cell

osteocyte: a bone cell

paralysis: the loss of power of voluntary movement or other function of a muscle as a result of disease or injury to its nerve supply

petechiae: minute spots caused by hemorrhage or bleeding into the skin; the spots are the size of pinheads

prone: the position of the body when face downward, on one's stomach and abdomen

pulse: the rhythmical dilation of an artery, produced by the increased volume of blood forced into the vessel by the contraction of the heart

transection: a partial or complete severance of the spinal cord

CAUSES AND SYMPTOMS

A fracture is a linear deformation or discontinuity of a bone produced by the application of a force that ex-

ceeds the modulus of elasticity (ability to bend) of a bone. Normal bones require excessive force to fracture. Bones may be weakened by disease or other pathology such as a tumor or tumor-related disease that reduces their ability to withstand an impact. Bones respond to stresses made upon them and can thus be strengthened through physical conditioning and made more resistant to fracture. This is a normal part of training in many athletic activities.

Fractures are classified according to the type of break or, more correctly, by the plane or surface that is fractured. A break that is at a right angle to the axis of the bone is called transverse. A fracture that is similar but at an angle, rather than perpendicular to the main axis of the bone, is called oblique. If a twisting force is applied, the break may be spiral, or twisted. A comminuted fracture is a break that results in two or more fragments of bone. If the pieces of bone remain in their original positions, the fracture is undisplaced. In a displaced fracture, the portions of bone are not properly aligned.

If bones do not penetrate the skin, the fracture is called closed, or simple. When bones protrude through the skin, the result is an open, or compound, fracture. Other types of fractures are associated with pathologic or disease processes. A stress fracture results from repeated stress or trauma to the same site of a bone. None of the individual stresses is sufficient to cause a break. If these stresses cause a callus to form, the bone will be strengthened and actual separation of fragments will not occur. A pathologic fracture occurs at the site of a tumor, infection, or other bone disease. A compression fracture results when bone is crushed; the force applied is greater than the ability of the bone to withstand it. A greenstick fracture is an incomplete separation of bone.

The diagnosis of a fracture is based on several criteria: instability, pain, swelling, deformity, and ecchy-

---

INFORMATION ON FRACTURE AND DISLOCATION

CAUSES: Usually injury, sometimes disease or infection

SYMPTOMS: Varies widely; typically pain, swelling, deformity, bruising

DURATION: Acute

TREATMENTS: Reduction (return of fractured bone to normal position), immobilization, surgery, orthopedic appliances

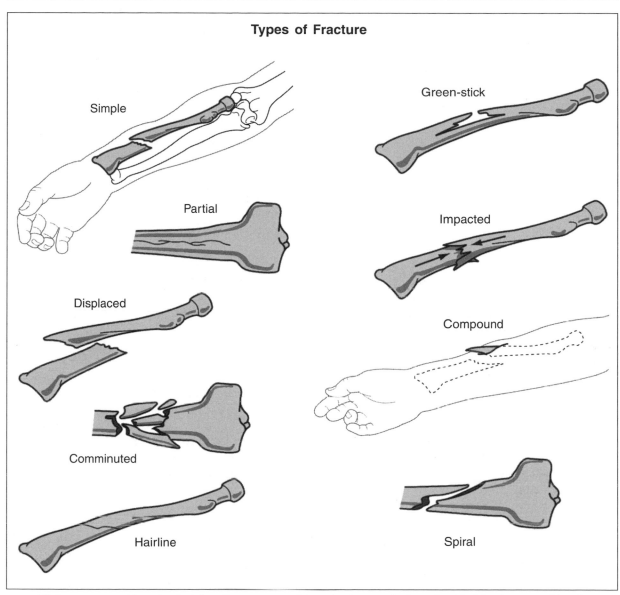

Types of Fracture

Simple

Green-stick

Partial

Impacted

Displaced

Compound

Comminuted

Hairline

Spiral

All fractures are either simple (closed) or compound (open); they are further classified by the type of break.

mosis. The most reliable diagnostic criterion is instability. Pain is not universally present at a fracture site. Swelling may be delayed and occur at some time after a fracture is sustained. Deformity is obvious with open fractures but may not be apparent with other, undisplaced breaks.

Ecchymosis is a purplish patch caused by bleeding into skin; it will not be present if blood vessels are not broken. A definitive diagnosis is made with two plane film X rays taken at the site of a fracture and at right angles to each other. If the fracture site is visually examined and palpated shortly after the injury occurs, an ac-

curate tentative diagnosis may be made; this should be confirmed with X rays as soon as is convenient. Occasionally, an X ray will not show undisplaced or chip fractures. If a patient experiences symptoms of pain, swelling, or ecchymosis but has a negative X ray for fracture, the site should be immobilized and X-rayed again in two to three weeks.

Fractures occur most commonly in extremities: arms or legs. Such fractures must be evaluated to determine if injuries have occurred to other tissues such as nerves or blood vessels. The presence of bruising or ecchymosis indicates blood vessel damage. The existence of peripheral pulses indicates that arteries are not injured. Venous flow is more difficult to evaluate. For a relatively short period of time, however, venous bleeding may be of lesser importance and therefore tolerated.

Neurologic functioning may be assessed by the ability of the patient to contract muscles or sense skin touches or pinpricks. Temporary immobilization may be necessary before nerve status can be evaluated accurately.

An open fracture creates a direct pathway between the skin surface and underlying tissues. If the site becomes contaminated by bacteria, an opportunity for osteomyelitis (infection of the bone) is created. Inadequate treatment by the initial surgeon may result in skin loss, delayed union, loss of joint mobility, osteomyelitis, and even amputation.

Skin damage may or may not be related to a fracture. When skin integrity is broken over or near a fracture site, bone involvement must be assumed. The problem is infection of the fracture site; appropriate antibiotics are normally administered. If skin damage is extensive, final surgical reduction of the underlying fracture may have to be delayed until the skin is healed.

Delayed union refers to the inability of a fractured bone to heal. This is a potentially serious problem, as normal stability is not possible as long as a fracture exists. Joints may not function normally in the presence of a fracture. If a fracture heals improperly, bones may be misaligned and cause pain with movement, leading to limitations of motion. If the bones are affected by osteomyelitis, the infection may spread to the joint capsule and reduce the normal range of motion for the bones or the joint. Amputation may become necessary if infection becomes extensive in the area of a fracture. An infection which becomes firmly established in bones or spreads widely into adjacent muscle tissue may lead to cellulitis or gangrene and may compromise a portion of an extremity. Amputation may be performed if the pathologic process cannot be treated with antibiotics.

Adequate blood supply to tissues is critical for survival. In an extremity, the maximum time limit for complete ischemia (lack of blood flow) is six to eight hours; after that time, the likelihood of later amputation increases. Pain, pallor, pulselessness, and paralysis are indicators of impaired circulation associated with a fracture. When two of these signs are present, the possibility of vascular damage must be thoroughly explored.

Dislocations occur at joints and are caused by an applied force that is greater than the strength of the liga-

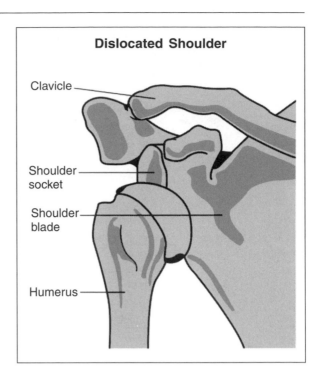

Dislocated Shoulder

Clavicle

Shoulder socket

Shoulder blade

Humerus

ments and muscles that keep a joint intact. The result is a stretching deformity or injury to a joint and abnormal movement of a bone out of the joint. Accidental trauma, commonly the result of an athletic injury or automobile accident, is the most common cause of a dislocation. Joints that are frequently dislocated include the shoulder and digits (fingers and toes). Dislocations of the ankle and hip are infrequent but serious; they require immediate management. Dislocations may accompany fractures, but the two injuries need not occur together.

When dislocations are reduced, the bones of the joint are returned to normal position. Reduction is accomplished by relaxing adjacent muscles and applying traction or a pulling force to the bone until it returns to its normal position in the joint. For most dislocations of the shoulder, the victim lies in a prone position and the dislocated arm hangs down freely. Gradual traction is applied until reduction occurs. This can be accomplished by bandaging a pail to the arm and slowly filling it with water. Alternatively, a heavy book can be held by the victim and the muscles of the arm allowed to relax until the dislocation is reduced. Such treatments are usually reserved for situations in which medical assistance is unavailable. Digits are reduced in a similar manner, by gentle pulling of the end of the finger or toe. Ankle and hip dislocations are potentially more serious because these joints are more complex and have extensive blood supplies. Reduction of dislocated ankles and hips should be undertaken by qualified medical personnel in an expedited manner.

After reduction, all dislocations should be evaluated by competent medical personnel. With dislocated digits, later damage is relatively unlikely but can occur because of ligament damage sustained in the initial injury. Dislocations of the shoulder may be accompanied by a fracture of the clavicle or collar bone and may involve nerve damage in the shoulder joint. Dislocations of the ankle and hip may lead to avascular necrosis (damage to the bone as a result of inadequate blood supply) if not evaluated and reduced promptly.

TREATMENT AND THERAPY

Fractures are usually treated by reduction and immobilization. Reduction, which refers to the process of returning the fractured bones to normal position, may be either closed or open. Closed reduction is accomplished without surgery by manipulating the broken bone through overlying skin and muscles. Open reduction requires surgical intervention in which the broken pieces are exposed and returned to normal position. Orthopedic appliances may be used to hold the bones in correct position. The most common of these appliances are pins and screws, but metal plates and wires may also be employed. Orthopedic appliances are usually made of stainless steel. These may be left in the body indefinitely or may be surgically removed after healing is complete. Local anesthesia is usually used with closed reductions; open reductions are performed in an operating room, under sterile conditions using general anesthesia.

Immobilization is generally accomplished by the use of a cast. Casts are often made of plaster, but they may be constructed of inflatable plastic. It is important to hold bones in a rigid, fixed position for a sufficient length of time for the broken ends to unite and heal. The cast must be loose enough, however, to allow blood to circulate. Padding is usually put in place before plaster is applied to form a cast. Whenever possible, the newly immobilized body part is elevated to reduce the chance of swelling in the cast, which would compromise the blood supply to the fracture site and body portion beyond the cast. Casts should be checked periodically to ensure that they do not impair circulation.

The broken bone and accompanying body part must be placed in an anatomically neutral position. This is done to minimize postfracture disability and improve the prospect for rehabilitation. The length of time that a fractured bone is immobilized is highly variable and dependent on a number of factors.

Traction may also be used to immobilize a fracture. Traction is the external application of force to overcome muscular resistance and hold bones in a desired position. Commonly, holes are drilled through bones and pins are inserted; the ends of these pins extend through the surface of the skin. Part of the body is fixed in position through the use of a strap or weights, and wires are attached to the pins in the body part to be stretched. Weights or tension is applied to the wires until the broken bone parts move into the desired position. Traction is maintained until healing has occurred.

Individual ends of a single fractured bone are sometimes held in position by external pins and screws. Holes are drilled through the bone, and pins are inserted. The pins on opposite sides of the fracture site are then attached to each other with threaded rods and locked in position by nuts. This process allows a fractured bone to be immobilized without using a cast.

Different bones require different amounts of time to heal. Further, age is a factor in fracture healing. Fractures in young children heal more quickly than do broken bones in adults. Older adults typically require even more time for healing. The availability of calcium and other nutrients also affects the speed with which a fracture heals.

Delayed union of fractures is a term applied to fractures that either do not heal or take longer than normal to heal; there is no precise time frame associated with delayed union. Nonunion refers to fractures in which healing is not observed and cannot be expected even with prolonged immobilization. X-ray analysis of a nonunion will show that the bone ends have hardened (sclerosed), that the ends of the marrow canal have become plugged, and that a gap persists between the ends of a fractured bone. Nonunion may be caused by inadequate blood supply to the fracture site, which leads to the formation of cartilage instead of new bone between the broken pieces of bone. Nonunion may also be caused by injury to the soft tissues that surround a fracture site. This damage impairs the formation of a callus and the reestablishment of an adequate blood supply to the fracture site; it is frequently seen in young children. Inadequate immobilization may also allow soft tissue to enter the fracture site by slipping between the bone fragments, and may lead to nonunion. Respect for tissue and minimizing damage in the vicinity of a fracture, especially with open reduction, will minimize problems of nonunion. Subjecting the nonuniting fracture site to a low-level electromagnetic field will usually stimulate osteoblastic activity and lead to healing.

The epiphyseal plate is the portion of bone where growth occurs. Bony epiphyses are active in children until they attain their adult height, at which time the epiphyses become inactive and close. Once an epiphysis ceases to function, further growth does not occur. In children, a fracture involving the epiphyseal plate is potentially dangerous because bone growth may be interrupted or halted. This situation can lead to inequalities in the length of extremities or impaired range of movement in joints. Accurate reduction of injuries involving an epiphyseal plate is necessary to minimize subsequent deformity. A key factor is blood supply to the injured area: If adequate blood supply is maintained, epiphyseal plate damage is minimized.

Fractures of the spinal vertebrae are potentially very dangerous because they can cause injury to the nerves and tracts of the spinal cord. Fractures of the vertebrae are commonly sustained in automobile accidents, athletic injuries, falls from heights, and other situations involving rapid deceleration. When vertebrae are fractured, the spinal cord can be compromised. Spinal cord injury can be direct and cut all or a portion of the spinal nerves at the site of the fracture. The extent of the damage is dependent on the level of the injury. An accident that completely severs the spinal cord will lead to a complete loss of function for all structures below the level of injury. Since spinal nerves are arranged segmentally, cord damage at a lower level involves compromise of fewer structures. As the level of injury becomes higher in the spinal cord, more vital structures are involved. Transection of the spinal cord in the neck usually leads to complete paralysis of the entire body; it can cause death if high enough to cut the nerves controlling the lungs. Individuals in whom vertebral fractures and thus spinal cord injuries are suspected must have the spinal column immobilized before they are moved. Reduction of spinal cord fractures must be undertaken by a highly skilled person.

When bones having large marrow cavities such as the femur (thigh bone) are fractured, fat globules may escape from the marrow and enter the bloodstream. Such a fat globule is then called an embolus (plural is emboli). Fat emboli are potentially dangerous in that they can become lodged in the capillaries of the lungs. This causes pain and can lead to impaired oxygenation of blood, a condition called hypoxemia. About 10 to 20 percent of individuals sustaining a fractured femur also have central nervous system depression and skin petechiae (minute spots caused by hemorrhage or bleeding into the skin) in addition to hypoxemia in the

two to three days after the injury. This triad of signs is called fat embolism syndrome. It is treated medically with oxygen, steroids, and anticoagulant drugs.

Perspective and Prospects

Fractures rarely threaten a patient's life directly, and injuries to the brain, heart, circulatory system, and abdominal cavity must receive priority of treatment. It is imperative, however, not to move a patient in whom a fracture is suspected without first immobilizing the potential fracture site. This is especially true with suspected fractures of the spine. Instability may not be apparent when a patient is lying down but can become catastrophic if the person is moved without proper preparation and immobilization.

Crush injuries of the spinal cord are relatively common among victims of osteoporosis. Osteoporosis is a pathological syndrome defined by a decrease in the density of a bone below the level required for mechanical support and is frequently associated with a deficiency of calcium, problems related to calcium in the body, or a rate of bone cell breakdown that is greater than the rate of bone cell remodeling. Crush fractures occur when the bones become so weak that the weight of the upper portion of the body is greater than the ability of the vertebrae to support it. These crush injuries may occur slowly over time and cause no serious injury to the underlying spinal cord. The resulting deformity of the spine, however, impairs movement. There is no treatment for osteoporotic crush fractures of the vertebrae.

Occupational exposures may lead to fractures and dislocations. Professional athletes are clearly at increased risk for skeletal injuries. These individuals are also usually well conditioned, however, and so can withstand increased impacts and blows to the body. Many are also trained in methods that minimize the force of impact; they know how to fall properly.

The vast proportion of workers are not conditioned and are given minimal training to avoid situations that lead to fractures. Accident analysis reveals that carelessness is the most common predisposing factor. Workers operating without safety equipment such as belaying lines or belts may become overconfident. In such a situation, slips or falls can occur, and fractures result. Unsafe equipment can lead to hazardous situations and cause fractures or dislocations. Machinery that is not properly maintained can fail; parts may become detached, hit nearby workers, and cause fractures.

Recreational activities also result in fractures. Individuals who once were well conditioned may engage in sports without proper equipment and sustain fractures or dislocations. Contact sports such as football, hockey, and basketball are primary examples of such activities. Riding bicycles and motorized recreational vehicles without proper safety equipment can lead to serious skeletal injuries. Activities such as rock climbing are inherently dangerous. With proper training and use of safety equipment, accidents can be reduced or their severity minimized. The keys to avoiding fractures and dislocations when participating in recreational activities are receiving proper instruction and training, employing adequate safety equipment, and using common sense by avoiding difficult or hazardous situations that are beyond one's physical abilities or skill level.

—*L. Fleming Fallon, Jr., M.D., Ph.D., M.P.H.*

See also Bone disorders; Bone grafting; Bones and the skeleton; Fracture repair; Head and neck disorders; Hip fracture repair; Orthopedic surgery; Orthopedics; Orthopedics, pediatric; Osteoporosis; Physical rehabilitation; Spinal cord disorders; Spine, vertebrae, and disks; Wounds.

FOR FURTHER INFORMATION:

Currey, John D. *Bones: Structures and Mechanics.* Princeton, N.J.: Princeton University Press, 2002. Very accessible overview of a range of information related to whole bones, bone tissue, and dentin and enamel. Topics include stiffness, strength, viscoelasticity, fatigue, fracture mechanics properties, buckling, impact fracture, and properties of cancellous bone.

Marieb, Elaine N. *Human Anatomy and Physiology.* 6th ed. Redwood City, Calif.: Benjamin/Cummings, 2003. Nonscientists at the advanced high school level or above will be able to understand this fine textbook. The chapters titled "Bones and Bone Tissue," "The Skeleton," and "Joints" are very well illustrated.

Sabiston, David C., Jr., ed. *Textbook of Surgery: The Biological Basis of Modern Surgical Practice.* 16th ed. Philadelphia: W. B. Saunders, 2001. A standard textbook of surgery which contains an extensive discussion of different types of fractures and dislocations and how they are treated. Intended for practicing professionals but can be generally understood by the layperson.

Schwartz, Seymour I., ed. *Principles of Surgery.* 7th ed. New York: McGraw-Hill, 1999. A standard textbook of surgery containing sections on fractures and dislocations. Its intended audience is practicing surgeons, and thus the language is sometimes technical. Nevertheless, the serious reader can obtain much useful detail from this work.

Way, Lawrence W., and Gerard M. Doherty, eds. *Current Surgical Diagnosis and Treatment.* 11th ed. New York: Lange Medical Books/McGraw Hill, 2003. The diagnosis and treatment of fractures and dislocations is discussed in a brief and concise format emphasizing treatment modalities. The different section authors are recognized experts in their fields. The material is accessible to the general reader, but the sections are brief.

Wilmore, Douglas W., et al., eds. *Care of the Surgical Patient.* New York: Scientific American, 1992. This book should be understandable to laypersons even though it is written for professionals. Sections in part 1 discuss fractures and dislocations. The reputation of *Scientific American* for style and clarity is evident in this book. A good source for the general reader.

FRACTURE REPAIR
PROCEDURE

ANATOMY OR SYSTEM AFFECTED: Arms, bones, hips, legs, musculoskeletal system, teeth

SPECIALTIES AND RELATED FIELDS: Dentistry, orthopedics

DEFINITION: The placement and fixation of broken portions of bones in their correct positions until they have grown together.

INDICATIONS AND PROCEDURES

A fracture is a break in a bone, either partial or complete, resulting from an applied force that is greater than the bone's internal strength. The most common causes of fractures are accidents or trauma.

Fractures are usually treated by reduction and immobilization. Reduction, which may be either closed or open, refers to the process of returning the fractured bones to normal position. Closed reduction is accomplished without surgery by manipulating the broken bone through overlying skin and muscles. Open reduction requires surgical intervention. The broken pieces are exposed and returned to their normal positions. Orthopedic appliances may be used to hold the bones in the proper position (internal fixation); the most common appliances are stainless steel pins and screws, but metal plates and wires may also be employed. These devices can be left in the body indefinitely or may be surgically removed after healing is complete. Local anesthesia is usually used with closed reductions; open reductions are performed in an operating room under sterile conditions, using general anesthesia.

After reduction, the broken bone and accompanying body part must be placed in an anatomically neutral po-

sition. Immobilization is generally accomplished by the use of a cast. Casts are usually made of plaster, but they may be constructed of inflatable plastic.

Individual ends of a single fractured bone are some-times held in position by external pins and screws (ex-

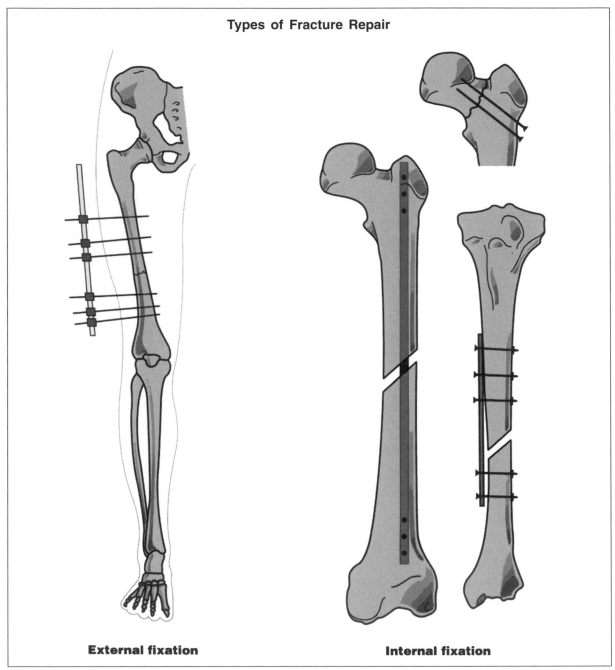

Types of Fracture Repair

External fixation

Internal fixation

Severe leg fractures can be immobilized through external fixation or internal fixation. External fixation involves the use of long pins that are inserted through the bone and held in place with a steel rod on the outside of the body. Internal fixation involves the use of screws, pins, and plates that are attached directly to the bones and often left there permanently.

ternal fixation). Holes are drilled through the bone, and pins are inserted as described above. The pins on opposite sides of the fracture site are then attached to each other with threaded rods and locked in position by nuts. This process allows a fractured bone to be immobilized without using a cast.

Traction, the external application of force to overcome muscular resistance and hold bones in a desired position, may also be used to immobilize a fracture. Commonly, holes are drilled through bones and pins are inserted; the ends of these pins extend through the surface of the skin. Part of the body is fixed in position through the use of a strap or weights. Wires are attached to the pins in the body part to be stretched. Force through weights or tension is applied to the wires until the broken bone parts are in the desired position. Traction is maintained until complete healing has occurred.

USES AND COMPLICATIONS

All broken bones must be held in position until healing takes place. The complications associated with repairing fractures include infection, which is rare, and loss of function. The potential for loss of function is minimized by placing the limb into an anatomically neutral position prior to the application of a cast.

The techniques of fracture repair have not changed radically in decades. New methods, however, are being tried. For example, electromagnetic fields are used with fractures that do not heal spontaneously. Such a field induces the growth of osteoblasts, which are bone-forming cells.

—*L. Fleming Fallon, Jr., M.D., Ph.D., M.P.H.*

See also Bone grafting; Bones and the skeleton; Dentistry; Emergency medicine; Fracture and dislocation; Hip fracture repair; Jaw wiring; Orthopedic surgery; Orthopedics; Orthopedics, pediatric; Osteoporosis; Teeth.

FOR FURTHER INFORMATION:

Browner, Bruce D. *Skeletal Trauma: Fractures, Dislocations, Ligamentous Injuries.* Philadelphia: W. B. Saunders, 1998.

Eiff, M. Patrice, Robert L. Hatch, Walter L. Calmbach. *Fracture Management for Primary Care.* Philadelphia: W. B. Saunders, 1998.

Gregg, Paul J., Jack Stevens, and Peter H. Worlock. *Fractures and Dislocations: Principles of Management.* Cambridge, Mass.: Blackwell Science, 1996.

Gustilo, Ramon B., Richard F. Kyle, and David C. Templeman, eds. *Fractures and Dislocations.* St. Louis: C. V. Mosby, 1993.

Hodgson, Stephen F. *Mayo Clinic on Osteoporosis: Keeping Bones Healthy and Strong and Reducing the Risk of Fractures.* New York: Kensington, 2003.

Magee, David J. *Orthopedic Physical Assessment.* 4th ed. New York: Elsevier, 2002.

Ruiz, Ernest, and James J. Cicero, eds. *Emergency Management of Skeletal Injuries.* St. Louis: C. V. Mosby, 1995.

Salter, Robert B. *Textbook of Disorders and Injuries of the Musculoskeletal System.* 3d ed. Philadelphia: Lippincott Williams & Wilkins, 1998.

FRAGILE X SYNDROME
DISEASE/DISORDER

ALSO KNOWN AS: Martin-Bell syndrome

ANATOMY OR SYSTEM AFFECTED: Brain, ears, feet, genitals, hands, joints

SPECIALTIES AND RELATED FIELDS: Genetics

DEFINITION: A genetic disorder of variable expression, with mental retardation being the most common feature.

CAUSES AND SYMPTOMS

Fragile X syndrome is caused by a change in a gene located on the long arm of the X chromosome. It is a sex-linked inherited disease, transmitted from parent to child, with boys being affected much more often and more severely than girls. The prevalence of the disorder is estimated to be 1 in 1,200 males and 1 in 2,500 females.

While symptoms and their severity vary widely, common physical features of fragile X syndrome include a long, thin face, a prominent jaw and ears, a

---

INFORMATION ON FRAGILE X SYNDROME

CAUSES: Genetic

SYMPTOMS: Thin face, prominent jaw and ears, broad nose, large testicles in males, large hands with loose finger joints, mental impairment ranging from severe retardation to learning disabilities, unusual speech patterns, problems with attention span and hyperactivity, motor delays, occasional autistic-type behaviors

DURATION: Chronic

TREATMENTS: None; alleviation of symptoms

broad nose, a high palate, large testicles (macroorchidism) in males, and large hands with loose finger joints. Physical features are more subtle in females. Nonphysical features include mental impairment ranging from severe retardation to learning disabilities, with the majority of affected males demonstrating a mental impairment ranging from low-normal intelligence to severe retardation. More recent research has found that the intelligence quotients (IQs) of males with fragile X syndrome appear to decline throughout childhood. Associated behavioral symptoms include unusual speech patterns, problems with attention span, hyperactivity, motor delays, and occasional autistic-type behaviors, such as poor eye contact, hand-flapping, or hand-biting.

TREATMENT AND THERAPY

While there is no cure for fragile X syndrome, a number of possible interventions can address various symptoms. Medications can be administered to assist with attention span and hyperactivity, as well as with aggressive behavior. Schools can provide children with assistance in speech, physical therapy, and vocational planning. Early childhood special education services for children prior to school age can provide necessary early intervention that may prove most helpful if indeed the rate of learning for children with fragile X syndrome slows with age. Genetic counseling is advised for families who carry the gene.

PERSPECTIVE AND PROSPECTS

In 1969, the discovery was made of a break or fragile site on the long arm of the X chromosome. It was not until the 1980's, however, that consistent diagnoses of fragile X syndrome were made. In 1991, the responsible gene was sequenced and named the FMR-1 (fragile X mental retardation 1) gene. Cytogenetic and deoxyribonucleic acid (DNA) testing are now available to identify affected persons.

—*Robin Hasslen, Ph.D.*

See also Genetic diseases; Genetics and inheritance; Learning disabilities; Mental retardation; Motor skill development; Speech disorders.

FOR FURTHER INFORMATION:

Fraxa Research Foundation. http://www.fraxa.org/.

Hagerman, Randi Jensen, and Paul J. Henssen. *Fragile X Syndrome: Diagnosis, Treatment, and Research.* 3d ed. Baltimore: Johns Hopkins University Press, 2002.

Maxon, Linda, and Charles Daugherty. *Genetics: A Human Perspective.* Dubuque, Iowa: Wm. C. Brown, 1992.

Moore, Keith L., and T. V. N. Persaud. *The Developing Human.* 7th ed. Philadelphia: W. B. Saunders, 2003.

Parker, James N., and Philip M. Parker, eds. *The 2002 Official Parent's Sourcebook on Fragile X Syndrome.* San Diego, Calif.: Icon Health, 2002.

Sherwood, Lauralee. *Human Physiology: From Cells to Systems.* 4th ed. Belmont, Calif.: Wadsworth, 2001.

Webb, Jayne Dixon. *Children with Fragile X Syndrome: A Parents' Guide.* Bethesda, Md.: Woodbine House, 2000.

FROSTBITE

DISEASE/DISORDER

ANATOMY OR SYSTEM AFFECTED: Hands, feet, skin and adjacent tissues

SPECIALTIES AND RELATED FIELDS: Emergency medicine, environmental health

DEFINITION: Frostbite is localized freezing of tissue, usually of extremities exposed to low temperatures and resulting in ice crystals forming within cells, thereby killing them.

KEY TERMS:

anticoagulant: a drug that reduces the clotting of the blood

basal metabolic rate: the rate at which the body burns calories and produces heat energy while the body is at rest or not active

gangrene: the death of part of the body (such as an arm or leg) caused by the death of the cells in that structure

hypothermia: the process by which the body core temperature falls below that needed for the body to function normally

hypoxia: a lack of an adequate amount of oxygen to the tissues; results in a reduction of mental and physical capabilities

maceration: the process of breaking down tissue to a soft mass, either by soaking it or through infection or gangrene

necrosis: the death of body tissue cells

sludging: an increase in red blood cell structures, known as platelets, which slows down the blood flow through vessels and promotes clotting of the blood

sympathectomy: the surgical process of removing or destroying nerves that may be afflicted by frostbite or other injury

vascoconstriction: a decrease in the diameter of vessels transporting blood throughout the body, reducing blood flow and oxygen transport

windchill: the effect of wind blowing across exposed flesh; increased heat is lost from the skin's surface, as if the air were much colder than the actual temperature indicates

CAUSES AND SYMPTOMS

The effect of cold on the human body is to reduce the circulation of blood to surface areas, such as the feet, hands, and face. This reduction restricts the amount of heat lost by the body and helps to prevent the development of hypothermia. Blood constriction may become so severe in severely chilled areas of the body, however, that circulation almost totally ceases. People with poorer circulation, such as the elderly and the exhausted, are not as resistant to low temperatures as are fit or younger people.

If the skin's temperature falls below –0.53 degree Celsius, the tissue actually freezes and frostbite occurs. Rapid freezing causes ice crystals to form within a cell. These crystals rupture the cell wall and destroy structures within the cell, effectively killing it. If freezing is slow, ice crystals form between the cells; they grow by extracting water from the cells. The tissue may be injured physically by the ice crystals or by dehydration and the resulting disruption of osmotic and chemical balance within the cells; however, tissue death following frostbite is more likely to be attributable to interruption of the blood supply to the tissue than to the direct action of freezing. Cold also damages the capillaries in the affected areas, causing blood plasma to leak through their walls, thus adding to tissue injury and further impairing circulation by allowing the blood to

---

INFORMATION ON FROSTBITE

CAUSES: Exposure to freezing temperatures, causing impaired circulation to nearly cease

SYMPTOMS: Tingling and pain in afflicted tissues, slightly flushed skin before freezing begins followed by white or blotchy blue color, skin that is firm and insensitive to the touch

DURATION: Acute

TREATMENTS: Manual or medical rewarming, antibiotics, hyperbaric oxygen, occasionally surgery

---

sludge (to clot because of an increase in red blood cells) inside the vessels. All sensation of cold or pain is lost as circulation becomes seriously impaired. Unless the tissue is warmed quickly, the skin and superficial tissues actually begin to freeze. With continual chilling, the frozen area enlarges and extends to deeper areas. This condition is known as frostbite.

Frostbite was common among soldiers during Napoleon's campaign in Russia in the early 1800's, during World War II in Northern Europe, in the Korean War, and in fighting between Indian and Chinese troops in the Himalayas. Air crews, especially waist-gunners in the U.S. Air Force in World War II, were particularly prone to frostbite. In 1943, frostbite injuries among these bomber crews were greater than all other casualties combined.

Polar travelers before the 1920's suffered severely from frostbite. Mountain climbers are at risk from frostbite at higher elevations. Lower oxygen availability increases the danger of frostbite because the body cannot take in sufficient oxygen in this thinner air. The resulting condition, called hypoxia, reduces mental abilities, and precautions normally taken against the cold may be either inadequate or neglected altogether. High winds, often experienced in the mountains, speed heat loss from exposed skin surfaces. This windchill can be deadly to mountaineers and often produces hypothermia. Poor appetite at high elevations reduces the energy available for the production of body heat. The insulating layer of subcutaneous fat also decreases with longer periods of time spent at higher elevations; this in turn decreases the insulation of the surface areas of the body against freezing. Inadequate food intake while mountain climbing increases the danger of frostbite, as the body does not have enough calories to keep its temperature constant. The occurrence of hypothermia also increases the risk of frostbite as heat is drawn away from extremities to protect the body's core temperature. At higher elevations, most humans function at only about 60 percent of the physiological efficiency that they have at sea level. Women have more resistance to cold and may be less likely to experience frostbite than are men.

Frostbite at high altitudes seems to be more common for the same temperature than at lower altitudes. More red blood cells are found in the blood of persons working at higher elevations, thickening the blood and reducing circulation to the extremities. This reduced circulation lowers the temperature of these extremities. The basal metabolic rate and cardiac output of the body also decrease as one goes higher; both of these actions reduce the body's ability to keep its feet, hands, and face warm.

Blood vessels move heat from the central body core to the skin; it radiates into the air from exposed surfaces. This heat loss is greatest in the hands, feet, and head, where the vessels are close to the skin's surface. Respiration loses body heat when cold air is inhaled into the lungs and body heat warms it; this heat is lost when the air is exhaled. Evaporation, moisture leaving the skin's surface, also draws heat from the body. In low temperatures, spilling gasoline on exposed skin will create frostbite because the evaporation of the fuel draws heat away from the body quickly. Convection carries body heat away by wind currents. This wind-chill factor, calculated for Fahrenheit temperatures by subtracting two times the windspeed from the air temperature, determines the amount of heat energy lost from the body's surface. Conduction transfers heat from one substance to another; for example, contact between the body and snow or metal will cause the skin to lose heat. Although many people work and live in subzero temperatures, frostbite is uncommon. Nevertheless, an accident that prevents one from moving, loss of the ability to shiver in order to generate heat, or inactivity may increase the chance of developing frostbite. Frostbite can occur in any cold environment. Warning symptoms of frostbite initially include tingling and pain in the afflicted tissues. The skin may be slightly flushed before freezing. It then turns white or a blotchy blue in color and is firm and insensitive to the touch. Tissue that is painful and then becomes numb and insensitive is frozen.

TREATMENT AND THERAPY

Slight cases of frostbite, often termed frostnip or superficial frostbite, can be treated outdoors or in the field with little or no medical help. Such cases are usually reversible, with no permanent damage, as only skin and subcutaneous tissues are involved. The frozen part, although white and frozen on the surface, is soft and pliable when pressed gently before thawing. The area is often a cheek or the tip of the nose or the fingers. The frozen area, usually small, can be warmed manually. A hand is placed over the frostnipped area if it is a cheek or nose, and frozen fingers can be placed under the armpit or on a partner's bare stomach for warming. Tissue that has had only a minor amount of frostnip soon returns to normal color. A tingling sensation is felt when frostnipped tissue is thawed. After thawing, areas that

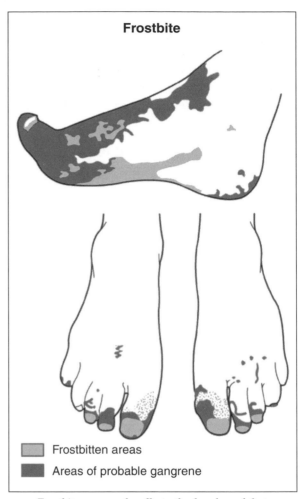

Frostbite

☐ Frostbitten areas
■ Areas of probable gangrene

Frostbite commonly affects the hands and feet.

have had more serious superficial frostbite become numb, mottled, or blue or purple in color and then will sting, burn, or swell for a period of time. Blisters, small ones called blebs, may occur within twenty-four to forty-eight hours. Blistering is more common where the skin is loose. Blister fluid is absorbed slowly; the skin may harden, become black (from gangrene), and be insensitive to touch. Throbbing or aching may persist for weeks. Gangrene occurring after frostnip is essentially superficial and extends only a few millimeters deep into the tissue. In two or three months, this type of frostbite will be mostly healed. With immediate treatment, frostnipped tissue will not progress to the much more serious injury of deep frostbite.

Tissues vary in their resistance to frostbite. Skin freezes at −0.53 Celsius, while muscles, blood vessels, and nerves are also highly subject to freezing. Connective tissue, tendons, and bones are relatively resistant to freezing, which explains why the blackened extremities of a frostbitten hand or foot can be moved: The tendons under the gangrenous skin remain intact and functional.

Deep frostbite includes not only skin and subcutaneous tissue but also deeper structures, including muscle, bone, and tendons. The affected area becomes cold, mottled, and blue or gray in color and may remain swollen for months. With deep frostbite, the tissues become quite hard to the touch. One to three days after thawing, the affected area becomes quite painful. Blisters, initially small blebs and then large, coalescing ones, may take weeks to develop. The patient should not be allowed to become alarmed about his or her condition; even mild cases of frostbite have a frightening appearance during blistering. Initially, the frozen part may be painless, but shooting and throbbing pains may occur for several months after thawing. Permanent loss of tissue is almost inevitable with deep frostbite. The affected extremity has a severely shriveled look. A limb may return to almost normal over some months, however, and amputation should never be carried out until a considerable period, probably at least six to nine months, has elapsed.

In cases of frostbite, surgical intervention must be minimal. Blackened frostbitten tissue will gradually separate itself from healthy, unfrozen tissue without interference; no efforts should be taken to hasten separation. Most cases of deep frostbite seem to heal in six to twelve months, and the gangrenous tissue, if it has not become infected with bacteria, is essentially superficial. Many unnecessary amputations have been carried out because of impatience at the slow recovery rate of tissue that has suffered deep frostbite; amputation is only necessary when infection has set in and it cannot be controlled with antibiotics.

If possible, deep frostbite should be treated under hospital care, not in the field or outdoors. The deep frozen tissue should remain frozen until hospital care is available. If frozen tissues are thawed, the patient will most likely be unable to move as the pain will be severe with any movement. Walking on feet that have been thawed after being frozen will cause permanent damage; however, walking on a frozen foot for twelve to eighteen hours or even longer produces less damage than inadequate warming. As frozen tissue thaws, cells exude fluid. If this tissue is refrozen, ice crystals form and cause more extensive, irreparable damage.

Rapid rewarming is the recommended treatment for deep frostbite and is a proven method of reducing tissue loss. Rubbing the frostbitten area with the hand or snow—akin to rubbing the area with broken glass—should never be done. This treatment does not melt the intracellular ice crystals, nor does it increase circulation to the frozen area. It breaks the skin and allows infection to enter into the system. Vasodilator agents do not improve tissue survival. Local antibiotics in aerosol form can be used, but it is unwise to rely on this method alone for combating infection. Sympathectomy, the removal or destruction of affected nerves, does not improve cell survival. The use of the drug dextran early to prevent sludging has limited use and may have dangerous side effects. The use of hyperbaric oxygen or supplementary oxygen may increase the tissue tension of oxygen and save some cells partially damaged by cold injury.

Rewarming should be carried out in a water bath with water temperatures ranging from 37.7 to 42.2 degrees Celsius (100 to 108 degrees Fahrenheit). Higher temperatures will further damage already injured tissues. Rewarming in a large bathtub warms the frozen extremity more rapidly, resulting in less tissue loss in many cases, particularly where frostbite has been deep and extensive. A large container also permits more accurate control of the water temperature. If a bathtub is not available, a bucket, large wastebasket, dishpan, or other similar container can be used. During rewarming, hot water usually must be added to the bath occasionally to keep the temperature correct; in such cases the injured extremity should be removed from the bath and not returned to it until the water has been thoroughly mixed and its temperature measured. An open flame must not come into contact with the area to which heat is applied, since sensation is lost as a result of the frostbite and the tissue could be seriously burned.

For rewarming, the extremity should be stripped of all clothing, and any constricting bands, straps, or other objects that might stop circulation should be removed. The injured area should be suspended in the center of the water and not permitted to rest against the side or bottom. Warming should continue for thirty to forty minutes. The frostbitten tissues may become quite painful during this process, so it may be necessary to give painkillers to the patient in order to reduce discomfort during or after thawing of the frostbitten area. Aspirin (as well as codeine, morphine, or meperidine, if needed) may be given for pain. Aspirin or an anticoagulant increases blood circulation by reducing red blood cell platelet formation and thus reducing sludging. Phenoxybenzamine reduces vasoconstriction.

Following rewarming, the patient must be kept warm and the injured tissue elevated and protected from any kind of trauma. One should avoid rupturing blisters that have formed. Blankets or bedclothes should be supported by a framework to avoid pressure or rubbing of the injured area.

Subsequent care is directed primarily toward preventing infection. Cleanliness of the frostbitten area is extremely important. It should be soaked daily in a water bath at body temperature to which a germicidal soap has been added. If contamination of the water supply is a possibility, the bath water should be boiled and cooled before use. Dead tissue should not be cut or pulled away; the water baths remove such tissue more efficiently.

The afflicted area should be immobilized and kept sterile. Even contact with sheets can be damaging to a frostbitten limb. Sterile, dry cotton may be placed between the fingers or toes to avoid maceration. If infection appears present, as indicated by the area between the frostbitten tissue and healthy tissue becoming inflamed and feeling tender or throbbing, antibiotics such as ampicillin or cloxicillin should be given every six hours. Wet, antiseptic dressings should be applied if gangrene occurs in the damaged tissue. A tetanus toxoid booster shot, or human antitoxin if the patient has not been previously immunized against tetanus, should be given. Complete rest and a diet high in protein will help healing. Moderate movement of the afflicted area should be encouraged but should be limited to that done by a physical therapist, without assistance by the patient. Considerable reassurance and emotional support may be required by the patient, as the appearance of the frostbitten area can be alarming.

Amputation in response to infected, spreading gangrene may be needed eventually, but it should be delayed until the natural separation of dead from living tissue and bone has taken place. Radionucleotide scanning helps save frostbitten limbs. These scans accurately demonstrate blood flow in frostbitten extremities, thus predicting what tissue will survive.

PERSPECTIVE AND PROSPECTS

Frostbite is an injury that can affect anyone who works or plays under cold conditions. Increased knowledge about what causes this injury, better equipment, and techniques that minimize its effect, however, have reduced its occurrence. Advances in medical knowledge regarding how the injury occurs within the afflicted tissues have produced treatment protocols that reduce the extent of permanent injury from frostbite.

Prevention is the most effective treatment for frostbite, which can occur only when the body lacks enough heat to keep the extremities above freezing. The overall body heat deficit results from inadequate clothing or equipment, reduced food consumption, exhaustion, injury or inactivity causing a lack of body movement, or some combination of these factors. Those playing or working in a cold environment should know the conditions under which frostbite may develop. For frostnip to occur, the windchill index must exceed 1,400 and the air temperature must be below the freezing point of exposed skin (−0.53 degree Celsius). An ambient temperature of −10 to −15 degrees Celsius is usually necessary for deep frostbite to develop.

Adequate clothing—especially boots that allow circulation to occur freely, mittens (not gloves) that cover the hands, and a head covering that protects the face, ears, and neck—must be worn. Boots should be well broken in and large enough to fit comfortably with several pairs of socks. The laces at the top of the boots should not be tight. Gaiters or overboots should be worn if deep or wet snow is anticipated. Windproof or insulated pants protect the legs from cold and help keep the feet warm. Dry socks and mitten liners should be carried. Moisture greatly reduces the insulative value of clothing, so it is necessary to stay dry; if clothing becomes wet or damp, one should change into dry items. Plastic bags, worn over bare feet, provide a vapor barrier liner that is effective in helping keep one's feet dry and warm under cold conditions. Adequate ventilation avoids dampness from excessive perspiration. Dressing in layers—having several light shirts, jackets, or a windbreaker—is better than wearing only one heavy jacket.

Heat production, resulting from exercise or the protective mechanism of shivering, is just as important as clothing in maintaining body temperature. Injuries that cause the victim to go into shock or lie immobilized, even though adequate clothing may be worn, predispose the victim to frostbite.

Eating high-energy foods and taking in 6,000 or more kilocalories (Calories) a day may be necessary to keep body temperatures constant under very cold or physically demanding conditions. Adequate rest, including eight or more hours of sleep, helps to reduce fatigue, which in turn increases the body's ability to produce heat. Alcohol and tobacco should be strictly avoided. Alcohol dilates the blood vessels and, although this action temporarily warms the skin, results in increased loss of total body heat. Smoking constricts the blood vessels in the skin and so reduces heat flow to surface areas; this may be sufficient to initiate frostbite in exposed tissue. A person who has sustained frostbite in the past is usually more susceptible to more cold injury. Problems with arthritis may develop in extremities that have been frostbitten.

—*David L. Chesemore, Ph.D.*

See also Amputation; Cyanosis; Gangrene; Hyperthermia and hypothermia; Skin; Skin disorders.

FOR FURTHER INFORMATION:

Calvert, John H., Jr. "Frostbite." *Flying Safety* 54, no. 10 (October, 1998): 24-25. Frostbite can be a painful and disfiguring injury, caused by the freezing of the moisture in one's body tissues. Steps for taking care of frostbite injuries are presented.

Phillips, David. "How Frostbite Performs Its Misery." *Canadian Geographic* 115, no. 1 (January/February, 1995): 20-21. This article explains the progression of frostbite and discusses its causes. Illustrated with photographs.

Tilton, Buck. *Backcountry First Aid and Extended Care.* 4th ed. Old Saybrook, Conn.: Globe Pequot Press, 2002. A small, portable guide to the myriad emergencies and medical problems encountered in the wilderness.

_____. "The Chill That Bites." *Backpacker* 28, no. 7 (September, 2000): 27. Tilton offers important information about windchill, frostbite, and appropriate attire for braving the cold.

Tredget, Edward E., ed. *Thermal Injuries.* Philadelphia: W. B. Saunders, 2000. Examines wounds, such as burns and frostbite, and their surgical treatments.

Wilkerson, James A., ed. *Medicine for Mountaineering and Other Wilderness Activities.* 5th ed. Seattle: The Mountaineers, 2001. This book is a first-aid manual that goes beyond traditional treatment protocols. It was written for those who need information to care for serious injuries when organized medical help is not available.

FRUCTOSEMIA

DISEASE/DISORDER

ANATOMY OR SYSTEM AFFECTED: Gastrointestinal system, intestines, kidneys, liver

SPECIALTIES AND RELATED FIELDS: Biochemistry, genetics, nutrition, pediatrics

DEFINITION: An inborn error of metabolism in which eating foods containing fructose or sucrose will result in high blood fructose levels.

CAUSES AND SYMPTOMS

Fructosemia may also be called hereditary fructose intolerance; it literally means "fructose in the blood." Fructosemia occurs as a result of a hereditary lack of an enzyme called fructose-1-phosphate aldolase B. This autosomal recessive disease is rare, although some researchers suspect that more people have the disorder than are diagnosed. These individuals may naturally avoid fructose after becoming ill following the consumption of fructose-containing foods. The infant, child, or adult with undiagnosed fructosemia will be normal unless foods containing fructose, sucrose, or sorbitol are eaten. If foods containing these carbohydrates are eaten, then fructose levels will increase in the patient's blood and urine and the person will become ill. Symptoms include vomiting and low blood glucose and may progress to failure to thrive and/or coma. The severity of the disease appears to be variable, being rather mild in some individuals and causing death in others. In severe cases, the liver, kidneys, and intestines may be affected, although this damage usually reverses with the elimination of dietary fructose.

TREATMENT AND THERAPY

Treatment for this disorder is entirely dietary. Foods containing fructose, sucrose, or sorbitol must be eliminated from the diet. Fructose is often thought of as "fruit sugar," but far more foods than fruits and juices must be eliminated. Honey contains fructose. Because half of sucrose becomes fructose when sucrose is metabolized, all foods containing sucrose (sugar) must be eliminated as well. This includes all sugar, whether from cane, beets, or sorghum. Sucrose is also part of maple syrup. Sorbitol metabolism also produces fructose, and so this sugar substitute must be avoided as well. Some infant formulas and baby foods may contain fructose, and many sweetened fruit beverages do.

INFORMATION ON FRUCTOSEMIA

CAUSES: Genetic enzyme deficiency

SYMPTOMS: Variable; may include vomiting, low blood glucose, failure to thrive, and coma if foods containing fructose, sucrose, or sorbitol are eaten

DURATION: Chronic

TREATMENTS: Avoidance of foods containing fructose, sucrose, or sorbitol

Reading food labels and being familiar with the ingredients of restaurant food is imperative for those with fructosemia.

Perspective and Prospects

Cases of fructosemia were first described in the mid-1950's. Soon after, the biochemical pathway defect was discovered. Today, genetic counseling may be of benefit to those who have fructosemia and want to have children, although strict avoidance of the three carbohydrates fructose, sucrose, and sorbitol will prevent symptoms.

—*Karen Chapman-Novakofski, R.D., L.D., Ph.D.*

See also Endocrine disorders; Endocrinology; Endocrinology, pediatric; Enzyme therapy; Enzymes; Galactosemia; Genetic diseases; Lactose intolerance; Metabolism; Nutrition.

For Further Information:

Ali, M., et al. "Hereditary Fructose Intolerance." *Journal of Medical Genetics* 35, no. 5 (May, 1998): 353-365.

Cox, T. M. "Aldolase B and Fructose Intolerance." *FASEB Journal* 8, no. 1 (January, 1994): 62-71.

Van den Berghe, G. "Disorders of Fructose Metabolism." In *Inborn Metabolic Diseases: Diagnosis and Treatment*, edited by J. Fernandes, J.-M. Saudubray, and Van den Berghe. 3d rev. ed. New York: Springer, 2000.

Fungal infections
Disease/disorder

Anatomy or system affected: Immune system, nails, respiratory system, skin

Specialties and related fields: Dermatology, family practice, immunology, internal medicine, microbiology, pulmonary medicine

Definition: Infections caused by fungi—simple, plantlike organisms—that range from minor skin diseases to serious, disseminated diseases of the lungs and other organs; patients whose immune systems are impaired are at greater risk of serious fungal infections.

Key terms:

asexual reproduction: the production of new individuals without the mating of two parents of unlike genotype, such as by budding

mycelium: a collection of threadlike fungal strands (hyphae) making up the thallus, or nonreproductive portion, of a fungus

mycosis: a disease of humans, plants, or animals caused by a fungus; the prefix *myco-* means "fungus," hence mycology (the study of fungi)

pleomorphic fungus: a fungus whose morphology changes markedly from one phase of its life cycle to another, or according to changes in environmental conditions

tinea: a medical term for fungal skin diseases, such as ringworm and athlete's foot, caused by a variety of fungi

yeast: a unicellular fungus which reproduces by budding off smaller cells from the parent cell; yeasts belong to several different groups of fungi, and some fungi are capable of growing either as a yeast or as a filamentous fungus

Types of Fungus

The term "fungus" is a general one for plantlike organisms that do not produce their own food through photosynthesis but live as heterotrophs, absorbing complex carbon compounds from other living or dead organisms. Fungi were formerly classified in the plant kingdom (together with bacteria, all algae, mosses, and green plants); more recently, biologists have realized that there are fundamental differences in cell structure and organization separating the lower plants into a number of groups which merit recognition as kingdoms. Fungi differ from bacteria and actinomycetes in being eukaryotic, that is, in having an organized nucleus with chromosomes within the cell. One division of fungi, which is believed to be distantly related to certain aquatic algae, has spores that swim by means of flagella. These water molds include pathogens of fish and aquatic insect larvae and a few economically important plant pathogens, but none have yet been recorded as causing a defined, nonopportunistic human disease. The other division of fungi lacks flagellated spores at any stage in its life cycle. It encompasses most familiar fungi, including molds, mushrooms, yeasts, wood-rotting fungi, leaf spots, and all fungi reliably reported to cause disease in humans.

Fungi that lack flagellated stages in their life cycles are further divided into three classes and one form-class according to the manner in which the spores are produced. The first of these, the Zygomycetes (for example *Rhizopus*, the black bread mold), produce thick-walled, solitary sexual spores as a result of hyphal fusion; they are a diverse assemblage including many parasites of insects. Species in the genus *Mucor* cause a rare, fulminating, rapidly fatal systemic disease called mucormycosis, generally in acidotic diabetic patients. The Basidiomycetes, characterized by the production of sexual spores externally on a club-shaped structure called a basidium, includes mushrooms, plant rusts (such as stem rust of wheat), and most wood-rotting fungi. There is one important basidiomycetous human pathogen (*Filobasidiella neoformans*) and a few confirmed opportunists. The Ascomycetes, including most yeasts and lichens, many plant pathogens (such as Dutch elm disease and chestnut blight), and a great diversity of saprophytes growing on wood and herbaceous material, produce sexual spores in a saclike structure called an ascus. One ascomycete, *Piedraia nigra*, regularly produces its characteristic fruiting bodies on its human host; others do so in culture. In addition, there is a form-class Deuteromycetes consisting of fungi that produce only asexual spores. Most are suspected of being stages in the life cycle of Ascomycetes, but some are Basidiomycetes or are of uncertain affinity. Human pathogens, at least as they occur on the host or in typical laboratory culture, are mostly Deuteromycetes.

Medical mycology would occupy only a single chapter in a book on the relationship of fungi to human affairs. Relatively few fungi have become adapted to living as parasites of human (or even mammalian) hosts, and of these, the most common ones cause superficial and cutaneous mycoses with annoying but scarcely life-threatening effects. Serious fungal diseases are mercifully rare among people with normally functioning immune systems.

The majority of fungi are directly dependent on green plants, as parasites, as symbionts living in a mutually beneficial association with a plant, or as sapro-phytes on dead plant material. One large, successful group of Ascomycetes lives in symbiotic association with algae, forming lichens. Fungi play a critical ecological role in maintaining stable plant communities. As plant pathogens, they cause serious economic loss, leading in extreme cases to famine. The ability of saprophytic fungi to transform chemically the substrate on which they are growing has been exploited by the brewing industry since antiquity and has been expanded to other industrial processes. Penicillin, other antibiotics, and some vitamins are extracted from fungi, which produce a vast array of complex organic compounds whose potential is only beginning to be explored and which constitutes a fertile field for those interested in genetic engineering.

This same chemical diversity and complexity also enable fungi to produce mycotoxins—chemicals that have an adverse effect on humans and animals. Saprophytic fungi growing on improperly stored food are a troublesome source of toxic compounds, some of which are carcinogenic. The old adage that "a little mold won't hurt you" is true in the sense that common molds do not cause acute illness when ingested, but it is poor advice in terms of long-term health.

A mycotoxicity problem of considerable medical and veterinary interest is posed by Ascomycetes of the order Clavicipitales, which are widespread on grasses. Some species of grasses routinely harbor systemic, asymptomatic infections by these fungi, which produce compounds toxic to animals that graze on them. From the point of view of the grass, the relationship is symbiotic, since it discourages grazing; from the point of view of range management, the relationship is deleterious to stock. *Claviceps purpurea*, a pathogen of rye, causes a condition known as ergotism in humans, with symptoms including miscarriage, vascular constriction leading to gangrene of the limbs, and hallucinations. Outbreaks of hallucinatory ergotism are thought by some authors to be responsible for some of the more spectacular perceptions of witchcraft in premodern times. Better control of plant disease and a decreased reliance on rye as a staple grain have virtually eliminated ergotism as a human disease in the twentieth century.

Fungi exhibit a bewildering variety of forms and life cycles; nevertheless, certain generalizations can be made. A fungus starts life as a spore, which may be a single cell or a cluster of cells and is usually microscopic. Under proper conditions, the spore germinates, producing a filament of fungal cells oriented end to end, called a hypha. Hyphae grow into the substrate, secreting enzymes that dissolve structures to provide food for the growing fungus and to provide holes through which the fungus can grow. In an asexually reproducing fungus, some of the hyphae become differentiated, producing specialized cells (spores) which differ from the parent hypha in size and pigmentation and are adapted for dispersal, but which are genetically identical to the parent. In a sexually reproducing fungus, two hyphae (or a hypha and a spore from different individuals) fuse, their nuclei fuse, and meiosis takes place before spores are formed. Spores are often produced in a specialized fruiting body, such as a mushroom.

Fungus spores are ubiquitous. Common saprophytic fungi produce airborne spores in enormous quantities; thus it is difficult to avoid contact with them in all but the most hypersterile environments. In culture, fungi (including pathogenic species) produce large numbers of dry spores that can be transmitted in the air from host to host, making working with fungi in a medical laboratory potentially hazardous.

Fungal Diseases and Treatments

Human fungal diseases are generally placed in four broad categories according to the tissues they attack, and they are further subdivided according to specific pathologies and the organisms involved. The categories of disease are superficial mycoses, cutaneous mycoses, subcutaneous mycoses, and systemic mycoses.

Superficial mycoses affect hair and the outermost layer of the epidermis and do not evoke a cellular response. They include tinea versicolor and tinea nigra, deutermycete infections that cause discolored patches on skin, and black piedra, caused by an ascomycete growing on hair shafts. They can be treated with a topical fungicide, such as nystatin, or, in the case of piedra, by shaving off the affected hair.

Cutaneous mycoses involve living cells of the skin or mucous membrane and evoke a cellular response, generally localized inflammation. Dermatomycoses (dermatophytes), which affect skin and hair, include tinea capitis (ringworm of the scalp), tinea pedis (athlete's foot), and favus, a scaly infection of the scalp. Domestic animals serve as a reservoir for some cutaneous mycoses. The organisms responsible are generally fungi imperfecti in the genera *Microsporon* and *Trichophyton*. Cutaneous mycoses can be successfully treated with topical nystatin or oral griseofulvin.

Candida albicans, a ubiquitous pleomorphic fungus with both a yeast and a mycelial form, causes a variety of cutaneous mycoses as well as systemic infections collectively named candidiasis. Thrush is a *Candida* yeast infection of the mouth which is most common in infants, especially in infants born to mothers with vaginal candidiasis. Vaginal yeast infections periodically affect 18 to 20 percent of the adult female population and more than 30 percent of pregnant women. *Candida* also causes paronychia, a nailbed infection. Small populations of *Candida* are normally present in the alimentary tract and genital tract of healthy individuals; candidiasis of the mucous membranes tends to develop in response to antibiotic treatment, which disturbs the normal bacterial flora of the body, or in response to metabolic changes or decreasing immune function.

None of the organisms causing cutaneous mycoses elicits a lasting immune response, so recurring infections by these agents is the rule rather than the exception. Even in temperate climates, under modern standards of hygiene, cutaneous mycoses are extremely common.

Subcutaneous mycoses, affecting skin and muscle tissue, are predominantly tropical in distribution and not particularly common. Chromomycosis and maduromycosis are caused by soil fungi that enter the skin through wounds, causing chronic localized tumors, usually on the feet. Sporotrichosis enters through wounds and spreads through the lymphatic system, causing skin ulcers associated with lymph nodes. Amphotericin B, a highly toxic systemic antifungal agent, has been used to treat all three conditions; potassium iodide is used to treat sporotrichosis, and localized chromomycosis and maduromycosis lesions can be surgically removed.

Systemic mycoses, the most serious of fungal infections, have the ability to become generally disseminated in the body. The main nonopportunistic systemic mycoses known in North America are histoplasmosis, caused by *Histoplasma capsulatum*; coccidiomycosis, caused by *Coccidioides immitis;* blastomycosis, caused by *Ajellomyces* (or *Blastomyces*) *dermatidis*; and cryptococcosis, caused by *Cryptococcus* (or *Filobasidiella*) *neoformans*. Similar infections, caused by related species, occur in other parts of the world.

Coccidiomycosis, also called San Joaquin Valley fever or valley fever, will serve as an example of the etiology of systemic mycoses. The causative organism lives in arid soils in the American southwest; its spores are wind-disseminated. When inhaled, the fungus grows in the lungs, producing a mild respiratory infection which is self-limiting in perhaps 95 percent of the cases. The mild form of the disease is common in rural areas. In a minority of cases, a chronic lung disease whose symptoms resemble tuberculosis develops. There is also a disseminated form of the disease producing meningitis; chronic cutaneous disease, with the production of ulcers and granulomas; and attack of the bones, internal organs, and lymphatic system. A chronic pulmonary infection may become systemic in response to factors that undermine the body's immune system. Factors involved in individual susceptibility among individuals with intact immune systems are poorly understood.

Histoplasmosis (also known as summer fever, cave fever, or Mississippi Valley fever) is even more common; 90 percent of people tested in the southern Mississippi Valley show a positive reaction to this fungus, indicating prior, self-limiting lung infection. The fungus is associated with bird and bat droppings, and severe cases sometimes occur when previously unexposed individuals are exposed to high levels of innoculum in caves where bats roost. A related organism, *Histoplasma duboisii*, occurs in central Africa. Blastomycosis causes chronic pulmonary disease, chronic cutaneous disease, and systemic disease, all of which were usually fatal until the advent of chemotherapy with amphotericin B. The natural habitat of the fungus is unclear. *Cryptococcus neoformans* occurs in pigeon droppings and is worldwide in distribution. The subclinical pulmonary form of the disease is probably common; invasive disease occurs in patients with collagen diseases, such as lupus, and in patients with weakened immune systems. It is the leading cause of invasive fungal disease in patients with acquired immunodeficiency syndrome (AIDS).

Systemic fungal diseases are notoriously difficult to treat. Chemotherapy of systemic, organismally caused diseases depends on finding a chemical compound which will selectively kill or inhibit the invading organism without damaging the host. Therefore, the more closely the parasite species is related biologically to the host species, the more difficult it is to find a compound which will act in such a selective manner. Fungi are, from a biological standpoint, more like humans than they are like bacteria, and antibacterial antibiotics are ineffective against them. If a fungus has invaded the skin or the digestive tract, it can be attacked with toxic substances that are not readily absorbed into the bloodstream, but this approach is not appropriate for a systemic infection. Amphotericin, intraconazole, and fluconazole, the drugs of choice for systemic fungal infections, are highly toxic to humans. Thus, dosage is critical, close clinical supervision is necessary, and long-term therapy may not be feasible.

PERSPECTIVE AND PROSPECTS

Medical mycology textbooks written before 1980 tended to focus on two categories of fungal infection: the common, ubiquitous, and comparatively benign superficial and cutaneous mycoses, frequently seen in clinical practice in the industrialized world, and the subcutaneous and deep mycoses, treated as a rare and/or predominantly tropical problem. Opportunistic systemic infections, if mentioned at all, were regarded as a rare curiosity.

The rising population of patients with compromised immune systems, including cancer patients undergoing chemotherapy, people being treated with steroids for various conditions, transplant patients, and people with AIDS, has dramatically changed this clinical picture. Between 1980 and 1986, more than a hundred fungi, a few previously unknown and the majority common inhabitants of crop plants, rotting vegetable debris, and soil, were identified as causing human disease. The number continues to increase steadily. Compared to organisms routinely isolated from soil and plants, these opportunistic fungi do not seem to have any special characteristics other than the ability to grow at human

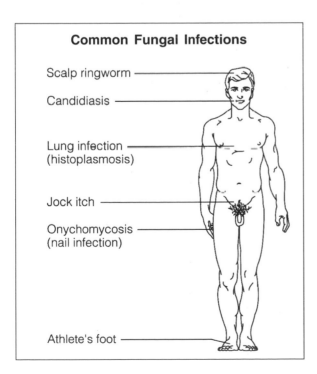

Common Fungal Infections

Scalp ringworm

Candidiasis

Lung infection (histoplasmosis)

Jock itch

Onychomycosis (nail infection)

Athlete's foot

body temperature; however, the possibility that an opportunistic pathogen might mutate into a form capable of attacking healthy humans is worrisome.

Systemic opportunistic human infections have been attributed to *Alternaria alternata* and *Fusarium oxysporum*, common plant pathogens that cause diseases of tomatoes and strawberries, respectively. Several species of *Aspergillus*, saprophytic molds (many of them thermophilic), have long been implicated in human disease. Colonizing aspergillosis, involving localized growth in the lungs of people exposed to high levels of aspergillus spores (notably agricultural workers working with silage), is not particularly rare among people with normal immune systems, but the more severe invasive form of the disease, in which massive lung lesions form, and disseminated aspergillosis, in which other organs are attacked, almost always involve immunocompromised patients. *Ramichloridium schulzeri*, described originally from wheat roots, causes "golden tongue" in leukemia patients; fortunately this infection responds to amphotericin B. *Scelidosporium inflatum*, first isolated from a serious bone infection in an immunocompromised patient in 1984, is being isolated with increasing frequency in cases of disseminated mycosis; it resists standard drug treatment.

Oral colonization by strains of *Candida* is often the first sign of AIDS-related complex or full-blown AIDS in an individual harboring the human immunodeficiency virus (HIV). Drug therapy with fluconazole is effective against oral candidiasis, but relapse rates of up to 50 percent within a month of the cessation of drug therapy are reported. Reported rates of disseminated candidiasis in AIDS patients range from 1 to 10 percent. Invasive procedures such as intravenous catheters represent a significant risk of introducing *Candida* and other common fungi into the bloodstream of patients.

Pneumocystis carinii, the organism causing a form of pneumonia which is the single most important cause of death in patients with AIDS, was originally classified as a sporozoan—that is, as a parasitic protozoan—but detailed investigations of the life cycle, metabolism, and genetic material of *Pneumocystis* have convinced some biologists that it is actually an ascomycete, although an anomalous one that lacks a cell wall. Unfortunately, it does not respond to therapy with the antifungal drugs currently in use.

In general, antifungal drug therapy for mycoses in AIDS patients is not very successful. In the absence of significant patient immunity, it is difficult to eradicate a disseminated infection from the body entirely, making a resurgence likely once drug therapy is discontinued. Reinfection is also likely if the organism is a common component of the patient's environment.

Given the increasing number of lethal systemic fungal infections seen in clinical practice, there is substantial impetus for a search for more effective, less toxic antifungal drugs. A number of compounds, produced by bacteria and chemically dissimilar to both antibacterial antibiotics and the most widely used antifungal compounds, have been identified and are being tested. It is also possible that the plant kingdom, which has been under assault by fungi for all its long geologic history, may prove a source for medically useful antifungal compounds.

—Martha Sherwood-Pike, Ph.D.

See also Acquired immunodeficiency syndrome (AIDS); Athlete's foot; Candidiasis; Diaper rash; Food poisoning; Immune system; Immunodeficiency disorders; Immunology; Immunopathology; Microbiology; Mold and mildew; Nail removal; Nails; Pneumonia; Poisonous plants; Ringworm; Skin; Skin disorders.

FOR FURTHER INFORMATION:

Alcamo, I. Edward. *Microbes and Society: An Introduction to Microbiology.* Sudbury, Mass.: Jones and Bartlett, 2002. A nonscientific text for the liberal arts student that explores the importance of microbes to human life and their role in food production and agriculture, in biotechnology and industry, in ecology and the environment, and in disease and bioterrorism.

Biddle, Wayne. *Field Guide to Germs.* 2d ed. New York: Anchor Books, 2002. This comprehensive book is easily accessible to the nonspecialist and includes a discussion of nearly every virus, bacterium, and fungus known to cause human and nonhuman animal disease. The history of the microbe and the treatment of diseases are included.

British Society for Antimicrobial Chemotherapy Working Party. "Antifungal Chemotherapy in Patients with Acquired Immunodeficiency Syndrome." *The Lancet* 340, no. 8820 (September 12, 1992): 648-650. Provides an overview of occurrence and therapies for the use of physicians in the British Isles. The article emphasizes candidiasis, cryptococcosis, histoplasmosis, and coccidiomycosis.

Crissey, John Thorne, Heidi Lang, and Lawrence Charles Parish. *Manual of Medical Mycology.* Cambridge, Mass.: Blackwell Scientific, 1995. This handbook discusses the diagnosis and treatment of fungal infections. Includes a bibliography and an index.

Mandell, Gerald L., R. Gordon Douglas, Jr., and John E. Bennett, eds. *Principles and Practice of Infectious Diseases*. 5th ed. New York: Churchill Livingstone, 2000. An outstanding textbook on infectious diseases, with chapters on the various diseases caused by *Candida*, illnesses and conditions associated with this fungus, and antifungal agents.

Murray, P. R., et al. *Medical Microbiology*. 4th Ed. New York: Elsevier, 2001. Focuses on microbes that cause disease in humans. Each chapter consistently presents the etiology, epidemiology, host defenses, identification, diagnosis, prevention, and control of each disease.

Rippon, John W. *Medical Mycology: The Pathogenic Fungi and Pathogenic Actinomycetes*. 3d ed. Philadelphia: W. B. Saunders, 1987. A standard medical mycology textbook for students of medicine and microbiology, with detailed descriptions of common mycoses and the organisms that cause them, as an aid to clinical diagnosis.

Robbins, Stanley L., Ramzi S. Cotran, and Vinay Kumar, eds. *Robbins' Pathologic Basis of Disease*. 6th ed. Philadelphia: W. B. Saunders, 1999. A leading medical textbook that covers the major topics of general and systemic pathology.

Shaw, Michael, ed. *Everything You Need to Know About Diseases*. Springhouse, Pa.: Springhouse Press, 1996. This well-illustrated consumer reference, compiled by more than one hundred doctors and medical experts, describes five hundred illnesses and conditions, their causes, symptoms, diagnosis, treatment, and prevention. Of particular interest is chapter 19, "Infection."

Watkinson, Sarah, and Graham W. Gooday. *Fungi*. 2d ed. New York: Elsevier, 2001. Text that takes a microbiological perspective and introduces the importance of fungi in the natural world and in practical applications. The diversity of fungi as organisms and their roles in relation to people, animals, and plants are clearly described.

Weedon, David. *Skin Pathology*. 2d ed. New York: Harcourt, 2002. Text with extensive photographs, covering tissue reaction patterns; the epidermis, dermis and subcutis; the skin in systemic and miscellaneous diseases; infections and infestations; and tumors, among other topics.

GALACTOSEMIA

DISEASE/DISORDER

ANATOMY OR SYSTEM AFFECTED: Eyes, liver

SPECIALTIES AND RELATED FIELDS: Biochemistry, genetics, nutrition, pediatrics

DEFINITION: An inherited disorder of carbohydrate metabolism in which an infant is unable to utilize galactose from food.

INFORMATION ON GALACTOSEMIA

CAUSES: Genetic enzyme deficiency

SYMPTOMS: Varies; may include jaundice, vomiting, liver enlargement, cataracts, failure to thrive, and mental retardation if foods containing galactose (milk sugar) are eaten

DURATION: Chronic

TREATMENTS: Avoidance of foods containing galactose

CAUSES AND SYMPTOMS

In classic I galactosemia, a congenital deficiency of the enzyme galactose-1-phosphate uridyl transferase (GALT) causes galactose to accumulate instead of being converted to glucose for energy production. As galactose accumulates in the child's tissues and organs, it will have a toxic effect and cause various signs and symptoms. Galactosemia means "galactose in the blood." Galactose is a sugar that may be found alone in foods but is usually associated with lactose, a milk sugar.

A gene mutation on the short arm of chromosome 9 has been identified in babies with galactosemia. About 1 in 40,000 newborns is affected with this autosomal recessive disorder. Both parents serve as carriers; they are not themselves affected, but there is a one in four chance that one of their children will be born with galactosemia. Prenatal diagnosis is possible in cultured fibroblasts from amniotic fluid. Mandatory screening programs in many states test all newborns for galactosemia during the first week of life.

Galactosemia is an example of a multiple-allele system. In addition to the normal allele (G) and the recessive allele (g), a third allele, known as G^D, has been found. The D allele is named after Duarte, California, where it was discovered. The existence of three alleles produces six possible genotypic combinations in the deoxyribonucleic acid (DNA). These enzymatic activities may range from 0 to 100 percent. Consequently, it is very important to monitor each patient with biochemical studies.

Homozygous recessive infants (gg) are unaffected at birth but develop symptoms a few days later, including jaundice, vomiting, an enlarged liver from extensive fatty deposits, cataracts, and failure to thrive. Mental retardation and death may also occur if dietary treatment has not been started.

TREATMENT AND THERAPY

Galactosemia is treated by removing foods that contain galactose from the diet. Since milk and milk products are the most common source of galactose, infants with galactosemia should not be given these foods. Serious problems can be prevented through this early exclusion of galactose.

While it is not possible for a child with galactosemia to have an entirely galactose-free diet, all persons with galactosemia should limit galactose intake from foods to a very low level. The galactose-1-phosphate levels determine the degree of dietary restriction for each individual. Advice from a dietician is needed.

—*Phillip A. Farber, Ph.D.*

See also Endocrine system; Endocrinology; Endocrinology, pediatric; Enzyme therapy; Enzymes; Fructosemia; Gaucher's disease; Genetic diseases; Glycogen storage diseases; Lactose intolerance; Mental retardation; Metabolism; Nutrition.

FOR FURTHER INFORMATION:

Cummings, Michael R. *Human Heredity: Principles and Issues*. 6th ed. Pacific Grove, Calif.: Thomson/Brooks/Cole, 2003.

Miesfeldt, Susan, and J. Larry Jameson. "Screening, Counseling, and Prevention of Genetic Disorders." In *Harrison's Principles of Internal Medicine*, edited by Eugene Braunwald et al. 15th ed. New York: McGraw-Hill, 2001.

Rudolph, Colin D., et al., eds. *Rudolph's Pediatrics*. 21st ed. New York: McGraw-Hill, 2003.

GALLBLADDER DISEASES

DISEASE/DISORDER

ANATOMY OR SYSTEM AFFECTED: Abdomen, gallbladder, gastrointestinal system

SPECIALTIES AND RELATED FIELDS: Gastroenterology, internal medicine

DEFINITION: A family of disorders affecting the gallbladder and causing abdominal pain or occasionally symptomless.

KEY TERMS:

bile: a complex solution formed by liver cells which is composed mainly of bile salts, fats, and cholesterol, which aids in fat digestion; it is secreted by the liver into a system of ducts connecting the liver, gallbladder, and intestinal tract

biliary colic: a distinct pain syndrome characterized by severe intermittent waves of right-sided, upper abdominal pain, often brought on by the ingestion of fatty foods; pain occurs when a gallstone obstructs the outflow of bile and usually resolves when the gallstone moves away from the outflow area

cholecystectomy: the surgical procedure that results in the removal of the gallbladder in its entirety; the two main techniques are the traditional open method and the laparoscopically aided method

cholecystitis: the disease that occurs when the gallbladder becomes inflamed or infected, which produces severe right-sided, upper abdominal pain, fever, and other signs of infection; a frequent indication for removal of the gallbladder

cholelithiasis: the presence of gallstones in the gallbladder

gallbladder: a muscular, walled sac located on the under surface of the liver which stores and concentrates bile; under stimulus from the intestine in response to a meal, the gallbladder contracts and expels bile into the digestive tract to aid in fat digestion

gallstones: particles that form in the gallbladder when the solubility of the components of bile is somehow altered, also resulting in the precipitation of cholesterol; the gallstones, which can grow very large, are made up mostly of cholesterol but can be pigmented or contain other substances

laparoscopic cholecystectomy: a procedure in which the gallbladder is removed with the help of a telescopic eyepiece which is attached to a tube inserted into the patient's body; the surgery is done using four small incisions and allows the patient to recover much faster than the traditional method of open surgery

CAUSES AND SYMPTOMS

Gallbladder diseases affect a large number of patients and are among the most common causes of abdominal pain. Most gallbladder problems stem from the presence of gallstones, which may be present in as many as one of every ten adults. In the past, anyone with gallstones was advised to have the gallbladder taken out, but this is no longer the case. It is now known that many people with gallstones never experience difficulty because of them.

A very common gallbladder disease is biliary colic. This is usually manifested by severe right-sided, upper abdominal pain which is fairly repetitive in nature. The pain may literally take the patient's breath away, but an episode usually lasts less than thirty minutes. The patient may also complain of right-sided shoulder or back pain, often caused by irritation of the diaphragmatic nerves, which are located just above the liver on the right side. Many people may confuse the pain of biliary colic with indigestion, because in some patients it may be experienced in the middle of the upper abdomen. This pain is almost always brought on by eating, since the gallbladder contracts in response to food in the intestinal tract. The meal triggering such an episode often is described as rich and fatty, and many patients soon learn what types of food to avoid. Biliary colic does not occur unless gallstones are present, because they tend to obstruct the outflow of bile from the gallbladder. The treatment for biliary colic usually consists of dietary manipulation, that is, the avoidance of fatty foods or other foods known to trigger the pain. Surgery is performed if the patient so desires, and removing the gallbladder should cure the problem.

When a diagnosis of gallstones is suspected, the physician will take down the patient's medical history and perform a physical examination. In most cases, however, such actions will yield no physical findings that are indicative of gallstone disease. Thus the diagnosis is usually confirmed by an imaging study of the gallbladder, in which the gallstones are either directly or indirectly visualized. The most commonly used imaging modality is the ultrasound test, which can be easily and rapidly performed with very reliable results. While the gallstones cannot actually be seen, they have a density which reflects, rather than transmits, sound waves. As a result, they create specific echoes and shadows that can be interpreted by the radiologists as gallstones. No patient should be treated for gallstone

---

INFORMATION ON GALLBLADDER DISEASES

CAUSES: Presence of gallstones

SYMPTOMS: Varies; often includes severe and repetitive right-sided, upper abdominal pain; inflammation and infection; chills or fever

DURATION: Acute

TREATMENTS: Surgery, dietary management

disease without such imaging to confirm the presence of gallstones.

A potentially serious type of gallbladder disease caused by gallstones is acute cholecystitis. In this condition, the outflow of bile is obstructed, usually by a gallstone that is stuck in the outflow tract, and severe inflammation and infection may develop. A patient with acute cholecystitis often complains of pain that does not go away promptly, may have chills or fever, and is usually found to have a very tender abdomen on the upper right side. The treatment of this condition is not controversial, and most physicians would probably recommend removing the gallbladder surgically. The only question remaining is whether the gallbladder should be removed immediately or electively, at a later date, if the patient recovers from acute cholecystitis with conservative management, including the use of antibiotics and the avoidance of eating until the inflammation subsides.

Inflammation and infection can also occur, although rarely, in gallbladders that do not produce gallstones. This happens in very select circumstances and is called acute acalculous cholecystitis. It usually afflicts very ill patients who have been in an intensive care unit for a long time, patients who have needed a heart-lung machine as a result of open heart surgery, or patients who are unable to eat for an extended period of time because of other problems. These patients are often fed only intravenously, which can lead to severe gallbladder problems. The exact mechanisms are not entirely known, but alterations in blood flow and an impaired ability to fight infection may play a role. Whatever the cause, the treatment often remains the same: removal of the gallbladder that does not respond to conservative therapy.

Gallstones can also move out of the gallbladder and cause serious problems. The main outflow tract of bile from the gallbladder and liver is the common bile duct, and this is a place gallstones frequently lodge. The end of this duct is surrounded by a small muscle called the sphincter of Oddi, which may not allow the passage of gallstones. If they become stuck there, they can completely obstruct the biliary system, and the patient will appear jaundiced. Removal of the gallstones will cure the problem. The presence of gallstones in the common bile duct is also associated with the development of pancreatitis, an inflammation of the pancreas which can be severe and life-threatening. Removal of the gallbladder at an appropriate time will prevent future bouts of pancreatitis.

The gallbladder can also be a source of cancer. Although cancer of the gallbladder is not common, it is estimated that one out of every one hundred gallbladders removed will contain cancer. Therefore, all specimens removed must be examined by a qualified pathologist and all reports must be reviewed in their entirety by the surgeon. If the disease is limited to a minor thickness of the gallbladder, no further therapy is needed, but if the tumor is larger, further surgery—including removal of part of the liver—may be necessary. Gallbladder cancer grows silently in many patients, and it is often not detected until late in its course.

TREATMENT AND THERAPY

Because there is no simple way to prevent gallbladder problems, surgery plays a large role in their manage-

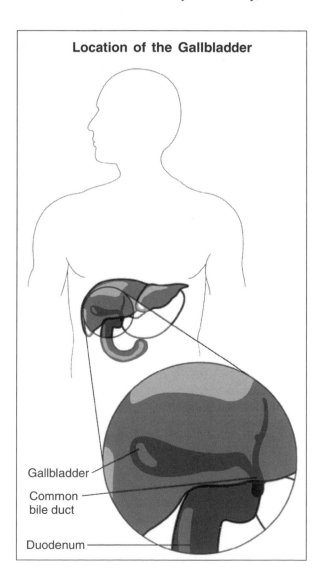

Location of the Gallbladder

Gallbladder

Common bile duct

Duodenum

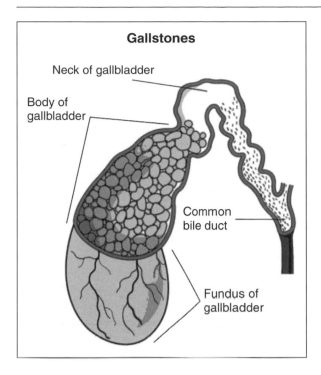

Gallstones

Neck of gallbladder

Body of gallbladder

Common bile duct

Fundus of gallbladder

ment. Removing the gallbladder, a relatively routine operation, results in a complete cure, with acceptably low complication rates and few long-term problems. While several exciting new ways of treating gallbladder and gallstone problems have been developed, the classic and standard method of therapy for gallbladder disease has been open cholecystectomy. This procedure entails making an incision across the upper right side of the abdomen a few inches below and parallel to the bottom of the rib cage. The muscles of the abdominal wall are cut, and the abdominal cavity is opened. The gallbladder, which is usually located right under this incision, is then removed and the incision closed in layers. This method of gallbladder removal has acceptable complication rates and is relatively safe and extremely effective. It allows the surgeon to inspect the entire abdomen and rule out other problems. One must consider, however, that this procedure constitutes major surgery. Most patients need to be in the hospital for a minimum of three to five days, and there is a considerable amount of pain with this incision. These problems have prompted surgeons to find a less invasive way of removing the gallbladder, thereby achieving better pain control and reducing the length of the hospital stay and the time lost from work and other activities.

A laparoscope is an optical instrument, composed of a tube connected to a telescopic eyepiece, that allows the surgeon to perform a procedure inside the patient's body. Although it has been employed in surgeries for many years, mainly in gynecological procedures, it was adapted only recently for removal of the gallbladder, as well as in other types of surgeries. Since then, laparoscopic cholecystectomy has become a procedure that all surgeons must know in order to stay current with the profession. The laparoscope and other surgical instruments are inserted directly into the abdomen through several small incisions, and the gallbladder is removed without a large incision having been made. The patients are often discharged the same day of the surgery, and they return to work much faster than with the open technique.

Despite its advantages, there are some pitfalls with laparoscopic cholecystectomy, and it cannot be used for all patients. There is an increased incidence of certain injuries to other organs and bile ducts at the time of the operation because less of the area can be seen than with an open operation. In addition, patients who have had previous upper abdominal surgery are not candidates for this procedure, and for those with acute cholecystitis, severe inflammation may make this technique unsafe. For most patients, however, laparoscopic cholecystectomy can be performed easily and safely with minimal complications and excellent results. It is becoming the standard of care and will continue to change the way gallbladder surgery is performed. The laparoscope is also being used to perform appendectomies, ulcer surgeries, cancer surveillance, and all types of intra-abdominal surgery.

Radiologists and internists may play an important role in the management of gallbladder disease. In certain circumstances, the techniques performed by these specialists may be indicated for extremely ill patients who might not be able to tolerate an operation, or for whom the anesthesia might be too hazardous. Invasive radiologists can actually place a tube into the gallbladder with help from their imaging equipment and remove infection or troublesome gallstones from the gallbladder. This procedure can alleviate symptoms in some patients, who may not even require any additional intervention. These practices are not common, however, and they are usually reserved for the very ill patient who might not survive an open operation or is at extremely high risk to develop a certain complication.

Gallstones can migrate out of the gallbladder and cause problems if they lodge in and obstruct the common bile duct. This places the patient at high risk for developing jaundice and infection in the biliary system. The standard method for dealing with this problem continues to be open surgery. In this procedure, the gallbladder is removed through an incision and the common bile duct is also opened. The gallstones are removed through a variety of techniques, and the duct is then closed. A tube is placed in the duct to keep it open, because otherwise it could scar and become narrowed. Many of these patients must be hospitalized for a number of days, making this surgery an expensive one.

Internists who specialize in the diseases of the abdomen have become proficient at performing endoscopic techniques. These techniques came about after the development of fiberoptics, which allow one to see through a tube, even if it is bent at a variety of angles. An endoscope, composed of surgical instruments, a light source, and fiberoptic cables, can be used to examine the lining of the stomach and intestines, allowing the diagnosis of many conditions.

Endoscopy is performed by inserting the endoscope through the mouth and into the patient's stomach and the first part of the intestines. From this location, the area where the common bile duct opens into the intestines can be seen, and this is often where gallstones become lodged. The gallstones can be removed with instruments attached to the scope, thus solving the patient's problem. Unfortunately, this technique does not remove the gallbladder, the source of the gallstones, and the patient is at some risk for a recurrence. This risk can be minimized by enlarging the opening where the duct enters the intestinal tract. This technique, too, is advantageous for patients who are elderly or ill and cannot withstand the trauma of surgery and anesthesia.

There are other options besides surgery or dietary changes for the treatment of patients with gallstones. Medicines are available that can dissolve the gallstones by changing the chemical nature and solubility of bile. Such drugs, however, are not ideal: They work only for certain types of gallstones, are expensive, and may produce side effects. In addition, there may be a recurrence of the gallstones when a patient stops taking these medicines. Such a result indicates that the bile-concentrating action of the gallbladder combines with a given patient's bile composition to create a gallstone-forming environment. Thus, gallstones will continue to form unless the gallbladder is removed or the bile is again altered when the taking of such medicines is resumed. Patients can also have the gallstones broken up into very small pieces, as is often done with kidney stones, by high-frequency sound waves aimed at the gallstones. This procedure, however, known as lithotripsy, has drawbacks: It works in only a small percentage of

patients (those with a limited number of small gallstones), and the results have not been uniformly consistent or satisfactory.

PERSPECTIVE AND PROSPECTS

Diseases of the gallbladder and biliary system are common in modern industrialized societies. The exact etiologies are not entirely clear, but they may involve dietary mechanisms or other customs of the Western lifestyle. There is also evidence that genetic factors are important, as gallbladder disease often runs in families. Traditionally, the treatment of non-life-threatening gallbladder disease has been conservative, with dietary discretion being the most important factor. When that failed, or if the condition was more serious, the gallbladder was removed. Open cholecystectomy was long considered the best method for dealing with these problems. This operation has been recently challenged by endoscopic and laparoscopic techniques, which have become widely available and enjoyed great success. These new treatment options will become more important as increasing medical costs promote the refinement of less invasive and better techniques. Nevertheless, open cholecystectomy is sometimes the only option for a patient, and less invasive techniques can have limitations as well as complications.

Basic scientific research is also important in this field. Investigations into the mechanisms of gallstone formation are critical to the understanding of gallbladder diseases, as gallstones are the cause of many of these problems. As with many other diseases, prevention might be the key to eliminating many gallbladder diseases, making biliary colic, cholecystitis, and common bile duct diseases rare.

—*Mark Wengrovitz, M.D.*

See also Abdomen; Abdominal disorders; Cholecystectomy; Cholecystitis; Gastroenterology; Gastroenterology, pediatric; Gastrointestinal disorders; Internal medicine; Jaundice; Kidney stones; Laparoscopy; Liver; Liver cancer; Liver disorders; Liver transplantation; Obesity; Pain; Pancreatitis; Stone removal; Stones; Ultrasonography.

FOR FURTHER INFORMATION:

Blumgart, L. H., ed. *Surgery of the Liver and Biliary Tract*. 3d ed. 2 vols. Edinburgh, Scotland: Churchill Livingstone, 2000. This authoritative text offers a comprehensive, detailed description of the subject.
Cameron, John L., ed. *Current Surgical Therapy*. 6th ed. St. Louis: C. V. Mosby, 1998. An excellent text-

book that covers all surgical problems, including those related to gallbladder and gallstone removal.

Krames Communications. *The Gallbladder Surgery Book*. San Bruno, Calif.: Author, 1991. This helpful book provides the general reader with an understanding of the symptoms of gallbladder diseases, their most common causes, and treatment options.

_____. *Laparoscopic Gallbladder Surgery*. San Bruno, Calif.: Author, 1991. This work offers information regarding laparoscopic cholecystectomy to patients who are facing gallbladder surgery.

Zinner, Michael J., et al., eds. *Maingot's Abdominal Operations*. 10th ed. Stamford, Conn.: Appleton & Lange, 1997. This textbook has long been considered the classic work on all surgical disciplines. Contains an excellent section on gallbladder diseases.

GALLBLADDER REMOVAL. *See* CHOLECYSTECTOMY.

GALLSTONES. *See* GALLBLADDER DISEASES; STONE REMOVAL; STONES.

GAMETE INTRAFALLOPIAN TRANSFER (GIFT)

PROCEDURE

ALSO KNOWN AS: Gamete intrafallopian tube transfer

ANATOMY OR SYSTEM AFFECTED: Reproductive system

SPECIALTIES AND RELATED FIELDS: Embryology, endocrinology, obstetrics

DEFINITION: A treatment for infertility in which sperm and eggs are introduced surgically into a Fallopian tube, where fertilization (and subsequent implantation in the uterus) are expected to occur naturally.

KEY TERMS:

assisted reproductive technology: any treatment or procedure involving the manipulation of sperm or eggs outside the body in order to achieve pregnancy

Fallopian tube: one of the pair of open-ended ducts branching from the top of the uterus which collects eggs released from the ovary and in which fertilization usually occurs

fertilization: the union of egg and sperm

gamete: any reproductive cell, either egg or sperm

in vitro fertilization (IVF): the fertilization of eggs outside the body with subsequent implantation of embryos in the uterus

laparoscope: a thin, needlelike medical instrument containing a fiber-optic light source that is inserted through the skin and used both to visualize internal organs and to perform certain surgical procedures

ovulation: the release of a mature egg from an ovary

uterus: the female organ in which the embryo/fetus develops

zygote: a fertilized egg before cell division occurs; after the first division, it is called an embryo

INDICATIONS AND PROCEDURES

Couples who have sexual intercourse for a year without contraception and do not achieve pregnancy are defined as infertile. So too are couples who conceive but, because of repeated miscarriages, have not had a child. There are many possible causes of infertility. In the female, they include abnormal or irregular ovulation, blocked or constricted Fallopian tubes, and growths, scarring, or abnormalities of the uterus. In the male, infertility may result from failure to ejaculate, low sperm count, abnormalities in sperm cells, or a blocked sperm tube. In many cases, no cause of infertility can be determined.

In order to have a child, some infertile couples turn to clinics offering assisted reproductive technology (ART) services. The most common form of ART is in vitro fertilization (IVF). Gamete intrafallopian transfer (GIFT) is similar to IVF, but it does not involve fertilization outside the body. Gametes (sperm and egg) are collected and then surgically introduced into a Fallopian tube, where fertilization and subsequent implantation in the uterus are expected to occur naturally. GIFT is the least frequently done of all ARTs. In 2000, it accounted for less than 1 percent of the ART procedures performed in the United States.

Women who have at least one Fallopian tube open are considered candidates for any of the ARTs, if sufficient numbers of healthy sperm can be collected from the male. (Women with blocked Fallopian tubes are candidates for IVF.) GIFT may be the ART of choice for young women who have never undergone laparoscopy and for men with weak or few sperm. GIFT is sometimes employed in cases of unexplained infertility.

To perform the procedure, egg maturation in the ovaries is stimulated with fertility drugs. With ultrasound guiding the probe, the physician retrieves eggs using a laparoscope. Sperm are collected several hours before the procedure. A laparoscope is also used to inject eggs and sperm into a Fallopian tube. The patient may be awake or under general anesthesia for GIFT, which is typically done as a same-day, outpatient procedure. The American Society for Reproductive Medicine recommends that GIFT be performed only in a facility capable of performing IVF, in case GIFT fails or excess eggs are recovered.

USES AND COMPLICATIONS

All ART procedures involve risks, including general surgical risks, pregnancy complications, multiple fetuses, low birth weight, and possibly certain birth defects. The rate of ectopic pregnancy (implantation outside the uterus) is also slightly higher. Multiple fetuses, which are present in nearly one-third of ART pregnancies, are associated with increased risk of prematurity, low birth weight, and neonatal death in the infant and of cesarean section and hemorrhage in the mother. Although ARTs are emotionally taxing, physically demanding, and expensive, thousands of infertile couples seek them annually. In 2000, more than 35,000 babies were born in the United States as a result of ART.

The possible side effects of the hormonal drugs used to induce ovulation include hot flashes, changes in vision, ovarian cysts (sacs of fluid forming in the ovary), ovarian enlargement, and leakage of fluid into the abdominal cavity, which can trigger kidney failure, strokes, and heart attacks if not treated. IVF entails a slightly increased risk of chromosomal birth defects; whether GIFT carries a similar risk is unknown. Some studies conclude that ART increases a woman's risk of ovarian cancer, but other studies dispute that claim. ARTs do not appear to increase the overall risk of birth defects, although specific defects, such as vision problems, have been uncovered in some studies. While some experts claim that the risk of miscarriage increases, others refute that assertion.

Some couples want GIFT because they consider it more "natural" than IVF. However, GIFT is a riskier procedure than IVF, because laparoscopic surgery is required. Also, because fertilization is not confirmed before the injection of gametes, there is no way of knowing whether it occurred unless pregnancy is achieved. Nevertheless, GIFT carries a success rate approximately equal to that of other ARTs—roughly one in every four attempts. The mother's age is an important factor: the younger the mother, the better the chance of success.

PERSPECTIVE AND PROSPECTS

Before the 1970's, infertility treatment was limited mostly to the surgical repair of blocked Fallopian tubes and the insertion of sperm into the uterus (artificial insemination). In the early 1960's, Min Chang, a scientist at the Worcester Foundation in Shrewsbury, Massachusetts, performed the first IVF. He used sperm and eggs from black rabbits to grow embryos in vitro (meaning literally "in glass," or in a laboratory dish). He then placed the embryos in the uterus of a white rabbit. A litter of black pups was born.

In 1969, English physician Robert G. Edwards successfully fertilized human eggs in vitro. Cell division was achieved a year later. He next collaborated with English physician Patrick Steptoe, who specialized in laparoscopic surgery. Together, they developed reliable techniques for retrieving eggs and maintaining embryos. The result was Louise Brown, the first "test tube baby." She was born in England in 1978. In 1981, the breakthrough was replicated in the United States. During the following twenty years, more than one million IVF babies were born.

After that, the field of reproductive endocrinology flourished, as did the development of ART techniques. Dr. Ricardo H. Asch of the University of Texas at San Antonio performed the first successful GIFT in 1984. Another, similar development was zygote intrafallopian transfer (ZIFT), first successfully performed in 1986. ZIFT involves mixing sperm and eggs together outside the body, then confirming fertilization before the zygote is surgically placed in a Fallopian tube. Another ART, intracytoplasmic sperm injection (ICSI), was introduced in 1992. It involves injecting a single sperm directly into an egg. It is often used in conjunction with IVF to fertilize eggs before embryo transplantation.

Research and development activities continue to improve ART methods and techniques. Certain conditions within the Fallopian tube that interfere with ART can now be treated, and better culture media have been developed for growing and maintaining embryos. The selection of smaller numbers of higher-quality embryos may cut the rate of multiple pregnancies, and improved methods for identifying those couples most likely to benefit from ART are being perfected. New blastocyst culture methods allow laboratories to grow embryos through the sixth day of development, when they contain one hundred fifty to two hundred cells. Researchers hope that implanting smaller numbers of more mature embryos will reduce the number of multiple births and diminish the risks that they entail.

ARTs raise ethical and social issues. Some churches

and religious leaders oppose ARTs, because they are "unnatural" or because some of the embryos produced in vitro are subsequently destroyed. Other controversies include pregnancies achieved in women past their natural reproductive age and legal issues surrounding the ownership of reproductive cells and frozen embryos.

—*Faith Hickman Brynie, Ph.D.*

See also Assisted reproductive technologies; Conception; Embryology; Ethics; Genetic engineering; Gynecology; In vitro fertilization; Infertility in females; Infertility in males; Multiple births; Obstetrics; Pregnancy and gestation; Reproductive system.

FOR FURTHER INFORMATION:

Centers for Disease Control and Prevention. *2000 Assisted Reproductive Technology Success Rates: National Summary and Fertility Clinic Reports.* Atlanta: Author, 2002.

Meniru, Godwin I. *Cambridge Guide to Infertility Management and Assisted Reproduction.* New York: Cambridge University Press, 2001.

Peoples, Debby, and Harriette Rovner Ferguson. *Experiencing Infertility: An Essential Resource.* New York: Norton, 1998.

GANGLION REMOVAL
PROCEDURE

ANATOMY OR SYSTEM AFFECTED: Feet, hands, tendons

SPECIALTIES AND RELATED FIELDS: Dermatology, family practice, general surgery

DEFINITION: The removal of fluid-filled sacs which usually develop on the tendons of the wrists, fingers, or feet.

INDICATIONS AND PROCEDURES

Sacs containing synovial fluid surround tendons to reduce the friction on adjacent tissues during movement. These sacs can form cysts, known as ganglions, that range in size from a pea to a golf ball. Smaller ganglions are more common and often spontaneously disappear. A ganglion is not harmful unless it causes pain or the patient desires its removal for cosmetic reasons. Ganglion formation typically occurs around the tendons of the wrist.

In order to remove a ganglion, the physician will disinfect the skin overlying the cyst and insert a needle attached to a syringe in order to aspirate the fluid from the ganglion. Unfortunately, this procedure usually reduces the ganglion's size only temporarily. Some physicians will make an incision into the skin and remove the whole ganglion. This procedure requires thorough disinfection of the skin using alcohol and/or povidone-iodine and may require a local anesthetic such as lidocaine to be injected under the skin. Surgical instruments are used to dissect the cyst wall from the tendon and surrounding tissues. The total removal of the ganglion usually prevents recurrence.

USES AND COMPLICATIONS

As with any invasive procedure, the physician performing the surgical removal of a ganglion must be cautious so as to prevent infections or damage to surrounding healthy tissues.

The larger the ganglion, the greater are the potential complications. A longer incision must be made, which allows a large site for potential bacterial invasion and infection. The larger ganglion also requires more extensive dissection from surrounding tissues, which increases the possibility of injury to these structures. Although it is rare, tendons, ligaments, and nerves can be permanently damaged in ganglion removal. For example, if the ganglion was located in the wrist and the underlying tendons and nerves were severely damaged, the result may be a limited use or loss of use of the hand.

—*Matthew Berria, Ph.D., and Douglas Reinhart, M.D.*

See also Abscess removal; Abscesses; Cyst removal; Cysts; Nervous system; Neurology; Tendon disorders; Tendon repair.

FOR FURTHER INFORMATION:

Breslau, R. C. "Ganglion of the Glenohumeral Joint: An Unusual Axillary Tumor." *Southern Medical Journal* 59, no. 5 (May, 1966): 566.

Kikuchi, Kenji, and Masahiro Saito. "Ganglion-Cell Tumor of the Filum Terminale: Immunohistochemical Characterization." *Tohoku Journal of Experimental Medicine* 188, no. 3 (July, 1999): 245-256.

Lenfant, C., R. Paoletti, and A. Albertini, eds. *Biotechnology of Growth Factors: Vascular and Nervous Systems.* New York: Karger, 1992.

McLendon, Roger E. *Pathology of Tumors of the Central Nervous System: A Guide to Histological Diagnosis.* New York: Oxford University Press, 2000.

GANGLIONS. *See* CYSTS; GANGLION REMOVAL.

Gangrene

Disease/disorder

Anatomy or system affected: All

Specialties and related fields: Bacteriology, internal medicine, microbiology

Definition: Necrosis (death of tissue) resulting from blood loss and bacterial invasion followed by putrefaction; may be initiated by a variety of diseases and conditions, and if left untreated may result in need for amputation or in death.

Key terms:

anaerobic: referring to conditions that favor the growth of an organism in the absence of oxygen

cellulitis: an infection of the skin which, if left untreated, can abscess and kill the affected tissue

collagenase: an enzyme that breaks down the proteins of collagen tissue, a primary component of connective tissue (ligaments and tendons)

debridement: cleansing of a wound by removal of dirt, foreign objects, damaged tissue, and cellular debris, in order to promote healing

exotoxin: a toxic protein, such as an enzyme, excreted by microorganisms into the environment

Gram's stain: a stain used to classify bacteria as either gram-positive (they retain the primary stain of crystal violet when subjected to treatment with a decolorizer) or gram-negative (no coloration)

hemolysis: the premature breakdown of red blood cells

hyaluronidase: an enzyme that breaks down hyaluronic acid, the gel-like matrix of connective tissue

lecithinase: an enzyme that breaks down lecithin, a kind of phospholipid that is a component of human cells (such as red blood cells)

necrosis: localized tissue death that occurs in groups of cells in response to disease or injury

Causes and Symptoms

The term "gangrene" is used when wounded or traumatized tissue has become so badly infected by bacteria that the tissue dies. The infection can be localized, but the threat of the gangrene spreading to other tissue is very serious: It can rapidly become fatal to the patient.

There are approximately thirty different clostridial bacteria species that can cause infection in the human body as they release toxins into the system. Five species of clostridia can cause gangrene. *Clostridium perfringens* is the most common culprit: This species is responsible for about 90 percent of invasive infections in damaged tissue. The other four species are *C. novyi*, *C. septicum*, *C. sordellii*, and *C. histolyticum*. Clostridia

are bacilli (rod-shaped bacteria). They are anaerobic and form spores that are heat-resistant. These spores are larger than the cells that produce them, but they are not motile.

C. perfringens is found in all types of soil, including desert sand and marine sediments. The spores produced by these bacteria can survive for years until conditions are right for germination. In addition to the soil, these bacteria are found in the mouth, vaginal tract, and intestinal tract. While these species can go undetected and be innocuous for a lifetime, they can cause gangrene in the intestinal tract and the adjoining peritoneum in persons with a bowel obstruction. They can also become dangerously active if freed into the abdominal cavity during invasive surgery or postoperatively if some of the intestine is isolated from the blood supply (ischemia). A type of gangrene, anaerobic puerperal sepsis, may result if the uterus is traumatized by surgical procedures such as septic instrumental abortions. This gangrene is especially dangerous, as mortality is high even with immediate treatment.

C. perfringens works anaerobically in tissue that has been deprived of oxygen. This deprivation can result from a decreased blood supply caused by damaged or crushed blood vessels or clots that block the flow of blood; the release of sulfhydryl groups or oxidases (oxygen-consuming enzymes) by traumatized tissue (from a wound, tourniquet, or foreign body); diseases that may damage the circulatory system, such as diabetes or arteriosclerosis; aerobic bacteria that use up the available oxygen in a given area; or chemicals introduced by soil or dirt that kill cells. Without living cells, there is no tissue to receive oxygen from the circulatory system. The anaerobes thrive in this oxygen-poor environment, since they also take advantage of and use the vitamins, amino acids, salts, and carbohydrates of damaged and dying cells. As the bacteria grow and re-

---

Information on Gangrene

Causes: Bacterial infection, blood loss, frostbite, disease

Symptoms: Varies with severity; can include inflammation and pain, fever, and feeling of increased weight in affected area

Duration: Acute

Treatments: Surgery, amputation, antibiotics, hyperbaric oxygen chamber

produce in this environment, they infect neighboring tissue, including the lymphatic system. More cells are killed, which in turn provides a larger anaerobic environment in which the bacteria can increase in number. This spreading process can be very quick; a whole limb can become affected within a matter of hours. Bacteremia, toxemia, and hemolysis then develop, followed by circulatory failure, renal shutdown, and death.

Types of wounds that have a greater likelihood of developing anaerobic infections are jagged shrapnel wounds in soldiers on the battlefield, crushed or torn limbs resulting from accidents (such as car wrecks), wounds contaminated by dirty hands or instruments, and wounds resulting from human or animal bites. These wounds can be jeopardized by clostridial spores that are in the soil, or, as in the case of abdominal surgery, perforation of the large intestine may liberate clostridia into the area. The spores germinate only under anaerobic conditions; once they begin reproducing, however, they can maintain their own anaerobic environment.

Gangrenous infections can be divided into three categories: simple contamination, cellulitis, and gas gangrene. Simple contamination is infection with clostridia and/or streptococcal bacteria. Visible signs of simple contamination include a brown discharge of pus with a putrid odor. While this infection may increase in severity, it is possible that healing may result instead.

The second category of gangrenous infection is anaerobic cellulitis. Anaerobic cellulitis may be a worsened condition of simple contamination or may be the initial contamination of clostridia. It can develop within three or four days of exposure. Typically, the bacteria will multiply within connective tissue spaces and release gas. As gas is produced, the resulting pressure keeps the wound open and allows seepage of a foul-smelling discharge. This infection may remain localized or may spread, but little pain is associated with this form.

Gas gangrene, the most dangerous form of this type of infection, is also known as malignant edema. Its incubation period may be a mere four to six hours or may be as long as six weeks. Gas gangrene is not painless; the onset is sudden, with a feeling of increased weight in the affected area. The sufferer will feel critically ill, look pale, sweat, and be delirious, maniacal, or totally apathetic. The patient should be monitored for shock. The wound has not changed in appearance, but there may be an odorless discharge. Gas released is trapped between muscle fibers and can be found by palpitation.

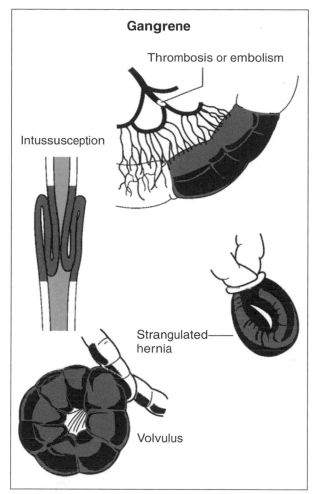

Gangrene

Thrombosis or embolism

Intussusception

Strangulated hernia

Volvulus

Gangrene may occur as a result of obstruction of the organs through a variety of means: strangulation, thrombosis, embolism, intussusception, volvulus, or other obstruction. The most dangerous form of gangrene, however (not pictured here), is gas gangrene, which results from infection by clostridial bacteria and usually occurs as a result of war wounds or other severe trauma.

If treatment is not begun, toxemia, hemolytic anemia, and renal failure (caused by tubular necrosis) may occur; death then follows.

The seriousness of the invasion is determined by the location of the infection. The least worrisome is an infection of the subcutaneous skin layers that develops slowly, producing little pain with its inflammation. Even so, gas released from the bacteria may be trapped within the affected area and can be palpated (a sensation known as crepitance). This localized infection, referred to as clostridial anaerobic cellulitis, is not particularly dangerous.

Gas gangrene will more likely occur when the affected area is a deep infection of the muscle layers. The muscle cells are abundant in carbohydrates, a rich energy source for the pervasive bacteria. The bacteria release two by-products as they consume cells: hydrogen gas and toxins. The gas collects and puts so much pressure on the sheets of muscles that the fibers begin to separate. In these gaps between fibers, the fluid accumulates and can further decrease the likelihood of the tissue's survival. The toxins emitted by the bacteria move quickly into more muscle cells, causing necrosis. This form of infection causes intense pain, and the rapid spread of the bacteria magnifies the symptoms. Affected muscle becomes pale, then fails to respond to stimuli. Following this stage, the muscle turns deep red and then black as the gangrene progresses. The skin covering the muscle also undergoes discoloration; a bronze tint colors the taut skin, and blisters filled with dark fluid appear. Eventually, even the skin blackens. The area is so inflamed that crepitance is hard to ascertain.

Though usually associated with skin and muscle, gangrene can also involve the lungs, pleural cavity, eye, brain, liver, or uterus.

TREATMENT AND THERAPY

When gas gangrene occurs, it should be considered a medical emergency. Because gas gangrene spreads and infects so rapidly and endangers either a limb or the patient's life, the use of the laboratory in diagnosis is minimal before treatment: If the physician waits two or three days while the bacteria are cultivated and identified, the patient will likely lose a limb or may die.

The surest way to detect the presence of *C. perfringens* to diagnose gas gangrene is to aspirate some of the fluid that is seeping from the wound. Since these bacteria may normally inhabit the human environment, care must be taken not to contaminate the sample. Using needle and syringe aspiration rather than swabs will help keep the sample clean. If a section of tissue is removed to study, it must not be exposed to air; the bacteria would not survive the oxygen bath, and the readings would therefore be inaccurate. To ensure that no oxygen contamination has occurred, the syringe used to collect the fluid should be capped off and the sample should be injected into a transport container that is oxygen-free. This container would be a vial filled with nitrogen gas or carbon dioxide, filled with a reducing agent, or filled with a solution containing thioglycolate or cysteine.

Once the specimen has reached the laboratory, it should first be examined by microscope. In order for the bacteria to be seen in the microscope, a Gram's stain should be done. It is important to pinpoint the genus and species of bacteria so that proper treatment can begin as soon as possible. Since *C. perfringens* is gram-positive, the stain pattern and the bacterial size and shape immediately identify this bacteria as an anaerobe. Identifying characteristics would be a rod shape (either large and blunt-ended or long, skinny, and pointed), irregular staining, or the presence of cocci of different sizes. Not only can shape and size be detected, but an estimate of bacterial number can indicate the extent of the infection as well.

After a preliminary identification of the bacteria has been accomplished with staining and microscopy, cultivation and definitive identification follow. The specimen is inoculated onto several media (such as meat glucose, thioglycolate, and blood agar) and allowed to incubate anaerobically for forty-eight to seventy-two hours at 35 to 37 degrees Celsius. Then the samples are examined to detect colonization and the presence or absence of hemolysis. Final identification is made by compiling information about the results of the Gram's stain, the structure of the colony, biochemical reactions, and a determination of the end products released as glucose is fermented. This determination is made by infusing the colony with a glucose broth and monitoring the end products that are released using gas chromatography. Another test to detect *C. perfringens* measures lecithinase production. There is no value in examining the blood serum in a gangrene patient's blood.

Mortality rates for cases of gas gangrene that do not receive treatment range from 40 to 60 percent. Therefore, if signs indicate the presence of clostridia, immediate surgery is important to examine the affected tissue. The wound (and all tissue showing signs of bacterial invasion) should be thoroughly and aggressively debrided (cleansed) and the infected area removed. Depending on the extent of the infection, amputation of the area may be indicated to prevent further spread of the disease. Antibiotic therapy is also given in an attempt to stop bacterial growth; penicillin is the drug of choice.

If the infection has not progressed to the point that amputation is necessary, hyperbaric oxygen can sometimes be used for successful treatment. This treatment consists of putting the patient in a chamber of pure oxygen for a brief period several times a day. This environment is too rich for the bacteria to survive. The exposure to these conditions does not alter the oxygen-carrying capabilities or saturation of red blood cells. It does result in an important difference in the oxygen tension of the serum (and thereby the lymph in the interstitial tissue). The significance of this variation is that it may interrupt toxin synthesis and bacteria growth. This enhances the body's ability to combat the infection in that it allows normal phagocytic and host defense mechanisms to take control.

Although clostridial infections are not usually transmissible from one person to another, patients diagnosed with gas gangrene should be placed on drainage/secretion precautions. This simply means that those in contact with the patient should wear gowns and gloves and should wash their hands thoroughly after touching the patient or any contaminated articles. Those articles that are contaminated should be disposed of or cleaned thoroughly. Autoclaving of instruments and equipment should ensure adequate sterilization. Boiling and chemical disinfection is not enough to kill resistant spores contaminating other articles. To be rid of the infective organisms completely, dressings should be burned, bed linens autoclaved, and mattresses and pillows sterilized in an ethylene oxide chamber. The relatively small danger of transmission is to other patients with surgical or traumatic wounds.

Antitoxins have been developed for gas gangrene, but they are not reliable and have not come into practical use. Since there is no effective antitoxin against gangrene induced by *C. perfringens*, prevention lies in how the wound is treated. There must be a thorough debridement and an adequate dosage of antibiotics. In addition, final closure of the wound should be delayed for two or three days to allow complete drainage of the area. Any bandage or cast that must be applied should allow adequate circulation of air (an airless environment would encourage growth of *C. perfringens*).

Perspective and Prospects

The first anecdotes describing gangrene were in the seventeenth century. Since the Napoleonic Wars, gas gangrene has caused much death and disfigurement. In World War I, this was especially the case; as many as 10 percent of all wounded soldiers were infected. Many who would have survived their injuries succumbed to gas gangrene. In most of these cases, infection came through contaminated soil that had been fertilized with human and animal waste. The contamination most often was by several clostridial species.

Early surgical procedures carried the same risk; lack of sanitary conditions and poor (or absent) disinfection techniques led to far more deaths than injuries warranted. By the late 1800's, anaerobes were identified as the culprits causing putrefaction and infections associated with tissue necrosis, gas emissions in tissue, and a foul odor. The scientists credited with first isolating *C. perfringens* as the causative bacteria in gas gangrene were George Nuttall and William Welch in 1892. Though these bacteria were extensively studied, it was not until the 1960's that adequate diagnostic technology was available for clinical use. Because of this technology, there was a far smaller impact of gangrene on the battlefields of the Vietnam War. The threat of gangrene is still a reality, however, in the postoperative patient.

C. perfringens is also implicated in another common health hazard: food poisoning. This species is responsible for 3 percent of food poisoning outbreaks and 11 percent of single cases. Such food poisoning usually occurs with ingestion of meat, poultry, and gravies that are contaminated with *C. perfringens*. Most outbreaks are associated with restaurant, dormitory, or bulk food preparation and not with home cooking. Once the bacteria enter the intestinal tract, they make their presence obvious within eight to twenty-four hours. Typically, the disease is mild, producing discomfort in the form of abdominal pain and diarrhea. It usually runs its course in twenty-four hours. Medicinal treatment is unwarranted; the manifestations of this disease are often mild enough that the infection is undiagnosed.

C. perfringens may have the opportunity to multiply before the food is eaten. Contaminated dishes should be thoroughly reheated to prevent illness. Since *C. perfringens* produces endospores that are heat resistant, simply cooking or heating the food may be insufficient. Contamination is reinforced because heating also drives off oxygen, creating an environment in which the bacteria thrive. Therefore, those spores that survive the heating process are encouraged in this oxygen-poor medium to reproduce and grow quickly. Clostridial food poisoning can be avoided by refraining from eating foods that have been sitting out for prolonged periods. When there is a delay between preparation and eating, then food should be kept at very warm or very cool temperatures (above 60 degrees Celsius or below 5 degrees Celsius).

—*Iona C. Baldridge*

See also Amputation; Bacterial infections; Embolism; Food poisoning; Frostbite; Hernia; Hernia repair; Infection; Poisoning; Thrombosis and thrombus; Wounds.

FOR FURTHER INFORMATION:

Jawetz, Ernest, Joseph L. Melnick, and Edward A. Adelberg. *Medical Microbiology.* 19th ed. Norwalk, Conn.: Appleton and Lange, 1991. A comprehensive microbiology text written primarily for medical students but also used by physicians and health science students. Some background is helpful in reading through the sections on microbiological principles, immunology, pathogenesis, and chemotherapy.

Morello, Josephine A., Helen Eckel Mizer, Marion E. Wilson, and Paul A. Granato. *Microbiology in Patient Care.* 6th ed. Dubuque, Iowa: Wm. C. Brown, 1998. This text is addressed to beginning students of health-related fields. It is divided into a section introducing the principles of microbiology and a section relating microbial diseases and their epidemiology. Well written and illustrated.

Pelczar, Michael J., Jr., E. C. S. Chan, and Noel R. Krieg. *Microbiology: Concepts and Applications.* New York: McGraw-Hill, 1993. After the history of microbiology is presented, fundamental concepts of microbiology are balanced with medical microbiology, environmental microbiology, and microbial genetics.

Schaechter, Moselio, Gerald Medoff, and Barry I. Eisenstein, eds. *Mechanisms of Microbial Disease.* 3d ed. Baltimore: Williams & Wilkins, 1999. A readable textbook designed for medical students, graduate students, and advanced undergraduate students. Combines microbiology with the study of infectious diseases, relating both subjects to the major human systems.

GASTRECTOMY

PROCEDURE

ANATOMY OR SYSTEM AFFECTED: Abdomen, gastrointestinal system, stomach

SPECIALTIES AND RELATED FIELDS: Gastroenterology, general surgery, oncology

DEFINITION: The surgical removal of all or part of the stomach.

KEY TERMS:

anesthesia: the use of drugs to inhibit pain and alter consciousness

duodenum: the first part of the small intestine, located just after the stomach and before the jejunum

hemostasis: the control of bleeding

incision: a cut made with a scalpel

jejunum: a region of the small intestine located after the duodenum

suture: a thread used to unite parts of the body

INDICATIONS AND PROCEDURES

The stomach is an important organ in the gastrointestinal system. It receives the food that has been swallowed from the esophagus and immediately begins to process it. The stomach produces and secretes gastric juices, which include hydrochloric acid and an enzyme called pepsin for digestion. As the stomach collects it, food is churned and mixed with the gastric fluid before it is passed to the first region of the small intestine, the duodenum. Occasionally, the stomach becomes cancerous or has an ulcer that will not heal and thus must be surgically removed.

Complete removal of the stomach, a total gastrectomy, is a relatively rare operation usually performed to treat stomach cancer. Partial gastrectomy, however, in which only the diseased portion of the stomach is removed surgically, is fairly common. A partial gastrectomy is often performed to treat a peptic ulcer that fails to heal after medical treatment. Peptic ulcers, which include gastric and more commonly duodenal ulcers, may not respond to drug therapy and can place the patient at risk for bleeding into the gastrointestinal tract or even complete perforation of the stomach or duodenal wall. Therefore, the indications for gastrectomy include perforation, obstruction, massive bleeding, and severe abdominal pain.

Gastrectomy requires hospitalization, general anesthesia, and postoperative care. An anesthesiologist will administer a general anesthetic rendering the patient unconscious and insensible to pain during the operation. A nasogastric tube is passed into the stomach via the nose and nasal cavity so that any stomach contents can be removed using suction before an incision is made into the stomach.

During total gastrectomy, the whole stomach is removed and the esophagus is attached to the jejunum. The two most common types of partial gastrectomy surgeries are the Billroth I and Billroth II. A surgeon performing a Billroth I will remove the diseased part of the stomach and attach the remaining healthy stomach to the duodenum. The Billroth I is also known as gastroduodenostomy. This operation preserves most of the digestive functions. Billroth II gastrectomy requires the surgeon to perform a gastrojejunostomy in which the remaining stomach is joined with the jejunum and bypasses the duodenum. Thus the opening of the duodenum must be closed to prevent the digestive contents from escaping into the abdominal cavity.

During the recovery period, the nasogastric tube is left in place to help drain the secretions from the gastro-

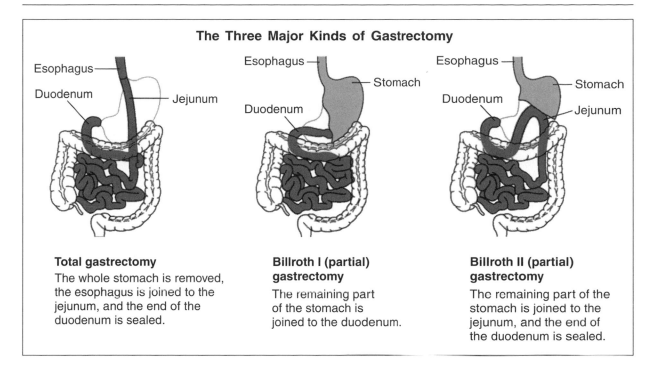

The Three Major Kinds of Gastrectomy

Total gastrectomy
The whole stomach is removed, the esophagus is joined to the jejunum, and the end of the duodenum is sealed.

Billroth I (partial) gastrectomy
The remaining part of the stomach is joined to the duodenum.

Billroth II (partial) gastrectomy
The remaining part of the stomach is joined to the jejunum, and the end of the duodenum is sealed.

intestinal system until the body is recovered enough to eliminate these secretions normally. Once the normal movement of the digestive tract (peristalsis) is detected, the patient is given very small amounts of fluid. If the intestines can process the ingested fluids, then the nasogastric tube is removed and the amount of fluid ingested is gradually increased. Typically, if there is no pain or nausea and vomiting, the patient can be started on a diet containing small amounts of solid food.

USES AND COMPLICATIONS

The risk of complications is relatively high in a total gastrectomy and lessens if smaller portions of the stomach are removed. The overall rate of complications is approximately 10 percent.

Since the stomach has such an important role in the process of digestion, it is not surprising that complications and adverse effects occur postsurgically. Some of the most common symptoms noted after gastrectomy include a feeling of discomfort and fullness after ingesting a relatively small meal. This feeling is attributable to the fact that the stomach volume has been reduced in a partial gastrectomy or eliminated in a total gastrectomy. New ulcers may also form and necessitate further drug treatment. Gastritis (inflammation of the stomach lining) may also occur after surgery, as well as a condition called dumping syndrome. Patients with dumping syndrome feel weak, nauseated, and light-

headed after a meal because the food moves too rapidly out of the stomach. Most of these side effects can be treated effectively with medications and dietary changes.

Long-term complications include malabsorption problems. Occasionally after gastrectomy, the digestive system cannot compensate adequately for the loss of the stomach, leading to poor digestion and absorption of nutrients. The most common malabsorptive disorder following gastrectomy is the inability to absorb vitamin B_{12}. The stomach produces a substance called intrinsic factor which is required for the absorption of this essential vitamin. Without intrinsic factor and the ability to absorb vitamin B_{12}, the patient must receive monthly injections of the vitamin for the rest of his or her life.

PERSPECTIVE AND PROSPECTS

Early detection of stomach cancers and ulcers may help reduce the need for gastrectomies. Endoscopic examinations in which the physician can observe the lining of the stomach through a surgical tube passed into the patient's mouth and down the esophagus may aid in the early detection of stomach problems such as cancer and ulcers that are failing to heal.

Aggressive medical management of gastrointestinal ulcers will likely reduce the chance that an ulcer will perforate and require gastrectomy. Antiulcer medications are available to reduce the amount of stomach acid released, to add to the protective barrier of the stomach, and to eradicate the bacteria known to cause many ulcers. Destroying the bacteria, *Helicobacter pylori*, increases the likelihood of curing the patient of ulcer formation.

—*Matthew Berria, Ph.D., and Douglas Reinhart, M.D.*

See also Bariatric surgery; Cancer; Digestion; Gastroenterology; Gastrointestinal disorders; Gastrointestinal system; Ileostomy and colostomy; Oncology; Stomach, intestinal, and pancreatic cancers; Ulcer surgery; Ulcers; Vitamins and minerals.

FOR FURTHER INFORMATION:

Clayman, Charles B., ed. *The American Medical Association Encyclopedia of Medicine.* New York: Random House, 1994. A concise presentation of numerous medical terms and illnesses. A good general reference.

Schwartz, Seymour I., ed. *Principles of Surgery.* 7th ed. New York: McGraw-Hill, 1999. A standard textbook on the topic. Intended for practicing surgeons, but valuable to general readers for its details.

GASTRITIS. *See* ABDOMINAL DISORDERS; GASTROINTESTINAL DISORDERS.

GASTROENTERITIS. *See* ABDOMINAL DISORDERS; GASTROINTESTINAL DISORDERS.

GASTROENTEROLOGY

SPECIALTY

ANATOMY OR SYSTEM AFFECTED: Abdomen, gallbladder, gastrointestinal system, intestines, liver, pancreas, stomach, throat

SPECIALTIES AND RELATED FIELDS: Internal medicine, microbiology, nutrition, oncology

DEFINITION: The subspecialty of internal medicine devoted to the digestive tract and the organs aiding digestion.

KEY TERMS:

biopsy: the use of special needles, forceps, and suction capsules to remove tissue samples for examination

endoscope: a long, maneuverable tube containing fiber optics through which physicians can view the gastrointestinal tract directly

enzyme: any of a large group of cell-produced proteins that act as catalysts for the chemical reactions necessary for digestion

motility: the spontaneous motion of the gastrointestinal tract's organs

peristalsis: the rhythmic waves of muscle contraction that move food through the esophagus, stomach, and intestines

procedure: any medical treatment which involves physical manipulation or invasion of the body

sphincter: a ringlike muscle that acts as a one-way valve to control the flow of fluids and waste

stool: the food wastes, mixed with bile and bacteria, that are eliminated through the anus

stricture: the narrowing of a passageway

SCIENCE AND PROFESSION

The gastrointestinal (GI), or digestive or alimentary, tract is a hose of layered membranes, about seven to nine meters long, that runs from the throat to the anus, allowing matter from the external world to pass through the human body. Along with its allied organs, glands, and nerve networks, the GI passage extracts the nutrients from food that are needed to fuel the body and excretes any substances that are left over. Physicians specializing in the GI system, gastroenterologists, care for everything from the upper esophageal sphincter to the anus; other specialists care for the mouth.

The GI tract has five major sections, each performing a different service: the esophagus, the stomach, the small intestine, the colon, and the anorectum. The esophagus begins where the throat ends, just below the vocal cords. It is a straight tube, about 20 to 22 centimeters long, with a valve at the top (upper esophageal sphincter). When food, formed into a ball and softened by chewing, enters from the mouth, rhythmic waves of muscle contractions (peristalsis) squeeze it smoothly toward the stomach, a trip that lasts about seven seconds. Peristaltic pressure triggers the lower esophageal sphincter to open, dropping the ball of food into the stomach; the sphincter immediately closes so that no stomach acids wash up into the esophagus.

The stomach, an ear-shaped bag that holds one to two liters of material, has three adjoining sections. First, the fundus, just below the lower esophageal sphincter, stores food. Second, the body mixes hydrochloric acid into the food, which breaks down proteins and kills bacteria, as well as a variety of enzymes, most of which also attack protein; a chemical is also introduced that prepares vitamin B_{12} for absorption in the small intestine. Third, the antrum grinds the food and pumps it through a sphincter (the pylorus) into the small intestine. Food usually takes from one to six hours to pass through the stomach.

The small intestine, about 3 meters long, loops and coils in the region from the rib cage to the pelvis. The first major loop, a squared U-shape, is the duodenum. Here bile from the liver and the gallbladder breaks down fats; water may come in from the blood if the food is salty, and enzymes from the pancreas and intestinal membrane glands continue digestion. The next section, the jejunum, absorbs most of the juices mixed with the food during digestion—up to 8 liters—as well as minerals and nutrients. The last section, the ileum, takes out bile salts and vitamin B_{12}. After about three to five hours, the remnants of food, moved by peristalsis, reach another sphincter, the ileocecal valve.

The ileocecal valve admits the remaining contents into the colon, which is wider and has segments like a caterpillar. Also called the large intestine, it rises along the right side of the body in the ascending colon; turns ninety degrees into the transverse colon, which crosses to the left side of the body; and turns another ninety degrees into the descending colon, which drops to the sigmoid (S-shaped) colon—altogether a passage of more than a meter. The colon receives watery matter from the small intestine each day, and colon bacteria, of which there is a great variety, mix with the solids and complete digestion. The colon absorbs most of this remaining water.

The anorectum is the last stop. The rectum stores fecal matter, the waste products of digestion: bile, bacteria, undigested fiber, cells sloughed from intestinal linings, and mucus. When a sufficient mass has built up, about 100 to 200 grams, pressure signals the time for defecation. The puborectalis muscle, which is under conscious control after toilet training, relaxes, tilting the feces into a vertical position. The anal sphincter opens, and the feces exit the body as stool. It normally takes from four to seventy-two hours for wastes to pass through the colon.

Three organs attached to the GI tract participate in digestion: the liver, the gallbladder, and the pancreas. The liver makes bile, an oily green liquid which aids the absorption of fats and fat-soluble vitamins and which stores and processes absorbed nutrients, as well as removing toxic substances from food. Bile travels from the liver through the common bile duct into the duodenum; along the way, the gallbladder, a small pouch, stores the bile until it is needed. In addition to making insulin, the pancreas secretes various enzymes for digestion into the duodenum via the pancreatic duct.

The enteric nervous system (ENS), or "gut brain," regulates peristalsis, secretions, and some immune responses throughout the digestive tract, although its mechanisms are not completely understood. The ENS comprises an intricate network of nerves and ganglia laced through the linings of the gut membranes and muscles, and it senses the presence of food through various hormones and neurotransmitters. The vagus nerve connects the esophagus and stomach to the base of the brain; sacral nerves do the same job for the colon. Other nerves reach from the GI tract to the spinal cord.

Mark Twain advised people to eat whatever they liked and then let the foods fight it out in the stomach. When the GI tract reacts to disagreeable foods, however, the result can be pain; in fact, because of the great number of possible malfunctions (deadly or not), the GI tract is responsible for more discomfort and misery than any other major system.

Gastroenterologists spend the largest percentage of their time treating maladies that cause pain but do no lasting harm. For example, gas, a perennial problem for people of all ages, causes bloating, and its pain is sometimes so severe that it is mistaken for a heart attack. An array of poorly understood functional disorders of the colon, called irritable bowel syndrome (IBS), affects 15 to 20 percent of Americans who have nausea, diarrhea or constipation, and abdominal distress; this condition is popularly known as "nervous stomach." Although not dangerous, it produces a bewildering variety of stomachaches. Likewise, chronic stomach and motility irregularities in the esophagus can affect digestion. Proctalgia fugax is intermittent, intense pain in the rectum.

Many GI diseases, however, are deadly. Various cancers grow in the stomach, esophagus, and, most commonly among Americans, colon. (Cancers rarely begin in the small intestine.) Gastroesophageal reflux disease (GERD) occurs when stomach juices repeatedly sluice into the esophagus, where they irritate and inflame the membrane. Aside from causing a burning sensation, the juices can erode through the membrane, creating ulcers. If the membrane is eaten through entirely, a hole opens into the body cavity around the gut, spilling food, blood, and digestive juices. Emergency surgery is then needed. Ulcers can also occur in the stomach and duodenum as a result of motility disorders, excess acid, or drugs, especially alcohol and aspirin, that irritate the membrane. Colitis and Crohn's disease are serious inflammations of the gut lining, especially in the colon; except for some forms of colitis that are caused by bacteria, the mechanism behind such inflammation remains unknown, but the disorders frequently require surgery to remove damaged and inflamed areas.

Similarly, tears in the gut lining, strictures, passages blocked by chunks of food, exposed veins (varices), infected sacs in the colon (diverticula), and communicable diseases such as dysentery and hepatitis produce potentially deadly symptoms.

Diagnostic and Treatment Techniques

An extensive battery of tests, procedures, and medications enable gastroenterologists to cure or palliate many GI diseases. In addition to the traditional physician's tools of the physical examination and the patient's medical history, high-tech instruments let gastroenterologists see inside parts of the gut, produce images of it, remove tissue and stones, stop bleeding, and destroy tumors. Medicines kill bacteria, help regulate motility, speed the healing of damaged tissue, and control diarrhea and constipation. Yet the GI tract is a very intricate system, and at times the gastroenterologist's most effective remedy is sympathy and advice about changing patients' behavior or diet so that they learn to live with their diseases.

Before treatment can begin, the disease must be identified. An interview with the patient and a medical examination constitute the first step in narrowing the range of possible causes of distressing symptoms. Symptoms described by the patient or discovered by the physician are clues to the underlying causes and suggest the kinds of tests that will most likely isolate the actions of a specific disease. Blood tests can reveal abnormal levels of white cells or chemicals and the presence of infection. Samples of digestive juices likewise can show chemical imbalances, infections, and bleeding, as can stool samples. Biopsies of the gut membrane, liver, and tumors allow pathologists to inspect tissue damage and look for viruses or bacteria. For example, a patient with yellowish skin (jaundice) and a tender liver who complains of nausea and chills may lead a physician to suspect hepatitis. The physician will then order a blood serum test, looking for specific proteins typical of hepatitis infection, and a liver biopsy to learn the type of hepatitis.

Some diseases, especially those destroying or inflaming tissue or involving motility problems, require imaging to identify, as do blockages and strictures. To obtain pictures of the gut, physicians use ultrasonography, X rays, magnetic resonance imaging (MRI), and computed tomography (CT) scans. Ultrasonographs transmit sound waves through the body and judge the density of tissues by the intensity and pattern of reflection; they are particularly useful for spotting gallstones. X rays, MRIs, and CT scans pass radiation through the body, which is recorded on film or by sensors that feed data to a computer to construct an image. Plain X rays show the pattern of air and gas distribution in the digestive tract and can detect obstructions; X rays may also be taken after barium, a radiopaque element, has been swallowed or inserted in the colon so that it coats the GI tract's walls and makes them easier to see. Such imaging helps the physician to locate strictures, perforations, cancers, diverticula, blockages, and distended areas.

Few tests are more revealing, however, than a direct look inside the GI tract. Until the 1960's, this could not be done without exploratory surgery. At that time, the endoscope became widely available. Developed by British, American, and Japanese scientists, the endoscope is a long, flexible, maneuverable tube filled with fiber optic strands and a central channel for inserting various instruments. A light source at its tip illuminates the area ahead of the scope; the fiber optics collect the reflected light and pass it directly to the eye of the examining physician at the scope's opposite end, to a television monitor, or to a camera. There are many types of endoscopes, of which three are most common: The meter-long upper gastrointestinal panendoscope (or gastroscope), inserted through the mouth, can be used for seeing well into the duodenum; the 60-centimeter flexible sigmoidoscope is used in the rectum and sigmoid colon; and the lower panendoscope (or colonoscope)—180, 140, 100, or 70 centimeters long—inserted through the anus, can be worked through the entire colon and as much as 30 centimeters into the ileum. Most of the small intestine cannot be seen by endoscopy.

With endoscopy, gastroenterologists can spot and examine a diseased or damaged area of the gut and perform a biopsy so that tissue can be examined under a microscope. Yet endoscopes can do even more than that. They can push a wad of food obstructing the esophagus into the stomach, stretch open a stricture, or clear a clogged duct with wires inserted through the scope's channel; small balloons can be inflated inside the gut to widen constricted passages. Similarly, endoscopes with wire attachments can open a passage between the surface skin and the stomach, allowing food to be put directly in the stomach for patients incapable of swallowing, a procedure called percutaneous endoscopic gastrostomy (PEG). With looped and electrified wires, they can remove polyps, cut away tissue, and cauterize bleeding vessels and ulcers. One such procedure, endoscopic retrograde-cholangiopancreatography (ERCP), can image the biliary and pancreatic ducts and allow removal of gallstones without surgery. Drugs may also be injected through the endoscope to control bleeding from varicose veins (sclerotherapy), and fiber optics permit the use of lasers to vaporize cancerous tissue.

Gastroenterologists use drugs to sedate patients during procedures and to treat dysfunctions and diseases. Other medications available are too numerous and their administration too complex to describe in detail, but basically they ease pain, check diarrhea and vomiting, decrease acid production to permit ulcers to heal, soften the stool of constipated patients, control motility problems (such as spasms), regulate secretions, speed coagulation at bleeding sites, or kill harmful bacteria and parasites. GI pain, especially from irritable bowel syndrome, is notoriously difficult to treat because of the diversity of contributing causes, including emotional problems. Researchers turn out a steady supply of new drugs each year, but improvements are slow, and new drugs require extensive clinical trials to determine proper dosage and detect harmful side effects. Sometimes, a placebo—that is, a pill with no active ingredient, a "sugar pill"—is enough to make a patient feel better. The interaction between a patient's gut, nervous system, and personality is intricate and sometimes highly idiosyncratic.

Gastroenterologists do not simply react to disease and trauma with treatments; they also try to prevent trouble from starting in the first place. A large part of their job involves educating patients. They discuss diets that can reduce GI pain and warn against the abuse of drugs, especially alcohol and tobacco, that are known to contribute to heartburn and ulcers. They routinely screen patients over the age of fifty for cancer, sometimes by endoscopic examination, especially if there is a family history of cancer.

PERSPECTIVE AND PROSPECTS

Jan Baptista van Helmont, a seventeenth century medical chemist, was the first to describe the diseases and digestive juices of the GI tract scientifically. Gastroenterology can be said to have started with his studies (he also coined the word "gas"). Yet no one directly observed the operations of digestion until 1833, when U.S. Army surgeon William Beaumont cared for a French Canadian with a bullet wound to the stomach.

The wound remained open, and Beaumont could watch the action of gastric juices and the stomach's mixing and grinding action. Throughout the nineteenth century, there were advances in the understanding and treatment of the GI tract, including the introduction of enemas and gastric lavage (washing out), X rays, and an early form of endoscopy.

As it did for most branches of medicine, twentieth century technology greatly expanded the role of gastroenterology in diagnosing, preventing, and treating disease. Imaging and endoscopy especially have revolutionized the field. In 1932, Rudolph Schindler developed a flexible gastroscope, and in 1943, Lester Dragstedt performed the first vagotomy (surgically cutting the vagus nerve) to reduce stomach acid secretions. Advances were also made to heal peptic ulcers with a special diet. The second half of the twentieth century saw an escalating number of refinements and innovations in procedures but was most remarkable for the development of drugs.

This progress has meant that far fewer surgical procedures are needed for common GI diseases. Because of new medicines, ulcer disease rarely requires surgery. Gallstones in the common bile duct that once necessitated surgical removal now may be taken out during an ERCP; a stent (perforated tube) can be inserted into a blocked bile duct under a gastroenterologist's guidance to keep bile flowing from the liver. Screenings for colon cancer and the removal of polyps, which can become cancerous, often identify cancerous or precancerous areas early and permit surgeons to remove tumors before the cancer spreads, sometimes making surgery unnecessary. Patients who once might have died because of a blocked or strictured esophagus can now be relieved and quickly released from the hospital. The overall trend has been shorter hospital stays and lower medical costs for common ailments. The sophistication of equipment and the training needed to treat difficult problems, however, have correspondingly inflated costs, as has the tendency to medicate painful ailments that sufferers once had to steel themselves to endure, such as irritable bowel syndrome.

Despite the expansion of gastroenterology's procedures and knowledge, it is far from an independent field. Gastroenterologists typically act as consultants, caring for patients only after they have been screened by family practitioners, emergency room doctors, and internists. Moreover, gastroenterologists rely on pathologists to decipher the information in biopsied tissue samples, radiologists to interpret imaging, neurologists to trace nervous system problems, and surgeons to repair perforated gut walls and remove diseased organs or transplant new ones. Finally, specially trained nurses and technicians must help them with many procedures and ensure that patients follow prescribed dietary and drug regimens.

—Roger Smith, Ph.D.

See also Abdomen; Abdominal disorders; Acid reflux disease; Appendectomy; Appendicitis; Bariatric surgery; Bulimia; Bypass surgery; Celiac sprue; Cholecystectomy; Cholecystitis; Cholera; Colic; Colitis; Colon and rectal polyp removal; Colon and rectal surgery; Colon cancer; Colonoscopy and sigmoidoscopy; Constipation; Crohn's disease; Diarrhea and dysentery; Digestion; Diverticulitis and diverticulosis; *E. coli* infection; Emergency medicine; Endoscopy; Enemas; Enzymes; Fistula repair; Food biochemistry; Food poisoning; Gallbladder diseases; Gastrectomy; Gastroenterology, pediatric; Gastrointestinal disorders; Gastrointestinal system; Gastrostomy; Glands; Heartburn; Hemorrhoid banding and removal; Hemorrhoids; Hernia; Hernia repair; Hirschsprung's disease; Ileostomy and colostomy; Indigestion; Internal medicine; Intestinal disorders; Intestines; Irritable bowel syndrome (IBS); Lactose intolerance; Liver; Liver cancer; Liver disorders; Liver transplantation; Malabsorption; Malnutrition; Metabolism; Nausea and vomiting; Nutrition; Obstruction; Pancreas; Pancreatitis; Peristalsis; Pinworms; Poisonous plants; Proctology; Pyloric stenosis; Roundworms; Salmonella infection; Shigellosis; Soiling; Stomach, intestinal, and pancreatic cancers; Stone removal; Stones; Tapeworms; Taste; Toilet training; Trichinosis; Ulcer surgery; Ulcers; Vagotomy; Weight loss and gain; Worms.

FOR FURTHER INFORMATION:

Brandt, Lawrence J. *The Clinical Practice of Gastroenterology.* 2 vols. Edinburgh, Scotland: Churchill Livingstone, 1999. Details virtually all of the adult and pediatric gastroenterologic problems encountered in practice. Features a full section on liver disease and synthesizes new advances in molecular immunology and imaging techniques.

Heuman, Douglas M., A. Scott Mills, and Hunter H. McGuire, Jr. *Gastroenterology.* Philadelphia: W. B. Saunders, 1997. This volume in the Saunders text and review series discusses digestive system diseases, the physiology of the digestive system, and the methods employed in the field of gastroenterology. Includes a bibliography and an index.

Janowitz, Henry D. *Indigestion: Living Better with Upper Intestinal Problems from Heartburn to Ulcers and Gallstones.* New York: Oxford University Press, 1994. Janowitz discusses common ailments of the upper GI tract with special attention to degenerative diseases afflicting people as they age. His style is clear and straightforward, aimed at general readers who want to prevent illness or to manage an existing one. Accompanied by charts and illustrations.

Massoni, Margaret. "Nurses' GI Handbook." *Nursing 20* (November, 1990): 65-80. Intended as a primer on GI problems for nurses, this article contains many illustrations of the gut, surgical techniques, and physical examination methods; lists of symptoms and the disorders they suggest; and tables of biochemical tests.

Morrissey, John F., and Mark Reichelderfer. "Medical Progress: Gastrointestinal Endoscopy." *The New England Journal of Medicine* 325 (October 17 and 24, 1991): 1142-1150, 1214-1223. This two-part review article presumes a sophisticated understanding of medicine; however, it is readable, if difficult, and clearly defines medical standards for using endoscopy in detecting, preventing, and treating most GI disorders.

Peikin, Steven. *Gastrointestinal Health.* Rev. ed. New York: HarperCollins, 1999. Concerned almost completely with the effect of nutrition on GI maladies, the author offers a self-help guide for the afflicted. After explaining the GI tract's workings and describing common symptoms, Peikin specifies diets that he argues will relieve symptoms.

Steiner-Grossman, Penny, Peter A. Banks, and Daniel H. Present, eds. *People . . . Not Patients: A Source Book for Living with Inflammatory Bowel Disease.* Rev. ed. Dubuque, Iowa: Kendall/Hunt, 1997. This book is for those suffering from ulcerative colitis or Crohn's disease. Easy-to-understand, detailed discussions of the diseases are accompanied by illustrations and photographs.

GASTROENTEROLOGY, PEDIATRIC
SPECIALTY

ANATOMY OR SYSTEM AFFECTED: Abdomen, gallbladder, gastrointestinal system, intestines, liver, pancreas, stomach, throat

SPECIALTIES AND RELATED FIELDS: Internal medicine, neonatology, nutrition, pediatrics

DEFINITION: The diagnosis and treatment of diseases and disorders of the digestive tract in infants and children.

KEY TERMS:

biopsy: a small sample of tissue, such as from the lining of the gastrointestinal tract, which is removed for laboratory study to aid in diagnosis

endoscopy: the use of a small-diameter, flexible tube of optical fibers with an external light source to examine visually the interior of the body, such as the gastrointestinal tract

SCIENCE AND PROFESSION

The pediatric gastroenterologist is a pediatrician who has received extra training in the diagnosis and treatment of gastrointestinal diseases and disorders. The full course of training requires a medical degree followed by three years of pediatric residency, plus an additional three years of solely studying children's gastrointestinal diseases. The six years of postdoctoral training are almost always conducted at a large teaching hospital.

The gastrointestinal tract extends from the mouth to the anus. It is responsible for the ingestion, digestion, and absorption of food and for the elimination of unusable waste from the diet. Its principal parts are the esophagus, the stomach, the small intestine and colon, and the liver, gallbladder, and pancreas.

Children suffer the same wide range of gastrointestinal problems that afflict adults. Each age group, however, has its own special problems. For example, children very rarely have stomach or colon cancer, both relatively common in adults. On the other hand, diarrhea is a very common cause of infant death worldwide but is seldom life-threatening for adults.

Childhood gastrointestinal disease varies widely in its severity, from simple constipation needing only a change in diet to liver disease so severe that the child must undergo a liver transplant in order to survive. Common problems that a pediatric gastroenterologist might treat include gastroenteritis, constipation, chronic diarrhea, gastroesophageal reflux (especially in infants), and infections such as bacterial dysentery or viral hepatitis. Less common disorders are peptic ulcers, inflammatory bowel diseases (IBDs) such as ulcerative colitis and Crohn's disease, and malabsorption disorders involving the ability of the intestines to absorb nutrients from digested food.

The liver, gallbladder, and pancreas are abdominal organs that connect directly with the gastrointestinal tract. They are important in the digestion and absorption of food and in the metabolism of the basic sugars, fats, and proteins that are absorbed by the intestines.

The diagnosis and treatment of disorders of these organs are part of gastroenterology.

Anatomical defects of the gastrointestinal tract can occur, such as intestinal malformations, obstructions, imperforate anus, and congenital fistulas between the trachea and esophagus. They are generally treated both by the gastroenterologist and by a general or pediatric surgeon, who performs any necessary surgery.

Since the gastrointestinal tract is critical in the digestion and absorption of food, a pediatric gastroenterologist must know much about nutrition. The physician will often prescribe the proper diet for a particular ailment. Occasionally, this program includes parenteral nutrition, in which a patient is fed intravenously with a complex solution of nutrients.

Most of the gastroenterologist's time is spent in the clinic, examining patients and prescribing medications, or performing procedures such as endoscopy of the stomach or colon. A minority of this specialist's patients require hospitalization, few of whom will be seriously or terminally ill.

A child's intestinal disease, especially if serious, can be very stressful for the patient's parents. The pediatric gastroenterologist must be able to communicate clearly with parents and to support them emotionally during the child's illness.

DIAGNOSTIC AND TREATMENT TECHNIQUES

Much of the pediatric gastroenterologist's work involves obtaining a thorough, detailed history of the ailment from the child and parent. Often, skillful questioning will lead to the proper diagnosis and suggest the best treatment. A careful physical examination of the entire child, not simply the abdomen, is also important.

The pediatric gastroenterologist conducts a wide variety of laboratory tests in evaluating the nature and severity of the illness, such as complete blood counts and liver enzyme measurements. Bowel movement specimens often provide important data, such as the presence of blood or infectious bacteria in the intestines.

The pediatric gastroenterologist performs several diagnostic and therapeutic procedures. Flexible endoscopy is the use of a thin, bendable tube of optic fibers to view the interior of the esophagus, stomach, or colon. The physician can obtain biopsies, small samples of gastric or intestinal tissue, through the endoscope and can remove benign intestinal growths called polyps. The gastroenterologist may place a pH probe, a small electrode on a wire, in the esophagus to test acidity levels for periods as long as twenty-four hours. This probe is used to monitor acid reflux from the stomach into the esophagus. This disease, called gastroesophageal reflux, can lead to weight loss, recurrent pneumonia, or a scarred esophagus if left untreated.

Liver transplantation may be necessary when a child suffers irreversible liver failure as a result of severe hepatitis, congenital abnormalities such as biliary atresia (failure of the bile ducts to form properly), or some disorders of the body's metabolism. The pediatric gastroenterologist is an important member of the transplant team.

PERSPECTIVE AND PROSPECTS

Subspecialties of pediatrics began to be recognized in the middle of the twentieth century. The first organization for pediatricians interested in gastroenterology was formed in the early 1970's.

In adult gastroenterology, diagnostic tools such as endoscopy and therapies such as antirejection medications for transplantation procedures improved rapidly in the last quarter of the twentieth century. Taking advantage of this new knowledge, pediatric gastroenterologists were also able to diagnose accurately more disorders in their own patients and to treat them effectively.

—*Thomas C. Jefferson, M.D.*

See also Abdomen; Abdominal disorders; Appendectomy; Appendicitis; Bulimia; Bypass surgery; Celiac sprue; Cholera; Colic; Colitis; Colon and rectal surgery; Constipation; Crohn's disease; Diarrhea and dysentery; Digestion; *E. coli* infection; Emergency medicine; Endoscopy; Enemas; Enzymes; Fistula repair; Food biochemistry; Food poisoning; Gastroenterology; Gastrointestinal disorders; Gastrointestinal system; Glands; Heartburn; Hernia; Hernia repair; Hirschsprung's disease; Ileostomy and colostomy; Indigestion; Internal medicine; Intestinal disorders; Intestines; Lactose intolerance; Liver; Liver disorders; Malabsorption; Malnutrition; Metabolism; Nausea and vomiting; Nutrition; Obstruction; Pancreas; Pancreatitis; Pediatrics; Peristalsis; Pinworms; Poisonous plants; Proctology; Pyloric stenosis; Roundworms; Salmonella infection; Shigellosis; Soiling; Tapeworms; Taste; Toilet training; Trichinosis; Weight loss and gain; Worms.

FOR FURTHER INFORMATION:

Kirschner, Barbara S., and Dennis D. Black. "The Gastrointestinal Tract." In *Nelson Essentials of Pediatrics*, edited by Richard E. Behrman and Robert M. Kliegman. 3d ed. Philadelphia: W. B. Saunders,

2000. A chapter in a great text for medical students rotating through pediatrics. It has thorough explanations of diseases and treatments.

Walker, W. Allan, et al., eds. *Pediatric Gastrointestinal Disease: Pathophysiology, Diagnosis, Management.* 3d ed. St. Louis: C. V. Mosby, 2000. This reference textbook deals extensively with the pathophysiologic basis of gastrointestinal disease in children of all ages. An approach to dealing with the families of children with gastrointestinal diseases augments the in-depth approach to disease manifestations and management. A careful approach to diagnosis follows.

GASTROINTESTINAL DISORDERS

DISEASE/DISORDER

ANATOMY OR SYSTEM AFFECTED: Abdomen, gastrointestinal system, intestines, stomach

SPECIALTIES AND RELATED FIELDS: Gastroenterology, internal medicine, microbiology

DEFINITION: The many problems that can affect the gastrointestinal tract, such as infections, injuries, dysfunctions, tumors, congenital defects, and genetic abnormalities.

KEY TERMS:

gastroenterologist: a medical specialist in diseases of the gut

endoscope: any of several flexible fiber-optic scopes used to examine the inside of the gut; it is equipped with tools to cauterize wounds or remove tissue or gallstones

intestines: the section of the gut between the anus and the stomach, consisting of the rectum, colon, and small bowel (subdivided into the ileus, jejunum, and duodenum)

motility: the spontaneous movements of the gut during swallowing, digestion, and elimination

mucosa: the tissue lining the interior of the gastrointestinal tract, through which nutrients pass into the bloodstream

stool: the waste products excreted from the body upon defecation; feces

tumor: a mass of abnormal cells that can be cancerous

CAUSES AND SYMPTOMS

What and how people eat, their digestion, and their toilet habits affect their health more than any other voluntary daily activity. Breathing, circulation, the brain's control of most bodily functions—these normally take place without conscious thought. The intake of nourishment and elimination of wastes, by contrast, afford a great variety of choices. Accordingly, poor or self-destructive eating and toilet habits lie behind many gastrointestinal (GI) disorders. Yet not all disorders result from an individual's habits. Many arise because of a person's cultural or physical environment, some are hereditary or congenital, and a fair amount have no known cause. All told, more than one hundred disorders may originate in the GI tract and its organs, including infections, cancer, dysfunctions, obstructions, autoimmune diseases, malabsorption of nutrients, and reactions to toxins taken in during eating, drinking, or breathing. Furthermore, diseases in other organs, systemic infections such as lupus, immune suppression such as that caused by acquired immunodeficiency syndrome (AIDS), reactions to altered body conditions as during pregnancy, and psychiatric problems can all reverberate to the gut.

The symptoms of GI disorders range from mildly annoying to life-threatening, although seldom does any single symptom except massive bleeding lead quickly to death. Indigestion, bloating, and gas send more people to gastroenterologists than any other set of symptoms, and they often reflect nothing more than overeating. Pain anywhere along the gut, aversion to food (anorexia), and nausea are general symptoms common to many disorders, although pain in the chest is likely to come from the esophagus while pain in the abdomen points to a stomach or intestinal problem. Red blood in the stool indicates bleeding in the intestines, black (digested) blood suggests bleeding in the upper small bowel or stomach, and vomited blood indicates injury to the stomach or esophagus—all dangerous signs indeed. Chronic diarrhea, fatty stool, constipation, difficulty in swallowing, hiccuping, vomiting, and cramps point to disturbances in the GI tract's orderly, wavelike contractions or absorption of nutrients and fluid. Pruritus (intense itching) can come from something as transient as a mild drug reaction or as serious as cancer. Dysentery (bloody diarrhea) usually comes from severe inflammation or lesions caused by viruses, bacteria, or other parasites. Malnourishment is a sign of badly disordered digestion, and ascites (fluid accumulation in body cavities) can result from serious disease in the liver or pancreas. Likewise, jaundice, the yellowing of the skin or eyes because of excess bile, signals problems in the liver, pancreas, or their ducts.

The large number and complexity of GI disorders do not allow a quick, comprehensive summary. Fortunately, many are uncommon, and the most frequent problems can be described through a tour of the GI tract. The GI tract is basically a tube that moves food from one end to the other, extracting energy and biochemical building blocks for the body along the way. So a disorder that interrupts the flow in one section of the intestines can have secondary effects on other parts of the gut. Disorders seldom affect one area alone.

The esophagus. The GI tract's first section, the esophagus, is simply a passageway from the mouth to the stomach. Although it rarely gets infected, the esophagus is the site of several common problems, usually relatively minor, if painful. Muscle dysfunctions, including slow, weak, or spasmodic muscular movement, can impair motility and make swallowing difficult, as can strictures, which usually occur at the sphincter to the stomach. The mucosal lining of the esophagus is not as hardy as in other parts of the gut. When acid backflushes from the stomach into the esophagus, it inflames tissue there and can cause burning and even bleeding, a condition popularly known as heartburn and technically called gastroesophageal reflux disease (GERD). Retching and vomiting, usually resulting from alcohol abuse or associated with a hiatal hernia, can tear the mucosa. Smokers and drinkers run the risk of esophageal cancer, which can spread down into the gut early in its development and then becomes deadly; however, it accounts for only about 1 percent of cancers. Most of these conditions can be cured or controlled if diagnosed early enough.

The stomach. In order to store food and prepare it for digestion lower in the gut, the stomach churns it into a homogenous mass and releases it in small portions into

---

INFORMATION ON GASTROINTESTINAL DISORDERS

CAUSES: Congenital and hereditary factors, infection, cancer, obstructions, autoimmune diseases, malabsorption of nutrients, reactions to toxins

SYMPTOMS: Varies; can include abdominal discomfort and pain, constipation, diarrhea, fever, nausea, weight loss, fatigue, indigestion, bloating, aversion to food, difficulty swallowing

DURATION: Ranges from acute to chronic

TREATMENTS: Drug therapy, surgery, dietary regulation, lifestyle changes

the small bowel; meanwhile, the stomach also secretes acid to kill bacteria. Bacteria that are acid-resistant, however, can multiply there. One type, *Helicobacter pylori*, is thought to be involved in the development of ulcers and perhaps cancer. Overuse of aspirins and other nonsteroidal anti-inflammatory drugs (NSAIDs) can also cause stomach ulcers. A variety of substances, including alcohol, can prompt inflammation and even hemorrhaging. Stomach cancer has been shown to strike those who have a diet high in salted, smoked, or pickled foods; the most common cancer in the world, although not in the United States, it has a low survival rate. When stomach muscle function fails, food accumulates until the stomach overstretches and rebounds, causing vomiting. Some foods can coalesce into an indigestible lump, and hair and food fibers can roll into a ball, called a bezoar; such masses can interfere with digestion.

The small intestine. The five to six meters of looped gut between the stomach and colon is called the small intestine. It secretes fluids, hormones, and enzymes into food passing through, breaking it down chemically and absorbing nutrients. Although cancers seldom develop in the small intestine itself, they frequently do so in the organs connected to it, the liver and pancreas. The major problem in the small bowel is the multitude of diseases causing diarrhea, dysentery, or ulceration: They include bacterial, viral, and parasitic disease; motility disorders; and the chronic, progressive inflammatory illness called Crohn's disease, which also ulcerates the bowel wall. Although most diarrhea is temporary, if it persists diarrhea severely weakens patients through dehydration and malnourishment. For this reason, diarrheal diseases caused by toxins in water or food are the leading cause of childhood death worldwide. Furthermore, the small bowel can become paralyzed, twisted, or kinked, thereby obstructing the passage of food. Sometimes its contents rush through too fast, a condition called dumping syndrome. All these disorders reduce digestion, and if they are chronic, then malnutrition, vitamin deficiency, and weight loss ensue.

The large intestine. The small intestine empties into the large intestine, or colon, the last meter of the GI tract; here the water content of digestive waste matter (about a liter a day) is reabsorbed, and the waste becomes increasingly solid along the way to the rectum, forming feces. Unlike the small bowel, which is nearly sterile under normal conditions, the colon hosts a large population of bacteria that ferments the indigestible fiber in waste matter, and some of the by-products are ab-

sorbed through the colon's mucosa. Bacteria or parasites gaining access from the outside world can cause diarrhea by interfering with this absorption (a condition called malabsorption) or by irritating the mucosa and speeding up muscle action. For unknown reasons, the colon can also become chronically inflamed, resulting in cramps and bloody diarrhea, an illness known as ulcerative colitis; Crohn's disease also can affect the colon. Probably because it is so often exposed to a variety of toxins, the colon is particularly susceptible to cancer in people over fifty years old: Colorectal cancer accounted for the second highest number of cancer deaths in 1993, with an equal proportion of men and women. As people age, the muscles controlling the colon deteriorate, sometimes forming small pouches in the bowel wall, called diverticula, that can become infected (diverticulitis). In addition, small knobs called polyps can grow, and they may become cancerous. One of the most common lower GI disorders is constipation, which may derive from a poor diet, motility malfunction, or both.

The rectum. The last segment of the colon, the rectum collects and holds feces for defecation through the anus. The rectum is susceptible to many of the diseases affecting the colon, including cancer and chronic inflammation. The powerful anal sphincter muscle, which controls defecation, can be the site of brief but intensely painful spasms called proctalgia fugax, which strikes for unknown reasons. The tissue lining the anal canal contains a dense network of blood vessels; straining to eliminate stool because of constipation or diarrhea or simply sitting too long on a toilet can distend these blood vessels, creating hemorrhoids, which may burn, itch, bleed, and become remarkably annoying. If infected, hemorrhoids or anal fissures may develop painful abscesses (sacs of pus). Extreme straining can cause the rectum to turn inside out through the anus, or prolapse.

The liver. The GI tract's organs figure prominently in many disorders. The liver is a large spongy organ that filters the blood, removing toxins and dumping them with bile into the duodenum. A number of viruses can invade the liver and inflame it, a malady called hepatitis. Acute forms of the disease have flulike symptoms and are self-limited. Some viruses, however, as well as alcohol or drug abuse and worms, cause extensive cirrhosis (the formation of abnormal, scarlike tissue) and chronic hepatitis. Although only recently common in the United States, viral hepatitis has long affected a large percentage of people in Southeast Asia; because hepatitis can trigger the mutation of normal cells, liver cancer is among the most common cancers worldwide. Hepatitis patients often have jaundice, as do those who, as a result of drug reactions, cancer, or stones, have blocked bile flow. Because of congenital or inherited errors of metabolism, excess fat, iron, and copper can build up in the liver, causing upper abdominal pain, skin discolorations, weakness, and behavioral changes; complications can include cirrhosis, diabetes mellitus, and heart disease.

The gallbladder. A small sac that concentrates and stores bile from the liver, the gallbladder is connected to the liver and duodenum by ducts. The concentrate often coalesces into stones, which seldom cause problems if they stay in one place. If they block the opening to the gallbladder or lodge in a duct, however, they can cause pain, fever, and jaundice. Although rare, tumors may also grow in the gallbladder or ducts, perhaps as a result of gallstone obstruction.

The pancreas. Lying just behind the stomach, the pancreas produces enzymes to break down fats and proteins for absorption and insulin to metabolize sugar; a duct joins it to the duodenum. The pancreas can become inflamed, either because of toxins (largely alcohol) or blockage of its duct, usually by gallstones. Either cause precipitates a painful condition, pancreatitis, that may last a few days, with full recovery, or turn into a life-threatening disease. If the source of inflammation is not eliminated, then chronic pancreatitis may develop and with it the gradual loss of the pancreas' ability to make enzymes and insulin. Severe abdominal pain, malnutrition, diarrhea, and diabetes may develop. Pancreatic cancer, once rare in the United States, ranked fifth among cancers causing death during 1993. Scientists are unsure of the causes; pancreatitis, gallstones, diabetes, and alcohol have been implicated, but only smoking is well attested to increase the risk of contracting pancreatic cancer, which is very lethal and difficult to treat. Only about 1 percent of patients live more than a year after diagnosis.

Functional diseases. Finally, some disorders appear to upset several parts of the GI tract at the same time, often with no identifiable cause but with chronic or recurrent symptoms. Gastroenterologists call them functional diseases, and they afflict as much as 30 percent of the population in Western countries. People with irritable bowel syndrome (IBS) complain of abdominal pain, urgency in defecation, and bloating from intestinal gas; they often feel that they cannot empty their rectums completely, even after straining. Functional dyspepsia manifests itself as upper abdominal pain, bloating, early feelings of fullness during a meal, and nausea. Also included in this group are various motility disorders in the esophagus and stomach, whose typical symptom is vomiting, and pseudo-obstruction, a condition in which the small bowel acts as if it is blocked but no lesion can be found. Many gastroenterologists believe that emotional disturbance plays a part in some of these diseases.

Treatment and Therapy

The majority of GI disorders are transient and pose no short-term or long-term threat to life. The body's natural defenses can combat most bacterial and viral infections in the gut without help. Even potentially dangerous noninfectious conditions, such as pancreatitis, resolve on their own if the irritating agent is eliminated. Many disorders require a gastroenterologist's help, however, and even despite help can make people semi-invalids. Regulation of diet and the use of drugs to combat infections or relieve pain are important treatments. If these fail, as is likely to happen in such serious conditions as chronic inflammatory disease and cancer, cures or palliation is yet possible because of gastroenterological technology, particularly endoscopy, and surgical techniques developed in the twentieth century.

While it is not true that GI disorders would necessarily disappear with improved diet, since genetic disorders would remain, gastroenterologists stress that proper nourishment is the first line of defense against trouble. For example, incidence of stomach cancer plummets in countries where people eat fresh foods and use refrigeration rather than salting and smoking to preserve food. Regions where fiber makes up a high percentage of the diet, such as Africa, have a far lower incidence of inflammatory bowel disease. Last, and certainly not least, groups that do not drink alcohol or smoke (such as Mormons) have far lower incidences of cancer and inflammatory disease throughout the GI tract.

—*Roger Smith, Ph.D.*

See also Abdomen; Abdominal disorders; Acid reflux disease; Appendectomy; Appendicitis; Bacterial infections; Bariatric surgery; Botulism; Bypass surgery; Candidiasis; Celiac sprue; Cholecystitis; Cholera; Cirrhosis; Colic; Colitis; Colon and rectal polyp removal; Colon and rectal surgery; Colon cancer; Colon therapy; Colonoscopy and sigmoidoscopy; Constipation; Crohn's disease; Diabetes mellitus; Diarrhea and dysentery; Digestion; Diverticulitis and diverticulosis; Enemas; Fistula repair; Food poisoning; Gallbladder diseases; Gastrectomy; Gastroenterology; Gastroenterology, pediatric; Gastrointestinal system; Gastrostomy; Heartburn; Hemorrhoid banding and removal; Hemorrhoids; Hernia; Hernia repair; Hirschsprung's disease; Ileostomy and colostomy; Incontinence; Indigestion; Internal medicine; Intestinal disorders; Intestines; Irritable bowel syndrome (IBS); Jaundice; Kwashiorkor; Lactose intolerance; Liver; Liver cancer; Liver disorders; Malabsorption; Malnutrition; Metabolism; Nausea and vomiting; Nutrition; Obstruction; Pancreas; Pancreatitis; Peristalsis; Peritonitis; Pinworms; Poisoning; Poisonous plants; Proctology; Protozoan diseases; Pyloric stenosis; Roundworms; Salmonella infection; Shigellosis; Soiling; Stomach, intestinal, and pancreatic cancers; Tapeworms; Toilet training; Trichinosis; Tumor removal; Tumors; Typhoid fever and typhus; Ulcer surgery; Ulcers; Vagotomy; Weight loss and gain; Worms.

FOR FURTHER INFORMATION:

Heuman, Douglas M., A. Scott Mills, and Hunter H. McGuire, Jr. *Gastroenterology*. Philadephia: W. B. Saunders, 1997. A review of digestive system diseases and methods of treating them. Includes a bibliography and an index.

Janowitz, Henry D. *Indigestion: Living Better with Upper Intestinal Problems from Heartburn to Ulcers and Gallstones*. New York: Oxford University Press, 1994. Clear explanations of common ailments, especially those related to aging, to help people prevent or manage GI disorders. With charts and illustrations.

Sachar, David B., Jerome D. Waye, and Blair S. Lewis, eds. *Pocket Guide to Gastroenterology*. Rev. ed. Baltimore: Williams & Wilkins, 1991. In detailed outlines intended for physicians, this handbook contains a wealth of information from which general readers can profit despite the extensive use of medical terminology.

Sleisenger, Marvin H., and John S. Fordtran, eds. *Sleisenger and Fordtran's Gastrointestinal and Liver Disease: Pathophysiology, Diagnosis, Management*. 7th ed. 2 vols. Philadelphia: W. B. Saunders, 2002. A comprehensive textbook of gastrointestinal diseases and physiology. Contains excellent chapters on all disorders mentioned in the text, as well as some beautiful endoscopic photographs.

Thompson, W. Grant. *The Angry Gut: Coping with Colitis and Crohn's Disease*. New York: Plenum Press, 1993. In addition to highlighting the significant similarities and differences of these two syndromes and stressing the importance of a correct diagnosis, Thompson broaches more sensitive topics that seem to be ignored by the medical profession.

GASTROINTESTINAL SYSTEM
ANATOMY

ANATOMY OR SYSTEM AFFECTED: Abdomen, gallbladder, intestines, liver, pancreas, stomach, teeth, throat

SPECIALTIES AND RELATED FIELDS: Dentistry, gastroenterology, internal medicine, nutrition, oncology, otorhinolaryngology

DEFINITION: A compartmentalized tube that is equipped to reduce food, both mechanically and chemically, to a state in which it is absorbed and used by the body; this system includes the mouth, esophagus, stomach, small intestine, and colon (large intestine), as well as the salivary glands, pancreas, liver, and gallbladder.

KEY TERMS:

absorption: the movement of digested food from the small intestine into blood vessels and from blood into body cells

bolus: food that has been mixed with saliva and formed into a ball; the bolus passes from the mouth to the stomach through a process called swallowing or deglutition

chyme: the semiliquid state of food as it is found in the stomach and first part of the small intestine

digestion: the mechanical and chemical breakdown of food into physical and molecular units that can be absorbed and used by cells

enzymes: substances that aid in the chemical digestion of food; enzymes are produced and secreted by glands found in digestive organs

peristalsis: a muscular contraction that helps to move food through the digestive tube

sphincter: a circular muscle that controls the opening and closing of an orifice

villus: a fingerlike projection in the small intestine that provides a site for the absorption of digested food into the circulatory and lymph systems

STRUCTURE AND FUNCTIONS

The gastrointestinal system or alimentary canal exists as a tube which runs through the body from mouth to anus. The wall of the tube is composed of four layers of tissue. The outermost layer, the serosa, is part of a large tissue called the peritoneum, which covers internal organs and lines body cavities. Extensions of the perito-neum called mesenteries anchor the organs of digestion to the body wall. Fatty, apronlike structures that hang in front of the abdominal organs are also modifications of the peritoneum. They are called the lesser and the greater omentum. The muscular layer, composed of circular and longitudinal muscles, makes up the bulk of the wall of the tube. The contractions of this layer aid in moving materials through the tube. Nerves, blood ves-sels, and lymph vessels are found in the third layer, the submucosa. The innermost or mucous layer has glands for secretion and modifications for absorption.

The tube is compartmentalized, and each section is equipped to accomplish some part of the digestive pro-cess. The mechanical phase of digestion involves the physical reduction of food to a semiliquid state; this is accomplished by tearing, chewing, and churning the food. Chemical digestion utilizes enzymes to reduce food to simple molecules that can be absorbed and used by the body to provide energy and to build and repair tissue.

The mouth (also called the buccal or oral cavity) marks the beginning of the gastrointestinal system and the digestive process. The mouth is divided into two ar-eas. The vestibule is the space between the lips, cheeks, gums, and teeth. Lips, or labia, are the fleshy folds that surround the opening to the mouth. The skin covers the outside, while the inside is lined with mucous mem-brane. The colored part of the lips, called the vermilion, is a juncture of these two tissues. Because the tissue at this point is unclouded, underlying blood vessels can be seen. A membrane called the labial frenulum attaches each lip to the gum, or gingivalum.

The oral cavity occupies the space posterior to the teeth and anterior to the fauces or opening to the throat. It is bounded on the sides by cheeks and on the roof by an anterior bony structure called the hard palate and a posterior muscular area, the soft palate. The uvula, a cone-shaped extension of the soft palate, can be seen hanging down in front of the fauces. The floor of the oral cavity is formed by the tongue and associated mus-cles. Taste buds are found on the surface of the tongue. The bottom of the tongue is anchored posteriorly to the hyoid bone. Anteriorly, the membranous frenulum lin-gua anchors the tongue to the floor of the mouth. The tongue's movement is controlled by extrinsic muscles that form the floor of the mouth and by intrinsic mus-cles that are part of the tongue itself. The movements of the tongue assist in speaking, swallowing, and forming food into a bolus.

Teeth, found in gum sockets, are the principal means of mechanical digestion in the mouth. Human teeth ap-pear in two sets. The deciduous or milk teeth are the first to appear. There are usually ten in each jaw, and they are replaced by the second, permanent set during childhood. The permanent set consists of sixteen teeth in each jaw. The four incisors and two canines have sharp chiseled edges, which permit biting and tearing of food. The four premolars and six molars have flat surfaces that are used in grinding the food. Frequently, the third pair of molars or wisdom teeth do not erupt un-til later in adolescence. The crown of a tooth appears above the gum line while the roots are embedded in the gum socket. The small area between the crown and the root is called the neck. The crown is covered with enamel and the root with cementum. Dentin is beneath the covering in both areas and forms the bulk of the tooth. The central cavity of the tooth is filled with a soft membrane called pulp. Blood vessels and nerves are embedded in the pulp.

At the rear of the mouth, the fauces or opening leads to the pharynx. The pharynx is a common passageway for the movement of air from nasal cavity to trachea and food from mouth to esophagus. The esophagus is a tube approximately 25 centimeters long. Most of the esoph-agus is located within the thoracic cavity, although the lower end of the tube pierces the diaphragm and con-nects with the stomach in the abdominal cavity. Both ends of the esophagus are controlled by a circular mus-cle called a sphincter. The movement of food through the esophagus is assisted by gravity and the contrac-tions of the muscularis layer. No digestion is accom-plished in either the pharynx or the esophagus.

The stomach, a J-shaped organ, is divided into four areas: the cardia, fundus, body, and pyloris. The cardia lies just below the sphincter at the juncture of esopha-gus and stomach, while the fundus is a pouch that pushes upward and to the left of the cardia. The large central area is the body, and the lower end of the stom-ach is the pyloris. Here another sphincter, the pyloric valve, controls the opening between stomach and intes-tine. The mucosa of the stomach is arranged in folds called rugae. The rugae permit distension of the organ as it fills. Gastric and mucus glands are present in the mucosa. The gastric glands produce and secrete en-zymes that are specific for protein digestion, as well as hydrochloric acid, which creates the proper acid envi-ronment for enzyme action. The muscularis of the stomach wall has three layers of muscle with a circular, longitudinal, and oblique arrangement. The muscle arrangement facilitates the churning action that reduces the food to a semiliquid called chyme. The pyloric valve relaxes under neuronal and hormonal influence, and the chyme is moved into the small intestine.

The site for the completion of digestion and the absorption of digested material is the small intestine. This tube, with a 2.5-centimeter diameter and a length of 6.4 meters, is coiled into the mid and lower abdomen. The first 25 centimeters of the small intestine constitute the duodenum. This is followed by the jejunum, which is 2.5 meters long. The ileum, at 3.6 meters, terminates at the ileocecal valve, which connects the small to the large intestine. The interior of the small intestine is characterized by the presence of fingerlike projections of the mucosa called villi that contain blood and lymph capillaries and circular folds of submucosa (the plicae circularis), both of which provide absorption surface for the digested food. Mucosal glands produce enzymes that contribute to the digestion of carbohydrates, lipids, and proteins. Enzymes from the pancreas and bile from the liver enter the small intestine at the duodenum and aid the chemical digestion.

The final compartment in the gastrointestinal system is the large intestine, sometimes called the bowel or colon. This tube, with a diameter of 6.5 centimeters and a length of 1.5 meters, is divided into the cecum; the as-

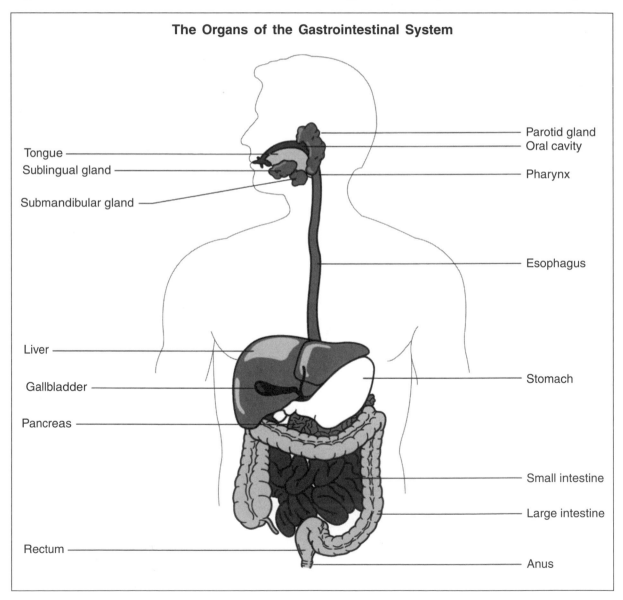

The Organs of the Gastrointestinal System

Tongue

Sublingual gland

Submandibular gland

Parotid gland

Oral cavity

Pharynx

Esophagus

Liver

Gallbladder

Pancreas

Stomach

Small intestine

Large intestine

Rectum

Anus

cending, transverse, and descending colon; the rectum; and the anal canal. The cecum is a blind pouch located just below the ileocecal valve. The fingerlike appendix is attached to the cecum. The ascending colon extends from the cecum up the right side of the abdomen to the underside of the liver, where it turns and runs across the body. The colon descends along the left side of the abdomen. The last few centimeters of colon form an S-shaped curve which gives the section its name, sigmoid colon. Three bands of longitudinal muscle called taeniae coli run the length of the colon. Contraction of these bands causes pouches or haustra to form in the colon, giving the tube a puckered appearance. The sigmoid colon leads into the rectum, a 20-centimeter segment which terminates in a short anal canal. The anus is the opening from the anal canal to the exterior of the body.

DISORDERS AND DISEASES

Because the primary function performed in the gastrointestinal system is the physical and chemical preparation of food for cellular absorption and use, any malfunction of the process has implications for the overall metabolism of the body. Structural changes or abnormalities in the anatomy of the system interfere with the proper mechanical and chemical preparation of the food.

Teeth are the principal agents of mechanical digestion or mastication in the mouth. Dental caries or tooth decay involves a demineralization of the enamel through bacterial action. Disrupted enamel provides an entrance for bacteria to underlying tissues, resulting in infection and inflammation of the tissues. The resulting pain and discomfort interfere with the biting, chewing, and grinding of food. Three pairs of salivary glands secrete the water-based, enzyme-containing fluid called saliva. These glands can be the target of the virus that causes mumps. (Although the pain and swelling that are typical of this disease can prevent swallowing, the more important effect of the virus in males is the possible inflammation of the testes and subsequent sterility.)

The gastroesophageal sphincter at the lower end of the esophagus controls the movement of materials from the stomach into the esophagus. Relaxation of this sphincter allows a backflow of food (gastroesophageal reflux) to occur. The acidity of the stomach contents damages the esophageal lining, and a burning sensation is experienced. Substances such as citric fruits, chocolate, tomatoes, alcohol, and nicotine as well as body positions that increase abdominal pressure, such as bending or lying on the side, induce heartburn or indi-gestion. A hiatal hernia occurs when a defect of the diaphragm allows the lower portion of the esophagus and the upper portion of the stomach to enter the chest cavity; it causes heartburn and difficulty in swallowing.

Pathologies and abnormalities of the stomach and intestines are studied in the medical science called gastroenterology. The stomach is the site of both mechanical and chemical digestion. Although small amounts of digested food begin to pass into the small intestine within minutes following a meal, the chyme usually remains in the stomach for three to five hours. Relaxation of the gastroesophageal sphincter will result in reflux; and stimulation by nerves from the medulla of the brain can cause the forceful emptying of stomach contents through the mouth. This is called vomiting and may be brought about by irritation, overdistension, certain foods, or drugs. Excessive vomiting results in dehydration, which in turn upsets electrolyte and fluid balance.

Chemical digestion in the stomach requires an acidic environment. This is provided by gastric glands, which secrete hydrochloric acid. The tissue lining the stomach protects it from this acidity and prevents self-digestion. Oversecretion of the gastric juices or a breakdown of the stomach lining can cause lesions or peptic ulcers to form in the mucosal lining. Gastritis, the inflammation of the stomach mucosa brought on by the ingestion of irritants such as alcohol and aspirin or an overactive nervous stimulation of the gastric glands, may be the underlying cause of ulcer formation. Ulcers can form in the lower esophagus, stomach, and duodenum because these are the organs that come in contact with gastric juice. The terms "gastric ulcer" and "duodenal ulcer" refer to peptic ulcers located in the stomach and the first portion of the small intestine, respectively.

Gastroenteritis could involve the stomach, the small intestine, or the large intestine. It is a disorder marked by nausea, vomiting, abdominal discomfort, and diarrhea. The condition has various causes and is known by several names. Bacteria are a common cause of the condition known as food poisoning. Amoebas, parasites, and viruses can bring about the symptoms associated with intestinal influenza or travelers' diarrhea. Allergic reactions to food or drugs may cause gastroenteritis.

Although diverticulitis may be found anywhere along the gastrointestinal tract, it is most commonly found in the sigmoid colon. This disorder results from the formation of pouches or diverticula in the wall of the tract. Undigested food and bacteria collect in the diverticula and react to form a hard mass. The mass interferes with the blood supply to the area and ultimately irritates and inflames surrounding tissue. Abscess, obstruction, and hemorrhage may develop. A diet lacking in fiber appears to be the major contributor to this disorder.

Colitis, or inflammation of the bowel, is accompanied by abdominal cramps, diarrhea, and constipation. It may be brought about by psychological stress, as in irritable bowel syndrome, or may be a manifestation of such disorders as chronic ulcerative colitis and Crohn's disease.

A change in the rate of motility through the colon or large intestine results in one of two disorders: diarrhea or constipation. As food passes through the colon, water is reabsorbed by the body. If the food moves too quickly through the colon, then much of the water will remain in the feces and diarrhea results. Severe diarrhea affects electrolyte balance. Viral, bacterial, and parasitic organisms may initiate the rapid motility of substances through the colon. Another condition, called constipation, develops from sluggish motility. When the food remains for too long a time in the bowel, too much water is reabsorbed by the body. The feces then become dry and hard, and defecation is difficult. Lack of fiber in the diet and lack of exercise are the leading causes of constipation.

Hemorrhoids are varicose veins that develop in the rectum or anal canal. Varicose veins are the result of weakened venous valves. Factors such as pressure, lack of muscle tone as a result of aging, straining at defecation, pregnancy, and obesity are among the common contributors. Hemorrhoids become irritated and bleed when hard stools are passed.

Disorders in the accessory organs contribute to the malfunctioning of the gastrointestinal system. Gallstones, cirrhosis of the liver, pancreatitis, and pancreatic cancer are among the major diseases affecting the digestive process. These disorders generally involve the obstruction of tubes or the destruction of glands, so that enzymes do not reach the intended site of digestion.

PERSPECTIVE AND PROSPECTS

The proper functioning of the gastrointestinal system is dependent on the anatomical structure and health of the organs. The organs provide the site for the mechanical and chemical digestion of food, the absorption of food and water, and the elimination of waste material. Two factors play a primary role in causing anatomical abnormalities in digestion: aging and eating disorders.

The aging process gradually changes anatomical structure. In order for food to be chewed properly, teeth must be in good health. Dental caries, periodontal dis-

ease, and missing teeth prevent the proper mastication of food. Because of these problems, older people tend to avoid foods that require chewing. This may lead to an unbalanced diet. Another age-related change in the mouth is the atrophy of the salivary glands and other secretory glands, which interferes with chemical digestion and swallowing. A loss of muscle tone in the organ walls impedes mechanical digestion and slows down the movement of food through the system. Often, the elimination of waste material becomes difficult and constipation results.

Eating disorders such as anorexia nervosa and bulimia contribute to digestive malfunctioning. These disorders are most often associated with but are not limited to young women. Anorexia is self-imposed starvation, while bulimia is characterized by a binge-purge cycle which incorporates vomiting and/or an abusive use of laxatives. Both conditions induce nutrient deficiencies and upset water and electrolyte balances. The vomiting of the acid contents of the stomach damages esophageal, pharyngeal, and mouth tissue. It also destroys tooth enamel. In addition to the harm done to the gastrointestinal system, eating disorders affect several other systems, such as the reproductive system.

The field of medical science that studies and diagnoses digestive system disorders is gastroenterology. Gastroenterologists use several investigative techniques. Blood tests and stool examination are used to detect internal bleeding and deficiency disorders. For a time, X rays were the only nonsurgical means of obtaining information on the structure of internal organs. The advent of nuclear medicine in the 1950's led to the use of radioisotopes in body scanning procedures. Instruments capable of a more detailed and direct visualization were developed, such as fiber optics and the fluoroscope. Fiber optics involves the use of long, threadlike fibers of glass or plastic that transmit light into the organ and reflect the image back to the viewer; this method allows the physician to detect ulcers, lesions, neoplasms, and structural abnormalities. The fluoroscope uses X rays to permit continuous observation of motion within the organs.

The 1970's saw the development of more sophisticated scanning and imaging techniques. Computed tomography (CT) scanning uses X-ray techniques to scan very thin slices of tissue and presents a defined, unobstructed view. Magnetic resonance imaging (MRI) can provide detailed information even to the molecular level; energies from powerful magnetic fields are translated into a visual representation of the structure being studied. Another technique, ultrasonography, passes sound waves through a body area, intercepts the echoes that are produced, and translates them into electrical impulses, which are recorded and interpreted by the physician.

—*Rosemary Scheirer, Ed.D.*

See also Abdomen; Acid reflux disease; Bariatric surgery; Constipation; Diarrhea and dysentery; Digestion; Endoscopy; Enzymes; Food biochemistry; Gastroenterology; Gastroenterology, pediatric; Gastrointestinal disorders; Glands; Hemorrhoids; Hernia; Host-defense mechanisms; Indigestion; Internal medicine; Intestinal disorders; Intestines; Laparoscopy; Lipids; Liver; Malnutrition; Metabolism; Muscles; Nausea and vomiting; Nutrition; Obstruction; Peristalsis; Proctology; Sense organs; Systems and organs; Taste; Teeth.

FOR FURTHER INFORMATION:
McMinn, R. M. H., and R. T. Hutchings. *McMinn's Color Atlas of Human Anatomy.* 4th ed. St. Louis: Mosby Year Book, 1998. Although this atlas is intended for an advanced student of human anatomy, the average reader can profit from the marvelous diagrams and pictures. The pictures are especially helpful in visualizing the organs as they actually appear in the human body.

Moog, Florence. "The Lining of the Small Intestine." *Scientific American* 245 (November, 1981): 154-176. This article incorporates a historical perspective in the detailed explanation of absorption as it occurs in the small intestine. The article requires some scientific literacy but is not beyond the comprehension of a reader with a high school science background.

Tortora, Gerard J., and Sandra R. Grabowski. *Principles of Human Anatomy and Physiology.* 10th ed. New York: John Wiley & Sons, 2003. This highly readable text gives a clear and accurate description of the anatomy and physiology of the gastrointestinal system. The illustrations and diagrams are excellent. The authors include descriptions of major disorders and clinical applications.

GASTROSTOMY
PROCEDURE
ANATOMY OR SYSTEM AFFECTED: Abdomen, gastrointestinal system, stomach

SPECIALTIES AND RELATED FIELDS: Gastroenterology, oncology

DEFINITION: The creation of a hole through the wall of the abdomen into the stomach in order to feed a patient who is unable to swallow.

INDICATIONS AND PROCEDURES
Gastrostomies are carried out during situations in which a patient is unable to swallow food. This condition may result from cancer or strictures of the esophagus; when an esophageal fistula is present, causing the diversion of swallowed food; or when a patient is unconscious. In some cases, the patient is a child who has swallowed a caustic substance, causing damage to the esophagus. Under such circumstances in which a gastrostomy is warranted, an artificial opening is prepared through the abdominal wall into the stomach, and a tube is inserted through the opening.

The gastrostomy tube, which is usually made of plastic or nylon, may be permanently inserted or removed after each feeding. The development of the Barnes-Redo prosthesis has alleviated some of the problems associated with permanent gastrostomies. The device, which is permanently installed, has a cap placed over the opening between feedings. When it is time to eat, the cap is removed, and a catheter is placed through the tube into the stomach, allowing food or liquids to be fed to the patient. When the meal is finished, the catheter is removed and the cap replaced on the gastrostomy tube.

Food for gastrostomy patients cannot be solid. It is recommended that any food first be thoroughly cooked and then blended into a mushy consistency. Patients should smell and taste the food prior to feeding, both to minimize difficulty in adjustment to the situation and to stimulate gastric secretions, which will aid in digestion.

USES AND COMPLICATIONS
Care must be taken with gastrostomy patients to minimize the chance of infection. Any tubes that will be inserted into the stomach must be sterilized prior to use. In addition, the skin around the gastrostomy tube must be protected from gastric juices such as stomach acid, which could cause irritation. The major adjustment for these patients, however, is often psychological—particularly for those with permanent gastrostomies, since meals are often times for social gatherings.

—*Richard Adler, Ph.D.*

See also Cancer; Catheterization; Critical care; Critical care, pediatric; Gastroenterology; Gastroenterology, pediatric; Gastrointestinal disorders; Gastrointestinal system; Nutrition; Poisoning; Stomach, intestinal, and pancreatic cancers.

FOR FURTHER INFORMATION:
Broadwell, Debra C., and Bettie S. Jackson, eds. *Principles of Ostomy Care.* St. Louis: Mosby, 1982.

Gauderer, Michael W. L., and Thomas A. Stellato. *Gastrostomies: Evolution, Techniques, Indications, and Complications.* Chicago: Year Book Medical, 1986.

Ponsky, Jeffrey L., ed. *Techniques of Percutaneous Gastrostomy.* New York: Igaku-Shoin, 1988.

GAUCHER'S DISEASE

DISEASE/DISORDER

ANATOMY OR SYSTEM AFFECTED: Abdomen, bones, cells, liver, lymphatic system, spleen

SPECIALTIES AND RELATED FIELDS: Biochemistry, cytology, genetics, internal medicine, pediatrics, toxicology

DEFINITION: A congenital disorder caused by a defect in lipid metabolism and characterized by cell hyperplasia in the liver, spleen, and bone marrow.

KEY TERMS:

enzyme: a protein that catalyzes a biological reaction in the body

hyperplasia: enlargement

CAUSES AND SYMPTOMS

Gaucher's disease is an inherited disorder resulting from a mutation in the gene that encodes the enzyme glucocerebrosidase, one of a class of enzymes that functions in the breakdown (hydrolysis) of glucosyl ceramide lipids. The result is an accumulation of a class of lipids known as glucosyl ceramide sphingolipids, primarily in cells of the liver, spleen, or bone marrow. Normally, these lipids are hydrolyzed within digestive organelles called lysosomes, found within these cells. The buildup of lipids within these structures classifies Gaucher's disease as a form of lysosomal storage disease; cells in which these pathologies are presented are known as Gaucher cells.

Gaucher's disease is not common in the general population, affecting approximately 1 in 100,000 persons, although three to four times that number probably carry one copy of the defective gene. However, in the ethnic population of Ashkenazi (Eastern European) Jews, approximately 1 in 450 persons is afflicted with the disease, making it among the most common genetic disorders in this group. In 2003, the National Gaucher Foundation, an organization that monitors the disorder, estimated that approximately 2,500 Americans had the disease.

Three different types of Gaucher's disease have been described, differing in their severity, in the presence or absence of neurological defects, and in the general de-

mographics of the disorder. The most common form is type I, characterized by hyperplasia of the liver and spleen and accompanied by bone marrow abnormalities; neurological problems are not observed in this form. Its symptoms include severe anemia, attributable to pathological events among the bone marrow precursors; low numbers of platelets, resulting in severe bleeding; and significant hyperplasia in the spleen and liver. The disease, when observed, is generally found in the adult population, though not all persons with this genetic mutation actually experience all, or even any, of the symptoms. Type II (infantile) disorder, a neuropathic or malignant presentation, is a significantly more severe form that affects children under the age of six months; rarely do these children survive beyond two years as a result of significant central nervous system damage, especially among the cranial nerves. The third form, type III (juvenile), is less severe than Type II, and significantly more variable in its prognosis; children can usually grow into their adult years.

TREATMENT AND THERAPY

Until the 1990's, control of Gaucher's disease involved a combination of splenectomy and repeated blood transfusions. The development of enzyme replacement therapy in 1991 provided a means of controlling the disease through the direct presentation of the missing enzyme glucocerebrosidase to the patient's system. The enzyme was obtained and purified from human placentas collected following hospital births. The initial studies using the natural form of glucocerebrosidase were disappointing, but a chemically modified product proved more successful. The modified form of the enzyme was presented intravenously to persons on an outpatient basis approximately twice each month.

INFORMATION ON GAUCHER'S DISEASE

CAUSES: Genetic enzyme deficiency

SYMPTOMS: Varies with type; may include liver and spleen enlargement, bone marrow abnormalities, severe anemia, severe bleeding, central nervous system damage

DURATION: Chronic

TREATMENTS: Enzyme replacement therapy, genetically engineered drugs

Though costly, the process proved effective in controlling most forms of type I disease, the most common, but less effective for other forms of the disease. In those patients for whom therapy had proven effective, other aspects of the disorder such as cell hyperplasia were often reversed.

Treatments developed in the late 1990's included genetically engineered forms of drugs that could be taken orally. This form of treatment has proven highly effective with those expressing the type I form and to a lesser extent the type III form. In addition to replacement of the defective enzyme, a new class of drugs was also developed that inhibited the actual synthesis of the potentially toxic lipids by blocking the action of the enzyme glucosylceramide synthase.

No effective treatment exists for the type II form of Gaucher's disease, and central nervous system damage is not reversible, even if the disease does respond to therapy.

PERSPECTIVE AND PROSPECTS

Since the chromosomal site of Gaucher's disease is known—chromosome 1q21, or the long arm of chromosome number 1—prenatal testing is possible to determine whether the developing fetus carries the defective gene. The course, or any decision with regard to treatment, is difficult because of the variable nature of many forms of the disease. Carriers can be observed through the use of molecular techniques, such as restriction fragment length polymorphisms (RFLPs), which detect the presence of abnormal forms of the affected gene. However, even within the population affected, such as Ashkenazi Jews, multiple forms of mutations can be found. The significance of different mutations within the same gene remains confusing, in that different persons with even similar defects may manifest the disease in a variety of forms. Clearly, the role of other factors in the expression of Gaucher's disease remains to be clarified.

The disease is not manifested in every individual carrying the mutation; genetic testing of parents in at-risk groups, or the testing of normal parents who have a child with the disorder, may also provide a means of screening during pregnancy for the possibility of illness in the developing child. Given the variable nature of the disease, the issue of screening remains controversial.

Ideally, gene replacement remains the only method, in theory, which could cure the disease. The systemic aspect of the disorder, however, means that even if pos-sible, replacement would have to be carried out at the level of the fetus. For the near future, treatment and control rest upon an increasingly effective use of oral drugs to compensate for the absent enzyme.

—*Richard Adler, Ph.D.*

See also Enzyme therapy; Enzymes; Genetic counseling; Genetic diseases; Glycogen storage diseases; Lipids; Metabolism; Mucopolysaccharidosis (MPS); Niemann-Pick disease; Screening; Tay-Sachs disease.

FOR FURTHER INFORMATION:

Desnick, Robert, Shimon Gatt, and Gregory A. Grabowski, eds. *Gaucher Disease: A Century of Delineation and Research.* New York: A. R. Liss, 1982.

Massimini, Kathy, ed. *Genetic Disorders Sourcebook.* 2d ed. Detroit: Omnigraphics, 2000.

Parker, James N., and Philip M. Parker, eds. *The Official Parent's Sourcebook on Gaucher's Disease.* San Diego, Calif.: Icon Health, 2002.

GENE THERAPY

PROCEDURE

ALSO KNOWN AS: Gene transfer

ANATOMY OR SYSTEM AFFECTED: Cells

SPECIALTIES AND RELATED FIELDS: Biotechnology, cytology, genetics

DEFINITION: The delivery of genetic material into a cell for the purpose of either correcting a genetic problem or giving the cell a new biochemical function.

KEY TERMS:

gene: the deoxyribonucleic acid (DNA) instructions necessary for the manufacture of a functional protein in a cell

genome: the total genetic information found within a virus, cell, or organism

germ cells: cells involved in the process of sexual reproduction and inheritance; also called gametes

somatic cells: cells that make up the majority of the human body and that are not passed on from generation to generation

stem cells: cells that are undifferentiated, meaning that they have the potential to develop into a variety of cell and tissue types

vector: in genetics, a system (usually a virus) that is used to carry a gene into the cell for gene therapy

virus: an infectious agent that consists of a protein coat enclosing a small piece of genetic material; viruses are usually less than one-thousandth the size of the living cell

INDICATIONS AND PROCEDURES

The overall goal of gene therapy is to correct an undesirable trait or disease by introducing a modified copy of a gene into a target cell. In most cases, the purpose is not to replace a defective gene in the host cell but rather to provide a new copy so that the correct protein can be expressed and the detrimental effects of the defective gene neutralized. While technically any genetic disorder may be treated by gene therapy, currently there are some limitations. First, the precise genetic mechanism of the disorder must be known, and it must be a single-gene defect. Second, scientists must know the complete genetic sequence of the gene, including regulatory regions, so that a functional copy can be delivered to the cell. Third, there needs to be an effective vector, or delivery system, for administering the correct copy to the target cells.

Generally, scientists classify forms of gene therapy as belonging to one of three types. Theoretically, the most effective form of this procedure is in situ gene therapy, which means that the genetic material is administered directly to the target cells. Unfortunately, it has been difficult to ensure that only target cells receive the genetic material, but there have been some successes. A second method injects the vector containing the genetic material into the fluids of the body. In this method, called in vivo gene therapy, the vector travels throughout the body until it reaches the target cells. A third mechanism, called ex vivo gene therapy, removes cells from the body to be exposed to the vector and then reintroduced back into the body. This method works especially well with undifferentiated stem cells.

Scientists have developed several mechanisms by which the genetic information can be introduced into the target cell. The most common is the viral vector. Viruses are used because typically they are very specific in the types of cells that they infect. Furthermore, their genomes are usually very small and well understood by scientists. The viruses that are chosen are derived almost exclusively from nonpathogenic strains or have been genetically engineered so that pathogenic portions of the genome have been removed. Common viral vectors are adenoviruses, retroviruses, and herpes simplex viruses. The choice of vector depends on the target and size of gene to be replaced. In each case, after the virus infects the target cell, the DNA is either incorporated directly into the host genome or becomes extrachromosomal.

Medical researchers are also investigating the use of nonviral vectors to deliver DNA into target cells. As is the case with viral vectors, these mechanisms must not disrupt the normal metabolic machinery of the target cell. One system, called plasmid DNA, utilizes small circular pieces of DNA called plasmids to deliver the genetic material. If small enough, the plasmids can pass through the cell membrane. Although they do not integrate into the host genome in the same way as viral vectors do, they are a simple mechanism and lack the potential problems associated with viral vectors. Another mechanism being studied is the packaging of the genetic material within a lipid-based vector called a liposome to ease transport across the membrane. In trials, however, both liposomes and plasmids have displayed a low efficiency in delivering genetic material into target cells.

USES AND COMPLICATIONS

Since the early 1990's, numerous scientific studies have examined the potential effectiveness of gene therapy in treating diseases in mammalian model species, such as mice and monkeys. Using gene therapy, researchers have demonstrated that it may be possible to treat diseases such as Parkinson's disease, sickle cell anemia, and some forms of cancer. Weekly scientific journals such as *Gene Therapy* report the status of these tests. Gene therapy trials in humans are a relatively recent development and represent the next stage in the treatment of human diseases. Diseases such as Canavan disease, severe combined immunodeficiency syndrome (SCID), and adenosine deaminase (ADA) deficiency have already begun trials in humans. Medical researchers have suggested that, in the future, almost any genetic defect may be treatable using gene therapy.

While gene therapy may appear to be the "silver bullet" for diseases such as cancer and Parkinson's disease, the procedure is not without its risks. Since gene therapy using viral vectors was first proposed, scientists have recognized the inherent problems with the procedure. Since the technology does not yet exist to target the specific gene, the chances are that the viral vector will integrate the genetic information into the genome at some site other than the location of the defective gene. This means that the potential exists for the virus to insert itself into a regulatory or structural region of a gene and either render it unusable or impart a new function to the protein. Because of the size of the human genome (more than three billion bases) and the fact that less than 2 percent of the genome is believed to produce functional proteins, the odds of such an event occurring are relatively low. Given the large numbers of vectors used, however, this risk remains a real possibility.

Two cases illustrate the dangers associated with viral vectors. First was the death of a gene therapy trial volunteer at the University of Pennsylvania in 1999. The volunteer, Jesse Gelsinger, suffered from a form of liver disorder called ornithine transcarbamylase deficiency (OTC). OTC is identified as being the result of a single defective gene in a five-step metabolic pathway. Using an adenovirus, researchers sought to replace the defective gene causing OTC in Gelsinger. Shortly after the gene therapy was begun, Gelsinger developed a systemic immune response to the vector and died.

The second case is actually a story of both success and failure. A French research team at the Necker Hospital for Sick Children in Paris effectively used a retrovirus vector to treat a group of young boys with SCID. Also called "bubble boy disease," SCID is a rare disorder in which the immune system is rendered inoperative. One form of the disease has been traced to a gene on the X chromosome. Using the procedure of ex vivo gene therapy, the researchers removed stem cells from the bone marrow of the boys and, using a retrovirus vector, delivered a functional copy of the defective gene into the cells. The cells were then reinserted back into the bone marrow. The procedure was successful in that all boys were cured of the disease. Thirty months later, however, one of the boys developed leukemia, which was followed four months later by a second case. Analysis of the boys' DNA indicated that the inserted gene had disrupted a gene in which mutations had previously been shown to cause cancer.

While the number of individuals that have developed complications from gene therapy is relatively small, these cases do indicate the potential hazards of using a viral system and have accelerated the research into using nonviral systems such as liposomes and plasmids. Additional research is underway to develop a means of targeting a specific gene. Scientists are also investigating the possibility of developing a so-called suicide gene, or "off switch," for the procedure that could terminate treatment if an error in insertion were detected.

PERSPECTIVE AND PROSPECTS

The process of gene therapy represents one of the more recent advances in the life sciences. Since James Watson and Francis Crick proposed the structure of DNA in 1953, scientists have been suggesting the possibility of correcting genetic defects in a cell. It has been only since the early 1990's, however, that advances in biotechnology have enabled the actual procedure to be conducted.

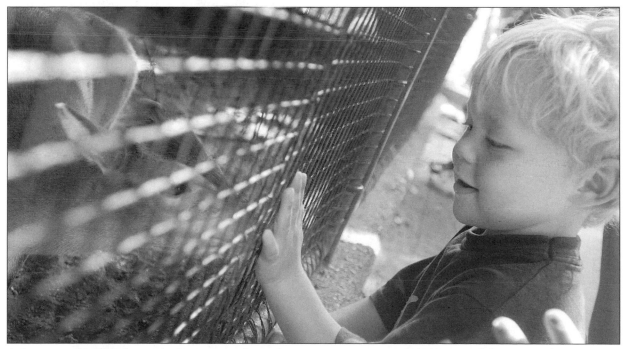

A three-year-old child who received experimental gene therapy to cure severe combined immunodeficiency syndrome (SCID), so-called bubble boy disease, visits a zoo in Amsterdam in 2002. (AP/Wide World Photos)

The science of gene therapy actually began as enzyme replacement therapy. For patients suffering from diseases in which an enzyme in a metabolic pathway is defective, enzyme replacement therapy provides a temporary cure. In these cases, however, the therapy must be administrated continuously since presence of a defective gene means that the body lacks the ability to manufacture new enzymes.

In the 1980's, enzyme replacement therapy was being used to treat a number of diseases including ADA deficiency, in which an enzyme in a biochemical pathway that converts toxins in the body to uric acid is defective. As a result, the toxins accumulate and eventually render the immune system ineffective. The modern era for gene therapy began in the early 1990's as scientists began to treat ADA deficiency with gene therapy. Through a series of trials, researchers learned that ex vivo treatment of stem cells proved to be the most effective mechanism for treating ADA deficiency with gene therapy. In 1993, researchers obtained stem cells from the umbilical cord of three babies that were born with ADA deficiency. After the correct genes were inserted into these stem cells, the altered cells were inserted back into the donor babies. After years of monitoring, it appears that the process has worked and the potentially fatal effects of ADA deficiency in these children has been reversed.

Another promising area of gene therapy is the treatment of cancer. Cancer treatment using gene therapy would probably not involve replacing defective genes but rather "knocking out" those genes that are causing uncontrolled cell division within cancer cells. By arresting cell division, scientists can halt the spread of the cancer. This treatment would be especially useful in areas of the body where surgery is risky, such as brain tumors. The primary challenge at this stage is the targeting of the vector. A knockout vector would need to infect only cancer cells and not the other dividing cells of the human body.

A potential area of gene therapy that has yet to be exploited is germ-line gene therapy. Germ cells are those that are responsible for the formation of gametes, or egg and sperm cells. Since a germ cell contains only half the genetic information of an adult cell, it is relatively easy to replace genes using available procedures learned from biotechnology. Furthermore, since following fertilization the genetic material in the germ cells is responsible for the formation of all the remaining more than sixty-three trillion cells in the human body, any genetic change in the germ cells has the ability to be inherited by subsequent generations. Somatic cell therapy, such as that used to treat ADA deficiency and SCID, has the ability to influence only the affected individual, since these cells are not normally part of the reproductive process. Gene therapy in germ cells is currently considered unethical, but many consider it to be the mechanism of eliminating certain diseases from the human species.

While the use of gene therapy to correct human diseases may be stalled temporarily until technical obstacles are overcome, little doubt exists in the biomedical community that gene therapy represents the procedure of the future. At a fundamental level, gene therapy has the potential to be the ultimate cure for many ailments and diseases of humankind. For most of recorded history, medicine has been confined to the treatment of symptoms. Since the start of the twentieth century, advances have enabled enhanced surgical procedures, pharmaceutical drugs that alter or interact with the biochemistry of the cell, improved diagnostic techniques, and a deeper understanding of genetic inheritance. Gene therapy represents the ultimate preventive procedure.

—*Michael Windelspecht, Ph.D.*

See also Bionics and biotechnology; Cancer; Cells; Clinical trials; DNA and RNA; Enzyme therapy; Enzymes; Ethics; Genetic diseases; Genetic engineering; Genetics and inheritance; Genomics; Mutation; Severe combined immunodeficiency syndrome (SCID); Stem cells; Viral infections.

FOR FURTHER INFORMATION:

Gorman, Jessica. "Delivering the Goods: Gene Therapy Without the Virus." *Science News* 163 (January, 2003): 43-44. A short but informative examination of research into nonviral mechanisms of gene therapy, including bioengineered liposomes and naked DNA.

Kresina, Thomas F., ed. *An Introduction to Molecular Medicine and Gene Therapy.* New York: Wiley-Liss, 2001. Covers the entire spectrum of the evolving field of molecular medicine, from nuclear transplantation to gene therapy. Includes specific discussions of cancer and human immunodeficiency virus (HIV), as well as other diseases. Sections also cover ethical considerations and federal regulation.

Lemoine, N. R., ed. *Understanding Gene Therapy.* New York: Springer, 1999. Contains a series of articles that cover most aspects of gene therapy, from diseases that show potential for therapy to vectors to deliver the genetic information to target cells. Also discusses the ethical issues of gene therapy and prospects for the future.

Lewis, Ricki. *Human Genetics: Concepts and Applications.* 5th ed. New York: McGraw-Hill, 2002. This clearly written text contains an entire chapter dedicated to the history of gene therapy, including specific examples of successes and setbacks.

Templeton, Nancy Smyth, and Danilo D. Lasic, eds. *Gene Therapy: Therapeutic Mechanisms and Strategies.* New York: Marcel Dekker, 2000. Provides a review of the various mechanisms of gene therapy, from the established viral vectors to research into less risky systems. Slightly more advanced than some titles, it can be used as a reference for both the general public and scientists.

GENETIC COUNSELING

SPECIALTY

ANATOMY OR SYSTEM AFFECTED: Cells, reproductive system, uterus

SPECIALTIES AND RELATED FIELDS: Cytology, embryology, genetics, obstetrics, preventive medicine, psychology

DEFINITION: The scientific field that uses several biochemical and imaging techniques, as well as family histories, to provide information about genetic conditions or diseases in order to help individuals make medical and reproductive decisions.

KEY TERMS:

chromosomal abnormality: any change to the number, shape, or appearance of the forty-six chromosomes in each human cell; the presence of many such abnormalities will prevent the normal development of an individual and lead to a miscarriage

dominant genetic disease: a disease caused by a mutation in a gene that can be inherited from only one parent

genetic screening: a program designed to determine whether individuals are carriers of or are affected by a particular genetic disease

karyotype: a photograph of the chromosomes taken from the cells of an individual; a karyotype can be used to predict the sex of a fetus or the presence of a large chromosomal abnormality

mutation: an alteration in the DNA sequence of a gene that usually leads to the production of a nonfunctional enzyme or protein and, thus, a lack of a normal metabolic function; this defect may cause a medical condition called a genetic disease

recessive genetic disease: a disease caused by a mutation in a gene that must be inherited from both parents in order for an individual to show the symptoms of the disease; such a disease may show up only occasionally in a family history, especially if the mutation is rare

SCIENCE AND PROFESSION

Genetic counseling is a process of communicating to a couple the medical problems associated with the occurrence of an inherited disorder or birth defect in a family. Included in this process is a discussion of the prognosis and treatment of the problem. Specific reproductive options include abortion of an ongoing pregnancy, birth control or sterilization to prevent additional pregnancies, artificial insemination, the use of surrogate mothers, embryo transplantation, and adoption.

In all cases, the role of the counselor is to provide unbiased information and options to the couple seeking advice. The counselor must not only discuss the medical implications of a condition but also help to alleviate the emotional impact of positive diagnoses and, in particular, to assuage the guilt or denial that a diagnosis may elicit in parents.

The two major categories of medical problems covered by counselors are birth defects and genetic diseases. The first group includes Down syndrome and spina bifida, while the latter includes hemophilia, sickle cell disease, and Tay-Sachs disease. Although the distinction between these two categories can sometimes blur, the key difference involves the clear pattern of inheritance shown by the genetic diseases.

Humans have between thirty thousand and thirty-five thousand genes. Genes are segments of deoxyribonucleic acid (DNA) that are arranged in linear fashion along the forty-six chromosomes. Most genes contain the information necessary for the cells to produce a specific protein, which often is involved in controlling some critical physiological function. For example, the beta globin gene produces a protein called beta globin that makes up half of the hemoglobin that carries oxygen in the red blood cells.

A genetic disease can occur when the DNA changes in structure. Such a change is also known as a mutation. A mutation can lead to the production of a defective protein that cannot carry out its normal function, thus causing a physiological defect. In the case of beta globin, changing only one of the 106 molecules that make up this protein leads to a form of hemoglobin that can produce nonfunctional protein aggregates in red blood cells. These aggregates can cause the red blood cells to collapse and take on a sickle shape. Such cells lose their function, and the tissues are starved for oxygen—a condition known as anemia. This defect, which is called sickle cell disease, is a fatal, heritable disease. As with all genetic disease, such mutations are relatively rare. Certain diseases may, however, be more prevalent within certain ethnic groups; for example, African Americans have a high incidence of sickle cell disease, and Ashkenazic Jews have a high incidence of Tay-Sachs disease.

Humans have two of each kind of chromosome; one set of twenty-three is inherited from the mother, and the other set of twenty-three is inherited from the father. Thus, each person has two copies of each gene, one located on a maternal chromosome, the other on a paternal one. Many types of defects, such as sickle cell disease, require that both genes have mutations in order for the disease to have an effect. Individuals who have one normal gene and one with a mutation are normal but carry the disease; they can pass the mutation on to the next generation in their eggs and sperm. This type of disease is called a recessive genetic disease. The only way a child can have sickle cell disease is if both parents are carriers, since it is unlikely that a person affected by the disease will live long enough to have children.

Since it is equally likely for each parent to pass on the normal gene in eggs or sperm as to pass on the mutation, the laws of probability predict that, on the average, one-fourth of such a couple's offspring should have the disease. One of the major tasks of a genetic counselor is to advise couples of these probabilities if the diagnoses and family histories suggest that they are carriers. Since the laws of genetics involve random occurrences, however, it is possible that in a family with three or four children, all the children will be normal, or that in another family, all the children will have the disease. This degree of uncertainty produces stress and anxiety in couples who seek counseling only to hear that they indeed are at risk. Discussing concepts that involve sophisticated genetic or biochemical themes or issues of probable risk with couples untrained in scientific thinking is difficult, especially considering the highly emotional atmosphere of such discussions.

Other diseases, such as Huntington's chorea, also known as Woody Guthrie's disease for the folksinger who was afflicted by it, are caused by a dominant mutation. A mutation is dominant when an individual needs to inherit only one copy of the mutation in order to have the disease. Unlike recessive diseases that can disappear from a family for generations, a dominant mutation can be inherited only from a person who has the disease. In most cases, such a person has one normal gene and one with the mutation, which means that there is a 50 percent chance that the gene will be passed on. Huntington's chorea is a particularly insidious genetic disease, because the symptoms usually begin to show only in middle age, often after childbearing decisions have been made. Thus, the children of an afflicted parent must decide whether they will marry and have children before they know whether they have inherited the mutation from their parents.

There are no cures for the permanent physiological defects that result from genetic disease. In some cases, the disease symptoms can be controlled by supplementing the protein that is lacking. Some forms of insulin-dependent diabetes and most cases of hemophilia can be treated in this way. In other cases, as with the disease phenylketonuria (PKU), special diets can prevent the severe neurological problems that inevitably lead to childhood death if the disease is left untreated.

DNA technology and genetic engineering offer potential cures for some diseases in which the primary defect caused by the mutation is well understood. Gene therapy is a process by which an additional copy of a normal gene is inserted into the cells of an affected individual or the defective gene is replaced by a normal one. Successful experiments with animals have given scientists confidence that these techniques will provide cures for many genetic diseases. These same DNA technologies are making better diagnosis possible and, as in the case of cystic fibrosis, are helping to extend the lives and enhance the quality of life of individuals afflicted with incurable diseases.

One of the more controversial aspects of genetic counseling is the procedure of screening. In this procedure, individuals suspected to be at risk are tested for the presence of a mutation. Screening can let people know whether they have a disease as well as whether they are carriers of the disease and therefore can pass the disease on to their children. Screening can be extended to all individuals, regardless of family or ethnic history. For example, in the United States, most states require that all newborn infants undergo a PKU test. This simple test involves taking a small sample of blood by pricking the heel of the baby. Although the costs of this screening are not insignificant, the benefit is that those infants found to have the disease can be treated immediately by being placed on a special diet so as to avoid the debilitating effects of the disease.

Other screening procedures are targeted at specific groups. The screening program for Tay-Sachs disease focuses on ethnic Jewish populations. This successful, voluntary program has reduced the incidence of Tay-Sachs disease significantly in the United States. The key to the success of the program was the money spent to educate the targeted group. In addition, key members of the population played a leading role in designing the overall program. Because of the much larger size of the potential group at risk, similar efforts to screen African American populations for sickle cell disease have been much less successful. Ethical concerns about the motivations behind government-sponsored or government-encouraged screening of minority populations make these programs difficult to implement. In addition, in mandatory programs, concerns about confidentiality and information release become major obstacles.

DIAGNOSTIC AND TREATMENT TECHNIQUES

Genetic counseling usually begins when a couple or an individual seeks the advice of a family physician or obstetrician regarding the medical risks associated with having a child. Motivating this request may be a previous birth of a child with a defect, a general uneasiness on the part of a couple worried about environmental exposure to potentially harmful agents, a family history of genetic disease, or advanced maternal age (which can be a factor in certain chromosomal abnormalities). Often, the family is referred to a genetic counseling clinic where most of the actual diagnosis and counseling will occur.

Arriving at a proper diagnosis for any obvious condition, as well as giving advice about potential risks, involves obtaining as much family history as possible with respect to the trait, as well as diagnostic information from the couple. If pregnant already, the woman may undergo a prenatal diagnostic procedure that could include ultrasound, blood tests, amniocentesis, and chorionic villus sampling.

Ultrasound is a technique that uses sound waves to visualize the exterior of the developing fetus. This widely used procedure is almost routine in many large urban hospitals. Ultrasound can be used to detect the presence of twins as well as of some profound birth defects such as hydrocephalus (water on the brain) or spina bifida. The latter defect, which involves the failure of the neural tube to close properly during development, leads to weakness, paralysis, and lack of function in lower body areas. The severity of the defect is hard to predict, and,

unlike genetic disease, the incidence of recurrence is no higher than normal for subsequent children.

Supplementing ultrasound in the detection of spina bifida is a simple blood test that looks for a protein that the fetus spills into the amniotic fluid in higher quantities if the neural tube fails to close properly. The protein, which is called alpha-fetoprotein, crosses the placenta to circulate in the mother's blood. The amount of this normal protein in the mother's blood correlates with the developmental age of the fetus; therefore, an abnormal level might indicate a problem. Older-than-calculated fetuses and twins can both cause increased levels of alpha-fetoprotein, so care must be taken in this diagnosis. If abnormally high levels of the protein are found, amniocentesis would then be used to measure the protein level in the amniotic fluid, thus increasing the reliability of the diagnosis. In amniocentesis, a few teaspoonfuls of amniotic fluid are removed from the sac that surrounds and protects the developing fetus. Ultrasound is used to visualize the exterior of the fetus to allow the safe removal of this fluid, which contains some fetal cells. Biochemical tests can be performed directly on the fluid and results obtained quickly. Tay-Sachs disease is an example of a genetic disease that can be detected in this fashion, since fetuses with the disease fail to make an enzyme that their normal counterparts do make.

Many techniques, however, require obtaining large numbers of fetal cells and/or DNA. In these cases, the cells must be cultured for one to two weeks in a laboratory in order to get enough material to test. The delay between taking the sample and discussing the results with the clients is a source of stress and anxiety for parents undergoing counseling.

Preparing a karyotype, a photograph showing the numbers and sizes of the chromosomes of the fetus, is a commonly performed procedure following amniocentesis. Normal fetuses contain forty-six chromosomes, and any change in chromosome number, shape, or size can be detected by a skilled clinician. A large percentage of miscarriages involve fetuses with chromosomal abnormalities, so this diagnosis can be critical. A relatively common type of birth defect that can be diagnosed with a karyotype is Down syndrome. Most children born with Down syndrome have forty-seven chromosomes instead of forty-six; thus, this diagnosis is very accurate. In addition, the sex of the fetus can be determined from a karyotype, since male fetuses have an X and a Y chromosome while females have two X chromosomes. This information can be valuable to couples who are at risk for carrying a sex-linked genetic disease such as hemophilia, which could not affect any female offspring. Such information could potentially be used inappropriately for sexual selection of offspring, however, and the counselor must provide this information cautiously.

Amniocentesis is usually performed in the sixteenth week of pregnancy to allow the fetus to grow to a size at which the removal of a small amount of amniotic fluid would not be harmful. Although there is little risk to mother or fetus in this procedure, the delay associated with laboratory culturing means that results are often known in the eighteenth week of pregnancy or even later. At this stage, abortion becomes a more traumatic medical procedure. Chorionic villus sampling, on the other hand, can actually sample small amounts of fetal tissue directly. Since the procedure can safely obtain enough tissue to diagnose most problems and can be performed as early as the ninth or tenth week of pregnancy, abortion becomes a medically less traumatic option.

DNA technology provides the counselor with a battery of new diagnostic procedures that can look directly for the presence of a mutation in the DNA of the fetus. These tests can be performed on parents who are worried about being carriers for a particular disease or can be used on DNA obtained from fetal cells grown in a laboratory. Such tests have very high reliability and can give information about diseases such as sickle cell disease, Huntington's chorea, muscular dystrophy, and cystic fibrosis.

The counselor's task is to take the diagnostic results and interpret them in the context of the medical history and particular family situation. The counselor must point out the options available, both for further diagnosis to confirm or rebut less-sensitive preliminary tests and to discuss potential medical interventions such as the special diets available for children born with PKU. In cases in which no medical intervention is possible, the severity of the problem should be discussed honestly so that the parents can choose either to continue or to abort the pregnancy. Other options, including adoption, artificial insemination, and embryo transplants, can also be evaluated. Finally, the risk of recurrence of the problem in future pregnancies should be discussed.

Counselors need to realize that their clients are often in emotionally fragile states. They must guard against using bias or interjecting their own personal beliefs or values when counseling their clients. Full disclosure of information, both verbally and in a carefully written report, is usually provided.

Compounding the tasks of the counselor is the fact that, in many cases, exact diagnoses are not yet possible. Sometimes, only the relative risks associated with another pregnancy can be determined. Different couples will perceive risks very differently depending on their own religious and moral backgrounds, as well as on the expected severity of the defect. In the case of a genetic disease such as Tay-Sachs, which is 100 percent fatal and requires extensive hospitalization of the child, a modest risk may be considered unacceptable, while in the case of a birth defect such as Down syndrome, whose severity cannot be predicted, and in which case the child may lead a long and rich life, a modest risk may be considered quite differently.

PERSPECTIVE AND PROSPECTS

The need for centers specializing in genetic counseling arose when it became clear that certain diseases and birth defects had a hereditary component. Many families request the services of counselors from these centers, and the centers are also involved in both voluntary and mandatory screening programs. In the United States, about 4 percent of all newborns suffer from a defect that is recognized either at birth or shortly thereafter. This group includes 0.5 percent who have a chromosomal abnormality that results in an obvious medical problem, 0.5 to 1 percent who have classical genetic diseases, and 2 percent who suffer from a birth defect that may have a heritable component. Estimates vary, but more than one-third of all children in pediatric hospitals are there because of some association with a genetic disease.

Physicians have always served as counselors to families, but the rapid advances made in genetics and molecular science during the second half of the twentieth century have clearly surpassed the abilities of most physicians to keep current with treatments and diagnoses. The first formal clinic for genetic counseling was established at the University of Michigan in the 1940's. Most clinics specializing in this field were based at large medical centers; first in major metropolitan areas, and later in smaller population centers.

Genetic counseling clinics usually employ a range of specialists, including clinicians, geneticists, laboratory personnel for performing diagnostic testing, and public health and social workers. In 1969, Sarah Lawrence College instituted a master's-level program in genetic counseling to train candidates formally in the scientific, medical, and counseling skills required for this profession. Since that time, many other programs have been established in the United States. Today, most large counseling programs at medical centers use these specially trained personnel. In rural areas, however, family physicians are still a primary source of counseling; thus, genetic training is an important component of basic medical education.

The sophisticated medical diagnostic tools described above allow a counselor to provide abundant information to couples requesting counseling, but the power of DNA technology has expanded and will continue to expand the scope of current practice. Soon, counselors will not have to give advice in terms of probabilities and likelihoods of risk; molecular detection techniques will make possible the absolute identification of not only individuals with a disease but also related carriers.

As these DNA tools become more widely available, counseling will become a more integral part of preventive medicine. A DNA diagnostic procedure for a heritable form of breast cancer is available that allows women who have the mutation to monitor their health closely in order to receive prompt, lifesaving medical intervention. An important ethical issue here is that some women who have been diagnosed as having the mutation are undergoing preventive mastectomies without having developed any growths in order to ensure that they will not develop cancer. This radical therapy carries with it considerable emotional stress and should be undertaken only after consultation with a physician. As DNA-based diagnostic procedures, perhaps coupled with mandatory screening, become more commonplace, concerns about the release of this information to potential employers or health insurers will become more critical.

—*Joseph G. Pelliccia, Ph.D.*

See also Abortion; Amniocentesis; Birth defects; Blood testing; Chorionic villus sampling; DNA and RNA; Down syndrome; Ethics; Gene therapy; Genetic diseases; Genetic engineering; Genetics and inheritance; Hemophilia; Laboratory tests; Mutation; Niemann-Pick disease; Phenylketonuria (PKU); Screening; Sickle cell disease; Spina bifida; Tay-Sachs disease; Ultrasonography.

FOR FURTHER INFORMATION:

Davis, Dena S. *Genetic Dilemmas: Reproductive Technologies, Parental Choices, and Children's Future*. London: Routledge, 2000. Explores real-life medical cases as a means to discuss ethical dilemmas raised by the availability of new reproductive technologies.

Fanaroff, Avroy A., and Richard J. Martin. *Neonatal-Perinatal Medicine: Diseases of the Fetus and Infant*. 2 vols. 7th ed. New York: Elsevier, 2001. Comprehensively covers the fetus, pregnancy disorders, provisions for neonatal care, risk factors, and development and disorders of organ systems, among many other topics.

Filkins, Karen, and Joseph F. Russo, eds. *Human Prenatal Diagnosis*. Rev. 2d ed. New York: Marcel Dekker, 1990. An advanced sourcebook that describes the procedures of prenatal diagnosis in great detail. Contains information on such issues as risk, reliability, and cost.

Harper, Peter S. *Practical Genetic Counselling*. 5th ed. Boston: Butterworth-Heinemann, 1998. A good overview of all aspects of genetic counseling, including a discussion of the types of diagnoses, treatments, risks, and emotional strains associated with counseling. Also gives a history of counseling as a discipline.

Jorde, Lynn B., John Carrey, and Michael J. Bamshed. *Medical Genetics*. 3d ed. New York: Elsevier, 2003. An introductory text that covers basic molecular genetics, chromosomal and single gene disorders, immunogenetics, cancer genetics, multifactorial disorders, and fetal therapy.

King, Richard A., et al., eds. *Genetic Basis of Common Diseases*. 2d ed. New York: Oxford University Press, 2002. Covers advances in the understanding of molecular processes involved in genetic susceptibility and disease mechanisms. Examines a range of diseases in detail and includes a chapter on genetic counseling.

Lewis, Ricki. *Human Genetics: Concepts and Applications*. 5th ed. New York: McGraw-Hill, 2002. A very accessible undergraduate text that covers the fundamentals, transmission genetics, DNA and chromosomes, and the latest genetic technology, among other topics.

Mange, Arthur P., and Elaine J. Mange. *Genetics: Human Aspects*. 2d ed. Sunderland, Mass.: Sinauer Associates, 1997. An excellent advanced high school or college text that introduces most of the concepts relevant to genetic counseling, from basic theory to practical applications.

Moore, Keith L., and T. V. N. Persaud. *The Developing Human*. 7th ed. Philadelphia: W. B. Saunders, 2003. An outstanding textbook on human embryonic development, with specific information about the causes of congenital malformations and common defects occurring in each of the body's systems.

Pierce, Benjamin A. *The Family Genetic Sourcebook.* New York: John Wiley & Sons, 1990. Good background reading on genetics and genetic diseases. The book gives short, clear descriptions of a number of genetic diseases, along with their diagnosis and treatment.

U.S. Congress. Office of Technology Assessment. *Genetic Counseling and Cystic Fibrosis Carrier Screening: Results of a Survey-Background Paper.* Washington, D.C.: Government Printing Office, 1992. Genetic screening is a controversial subject. This source discusses the problems and successes associated with one such effort.

GENETIC DISEASES

DISEASE/DISORDER

ANATOMY OR SYSTEM AFFECTED: All

SPECIALTIES AND RELATED FIELDS: Embryology, genetics, internal medicine, neonatology, obstetrics, pediatrics

DEFINITION: A variety of disorders transmitted from parent to child through chromosomal material; most people experience disease related to genetics in some form, and research into this area is yielding greater understanding of the relationship between disease and hereditary proclivities toward disease, as well as new strategies for early detection and prevention or therapy.

KEY TERMS:

autosomal recessive disease: a disease which is expressed only when two copies of a defective gene are inherited, one from each parent; present on non-sex-determining chromosomes

chromosomes: rod-shaped structures in each cell which contain genes, the chemical elements that determine traits

deoxyribonucleic acid (DNA): the chemical molecule that transmits hereditary information from generation to generation

dominant gene: a gene which can express its effect when an individual has only one copy of it

gene: the hereditary unit, composed of DNA, that resides on chromosomes

inheritance: the passing down of traits from generation to generation

X-linked: a term used to describe genes or traits that are located on the X chromosome; a male needs only one copy of an X-linked gene for it to be expressed

CAUSES AND SYMPTOMS

Hereditary units called genes determine the majority of the physical and biochemical characteristics of an organism. Genes are composed of a chemical compound called deoxyribonucleic acid (DNA) and are organized into rod-shaped structures called chromosomes that reside in each cell of the body. Each human cell carries forty-six chromosomes organized as twenty-three pairs, each composed of several thousand genes. Twenty-two of the chromosome pairs are homologous pairs; that is, similar genes are located at similar sites on each chromosome. The remaining chromosomes are the sex chromosomes. Human females bear two X chromosomes, and human males possess one X and one Y chromosome.

During the formation of the reproductive cells, the chromosome pairs separate and one copy of each pair is randomly included in the egg or sperm. Each egg will contain twenty-two autosomes (non-sex chromosomes) and one X chromosome. Each sperm will contain twenty-two autosomes and either one X or one Y chromosome. The egg and sperm fuse at fertilization, which restores the proper number of chromosomes, and the genes inherited from the baby's parents will determine its sex and much of its physical appearance and future health and well-being.

Genetic diseases are inherited as a result of the presence of abnormal genes in the reproductive cells of one or both parents of an affected individual. There are two broad classifications of genetic disease: those caused by defects in chromosome number or structure, and those resulting from a much smaller flaw within a gene. Within the latter category, there are four predominant mechanisms by which the disorders can be transmitted from generation to generation: autosomal dominant inheritance, in which the defective gene is inherited from one parent; autosomal recessive inheritance, in which one defective gene is inherited from each parent, who themselves show no signs of the disorder; X-linked chromosomal inheritance (often called sex-linked), in which the flawed gene has been determined to reside on the X chromosome; and multifactorial inheritance, in which genes interact with each other and/or environmental factors.

Errors in chromosome number include extra and missing chromosomes. The most common chromosomal defect observed in humans is Down syndrome, which is caused by the presence of three copies of chromosome 21, instead of the usual two. Down syndrome occurs at a frequency of about one in eight hundred live births, this frequency increasing with increasing maternal age. The symptoms of this disorder include mental retardation, short stature, and numerous other medical problems. The most common form of Down syndrome results from the failure of the two copies of chromosome 21 to separate during reproductive cell formation, which upon fusion with a normal reproductive cell at fertilization produces an embryo containing three copies of chromosome 21.

Gross defects in chromosome structure include duplicated and deleted portions of chromosomes and broken and rearranged chromosome fragments. Prader-Willi syndrome results from a deletion of a small portion of chromosome 15. Children affected with this disorder are mentally retarded, obese, and diabetic. Cri du chat (literally, cat cry) syndrome is associated with a large deletion in chromosome 5. Affected infants exhibit facial abnormalities, are severely retarded, and produce a high-pitched, kittenlike wail.

Genetic diseases caused by defects in individual genes result when defective genes are propagated through many generations or a new genetic flaw develops in a reproductive cell. New genetic defects arise from a variety of causes, including environmental assaults such as radiation, toxins, or drugs. More than four thousand such gene disorders have been identified.

Manifestation of an autosomal dominant disorder requires the inheritance of only one defective gene from one parent who is afflicted with the disease. Inheritance of two dominant defective genes, one from each parent, is possible but generally creates such severe consequences that the child dies while still in the womb or shortly after birth. An individual who bears one copy of

the gene has a 50 percent chance of transmitting that gene and the disease to his or her offspring.

Among the most common autosomal dominant diseases are hyperlipidemia and hypercholesterolemia. Elevated levels of lipids and cholesterol in the blood, which contribute to artery and heart disease, are the consequences of these disorders, respectively. Onset of the symptoms is usually in adulthood, frequently after the affected individual has had children and potentially transmitted the faulty gene to them.

Huntington's chorea causes untreatable neurological deterioration and death, and symptoms do not appear until affected individuals are at least in their forties. Children of parents afflicted with Huntington's chorea may have already made reproductive decisions without the knowledge that they might carry the defective gene; they risk a 50 percent chance of transmitting the dread disease to their offspring.

Autosomal recessive genetic diseases require that an affected individual bear two copies of a defective gene, inheriting one from each parent. Usually the parents are simply carriers of the defective gene; their one normal copy masks the effect of the one flawed copy. If two carriers have offspring, 25 percent will receive two copies of the flawed gene and inherit the disease, and 50 percent will be asymptomatic carriers.

Cystic fibrosis is an autosomal recessive disease which occurs at a rate of about one in two thousand live births among Caucasians. The defective gene product causes improper chloride transport in cells and results in thick mucous secretions in lungs and other organs. Sickle cell disease, another autosomal recessive disorder, is the most common genetic disease among African Americans in the United States. Abnormality in the protein hemoglobin, the component of red blood cells that carries oxygen to all the body's tissues, leads to deformed blood cells that are fragile and easily destroyed.

X-linked genetic diseases are transmitted by faulty genes located on the X chromosome. Females need two copies of the defective gene to acquire such a disease, and in general women carry only one flawed copy, making them asymptomatic carriers of the disorder. Males, having only a single X chromosome, need only one copy of the defective gene to express an X-linked disease. Males with X-linked disorders inherit the defective gene from their mothers, since fathers must contribute a Y chromosome to male offspring. Half of the male offspring of a carrier female will inherit the defective gene and develop the disease. In the rare case of a female with two defective X-linked genes, 100 percent of her male offspring will inherit the disease gene, and, assuming that the father does not carry the defective gene, 50 percent of her female offspring will be carriers. There are more than 250 X-linked disorders, some of the more common being Duchenne's muscular dystrophy, which results in progressive muscle deterioration and early death; hemophilia; and red-green color blindness, which affects about 8 percent of Caucasian males.

Multifactorial inheritance, which accounts for a number of genetic diseases, is caused by the complex interaction of one or more genes with each other and with environmental factors. This group of diseases includes many disorders which, anecdotally, "run in families." Representative disorders include cleft palate, spina bifida, anencephaly, and some inherited heart abnormalities. Other diseases appear to have a genetic component predisposing an individual to be susceptible to environmental stimuli that trigger the disease. These include cancer, hypertension, diabetes, schizophrenia, alcoholism, depression, and obesity.

Diagnosis and Detection

Most, but not all, genetic diseases manifest their symptoms immediately or soon after the birth of an affected child. Rapid recognition of such a medical condition and its accurate diagnosis are essential for the proper treatment and management of the disease by parents and medical personnel. Medical technology has developed swift and accurate diagnostic methods, in many cases allowing testing of the fetus prior to birth. In addition, tests are available that determine the carrier status of an individual for many autosomal recessive and X-linked diseases. These test results are used in conjunction with genetic counseling of individuals and couples who are at risk of transmitting a genetic disease to their offspring. Thus, such individuals can make informed decisions when planning their reproductive futures.

Errors in chromosome number and structure are detected in an individual by analyzing his or her chromosomes. A small piece of skin or a blood sample is taken, the cells in the sample are grown to a sufficient number, and the chromosomes within each cell are stained with special dyes so that they may be viewed with a microscope. A picture of the chromosomes, called a karyotype, is taken, and the patient's chromosome array is compared with that of a normal individual. Extra or missing chromosomes or alterations in chromosome structure are determined, thus identifying the genetic

disease. The analysis of karyotypes is the method used to determine the presence of Down, Prader-Willi, and cri du chat syndromes, among others.

Defects in chromosome number and structure can also be identified in the fetus, prior to birth, using two different sample collecting methods: amniocentesis and chorionic villus sampling. In amniocentesis, a needle is inserted through the pregnant woman's abdomen and uterus, into the fluid-filled sac surrounding the fetus. A sample of this fluid, the amniotic fluid, is withdrawn. The amniotic fluid contains fetal cells sloughed off by the fetus. The cells are grown for several weeks until there are enough to perform chromosome analysis. This procedure is performed only after sixteen

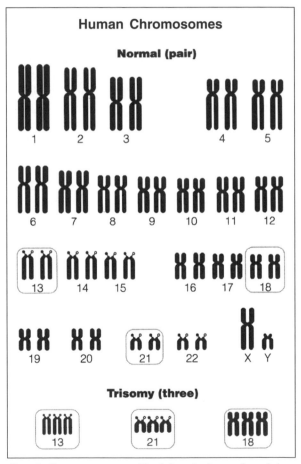

Genetic diseases are caused by defects in the number of chromosomes, in their structure, or in the genes on the chromosome (mutation). Shown here is the human complement of chromosomes (23 pairs) and three errors of chromosome number (trisomies) that lead to the genetic disorders Patau's syndrome (trisomy no. 13), Edward's syndrome (trisomy no. 18), and the more common Down syndrome (trisomy no. 21).

weeks' gestation, in order to ensure adequate amniotic fluid for sampling.

Chorionic villus sampling relies on a biopsy of the fetal chorion, a membrane surrounding the fetus which is composed of cells that have the same genetic constitution as the fetus. A catheter is inserted through the pregnant woman's vagina and into the uterus until it is in contact with the chorion. The small sample of this tissue that is removed contains enough cells to perform karyotyping immediately, permitting diagnosis by the next day. Chorionic villus sampling can be performed between the eighth and ninth week of pregnancy. This earlier testing gives the procedure an advantage over amniocentesis, since the earlier determination of whether a fetus is carrying a genetic disease allows safer pregnancy termination if the parents choose this course.

Karyotype analysis is limited to the diagnosis of genetic diseases caused by very large chromosome abnormalities. The majority of hereditary disorders are caused by gene flaws that are too small to see microscopically. For many of these diseases, diagnosis is available through either biochemical testing or DNA analysis.

Many genetic disorders cause a lack of a specific biochemical which is necessary for normal metabolism. These types of disorders are frequently referred to as "inborn errors of metabolism." Many of these errors can be detected by the chemical analysis of fetal tissue. For example, galactosemia is a disease which results from the lack of galactose-1-phosphate uridyl transferase. Infants with this disorder cannot break down galactose, one of the major sugars in milk. If left untreated, galactosemia can lead to mental retardation, cataracts, kidney and liver failure, and death. By analyzing fetal cells obtained from amniocentesis or chorionic villus sampling, the level of this important chemical can be assessed, and, if necessary, the infant can be placed on a galactose-free diet immediately after birth.

DNA analysis can be used to determine whether a genetic disease has been inherited when the chromosomal location of the gene is known, when the chemical sequence of the DNA is known, and/or when particular DNA sequences commonly associated with the gene in question, called markers, are known.

A sequence of four chemical elements of DNA—adenine (A), guanine (G), thymine (T), and cytosine (C)—make up genes. Sometimes the proper DNA sequence of a gene is known, as well as the changes in the sequence that cause disease. Direct analysis of the DNA of the individual suspected of carrying a certain genetic disorder is possible in these cases. For example,

in sickle cell disease, it is known that a change in a single DNA chemical element leads to the disorder. To test for this disease, a tissue sample is obtained from prenatal sources (amniocentesis or chorionic villus sampling). The DNA is isolated from the cells and analyzed with highly specific probes that can detect the presence of the defective gene which will lead to sickle cell disease. Informed action may be taken regarding the future of the fetus or the care of an affected child.

Occasionally a disease gene itself has not been precisely isolated and its DNA sequence determined, but sequences very near the gene of interest have been analyzed. If specific variations within these neighboring sequences are always present when the gene of interest is flawed, these nearby sequences can then be used as a marker for the presence of the defective gene. When the variant sequences, called restriction fragment length polymorphisms, are present, so is the disease gene. Prenatal testing for cystic fibrosis has been done using restriction fragment length polymorphisms.

Individuals who come from families in which genetic diseases tend to occur can be tested as carriers. In this way, they will know the risk of passing a certain disease to offspring. For example, individuals whose families have a history of cystic fibrosis, but who themselves are not affected, may be asymptomatic carriers. If they have children with individuals who are also cystic fibrosis carriers, they have a 25 percent chance of passing two copies of the defective gene to their offspring. DNA samples from the potential parents can be analyzed for the presence of one defective gene. If both partners are carriers, their decision about whether to have children will be made with knowledge of the possible risk to their offspring. If only one or neither of them is a carrier, their offspring will not be at risk of inheriting cystic fibrosis, an autosomal recessive disease. Carrier testing is possible for many genetic diseases, as well as for disorders which appear late in life, such as Huntington's chorea.

Many of the gene flaws of multifactorial diseases, those that interact with environmental factors to produce disease, have been identified and are testable. Individuals armed with the knowledge of having a gene which puts them at risk for certain disorders can incorporate preventive measures into their lifestyle, thus minimizing the chances of developing the disease. For example, certain cancers, such as colon and breast cancer, have a genetic component. Individuals who test positive for the genes that predispose them to develop cancer can modify their diets to include cancer-fighting foods and receive frequent medical checkups to detect cancer development at its earliest, most treatable stage. Those with genes that contribute to arteriosclerosis and heart disease can modify their diets and increase exercise, and those with a genetic predisposition for alcoholism could avoid the consumption of alcohol.

PERSPECTIVE AND PROSPECTS

The scientific study of human genetics and genetic disease is relatively new, having begun in the early twentieth century. There are many early historical records, however, which recognize that certain traits are hereditarily transmitted. Ancient Greek literature is peppered with references to heredity, and the Jewish book of religious and civil laws, the Talmud, describes in detail the inheritance pattern of hemophilia and its ramifications upon circumcision.

The Augustinian monk Gregor Mendel worked out many of the principles of heredity by manipulating the pollen and eggs of pea plants over many generations. His work was conducted from the 1860's to the 1870's but was unrecognized by the scientific community until 1900.

At about this time, many disorders were being recognized as genetic diseases. Pedigree analysis, a way to trace inheritance patterns through a family tree, was used since the mid-1800's to track the incidence of hemophilia in European royal families. This analysis indicated that the disease was transmitted through females (indeed, hemophilia is an X-linked disorder). In the early 1900's, Sir Archibald Garrod, a British physician, recognized certain biochemical disorders as genetic diseases and proposed accurate mechanisms for their transmission.

In 1953, Francis Crick and James D. Watson discovered the structure of DNA; thus began studies on the molecular biology of genes. This research resulted in the monumental discovery in 1973 that pieces of DNA from animals and bacteria could be cut and spliced together into a functional molecule. This recombinant DNA technology fostered a revolution in genetic analysis, in which pieces of human DNA could be removed and put into bacteria. The bacteria then replicate millions of copies of the human DNA, permitting detailed analysis. These recombinant molecules also produced the human gene product, thereby facilitating the analysis of normal and aberrant genes.

The recombinant DNA revolution spawned the development of the DNA tests for genetic diseases and carrier status. Knowledge of what a normal gene product is and does is exceptionally helpful in the treatment of genetic diseases. For example, Duchenne's muscular dystrophy is known to be caused by the lack of a protein called dystrophin. This suggests that a possible treatment of the disease is to provide functional dystrophin to the affected individual. Ultimately, medical science seeks to treat genetic diseases by providing a functional copy of the flawed gene to the affected individual. While such gene therapy would not affect the reproductive cells—the introduced gene copy would not be passed down to future generations—the normal gene product would alleviate the genetic disorder.

—*Karen E. Kalumuck, Ph.D.*

See also Albinos; Amniocentesis; Batten's disease; Birth defects; Breast cancer; Cerebral palsy; Chorionic villus sampling; Colon cancer; Color blindness; Congenital heart disease; Cornelia de Lange syndrome; Cystic fibrosis; Diabetes mellitus; DiGeorge syndrome; DNA and RNA; Down syndrome; Dwarfism; Embryology; Environmental diseases; Fragile X syndrome; Fructosemia; Gaucher's disease; Gene therapy; Genetic counseling; Genetic engineering; Genetics and inheritance; Genomics; Gigantism; Glycogen storage diseases; Hemochromatosis; Hemophilia; Huntington's disease; Immunodeficiency disorders; Klinefelter syndrome; Klippel-Trenaunay syndrome; Laboratory tests; Leukodystrophy; Maple syrup urine disease (MSUD); Marfan syndrome; Mental retardation; Mucopolysaccharidosis (MPS); Muscular dystrophy; Mutation; Neonatology; Neurofibromatosis; Niemann-Pick disease; Oncology; Pediatrics; Phenylketonuria (PKU); Polycystic kidney disease; Porphyria; Prader-Willi syndrome; Progeria; Proteomics; Rubinstein-Taybi syndrome; Screening; Severe combined immunodeficiency syndrome (SCID); Sickle cell disease; Spina bifida; Tay-Sachs disease; Thalassemia; Thrombocytopenia; Turner syndrome; Von Willebrand's disease; Wilson's disease; Wiskott-Aldrich syndrome.

FOR FURTHER INFORMATION:

Alliance of Genetic Support Groups. http://www .geneticalliance.org. Site provides information on an international coalition of individuals, professionals, and genetic support organizations working together to enhance the lives of everyone affected by genetic conditions.

GeneClinics. http://www.geneclinics.org/home.html. Site contains genetics disease database and information relating genetic testing to diagnosis, management, and counseling of individuals and families with inherited disorders.

Gormley, Myra Vanderpool. *Family Diseases: Are You at Risk?* Reprint. Baltimore: Genealogical, 1998. The author, a certified genealogist and syndicated columnist, explores the relationship between family trees and genetic diseases. Written in popular language, this book gives instruction on how to assess a family's genetic risk, information on the latest scientific breakthroughs, and directions for obtaining further information.

Grant Cooper, Necia, ed. *The Human Genome Project: Deciphering the Blueprint of Heredity.* Rev. ed. Mill Valley, Calif.: University Science Books, 1994. Written to be accessible to the general reader, this book provides a basic introduction to the ideas underlying classical and molecular genetics before going on to describe the purpose of the Human Genome Project.

Hereditary Disease Foundation. http://www.hdfoundation.org. Site describes the mission of this nonprofit, basic science organization dedicated to the cure of genetic disease.

Jorde, Lynn B., John Carrey, and Michael J. Bamshed. *Medical Genetics.* 3d ed. New York: Elsevier, 2003. An introductory text that covers basic molecular genetics, chromosomal and single gene disorders, immunogenetics, cancer genetics, multifactorial disorders, and fetal therapy.

King, Richard A., et al., eds. *Genetic Basis of Common Diseases.* 2d ed. New York: Oxford University Press, 2002. Covers advances in the understanding of molecular processes involved in genetic susceptibility and diseases mechanisms. Examines a range of diseases in detail and includes a chapter on genetic counseling.

Lewis, Ricki. *Human Genetics: Concepts and Applications.* 5th ed. New York: McGraw-Hill, 2002. A very accessible undergraduate text that covers the fundamentals, transmission genetics, DNA and chromosomes, and the latest genetic technology, among other topics.

McCance, Kathryn L., and Sue M. Huether. *Pathophysiology: The Biologic Basis for Disease in Adults and Children.* 4th ed. New York: Elsevier, 2001. A text that explores the myriad cellular and genetic causes of disease. Topics include cell injury, immunity, inflammation and wound healing, coping and illness, and ontogenesis.

Marshall, Elizabeth L. *The Human Genome Project: Cracking the Code Within Us.* New York: Franklin Watts, 1997. Describes the Human Genome Project and its process of gene mapping, including concerns of critics of the project. Suitable for grades eight through twelve. Includes an extensive glossary and a bibliography.

Massimini, Kathy, ed. *Genetic Disorders Sourcebook: Basic Consumer Information About Hereditary Diseases and Disorders, Including Cystic Fibrosis, Down Syndrome, Hemophilia, Huntington's Disease, Sickle Cell Anemia, and More.* 2d ed. Detroit: Omnigraphics, 2000. This nontechnical sourcebook offers basic information about lifestyle expectations, disease management techniques, and current research initiatives for the most common types of genetic disorders, including a resource list of three hundred genetic disorders and related topics.

Millunsky, Aubrey, ed. *Genetic Disorders of the Fetus: Diagnosis, Prevention, and Treatment.* 4th ed. Baltimore: Johns Hopkins University Press, 1998. This source treats a number of issues, from fetal cells in the maternal circulation to ethical issues surrounding a misdiagnosis, in chapters written by experts in the field. Recommended for clinicians in training and scientists working on the laboratory side of prenatal genetic testing.

Shaw, Michael, ed. *Everything You Need to Know About Diseases.* Springhouse, Pa.: Springhouse Press, 1996. This well-illustrated consumer reference, compiled by more than one hundred doctors and medical experts, describes five hundred illnesses and conditions, their causes, symptoms, diagnosis, treatment, and prevention. A valuable reference book for everyone interested in health and disease. Of particular interest is chapter 21, "Genetic Disorders."

Wingerson, Lois. *Mapping Our Genes.* New York: E. P. Dutton, 1990. Using an engaging narrative style and many anecdotal stories as illustrations, Wingerson provides an account of the history of scientific discoveries that led to the human genome initiative, the mapping of the chromosomal location of all human genes.

GENETIC ENGINEERING
PROCEDURE

ALSO KNOWN AS: Biotechnology, gene splicing, recombinant DNA technology

ANATOMY OR SYSTEM AFFECTED: All

SPECIALTIES AND RELATED FIELDS: Alternative medicine, biochemistry, biotechnology, dermatology, embryology, ethics, forensic medicine, genetics, pharmacology, preventive medicine

Definition: A wide array of techniques that alter the genetic constitution of cells or individuals by selective removal, insertion, or modification of individual genes or gene sets.

Key terms:

gene cloning: the development of a line of genetically identical organisms which contain identical copies of the same gene or deoxyribonucleic acid (DNA) fragments

gene therapy: the insertion of a functional gene or genes into a cell, tissue, or organ to correct a genetic abnormality

polymerase chain reaction (PCR): an in vitro process by which specific parts of a DNA molecule or a gene can be made into millions or billions of copies within a short time

recombinant DNA: a hybrid DNA molecule created in the test tube by joining a DNA fragment of interest with a carrier DNA

southern blot: a procedure used to transfer DNA from a gel to a nylon membrane, which in turn allows the finding of genes that are complementary to particular DNA sequences called probes

Genetic Engineering and Human Health

Genetic engineering, recombinant DNA technology, and biotechnology constitute a set of techniques used to achieve one or more of three goals: to reveal the complex processes of how genes are inherited and expressed, to provide better understanding and effective treatment for various diseases (particularly genetic disorders), and to generate economic benefits, which include improved plants and animals for agriculture and the efficient production of valuable biopharmaceuticals. The characteristics of genetic engineering possess both vast promise and potential threats to humankind. It is an understatement to say that genetic engineering will revolutionize the medicine and agriculture in the twenty-first century. As this technology unleashes its power to have an impact on daily life, it will also bring challenges to ethical systems and religious beliefs.

Soon after the publication of the short essay by Francis Crick and James Watson on DNA structure in 1953, research began to uncover the way by which DNA molecules can be cut and spliced back together. With the discovery of the first restriction endonuclease by Hamilton Smith and colleagues in 1970, the real story of genetic engineering began to unfold. The creation of the first engineered DNA molecule through the splicing together of DNA fragments from two unrelated species was made public in 1972. What soon followed was an array of recombinant DNA molecules and genetically modified bacteria, viruses, fungi, plants, and animals. The debate over the issues of "tinkering with God" heated up, and public outcry over genetic engineering was widespread. In 1996, the birth of Dolly, a ewe that was the first mammal cloned from an adult body cell, elevated the debate over the impact of biological research to a new level. Furthermore, a number of genetically modified organisms (GMOs) have been released commercially since 1996. In 2003, it was estimated that more than 70 percent of foods in the United States contained some ingredients from GMOs.

Genetic engineering holds tremendous promise for medicine and human well-being. Medical applications of genetic engineering include the diagnosis of genetic and other diseases, treatment for genetic disorders, regenerative medicine using pluripotent (stem) cells, the production of safer and more effective vaccines and pharmaceuticals, and the prospect of curing genetic disorders through gene therapy. Many human diseases such as cystic fibrosis, Down syndrome, fragile X syndrome, Huntington's disease, muscular dystrophy, sickle cell anemia, and Tay-Sachs disease are inherited. There are usually no conventional treatments for these disorders because they do not respond to antibiotics or other conventional drugs. Another area is the commercial production of vaccines and pharmaceuticals through genetic engineering, which has emerged as a rapidly developing field. The potential of embryonic stem cells to become any cell, tissue, or organ under adequate conditions holds enormous promise for regenerative medicine.

Prevention of genetic disorders. Although prevention may be achieved by avoiding any environmental factors that cause an abnormality, the most effective prevention, when possible, is to reduce the frequency of or eliminate entirely the harmful genes (mutations) from the general population. As more precise tools and procedures for manipulating individual genes are optimized, this will eventually become a reality. The prevention of genetic disorders at present is usually achieved by ascertaining those individuals in the population who are at risk for passing a serious genetic disorder to their offspring and then offering them genetic counseling and prenatal screening, followed with the selective abortion of affected fetuses.

Genetic counseling is the process of communicating information gained through classic genetic studies and contemporary research to those individuals who are themselves at risk or have a high likelihood of passing defects to their offspring. During counseling, information about the disease itself—its severity and prognosis, whether effective therapies exist, and the risks of recurrence—is generally presented. For those couples who find the risks unacceptably high, counseling may also include discussions of contraceptive methods, adoption, prenatal diagnosis, possible abortion, and artificial insemination by a donor. The final decision must still rest with the couple themselves, but the significant increase in the accuracy of risk assessment through genetic technology has made it easier for parents to make well-informed decisions.

For those couples who find the burden of having an affected child unbearable, prenatal diagnosis may solve their dilemma. Prenatal screening could be performed for a variety of genetic disorders. It requires samples, acquired through either amniocentesis or chorionic villus sampling, of fetal cells or chemicals produced by the fetus. After sampling, several analyses can be performed. First, biochemical analysis is used to determine the concentration of chemicals in the sample and therefore to diagnose whether a particular fetus is deficient or low in enzymes that facilitate specific biological reactions. Next, analysis of the chromosomes of the fetal cells can show if all the chromosomes are present and whether there are structural abnormalities in any of them. Finally, the most effective means of detecting the defective genes is through recombinant DNA techniques. This has become possible with the rapid increase of DNA copies through a technique called polymerase chain reaction (PCR), which can produce virtually unlimited copies of a specific gene or DNA fragment, starting with as little as a single copy. Routine prenatal diagnosis can be performed to screen a fetus for Down syndrome, Huntington's disease, sickle cell anemia, and Tay-Sachs disease. Procedures are being developed for prenatal diagnosis of more, and more severe, genetic disorders. Thus, an effective roadblock to the passing of defective genes from one generation to another in the population is possible.

Treatment of diseases and genetic disorders. Genetic engineering may be used for direct treatments of diseases or genetic disorders through various means, including the production of possible vaccines for acquired immunodeficiency syndrome (AIDS), the treatment of various cancers, and the synthesis of biopharmaceuticals for a variety of metabolic, growth, and development diseases. In general, biosynthesis is a process in which gene coding for a particular product is isolated, cloned into another organism (mostly bacteria), and later expressed in that organism (the host). By cultivating host organism, large quantities of the gene products can be harvested and purified. A few examples can illustrate the useful features of biosynthesis.

Insulin is essential for the treatment of insulin-dependent diabetes mellitus, the most severe form of diabetes. Historically, insulin was obtained from a cow or pig pancreas. Two problems exist for this traditional supply of insulin. First, large quantities of the pancreas are needed

The Use of Genetic Engineering

Bacterium

Gene for insulin is synthesized

Synthetic gene is inserted into bacterial DNA

DNA strand

Bacterium produces insulin and multiplies

Insulin is extracted

Genetic engineering, the manipulation of genetic material, can be used to synthesize large quantities of drugs or hormones, such as insulin.

to extract enough insulin for continuous treatment of one patient. Second, insulin so obtained is not chemically identical to human insulin, hence some patients may produce antibodies that can seriously interfere with treatment. Human insulin produced through genetic engineering is quite effective yet without any side effects. It has been produced commercially and made available to patients since 1982.

Another successful story in biosynthesis is the production of human growth hormone (HGH), which is used in the treatment of children with growth retardation called pituitary dwarfism. The successful biosynthesis of HGH is important for several reasons. The conventional source of HGH was human pituitary glands removed at autopsy. Each child afflicted with pituitary dwarfism needs twice-a-week injections until the age of twenty. Such a treatment regime requires more than a thousand pituitary glands. The autopsy supply could hardly keep up with the demand. Furthermore, as a result of a small amount of virus contamination in the extracted HGH, many children receiving this treatment developed virus-related diseases.

Other biopharmaceuticals under development or in preclinical or clinical trials through genetic engineering include anticancer drugs, antiaging agents and possible vaccines for AIDS and malaria.

Broadly speaking, three types of gene therapy exist: germ line therapy, enhancement gene therapy, and somatic gene therapy. All gene therapy trials currently underway or in the pipeline are restricted to the somatic cells as targets for gene transfer. Germ line therapy involves the introduction of novel genes into germ cells, such as eggs or in early embryos. Although it has the potential for correcting defective genes completely, germ line therapy is highly controversial. Enhancement gene therapy, through which human potential might be enhanced for some desired traits, raises an even greater ethical dilemma. Both germ line and enhancement gene therapies have been banned based on the unresolved ethical issues surrounding them.

Somatic gene therapy is designed to introduce functional genes into body cells, thus enabling the body to perform normal functions and providing temporary correction for genetic abnormalities. The cloned human gene is first transferred into a viral vector, which is used to infect white blood cells removed from the patient. The transferred normal gene is then inserted into a chromosome and becomes active. After growth to enhance their numbers under sterile conditions, the cells are reimplanted into the patient, where they produce a gene product that is missing in the untreated patient, allowing the individual to function normally. Several disorders are currently being treated with this technique, including severe combined immunodeficiency disease (SCID). Individuals with SCID have no functional immune system and usually die from infections that would be minor in normal people. Gene therapy is also being used or tested as a treatment for cystic fibrosis, skin cancer, breast cancer, brain cancer, and AIDS.

Most of these treatments are only partially successful, and they are prohibitively expensive. Over a ten-year period, from 1990 to 2000, more than four thousand people were treated through gene therapy. Unfortunately, most of these trials were failures that led to some loss of confidence in gene therapy. These failures have been attributed to inefficient vectors. In the future, as more efficient vectors are engineered, gene therapy is expected to be a common method for treating a large number of genetic disorders.

GENETIC ENGINEERING IN AGRICULTURE, FORENSICS, AND ENVIRONMENTAL SCIENCE

As the use of genetic engineering expands rapidly, it is difficult to generate an exhaustive list of all possible applications, but three other areas are worth noting: forensic, environmental, and agricultural applications. Although these areas are not directly related to medicine, they certainly have profound impacts on human well-being. There are numerous ways that genetic engineering may be used to benefit agriculture and food production. First, the production of vaccines and the application of methods for transferring genes is likely to benefit animal husbandry, as scientists can alter commercially important traits such as milk yield, butter fat, and proportion of lean meat. For example, the bovine growth hormone produced through genetic engineering has been used since the late 1980's to boost milk production by cows. A mutant form of the myostatin gene has been identified and found to cause heavy muscling after this gene was introduced first into a mouse and later into the Belgian Blue bull. This technique marks the first step toward breeding cows and meat animals with lower fat and a higher proportion of lean meat. Other examples of using genetic engineering in animal husbandry include hormones for a faster growth rate in poultry and the production of recombinant human proteins in the milk of livestock.

Second, genetic engineering is expected to alter dramatically the conventional approaches of developing new strains of crops through breeding. The technology allows the transferring of genes for nitrogen fixation; the improvement of photosynthesis (and therefore yield); the promotion of resistance to pests, pathogens, and herbicides and tolerance to frost, drought, and increased salinity; and the improvement of nutritional value and consumer acceptability. Genetically engineered tobacco plants have been grown to produce protein phaseolin, which is naturally synthesized by soybeans and other legume crops.

The first genetically engineered potato was approved for human consumption by the U.S. government in 1995 and by Canada in 1996. This NewLeaf potato, developed by corporate giant Monsanto, carries a gene from the bacterium *Bacillus thuringiensis*. This gene produces a protein toxic to the Colorado potato beetle, an insect which causes substantial loss of the crop if left uncontrolled. The production of this protein by potato plants equips them with resistance to beetles, hence alleviating crop loss, saving on the cost on pesticides, and reducing the risk of environment contamination.

Antiviral genes have been successfully transferred and expressed into cotton, and the release of new cotton strains with resistance to multiple viruses is a matter of time. At least five transgenic corn strains with resistance to herbicides or pathogens had been developed and commercially produced by U.S. farmers by 2002. Some genes coding tolerance to drought and to subfreezing temperatures have been cloned and transferred into or among crop plants, some of which have already made a great impact on agriculture in developing countries. Initial effort has been made to replace chemical fertilizers with more environment-friendly biofertilizers. Secondary metabolites produced naturally by plants have also been purified and used as biopesticides. Soon, there will be more grain, produce, milk, and meat produced by animals or plants that have been genetically engineered in some manner.

Genetic engineering is also useful in forensics. DNA fingerprints from samples collected at crime scenes provide strong evidence in trials, thus helping to solve many violent crimes. DNA can be isolated easily from tissue left at a crime scene, a splattering of blood, a hair sample, or even skin left under a victim's fingernails. A variety of techniques can be used routinely to determine the probability of matching between sample DNA and that of a suspect. DNA fingerprints are also useful in paternity and property disputes and in the study of the genealogy of various species.

The metabolism of microorganisms can be altered through genetic engineering, which enables them to absorb and degrade waste and hazardous material from the environment. The growth rate and metabolic capabilities of microorganisms offer great potential for coping with some environmental problems. Sewage plants can use engineered bacteria to degrade many organic compounds into nontoxic substances. Microbes may be engineered to detoxify specific substances in waste dumps or oil spills. Many bacteria can extract heavy metals (such as lead and copper) from their surroundings and incorporate them into compounds that are recoverable, thus cleaning them from the environment. Many more such applications have yet to be tested or discovered.

PERSPECTIVE AND PROSPECTS

Since the discovery of the double-helical structure of DNA by Francis Crick and James Watson in 1953, human curiosity regarding this amazing molecule has propelled the advancement of biological sciences in an unprecedented fashion. The first successful experiment in genetic engineering was described in 1972 when DNA fragments from two different organisms were joined together to produce a biologically functional hybrid DNA molecule. The next milestone came in 1975, when Dr. Edward Southern introduced Southern blotting, a technique that has many applications and has proved invaluable for the subsequent development of genetic engineering. This technique is used to identify a particular gene or DNA fragment from a mixture of thousands of different genes or DNA fragments. Later, the automated DNA sequencers, which can rapidly churn out letter sequences from DNA fragments, and the discovery of reverse transcriptase and PCR further improved the capabilities of scientists in studying and manipulating DNA molecules and the genes that they carry.

Using these techniques, the first prenatal diagnosis of a genetic disease was made in 1976 for alpha-thalassemia, a genetic disorder caused by the absence of globin genes. This represented a monumental step forward in the use of genetic tools in the medical field. It paved the way for the later development in which mutations in many genes could be detected in early pregnancy. Three years later, insulin was first synthesized through genetic engineering. In 1982, the commercial production of genetically engineered human insulin became a reality.

Gene therapy trials began in 1990, first with SCID. The first complete human genetic map was published in 1993, and various new techniques in DNA fingerprinting and the isolation of specific genes were developed. Also, an increasing number of pharmaceuticals have been produced through genetic engineering. Two versions of the draft copy of the human genome were published in 2001, launching the genomic revolution. In the twenty-first century, genetic engineering will continue to offer more benefits in medicine and in agriculture in undreamed of ways.

In retrospect, genetic engineering presents a mixed blessing of invaluable benefits and dilemmas that science and technology have always offered humankind. There are those who would like to restrict the uses of genetic engineering and who might prefer that such technology had never been developed. Others believe that the benefits far outweigh the possible risks and that any potential threat can be overcome easily through government regulation or legislation. Others do not take sides on the debate in general but are greatly concerned with some specific applications.

Obviously, the power of genetic engineering demands a new set of decisions, both ethical and economical, by individuals, government, and society. Considerable concern has been expressed by both scientists and the general public regarding possible biohazards from genetic engineering. What if engineered organisms prove resistant to all known antibiotics or carry cancer genes that might spread throughout the community? What if a genetically engineered plant becomes an uncontrollable super weed? Would these kinds of risks outweigh the potential benefits? On the other hand, others argue that the risk has been exaggerated and therefore do not want to impose limits on research. Genetic engineering has also generated legal issues concerning intellectual properties and patents for different aspects of the technology.

Even more controversial are the many ethical issues. Perhaps the most obvious ethical issue surrounding genetic engineering is the objection to some applications that are considered socially undesirable and morally wrong. One example is bovine growth hormone. Some vigorously opposed its use in boosting milk production for two main reasons. First, the recombinant hormone could change the composition of the milk. However, this view was dismissed by experts from the National Institutes of Health (NIH) and the Food and Drug Administration (FDA) after a thorough study. Second, many dairy farmers feared that greater milk production per cow would drive prices down even further and put some small farmers out of business.

Numerous aspects of the application of genetic engineering to humans also present ethical challenges. In some couples, both people carry a defective gene and have an appreciable chance of having an affected child. Should they refrain entirely from having children of their own? For genetic disorders caused by chromosomal abnormalities, such as Tay-Sachs disease, prenatal diagnosis can detect the defect in a fetus with great precision. Should the fetus be aborted if the screening result is positive? Should screening tests of infants for genetic disorders be required? If so, would such a requirement infringe the rights of the individual by the government? Perhaps the greatest concern of all is the possibility to design or clone a human being through genetic engineering. The debate over the ethical, legal, and social implications of genetic engineering should help in the formulation and optimization of public policy and laws regarding this technology, and genetic engineering research and its applications should proceed with caution.

—*Ming Y. Zheng, Ph.D.*

See also Bacteriology; Bionics and biotechnology; Cancer; Cells; Chemotherapy; Cloning; Cytology; Diabetes mellitus; DNA and RNA; Enzyme therapy; Enzymes; Ethics; Fetal tissue transplantation; Gene therapy; Genetic counseling; Genetics and inheritance; Genomics; Hormones; Immunization and vaccination; Mutation; Pharmacology; Screening; Stem cells.

FOR FURTHER INFORMATION:

Brungs, Robert S. J., and R. S. M. Postiglione, eds. *The Genome: Plant, Animal, Human.* St. Louis: ITEST Faith/Science Press, 2000. A collection of excellent scientific, ethical, educational, and theological papers focuses on the genomic revolution and the application of genetic engineering to plants, humans, and other animals.

Daniell, H., S. J. Streatfield, and K. Wycoff. "Medical Molecular Farming: Production of Antibodies, Biopharmaceuticals, and Edible Vaccines in Plants." *Trends in Plant Science* 6 (2001): 219-226. A contemporary review on the production of plant-based medicinal products through genetic engineering and related biotechnology.

Dudley, William, ed. *Genetic Engineering: Opposing Viewpoints.* San Diego, Calif.: Greenhaven Press, 1990. Presents balanced and well-thought opposing views on genetic engineering by proponents and opponents from various angles.

Frankel, M. S., and A. Teich, eds. *The Genetic Frontier.* Washington, D.C.: American Association for the Advancement of Science, 1994. A wonderful collection of essays from many experts and organizations dealing with the ethics, laws, and policies of genetic engineering.

Holland, Suzanne, K. Lebacqz, and L. Zoloth, eds. *The Human Embryonic Stem Cell Debate*. Cambridge, Mass.: MIT Press, 2001. Very thoughtful reflections on debates regarding stem cell research and potential pros and cons by a number of extraordinary people from diverse disciplines.

Kilner, John F., R. D. Pentz, and F. E. Young, eds. *Genetic Ethics: Do the Ends Justify the Genes?* Grand Rapids, Mich.: Wm. B. Eerdmans, 1997. An assembly of experts addresses three dimensions of the genetic challenge: perspective, information, and intervention. A wonderful collection of useful and informative guiding principles on genetic engineering.

Kmiec, E. B. "Gene Therapy." *American Scientist* 87 (1999): 240-247. A good summary of trends in gene therapy.

Old, R. W., and S. B. Primrose. *Principles of Genetic Manipulation: An Introduction to Genetic Engineering*. Palo Alto, Calif.: Blackwell Science, 1994. A resource that provides foundational knowledge on the principle and process of genetic engineering.

Tal, J. "Adeno-Associated Virus-Based Vectors in Gene Therapy." *Journal of Biomedical Science* 7 (2000): 279-291. A good summary of gene therapy and the outlook on recent developments.

GENETICS AND INHERITANCE
BIOLOGY

ANATOMY OR SYSTEM AFFECTED: All

SPECIALTIES AND RELATED FIELDS: Embryology, forensic medicine, genetics, pediatrics

DEFINITION: The passage of traits from parents to offspring in discrete units called genes.

KEY TERMS:

allele: a version of a gene; different alleles of a gene have slightly different nucleotide sequences, resulting in differences in the protein encoded in the gene

chromosome: one of the DNA molecules of a nucleus; in humans, chromosomes occur in twenty-three pairs, with each member of a pair having the same genes but possibly having different alleles of the genes

deoxyribonucleic acid (DNA): the hereditary molecule, in which sequences of nucleic acids encode genetic information

dominant allele: the version of a gene that can produce a recognizable trait in offspring when present in only one of the two chromosomes of a pair

fertilization: the process by which chromosome pairs, separated in production of egg and sperm cells, are rejoined

gene: a sequence of nucleotides in DNA encoding a protein

meiosis: a division mechanism in which homologous chromosomes are separated and delivered singly to egg or sperm cells; as a part of meiosis, recombination generates new combinations of alleles

nucleotide: a chemical subunit of DNA; different sequences of linked nucleotides spell out instructions for the assembly of proteins

recessive allele: a version of a gene that must be present on both chromosomes of a pair in order to produce a recognizable trait in offspring

recombination: the reciprocal exchange of segments between the two chromosomes of a pair, producing new combinations of alleles

THE RULES OF INHERITANCE

The primary genes of interest to heredity consist of a set of coded directions for making proteins. Each gene codes for a protein; distinct versions of a gene, which encode slightly different versions of the protein, may be carried in the same or different individuals. The distinct versions of a gene, called alleles, are responsible for differences in hereditary traits among individuals. Each individual receives a combination of alleles encoding proteins that directly or indirectly determine traits such as eye, skin, and hair color; height; and, to a degree, characteristics such as personality, behavior, and intelligence.

In molecular terms, genes consist of a sequence of chemical units called nucleotides, linked end to end in long, linear deoxyribonucleic acid (DNA) molecules. There are four kinds of nucleotides in DNA; each gene has its own nucleotide sequence. The alleles of a gene differ slightly in nucleotide sequence—some alleles differ in the substitution of only a single nucleotide. There are many thousands of genes arranged in tandem on the DNA molecules of a human cell; each DNA molecule is known as a chromosome. In humans, the chromosomes occur in twenty-three pairs, for a total of forty-six chromosomes. The two members of a chromosome pair contain the same genes in the same order, but different alleles of a gene may be present in the two members of a pair. One member of a chromosome pair is derived from the female parent of the individual; the other member is derived from the male parent. These are called the maternal and paternal chromosomes of the pair.

Inheritance, and the variation in traits among individuals, depends on two processes that separate and rejoin the chromosome pairs in sexual reproduction. One is a division mechanism, meiosis, which occurs in cell lines leading to egg or sperm cells. Meiosis separates the chromosome pairs and places one member of each pair in an egg or sperm cell. The particular combination of maternal and paternal chromosomes delivered to an egg or sperm cell is random. This random segregation, as it is called, is one source of the variability between offspring in a family. Because there are so many chromosomes, the possibility that two egg or sperm cells produced by the same individual could receive the same combination of maternal and paternal chromo-

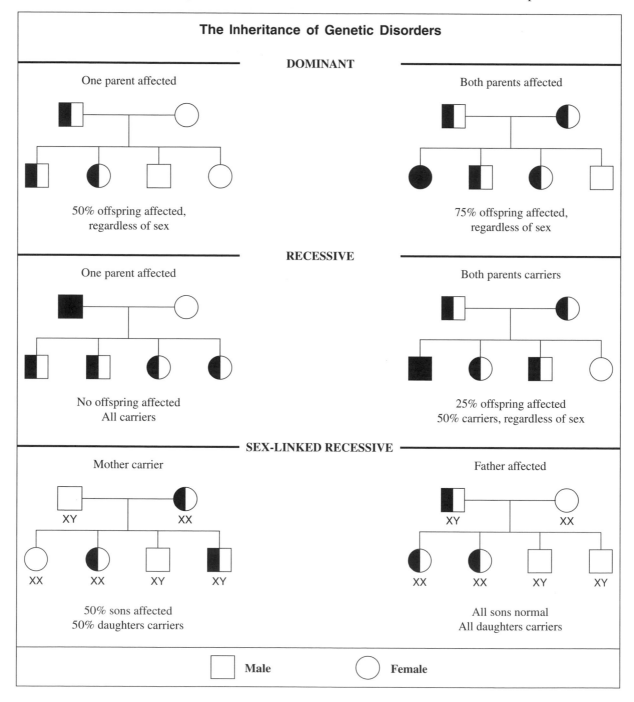

The Inheritance of Genetic Disorders

DOMINANT

One parent affected

50% offspring affected,
regardless of sex

Both parents affected

75% offspring affected,
regardless of sex

RECESSIVE

One parent affected

No offspring affected
All carriers

Both parents carriers

25% offspring affected
50% carriers, regardless of sex

SEX-LINKED RECESSIVE

Mother carrier

XY   XX

XX   XX   XY   XY

50% sons affected
50% daughters carriers

Father affected

XY   XX

XX   XX   XY   XY

All sons normal
All daughters carriers

☐ **Male**   ○ **Female**

somes is very small—equivalent to one chance in 8.4 million. Another important source of variability comes from a mechanism that occurs before the pairs are separated in meiosis. In this mechanism, called recombination, the two members of a chromosome pair line up side by side and exchange segments perfectly and reciprocally. As a result, alleles are exchanged between the pairs, generating new combinations of alleles. The variability generated by recombination adds to that produced by independent segregation of maternal and paternal chromosomes, so that it is essentially impossible for an individual to produce two egg or sperm cells that are genetically the same.

The second process underlying inheritance is fertilization, in which a sperm and an egg cell fuse, rejoining the twenty-three pairs of chromosomes. Fertilization is another random process, in which any of the millions of sperm cells ejaculated by a male and any of the hundreds of egg cells carried in a female may join. The total variability generated by independent segregation of alleles, recombination, and random union of gametes is such that each human individual, except identical twins, receives a unique combination of alleles. Thus the possibility that any individual has or will ever have a genetic double in the human population, except for an identical twin, is essentially zero. (In the case of identical twins, a single fertilized egg divides to produce two separate, genetically identical cells; instead of remaining together to produce a two-celled embryo, as is normally the case, the cells separate to create two embryos, which develop into genetically identical individuals.)

Because chromosomes occur in pairs, each individual receives two alleles of every gene of the human complement. The two alleles may be the same or different. Some alleles are dominant in their effects, so that one copy of the allele on either chromosome is sufficient to produce the trait encoded in the allele. Other alleles are recessive, so that both chromosomes of the pair must carry the allele for the trait to appear in offspring. In humans, few physical traits are determined by a single gene. Most are the result of complex interactions between several genes, as well as environmental influences. Nonetheless, some traits do tend to follow certain inheritance patterns, but there are exceptions. For example, brown eyes tend to be dominant to blue eyes. If either chromosome carries the brown eye allele, the individual will usually have brown eyes. To have blue eyes, an individual usually carries two genes for blue eyes. Human traits that tend toward dominant inheritance include nearsightedness and farsightedness,

astigmatism, dark or curly hair, early balding in males, normal body pigment (as compared to albinism), supernumerary fingers or toes, short fingers or toes, and webbing between fingers and toes. Alleles that tend to be expressed in a recessive fashion include blond hair, straight hair, and congenital deafness.

Although each individual normally carries a maximum of two alleles of any gene, several or many alleles of a gene may exist in the human population as a whole. The major histocompatibility complex (MHC), for example, occurs in hundreds of different alleles throughout the human population—so many that unrelated individuals are unlikely to carry the same combination of MHC alleles. The proteins encoded in these alleles are recognized by the immune system as "self" or "foreign." Unless the same, or a very similar, combination of MHC alleles is present, cells are recognized by the immune system as foreign, and the cells are destroyed. Therefore, MHC combinations recognized as foreign are the primary factor in the rejection of tissue or organ transplants among humans. If the transplant does not come from an individual with the same or a very similar MHC combination, rejection is likely unless the immune system is suppressed by drugs such as cyclosporine. The best donor for a transplant is a close relative, who is most likely to have a similar MHC combination. Because identical twins have the same MHC combination, tissues and organs can be transplanted between them with no danger of rejection.

Sex is determined by a pair of chromosomes that is different in males and females. Females have two members of the pair, the X chromosomes, which have the same genes in the same order but which may have different alleles of the genes. One member of the XX pair was derived from the female's father, and the other from her mother. Males have only one member of this pair, a single X. In addition, males have a small, single chromosome, the Y, which is not present in females. Thus females are XX, and males are XY. During meiosis in females, the XX pair is separated, so that an egg cell may receive either member of the pair. In males, the X and Y are separated, so that a sperm cell receives either an X or a Y. In fertilization, the X chromosome carried by the egg may be joined with an X-carrying sperm, producing a female (XX), or, the egg may be fertilized by a sperm cell carrying a Y, producing a male (XY). Thus in humans, the sex of the offspring is determined by the type of sperm cell, an X or a Y, fertilizing the egg. Most genes carried on an X chromosome have no counterparts on the Y chromosome. Therefore, traits encoded in genes on the X chromosomes (almost none are carried on the Y) are inherited differently from traits carried on other chromosomes of the set, in a pattern known as sex-linked inheritance.

Disorders and Diseases

Many human diseases, involving every system in the body, depend on the presence of particular dominant or recessive alleles and are directly inherited. Only the disposition for development of other diseases is inherited—that is, some individuals inherit a combination of alleles that increases the possibility that a genetically based disease will develop during their lifetimes.

The list of diseases contracted through inheritance of a dominant allele is long and impressive. Among the more important of these diseases are achondroplasia, in which individuals are short-statured; familial hypercholesterolemia, in which cholesterol concentration in the blood is abnormally high, leading to vascular disease, particularly of the coronary arteries; Huntington's disease, a disease characterized by dementia, delusion, paranoia, and abnormal movements that begins in persons between twenty and fifty years of age and progresses steadily to death in about fifteen years; Marfan syndrome, a disease of connective tissues involving the skeleton, eyes, and cardiovascular system, characterized by elongated limbs, abnormal position of the eye lens, and structural weakness of blood vessels, particularly of the aorta; neurofibromatosis, characterized by tumors dispersed throughout the body and coffee-colored skin lesions; polycystic kidney disease, in which dilated cysts grow in the kidneys and interfere with kidney function, leading to hypertension and chronic renal failure; spherocytosis, another disease in which blood cells are fragile and easily broken during travel through the circulatory system, producing anemia and jaundice; and thalassemia, a group of diseases most common in persons of Mediterranean descent in which hemoglobin production is faulty, leading to anemias that range from mild to severe.

Diseases caused by recessive genes also appear in the human population. Although many persons are carriers for these diseases, affected persons are rare because both alleles must be present in the recessive form for the disease to develop. Diseases in this category include albinism; sickle cell disease, common in persons of African descent, in which hemoglobin is faulty, leading to fragility of red blood cells, anemia, blockage of blood vessels, and susceptibility to infection; phenylketonuria (PKU), in which the amino acid phenylala-

nine accumulates in excess in the bloodstream, leading to nervous system damage including mental retardation; Tay-Sachs disease, most common in persons of Jewish descent, characterized by accumulation of lipid molecules in nerve cells leading to motor incoordination, blindness, and mental deterioration; and glycogen storage diseases, with symptoms ranging from cramps to serious muscular and cardiac disease and convulsions. Sickle cell disease is recessively inherited. A person with one copy of the sickle cell gene makes sufficient normal hemoglobin that symptoms of the disease occur only under extreme low oxygen conditions. Cystic fibrosis, one of the most common of genetically determined diseases in Caucasians, is probably also attributable to a recessive allele. In this disease, sweat and mucus-secreting glands are affected; the most serious effects are caused by the secretion of unusually thick and viscid mucus, leading to blockage of ducts in the lungs, liver, pancreas, and salivary glands. Most critical to survival is blockage of passages in the lungs, producing a chronic cough and persistent pulmonary infections. The average life expectancy of persons with cystic fibrosis is twenty years of age.

A number of diseases are caused by recessive genes carried on the X chromosomes and are inherited in sex-linked patterns. Among these are one form of diabetes (diabetes insipidus) in which glucose uptake by cells is faulty, leading to the accumulation of glucose in the blood; hemophilia, in which the blood-clotting mechanism is deficient, making afflicted persons subject to uncontrolled bleeding; and some forms of muscular dystrophy, characterized by progressive muscular weakness. The Duchenne muscular dystrophy appears early in life, progresses rapidly, and leads to death in most cases by the age of twenty.

Because males receive only one copy of the X chromosome, recessive genes are fully expressed in males—there is no chance for a normal allele to compensate for the effects of the recessive gene. For a sex-linked disease to appear in females, both X chromosomes must carry the recessive allele. For these reasons, sex-linked recessive diseases are much more common in males than in females; for some, appearance of the disease is limited almost exclusively to males.

The molecular basis for some genetically based diseases is known. In familial hypercholesterolemia, for example, receptors for cholesterol on cell surfaces are faulty or not produced, preventing the normal uptake of cholesterol from the bloodstream. As a result, cholesterol accumulates and reaches a dangerously high concentration in the blood. In persons carrying dominant alleles for familial hypercholesterolemia on both chromosomes of the pair, coronary arterial disease advances so rapidly that death from heart attack by the age of twenty is frequent. The disease is among the most common of genetically based defects—about 1 in 500 persons has at least one allele for hypercholesterolemia and develops premature coronary artery disease. In PKU, individuals lack an enzyme normally produced in the liver. The enzyme, phenylalanine hydroxylase, converts excess phenylalanine into another amino acid, tyrosine. Without the enzyme, phenylalanine taken in the diet accumulates to dangerously high levels in the body. Some forms of PKU are treatable by restricting dietary intake of phenylalanine from infancy onward.

Some persons have a genetically determined predisposition to develop certain cancers with greater frequency than the average in the population. About 5 percent of cancers are strongly predisposed—that is, individuals inherit a marked tendency to develop the cancer. Among these are familial retinoblastoma, in which retinal tumors develop; familial adenomatous polyps of the colon; and multiple endocrine neoplasia, in which tumors develop in the thyroid, adrenal medulla, and parathyroid glands. Often underlying these strongly predisposed cancers is the inheritance of a faulty gene (called an oncogene) that promotes uncontrolled cell division, or the opposite—inheritance of a faulty gene that in its normal form suppresses cell division (called a tumor suppressor gene). Typically, oncogenes are inherited as dominant genes, and tumor suppressor genes as recessives. In addition, some cancers, including breast, ovarian, and colon cancers other than familial adenomatous polyps, show a degree of predisposition in family lines.

PERSPECTIVE AND PROSPECTS

The primary features of meiosis and fertilization, random segregation of chromosome pairs in meiosis and random rejoining of pairs in fertilization, makes heredity subject to analysis by mathematical techniques. In fact, mathematical analysis of heredity was carried out successfully before there was any understanding concerning meiosis or DNA. The groundwork for this analysis was laid down in the 1860's by an Austrian monk, Gregor Mendel. Mendel's research approach and his conclusions were so advanced that they were misunderstood and unappreciated during his lifetime.

Mendel chose garden peas for his research because they could be grown easily and they possessed several hereditary traits that were known to breed true—that is, to appear dependably in offspring. Mendel crossed pea plants with different traits in various combinations. On analyzing the results of his crosses, Mendel realized that the numbers of offspring exhibiting different traits could be explained mathematically if he assumed that parents contain a pair of factors governing the inheritance of each trait. Furthermore, he concluded that the factors separate, or segregate, independently as gametes are formed and are reunited randomly at fertilization. He also discovered that some traits are inherited as dominant and some as recessive. Mendel's factors were later called genes.

Until Mendel's time, inheritance was commonly believed to occur through a blending of maternal and paternal characteristics. Mendel's work showed instead that traits are passed on as units; depending on whether a trait is dominant or recessive, it may appear in all offspring or only in a definite, predictable percentage. Some time after Mendel's discoveries, in the early 1900's, meiosis was discovered. At this time, Walter Sutton pointed out that Mendel's genes and chromosomes behave similarly in meiosis and fertilization: Both genes and chromosomes occur in pairs that separate randomly in meiosis and are rejoined at fertilization. Genes were therefore concluded to be carried on the chromosomes. Further genetic research confirmed that Mendel's findings with plant genes also apply to animals, including humans, and worked out many additional features of inheritance, including genetic recombination and sex linkage. Later, in the 1950's, almost one hundred years after Mendel's findings, James D. Watson and Francis Crick discovered the structure of DNA and deduced the fact that hereditary information is encoded in the sequence of nucleotides in DNA.

Research in human genetics differs from genetic investigation in other organisms because, for obvious reasons, it is impossible to set up experimental crosses to test whether particular diseases are inherited. Instead, human family lines are analyzed carefully in pedigrees to trace the appearance of disease over several generations. If a disease is genetically determined, it shows up in definite patterns as dominant, recessive, or sex-linked among parents and offspring in the pedigrees. On this basis, prospective parents can be counseled on the chances that their offspring will develop a hereditary disease.

In June of 2000, Francis Collins, director of the National Human Genome Research Initiative, and J. Craig

Venter, of Celera Genomics, announced that they had jointly sequenced the entire human genome and that the first working draft was available. Sequencing the human genome will allow scientists to directly compare healthy DNA to DNA harboring disease genes. Discovering the disease genes and studying them will lead to much more rapid understanding of disease processes, as well as the development of diagnostic procedures and potential therapy and cures, than allowed by the techniques available before the completion of this initiative.

—Stephen L. Wolfe, Ph.D.;
updated by Karen E. Kalumuck, Ph.D.

See also Aging; Amniocentesis; Bioinformatics; Biostatistics; Birth defects; Chorionic villus sampling; Cloning; DNA and RNA; Embryology; Environmental diseases; Gene therapy; Genetic counseling; Genetic diseases; Genetic engineering; Genomics; Laboratory tests; Multiple births; Mutation; Neonatology; Obstetrics; Oncology; Pediatrics; Pregnancy and gestation; Preventive medicine; Proteomics; Screening; Sexual differentiation; Sexuality.

FOR FURTHER INFORMATION:

Campbell, Neil A. *Biology: Concepts and Connections*. 6th ed. Redwood City, Calif.: Benjamin/Cummings, 2002. This classic introductory textbook provides an excellent discussion of essential biological structures and mechanisms. Of particular interest are the chapters entitled "Mendel and the Gene Idea," "The Chromosomal Basis of Inheritance," and "The Molecular Basis of Inheritance."

Lewin, Benjamin. *Genes: VIII.* New York: Oxford University Press, 2003. A college textbook that discusses the entire field of molecular biology and genetics, with many references to the structure and activity of the cell nucleus. Although written at the college level, it is readable and accessible to a general audience. Many highly informative illustrations and diagrams are included.

Lewis, Ricki. *Human Genetics: Concepts and Applications*. 5th ed. New York: McGraw-Hill, 2002. A very accessible undergraduate text that covers the fundamentals, transmission genetics, DNA and chromosomes, and the latest genetic technology, among other topics.

Marieb, Elaine N. *Essentials of Human Anatomy and Physiology.* 7th ed. Redwood City, Calif.: Benjamin/Cummings, 2003. This introductory anatomy and physiology textbook, easily accessible to those with little science background, is richly illustrated with diagrams and photographs, which help to illuminate body systems and processes. In-depth discussions of prevalent diseases and disorders and of current areas of research make this an all-around useful reference work.

Moore, Keith L., and T. V. N. Persaud. *The Developing Human.* 7th ed. Philadelphia: W. B. Saunders, 2003. An outstanding textbook on human embryonic development, with specific information about the causes of congenital malformations and common defects occurring in each of the body's systems.

Ridley, Matt. *Nature Via Nurture: Genes, Experience, and What Makes Us Human.* New York: Harper-Collins, 2003. Accessible, engaging discussion of genes, what they contribute to the development of the human brain and neurons, and how that contribution is changed or modified by the environment in which they are expressed.

Wolfe, Stephen L. *Molecular and Cellular Biology.* Belmont, Calif.: Wadsworth, 1993. Chapter 25, "Meiosis and Genetic Recombination," describes these mechanisms. The book, written at the college level, is highly readable and illustrated with many informative diagrams and photographs.

GENITAL DISORDERS, FEMALE
DISEASE/DISORDER

ANATOMY OR SYSTEM AFFECTED: Genitals, reproductive system, uterus

SPECIALTIES AND RELATED FIELDS: Family practice, gynecology, obstetrics, oncology, urology

DEFINITION: All maladies affecting the reproductive organs of women.

KEY TERMS:

cervix: the narrow portion of the uterus situated at the upper end of the vagina

cyst: a closed sac having a distinct border which develops abnormally within a body space or structure

estrogen: the hormone responsible for female sexual characteristics, produced primarily by the ovaries

Fallopian tubes: tiny tubes that connect the ovaries to the uterus; after ovulation, the egg travels through these tubes, and its fertilization by sperm occurs here

hormone: a chemical compound produced at one site in the body which travels to other parts of the body to exert its effect

hysterectomy: the surgical removal of the uterus; in a total hysterectomy, the uterus, ovaries, and Fallopian tubes are removed

laparoscopy: a surgical procedure in which an instrument is inserted into the body through tiny incisions; usually performed without hospitalization

CAUSES AND SYMPTOMS

Diseases and disorders of the female genitals, both internal organs and outward anatomical structures, encompass a huge number of different types of conditions that can range in severity from merely physically annoying to life-threatening. These disorders affect the vulva, vagina, uterus, ovaries, and Fallopian tubes. Many develop from unknown causes, and others have clear-cut origins, such as sexually transmitted diseases. Some have immediately recognizable symptoms, while others are silent until the disease has progressed to a serious stage. Early recognition of symptoms or abnormalities and proper treatment can alleviate pain and save lives.

Endometriosis is a chronic, recurring disease in which the tissue that lines the uterus grows into the abdominal cavity. This tissue normally thickens with blood vessels in preparation for receiving a fertilized egg. In endometriosis, the tissue overgrows the uterus, invades the Fallopian tubes, and reaches the abdominal cavity, where it continues to grow. This abnormally growing tissue will attach to any nearby internal organs, such as the ovaries, bladder, Fallopian tubes, and rectum. The endometrial tissue responds to the same hormonal cues that signal the sloughing off of the uterine lining during menstruation; however, the blood from the endometrial tissue cannot leave the abdominal cavity, leading to inflammation. As the inflammation subsides, it is replaced with scar tissue. This process will repeat with each menstrual cycle, and the scarring can result in infertility, organ malfunction, or adhesions that bind organs together. Some women with endometriosis experience no symptoms, while many experience severe abdominal pain before, during, and after their menstrual periods. Endometrial tissue sometimes can be diagnosed with a pelvic examination, but a definitive diagnosis can be reached only with laparoscopy. The cause of endometriosis is unknown, but some evidence suggests an inherited tendency to develop endometriosis.

Vaginitis is a general term for infections of the vagina. The most common of these is commonly called a yeast infection, caused by the fungus *Candida albicans.* This fungus is usually a harmless organism which lives in nearly everyone's intestinal tract and in the vagina of 20 to 40 percent of American women. Symp-

---

INFORMATION ON FEMALE GENITAL DISORDERS

CAUSES: Endometriosis, hormonal imbalances, infection, disease, uterine fibroids, sexually transmitted diseases

SYMPTOMS: Varies; can include abdominal pain, pain during menstruation or sexual intercourse, vaginal itching, vaginal discharge, burning upon urination

DURATION: Acute or chronic, often with recurrent episodes

TREATMENTS: Depends on cause; may include oral contraceptives, corticosteroids, hormone therapy, anti-inflammatory drugs, surgery, radiation therapy, chemotherapy, immunotherapy

---

toms are caused when the organism grows at an accelerated rate and include severe itching, vaginal discharge, and burning upon urination. Many situations may cause the enhanced growth of the fungus, including use of antibiotics which disturb the acid balance within the vagina, stress, use of oral contraceptives and corticosteroids, and the low estrogen levels that accompany the menopause.

Uterine fibroids are benign tumors made mainly of muscle tissue that can grow inside the uterus or along its outer surface. They grow slowly and are dependent on the hormone estrogen for continued growth. They are usually not problematic, but if they become very large they may cause extremely heavy bleeding during menstruation and can interfere with pregnancy and childbirth. Their cause is unknown, but they will shrink or disappear after the menopause.

Uterine prolapse occurs when the pelvic muscles are no longer able to support the pelvic organs, and the uterus "falls" into the vagina. A feeling of one's "insides falling out" is typical of this disorder, which is often precipitated by one or more difficult births.

Ovarian cysts form when an egg developing inside a follicle within the ovary does not ovulate but instead keeps growing. Small cysts will be painless, but larger ones (up to 7.5 centimeters in diameter) may cause abdominal pain. Most cysts will go away on their own, but some can rupture and cause severe pain.

The hallmark of cancer is uncontrolled cell growth. Cancer may prove fatal by causing destruction of a particular organ at the site of origin or by spreading throughout the body and damaging other organs and systems. All the organs of the female reproductive system can be affected by cancer. Cervical cancer begins in superficial layers of the cervix but may spread rapidly through the vagina and throughout the body. Cervical cancer can be detected in its early, most curable stages by a Pap smear. Endometrial cancer affects the glands which line the uterus. It can occur at any age, but the most common age of onset is sixty. Abnormal bleeding accompanies this disorder, which is diagnosed by examination of a biopsy of uterine tissue. Sarcomas of the uterus are malignant tumors of muscle tissue frequently confused with benign fibroids. This rare cancer is aggressive and difficult to treat. Ovarian cancer constitutes about 25 percent of female reproductive tract cancers, is difficult to detect and cure, and therefore has a high mortality rate. There are no early symptoms, and the cancer seems to occur frequently in those with a family history of the disease. Cancers of the Fallopian tubes and vagina are very rare, but vaginal cancer occurs with greater frequency in women whose mothers were treated with the synthetic estrogen diethylstilbestrol (DES) during the 1940's through the 1960's with the intent of preventing miscarriages. Cancer of the vulva, a form of skin cancer, is relatively easy to treat and has a high cure rate.

Sexually transmitted diseases (STDs) can involve any part of the female genital system. STDs of bacterial origin include gonorrhea and chlamydia, which are major precursors to pelvic inflammatory disease (PID) and syphilis. Untreated, these diseases can lead to serious complications. STDs with a viral cause include genital herpes, genital warts, and acquired immunodeficiency syndrome (AIDS). The causative agent of trichomoniasis is a protozoan. Each STD can be transmitted through direct sexual contact with an infected person, and each has its own set of symptoms and diagnostic criteria.

Treatment and Therapy

A variety of treatments are available for endometriosis, depending on the severity of the disorder. Over-the-counter or prescription anti-inflammatory drugs may give immediate relief of pain, but the condition itself is frequently treated with hormone therapy. Birth control pills that are high in the hormone progestin and low in estrogen can help shrink endometriosis. Danazol, a synthetic male hormone, suppresses the production of estrogen by the ovaries, thereby helping to eliminate the condition, but it has undesirable side effects. In

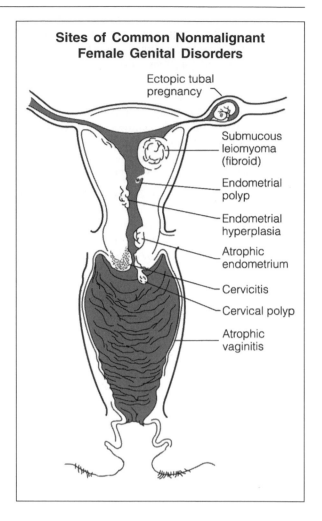

Sites of Common Nonmalignant Female Genital Disorders

Ectopic tubal pregnancy

Submucous leiomyoma (fibroid)

Endometrial polyp

Endometrial hyperplasia

Atrophic endometrium

Cervicitis

Cervical polyp

Atrophic vaginitis

some cases, surgical removal of the tissue is necessary. In laparoscopy, an instrument is inserted through tiny abdominal incisions and used to remove the tissue. In the most severe cases, a complete hysterectomy (removal of the uterus and ovaries) is performed.

Yeast infections that result in vaginitis must be properly diagnosed by a physician. Two medications for yeast infections are available without a prescription: miconazole and clotrimazole, available under brand names in most pharmacies. If a severe infection does not respond to this treatment, cortisone may be prescribed. Yeast infections have a tendency to recur, and taking precautions to prevent additional episodes is advised. Some ways in which to reduce the chance of reinfection include eating a cup of yogurt daily, avoiding sweets, reducing stress, wearing cotton underwear, avoiding tight-fitting clothing, avoiding feminine hygiene sprays, and using vinegar-and-water or povidone-iodine douches.

If no major discomfort is experienced by the woman when uterine fibroids are first detected, usually no treatment beyond regular observation is necessary. For those experiencing pain or difficulty in conception or pregnancy, the fibroids may be surgically removed in an operation called a myomectomy; in severe cases, a hysterectomy is performed. A laparoscope can be used to remove tumors on the outside of the uterus, or a hysteroscope can be inserted through the cervix, which uses a laser to burn away internal fibroids. Synthetic hormones called gonadotropin-releasing hormone agonists block the ovaries' production of estrogen, which leads to shrinking of the fibroids and the possible avoidance of surgery. Even with surgery, about 25 percent of fibroids grow back within five years.

A prolapsed uterus is frequently treated by hysterectomy, but other therapies are possible. Kegel exercises, designed to strengthen the muscles of the pelvic floor, are effective if done regularly for an extended period of time. A pessary, a ring-shaped device which fits around the cervix and props up the uterus, is another alternative, though an inconvenient one. Major surgery to resuspend the uterus is a surgical option to hysterectomy.

Ovarian cysts will usually be resorbed into the ovary within one to three menstrual cycles. Proper monitoring by a physician is needed to determine if the cysts have cleared. If the cyst does not disappear within three months or if it increases in size, ultrasound and/or laparoscopy will be used to determine if a different type of ovarian tumor is present, which would necessitate surgical removal.

Cancer treatment is highly specialized for the particular variety of the disease, its severity, and consideration of the affected individual. Typical treatments include surgical removal of the tumor and/or affected organ, radiation therapy, chemotherapy, and immunotherapy (the reinforcement of the immune system, generally administered after radiation or chemotherapy). When diagnosed in premalignant stages, cervical abnormalities may be treated by cryosurgery (freezing and killing the abnormal cells) or laser destruction of the abnormal cells. Advanced cervical cancer is treated by hysterectomy. Endometrial cancer is treated with total hysterectomy, including the uterus, ovaries, and Fallopian tubes, and if the cancer has spread, radiation and/or chemotherapy. The only known cure for uterine sarcoma is total hysterectomy, and removal of both the ovaries and the Fallopian tubes is performed for ovarian cancer. The tumors of vaginal cancer are eliminated surgically or with laser treatment.

Sexually transmitted diseases of bacterial origin are treated successfully with antibiotics. Drug therapy can also eliminate trichomoniasis. There are no cures for the virally transmitted STDs. Certain drugs can reduce the frequency of outbreaks of genital herpes, and genital warts may be removed by freezing, burning, or surgery. No cure exists for AIDS, and only experimental drugs are available to prolong life.

PERSPECTIVE AND PROSPECTS

The diagnosis and treatment of female genital disorders and diseases have evolved from a state of some being considered psychosomatic to a field which spurs the continued development and improvement of diagnostic and treatment technologies. It is also a field which has been a major force in the mass screening of diseases and in public health issues. Many conditions such as endometriosis have historically been misdiagnosed and the associated pain dismissed as nonexistent—to the dismay of the suffering woman. This and other conditions such as prolapsed uterus and fibroids were typically treated with the drastic surgery of hysterectomy. Women have demanded that more research into the causes of these disorders, and options to hysterectomy, be developed. Laparoscopy has replaced hysterectomy in many cases, preserving the uterus and childbearing capacity.

The treatment of all female cancers has benefited from research into the cause and treatment of these disorders. For decades, the Pap smear has been routinely used with American women on an annual basis, and it has been responsible for saving thousands of lives through early detection of abnormal cervical cells that may progress to a cancerous state. Public education about the necessity of early cancer detection has helped to improve the survival chances of individuals with cancer, and sensitive blood tests can detect some cancers at their most treatable stages, long before any symptoms occur. Discovery of the hereditary nature of female genital cancers has established routine monitoring of those at risk for the disease, again resulting in early detection. New, better radiation and chemotherapy treatments, as well as improved immune system support, benefit all cancer patients. The connection between certain "cancer-fighting" foods and good health has led to a revision of Americans' eating habits.

While some sexually transmitted diseases are easily cured with antibiotics if caught early, those of viral origin are not and may have fatal consequences. Information through such diverse means as television and grade-school programs has educated people about this problem and the best ways to protect themselves from becoming victims of an incurable STD. Continuing research into diagnostic methods and treatment regimes in this area will lead to improved health for everyone.

—*Karen E. Kalumuck, Ph.D.*

See also Amenorrhea; Aphrodisiacs; Behçet's disease; Candidiasis; Cervical, ovarian, and uterine cancers; Cervical procedures; Childbirth; Childbirth complications; Chlamydia; Circumcision, female, and genital mutilation; Conception; Contraception; Culdocentesis; Cystitis; Dysmenorrhea; Ectopic pregnancy; Electrocauterization; Endometrial biopsy; Endometriosis; Episiotomy; Gonorrhea; Gynecology; Herpes; Infertility in females; Menopause; Menorrhagia; Menstruation; Miscarriage; Ovarian cysts; Pap smear; Pelvic inflammatory disease (PID); Pregnancy and gestation; Premature birth; Premenstrual syndrome (PMS); Reproductive system; Sexual dysfunction; Sexuality; Sexually transmitted diseases (STDs); Sterilization; Stillbirth; Syphilis; Urology; Urology, pediatric; Warts.

FOR FURTHER INFORMATION:

Boston Women's Health Book Collective. *Our Bodies, Ourselves for the New Century.* New York: Simon & Schuster, 1998. Gives expanded and accessible information on a broad range of topics concerning women's health. An excellent reference book for all women. A listing of local, national, and international resources is included.

Carlson, Karen J., Stephanie A. Eisenstat, and Terra Ziporyn. *The Harvard Guide to Women's Health.* Cambridge, Mass.: Harvard University Press, 1996. Some three hundred clearly written, alphabetically arranged entries provide authoritative information for the lay public on both mental and physical diseases, tests, symptoms, and commonly asked questions.

Foley, Denise, and Eileen Nechas. *Women's Encyclopedia of Health and Emotional Healing: Top Women Doctors Share Their Unique Self-Help Advice on Your Body, Your Feelings, and Your Life.* Emmaus, Pa.: Rodale Press, 1993. A very readable and informative book filled with practical information and anecdotal examples covering all aspects of women's physical and emotional health.

Gray, Mary Jane, and Florence Haseltine. *The Woman's Guide to Good Health.* Yonkers, N.Y.: Consumer Reports Books, 1991. This practical and comprehensive guide is written by physicians and gives complete information about the myths, risks, and alternatives regarding female diseases, diagnosis, and treatment. A useful appendix includes a list of societies for support and further information.

Henderson, Gregory, et al. *Women at Risk: The HPV Epidemic and Your Cervical Health.* New York: Putnam, 2002. A candid and engaging examination of human papillomavirus (HPV) and the disorders it causes that affect cervical health, including genital warts, cervical dysplasia, and cervical cancer. Covers the importance of the Pap smear for early detection and treatment of HPV, the meaning of Pap test results, and ways of treating cervical disorders.

Novak, Emil, and Jonathan S. Berek, eds. *Novak's Gynecology.* 13th ed. Philadelphia: Lippincott Williams & Wilkins, 2002. A standard text covering all aspects of gynecology with an emphasis on diagnosis and treatment. Topics include biology and physiology, family planning, sexuality, evaluation of pelvic infections, early pregnancy loss, benign breast disease, benign gynecologic conditions, malignant diseases of the reproductive tract, and breast cancer.

Novotny, P. P. *What Women Should Know About Chronic Infections and Sexually Transmitted Diseases.* New York: Dell, 1991. This compact, easy-to-understand book gives complete and accurate information on the transmission, diagnosis, and prevention of all sexually transmitted diseases that affect women. A handy reference guide.

Rushing, Lynda, and Nancy Joste. *Abnormal Pap Smears: What Every Woman Needs to Know.* Amherst, N.Y.: Prometheus Books, 2001. Details what the Pap smear screens for, what women can do to ensure optimal results, how laboratory errors can affect results, what various diagnoses mean, and what to expect in follow-up and treatment procedures.

Shaw, Michael, ed. *Everything You Need to Know About Diseases.* Springhouse, Pa.: Springhouse Press, 1996. This well-illustrated consumer reference, compiled by more than one hundred doctors and medical experts, describes five hundred illnesses and conditions, their causes, symptoms, diagnosis, treatment, and prevention. Of particular interest is chapter 9, "Gynecologic Disorders."

Stewart, Elizabeth Gunther, and Paula Spencer. *V Book: A Doctor's Guide to Complete Vulvovaginal Health.* New York: Bantam Books, 2002. Covers a wealth of information related to vulvovaginal health, including picking a good gynecologist and how to ask the right questions, vulvovaginal hygiene, safe use of tampons, common ailments and their symptoms, and which medical tests to insist upon from one's doctor.

GENITAL DISORDERS, MALE

DISEASE/DISORDER

ANATOMY OR SYSTEM AFFECTED: Genitals, reproductive system

SPECIALTIES AND RELATED FIELDS: Family practice, oncology, proctology, urology

DEFINITION: Disorders and diseases of the male reproductive system, including sexual dysfunction, infertility, genital cancer, and sexually transmitted diseases.

KEY TERMS:

autonomic nervous system: the part of the vertebrate nervous system that controls involuntary actions

dysfunction: the disordered or impaired function of a body system or organ

endocrine: relating to the production or action of a hormone

hormone: a substance which creates a specific effect in an organ distant from its site of production

impotence: the inability to have or maintain an erection satisfactory for sexual intercourse

organic: pertaining to, arising from, or affecting a body organ

parasympathetic nervous system: the part of the autonomic nervous system that stimulates digestion, slows the heart, and dilates blood vessels, acting in opposition to sympathetic nerves

psychogenic: originating in the mind or in mental conditions and activities

spermatogonia: cells of the testes that become sperm during spermatogenesis

sphincter: a ringlike muscle which constricts or relaxes to close or open a body orifice or passage, as required by normal body function

sympathetic nervous system: the part of the autonomic nervous system that represses digestion, speeds up the heart, and constricts blood vessels, acting in opposition to parasympathetic nerves

PROCESS AND EFFECTS

Before discussion of male genital disorders and diseases, it is useful to describe the male genital system, which is composed of the scrotum, testes, epididymis, vas deferens, prostate and bulbourethral glands, seminal vesicles, penis, and urethra. The scrotum, composed of skin and underlying muscle, encloses the two testes and protects these sperm-making organs.

Each human testis is an ovoid structure about 5.0 centimeters long and 3.3 centimeters in width. A testis is composed of seminiferous tubules, a structure which surrounds the sperm-producing tubules, and accessory cells (the Leydig cells). The production of sperm, spermatogenesis, is controlled by hormones from the brain's hypothalamus and pituitary glands. It begins with the secretion of testosterone, the main male hormone, by Leydig cells. Brain hormone and testosterone actions cause the metamorphosis of cells called spermatogonia into sperm during a two-month passage through the seminiferous tubules.

The highly coiled seminiferous tubules, tiny in diameter and more than 200 meters long, coalesce into the efferent tubules, which release sperm into the epididymis. In a twelve-day trip through the highly coiled, 4.5-meter-long epididymis, sperm attain the ability to move (motility) and to fertilize a human egg cell, or ovum. Next, they enter the vas deferens, paired structures that connect the epididymis of each testis to its ejaculatory duct and the urethra. The only known vas function is to transport sperm, as a result of the action of nearby nerves and muscles, into the latter structures. The vas are cut in bilateral vasectomy surgery, which is often used for male sterilization.

The prostate, seminal vesicles, and bulbourethral glands produce the secretions that constitute most sperm-containing semen, which is ejaculated during intercourse. The prostate gland is situated immediately below the urinary bladder and surrounds the portion of the urethra closest to the bladder. It is a fibromuscular gland which empties into the male urethra on ejaculation. Prostate secretions contain important enzymes and make up a quarter of the seminal fluid.

The seminal vesicles are 7.5 centimeters long and empty into the ejaculatory ducts. They produce more than half of the liquid portion of semen, contributing fluid rich in fructose, the main nutrition source of sperm. The tiny, paired bulbourethral (or Cowper's) glands are located below the prostate. They secrete lubricants into the male urethra that ease semen passage.

The male urethra passes from the urinary bladder, through the prostate, and then through the penis. At the end of the penis, it reaches the outside of the body, to pass semen and urine. The penis, a cylindrical erectile organ, surrounds most of the male urethra and contains three cavernous regions. One, the corpus spongiosum, is found around the urethra. The others, the paired corpora cavernosa, are erectile tissues that fill with blood to produce an erection upon male sexual arousal. Erection is a complex reflex which involves both the sympathetic and parasympathetic portions of the human nervous system.

At the time of erection, nerve impulses dilate blood vessels that communicate with the corpora cavernosa and allow them to fill with blood. Sphincters then close off the portion of the urethra closest to the urinary bladder. At the same time, sperm, prostate secretions, bulbourethral gland secretions, and seminal vesicle secretions enter the urethra. Next, muscle contractions propel the ejaculate out of the urethra. The blood then leaves the corpora cavernosa, and the penis resumes its unexcited state.

Complications and Disorders

Proper male sexual function involves several closely coordinated hormone, nervous, and chemical processes. After a discussion of the male genital system, it thus becomes clear that many factors can cause male genital problems and diseases. Male infertility, for example, can be attributable to inadequate sperm production; undersecretion by the seminal vesicles, Cowper's glands, and/or prostate; malfunction of other endocrine glands or of the nervous system; and dysfunction or lack of the epididymis. Impotence, the inability to have or maintain a satisfactory erection for intercourse, is another frequent male genital problem. It may be psychogenic or caused by anatomic dysfunction, disease, or medications used to treat health problems.

The male sexual response cycle is mediated by the complex interplay of parasympathetic and sympathetic nerves. For example, penis erection is mostly parasympathetic, while ejaculation is largely attributable to sympathetic enervation. Dysfunction disorders include low sexual desire, impotence (erectile dysfunction), and lost orgiastic control (premature ejaculation). Impotence is the most frequent of these problems.

Erectile dysfunction is said to occur when the failure to complete successful intercourse occurs at least 25 to 30 percent of the time. Most often, it is short term (secondary impotence) and related to individual partners or to temporary damage to male self-esteem. Secondary impotence may also be caused by diseases such as diabetes mellitus, medications such as tranquilizers and amphetamines, alcoholism and other psychoactive drug addictions, and minor genital abnormalities. Aging is not necessarily a cause of impotence, even in octogenarians.

Long-lasting (or primary) impotence that occurs despite corrective medical treatment is generally attributable to severe psychopathology and must be treated by psychotherapy and counseling. Psychogenic impotence is implicated when an erection can be achieved by masturbation. The treatment of impotence caused by organic problems may include testosterone administration, the discontinuation of drug therapy or addictive drugs, or corrective surgery, which may include inflatable penis implants.

Male infertility is a problem found in about a third of all cases in which American couples are unable to have children. The problem is thus estimated to occur in 4 to 5 percent of American men. There are a wide number of causes for male infertility, which is always caused by the failure to deliver adequate numbers of mature sperm into the female reproductive tract as a result of organic problems. Impaired spermatogenesis, a frequent cause of male infertility, may have numerous causes. Examples include severe childhood mumps, brain and/or testicular hormone imbalances, drug abuse, obstruction or anatomic malformation of the seminal tract (especially the seminiferous tubules and epididymis), and a defective prostate gland.

Diagnosis includes careful physical examination by a urologist and evaluation of ejaculated semen to identify the number, activity, and potential for fertilization of its sperm. Blood tests will identify hormone imbalances and other possible causative agents. Many treatments are possible for male infertility, ranging from medications, to corrective surgery, to artificial insemination with sperm collected and frozen until enough are on hand to effect fertilization.

Cancer of the male genital organs may occur in the prostate, urethra, penis, or testis. The most important of

Information on Male Genital Disorders

Causes: Psychological factors, genital cancer, sexually transmitted diseases, anatomic dysfunction, various diseases, certain medications

Symptoms: Sexual dysfunction, infertility, impotence

Duration: Acute or chronic

Treatments: Depends on cause; may include psychotherapy, counseling, hormone therapy, discontinuation of medications or addictive drugs, corrective surgery (*e.g.*, penile implants), drug therapy, surgery, radiation, chemotherapy

these is prostate cancer. Urethral cancer is rare. More common is carcinoma of the penis, which occurs most often in uncircumcised men who practice poor genital hygiene. It is very often located beneath the foreskin and does not spread quickly. Total or partial removal of the penis is often required in advanced cases that have been ignored for long periods. Testicular cancers account for most solid genital malignancies in young men. These cancers appear as painful scrotal masses which increase rapidly in size. Any large, firm mass arising from a testis is suspicious and should be examined immediately by X ray, computed tomography (CT) scan, and tests for various tumor markers seen in the blood. Treatment of these tumors includes surgery, radiation, and chemotherapy. Survival rates vary greatly and depend upon the cancer type. Cancer of the prostate and other male genital organs is not clearly understood and may have hormonal and chemical bases. It is believed that periodic self-examination is the most valuable preventive methodology.

Common disorders of the male genital organs include priapism, hydrocele and spermatocele, testicular torsion, and varicocele. Priapism is persistent, painful erection not accompanied by sexual arousal. It is caused by a poorly understood mechanism and is characterized by both pain and much-thickened blood in the corpora cavernosa. Priapism often occurs after prolonged sexual activity and may accompany prostate problems, genital infections such as syphilis, and addictive drug use. Treatment of priapism includes spinal anesthesia, anticoagulants, and surgery. In the absence of prompt, effective treatment, priapism may end male sexual function permanently.

Hydrocele is a common, noncancerous scrotum lesion most common in men over forty. The problem is caused by fluid accumulation resulting from testis inflammation. Hydrocele is not painful and is removed surgically only if excessive in size. Closely related in appearance is a spermatocele, which contains sperm and occurs adjacent to an epididymis. Both hydroceles and spermatoceles are said to transilluminate: They are both so transparent that a flashlight beam will pass through them. Testicular torsion is a twisting of the vas deferens, which causes pain and swelling; surgery is required to return blood flow to the testis. Varicocele describes varicose veins of the testis, which is common and usually harmless.

Sexually transmitted diseases can also affect the male genitals. These diseases include herpes, gonorrhea, syphilis, chlamydia, and genital warts. For the prevention of sexually transmitted diseases, abstention, the careful choice of sexual partners, and the use of male or female condoms are useful.

PERSPECTIVE AND PROSPECTS
Treatment of the various types of male genital disorders and diseases has evolved greatly. Particularly valuable are the strides made in the treatment of impotence. It has been realized that such sexual dysfunction is often a consequence of organic problems that may be remedied by the cessation of causative medication use or by minor surgery. In addition, the utilization of inflatable penis implants in the cases where insoluble psychogenic or organic problems occur has been a milestone in the treatment of this emotionally devastating male genital problem.

Wide examination of the entire spectrum of male genital problems has led to numerous advantageous treatments and to an understanding that withholding unneeded medical treatments can be beneficial. For example, information regarding spermatoceles, hydroceles, and many related nonacute male genital problems has decreased the incidence of unnecessary male genital surgery, and its related risks, for patients.

Another important concept is that of frequent self-examination of the male genitals. This practice has led to a shortening of the time lag between the appearance of a suspicious mass in the scrotum, testes, or other male sex organ and medical attention from professionals (such as urologists) trained both to evaluate their seriousness and to treat them. Early detection has diminished the severity of many genital cancers and facilitated their treatment. Moreover, several clinical tests for such lesions have become more available and more widely used by the public.

It is hoped that these avenues and others, as well as further advances in both diagnostic techniques and treatment possibilities, will eventually eradicate male genital diseases and disorders. Two areas in need of advancements are priapism and prostate cancer, which is an effective killer.

—*Sanford S. Singer, Ph.D.*

See also Aphrodisiacs; Behçet's disease; Candidiasis; Chlamydia; Circumcision, male; Gonorrhea; Herpes; Hydrocelectomy; Hypospadias repair and urethroplasty; Infertility in males; Orchitis; Penile implant surgery; Prostate cancer; Prostate gland; Prostate gland removal; Reproductive system; Sexual dysfunction; Sexuality; Sexually transmitted diseases (STDs); Sterilization; Stones; Syphilis; Testicles, undescended;

Testicular surgery; Testicular torsion; Urology; Urology, pediatric; Vasectomy; Warts.

FOR FURTHER INFORMATION:

American Psychiatric Association. *Diagnostic and Statistical Manual of Mental Disorders: DSM-IV-TR.* Rev. 4th ed. Washington, D.C.: Author, 2000. This compilation includes diagnostic criteria and other useful facts about mental problems associated with male genital diseases. It thus provides insight into the psychogenic aspects of these afflictions.

Berkow, Robert, and Andrew J. Fletcher, eds. *The Merck Manual of Diagnosis and Therapy.* 17th ed. Rahway, N.J.: Merck Sharp & Dohme Research Laboratories, 1999. This book abounds with useful data on the characteristics, etiology, diagnosis, and treatment of male genital disorders and diseases. Written for physicians, it is also quite useful to general readers.

Ellsworth, Pamela, and Bob Stanley. *One Hundred Questions and Answers About Erectile Dysfunction.* Sudbury, Mass.: Jones and Bartlett, 2002. A patient-oriented guide that covers basic questions about the condition, such as causes, symptoms, and diagnosis; available treatments and how to choose among them; and ways of coping with common emotional and physical difficulties associated with the diagnosis and treatment.

Milsten, Richard, and Julian Slowinsky. *The Sexual Male: Problems and Solutions.* New York: W. W. Norton, 2001. Accessible discussion of impotence and its causes, effects, and treatments.

Montague, Drogo K. *Disorders of Male Sexual Function.* Chicago: Year Book Medical, 1988. This medical text is useful to all readers wishing detailed information on aspects of men's health, including male reproductive anatomy and physiology, terminology, clinical evaluation, pharmacology, and the treatment of male sexual diseases.

Parker, James N., and Philip M. Parker, eds. *The Official Patient's Sourcebook on Impotence.* San Diego, Calif.: Icon Health, 2002. Draws from public, academic, government, and peer-reviewed research to provide a wide-ranging handbook for patients with impotence.

_____. *The Official Patient's Sourcebook on Testicular Cancer: A Revised and Updated Directory for the Internet Age.* San Diego, Calif.: Icon Health, 2002. Draws from public, academic, government, and peer-reviewed research to provide a wide-ranging handbook for patients with testicular cancer.

Sherwood, Lauralee. *Human Physiology: From Cells to Systems.* 4th ed. Belmont, Calif.: Wadsworth, 2001. This college text contains useful information on the male genital system, background endocrinology, spermatogenesis, aspects of sexual dysfunction, and sexually transmitted diseases in men. Also a source of many explanatory illustrations.

Taguchi, Yosh, and Merrily Weisbord, eds. *Private Parts: An Owner's Guide to the Male Anatomy.* Toronto: McClelland & Stewart, 2003. A guide to male genital and sexual health, covering topics such as prostate trouble, erectile dysfunction, infertility, cancer, sexually transmitted diseases, vasectomies, and artificial insemination.

GENOMICS

SPECIALTY

ANATOMY OR SYSTEM AFFECTED: All

SPECIALTIES AND RELATED FIELDS: Bacteriology, biochemistry, biotechnology, cytology, embryology, ethics, genetics, microbiology, pharmacology

DEFINITION: The study of whole genomes; a genome is the complete set of genetic information found in a particular organism.

KEY TERMS:

bioinformatics: a computational discipline that provides the tools needed to study whole genomes and proteomes

DNA microarrays: solid supports which contain many or all genes from a given genome, enabling the expression of these genes to be monitored simultaneously

DNA sequencing: determining the order of deoxyribonucleic acid (DNA) bases in a particular unit of genetic information

orthologues: similar genes from different species that are thought to be related by evolution

proteomics: the study of proteomes; a proteome is the complete set of proteins in a particular cell type

synteny: when whole regions of chromosomes from different species are similar in structure

A NEW SCIENTIFIC DISCIPLINE

Genomics grew out of the field of genetics, the study of heredity. Until the late twentieth century, it had not been possible to study the complete set of hereditary information in a living organism. So, while the field of genetics traces its roots to the 1860's, when the Austrian monk Gregor Mendel performed experiments on the mechanism of heredity in pea plants, the field of genomics is much younger, dating from the 1980's, when American geneticist Thomas Roderick used this term to name a new scientific journal which dealt with the analysis of genomic information. In Mendel's time, while organisms were seen to exhibit certain traits, it was not known how these traits were determined. By the early 1900's, it was recognized that traits are inherited in units of information called genes, although the chemical nature of the gene was still unknown. It took until the middle of that century to recognize that genes were made up of deoxyribonucleic acid (DNA), the structure of which was first identified by American biologist James Watson and British biophysicist Francis Crick in 1953.

DNA is made up of four different deoxyribonucleotides, commonly referred to as bases: adenine (A), cytosine (C), guanine (G), and thymine (T). Together, they spell out a chemical code that is used by the cell to make proteins. Since it is the set of proteins contained within a cell which gives that cell its unique properties, determining the order of DNA bases in a given genetic unit will reveal what types of proteins are encoded by this information, a procedure known as DNA sequencing. While a gene has been defined as the amount of DNA needed to encode one protein, a genome is the entire set of genes found in an organism, including any noncoding DNA found between genes. The number of genes that have been found to be present in an organism varies between about five hundred (in a bacterium that causes venereal disease) to about twenty-three thousand (in the simple flowering plant *Arabidopsis*); humans were found to have slightly less than this number.

During the 1980's, a public consortium was formed with the goal of sequencing the human genome by 2005, the International Human Genome Sequencing Consortium. The Human Genome Project, as this effort was called, also had the goal of sequencing the genomes of a number of model organisms that have been used by scientists to help understand biological complexity. These model organisms, which included the *Escherichia coli* bacterium, yeast, *Caenorhabditis elegans* (a roundworm), *Drosophila* (the fruit fly), and mouse, also served as steps by which the efficiency of DNA sequencing could be improved over time. *E. coli*, like most bacteria, has a genome that numbers in the millions of bases—usually abbreviated bp (for base pair), since each base in DNA is paired with its complementary base, A to T and G to C—while yeast has a genome of approximately ten million bp and the next three organisms have genomes that number in the hun-

dreds of millions of bp. Mice, like humans, have genomes that are three billion bp in size. Around the turn of the twentieth century, steady progress was made on the genome efforts described above as the sequence of each respective genome was determined and made publicly available via computer databases. The completion of the human genome was announced in April, 2003, the month of the fiftieth anniversary of Watson and Crick's first description of the structure of DNA.

Does the field of genomics represent a new scientific discipline in and of itself, or is it just another extension of genetics? Other than the sheer size of hereditary information being analyzed in genomics, another major difference would support the former possibility. Ever since Mendel's time, genetics has taken a reductionist approach. Since Mendel could not have dreamed of understanding the pea plant as a whole, he limited his investigation to a number of easily characterized traits, such as plant height and seed color. Since that time, many scientists have sought to understand complex biological processes by breaking them into manageable pieces. Genomics attempts a different, expansionist approach. In the postgenomics era (as the twenty-first century has been called by some scientists), the questions being posed are holistic in nature: They attempt for the first time to understand organisms as a whole using their complete set of genetic information as a guide. In fact, genomics has spawned a new set of fields that end in "-omics," denoting the fact that they attempt to study the complete set of particular molecules in an organism or cell type. Proteomics is the study of the complete set of proteins in a cell type, while metabolomics is the study of the complete set of metabolic reactions in a cell.

New approaches to science call for new tools as well. The tools on which geneticists have relied over the years have largely proved to be insufficient for studying entire genomes. Bioinformatics is a subdiscipline of computational biology that has arisen to provide such tools. Bioinformatics includes the computational methods required to find patterns in the huge genomic databases that have been produced, to track the expression of genes using DNA microarrays, to identify all the proteins in a cell, and to model the protein interactions involved in cell metabolism, among other things.

DIVISIONS WITHIN THE FIELD

In addition to producing the "-omics" disciplines, the field of genomics can itself be subdivided. Although these divisions are somewhat artificial, they do help illustrate the different goals of genomics research. The main divisions of genomics are structural genomics, functional genomics, and comparative genomics.

Structural genomics is concerned with the structure of hereditary information. The determination of the number, location, and order of genes on a particular chromosome is one pursuit of this field. While bacterial genomes are typically contained within a single circular chromosome, humans have twenty-three pairs of chromosomes and some organisms have even more. Studying regions of DNA between genes, or intergenic regions, is also the realm of structural genomics. Intergenic regions are often composed of a highly repetitive DNA sequence that does not code for any type of protein. In the early twenty-first century, the precise function of these regions still eluded scientists. Although noncoding sequence is relatively rare in bacteria, it makes up a major portion of many multicellular organisms, including about 98 percent of the human genome. A separate goal of structural biology is the determination of the three-dimensional structure of all the proteins encoded by a genome, an endeavor called structural proteomics.

Functional genomics is less concerned with the structure of a genome and more concerned with its function. This division of genomics tends to be of more interest to pharmaceutical companies and the medical community as a whole. Functional genomics asks questions such as, "What do the products of individual genes do?" and "How does the perturbation of gene function lead to disease states?" Determining the function of a gene, however, is not as straightforward as it might appear. By the early twenty-first century, determining the structure of a given genome was the relatively easy part, but the function of up to half the genes in a typical sequenced genome remained undetermined. Even the determination of the three-dimensional structure of a protein which is produced by a specific gene does not guarantee that its function can be discerned, but scientists are always hopeful that this will lead to conjecture concerning its function.

Another clue concerning gene function can be derived by the determination of where and when a particular gene is expressed (activated to produce its corresponding protein). While gene expression has traditionally been monitored one gene at a time using molecular genetic techniques, around the turn of the twenty-first century researchers began experimenting with DNA microarrays. DNA microarrays, or "gene chips," include copies of many, if not all, genes from a given genome attached to a solid support such as a glass slide. The expression of these genes can be monitored at any given time by binding fluorescently tagged sequences of DNA that are complementary to the genes in question. An automated scanner then measures the fluorescence of each spot and records the data into a computer.

The final division of genomics, comparative genomics, encompasses the goals of the other two divisions but achieves these goals by making comparisons between two different genomes. For example, the structure of a given genome, by itself, may not appear significant until the same basic structure is detected in another species. Regions of chromosomes from two different species that are similar in structure are said to display synteny. Comparative genomics has also aided in the quest to determine gene function. One of the most common techniques of determining gene function is by looking for orthologues in related species. Orthologues are genes from different species that are thought to be related by evolution; they often encode similar, but not identical, proteins with related functions.

PERSPECTIVE AND PROSPECTS

Genomics can trace its origins to the development of techniques used to determine the sequence of DNA. In 1977, British biochemist Frederick Sanger and colleagues published a sequencing method based on the principle of chain termination. In this method, the sequence of target DNA is determined by enzymatically producing a complementary strand of DNA. In Sanger sequencing, as it is now called, a molecular "poison" is included in a given reaction mixture so that the newly synthesized complementary chain is terminated at specific bases. Sanger's method was then modified in the 1990's to include fluorescent dyes on the chain-terminating bases so that the DNA sequence could be read using a scanner and recorded directly into a computer. Some have claimed that Sanger and colleagues were actually the first group to sequence a genome, since they published the sequence of a viral genome in the same year that they described their revolutionary technique. Viruses, however, are not free-living organisms, and their genomes are thousands of times smaller than the typical bacterial genome.

The Human Genome Project was first proposed in 1986 and was funded two years later at an expected cost of three billion dollars. The project officially got underway in 1990 as sequencing began in earnest on some of the smaller model genomes. In 1995, as some of these sequencing efforts were nearing completion, American pharmacologist Craig Venter and his colleagues at a private not-for-profit institute, the Institute for Genome Research, published the genome sequence of the bacterium *Haemophilus influenzae*, the first free-living organism to have its genome sequenced.

While the public consortium had been working on sequences using established techniques, Venter and colleagues had developed a faster technique for determining the sequence of whole genomes. While this technique still used the basic Sanger-style chain termination procedure, it simplified an earlier step in the process in which large numbers of clones of genomic fragments were made before sequencing could begin. Venter had circumvented this cloning step; he called his approach whole-genome shotgun sequencing. During the next two years, the public consortium published the sequences of yeast and *E. coli*, respectively, and in 1998 announced that the sequence of *C. elegans* was complete. That same year, Venter announced that he was starting a for-profit company, Celera Genomics, which would complete the human genome within three years using shotgun sequencing. Up until this time, however, Venter had only demonstrated this approach using bacterial genomes. In order to demonstrate the validity of the shotgun approach on large genomes, and to gear up for sequencing the human genome, Celera sequenced the 170 million bp genome of the fruit fly in 2000, at that time the largest genome ever sequenced.

During the final years of the twentieth century, spurred on by the competition from the private sector, the public consortium had redoubled its efforts on the human genome. In February, 2001, the race to sequence the human genome ended in a tie. Both sequencing efforts, public and private, published their draft sequence of the human genome at this time, and in April, 2003, the two efforts together announced the final completed sequence. The mouse genome sequence was also published in 2003. In fact, by mid-2003, about 150 genomic sequences had been determined (the vast majority of which were bacterial genomes) and almost 600 more were underway, including many more multicellular organisms.

Are the time, effort, and money that have been spent on various genome-sequencing projects really worth it? One promise that genomics may hold for the future is the identification of all human disease genes. While this has been one of the main justifications for the Human Genome Project, one should keep in mind that identifying the gene which causes a particular disease is not always equivalent to finding a cure for that dis-

ease. Another potential benefit of genomic research is the development of better treatments for bacterial and parasitic infections. A number of disease-causing bacteria have already been the subject of genome sequencing efforts, including the causative agents of bubonic plague, anthrax, and tuberculosis, to name a few. Some indirect benefits of genomics (which may, in time, prove just as valuable) include a better understanding of evolutionary relationships between species as well as a firmer grasp on basic cellular function. In all, the field of genomics promises to be a powerful means of scientific inquiry well into the future.

—James S. Godde, Ph.D.

See also Bioinformatics; Biostatistics; Cloning; DNA and RNA; Gene therapy; Genetic counseling; Genetic diseases; Genetic engineering; Genetics and inheritance; Laboratory tests; Mutation; Screening.

FOR FURTHER INFORMATION:

Campbell, A. Malcolm, and Laurie J. Heyer. *Discovering Genomics, Proteomics, and Bioinformatics*. 1st ed. San Francisco: Benjamin/Cummings, 2003. An introduction to genomics and the techniques used to study genomic data. Contains many Internet-based exercises in bioinformatics.

Clark, M. S. "Comparative Genomics: The Key to Understanding the Human Genome Project." *BioEssays* 21 (1999): 121-130. An in-depth discussion of comparative genomics and its significance to the field as a whole.

Collins, Francis S., et al. "A Vision for the Future of Genomics Research." *Nature* 422 (April, 2003): 835-847. Upon the completion of the Human Genome Project, the director of the public consortium and his colleagues wrote this article, which presents a plan for the future of genomics.

DeRisi, Joseph L., and Vishwanath R. Iyer. "Genomics and Array Technology." *Current Opinion in Oncology* 11 (1999): 76-79. A review of how DNA microarrays are used in genomic research.

Klug, William S., and Michael R. Cummings. "Genomics, Bioinformatics, and Proteomics." In *Concepts of Genetics*. 7th ed. Upper Saddle River, N.J.: Prentice Hall, 2003. A chapter that details the differences between genomes among the various model organisms which have been sequenced.

Russell, Peter J. "Genome Analysis." In *Essential Genetics*. San Francisco: Benjamin/Cummings, 2003. A chapter in a text which is designed to serve as an introduction to genetics and genomics.

Snustad, D. Peter, and Michael J. Simmons. "Genomics." In *Principles of Genetics*. 3d ed. New York: John Wiley & Sons, 2003. A chapter from a textbook which describes the history of genomics as well as its various permutations.

Wei, Liping, et al. "Comparative Genomics Approaches to Study Organism Similarities and Differences." *Journal of Biomedical Informatics* 35 (2002): 142-150. A review of how comparative genomics has been used in both structural and functional studies.

GERIATRICS AND GERONTOLOGY

SPECIALTIES

ANATOMY OR SYSTEM AFFECTED: All

SPECIALTIES AND RELATED FIELDS: All

DEFINITION: Geriatrics refers to the social and health care of the elderly; gerontology is the study of the aging process.

KEY TERMS:

decubitus ulcer: ulceration of the skin and subcutaneous tissues, resulting from protein deficiency and prolonged, unrelieved pressure on bony prominences

dementia: a deterioration or loss of intellectual faculties, reasoning power, memory, and will that is caused by organic brain disease

glaucoma: an eye disease characterized by increased intraocular pressure, which can lead to degeneration of the optic nerve and ultimately blindness if left untreated

Medicare: the popular designation for 1965 amendments to the U.S. Social Security Act, providing hospitalization and certain other benefits to people over the age of sixty-five

polypharmacy: the prescription of many drugs at one time, often resulting in excessive use of medications and adverse drug interactions

prostate: in men, the organ surrounding the neck of the urinary bladder and beginning of the urethra; its secretions make up about 40 percent of semen

THE STUDY OF AGING

The field of geriatrics deals with the care of the elderly. The U.S. government's definition of elderly includes persons sixty-five years of age or older. Geriatricians are physicians with specialized training in geriatric medicine who restrict their practices to caring for persons seventy-five years of age or older. These patients are most likely to suffer from specific geriatric syndromes, including dementia, delirium, urinary incontinence, malnutrition, osteoporosis, falls and immobility, decubitus ulcers, polypharmacy, and sleep disorders. The majority of older persons in the United States live in family settings with their spouses or children. Approximately 30 percent of older persons live alone, the majority of them being women. The proportion of older persons (those over sixty-five) who live in nursing homes is about 5 percent; this number increases strikingly with age, with 22 percent of Americans aged eighty-five or older residing in a nursing home.

The focus of geriatric medicine is on improving functional disability and treating chronic disease conditions that impair a person's ability to perform such activities of daily living as bathing and dressing, maintaining urinary and bowel continence, and eating. A more objective measure of an older person's ability to live independently is the instrumental activities of daily living scale. This scale measures an individual's ability to use the telephone, obtain transportation, go shopping, prepare meals, do housework and laundry, self-administer medicines, and manage money.

The maximum life span of an organism is the theoretical longest duration of that organism's life, excluding premature, unnatural death. The maximum life span of humans is unknown, although most experts believe it to be approximately 120 years. Most people will die of disease or accident, however, before they reach this biological limit. Attempts to understand why this occurs have led to the development of several theories of aging. The aging process is controlled, in large part, by genetic mechanisms. Aging is a biologic process characterized by a progressive development and maturation leading to senescence and death. There are profound changes in cells, tissues, and organs as well as in physiological, cognitive, and psychological processes. Aging is not the acquisition of disease, although aging and disease can be related. In the absence of disease, normal aging is a slow process. It involves the steady decline of organ reserves and homeostatic control mechanisms, which is often not apparent unless there is maximal exertion or stress on an individual system or on the total organism.

Numerous changes in the body occur as people age. For example, one can expect to lose two inches in height from age forty to age eighty. This shrinkage results from a decrease in vertebral bone mass and in the thickness of intervertebral disks, as well as from postural alterations with increased flexion or bending at the hips and knees. Total body fat increases as one ages, accompanied by decreases in muscle mass and total body water. Such changes in body composition have important implications for drug treatments and nutritional plans. For example, fat-soluble medications exhibit a longer duration of action in the elderly. Older persons also experience a thinning of the dermal layer of the skin, with thinner blood vessels, decreased collagen, and less skin elasticity. Sun damage can accelerate these changes. Graying of the hair reflects a progressive loss of functional melanocytes from the hair bulbs. The number of hair follicles of the scalp decreases, as does the growth rate of remaining follicles. The brain also alters with age: The weight of the brain declines, blood flow to the brain decreases, and there is a loss of neurons in specific areas of the brain. These changes in brain structure are highly variable and do not necessarily affect thinking and behavior.

Many changes occur in the vision of the older person. Loss of elasticity in the lens leads to presbyopia, the most common visual problem associated with aging. Presbyopia is a condition in which the distance that is needed to focus on near objects increases. Cataracts increase in prevalence with age, although unprotected exposure of the eyes to ultraviolet rays has been implicated in the pathogenesis as well. Glaucoma also occurs more often in the elderly.

Older persons often experience hearing loss from degenerative processes, including atrophy of the external auditory canal and thickening of the tympanic membrane. The result is presbycusis, a bilateral hearing loss for pure tones. Higher frequencies are more affected than lower ones, and the condition is more severe in men than in women. Pitch discrimination also declines with age, which may account for an increased difficulty in speech discrimination.

The heart alters with age, although the significance of these changes is unclear in the absence of disease. There are declines in intrinsic contractile function and electrical activity. The resting heart rate and cardiac output do not change, but the maximum heart rate decreases in a linear fashion and may be estimated by subtracting a person's age from 220. There are also modest increases in systolic blood pressure.

Minor changes occur in the gastrointestinal system. The liver and pancreas maintain adequate function throughout life, although the metabolism of specific drugs is prolonged in older people. Kidney function declines with age, with a 30 percent loss in renal mass and a decrease in renal blood flow. A linear decline in the ability of the kidneys to filter blood after the age of forty can lead to a decrease in the clearance of some drugs from the body.

In the endocrine system, the blood glucose level before meals changes minimally after the age of forty, although the level of blood glucose after meals increases. These changes may be related to decreases in muscle mass and a decreased insulin secretion rate. Glucose intolerance with aging must be distinguished from the hyperglycemia that can accompany diabetes mellitus; the latter requires treatment. No clinically significant alterations in the levels of the thyroid hormone occur, although the end organ response to thyroid hormones may be decreased. The hypothalamic-pituitary-adrenal axis remains intact. Plasma basal and stimulated norepinephrine levels are higher in healthy elderly individuals than in the young. The secretion of hormones such as androgens and estrogens falls sharply as a result of the loss of endocrine cells.

DISEASES AFFECTING THE ELDERLY

One of the chronic diseases frequently seen in elderly people is osteoporosis. Osteoporosis is defined as a decreased amount of bone per unit of volume; mineralization of the bone remains normal. Many studies have shown that bone mass decreases with age. Vertebral fractures resulting from osteoporosis cause deformity of the spine, loss in height, and pain. The absolute number of vertebral fractures that occur in older persons has been difficult to estimate, as some of these fractures go undiagnosed. The approximately 200,000 hip fractures that the elderly in the United States suffer annually have much more serious consequences. The lifetime risk of hip fracture by the age of eighty is approximately 15 percent for white women and 7 percent for white men. The risk of hip fracture by this age is significantly less in African Americans, with a 6 percent risk for women and a 3 percent risk for men.

One approach to preventing osteoporosis is to maximize the amount of bone that is formed during adolescence. Under normal circumstances, people begin to experience a net bone loss after the age of thirty-five. In women, the onset of menopause accelerates bone loss because of the decline in estrogen levels. Relative calcium deficiency has also been implicated in age-related osteoporosis. By definition, age-related osteoporosis is a diagnosis of exclusion. An older patient who has suffered a fracture first should be evaluated for other causes of osteoporosis, including hyperparathyroidism, hyperthyroidism, diabetes, glucocorticoid excess, or, in men, hypogonadism. Other secondary causes of osteoporosis include malignancy, such as multiple myeloma, leukemia, or lymphoma, and the drug-related effects of alcohol or steroids. Any identifiable causes should be corrected.

People at increased risk for age-related osteoporosis include those with a family history of the disease; light hair, skin, and eyes; and a small body frame. Bone densitometry or quantitative computed tomography (CT) scanning can be performed to provide the most accurate estimates of the risk of an initial fracture. There are a number of prevention and treatment strategies for patients. One should ensure an adequate calcium intake; the current recommendation is a daily intake of 1,200 milligrams of calcium for postmenopausal women. Weight-bearing exercise should be performed throughout the life span. In postmenopausal women, estrogen treatment is often given. While estrogen has not been shown conclusively to increase bone density, it does prevent further bone loss. In patients who cannot take estrogen, an alternative treatment is the hormone calcitonin. Calcitonin works by inhibiting osteoclast function, thereby halting the otherwise normal breakdown of bone.

A disorder that is commonly seen in elderly men is benign prostatic hypertrophy. The incidence of this disease increases in a progressive fashion, with approximately 90 percent of men aged eighty affected by this condition. The pathogenesis of prostatic hypertrophy is hormonal, caused by increased levels of dihydrotestosterone formed from the testosterone within the gland itself. The usual symptoms are those of urinary obstruction, which include hesitancy, straining, and decreased force and dimension of the urinary stream. Screening for benign prostatic hypertrophy includes two parts. The first is a blood test for prostate-specific antigens. The second is a digital rectal exam to inspect the prostate gland. Patients with positive findings will require further evaluation. A significant increase in prostatic tissue may need to be removed surgically. In patients with minimal disease, drug treatment may be used. Finesteride is an inhibitor of the enzyme 5-alpha reductase that is responsible for the conversion of testosterone to dihydrotestosterone. It slows the rate of increase in prostate tissue mass.

Depression is a common problem in both men and women as they get older. The elderly can experience transient mood changes that are the result of an identifiable stress or loss. In older persons, however, depression may be related to some medical condition, particularly dementia, which is associated with multiple strokes or Parkinson's disease. Major depression is more common in hospital and long-term care settings,

where the prevalence is about 13 percent. The symptoms of depression include significant weight change, insomnia or hypersomnia, psychomotor agitation or retardation, decreased energy and easy fatigability, feelings of worthlessness or excessive guilt, decreased ability to think or concentrate, and recurrent thoughts of death or suicide. The diagnosis of major depression can be made if at least five of these symptoms are present for at least two weeks. Depressive symptoms must be taken seriously in the elderly. The rate of suicide in older persons is higher than for other groups, with older white males having the highest rates of any age, racial, or ethnic group.

Another depressive disorder experienced by the elderly is dysthymia. Dysthymic disorders are characterized by less severe symptoms than those associated with major depression and by a duration of at least two years. The symptoms generally include at least two of the following: poor appetite or overeating, insomnia or hypersomnia, low energy and fatigue, low self-esteem, poor concentration or difficulty in making decisions, and feelings of hopelessness. Dysthymia may be primary or secondary to a preexisting chronic psychiatric or medical illness, with accompanying loss of function and debilitation.

Adjustment disorders with depressed mood are also seen in older persons. Such disorders occur within three months of a stressful situation and last up to six months. The prototypical situation is the depressive reaction that follows an acute medical illness. In the elderly, the four most common stressors are physical illness, reactions to the death of family and friends, retirement, and moving to an institutional setting. In dealing with depressive symptoms, however, it is important to consider other diagnoses, such as underlying medical illnesses, drug reactions to prescribed or over-the-counter medicines, hypochondriasis, alcohol abuse, and dementias. In older patients, the disorder most often associated with depression is dementia.

A thorough diagnostic evaluation can help in the diagnosis of a depressive disorder and can rule out other complicating problems. A careful history is elicited from the patient and from a family member or caretaker. A formal mental status examination is conducted to uncover abnormalities in concentration, speech, psychomotor skills, cognitive ability, and memory. Laboratory blood tests often include a complete blood count, chemical analysis, and thyroid function tests. Abbreviated neuropsychological tests can differentiate between patients with dementia and those with depression alone. The treatment of depression includes psychotherapy and pharmacotherapy. Behavioral interventions, such as special weekly activities and assignments, can be helpful. Most often, some kind of antidepressant medication is effective.

PERSPECTIVE AND PROSPECTS

In the United States, there has been increasing interest in the fields of geriatrics and gerontology because of the country's changing demographics. In 2000, thirty-five million Americans were sixty-five years of age or older. Because of the very large numbers in the baby-boom age group—that is, people born between 1946 and 1964—it was expected that the number of elderly people would increase dramatically by the year 2030 to about sixty-five million elderly persons. The elderly will compose approximately 22 percent of the total U.S. population.

Another reason for the increase in the size of the older population in the United States is an increase in life expectancy. Life expectancy is defined as the average number of years a person is expected to live, given population mortality rates. It can be calculated for any age category but is usually given as life expectancy from birth. The life expectancy in the United States is much higher than in undeveloped countries and in most other developed countries as well. This figure rose steadily throughout the twentieth century. A child born in 2000 could expect to live seventy-five years, while someone born in 1900 could expect to live only fifty years. Most of this increase in life expectancy is attributable to a decreased death rate for infants and children resulting from improvements in sanitation, active immunization against childhood diseases, and advances in medical treatments. For persons aged sixty-five, there was an increase in life expectancy over that same time period of only five years, probably the result of improved medical therapies.

As Americans live longer, the length of time that older persons will rely on society for their care increases as well. This situation places a greater burden on those persons who are working, as they must support greater numbers of people receiving Social Security and Medicare benefits, and requires a rethinking of the age requirements to be eligible for these programs. In 1997, while older persons represented 13 percent of the population, they accounted for 38 percent of the total costs for health care. Other factors adding to the cost of health care include such new technologies as specialized imaging equipment, complex laboratory procedures, and new therapeutic drugs. The goal of much research in geriatric medicine is to prevent or slow down the effects of aging so that the elderly may live in good health. Further research to understand better the mechanisms involved in human aging will help to design preventive and treatment strategies.

—*RoseMarie Pasmantier, M.D.; updated by L. Fleming Fallon, Jr., M.D., Ph.D., M.P.H.*

See also Aging; Aging: Extended care; Alzheimer's disease; Arthritis; Bed-wetting; Blindness; Bone disorders; Brain disorders; Cataract surgery; Cataracts; Critical care; Death and dying; Dementias; Depression; Domestic violence; Emergency medicine; Endocrinology; Euthanasia; Family practice; Fatigue; Hearing loss; Hip fracture repair; Hormone replacement therapy (HRT); Hospitals; Incontinence; Memory loss; Nursing; Nutrition; Ophthalmology; Orthopedics; Osteoporosis; Pain management; Paramedics; Parkinson's disease; Pharmacology; Physician assistants; Polypharmacy; Psychiatry; Psychiatry, geriatric; Rheumatology; Sleep disorders; Spinal cord disorders; Spine, vertebrae, and disks; Suicide; Visual disorders.

FOR FURTHER INFORMATION:

Beerman, Susan, and Judith Rappaport-Musson. *Eldercare 911: The Caregiver's Complete Handbook for Making Decisions.* Amherst, N.Y.: Prometheus Books, 2002. A practical guide for elder care. Includes topics such as locating services, managing medications, understanding benefits, choosing a nursing home, coping with memory loss, hiring and handling in-home help, helping a parent who refuses help, and recognizing signs of elder abuse.

Birren, James E., and K. Warner Schaie, eds. *Handbook of the Psychology of Aging.* 5th ed. San Diego, Calif.: Academic Press, 2001. Twenty-four contributions from international researchers explore topics such as the genetics of behavioral aging, environmental influences on aging, gender roles, mental health, declining motor control, wisdom, and technological change and the older worker.

Coni, Nicholas, and Steven Webster. *Lecture Notes on Geriatrics.* 5th ed. Oxford, England: Blackwell Scientific, 1998. Easy-to-read study notes on geriatric medicine. Discusses the different changes that occur in the patient during the aging process and characterizes the different diseases seen in the elderly.

Ferri, Fred F., Marsha Fretwell, and Tom J. Wachtel. *Practical Guide to the Care of the Geriatric Patient.* 2d ed. St. Louis: Mosby Year Book, 1997. An excellent resource. The text is clearly written, and the index is especially useful. Nonprofessional readers will have no trouble understanding this book.

Hampton, Roy, and Charles Russell. *The Encyclopedia of Aging and the Elderly*. New York: Facts On File, 1992. Much well-stated information is presented. The scope is broad—lifestyle, myths and misconceptions, medical and legal concerns, death and dying. Statistical information is presented in charts and tables, appendices list organizations, and the bibliography is useful.

Hooyman, Nancy, and H. Asuman Kayak. *Social Gerontology: A Multidisciplinary Perspective*. 6th ed. Boston: Allyn and Bacon, 2002. Contributions from social workers, psychologists, gerontology professionals, and professors examine the ways in which age-related changes in the biological, functional, and psychological domains can influence the older person's interactions with his/her social and physical environment.

Hoyer, William, et al. *Adult Development and Aging*. 5th ed. New York: McGraw-Hill, 2002. An interdisciplinary exploration of the biological, social, and cultural contexts in which change occurs during the adult years.

Isaacs, Bernard. *The Challenge of Geriatric Medicine*. London: Oxford Medical, 1992. This volume presents the issues associated with geriatric medicine and the care of older citizens. It is well written and should be of interest to most readers who want additional information on this subject.

Margolis, Simeon, and Hamilton Moses III, eds. *The Johns Hopkins Medical Handbook: The One Hundred Major Medical Disorders of People over the Age of Fifty*. Rev. ed. Garden City, N.Y.: Random House, 1999. This definitive home medical reference for adults offers an in-depth guide to the most common medical problems occurring in adults over fifty. The directory of hospitals and other health care resources, from support groups to treatment centers, is comprehensive.

Schneider, Edward L., and John W. Rowe. *Handbook of the Biology of Aging*. 5th ed. San Diego, Calif.: Academic Press, 2001. Part of a three-volume series that includes the biological, psychological, and social aspects of aging. Focuses on research approaches to understanding aging, including genetic studies, cellular and molecular biology, neurobiology, and nutrition.

Stenchever, Morton A. *Health Care for the Older Woman*. New York: Chapman and Hall, 1996. A ref- erence that provides medical practitioners and students with comprehensive, current information specific to the care of middle-aged and advanced-aged women. It covers health maintenance issues, including diet, exercise, safety, psychological and psychosocial problems, social problems, and grief and loss.

GERMAN MEASLES. *See* CHILDHOOD INFECTIOUS DISEASES; RUBELLA.

GESTATION. *See* PREGNANCY AND GESTATION.

GESTATIONAL DIABETES
DISEASE/DISORDER

ANATOMY OR SYSTEM AFFECTED: Endocrine system

SPECIALTIES AND RELATED FIELDS: Endocrinology, nutrition, obstetrics

DEFINITION: A medical condition in which diabetes, or unregulated blood glucose, first occurs during pregnancy.

KEY TERMS:

diabetes: a group of disorders characterized by hyperglycemia caused by a lack of insulin secretion or ineffective insulin action

hyperglycemia: high blood glucose

insulin: a hormone secreted by the pancreas whose primary function is to maintain blood glucose levels within a normal range

CAUSES AND SYMPTOMS

Gestational diabetes is the medical term describing a type of diabetes mellitus that is first diagnosed during a woman's pregnancy. Diabetes is a condition where blood glucose is not kept within a normal range. Normally, insulin is a key regulator of blood glucose. In diabetes, insulin may be absent, be present in insufficient amounts, or be ineffective. Gestational diabetes occurs in about 4 percent of all pregnancies in the United States. There is variance in incidence rates as a result of ethnicity, age, and genetic predisposition. Hispanic and African American women have a higher incidence than do Asian and Caucasian women, and older women have a higher incidence than do those who are younger. In general, women with a family history of diabetes are more likely to develop gestational diabetes.

Gestational diabetes normally develops midway through pregnancy. A two-step approach is used to screen women who are not at high risk for diabetes. The first step is the 50-gram oral glucose tolerance test. For this test, the woman is given 50 grams of glucose in solution after having fasted overnight. Her blood glucose is tested one hour after drinking the solution. If her blood glucose is above a normal range, the next step is a 100-gram three-hour oral glucose tolerance test. Normally, a person's insulin would react to the ingested glucose to keep the blood glucose within a normal range. If that does not occur, and blood glucose remains high, then a diagnosis of gestational diabetes is made.

As maternal blood glucose rises, so does the risk of fetal complications. The most common complication is fetal macrosomia, or having a birth weight greater than or equal to 4,500 grams. Fetal macrosomia is associated with an increased risk of birth trauma, especially to the head, shoulders, and throat area. Infants born this large often require a cesarean section, which itself has greater health risks than a vaginal birth.

When maternal blood glucose levels are elevated above normal, the fetus is stimulated to increase production of insulin. Although this manages the problem of the increased blood glucose for the fetus, it also has negative consequences. If the mother's blood glucose has been elevated just preceding delivery, then the infant's insulin level will be elevated. After delivery, the infant's insulin level may remain elevated, although there is no longer a need for it. This can lead to hypoglycemia, or low blood glucose. Continued hypoglycemia can lead to coma or death for the newborn. In addition, high insulin levels and poor control of the mother's blood glucose is associated with problems with the infant's heart and lung function.

Treatment and Therapy

Diet is the primary treatment for gestational diabetes. Depending on the meal planning approach, a certain number of calories and/or a certain amount of carbohydrates is prescribed. The total carbohydrates to be eaten is about 40 to 45 percent of total daily calories. Calories should be prescribed to allow for recommended weight gain during pregnancy and to prevent blood glucose from being either too high or too low. If caloric intake is too high, then the blood glucose level will rise, which is detrimental to the fetus. If caloric intake is too low, then the body will break down the mother's body fat or protein reserves to supply the needed energy. When this occurs, breakdown products called ketones are produced. Ketones in the mother's blood are also detrimental to the fetus.

Consistency, in the form of eating the same amount of food at the same time each day, is important. The diet must support three outcomes: blood glucose levels within a target range, adequate nutrient intake to support the pregnancy, and appropriate weight gain for pregnancy. If these three outcomes cannot be achieved by diet alone, then insulin will be used to achieve the desired blood glucose level. Oral hypoglycemic medications have not been tested for use in pregnancy and are not recommended.

Because achieving a normal or near-normal blood glucose level is so critical, the woman will monitor her blood glucose at home using a fingerstick blood sample and a home glucometer. Blood glucose levels are usually tested three to four times a day, although some women will need to test their blood glucose six times each day. Decisions about adjustments in diet and insulin will be based on blood glucose levels.

Usually blood glucose levels normalize postpartum, and continued diet or medication therapy is not needed. However, women who develop gestational diabetes have a higher likelihood of developing type II diabetes mellitus later in life. For women who have developed gestational diabetes, an oral glucose tolerance test is administered six to eight weeks postpartum and then at three-year intervals. These women should maintain an optimal weight, since obesity is strongly associated with type II diabetes onset.

Perspective and Prospects

Observations in the 1950's and 1960's that infants born to mothers who had an elevated blood glucose level had a higher rate of morbidity and mortality led to the screening, diagnosis, and treatment guidelines used today. Adherence to these guidelines has greatly improved the health of infants born to mothers with gestational diabetes. However, these infants do have a greater risk of becoming obese and/or developing diabetes in adolescence. Additionally, daughters of mothers who have had gestational diabetes have a greater likelihood of developing gestational diabetes themselves.

—*Karen Chapman-Novakofski, R.D., L.D., Ph.D.*

See also Cesarean section; Childbirth; Childbirth complications; Diabetes mellitus; Endocrine disorders; Endocrinology; Endocrinology, pediatric; Hormones; Hypoglycemia; Insulin resistance syndrome; Neonatology; Obesity; Perinatology; Pregnancy and gestation.

FOR FURTHER INFORMATION:

American Diabetes Association. *Gestational Diabetes: What to Expect.* Alexandria, Va.: Author, 2000.

Holler, Harold J., and Joyce Green Pastors. *Diabetes Medical Nutrition Therapy: A Professional Guide to Management and Nutrition Education Resources.* Chicago: American Dietetic Association, 1997.

Jovanovic-Peterson, Lois. *Managing Your Gestational Diabetes: A Guide for You and Your Baby's Good Health.* New York: John Wiley & Sons, 1998.

GIARDIASIS
DISEASE/DISORDER

ANATOMY OR SYSTEM AFFECTED: Gastrointestinal system

SPECIALTIES AND RELATED FIELDS: Family practice, gastroenterology, pediatrics

DEFINITION: An acute or chronic parasitic infection of the gastrointestinal system.

CAUSES AND SYMPTOMS

The parasite *Giardia lamblia*, which causes giardiasis, is a protozoan acquired through the ingestion of contaminated food or water. This organism can also be spread by person-to-person contact involving fecal contamination. It is the most frequent parasite acquired by children in day care centers and preschools.

After exposure, the incubation period before the onset of symptoms is one to two weeks. After infection, only 25 to 50 percent of affected individuals become symptomatic. The disease is characterized by abdominal pain, cramps, flatulence, weight loss, and diarrhea, which in many cases may be chronic (of a duration longer than fifteen days).

TREATMENT AND THERAPY

Some cases of giardiasis are self-limited. Symptomatic cases, however, in which the diagnosis has been con-

---

INFORMATION ON GIARDIASIS

CAUSES: Parasitic infection

SYMPTOMS: Often asymptomatic; can include abdominal pain, cramps, flatulence, weight loss, diarrhea

DURATION: One to two weeks; occasionally chronic

TREATMENTS: Medication (furazolidone, metronidazole, paromomycin)

---

firmed by laboratory studies, need to be treated. Furazolidone, metronidazole, and paromomycin are effective drugs in the treatment of giardiasis. Furazolidone and metronidazole are equally efficacious; the first may be more practical in children because of its availability in liquid form.

Giardiasis can be prevented by strict hand-washing, especially in those individuals who are in close contact with patients with diarrhea or children in diapers at day care centers. Another important consideration in the prevention of giardiasis resides in the purification of drinking water, which can be achieved through boiling or chemical decontamination. It has been demonstrated that breast-feeding protects infants against symptomatic infection.

PERSPECTIVE AND PROSPECTS

G. lamblia was first observed by microscopist Antoni van Leeuwenhoek in 1675. It was once considered a harmless organism, but its pathogenic role was clearly established in the 1960's. This parasite is one of the most common protozoans able to infect humans in the United States and other developed countries.

—*Benjamin Estrada, M.D.*

See also Diarrhea and dysentery; Food poisoning; Gastroenterology; Gastroenterology, pediatric; Gastrointestinal system; Parasitic diseases; Protozoan diseases.

FOR FURTHER INFORMATION:

Biddle, Wayne. *Field Guide to Germs.* 2d ed. New York: Anchor Books, 2002.

Despommier, Dickson D., Robert W. Gwadz, and Peter J. Hotex. *Parasitic Diseases.* 4th ed. New York: Appletree Productions, 2000.

Gutteridge, W. E., and G. H. Coombs. *Biochemistry of Parasitic Protozoa.* Baltimore: University Park Press, 1977.

Roberts, Larry S., and John Janovy, Jr., eds. *Gerald D. Schmidt and Larry S. Roberts' Foundations of Parasitology.* Rev. 7th ed. Boston: McGraw-Hill, 2003.

GIGANTISM

DISEASE/DISORDER

ALSO KNOWN AS: Acromegaly

ANATOMY OR SYSTEM AFFECTED: Arms, bones, brain, circulatory system, endocrine system, eyes, hands, hair, legs, musculoskeletal system, reproductive system

SPECIALTIES AND RELATED FIELDS: Biochemistry, cardiology, endocrinology, family practice, general surgery, internal medicine, neurology

DEFINITION: A rare congenital disease that begins in children with pituitary gland tumors that make too much growth hormone, which yields pituitary giants who often die at relatively young ages. After adolescence, the disease is manifested as acromegaly, which is quite serious over the long term.

KEY TERMS:

acromegaly: a disease of adults initially characterized by pathological enlargement of bones of the hands, feet, and face; caused by chronic pituitary gland overproduction of growth hormone by tumors

congenital: referring to a condition (such as a health problem) present or occurring at birth

growth hormone: a hormone produced by the pituitary gland that mediates overall growth

pituitary gland: a peanut-sized gland at the base of the vertebrate brain; its hormone secretions control many other hormone-producing (endocrine) glands and hence control growth, gender maturation, and many other life processes

CAUSES AND SYMPTOMS

Gigantism is a rare disease caused by the presence of tumors of the peanut-sized pituitary gland, located at the base of the brain. Such tumors produce an excess of growth hormone, the biomolecule responsible for overall growth. In children or adolescents having these tumors, excess growth hormone results in overgrowth of all parts of the body. Gigantism occurs because the bones of the arms and legs have not yet calcified and can grow much longer than usual. Hence, an afflicted child becomes very large in size and very tall, often reaching a height of more than 6 feet, 6 inches.

A young child afflicted with pituitary gigantism grows in height as much as 6 inches per year. Thus, an important symptom that identifies the problem is that such children are much taller and larger than others of the same age. In many cases, this great size difference may lead to individuals who are more than twice the height of their playmates. Excessive growth of this sort should lead parents to seek the immediate advice of their family physician, who can aid in the selection of a specialist to identify the problem and develop an appropriate treatment.

As gigantism proceeds, pituitary tumors often invade and replace the rest of the pituitary gland. This is unfortunate, because the pituitary gland produces several other hormones—called trophic hormones—which control mental processes, gender maturation, and healthy overall growth. Consequently, prolonged, untreated gigantism may yield a huge individual who is mentally ill, possessed of various psychoses, sexually immature, and quite unhealthy. In addition, the human musculoskeletal system is not designed to accommodate individuals attaining the great heights of many postadolescent pituitary giants. Hence, it is fairly common that the giants have great difficulty standing and walking; some can do so only with the aid of canes. Moreover, the average life expectancy of a full-sized pituitary giant is shorter than that of individuals of normal stature, and many die by the middle of the third decade of their lives.

In cases where pituitary tumors that oversecrete growth hormone occur after calcification of the long bones is complete—after adolescence—gigantism will not occur. Such individuals develop acromegaly. This often-fatal disease, progressive throughout life, thickens bones and causes the overgrowth of all body organs. Hands and feet grow larger, and the lower jaw, brow ridges, nose, and ears enlarge, coarsening the features. More damaging is the development of headaches, high blood pressure that can lead to heart attacks, irritability,

---

INFORMATION ON GIGANTISM

CAUSES: Congenital endocrine disorder resulting in pituitary gland tumors

SYMPTOMS: Enlargement of bones of hands, feet, and face; excessive growth and height; sometimes mental illness; sexual immaturity; difficulty walking and standing

DURATION: Lifelong

TREATMENTS: Chemotherapy, antigrowth hormone drugs, surgery, radiation therapy

and even cancer over the long run. It should be noted that these disabilities are rarely seen in pediatric patients and most often begin in the fourth decade of life. Many medical scientists believe that pituitary gigantism and acromegaly are the basis for the legends about giants and ogres.

TREATMENT AND THERAPY

If a diagnosis of gigantism or acromegaly seems probable, the physician or specialist involved will order a blood test to identify the amount of growth hormone present in the body. Computed tomography (CT) and magnetic resonance imaging (MRI) scans will also be carried out, especially in those suspected of having acromegaly, to identify possible organ changes away from normal size. In cases where growth hormone levels are high and cannot be reduced by chemotherapy—for example, with antigrowth hormone drugs such as somatostatin and bromocriptine—and/or a tumor is identified as being present via CT and MRI, surgery or radiation therapy to destroy the tumor will be attempted.

PERSPECTIVE AND PROSPECTS

It must be recognized that the success of any therapeutic regimens or their combination will prevent additional gigantism or symptoms of acromegaly from occurring. It is not possible, however, to reverse preexisting consequences of the pituitary tumors on young children and adolescent pituitary giants or older giants and acromegalics.

For this reason, it is essential for worried parents or adult patients to visit an appropriate physician as quickly as possible. Such foresight will usually minimize problems associated with either manifestation of pituitary tumors and enable an afflicted individual to have the best possible future life. In addition to extirpating causative tumors, it will then become possible, after additional blood tests plus the thorough examination of CT and MRI data, to identify which body organs need to be treated and to arrest or minimize health complications, such as those associated with the reproductive, cardiovascular, and musculoskeletal systems.

—*Sanford S. Singer, Ph.D.*

See also Birth defects; Bones and the skeleton; Congenital heart disease; Dwarfism; Endocrine disorders; Endocrine system; Endocrinology; Endocrinology, pediatric; Growth; Hormones; Orthopedics, pediatric.

FOR FURTHER INFORMATION:

Berkow, Robert, and Andrew J. Fletcher, eds. *Merck Manual of Diagnosis and Therapy.* 17th ed. Rahway, N.J.: Merck Sharp & Dohme Research Laboratories, 1999. This book abounds with useful data on the characteristics, etiology, diagnosis, and treatment of gigantism. Written for physicians, it is also quite useful to general readers.

Brooks, S. J., and Robert S. Bar. *Early Diagnosis and Treatment of Endocrine Disorders.* Totowa, N.J.: Humana Press, 2003. Reviews the early signs and symptoms of endocrine diseases, surveys the clinical testing needed for a diagnosis, and presents recommendations for therapy.

Griffin, James E., and Sergio R. Ojeda, eds. *Textbook of Endocrine Physiology.* 5th ed. New York: Oxford University Press, 2004. A detailed account of normal and abnormal functioning of the endocrine system. Written by specialists.

Henry, Helen L., and Anthony W. Norman, eds. *Encyclopedia of Hormones.* 3 vols. San Diego, Calif.: Academic Press, 2003. A comprehensive overview of the role of hormones, the major physiological systems in which they operate, and the biological consequences of an excess or deficiency of a particular hormone.

Imura, Hiroo, ed. *The Pituitary Gland.* 2d ed. New York: Raven Press, 1994. Discusses such topics as the physiology of the pituitary gland, pituitary hormones, the hypothalamo-hypophyseal system, and the diagnosis of pituitary diseases.

Landau, Elaine. *Standing Tall: Unusually Tall People.* New York: Franklin Watts, 1997. This respectful treatment of a sensitive subject opens with actual, personal stories. It explores the role of unusually sized characters in folklore, then explains the causes and challenges of uncommon growth patterns.

Melmed, Schlomo, et al. *The Pituitary.* 2d ed. Boston: Blackwell Scientific, 2002. Text covering the biochemistry, molecular biology, physiology, pathophysiology, and clinical aspects of the pituitary. Sections include hypothalamic-pituitary function, hypothalamic-pituitary dysfunction, pituitary tumors, pituitary disease in systemic disorders, and diagnostic procedures.

GINGIVITIS

DISEASE/DISORDER

ANATOMY OR SYSTEM AFFECTED: Gums, mouth, teeth

SPECIALTIES AND RELATED FIELDS: Bacteriology, biochemistry, dentistry

DEFINITION: A gum disease that begins when plaque and calculus cause gum inflammation and bleeding. It can lead to periodontitis, which is associated with tooth loss, cardiovascular disease, and diabetes.

KEY TERMS:

collagen: a fibrous protein of bone, cartilage, and connective tissue

epithelium: a tissue made of closely arranged cells that covers most internal surfaces and organs

gingiva: tissue surrounding the teeth

periodontitis: gum disease that causes bone and tooth loss

INFORMATION ON GINGIVITIS

CAUSES: Irritation of the gums by dental plaque and tartar; sometimes occurs with colds and influenza or with hormonal changes

SYMPTOMS: Inflammation and bleeding of gums, which become red or reddish-purple

DURATION: Chronic; sometimes acute

TREATMENTS: Removal of plaque and tartar

CAUSES AND SYMPTOMS

Healthy pink gingiva (gums) end at tooth bases in epithelium-covered connective tissue, detached from teeth for 0.15 to 0.30 millimeter. This free gingiva is demarcated from the next gum portion, attached gingiva, by a gingival groove. The space between free gingiva and a tooth is the gingival sulcus. Attached gingiva is bound to the bone that it covers and is 3 to 6 millimeters deep. Free gingiva between teeth, interdental papillae, extend upward in the front of teeth and make the gums look scalloped. All gingival epithelium covers connective tissue holding collagen fibers. Gingival sulcus epithelium holds oral crevicular and junctional epithelium (JE). JE forms a tooth collar, joined to tooth surfaces. Each collar girdles the neck of a tooth and prevents marginal gingivitis and periodontitis.

Gingivitis begins when plaque and calculus irritate free gingiva, causing inflammation and bleeding. Unchecked, it leads to the more serious periodontitis, resulting in tooth loss, cardiovascular disease, and diabetes. Plaque starts as aggregates of bacteria and their capsules on tooth surfaces. It forms in a protein film deposited on the surfaces and thickens as bacteria become established in a growing matrix of protein and capsule polysaccharide, extending into attached gingiva. Plaque and bacterial toxins damage tissue, producing gingivitis by irritating free gingiva, loosening collars around teeth, and causing the detachment of attached gingiva. Plaque is best identified via disclosing solutions of dyes (such as erythrosin). Many view it as the main factor in initial gingival inflammation. Plaque calcification produces calculus, which is most problematic when it causes irritation if gingiva push up against it.

Acute gingivitis of several types is short term and of minor interest. Nonspecific acute gingivitis occurs with colds and influenza. It causes diffuse redness, swelling, and discomfort but resolves quickly upon recovery. Localized acute gingivitis arises from gingival trauma (such as hard food). Removing its causes promotes rapid healing. Ulcerative acute gingivitis, called trench mouth, occurs widely, mostly in the teens or twenties. Patients report soreness, eating difficulty, facile gum bleeds, and headache. It also occurs in heavy smokers as a result of chemical and thermal irritation.

Chronic marginal gingivitis, which accounts for most cases, begins with the reddening and swelling of interdental papilla and/or the gingival margin. Attempts to explore a sulcus cause bleeding. Enlargement, as a result of edema or hyperplasia, may be extensive and followed, after years of disease, by chronic periodontitis where supporting bone is lost. The initial symptoms of chronic marginal gingivitis reported most often are gingival bleeding, either spontaneous or caused by brushing or chewing; gingival margin recession; gums coming away from teeth; gingival enlargement; and color change to red or reddish-purple.

Three types of chronic marginal gingivitis are associated with sex hormones in people who do not practice good oral hygiene: chronic marginal gingivitis of puberty, pregnancy, and menopause. In the puberty type, the hormone changes come with approaching adulthood are causative. Puberty gingivitis is often accompanied by hyperplasia of interdental papillae. Pregnancy gingivitis occurs in women whose chronic marginal gingivitis worsens after the first trimester. The culprits here, changed blood-vessel permeability and increased inflammation, are the result of hormone changes. The condition produces severe inflammation, marked edema, gingival enlargement, and loose teeth. With good oral hygiene, these problems disappear by the third trimester or birth. Menopausal chronic marginal gingivitis, which can occur at and after the menopause, causes blotchy, reddened attached gingiva, starting as blisters. It may be immunological, the result of patients developing antibodies to their own epithelia.

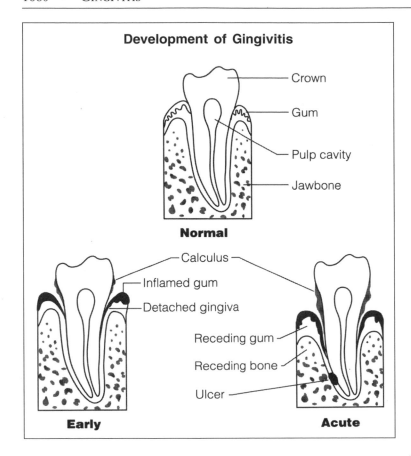

Development of Gingivitis

Crown

Gum

Pulp cavity

Jawbone

Normal

Calculus

Inflamed gum

Detached gingiva

Receding gum

Receding bone

Ulcer

Early

Acute

TREATMENT AND THERAPY

Trench mouth is treated with bacteria-killing penicillin or peroxide. The key to treating chronic marginal gingivitis begins by determining gum health from gingival sulcus depth. To obtain this measurement, a metal probe is inserted into the gingiva at several mouth sites until slight resistance is felt. Sulcus depths under 0.30 millimeter indicate healthy gums. Greater depths indicate chronic marginal gingivitis. The deeper the sulcus, the more serious is the gingivitis. The first gingivitis-related dental visit begins with sulcus examination.

When chronic marginal gingivitis is apparent, most plaque and calculus is removed, and the patient is quizzed on oral hygiene habits. The information gained is used to plan several more visits to prove that the patient practices good oral hygiene and to remove any remaining plaque and calculus. The larger and deeper the deposits and the longer exposure to poor hygiene, the more visits are required.

Most chronic marginal gingivitis disappears after dental cleaning and ensuing good oral hygiene. Calculus and plaque removal eliminates the source of irritation and causes healing. Gums become healthy in a few weeks. Mild periodontitis requires more extensive treatment: Bacterial pockets are cleaned out, and antiseptic mouthwash or toothpaste is prescribed. Severe periodontitis may require surgery.

PERSPECTIVE AND PROSPECTS

The best current way to treat gingivitis is preventing it via good oral hygiene, which consists of regular brushing and periodic dental cleaning to prevent plaque and calculus buildup. It is best to brush all teeth and gums with a soft-bristled brush and fluoride toothpaste. Brushing should be done at least twice daily, in the morning and at bedtime. Daily flossing is also recommended. Floss is used to scrape the underside of each tooth, just below the gum line, to remove interdental plaque and to massage the gums. In addition to good daily oral hygiene, annual or semiannual dental visits for cleaning and checkup are valuable.

Curing chronic marginal gingivitis and preventing periodontitis are now thought to diminish the risk of heart disease and stroke, as relationships between oral bacteria and clogged arteries have arisen from recent research. A relationship also exists between diabetes mellitus and chronic marginal gingivitis or periodontitis: Diabetes increases the risk of developing periodontitis, and oral infection makes blood glucose harder to control. People having serious periodontitis and lung problems may inhale mouth bacteria and develop pneumonia. It is believed that susceptibility to gingivitis differs between individuals, so study of the genetics and immunology of gingivitis may have the potential to provide better treatments as well as vaccines.

—*Sanford S. Singer, Ph.D.*

See also Cavities; Dental diseases; Dentistry; Endodontic disease; Gum disease; Periodontal surgery; Periodontitis; Root canal treatment; Teeth; Tooth extraction; Toothache.

FOR FURTHER INFORMATION:

Cook, Allan R. *Oral Health Sourcebook: Basic Information About Diseases and Concepts.* Detroit: Omnigraphics, 1998. Includes much information on oral disease, including gingivitis and periodontitis.

Cross, William G. *Gingivitis*. 2d ed. Bristol, England: J. Wright, 1977. This classic work contains many facts on the disease, as well as excellent illustrations.

Wilson, Thomas G., and Kenneth S. Kornman. *Fundamentals of Periodontics*. Chicago: Quintessence, 2003. A complete source on periodontics and periodontal diseases of all types.

GLANDS

ANATOMY

ANATOMY OR SYSTEM AFFECTED: Breasts, endocrine system, gastrointestinal system, genitals, nervous system, pancreas, reproductive system, skin

SPECIALTIES AND RELATED FIELDS: Biochemistry, dermatology, endocrinology, gastroenterology, gynecology, vascular medicine

DEFINITION: Organs or areas of the body that produce, store, and secrete fluids, exerting a profound effect on growth, energy production, chemical balance, reproduction, and health.

KEY TERMS:

adrenal glands: the endocrine glands on top of the kidneys, which produce a large number of hormones involved in metabolism and in response to stress

endocrine system: the system of glands located throughout the body that produces hormones and secretes them directly into the blood for delivery by the circulatory system

hormone: a product of the endocrine glands transported throughout the bloodstream which controls and regulates other glands or organs by chemical stimulation

pancreas: the gland located under the stomach that produces insulin and glucagon, the hormones responsible for control of the body's blood sugar level

parathyroid glands: four tiny structures on the back of the thyroid, chiefly concerned with the regulation of calcium and phosphorus

pituitary gland: a tiny gland located under the brain which controls the thyroid, adrenal, and sex glands

sex glands: the ovaries in the female and the testes in the male, which secrete hormones involved in reproduction

thyroid gland: an endocrine gland located in the neck, which regulates the rate of energy production throughout the body

STRUCTURE AND FUNCTIONS

A gland is any tissue or organ that produces and releases a fluid. Some, such as digestive or sweat glands, secrete their juices through a duct or tube. These glands are known as exocrine glands, meaning "externally secreting." Other glands pass their secretions directly into the blood that flows through them. Known as endocrine or "internally secreting" glands, these are the ones that produce hormones. This article will focus only on the endocrine glands and their hormones that control, stimulate, and regulate almost every important function in the body.

Although there are hundreds of known or suspected hormones, there are only several major endocrine glands to produce them. They include the pituitary, pineal gland, and hypothalamus in the brain; the thyroid, parathyroid glands, and thymus in the neck; and the adrenal glands and pancreas in the abdomen. In addition, the female ovaries in the pelvic cavity and the male testes in the scrotum contribute their hormones to the widespread work of the endocrine system.

The largest endocrine organ, the thyroid, is quite small, weighing only about an ounce. It is butterfly-shaped and wrapped around the windpipe in the throat. By means of the two iodine-containing hormones that it produces, called thyroxine (T_4) and triiodothyronine (T_3), this gland controls the rate of the body's metabolism; that is, these hormones control the speed at which energy-producing chemical reactions occur in all the cells of the body. They also play a crucial role in oxygen use, protein synthesis, and the development of the central nervous system. A third thyroid secretion, calcitonin, has a completely different role. By opposing the work of the parathyroids discussed below, it prevents the existence of too much calcium in the blood.

The four tiny parathyroid glands on the back of the thyroid are each only 0.25-inch wide. They supply parathyroid hormone, which maintains the proper balance of calcium in various parts of the body. It is very important to the bones, nerves, muscles, and blood that each contain the exact amount of calcium needed to function correctly. If there is not enough calcium, parathyroid hormone instructs the intestine to absorb more calcium and the kidneys to retain more. If the blood still has an insufficient level of calcium, parathyroid hormone causes it to be released from storage in the bones.

The pancreas, found behind the stomach, is unusual because it is both an exocrine gland, producing digestive enzymes for the intestine, and an important endocrine gland. Its major hormones, insulin and glucagon, are the major regulators of the blood sugar level. Soon after a meal is digested, insulin is released, enabling all cells in general but liver cells in particular to take excess sugar out of the blood at a rapid rate. The liver's stored sugar is then released steadily into the blood between meals because of the steady glucagon production in the pancreas. The careful balancing of these two hormones enables the body to have just the right sugar content in the blood at all times.

The hormones that bring about the most striking changes in both anatomy and behavior are known as the sex hormones. Because sex hormone levels are high in the fetus, they directly influence the development of its sex organs.

Somewhere around the age of eleven, the level of a girl's estrogens rises sharply, causing female puberty. These hormones, produced in the two ovaries (located in the pelvic cavity), cause breast development, the growth of pubic and underarm hair, and the broadening of hips and thighs. Each month of the woman's life until the menopause, the ovarian estrogen and progesterone levels rise and fall, controlling the release of an egg or ovum from her ovary. These same hormones have prepared the uterus to support and nourish a developing embryo if the egg is fertilized.

The two testes, located in the scrotal sac, by their production of testosterone and other androgens bring about male puberty around the age of thirteen. These hormones are responsible for such male secondary sex characteristics as facial hair, deepening of the voice, and heavier muscles and bones. The testes' secretions seem also to cause the greater aggressiveness of men compared to women. Their prime function, however, is aiding the production of healthy sperm.

The two-inch-long adrenal glands, perched on top of the kidneys, are actually two glands in one. The outer 80 percent is called the cortex, while the inner part is named the medulla. The adrenals produce dozens of hormones, most of which are involved in some way with one's ability to cope with stress. One of the major adrenal cortex hormones is cortisol. It helps maintain blood pressure, regulates fluid levels, directs protein and sugar metabolism, increases or decreases body fat reserves, and affects the immune system. A second area of the cortex secretes aldosterone, which directs the kidney to retain sodium and excrete potassium, controlling their levels in the blood. The third cortex area, surprisingly, produces some testosterone and estrogen in both males and females.

The adrenal medulla responds to sudden stress by pouring epinephrine, formerly called adrenaline, into the blood. Dramatic changes in the working of the heart, lungs, liver, muscles, and many other organs then enable the body to cope with sudden emergencies.

The thymus gland, behind the breastbone, is very unusual because it is quite large in a newborn, grows throughout childhood, but shrinks drastically from puberty onward. It is the source of several important secretions, including thymosin, which activates the T cells and B cells. These lymphocytes, a type of white blood cell, provide immunity to disease by destroying invading organisms.

The tiny pineal gland, less than a quarter of an inch long, is embedded close to the very center of the brain. Although the exact function of this pinecone-shaped structure is a mystery, it appears to be the only gland producing melatonin. Proven to be involved in seasonal reproduction in other mammals, melatonin seems to be related to puberty in humans.

The careful and precise control of most of these glands is the work of the pituitary, causing it to be called "the master gland." This small gland, about 0.5 inch in size, has three distinct parts: the front or anterior pituitary, the back or posterior pituitary, and a tiny middle section.

The anterior pituitary sends thyroid-stimulating hormone (TSH) to the thyroid, causing it to release T_3 and T_4. It also secretes adrenocorticotropic hormone (ACTH), which causes the adrenal cortex to give off its many secretions. In the female, the follicle-stimulating hormone (FSH) that the anterior pituitary sends to the ovary causes an egg to mature, while in the male it fosters sperm development. Luteinizing hormone (LH), from the anterior pituitary, triggers the monthly release of an egg and then coaxes the ovary to produce progesterone. The male's LH causes clusters of cells in the testes, called interstitial cells, to produce testosterone. As if these were not enough important jobs for the anterior pituitary to have, it also secretes growth hormone (GH) to stimulate body growth until maturity and secretes prolactin or lactogenic hormone to cause the female breast to produce milk for a nursing baby.

The posterior pituitary secretes only two hormones: oxytocin, which brings about labor and birth, and antidiuretic hormone (ADH), which is also known as vasopressin. ADH causes the kidney to reabsorb the proper amount of water needed by the body, a most important function.

Long after the anterior pituitary was named "the master gland," it was learned that the hypothalamus is the master of the master. This small area of tissue below the brain produces a number of releasing hormones and inhibiting hormones which, in turn, carefully control the anterior pituitary's secretion of FSH, LH, TSH,

ACTH, prolactin, and growth hormone. The hypothalamus is also the source of oxytocin and ADH, which is then stored by the posterior pituitary until it is needed by the body.

DISORDERS AND DISEASES

In 1970, only a few dozen hormones from the endocrine glands were known to medical science. By 1990, at least two hundred had been discovered. An understanding of their actions and interactions has generated numerous helpful medical applications.

These complex interactions, involving the concept of feedback, have made possible many treatments for defective glands. Feedback means that healthy glands are self-regulating. For example, more calcium in the blood causes less parathyroid hormone to be released, and then the lowered amount of blood calcium causes more parathyroid hormone production. All glands have

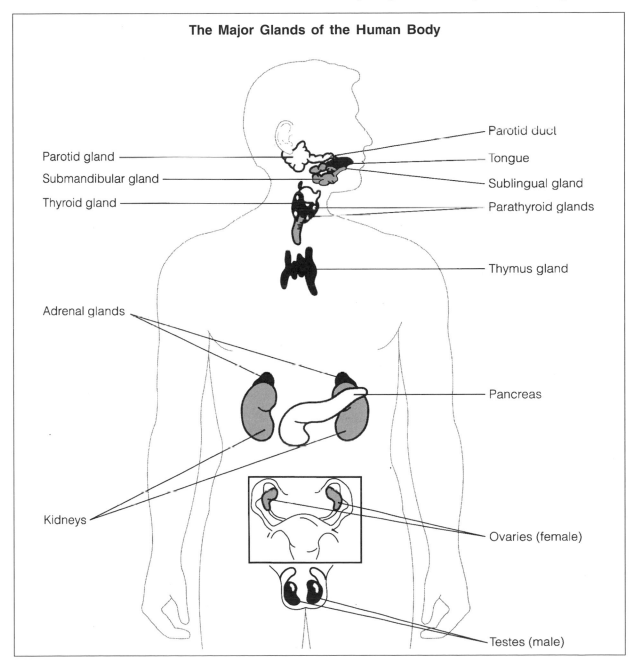

The Major Glands of the Human Body

Parotid gland
Submandibular gland
Thyroid gland
Adrenal glands
Kidneys

Parotid duct
Tongue
Sublingual gland
Parathyroid glands
Thymus gland
Pancreas
Ovaries (female)
Testes (male)

these feedback loops, but those involving the hypothalamus, pituitary, and one of its target glands are particularly complicated.

Appropriate medical treatment of thyroid disease, for example, requires careful understanding of its feedback mechanism. An increase in thyroid-stimulating hormone releasing hormones (TRH) from the hypothalamus normally causes the pituitary to give off its thyroid-stimulating hormone. This in turn triggers the production of thyroxine and triiodothyronine.

The type of thyroid disease in which insufficient thyroid hormones are produced is called hypothyroidism. It is quite common, with one in every one thousand men and two in every one hundred women afflicted at some time during life. It is often caused by an inability of the thyroid gland to produce enough hormone, the result of a disease of the pituitary that prevents it from producing TSH or a disease of the hypothalamus that prevents it from producing TRH. Surprisingly, an underactive thyroid is often enlarged but still unable to produce enough T_3 or T_4. This enlargement is called a goiter. In the type called Hashimoto's disease, the hypothyroidism develops because the body mistakenly produces antibodies that destroy the thyroid tissue.

Because of the complexity of the chemical feedback loop involved in thyroid gland control, many cases of hypothyroidism have been caused inadvertently by drugs given for other conditions. Among these medicines are lithium carbonate, used to treat manic depressives; expectorants containing potassium iodide, prescribed for respiratory infections; and a host of other drugs. Physicians prescribing these drugs and patients using them need to watch carefully for the development of symptoms such as intolerance to cold, puffy face and back of hands, weight gain, high blood pressure, yellowed skin, and loss of hair.

Adults afflicted with hypothyroidism, no matter what the cause, also commonly suffer some disturbances to their nervous system, experiencing lethargy, slowness of thought, poor memory, and slowness of reaction to events occurring around them. Even more disastrous are the effects of an underactive thyroid in infants, where it causes mental retardation and stunted physical growth. If diagnosed early enough, the infant can be successfully treated in the same manner as an adult, with lifelong daily doses of TSH, T_3, and T_4 in individually and carefully adjusted amounts.

In addition, like any gland, the thyroid can oversecrete as well as undersecrete. Hypersecretion is also quite common, with three or four out of one thousand people having this disease, the majority being women. The resulting excessive rate of metabolism causes many possible symptoms including intolerance to heat, irritability, excessive perspiration, heart palpitations, rapid weight loss, weakness, shortness of breath, and sore, bulging eyes.

There are two main types of hyperthyroidism. By far the most common is called Graves' disease. It is brought about when the patient's own immune system creates antibodies that cause continuous excess hormone production by the thyroid even though the pituitary is sending the normal amount of TSH. The less common cases of hyperthyroidism involve lumps or nodules that form in the thyroid and oversecrete T_3 and T_4 for no apparent reason. One of three treatments is usually used to cure hyperthyroidism: Radioactive iodine is given to destroy part of the overactive gland, surgery is used to remove part of the gland, or certain drugs are prescribed that prevent the thyroid from producing its hormones.

As common as thyroid disorders are, there is no endocrine disorder as common as diabetes mellitus, which afflicts one out of every one thousand people. When certain cells of the pancreas are destroyed and cannot produce insulin, the person is said to have insulin-dependent diabetes (IDD). This type is most often found in children and young adults. Non-insulin-dependent diabetes (NIDD) occurs more frequently in middle-aged and older people. This condition occurs because the person's tissues become resistant to the insulin; no matter how much the pancreas tries to produce it, sugar is not able to enter the tissues properly. IDD patients are suspected to have been born with genes that make their immune systems destroy their insulin-producing pancreatic cells by mistake, after they have been exposed to certain viruses. NIDD also seems to be inherited, but stress, various illnesses, and obesity rather than viruses trigger the lack of response to insulin as the person ages.

Patients who develop either type of diabetes mellitus usually soon exhibit some if not all of the following symptoms: constant thirst and urination; loss of weight, strength, and energy; frequent hunger pains; and the inability of cuts or bruises to heal. The long-term effects of the very high blood sugar level of diabetics vary from patient to patient. They often include heart disease and high blood pressure, unhealed wounds which become gangrenous, kidney failure, endless infections, nerve damage, and possible coma.

Treatment for diabetes attempts to make the body's

cells absorb sugar normally. This can often be achieved through diet, medicines that stimulate insulin production, other drugs that make the tissues more responsive to the work of insulin, and, if necessary, injections of insulin itself. These traditional methods may or may not ever be completely replaced by exciting possibilities explored in the early 1990's: insulin pumps to deliver a steady supply and full or partial pancreas transplants.

Although no one objects to attempts to aid sufferers of thyroid disorders or diabetes mellitus, ethical questions have arisen concerning defects in some endocrine glands. A striking example involves a lack of growth hormone from the pituitary. Doctors, parents, and youngsters often disagree over whether GH therapy should be given to a child who is noticeably shorter than peers at a given age. Because GH, like any hormone, may produce many unwanted side effects, there is much controversy over this particular medical application of endocrine gland research.

PERSPECTIVE AND PROSPECTS

Glands, together with the nervous system, are the body's means of control and coordination. Given this fact, the discovery of each gland's functions had ramifications for medical science as a whole.

Although the ancient Greeks, Romans, and Chinese suspected the importance of some glands, it was only in the seventeenth century that scientists began to acquire useful knowledge of them. At that time, the Englishman Thomas Wharton first recognized the difference between duct and ductless glands. In the 1660's, Théophile Bordeu, a Frenchman regarded by many as the founder of endocrinology, declared that some parts of the body gave off "emanations" that had dramatic effects on other parts of the body. Following Bordeu's lead, the Dutchman Fredrik Ruysch claimed in the 1690's that the thyroid poured important substances into the bloodstream.

Then, in 1775, Percival Platt made an unusual discovery in London while repairing a hernia in a female patient. When he inadvertently removed her ovaries, the woman's menstrual period ceased. This led John Davidge to realize the importance of the ovaries in controlling menstruation. Also in the late 1700's, doctors began to associate a swollen neck, bulging eyes, and a racing pulse with a swollen thyroid gland; they suspected a cause-and-effect relationship.

Thomas Addison, an English physician, found diseased adrenals by autopsy in a group of patients who had exhibited all the same symptoms. He published in 1849 that he definitely suspected another cause-and-effect relationship. That same year, the first experimental proof of the functions of a hormone was found by A. A. Berthold in Germany. Roosters whose testes he had removed lost all usual male characteristics. Testes that had been left free in the abdomens of other birds soon attached themselves, grew blood vessels, and produced the expected rooster characteristics.

Two major breakthroughs occurred in the late 1800's when Paul Langerhans found the actual pancreas cell clusters, called islets, that produce insulin and when Charles-Edouard Brown-Séquard developed a technique to use extracts from glands to determine their function.

The year 1900 brought three major discoveries: William Bayliss and Ernest Starling found that a chemical messenger from the intestine causes the pancreas to excrete digestive juice; Jokichi Takamine discovered that adrenaline increases heart rate and blood pressure; and Alfred Frölich described dwarfed individuals who had suffered previous pituitary damage.

In 1914, in Minnesota, Edward Kendall obtained the chemical he named thyroxine from animal thyroids. Similarly, in 1921, Frederick Banting and Charles Best isolated insulin from the pancreases of animals. By 1948, Kendall and many other workers had isolated two dozen adrenal cortex hormones; Philip Hench made medical news when he first used the one named cortisone to relieve, though not cure, arthritis.

By the mid-1970's, Rosalind Yalow and her colleagues had perfected a technique called radioimmunoassay, which uses radioactive materials to measure minute quantities of hormones. This enables physicians to measure the circulating level of nearly every hormone and diagnose anyone with an excess or deficiency. Many hormones such as insulin, growth hormone, and estrogen can then be given to supplement what the body is underproducing; they have been very expensive and hard to obtain in quantity from animals or deceased humans. By the 1980's, however, recombinant DNA technology and the polymerase chain reaction (PCR) offered unlimited, pure, and readily accessible hormones.

—Grace D. Matzen

See also Abscess drainage; Abscesses; Addison's disease; Adrenalectomy; Brain; Breasts, female; Corticosteroids; Cyst removal; Cysts; Diabetes mellitus; Dwarfism; Endocrine disorders; Endocrinology; Endocrinology, pediatric; Gigantism; Goiter; Hashimoto's thyroiditis; Hormone replacement therapy (HRT);

Hormones; Hyperparathyroidism and hypoparathyroidism; Hypoglycemia; Mastectomy and lumpectomy; Mumps; Pancreas; Parathyroidectomy; Prostate gland; Prostate gland removal; Sjögren's syndrome; Systems and organs; Testicular surgery; Thyroid disorders; Thyroid gland; Thyroidectomy.

FOR FURTHER INFORMATION:

Brook, Charles G. D., and Nicholas J. Marshall. *Essential Endocrinology*. Rev. 4th ed. Cambridge, Mass.: Blackwell Scientific, 2001. This text addresses the field of endocrinology, describing the physiology of the endocrine glands and the hormones that they produce. Includes an index.

Goodman, H. Maurice. *Basic Medical Endocrinology*. 3d ed. San Diego, Calif.: Academic Press, 2003. Focuses on research advances in the understanding of hormones involved in regulating most aspects of bodily functions. Includes in-depth coverage of individual glands and regulatory principles.

Henry, Helen L., and Anthony W. Norman, eds. *Encyclopedia of Hormones*. 3 vols. San Diego, Calif.: Academic Press, 2003. A comprehensive overview of the role of hormones, the major physiological systems in which they operate, and the biological consequences of an excess or deficiency of a particular hormone.

Little, Marjorie. *The Endocrine System*. Rev. ed. New York: Chelsea House, 2000. This volume is intended not only to provide basic knowledge but also to enable the general reader to pursue the subject through its lengthy bibliography. Also includes a helpful glossary and an extensive list of organizations which will provide further information.

Ruggieri, Paul. *A Simple Guide to Thyroid Disorders: From Diagnosis to Treatment*. Omaha, Nebr.: Addicus Books, 2003. A user-friendly guide that covers how the thyroid gland works, and explains common disorders, including hypothyroidism and hyperthyroidism. Special attention is given to how thyroid diseases affect specific populations such as women, children, and the elderly.

Scanlon, Valerie, et al. *Essentials of Anatomy and Physiology*. 4th ed. Philadelphia: F. A. Davis, 2002. A text designed around three themes: the relationship between physiology and anatomy, the interrelations among the organ systems, and the relationship of each organ system to homeostasis.

Wilson, Jean D. *Wilson's Textbook of Endocrinology*. 10th ed. New York: Elsevier, 2003. Text that covers the spectrum of information related to the endocrine system, including thyroid disorders, diabetes, endocrinology and aging, female reproduction and fertility control, sexual function and dysfunction, kidney stones, and endocrine hypertension.

GLAUCOMA
DISEASE/DISORDER
ANATOMY OR SYSTEM AFFECTED: Eyes
SPECIALTIES AND RELATED FIELDS: Ophthalmology, optometry
DEFINITION: A group of eye diseases characterized by an increase in the eye's intraocular pressure; early diagnosis through regular eye examinations can manage the effects of the disease, while late diagnosis may result in impaired vision or blindness.

KEY TERMS:
aqueous humor: the liquid filling the space between the lens and the cornea of the eye, which nourishes and lubricates them

ciliary body: a structure built of muscle and blood vessels which produces the aqueous humor

cornea: the curved, transparent membrane forming the front of the outer coat of the eyeball that serves primarily as protection and focuses light onto the lens

intraocular pressure: the degree of firmness of the eyeball, as controlled by the proper secretion and drainage of the aqueous humor

lens: a transparent, flexible structure, convex on both surfaces and lying directly behind the iris of the eye; it focuses light rays onto the retina

ophthalmic laser: a high-intensity beam of light which permits a surgeon to cut tissue precisely in the treatment of eye diseases

optic disc: the portion of the optic nerve at its point of entrance into the rear of the eye

peripheral vision: side vision, or the visual perception to all sides of the central object being viewed

retina: the thin, delicate, and transparent sheet of nerve tissue that receives visual stimuli and transmits them to the brain through the optic nerve

tonometer: an instrument used to measure the eye's intraocular pressure, thus checking for the presence of glaucoma

CAUSES AND SYMPTOMS
Glaucoma is an eye disease caused by higher-than-normal pressure inside the eye. The intraocular pressure can increase slowly or suddenly for various reasons but always with detrimental results. Of all the

possible causes of blindness, glaucoma is among the most common, but it is also the most preventable. If diagnosed early, it can be controlled and the loss of sight avoided. What complicates the problem is that the most common form of glaucoma shows no symptoms until extensive, irreversible damage has occurred.

To understand this disease, it is necessary to know what occurs within the eye when the intraocular pressure increases. The inner surface of the cornea is nourished by the aqueous humor, which is also called the aqueous fluid. This secretion from the ciliary body flows into the space behind the iris and then through the pupil into the space in front of the iris. Where the front of the iris joins the back of the cornea is a point called the venous sinus, at the anterior drainage angle. Here the aqueous humor is reabsorbed and transported to the bloodstream. In a normal eye, this drainage process works correctly and the balance between the amount secreted and the amount reabsorbed maintains a constant intraocular pressure. In glaucoma, the drainage part of the process works inefficiently. For a variety of reasons, some of which are not fully understood, the drainage mechanism is defective. The upset balance in secretion drainage causes the unwanted increase in intraocular pressure in one eye or, more commonly, in both. The iris is pushed forward, further inhibiting drainage of the aqueous fluid.

Even a very small elevation in intraocular pressure will affect the eye adversely, causing damage to its particularly delicate parts. Although the eye as a whole is quite tough, the optic nerve is vulnerable to increased pressure. This vital connection between the eye and the brain is damaged by the stress within the harder eyeball. The delicate nerve fibers and blood vessels of the optic disc, as the beginning of the optic nerve is called, then die. Once they die, they can never be regenerated or replaced, and blindness is the result. The destruction of the optic disc causes a condition called cupping. A normal optic disc is quite level with the retina. Glaucoma causes it to collapse, creating a genuine indentation. Thus, cupping is a definite sign of glaucoma.

The damage that glaucoma inflicts is progressive. The defect in drainage does not necessarily worsen, and the pressure, once elevated, does not necessarily continue to increase. Once begun, however, the killing of the optic nerve cells continues until the resulting loss of vision progresses to total blindness. The first nerve fibers to die are the ones near the outer edge of the optic disc, which originates near the periphery of the retina. The first decrease in vision, therefore, is in one's peripheral vision. Then, as each layer of nerve fibers dies, the visual field narrows and narrows.

This slow, progressive route to blindness is typical of the most common type of glaucoma, called chronic simple glaucoma. It is called "simple" because the rise in intraocular pressure does not result from any known underlying reason. Although individuals with a family history of glaucoma are more prone to the disease, it is not directly hereditary. Moreover, not everyone with a family history of glaucoma will develop the disease. For reasons that are not well understood, people of African ancestry have glaucoma in much greater numbers than those of European ancestry. In the United States, the incidence of glaucoma among African Americans is three times that of Caucasians.

In persons of all races, chronic simple glaucoma usually begins after the age of forty; however, the aging process does not seem to be a direct cause of glaucoma. Unlike the formation of senile cataracts, which result from inevitable eye changes as one grows older, glaucoma's development is not explained by the aging process. It can safely be said that glaucoma seems to occur in persons who have a tendency toward inadequate aqueous fluid drainage. As those persons grow older and their bodies lose their resiliency in general, the drainage problem reaches a point where it begins to raise the intraocular pressure beyond the normal range. Those with untreated chronic simple glaucoma are seldom aware of the disease before considerable damage has been done. The progressive death of nerve fibers is ordinarily very slow because the elevation of pressure is slight and causes no pain or blurriness of sight.

Chronic simple glaucoma makes up about 95 percent of all cases of the disease. Several other rare types together make up the other 5 percent. In chronic secondary glaucoma, the drainage defect is caused by some complication of a different eye problem. The causes

---

Information on Glaucoma

Causes: Congenital or hereditary factors

Symptoms: Often asymptomatic; eye pressure; slow progression toward blindness; at times, terrible pain, nausea, vomiting, severe headaches

Duration: Ranges from acute to chronic

Treatments: Eyedrops, ointments, pills, surgery

of chronic secondary glaucoma include inflammation from an eye infection, an allergic reaction, trauma to the eye, a tumor, or even the presence of a cataract. Medications such as corticosteroids can sometimes cause this type of glaucoma to develop. Whatever the cause, chronic secondary glaucoma exhibits the same increased pressure, slow nerve destruction, and ultimate loss of vision as chronic simple glaucoma.

A third variety, acute glaucoma, is both rare and dramatic in its onset. The increase in intraocular pressure is many times higher than that in chronic glaucoma. It also occurs very rapidly, sometimes within hours. The anterior drainage angle where drainage is accomplished is almost totally blocked. The eyeball becomes so hard that the elevated pressure can often be felt simply by touching the front of the eye. The great pressure causes terrible pain and immediate damage to the eye. When nausea, vomiting, and severe headaches accompany eye pressure, acute glaucoma should be suspected. Immediate treatment is required to prevent blindness. Acute glaucoma can be either simple or secondary. It is termed simple when a drainage area that has always been abnormally narrow suddenly becomes totally blocked. It is called secondary when it is precipitated by some other eye condition.

The rarest type of glaucoma, congenital glaucoma, is present at birth or develops during early infancy. It results from the incorrect formation of drainage canals while the eye is developing. Because a baby's eyeball is much smaller and softer than an adult's, this glaucoma is often recognized by the bulging of the eyes.

It is quite easy for an eye doctor to detect even the apparently symptomless chronic glaucoma, and the rate of successful treatment is high. It is unfortunate, then, that glaucoma is responsible for innumerable cases of permanent loss of vision. In the vast majority of these patients, the destruction of the eye could have been prevented. If everyone over the age of forty had an annual eye examination, blindness caused by glaucoma could essentially be eliminated.

TREATMENT AND THERAPY

The treatments available for glaucoma include eyedrops, ointments, pills, and surgery, using both scalpels and lasers. In both acute and congenital glaucoma, there is no time for the use of medications. Patients need to be admitted to the hospital and operated on immediately if their eyesight is to be saved.

If diagnosed early, cases of both chronic simple and chronic secondary glaucoma can often be effectively treated by medications. The first drug given in the form of eyedrops was discovered in the nineteenth century. Called pilocarpine, it is obtained from the leaves or roots of a South American bush. The drug is classified as a miotic because it constricts the pupil of the eye. Constriction of the pupil draws it away from the drainage angle, automatically increasing the drainage of aqueous fluid and therefore decreasing the pressure. To be effective, it is generally used four times a day. Other glaucoma drugs act to decrease the secretion of the fluid, which also decreases the intraocular pressure. Timolol maleate, the most frequently prescribed drug for glaucoma, works in this fashion. It usually needs to be used twice a day. Some ophthalmologists prefer to use some of both types of drops for the same patient, decreasing pressure by both mechanisms. Others prescribe one medication that produces both effects. Dipivefrin is one such medication.

In either case, to avoid possible unpleasant side effects the most dilute concentration, to be used the fewest times each day, is prescribed first. If this does not control the pressure, more concentrated drops, to be used more times daily, must then be prescribed. The medications in these eyedrops can often be used more easily by elderly patients in the form of a gel, an ointment, or a tiny disc which is placed on the cornea. Although considerably more costly than frequent drops, these methods are less of a nuisance. The gels and ointments need only be used once a day, while the discs are time-released over an entire week.

If drops or gels do not produce the desired reduction in pressure, pills can be used, not to replace the drops but to supplement them. These tablets are essentially diuretics that decrease the production of aqueous humor. Taken once a day, or less frequently in a time-release capsule, acetazolamide is the drug most often prescribed.

There are also several fast-acting drugs that can be injected into a vein to lower pressure by rapidly pulling some aqueous fluid into blood vessels in the eye, bypassing the drainage angle. These are not used in the treatment of chronic glaucoma except as preparation for a planned surgery. They are, however, often used when patients are admitted to the hospital for acute glaucoma to prevent damage until emergency surgery can be performed.

In the great number of patients, chronic glaucoma can be controlled by one of these medications. In those rare cases when it cannot, surgery must be performed. Although initially successful, such surgeries must of-

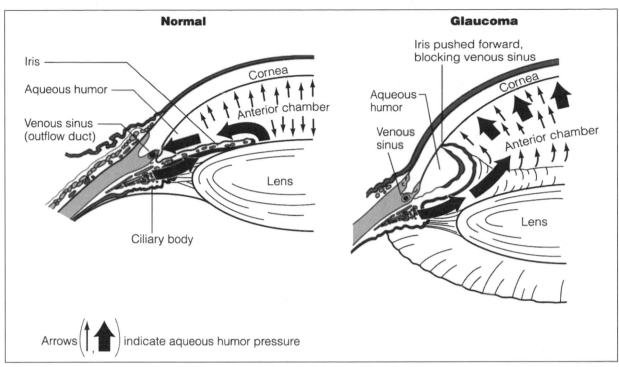

A normal eye versus an eye affected by glaucoma.

ten be repeated in the future. As with the above medications, glaucoma surgery aims to decrease the intraocular pressure by decreasing secretion or increasing effective drainage.

Although surgery can never reverse the optic nerve damage that has already occurred, it is often effective in preventing further destruction. The first of these surgical procedures was developed in the mid-nineteenth century. Called an iridectomy or iridotomy, it attempts to provide a better access to the patient's drainage angle by removing part of the iris. A second type of surgical procedure, known as a trabeculectomy or filtering operation, attempts to control intraocular pressure by creating a new, wider drainage outlet for the aqueous humor. Until the use of lasers, both of these operations were performed manually by a surgeon with steady hands using sharp blades on a tiny part of the eye.

To perform an iridectomy, the surgeon must cut a tiny hole into the edge of the iris with surgical scissors, allowing aqueous fluid to flow into the space between the iris and the cornea. Covered by the upper eyelid, this small hole is visible only by close examination and should not let in unwanted extra light or cause any discomfort to the patient.

The filtering operation, or trabeculectomy, can be performed in several different ways, but each involves the eye surgeon's use of a knife called a scalpel to create an artificial canal through the outer wall of the patient's eye. The passageway created, known as a fistula or filtering bleb, permits the aqueous humor to drain properly from the inner eye. By removing a part of the abnormal tissue from the drainage angle, the surgeon unclogs the drainage mechanism.

A different approach to glaucoma control does not involve cutting. It attempts to help the patient by destroying part of the source of the excess fluid, the oversecreting ciliary body. When a cold probe is applied to the ciliary body, the procedure is termed cryotherapy; when a hot probe is used, the method is called cyclodiathermy. No incision is required in either case because the probes are applied externally. A very common side effect of these two procedures, however, is fairly severe inflammation. Even when inflammation does not occur, the desired result may be only partially achieved. Both cryotherapy and cyclodiathermy are less commonly used than either iridectomy or trabeculectomy, and the procedures are usually performed only on older patients.

Many of these manual procedures are being replaced by several types of laser therapy. A laser is a precisely directed beam of high-intensity light that can function as a surgical knife. Laser surgery is generally safer than the older methods because it is less invasive to the body, as no incision is made in the eye. It can be done on an outpatient basis with only a local anesthetic. Recovery time, the likelihood of complications, and postoperative discomfort are all lessened. Patients with acute glaucoma, chronic simple glaucoma, and certain types of secondary glaucoma (depending on the cause) can be successfully treated with lasers.

Both iridotomy and trabeculectomy can be performed using an instrument called the argon laser. This particular laser is relatively low-powered, but it is efficient and very popular with ophthalmologists. After a drop of anesthetic is placed in the eye, the surgeon aims the highly focused argon beam at a precise location within the affected eye. The beam need only be directed into the eye for one-tenth of a second to achieve its effect. In an iridotomy, the laser simply drills a tiny hole in the iris for the fluid to circulate freely, while in a trabeculectomy several laser cuts are made on the clogged drainage angle to open it. A more sophisticated ophthalmic laser is the YAG laser. After a drop of anesthetic is placed on the eye, a weak "aiming beam" of helium-neon laser light is shone directly into the afflicted eye to pinpoint the area to be treated. This is followed by two to five bursts of the YAG laser, which drills a hole for better drainage.

All the above treatments for glaucoma, whether pharmaceutical or surgical, have the potential for serious side effects and complications. Consequently, research continues to seek therapies with better rates of success and fewer complications.

PERSPECTIVE AND PROSPECTS

The development of ways to diagnose glaucoma has paralleled the general development of the ophthalmologist's tools. These devices in turn reflect the links between the science of those branches of physics that study pressure, lenses, mirrors, and light and the science that studies the normal and abnormal functioning of the eye.

In 1851, the German doctor Hermann von Helmholtz invented the ophthalmoscope, which enables one to study the interior of the eye. His instrument focuses a beam of light into the patient's eye and then magnifies its reflection. If this test reveals early signs of cupping of the optic disc, glaucoma can be diagnosed long before other symptoms have appeared.

Intraocular pressure can be measured with an instrument called a tonometer. The two basic varieties are called Schiötz tonometry and applanation tonom-

etry. Both only became possible after biochemists developed anesthetic drops to put in the eye so that the patient would not feel the device touching the very sensitive cornea. The earlier of the two devices, developed in 1905 by the Norwegian physician Hjalmar Schiötz, is a very simple device that is still the most widely used tonometer in the world. With the patient lying down and looking upward, the physician places the hand-sized instrument directly on the cornea. A simple lever is moved by the pressure within the eye to indicate whether that pressure is within the normal range or dangerously high. The Goldman applanation tonometer is considered even more accurate and is often used to confirm the results of the simpler Schiötz device. An orange dye called fluorescein is added to the anesthetic. The patient, in a sitting position, rests the head against a bar to steady it. The doctor uses a tonometer to touch the cornea while simultaneously peering into it with a well-illuminated microscope.

More specialized glaucoma examination may require gonioscopy, visual field tests, or tonography. The gonioscope has mirrors and facets to provide an illuminated view of the drainage angle, a normally dark corner at a 90 degree angle from the examiner. Excessive narrowing of the angle is an indication of glaucoma. There are many kinds of visual field tests, but all give a map of the central area where vision is sharp and more acute, versus the peripheral area where it is weaker. Since damage to the optic nerve always causes a narrowing of the visual field, this mapping is very important. The ability to measure the field has grown from oculokinetic perimetry—using an inexpensive test chart, pencil, record sheet, and human examiner— to the expensive and sophisticated automated perimetry, which generates a computer analysis for the physician. Tonography does not measure the visual field but again attacks the problem by measuring the intraocular pressure. Unlike the ordinary use of tonometry, which involves momentary contact with the cornea, tonography uses the tonometer for four minutes to massage the eye. In a normal eye, pressure will drop; in a glaucoma patient, it will not.

All these tests, developed through years of ophthalmic research, have given medical science invaluable tools to diagnose glaucoma and prevent blindness.

—*Grace D. Matzen*

See also Blindness; Cataract surgery; Cataracts; Eye surgery; Eyes; Laser use in surgery; Ophthalmology; Optometry; Sense organs; Visual disorders.

FOR FURTHER INFORMATION:

Buettner, Helmut, ed. *Mayo Clinic on Vision and Eye Health: Practical Answers on Glaucoma, Cataracts, Macular Degeneration, and Other Conditions.* Rochester, Minn.: Mayo Foundation for Medical Education and Research, 2002. A helpful handbook on all the medical, social, and emotional facets of vision impairment.

Eden, John. *The Physician's Guide to Cataracts, Glaucoma, and Other Eye Problems.* Yonkers, N.Y.: Consumer Reports Books, 1992. This excellent book provides the reader with nontechnical yet truly accurate explanations of the functioning of the normal eye and of the disease conditions glaucoma and cataracts.

Epstein, David L., et al., eds. *Chandler and Grant's Glaucoma.* Rev. 4th ed. Baltimore: Williams & Wilkins, 1997. A standard text on glaucoma. Includes bibliographic references and an index.

Galloway, N. R. *Common Eye Diseases and Their Management.* 2d ed. New York: Springer-Verlag, 1999. While this text may be difficult for the general reader, it is useful for obtaining more precise medical information. Intended for medical students but accessible to nonscientists because of the author's writing style.

Glaucoma Research Foundation. http://www.glaucoma.org/. A group that strives to maintain the sight and independence of individuals with glaucoma through research and education with the ultimate goal of finding a cure.

Morrison, John C., and Irvin P. Pollack. *Glaucoma: A Clinical Guide.* New York: Thieme, 2003. A clinical text that is nonetheless helpful for the lay reader covering such topics as genetics, gonioscopy, perimetry, childhood glaucoma, retinal disorders, neuroprotection, and ocular hypotony.

Samz, Jane. *The Encyclopedia of Health: Vision.* New York: Chelsea House, 1990. Contains a rather brief treatment of the topic of glaucoma. This volume is useful for understanding the normal eye, eye tests in general, and a diversity of other eye diseases. Includes lists of helpful organizations and further readings, as well as a brief glossary.

Sutton, Amy, ed. *Eye Care Sourcebook: Basic Consumer Health Information About Eye Care and Eye Disorders.* 2d ed. Detroit: Omnigraphics, 2003. A complete guide to eye care that includes such topics as eye anatomy, preventive vision care, refractive disorders and eye diseases, current research and clinical trials, and a list of organizations.

GLOMERULONEPHRITIS. *See* NEPHRITIS.

GLYCOGEN STORAGE DISEASES
DISEASE/DISORDER
ANATOMY OR SYSTEM AFFECTED: Heart, liver, muscles

SPECIALTIES AND RELATED FIELDS: Biochemistry, biotechnology, nutrition, pediatrics, perinatology

DEFINITION: Inherited metabolic disorders that lead to the accumulation of an abnormal amount or type of glycogen in the liver, muscles, and heart.

KEY TERMS:

autosomal recessive trait: a genetic trait coded on an autosomal chromosome (not an X or Y chromosome) that is expressed only when two copies are inherited, one from each parent

cirrhosis: the abnormal formation of connective tissue in an organ, resulting in loss of function; usually refers to the liver

enzyme: a protein that catalyzes a biological reaction in the body

glycogen: the storage form of carbohydrate in the body; a polymer of glucose units that has a highly branched, treelike structure

lysosome: an organelle inside cells that contains a variety of enzymes for breaking down cellular constituents

nasogastric tube: a tube fed through the nose to the stomach

X-linked trait: a genetic trait coded on the X chromosome; predominantly affects males, who have only one X chromosome

CAUSES AND SYMPTOMS

Glycogen storage diseases are caused by inherited defects in the enzymes involved in the synthesis or break-

---

INFORMATION ON GLYCOGEN STORAGE DISEASES

CAUSES: Genetic enzyme defects

SYMPTOMS: In liver diseases, may include seizures, coma, growth retardation, kidney problems, and liver cancer; in muscle diseases, may include exercise intolerance, susceptibility to fatigue, heart enlargement, and heart failure

DURATION: Lifelong

TREATMENTS: Varies by type; includes continuous glucose intake

down of glycogen and are characterized by the accumulation of an abnormal type or amount of glycogen. At least twelve such diseases have been identified; they can be diagnosed by enzymatic analysis of a biopsy tissue sample. Prenatal diagnosis of most of these conditions is possible but, because their overall frequency is estimated at 1 in 20,000 to 25,000 live births, is generally not performed unless warranted. Most of these diseases are inherited as autosomal recessive traits, although phosphorylase kinase deficiency is X-linked. In many cases, the causative deoxyribonucleic acid (DNA) mutations have been identified. These diseases primarily affect the liver and muscles, which normally contain most of the glycogen in the body.

Maintaining normal blood glucose levels is essential for the function of various tissues and particularly the brain, which depends on blood glucose as a source of energy. In the fed state, when dietary carbohydrate is digested, blood glucose levels rise and are used to replenish liver glycogen. In the fasted state, when blood glucose levels otherwise fall, liver glycogen is broken down and used to maintain normal blood glucose levels. This cycling in the storage and breakdown of liver glycogen is essential to permit the body to survive periods without meals, especially overnight.

In liver glycogen storage diseases, this cycling is disrupted. Most cases are attributed to defects in four enzymes: glucose-6-phosphatase, glycogen branching enzyme, glycogen debrancher enzyme, and glycogen phosphorylase (or phosphorylase kinase). Because glucose-6-phosphatase is responsible for converting the breakdown product of glycogen (glucose-6-phosphate) to free glucose for release into the blood, its deficiency does not allow stored liver glycogen to restore depleted blood glucose, as during an overnight fast. If untreated, this condition, also known as von Gierke's disease, results in seizures, coma, and death. Inadequately treated patients may survive but experience growth retardation and develop kidney problems and liver cancer.

Muscle glycogen is also synthesized in the fed state, but it is broken down to provide energy for muscle contraction. Glycogen storage diseases of muscle usually cause intolerance to exercise and susceptibility to fatigue. Most of these cases are attributed to defects in three enzymes: lysosomal glucosidase, glycogen phosphorylase, and phosphofructokinase. The glucosidase found in lysosomes is responsible for breaking down any glycogen that accumulates in these intracellular organelles. When this enzyme is missing, the lysosomes become engorged with glycogen, disrupting

their normal function and other cellular metabolism. In the most severe cases, glycogen accumulation in the heart is pronounced, resulting in an enlarged heart and death from heart failure before age two. Glycogen phosphorylase in muscle breaks down glycogen for its use in contraction. When this enzyme is deficient, muscle tissues lack the fuel to provide for extensive exercise, resulting in cramping; the avoidance of heavy exercise prevents symptoms. Phosphofructokinase is a crucial enzyme in the metabolism of glucose; in the muscle, its deficiency has a consequence much like that of glycogen phosphorylase, namely the inability to engage in strenuous exercise.

When glycogen is synthesized, the branching enzyme inserts branchpoints to give it a treelike structure. A defect in this enzyme leads to an abnormal, long, unbranched glycogen. Because it folds back on itself in a way that makes it difficult for glycogen breakdown enzymes to act on it, it is not broken down. While this condition generally does not lead to low fasting

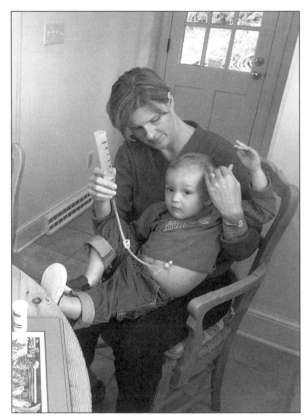

A mother pours liquid cornstarch solution into her young child's feeding tube. He has a rare glycogen storage disease and must have cornstarch every four hours in order to avoid seizures. (AP/Wide World Photos)

blood glucose, as alternative pathways are available, the accumulated abnormal glycogen, apparently considered a foreign object, leads to liver cirrhosis and death by age five; no treatment is available other than liver transplantation. A defect in the debranching enzyme that removes the branchpoints during the breakdown of glycogen severely restricts the yield of glucose to those units beyond a branchpoint. Glycogen phosphorylase is the main enzyme that breaks down glycogen to monomeric units, and its deficiency or that of an enzyme controlling its activity (phosphorylase kinase) result in variable manifestation, depending on the severity of the condition. Most patients with the latter diseases usually require no specific treatment.

TREATMENT AND THERAPY

A defect in glucose-6-phosphatase can be treated by providing continuous sources of glucose during the day (snacks between meals) and especially overnight (nightly nasogastric infusions of glucose or eating slowly digested carbohydrate, such as uncooked cornstarch, before sleep). If this condition is detected early and treated properly, then normal growth and development are observed. No effective treatment is available for muscle glycogen storage disease involving a defect in lysosomal glucosidases.

PERSPECTIVE AND PROSPECTS

The first observation of a defect in glycogen metabolism was made in 1928. In 1929, Edgar von Gierke first noted glucose-6-phosphatase deficiency and, in 1932, J. C. Pompe first reported the lysosomal glucosidase deficiency; their names remain associated with these conditions. As normal glycogen metabolism came to be understood, the enzymatic basis for at least twelve glycogen storage disorders were identified. Each is a candidate for enzyme replacement therapy or gene replacement therapy, although these treatments remained experimental at the beginning of the twenty-first century.

—*James L. Robinson, Ph.D.*

See also Enzyme therapy; Enzymes; Fatty acid oxidation disorders; Food biochemistry; Metabolism; Niemann-Pick disease.

FOR FURTHER INFORMATION:

Chen, Y.-T. "Glycogen Storage Diseases." In *The Metabolic and Molecular Bases of Inherited Disease*, edited by Charles R. Scriver et al. 8th ed. New York: McGraw-Hill, 2001.

Hirschhorn, R., and A. J. J. Reuser. "Glycogen Storage Disease Type II: Acid-Glucosidase (Acid Maltase) Deficiency." In *The Metabolic and Molecular Bases of Inherited Disease*, edited by Charles R. Scriver et al. 8th ed. New York: McGraw-Hill, 2001.

Professional Guide to Diseases. 7th ed. Springhouse, Pa.: Springhouse, 2001.

GLYCOLYSIS

BIOLOGY

ANATOMY OR SYSTEM AFFECTED: Cells, muscles, musculoskeletal system

SPECIALTIES AND RELATED FIELDS: Biochemistry, cytology, exercise physiology, pharmacology, sports medicine

DEFINITION: The chemical process of splitting a molecule of glucose in order to obtain energy for other cellular processes; at times of intense activity, glycolysis produces most of the energy used by muscles.

KEY TERMS:

adenosine triphosphate (ATP): an important biological molecule that represents the energy currency of the cell; the energy in a special high-energy bond in ATP is used to drive almost all cellular processes that require energy

aerobic: occurring in the presence of oxygen

anaerobic: occurring in the absence of oxygen

cellular respiration: a complex series of chemical reactions by which chemical energy stored in the bonds of food molecules is released and used to form ATP

chemical energy: the energy locked up in the chemical bonds that hold the atoms of a molecule together; food molecules, such as glucose, contain much energy in their bonds

creatine phosphate: an energy-containing molecule present in significant quantities in muscle tissue; energy is stored in a high-energy bond similar to that of ATP

enzyme: a biological catalyst that speeds up a chemical reaction without itself being used up; enzymes are made of protein, and a single enzyme can usually only catalyze a single chemical reaction

nicotinamide adenine dinucleotide (NAD): a molecule used to hold pairs of electrons when they have been removed from a molecule by some biological process; the empty molecule is denoted by NAD^+, while it is denoted as NADH when it is carrying electrons

STRUCTURE AND FUNCTIONS

Glycolysis is the first step in the process that cells use to extract energy from food molecules. Although energy can be extracted from most types of food molecule, glycolysis is usually considered to begin with glucose. In fact, the term "glycolysis" actually means the splitting (*lysis*) of glucose (*glyco*). This is a good description for the process, since the glucose molecule is split into two halves. The glucose molecule consists of a backbone of six carbon atoms to which are attached, in various ways, twelve hydrogen atoms and six oxygen atoms. The glucose molecule is inherently stable and unlikely to split spontaneously at any appreciable rate.

When the energy is extracted from a glucose molecule, it is stored, for the short term, in a much less stable molecule called adenosine triphosphate (ATP). The ATP molecule consists of a complex organic molecule (adenosine) to which are attached three simple phosphate groups. While the first phosphate is attached by what one could call a "normal" chemical bond, the second and third phosphates are attached by high-energy bonds. These are chemical bonds that require a considerable amount of energy to create. Therefore, the ATP molecule can store much energy. When one of the high-energy bonds of ATP is broken, a large amount of energy is released. Usually, only the bond holding the last phosphate is broken, producing a molecule of adenosine diphosphate (ADP) and a free phosphate group. The phosphate group is only split from ATP at the precise moment when energy is required by some other process in the cell. This breaking of ATP provides the energy to drive cellular processes. The processes include activities such as the synthesis of molecules, the movement of molecules, and the contraction of muscle. The third phosphate can be reattached to ADP using energy released from glycolysis, or by other components of cellular respiration. The production of ATP can be diagrammed as follows: "energy from glycolysis + ADP + phosphate → ATP." Similarly, the breakdown of ATP can be diagrammed as "ATP → ADP + phosphate + usable energy." With this understanding of how ATP works, one can look at how it is generated in the cell by glycolysis.

The first step in the production of energy from food is really an energy-consuming process. Since glucose is inherently a stable molecule, it must be activated before it will split. It is activated by attaching a phosphate group to each end of the six-carbon backbone. These phosphate groups are supplied by ATP. Therefore, glycolysis begins by using the energy from two ATP molecules. The atoms of the glucose molecule are also rearranged during the activation process so that it is changed into a very similar sugar, fructose. A fructose molecule with a phosphate group on either end is called fructose 1,6-diphosphate. Thus one can summarize the activation process as "glucose + 2 ATP → fructose 1,6-diphosphate + 2 ADP."

Fructose 1,6-diphosphate is a much more reactive molecule and can be readily encouraged to split by the appropriate enzyme. The split produces two identical molecules with the rather cumbersome name of phosphoglyceraldehyde, usually abbreviated to PGAL. Each PGAL consists of a three-carbon backbone with attached oxygen and hydrogen atoms, and a phosphate group at the end. Each PGAL molecule then undergoes several changes, only the important results of which will be mentioned. At one point, the PGAL molecule picks up a free phosphate group at the end opposite from where one is already attached. Various arrangements of the atoms convert the bonds holding the phosphate groups into high-energy bonds. These phosphate groups are then able to be transferred to ADP molecules producing ATP. Since each PGAL produces two ATPs, and two PGALs are produced from each original glucose, four ATP molecules are produced all together. Since two ATPs were used to activate the glucose, the cell has a net gain of two ATP molecules for each glucose molecule used.

The rearrangement of the atoms leaves them in a form called pyruvic acid. Pyruvic acid still contains much energy locked up in its chemical bonds. In most of the cells of the body and most of the time, pyruvic acid will be further broken down and all of its energy released. This further breakdown of pyruvic acid requires oxygen and is beyond the scope of this topic. It should be pointed out, however, that the complete breakdown of two molecules of pyruvic acid can produce more than thirty additional ATP molecules. With the addition of oxygen, the end products are the simple molecules of carbon dioxide and water.

Other products of the rearrangement of PGAL are energy-containing electrons. Electrons are highly energetic and have a negative electrical charge. They cannot be allowed simply to dart around the cell by themselves. Instead, they are picked up and carried by molecules specially designed for this purpose. These energy-carrying molecules have the rather intimidating name nicotinamide adenine dinucleotide, abbreviated to NAD. Biologists have more or less agreed to a conventional notation for this molecule, to allow the reader to know whether the molecule is carrying electrons or is empty. Since the empty molecule has a net positive charge, it is denoted as NAD^+. When full, it holds a pair of electrons. One electron would neutralize the positive charge, while two result in a negative charge. The negative charge attracts one of the many hydrogen ions (H^+) in the cell. Thus when carrying electrons the molecule is denoted NADH.

These energy-carrying electrons have little significance most of the time in most of the cells of the body. The NADH molecules are able to donate their electrons to systems that generate ATP from them. These systems, however, require the use of oxygen. Although the body has an excellent respiratory system and circulatory system to obtain and deliver oxygen to all parts of the body, there are times when it is inadequate. When a muscle is working very hard, there simply is not enough blood supply to bring all the oxygen that the muscle needs.

The oxidative pathways that completely break down pyruvic acid are limited by the lack of oxygen in very active muscles. The ability to deal with electrons from NADH is also drastically reduced. Glycolysis can continue even in the absence of oxygen, but the electrons produced by glycolysis must be dealt with.

There is a very limited amount of NAD^+ in each cell. NAD^+ is designed to hold electrons briefly, while they are transferred to some other system. In the absence of oxygen, the electrons are transferred to pyruvic acid. Since pyruvic acid cannot be broken down without oxygen, there is an ample supply. Transferring electrons from NADH to pyruvic acid allows the empty NAD^+ to pick up more electrons produced by glycolysis. Therefore, glycolysis can continue producing two ATP molecules from each glucose molecule used. While two ATPs per glucose molecule is a small amount compared to the more than thirty ATPs produced by oxidative metabolism, it is better than none at all.

The process of generating energy (ATPs) in the absence of oxygen is referred to as fermentation. Most people are familiar with the fermentation of grapes to produce wine. Yeast has the enzymes to transfer electrons from NADH to pyruvic acid and to convert the resulting molecule into alcohol and carbon dioxide. No further energy is obtained from this process. Alcohol still contains much of the energy that was in glucose. Humans and other mammals have different enzymes than yeast cells. These enzymes transfer the electrons from NADH to pyruvic acid, producing lactic acid.

GLYCOLYSIS AND MUSCLE ACTIVITY

When yeast is respiring anaerobically (without oxygen), it will continue producing alcohol until it poisons itself. Most yeast cannot tolerate more than about 12 percent alcohol, the concentration found in most wine. The lactic acid produced by fermentation in humans is also poisonous. People, however, do not respire completely anaerobically. The two ATPs produced per glucose molecule used are simply not enough to supply the energy needs of most human cells. Muscle cells have to be somewhat of an exception. There are times when one asks the muscle cells to use energy much faster than one can supply them with oxygen. One may consider a muscle working under various levels of physical activity and examine its oxygen requirements and waste products.

At rest, a muscle requires very little ATP energy. For an individual sitting on the couch watching television, energy demands are minimal. The lungs inhale and exhale slowly and take in enough oxygen to keep its concentration in the blood high. A relatively slow heart rate can pump enough of this oxygen-rich blood to the muscles to supply their very minimal needs. As soon as one uses a muscle, however, its ATP consumption increases dramatically. Even if an individual simply walks as far as the refrigerator, large quantities of ATP are required to cause the leg muscles to contract. Muscle cells maintain a constant level of ATP so that, as soon as one asks a muscle to contract, it can do so. The ATP that is broken down is almost instantly regenerated from an additional energy store peculiar to muscle cells. Creatine phosphate is a molecule similar to ATP, in that the phosphate group is attached by a high-energy bond. There is more creatine phosphate in muscle cells than ATP. As soon as ATP is broken down, phosphates, and their high-energy bonds, are transferred from creatine phosphate. Within the first few seconds of activity, the ATP concentration in a muscle cell remains almost constant, but the creatine phosphate level begins to drop.

As soon as the creatine phosphate concentration drops, the aerobic (oxygen-requiring) respiratory processes speed up. These processes break down glucose all the way to carbon dioxide and water and release plenty of ATP. This ATP can then be used for muscle contraction. If the muscle has now stopped contracting, the new ATP produced will be used to rebuild the store of creatine phosphate.

Within the first minute or so of muscle contraction, the use of oxygen can be quite high. The circulatory system has not yet responded to this increased oxygen demand. Muscle tissue, however, has a reserve of oxygen. The red color of most mammalian muscles is attributable to the presence of myoglobin, which is similar to hemoglobin in that it has a strong affinity for oxygen. The myoglobin stores oxygen directly in the muscle, so that the muscle can operate aerobically while the circulatory and respiratory systems adjust to the increased oxygen demand.

At low or moderate muscle activity, the carbon dioxide produced by aerobic respiration in muscles will trigger an increase in the activity of both the circulatory and the respiratory systems. The increased demand for oxygen by the muscles is supplied by an increased blood flow. Jogging around a track or participating in aerobic exercises would be considered low to moderate muscular activity. Respiration rate and pulse rate both increase with jogging. This increase in oxygen supply to the muscles provides all that they need. The level of creatine phosphate will be lower than that in resting muscles, but it will soon be replenished when the activity is stopped. The muscle cells have a good supply of food molecules in the form of glycogen. Glycogen is simply a long string of glucose molecules connected together for convenient storage. At a rate of activity such as that created by jogging, the glycogen supply can last for hours. Even after it is used up, glycogen stored in the liver can be broken down to glucose and carried to the muscles by the blood. An individual will probably want to stop jogging before his or her muscles will want to quit.

High levels of muscular activity pose a different set of problems. After more than about a minute of vigorous exercise, the muscles begin to use ATP faster than oxygen can be supplied to regenerate it. The additional ATP is supplied by lactic acid fermentation. Glucose is only broken down as far as pyruvic acid, then converted to lactic acid by the addition of electrons from NADH. Lactic acid begins to accumulate in the muscle tissue. Since the body is still using large amounts of ATP but not taking in enough oxygen, it is said to enter a state of oxygen debt. When the muscular activity ends, the oxygen debt is repaid.

One can use an example of someone running to catch a bus, sprinting for 50 yards at full speed. That is not enough time for the circulation and lungs to respond to the increased demand for oxygen. The muscles have made up the difference between supply and demand with lactic acid fermentation. The individual now sits down in the bus and pants—to repay his or her oxygen debt.

Some of the oxygen will go to replenish the store in muscle myoglobin. Some of it will be used in oxidative metabolism in the muscle to replenish the reserves of creatine phosphate. The rest will be used to deal with the accumulated lactic acid. The lactic acid is not all dealt with in the muscle where it was produced. Being a small molecule, it easily enters the bloodstream. In muscles throughout the body, it can be converted back to pyruvic acid. Pyruvic acid can then reenter the oxidative pathway and be used to generate ATP, with the use of oxygen. The lactic acid, then, is being used as a food molecule to supply the needs of resting muscle. Much of the lactic acid is metabolized in the liver. Some of it will be metabolized with oxygen to produce the energy to convert the rest of it back to glucose. The glucose can then be circulated in the blood or stored in the liver or muscles as glycogen. A minimal amount of lactic acid is excreted in the urine or in sweat.

If the subject of the preceding example kept running at full speed, having missed the bus and run all the way to the office, lactic acid would build up in the muscles and in the blood. If the office was far enough away, the subject would eventually reach the point of exhaustion and stop running. At that point, the level of lactic acid in the leg muscles would be high enough to inhibit the enzymes of glycolysis. Glycolysis would slow down so that lactic acid would not become any more concentrated. The muscles' supply of creatine phosphate would be almost exhausted, but the ATP supply would be only slightly lower than in a resting muscle. The body is protected from damaging itself: Too much lactic acid would lower the pH to dangerous levels, and the absolute lack of ATP causes muscles to lock, as in rigor mortis. The body's self-protection mechanisms force one to stop before either of these conditions exists. Once the subject stops running, and pants long enough, he or she can continue. The additional oxygen taken in by increased respiration will have metabolized a sufficient amount of lactic acid to allow the muscles to start working again.

PERSPECTIVE AND PROSPECTS

Cellular respiration is the process by which organisms harvest usable energy in the form of ATP molecules from food molecules. Lactic acid fermentation is the form of respiration used by human muscles when oxygen is in limited supply. Glycolysis is the energy-producing component of lactic acid fermentation, which is much less efficient than aerobic cellular respiration. Fermentation harvests only two molecules of ATP for every glucose molecule used, while aerobic respiration produces a yield of more than thirty molecules of ATP. Most forms of life will only resort to fermentation when oxygen is absent or in short supply.

While higher forms of life such as humans can obtain energy by fermentation for short periods, they incur an oxygen debt which must eventually be repaid. The yield of two molecules of ATP for each glucose molecule used is simply not enough to sustain their high demand for energy.

Nevertheless, lactic acid fermentation is an important source of ATP for humans during strenuous physical exercise. Even though it is an inefficient use of glucose, it can provide enough ATP for a short burst of activity. After the activity is over, the lactic acid produced must be dealt with, which usually requires the use of oxygen.

Most popular exercise programs focus on aerobic activity. Aerobic exercises do not place stress on muscles to the point where the blood cannot supply enough oxygen. These exercises are designed to improve the efficiency of the oxygen delivery system so that there is less need for anaerobic metabolism. Training programs in general attempt to tune the body so that the need for lactic acid fermentation is reduced. They concentrate on improving the delivery of oxygen to the muscles, storing oxygen in the muscles, or increasing the efficiency of muscular contraction.

—*James Waddell, Ph.D.*

See also Cells; Enzymes; Exercise physiology; Food biochemistry; Metabolism; Muscles; Sports medicine.

FOR FURTHER INFORMATION:

Alberts, Bruce, et al. *Molecular Biology of the Cell.* 4th ed. New York: Garland, 2002. Describes the evolution of cells and introduces cell structure and function. The text is clearly written at the college level and is illustrated by numerous diagrams and photographs.

Campbell, Neil A. *Biology: Concepts and Connections.* 6th ed. San Francisco: Benjamin/Cummings, 2002. This classic introductory textbook provides an excellent discussion of essential biological structures and mechanisms. Its extensive and detailed illustrations help to make even difficult concepts accessible to the nonspecialist.

Lehninger, Albert L. *Bioenergetics.* New York: W. A. Benjamin, 1971. Chapter 4, "Generation of ATP in Anaerobic Cells," provides a detailed but very readable account of the anaerobic portion of respiration. The chapter also provides a succinct account of enzyme action in general.

Sackheim, George I., and Dennis D. Lehman. *Chemistry for the Health Sciences.* 8th ed. Upper Saddle River, N.J.: Prentice-Hall, 1998. An accessible guide to the chemical processes involved in human health. Stresses the relationship between inorganic chemistry and the life processes.

Shephard, Roy J. *Biochemistry of Physical Activity.* Springfield, Ill.: Charles C Thomas, 1984. Chapter 3, "Carbohydrates and Phosphagen," provides a detailed description of energy production and use in muscles.

GOITER

DISEASE/DISORDER

ANATOMY OR SYSTEM AFFECTED: Endocrine system, glands, neck

SPECIALTIES AND RELATED FIELDS: Endocrinology

DEFINITION: An enlargement of the thyroid gland that is noncancerous and not caused by a temporary condition such as inflammation.

KEY TERMS:

goitrogenic: referring to a factor (typically food or chemicals) that produces goiter

hypersection: the excess production and secretion of a hormone or other chemical

CAUSES AND SYMPTOMS

Goiter is often a painless medical condition. Its only visible symptoms may be a slight but visible enlargement of the thyroid that creates a swelling at the base of the neck. In severe cases, the swelling becomes massive and the patient experiences difficulty breathing or swallowing as the enlarged thyroid compresses against the windpipe or esophagus. Other symptoms that may indicate goiter include weight loss, increased heart rate, elevated blood pressure, hair loss, and tremors. Goiter

---

INFORMATION ON GOITER

CAUSES: Of simple goiter, iodine deficiency or hormonal changes (adolescence, pregnancy); of toxic goiter, excessive production of thyroxine from oversecretion of thyroid-stimulating hormone by pituitary

SYMPTOMS: Thyroid enlargement ranging from slight to massive, with difficulty breathing or swallowing

DURATION: Acute or chronic

TREATMENTS: Iodine tablets, sometimes surgical removal of all or part of thyroid

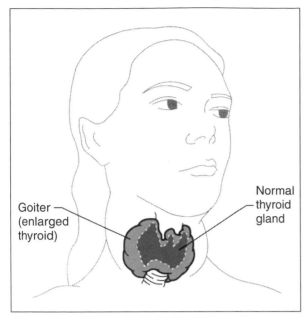

Goiter (enlarged thyroid); dashed lines show relative size of normal thyroid.

can be confirmed by ultrasound scan of the thyroid, blood tests for abnormal levels of thyroxine or thyroid-stimulating hormone, or low rates of iodine excretion in the urine.

The several types of medical goiter fall into two broad categories, simple goiter and toxic goiter. Simple goiter is caused by a dietary deficiency of iodine. In response, one or both lobes of the thyroid gland enlarge in an attempt to produce more of the iodine-containing hormone thyroxine. Two types of simple goiter are recognized, endemic goiter and sporadic goiter.

Endemic goiter typically occurs in land-locked geographic regions or in areas where farm soils are iodine-depleted. Simple goiter was once common in areas of central Asia, central Africa, and the so-called Goiter Belt of the United States, which extended from the Great Lakes to the Intermountain West (between the Rockies and the Sierras).

Simple goiter most often appears in adolescence, but it may sometimes occur during pregnancy. This condition should be corrected in pregnant women to ensure the healthy development of the fetus and the birth of a healthy infant. Simple goiter readily responds to treatment via iodine tablets, but in some patients surgical removal of all or part of the enlarged thyroid may be necessary. Public health measures undertaken to eliminate or prevent simple goiter include the addition of iodine to table salt and also to water reservoirs in certain areas.

Sporadic goiter occurs in some individuals because of an excessive consumption of goitrogenic (goiter-causing) foods, such as cabbage, soybeans, spinach, and radishes. Sporadic goiter has also been linked with exposure to certain medications, such as aminoglutethimide or lithium. Although this type of goiter is considered nontoxic, it does produce impaired thyroid activity. Sporadic goiter can be treated by limiting the consumption of goitrogenic foods.

Toxic goiter is caused by an excessive production of thyroxine hormone by the thyroid gland. This type of goiter is also called hyperthyroid goiter, exopthalmic goiter, or Graves' disease. Toxic goiter results from an oversecretion (hypersecretion) of thyroid-stimulating hormone by the pituitary. In turn, the thyroid gland responds by enlarging and secreting excess amounts of thyroxine, resulting in goiter. Symptoms of Graves' disease include elevated metabolic rate, higher body temperature, rapid weight loss, nervousness, and irritability. In some patients, this type of goiter results in protrusive eyeballs and the appearance of staring.

Euthyroid goiter occurs when dietary levels of iodine are only slightly below normal. The pituitary gland responds to lowered thyroxine levels in the blood by producing additional thyroid-stimulating hormone. The thyroid gland responds to the elevated thyroid-stimulating hormone by enlarging in an effort to increase thyroxine production.

TREATMENT AND THERAPY

Most goiters can be treated effectively through dietary supplements of iodine. The administration of iodine supplements must be very carefully regulated, however, to prevent a so-called thyroxin storm resulting from excess thyroxine production by the enlarged thyroid gland. Some patients may choose alternative natural herbal therapies taken in tablet form, but these substances should be used only in consultation with a physician.

—*Dwight G. Smith*

See also Endocrine disorders; Endocrinology; Endocrinology, pediatric; Hyperparathyroidism and Hypoparathyroidism; Malnutrition; Thyroid disorders; Thyroid gland; Thyroidectomy.

FOR FURTHER INFORMATION:

DeMaeyer, E. M. *The Control of Endemic Goiter.* Washington, D.C.: World Health Organization, 1988. Informational booklet published by the World Health Organization.

Gaitan, Eduardo, ed. *Environmental Goitrogenesis.* Boca Raton, Fla.: CRC Press, 1989. Comprehensive and balanced treatment of all forms of factors that affect thyroid condition and function.

Hall, R., ed. *Thyroid Disorders Associated with Iodine Deficiency and Excess.* Hagerstown, Md.: Lippincott Williams & Wilkins, 1985. Provides an extensive treatment of the types of goiter associated with dietary deficiency of iodine.

Hamburger, J. I. *Nontoxic Goiter: Concept and Controversy.* Springfield, Ill.: Charles C Thomas, 1973. A classic review of the medicinal science of goiter.

GONORRHEA
DISEASE/DISORDER

ANATOMY OR SYSTEM AFFECTED: Eyes, genitals, reproductive system, throat, urinary system

SPECIALTIES AND RELATED FIELDS: Gynecology, microbiology

DEFINITION: A common treatable sexually transmitted disease which primarily infects the reproductive tract and which is caused by the bacterium *Neisseria gonorrhea.*

KEY TERMS:

contact tracing: also known as partner referral; a process that consists of identifying the sexual partners of infected patients, informing these partners of their exposure to disease, and offering resources for counseling and treatment

screening procedures: tests that are carried out in populations which are usually asymptomatic and at high risk for a disease in order to identify those in need of treatment

sexually transmitted disease: an infection caused by organisms transferred through sexual contact (genital-genital, oral-genital, or anal-genital); the transmission of infection occurs through exposure to lesions or secretions that contain the organisms

CAUSES AND SYMPTOMS

Gonorrhea is the second most common sexually transmitted disease (STD) in the United States, the most common being chlamydia. In the United States, the incidence of gonorrhea has fallen. In 1995, the incidence was about 150 cases out of every 100,000 population, down from the mid-1970's of more than 400 cases. The highest incidence of gonorrhea is in sexually active men and women under twenty-five years of age.

Gonorrhea is caused by the bacterium *Neisseria gonorrhea,* a gram-negative diplococcus. The bacterium

---

INFORMATION ON GONORRHEA

CAUSES: Bacterial infection through intercourse
SYMPTOMS: In men, sometimes urinary discomfort and discharge, with long-term complications of epididymitis, prostatitis, and urethral scarring; in women, sometimes vaginal discharge, urinary discomfort, urethral discharge, lower abdominal discomfort, and pain with intercourse, with possible pelvic inflammatory disease, infertility, and increased risk of ectopic pregnancy
DURATION: Acute
TREATMENTS: Antibiotics, counseling regarding safe sex

---

infects the mucous membranes with which it comes in contact, most commonly the urethra and the cervix but also the throat, rectum, and eyes. Some men will be asymptomatic, but most will experience urinary discomfort and a purulent urethral discharge. Long-term complications of this infection in men include epididymitis, prostatitis, and urethral strictures (scarring). In women, the disease is more likely to be asymptomatic. Women with symptoms may have purulent vaginal discharge, urinary discomfort, urethral discharge, lower abdominal discomfort, or pain with intercourse. Pelvic inflammatory disease (PID) and its consequences may occur if gonorrheal infection ascends past the cervix into the upper genital tract (uterus, Fallopian tubes, ovaries, and pelvic cavity) in women. Complications of PID include infertility and an increased risk of ectopic pregnancy.

In rare cases, gonorrhea can enter the bloodstream and disseminate throughout the body, causing fever, joint pain, and skin lesions. Gonorrhea can infect the heart valves, pericardium, and meninges as well. When it infects the joints, a condition known as septic arthritis occurs, characterized by pain and swelling of the joints and potential destruction of the joints.

Gonorrhea can be transmitted to infants through the birth canal, leading to an eye infection that can damage the eye and impair vision. Fortunately, erythromycin eye drops are routinely given to newborns to prevent eye infection. These eyedrops are effective against *Neisseria gonorrhea* as well as *Chlamydia trachomatis.*

TREATMENT AND THERAPY

Treatment for gonorrhea consists of antibiotics. With the development of penicillin-resistant strains of gonorrhea, effective therapy relies on antibiotics to which gonorrhea remains susceptible, such as ceftriaxone. In uncomplicated cases of gonorrheal infection, such as cervicitis, a single dose is given.

A patient who has risk factors for STDs and a clinical picture suggestive of gonorrhea may receive treatment presumptively, before confirmatory laboratory test results for gonorrhea are available. Because a large number of patients with gonorrhea also have chlamydia, patients are treated concomitantly with an antibiotic directed against chlamydia, such as doxycycline. Once laboratory test results confirm the diagnosis of gonorrhea, the patient is tested for other STDs, such as human immunodeficiency virus (HIV), hepatitis B and C, and syphilis.

As with all STDs, a key component of therapy includes counseling regarding safe sex. This includes the use of barrier contraceptives, such as condoms, and the avoidance of high-risk sexual behaviors. Contact tracing is another important element to STD treatment. It notifies the patient's sexual partners of their exposure to gonorrhea or other STDs. Contact tracing also involves offering resources to these partners for medical attention. Contact tracing can prevent both reinfection of the patient through subsequent sexual encounters and the spread of STDs to other sexual partners that the patient's partner may have.

PERSPECTIVE AND PROSPECTS

The symptoms of gonorrhea have been described in numerous cultures in the past, including those dating back to the ancient Chinese, Egyptians, and Romans. The actual gonorrhea bacterium was first identified by Albert Neisser in the 1870's, and it was one of the first bacteria ever discovered. *Neisseria gonorrhea* has continued to be well-studied on both the molecular and the epidemiological level.

Antibiotic therapy, in the form of sulfanilamide, was first used to combat *N. gonorrhea* in the 1930's. By the 1940's, however, gonococcal strains resistant to this antibiotic appeared, and the therapy of choice became penicillin. Over the next several decades, *N. gonorrhea* evolved the ability to resist penicillin, forcing clinicians to use other drugs to combat the bacterium, such as ceftriaxone and ciprofloxacin. In the 1980's, the Centers for Disease Control instituted surveillance programs to monitor antibiotic resistance patterns in different United States cities. Continued success in combating *N. gonorrhea* will depend on the ability to minimize the development of antibiotic resistance.

Finally, since many patients with gonorrhea infection have no symptoms, screening programs of asymptomatic patients who are in high-risk groups (those younger than twenty-five and/or with multiple sexual partners) play a vital role in decreasing the incidence of *N. gonorrhea* infections.

—Anne Lynn S. Chang, M.D.

See also Blindness; Conjunctivitis; Eyes; Genital disorders, female; Genital disorders, male; Gynecology; Reproductive system; Sexually transmitted diseases (STDs); Urology.

FOR FURTHER INFORMATION:

Braunwald, Eugene, et al., eds. *Harrison's Principles of Internal Medicine.* 15th ed. New York: McGraw-Hill, 2001.

Centers for Disease Control. "1998 Guidelines for the Treatment of Sexually Transmitted Diseases." *Morbidity and Mortality Weekly Report* 47, no. RR-1 (January, 1997): 1-118.

Holmes, King K. *Sexually Transmitted Diseases.* 3d ed. New York: McGraw-Hill, 1999.

Ryan, Kenneth J., and C. George Ray, eds. *Sherris Medical Microbiology: An Introduction to Infectious Diseases.* 4th ed. New York: McGraw-Hill/Appleton & Lange, 2003.

GOUT

DISEASE/DISORDER

ALSO KNOWN AS: Gouty arthritis

ANATOMY OR SYSTEM AFFECTED: Feet, joints

SPECIALTIES AND RELATED FIELDS: Internal medicine, podiatry, rheumatology

DEFINITION: A form of arthritis of the peripheral joints, often characterized by painful, recurrent acute attacks and resulting from deposits of uric acid in joint spaces.

KEY TERMS:

acute gout: a very painful gout attack, most common in the left big toe; usually the first indicator of occurrence of the disease

arthritis: any of more than a hundred related diseases, including gout, that are characterized by joint inflammation

cartilage: a tough, white, fibrous connective tissue attached to the bone surfaces that is involved in movement

corticosteroid: a fatlike steroid hormone made by the adrenal glands, or similar synthetic chemicals manufactured by pharmaceutical companies *gene:* a piece of the hereditary material deoxyribonucleic acid (DNA) that carries the information needed to produce an inheritable characteristic

genetic engineering: also called recombinant DNA research; a group of scientific techniques that allow scientists to alter genes

hyperuricemia: the presence of abnormally high uric acid levels, which usually leads to gout symptoms

rheumatologist: a physician who studies rheumatoid arthritis and related diseases

secondary gout: gout symptoms caused by other diseases and by therapeutic drugs

synovial fluid: the thick, clear, lubricating fluid that bathes joints and helps them to move smoothly

tophaceous gout: chronic gout that may be characterized by tophi, severe joint degeneration, and/or serious kidney problems

tophi: lumps in the cartilage and joints of chronic gout sufferers, caused by crystals of uric acid

CAUSES AND SYMPTOMS

Gout, once called the affliction of kings, is a hereditary disease that causes inflammation of the peripheral joints. It is also called gouty arthritis because arthritis means joint inflammation and describes more than a hundred related diseases. Gout has afflicted humans since antiquity, and it was first described by Hippocrates in the fifth century B.C.E. It usually first presents itself as an extremely painful swelling of the big toe of the left foot in men over the age of forty. Gout attacks, termed acute gout, are quite rare in premenopausal women. In fact, more than 90 percent of all gout sufferers are men. The prevalence of gout is extremely high in Pacific Islanders, with 10 percent of adult males afflicted. One characteristic portrayal of gout sufferers, which may come from the "affliction of kings" concept, is of obese and obviously affluent individuals. This is partly a misconception because gout is a very

democratic disease, found in the poor as often as in the wealthy. Nevertheless, acute gout attacks are often brought on by very rich meals or by drinking sprees, so obesity is accurately portrayed as a contributing factor.

An acute gout attack may occur in almost any joint, with the most common sites after the big toe being the ankles, fingers, feet, wrists, elbows, and knees. Such attacks are not often seen in the shoulders, hips, or spine and, if they do occur, appear only after a gout sufferer has had many previous attacks in other joints. Acute gout of the big toe occurs so often that it has been given its own name, podagra. Common explanations for the very frequent occurrence of podagra are that considerable pressure is placed on the big toe in the process of walking and that most people are right-handed and are therefore "left-footed," putting more pressure on the left foot than on the right one in walking or in sports.

An acute gout attack is preceded by feelings of weakness, nausea, chills, and excessive urination. Then, the area that is affected becomes red to purple, swollen, and so tender that the slightest touch is very painful. This pain is so severe that many sufferers describe it as being crushing, or even excruciating. Acute gout attacks come on suddenly, and many victims report suddenly being jolted awake by pain in the night. Fortunately, such attacks are few and far between and usually last only from a few days to a week. In addition, more than half of those who have one attack of podagra will never have another gout attack.

The problems associated with acute gout are attributable to a chemical called uric acid. Uric acid does not dissolve well in the blood and other biological fluids, such as the synovial fluid in joints. When overproduced by the body or excreted too slowly in urine, undissolved uric acid forms sharp crystals. These crystals and their interactions with other joint components cause the pain felt by gout sufferers. It is interesting to note that gout is caused by the overproduction of uric acid in some individuals and by uric acid underexcretion in others. Many of the foods that seem to cause gout are rich in chemicals called purines, which are converted to uric acid in the course of preparation for excretion by the kidneys.

Much more dangerous to gout victims than the acute attacks is leaving the disease untreated. When this happens, crystals of uric acid produce lumps or masses in the joints throughout the body and in the kidneys. In the joints, the masses, called tophi, lead to inflammation, scarring, and deformity that can produce an irreversible degenerative process. Tophi are most common in the

---

INFORMATION ON GOUT

CAUSES: Heredity, female hormones, disease, medications (chemotherapy, diuretics, some antibiotics)

SYMPTOMS: Joint inflammation (particularly the big toe), scarring, and deformity

DURATION: Chronic with acute episodes

TREATMENTS: Drugs, surgery, dietary changes

fingers and the cartilage of various parts of the body, and external tophi are found in the cartilage of the ears of gout sufferers. The visible tophi, however, are only representative, and undetected uric acid masses may be widely spread throughout the body. Such untreated gout is called chronic or tophaceous gout.

Tophaceous gout is another disease with a long history. It was first described by the Greek physician Galen in the second century C.E. Another extremely dangerous aspect of tophaceous gout is unseen kidney stones, which will cause great pain on urination, produce high blood pressure, and even cause fatalities in 3 to 5 percent of afflicted persons.

The prime indicator of gout is high blood levels of uric acid, called hyperuricemia; however, this condition, without other symptoms, does not always signal existent, symptomatic gout. Therefore, the best indicator of the presence of the disease is a combination of hyperuricemia, acute attacks, and observed uric acid in the synovial fluid of all troublesome, gouty joints.

Some investigators propose that gout sufferers are highly intelligent because such famous individuals as Michelangelo, Leonardo da Vinci, Martin Luther, Charles Darwin, and Benjamin Franklin were afflicted with the disease. This trend, however, may indicate that famous people are usually able to afford a lifestyle that causes the predilection to high uric acid levels (for example, the eating of purine-rich foods and high alcohol consumption). Rheumatologists who have studied gout would argue that alcoholism is a better predictor for the disease because it is very common in heavy drinkers. In fact, studies in which gout patients were given purine-rich diets or purine-rich diets plus alcoholic beverages showed that alcohol increased the number and severity of gout attacks.

Gout is also associated with a number of other diseases, including Down syndrome, lead poisoning, some types of diabetes, psoriasis, and kidney disease. Furthermore, a number of therapeutic drugs used in chemotherapy for cancer, diuretics, and some antibiotics can cause acute gout symptoms. These types of gout are differentiated from the hereditary disease already described—so-called primary gout—by the term "secondary gout." Drug-induced secondary gout goes away quickly when administration of the offending drug is stopped.

Another group of diseases that have symptoms somewhat similar to gout are called pseudogout. They have an entirely different cause (mineral crystals in the joints), occur in men and women with equal frequency,

usually begin in extreme old age, and are treated quite differently.

It is also interesting that while premenopausal women are nearly gout-free, the disease becomes fairly common after the menopause. This fact supports a role for female hormones in preventing the disease. Primary gout in women is usually much more severe and destructive than gout in men. In those families in which maternal gout is observed, it is likely that occurrence of the disease in male offspring will occur earlier than is usual, such as near the age of thirty.

TREATMENT AND THERAPY

Once primary gout has been diagnosed, three methods are available for treating it: therapeutic drugs, surgery, and special diets. Most often, gout treatment uses therapeutic drugs, with the drug of choice being colchicine. Colchicine treatment can be traced back for thousands of years, to Egypt in 1500 B.C.E. Originally, it was given as an extract of the meadow saffron plant, *Colchicum autumnale*. In modern times, the pure chemical has been isolated for medicinal use.

Colchicine is reportedly a specific remedy for gout and has no effect on any other type of arthritis. In fact, the reversal of severe joint pain with colchicine is often used as a diagnostic tool that tells physicians that the joint disease being treated is indeed gout. Colchicine can be utilized to treat acute gout attacks or can be taken routinely for long periods of time. Its actions in the handling of acute attacks are quick and profound. In some cases, however, colchicine will have side effects, including severe stomach cramps, nausea, and diarrhea. When these effects occur, colchicine use is discontinued until they disappear and then its reuse is instituted.

Most of the basis for colchicine action is its decrease of the inflammation that causes the pain of gout attacks. This action is believed to be attributable to colchicine's interaction with white blood cells that destroy uric acid crystals and subsequent prevention of the cells from releasing inflammatory factors. Other drugs that work in this way are nonsteroidal anti-inflammatory drugs (NSAIDs) such as aspirin, ibuprofen, indomethacin, naproxin, and phenylbutazone. Colchicine and NSAIDs are usually given by mouth. In some cases, anti-inflammatory steroid hormones called corticosteroids, such as prednisone and prednisolone, are used to treat acute gout. The corticosteroids are given by injection into the gouty joint. Despite the rapid, almost miraculous effects of these steroids, they are best avoided

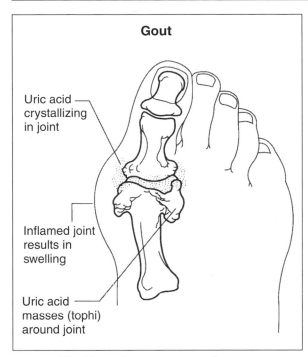

Gout

Uric acid crystallizing in joint

Inflamed joint results in swelling

Uric acid masses (tophi) around joint

The big toe is a common site for gout.

unless absolutely necessary because they can lead to serious medical problems.

Another group of antigout medications consists of the uricosuric drugs. Two favored examples of such drugs are probenecid (Benemid) and sulfinpyrazone (Anturane). The uricosuric drugs prevent the occurrence of hyperuricemia and eventual tophaceous gout by increasing uric acid excretion in the urine, therefore lowering the uric acid levels in the blood. This lowering has two effects: the prevention of the attainment of uric acid levels in the blood and joints that lead to crystal or tophus formation and the eventual dissolution of crystals and tophi as blood levels of uric acid drop.

Uricosuric drugs have no effect, however, on an acute gout attack and can sometimes make such attacks even more painful. For this reason, uricosuric drug therapy is always started after all acute gout attack symptoms have subsided. Aspirin blocks the effects of the uricosuric drugs and should be replaced with acetaminophen (for example, Tylenol) whenever they are utilized for chemotherapeutic purposes. Side effects of excessive doses of uricosuric drugs can include headache, nausea and vomiting, itching, and dizziness. Their use should be discontinued immediately when such symptoms occur. Later reuse of the uricosuric drugs is usually possible.

The third category of antigout drugs is a single chemical, allopurinol (usually, Lopurin or Zyloprim). This drug lowers the body's ability to produce uric acid. It is highly recommended for all gout-afflicted people who have kidney disease that is severe enough for kidney stones to form. It has undesired side effects, however, that include skin rashes, drowsiness, a diminished blood count, and severe allergic reactions. As a result, the use of allopurinol is disqualified for many patients. One advantage of allopurinol chemotherapy over the use of uricosuric agents is the fact that it can be taken along with aspirin.

The end result of a chemotherapeutic regimen with uricosuric drugs and/or allopurinol is the lowering of the blood and urinary uric acid levels so that crystals and tophi do not form or, where formed, redissolve. Often, their combination with colchicine is useful for preventing the occurrence of gout attacks during the initial chemotherapy period.

While surgery is not a common treatment for gout, people who have large tophi that have opened up, become infected, or interfere with joint mobility may elect to have them removed in this fashion. In some cases, severe disability or joint pain caused by the degenerative effects of long-term tophaceous gout is also corrected surgically. Care should be taken, however, to evaluate the consequences of such surgery carefully because the postoperative healing process is often quite slow and many other problems can be encountered.

Media sources often praise special diets in treating gout, without firm proof of their effectiveness. The finding that gout is usually a hereditary disease resulting from metabolic defects that either prevent uric acid excretion or cause its accumulation has pointed out that most dietary factors have a relatively small effect on the disease. Consequently, chemotherapy is much more effective than dietary intervention for diminishing gout symptoms. Nevertheless, there are several incontestable dietary aspects essential to the well-being of persons afflicted with gout.

First, dieting is quite useful, and overweight gout sufferers should lose weight. Such action is best taken slowly and under medical supervision. In fact, excessively fast weight loss can temporarily worsen gout symptoms by elevating blood uric acid levels. In addition, excesses of a number of foods should be avoided by gout sufferers because they are overly rich in the purines that give rise to uric acid when the body processes them. Some examples are the organ meats (liver, kidneys, and sweetbreads), mushrooms, anchovies, sardines, caviar, gravy and meat extracts, shellfish, wine, and beer. Modest intake of these foods is allowable. For example, the daily intake of one can of beer, a glass of wine, or an ounce or two of hard liquor is permissible. The gout sufferer should remember that excessive alcohol intake often brings on acute gout attacks and, even worse, will contribute to worsening tophus and kidney stone formation.

Another adjunct to the prevention or diminution of gout symptoms is the daily intake of at least a half gallon of water or other nonalcoholic beverages. This will help to flush uric acid out of the body, in the urine, and may help to dissipate both tophi and kidney stones. Plain water is best, as it contains no calories that will increase body weight, potentially aggravating gout and leading to other health problems.

PERSPECTIVE AND PROSPECTS

Many sources agree that primary gout is under control in most afflicted people, who can look forward to a normal life without permanent adverse effects of the disease. Those individuals who seek medical treatment at the first appearance of gout symptoms may combine chemotherapy, an appropriate diet regimen, and alcohol avoidance to prevent all but a few acute attacks of the disease. In addition, they will not develop tophi or kidney problems.

Even those afflicted persons who put off treatment until kidney stones or tophi appear can be helped easily. Again, an appropriate diet and the wise choice of chemotherapy agents will prevail. Only the patients who neglect all gout treatment until excessive joint damage and severe kidney disease occur are at serious risk, yet even with these individuals, remission of most severe symptoms is usually possible. The long-term neglect of gout symptoms is unwise, however, because severe tophaceous gout can be both deforming and fatal.

Currently, the eradication of most primary gout, not gout treatment, is seen as the desired goal of research. It is believed that a prime methodology for the eradication of gout will be the use of genetic engineering for gene replacement therapy. Primary gout sufferers are victims of gene lesion diseases: Their bodies lack the ability, because of defective genes, to control either the production or the excretion of uric acid. It is hoped that gene replacement technology will enable medical science to add the missing genes back into their bodies. Other research aspects viewed worthy of exploration in the attempts to vanquish primary gout are the understanding of how to cause white blood cells to destroy

uric acid crystals in the joints more effectively and safely and to decode the basis for the gout-preventing effects of female hormones related to their presence in premenopausal women.

—*Sanford S. Singer, Ph.D.*

See also Alcoholism; Arthritis; Down syndrome; Feet; Foot disorders; Lead poisoning; Obesity; Podiatry; Rheumatology; Urinary disorders.

FOR FURTHER INFORMATION:

Berkow, Robert, and Mark H. Beers, eds. *The Merck Manual of Diagnosis and Therapy.* 17th ed. Whitehouse Station, N.J.: Merck Research Laboratories, 1999. Contains a useful exposition of the characteristics, etiology, diagnosis, and treatment of gout and its relationship to other forms of arthritis. Designed for physicians, the material is also useful for less specialized readers. Information on related topics is also included.

Devlin, Thomas E. *Textbook of Biochemistry: With Clinical Correlations.* 5th ed. New York: Wiley-Liss, 2002. This college textbook presents considerable information on gout, hormones, genetic engineering, and related topics. Includes chemical structures, diagrams, and references useful to the reader. All descriptions are simple but scholarly.

Fries, James F. *Arthritis: A Take-Care-of-Yourself Health Guide for Understanding Your Arthritis.* 5th ed. Reading, Mass.: Addison-Wesley, 1999. Covers gout and pseudogout in a chapter on crystal arthritis, discussing the features, prognosis, and treatments of both problems. Crystal arthritis types are very well differentiated and integrated into the consideration of arthritis.

Parker, James N., and Philip M. Parker, eds. *The 2002 Official Patient's Sourcebook on Gout.* San Diego, Calif.: Icon Health, 2002. Draws from public, academic, government, and peer-reviewed research to provide a wide-ranging handbook for patients with gout.

Scriver, Charles R., et al., eds. *The Metabolic Basis of Inherited Disease.* 8th ed. 2 vols. New York: McGraw-Hill, 2001. This classic medical text contains excellent information on gout describing the symptoms, diagnosis, biochemistry, and genetics of the disease in great detail. Aimed at health science professionals, the book contains much important information for the diligent general reader as well. Pictures, diagrams, and large number of handy references are included.

2002 Physician's Desk Reference Companion Guide. Montvale, N.J.: Medical Economics, 2002. This atlas of prescription drugs includes those used against gout—their manufacturers, useful dose ranges, metabolism and toxicology, and contraindications. This text, found in most public libraries, is useful for both physicians and patients.

GRAFTS AND GRAFTING
PROCEDURE

ANATOMY OR SYSTEM AFFECTED: All

SPECIALTIES AND RELATED FIELDS: Critical care, dermatology, emergency medicine, general surgery, genetics, immunology, neurology, physical therapy, plastic surgery

DEFINITION: The transplantation of tissue from one part of the body to another or from one individual to another in order to treat disease or injury; such surgery requires careful genetic matching in order to avoid a harmful immune response.

KEY TERMS:

allograft: a graft of tissue from one individual to another individual (usually between close relatives)

autograft: a graft of tissue from one part of an individual's body to another part

graft-versus-host disease (GVHD): a genetic incompatibility between tissues in which immune system cells from the grafted tissue attacks host tissue

histocompatibility: tissue compatibility, as determined by histocompatibility protein antigens present on the cell membranes of all tissue cells

histology: the study of tissues and their development, roles, and locations within the body

host-versus-graft disease (HVGD): a tissue rejection in which the immune system cells of the graft recipient attack the grafted tissue from a donor individual

immune response: the reaction of an intricate system of cells, which identify, attack, immobilize, and remove foreign tissue from the body through chemical signals

leukocytes: white blood cells, immune system cells which either produce antibodies or phagocytically consume cells and tissues that are genetically foreign in nature

tissue: a specialized region of cells that forms organs within the body; the four principal types are epithelial, connective, nervous, and muscular

totipotence: the capacity for cells of a given tissue type to regenerate and replace killed or damaged cells within a given body region

INDICATIONS AND PROCEDURES

In medicine, a graft is a tissue region which is transferred from one part of the body to another body part (autograft) or from one individual to another individual (allograft). Grafts between individuals of differing species (xenografts) also are possible. The actual transfer of tissue is called a transplant. The identification and matching of appropriate tissue types and the surgical connection of the tissue constitute grafting.

Examples of autografts include the use of leg veins to reconstruct the coronary arteries during heart bypass surgery, skin transplants during reconstructive facial surgery, and thumb/big toe interposable transplants following the loss of a hand or foot digit. Examples of allografts include major organ transplantations (including that of the heart, liver, and kidney), bone marrow transplantation, and blood transfusions between two genetically matched individuals. Xenograft examples include the grafting of animal tissue such as skin or stomach epithelia to the equivalent body parts in humans.

Genetic matching of donor and recipient tissues in grafting and transplantation is critical to the success of the tissue graft. Thus, tissue compatibility, termed histocompatibility, is of primary importance for successful grafting. Autografts are the most successful grafts because they occur on the same individual, and consequently there is no genetic difference between donor and recipient cells. As the genetic difference between donors and graft recipients increases, however, the probability decreases that a graft will be successful.

For example, grafts between identical twins are highly successful because the donor and recipient are genetically identical; hence, the situation is the same as an autograft. Grafts between siblings are likely to succeed. Allografts between people having distinct genetic differences, however, are less likely to succeed. Xenografts are extremely difficult except for basic mammalian tissues, such as epithelial tissue.

Histology is the study of tissues and their development within the human body. The four principal tissue types within the human body and within other mammalian species are epithelial tissue, which lines the surfaces of organs inside and outside throughout the body; connective tissue (such as cartilage, bone, fat, and blood), which provides structure or transport throughout the body; nervous tissue, which conducts electrical impulses as information networks throughout the body; and muscular tissue, which provides contractility and movement for various body parts. All organs consist of a specific pattern of these four tissues: Epithelial tissue provides cover and protection, connective tissue provides support, nervous tissue provides information from the central control regions of the brain, and muscular tissue allows responses to localized change in the organ. In addition, the cells of tissues subspecialize for unique roles within the tissue of which they are a part. For example, nervous system cells may specialize to form receiving sensory neurons or transmitting motor neurons.

Regardless of tissue type, each of the thousand trillion cells in an individual possesses the same basic genes as the others, and therefore many of the same proteins are expressed throughout the body. All cells within an individual have proteins located within the lipid bilayers of their cell membranes. Several of these proteins are located on every single cell of the individual and thus serve as genetic identification markers for the individual's immune system. These cell surface identification proteins are called histocompatibility proteins.

The histocompatibility proteins, of which there are many, are encoded by a battery of human genes called the major histocompatibility complex (MHC). These proteins ensure tissue compatibility for all cells in an individual with respect to that individual's immune system. The cells of the immune system recognize the specific histocompatibility proteins of one's own cells as "self" markers. Foreign cells, which are missing a few or many of the individual's specific set of histocompatibility proteins, are recognized by the im-

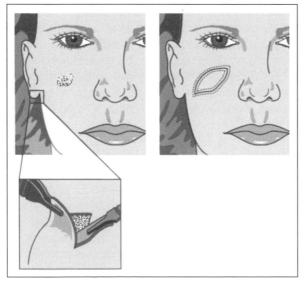

Skin grafting requires the excision of tissue from a less noticeable location, such as behind the ear, and its relocation to an injured or more cosmetically important area, such as the face.

mune system as "nonself" and are attacked. This self-versus-nonself reaction is how the immune system distinguishes its own cells from any invading foreign cells and tissues. Therefore, the histocompatibility proteins play a critical role in the successful identification of one's own cells and the destruction of infections, such as those caused by bacterial or fungal cells.

An immune response occurs when immune system cells called leukocytes (white blood cells) cannot locate the specific "self" histocompatibility proteins on a sampled cell. A type of leukocyte called a T lymphocyte will release a protein called immunoglobulin to immobilize the foreign "nonself" cell lacking the correct histocompatibility antigens (the proteins on the cell membranes). Immunoglobulins, also called antibodies, are proteins secreted by T lymphocytes to immobilize foreign antigens.

After the T lymphocyte antibodies have immobilized the antigens on the foreign cells, another type of leukocyte called a B lymphocyte produces antibodies that attack the foreign antigens. Furthermore, the B lymphocytes will multiply themselves, creating millions of copies to produce a clone army of B lymphocytes, all of which make the same antibodies targeted at the same foreign antigens. These specialized clones constitute a memory cell line, which will attack these antigens again if the organism is exposed to them in the future. This reaction is the basis of immunization.

Furthermore, after the T and B lymphocyte antibodies immobilize the foreign antigens, phagocytic leukocytes such as neutrophils and macrophages migrate to the region to ingest and completely destroy the foreign cells. This process will continue until either the foreign cells are vanquished or the immune system is exhausted.

The immune response just described may appear simple, but it is very complicated. In addition to the complex chemical identification of histocompatibility proteins on all of an individual's cells, the production of specific antibodies by T and B lymphocytes involves an extraordinary rearrangement of genes within these immune cells that is still poorly understood.

The immune response directly affects grafts and grafting. For transplants performed between two individuals, most tissues require a close genetic match between the donor and the recipient. They should be as closely related to each other as possible so that they share a common genetic heritage and, therefore, a high probability that their respective cells have most, if not all, of the same histocompatibility proteins. A close genetic relationship between the graft donor and recipient maximizes the chance that a graft will succeed and that an immune response against nonself tissues will not occur.

USES AND COMPLICATIONS

Grafts, grafting, and transplants between individuals are extremely important in the treatment of maiming or disfiguring accidents and life-threatening diseases. A huge demand exists for grafted tissue, not merely organ transplants, for use in a variety of medical conditions and procedures.

The most common and successful types of grafts are autografts from one part of an individual's body to another part, or from one identical twin to her or his sibling. In autograft cases, there is a perfect match for the histocompatibility proteins on all the cells and tissues. Thus, an immune response will not occur unless the immune system is abnormal in some way, as with such autoimmune diseases as lupus erythematosus and rheumatoid arthritis.

An example of an autograft is the transfer of a vein from the leg to the heart in a patient suffering from coronary artery disease; the grafted vein serves as a replacement coronary artery supplying blood, nutrients, and oxygen to the heart muscle. Another type of autograft is the transfer of skin from the abdomen or pelvic region to the face as part of reconstructive plastic surgery. A severed thumb can be replaced by the big toe, its equivalent digit on the foot.

Allografts, those between different individuals, can be successful if there is careful genetic matching between the donor and recipient tissues. Because of the specificity of matching for certain tissue and cell types, donor-recipient matching may mean an average of any two people out of a thousand or, with more critical tissue lines such as stem cells, two people out of ten million. Often, siblings will serve as tissue donors. Otherwise, the lengthy process of finding possible tissue donors and determining their specific histocompatibility profiles must be conducted before the graft can take place between a recipient and a matched tissue donor.

Grafts are simple between generalized surface tissue such as epithelial and connective tissues. Pig epithelial tissue has been used for skin and stomach tissue grafts on human recipients. Bone marrow transplants for aplastic anemia and leukemia patients, however, require more difficult histocompatibility matching. The use of fetal nervous tissue grafts into the brain tissue of Alzheimer's disease patients has yielded promising re-

sults in regenerating brain tissue and slowing the acceleration of this debilitating disease, which generally strikes the elderly.

Grafts are useful for tissue lines lacking totipotence, the ability to regenerate damaged or dead cells. The example cited above of fetal tissue being used to treat Alzheimer's disease is a clear illustration of such tissue-grafting applications. Mature brain tissue in adult humans cannot regenerate. Fetal tissue grafts, however, have facilitated the regenerative capacity of some brain tissue in these patients.

Likewise, stem cell lines such as the red bone marrow of flat bones, where white blood cells (leukocytes) and red blood cells (erythrocytes) are manufactured, are important targets for tissue grafting. In leukemia, a patient's bone marrow is rapidly producing malignant leukocytes. It is clear that the stem cell line producing these cells is aberrant in such patients. Consequently, a small graft of bone marrow tissue from a histocompatible donor's bone marrow may lead to the establishment of a healthy stem cell line in the patient to stop the overproduction of aberrant cells.

In any grafting process, the donor tissue is surgically inserted and secured into the recipient's tissue site. There, the tissue, if successful, can grow and expand into the localized organ region to perform its correct function in the individual's body. In the event that there is not a histocompatible match between the donor tissue within the recipient's body, two possible rejection mechanisms can ensue. In host-versus-graft disease (HVGD), which is the most common type, the recipient's immune system releases antibodies and eventually destroys the donor tissue. In graft-versus-host disease (GVHD), immune system cells transplanted with the donor tissue into the recipient migrate into the recipient's tissues and attack the cells; the recipient will become ill and may die. The grafted tissue has rejected the entire body into which it has been transferred.

PERSPECTIVE AND PROSPECTS

In 1990, the Nobel Prize in Physiology or Medicine was awarded to American medical researchers Joseph E. Murray of the Harvard Medical School and E. Donnall Thomas of Seattle's Fred Hutchinson Cancer Research Center. These two scientists were pioneers in the use of grafts, grafting, and tissue transplants to save people's lives. Murray performed the first successful kidney transplant, between two identical twins, in 1954. Murray teamed with Thomas at Harvard to study methods for preventing host-versus-graft rejections. During the 1960's at the University of Washington, Thomas developed the technique of destroying a potential bone marrow recipient's immune system using radiation, followed by the grafting of donor bone marrow tissue into the patient, thereby increasing the chances that the transplant will succeed before the patient's immune system can become active again. Both scientists also made important discoveries concerning the major histocompatibility proteins.

Grafts and grafting play a vital role in medicine. Grafts can save the lives of people with such diseases as leukemia, anemia, and cancer. Grafts also can be useful in reconstructing damaged organs and skin, especially for burn victims. Still, much research is needed to understand histocompatibility better and to reduce the chance of tissue rejection.

—David Wason Hollar, Jr., Ph.D.

See also Alzheimer's disease; Amputation; Bone grafting; Bone marrow transplantation; Breast surgery; Burns and scalds; Cleft lip and palate repair; Corneal transplantation; Critical care; Critical care, pediatric; Dermatology; Dermatopathology; Emergency medicine; Fetal tissue transplantation; Hair transplantation; Heart transplantation; Heart valve replacement; Immune system; Kidney transplantation; Laceration repair; Leukemia; Liver transplantation; Malignant melanoma removal; Pigmentation; Plastic surgery; Skin; Skin lesion removal; Transplantation; Xenotransplantation.

FOR FURTHER INFORMATION:

Adelman, Daniel C., et al., eds. *Manual of Allergy and Immunology*. Philadelphia: Lippincott Williams & Wilkins, 2002. Examines research developments and the clinical diagnosis and treatment of allergies and immune disorders. Covers transplantation immunology.

Alberts, Bruce, et al. *Molecular Biology of the Cell*. 4th ed. New York: Garland, 2002. Describes the evolution of cells and introduces cell structure and function. The text is clearly written at the college level and is illustrated by numerous diagrams and photographs. Section on the immune system contains an excellent discussion of the immune system, grafts, rejection, and histocompatibility.

Beck, William S., Karel F. Liem, and George Gaylord Simpson. *Life: An Introduction to Biology*. 3d ed. New York: HarperCollins, 1991. An outstanding introductory textbook for biology majors that is clearly written and beautifully illustrated. Chapter 23, "Immunity," is a good discussion of basic concepts, including descriptions of immune reactions and various types of transplants such as blood type ABO and Rh factor matchups.

Eisen, Herman N. *General Immunology: An Introduction to Molecular and Cellular Principles of the Immune Response*. 3d ed. Philadelphia: J. B. Lippincott, 1990. This incredibly thorough and concise work describes in great detail the various workings of animal immune systems, including types of antibodies, immune system cells, grafts, graft rejection, histocompatibility proteins, and the genetic basis of the immune response.

Kuby, Janis. *Immunology*. 4th ed. New York: W. H. Freeman, 2000. The section on hypersensitivity in this immunology textbook is well written and includes a mixture of detail and overview of the subject. Particularly useful are discussions of the various types of hypersensitivity reactions.

Memmler, Ruth L., Barbara J. Cohen, and Dena L. Wood. *Memmler's The Human Body in Health and Disease*. 9th ed. Philadelphia: J. B. Lippincott, 2000. This book is a thorough but brief introduction to human anatomy, physiology, and disease that is written specifically for the layperson. Chapter 17, "Body Defenses, Immunity, and Vaccines," describes the immune system, transplants, and graft rejection.

Palca, Joseph. "Overcoming Rejection to Win a Nobel Prize." *Science* 250 (October 19, 1990): 378. Palca's article is an announcement of the 1990 Nobel Prize in Physiology or Medicine awarded to Americans Joseph E. Murray and E. Donnall Thomas, pioneers in grafting and transplant medical research. Palca discusses the careers of these two scientists and the major experiments leading to their momentous discoveries.

GRAM STAINING
PROCEDURE

ANATOMY OR SYSTEM AFFECTED: Cells, immune system

SPECIALTIES AND RELATED FIELDS: Bacteriology, biochemistry, cytology, microbiology

DEFINITION: A staining process used as a means of differentiating microorganisms, which are classified as either gram-positive or gram-negative.

KEY TERMS:

cell wall: a structure outside the cell membrane of most bacteria, composed of varying amounts of carbohydrates, lipids, and amino acids *gram-negative:* referring to microorganisms that appear pink following the Gram-staining procedure

gram-positive: referring to microorganisms that appear violet following the Gram-staining procedure

Gram's stain: a method of staining bacteria as a primary means of differentiation and identification

lipopolysaccharide (LPS): a major component of the cell wall of gram-negative bacteria; the toxicity of LPS is associated with illnesses caused by gram-negative organisms

mordant: a chemical that acts to fix a stain within a physical structure; the role played by iodine in Gram's stain

peptidoglycans: repeating units of sugar derivatives that make up a rigid layer of bacterial cell walls; found in both gram-positive and gram-negative cells

INDICATIONS AND PROCEDURES

The observation and identification of bacteria are of obvious primary importance in the study of microorganisms. Even with the use of powerful microscopes, direct observation of unstained bacteria is difficult. The use of stains to increase their contrast with the background allows bacteria to be observed more easily.

As a result of resident acidic groups—polysaccharides or nucleic acids—the surfaces of bacteria tend to be negatively charged. Conversely, the dye portion of common stains such as methylene blue or crystal violet consists of positively charged ions. For staining purposes, a sample of bacteria is placed on a glass slide and allowed to dry. The solution of stain is flooded over the bacterial "smear" for about a minute, and the slide is then rinsed. The main purpose of such simple stains is to allow the cells to be observed.

In contrast with simple stains, differential staining methods do not stain all cells in the same manner. Bacteria grown under different environmental conditions, or bacteria that may differ from one another in their physical structure, will exhibit different staining properties when treated with differential stains. Gram staining (also called Gram's stain) is an example of a differential stain.

Gram staining is a relatively simple procedure and is among the first practices learned by students in microbiology laboratories. The process begins with the preparation of a bacterial smear on the slide. A stain, crystal violet, is allowed to flood the dried smear. The slide is rinsed, and a solution of iodine is dropped over the smear. The iodine functions as a mordant, fixing the crystal violet into a complex insoluble in water. Following another rinse, the smear is covered with either an alcohol or an acetone "destaining" solution for several seconds, rinsed again, and counterstained with the red dye safranin. After a last wash, the bacteria are observed with a microscope. If they were not destained by the alcohol step, retaining the blue or violet color, they are considered gram-positive; if they have stained pink because of the counterstain safranin, they are considered gram-negative.

The precise means by which Gram staining works is not entirely clear. The cell wall structure of gram-positive bacteria either prevents the alcohol/acetone solution from removing the crystal violet-iodine complex from the cell or prevents the solution from having access to the complex. Though the question remains whether the cell wall structure is the sole determining factor in the differential procedure, there is no doubt that the cell wall features are primary factors in the determination of Gram-staining results. Therefore, the structure of the cell wall in most bacteria reflects the Gram-staining characteristics.

The cell wall structure found in gram-positive bacteria differs significantly from that in gram-negative cells. While both contain a rigid layer called the peptidoglycan, the peptidoglycan layer is much thicker and makes up a significantly larger portion of the cell wall in gram-positive bacteria. In contrast, a significant portion of the cell wall found in gram-negative bacteria is composed of lipid derivatives.

The peptidoglycan portion of the cell is composed of repeating units of two sugar derivatives: N-acetylglucosamine and N-acetylmuramic acid. The peptidoglycan within the wall is in the form of sheets, layered on top of one another. In gram-positive bacteria, approximately 90 percent of the cell wall material consists of peptidoglycan; among gram-negative bacteria, about 10 percent of the wall is represented by this rigid layer.

These cell wall structures are stabilized by short chains of amino acids that cross-link the layers of peptidoglycan. Formation of the cross bridges is an enzymatic process called transpeptidation. The antibiotic penicillin inhibits the enzyme that carries out the formation of such cross-links. The result is a weakening in the cell wall, and possibly cell death. Since the peptidoglycan layer of gram-negative bacteria represents a much smaller proportion of the cell wall, such microorganisms are often more resistant to the action of penicillin than are gram-positive bacteria.

During the Gram-staining procedure, decolorization of the cell is carried out during the wash with alcohol or acetone. The thick peptidoglycan layer found in gram-positive bacteria, however, prevents movement of the crystal violet-iodine complex from the cell. Thus, the cells do not decolorize; they retain their violet appearance.

The peptidoglycan layer is a small proportion of the gram-negative cell wall. Much of the outer wall in these bacteria is a layer of lipopolysaccharide (LPS), which acts as a physical barrier but also contains pharmacological properties. The LPS layer is a complex structure containing a lipid portion (lipid A), a core polysaccharide consisting of a variety of sugars, and an outer layer of branched sugars called the O-region (O-polysaccharide). The LPS layer is anchored to the thin peptidoglycan portion of the cell wall through a lipoprotein complex. The LPS portion of gram-negative cell walls is often termed endotoxin because of its pharmacological activity. Release of LPS as a result of cell death during certain types of infection can result in high fever or shock.

Since the cell wall of gram-negative bacteria contains proportionately little peptidoglycan, the crystal violet-iodine complex is easily removed during the Gram-staining procedure. Following the alcohol step, the cells again appear colorless. Therefore, when they are counterstained with the safranin, the bacteria will appear pink.

An evaluation of Gram-staining characteristics is generally the first step in the identification of newly isolated bacteria. Most bacteria can be classified as either gram-positive or gram-negative, and this step, along with characterization of the shape of the organism, is of immense importance in narrowing down the possible identities of an isolate.

Further means of identification generally involve the use of selective or differential types of media. These processes utilize the biochemical properties of bacteria for their identification. A selective medium is one in which chemical compounds have been added that inhibit the growth of certain forms of bacteria but allow the growth of others. For example, the chemical dye cosin-methylene blue (EMB) inhibits the growth of gram-positive bacteria while allowing gram-negative bacteria to grow. If a mixed culture of bacteria is inoculated onto EMB medium, only the gram-negative microorganisms will grow. A differential medium will allow a variety of bacteria to grow, but different types of bacteria may produce different reactions on the medium. Since EMB agar contains lactose as a carbon source, it is also a differential medium. Bacteria that ferment lactose produce a green metallic color of colony on EMB; bacteria that do not ferment lactose produce a pink colony.

Biochemical tests are more useful for the identification of organisms that are gram-negative than for those that are gram-positive. Biochemical variations among both genera and species of gram-positive bacteria tend to be too variable for effective identification of these organisms. By contrast, such biochemical results among gram-negative bacteria generally do not vary significantly within the species and hence are useful means of further identification.

The biochemical tests used for identification of gram-negative bacteria can be summarized in the form of a flow chart. Such charts represent the series of tests that divide bacteria into smaller and smaller groups. For example, following a determination of morphological and Gram-staining characteristics, differential tests may be carried out to observe the ability of the bacteria to ferment various types of carbohydrates. A series of broths containing such sugars as glucose, lactose, or sucrose are inoculated. Generally, a pH indicator such as the chemical phenol red is included, as is an inverted glass tube (Durham tube) for observation of gas production. If the organism can ferment lactose and produces acid and gas, the broth tube of lactose will appear yellow and there will be a gas bubble in the Durham tube. If the organism does not ferment lactose, no growth or change from the red color of the broth will be observed in that tube.

Further differentiation of either lactose-positive or lactose-negative organisms, to continue with this particular example, can be carried out with other biochemical tests. Certain species of bacteria are capable of removing a molecule of carbon dioxide from amino acids; others are not. In some cases, multiple tests can be run at the same time. For example, a common differential test for gram-negative bacteria utilizes a medium called triple sugar iron (TSI) agar. TSI agar contains a small amount of glucose and larger amounts of lactose and sucrose, hence the designation of triple sugar. Iron is also contained in the medium. The agar is prepared in a test tube and allowed to harden on a slant. Organisms are inoculated onto the surface of the slant and stabbed into the butt of the slant. If glucose alone is fermented, only enough acid is produced to turn the butt yellow. If either lactose or sucrose is fermented, both the slant and butt of the agar will turn yellow. Production of hydrogen sulfide gas is indicated by a black precipitate from iron sulfide; other gas production is indicated by bubble formation in the region of the stab. In this manner, inoculation of a single type of medium can provide multiple tests for identification.

At one time, each of these differential tests had to be carried out individually. Beginning in the 1970's, however, a variety of media kits became available that allow fifteen to twenty tests to be run simultaneously. These kits consist of strips of miniaturized versions of biochemical tests that permit the rapid identification of gram-negative bacteria.

Even though some biochemical tests are less helpful in the identification of gram-positive bacteria, some characteristics of these organisms can be used. These organisms may be round (cocci) or rod-shaped (bacilli). If bacilli, they may be aerobic (they utilize oxygen) or anaerobic (they do not utilize oxygen). By testing for coagulase, an enzyme which will cause the coagulation of plasma, cocci can be further differentiated.

Finally, serological methods can be used in the identification of either gram-positive or gram-negative organisms. In these tests, a fluorescent dye is attached to molecules of antibodies, proteins directed against the surface molecules of specific bacteria. The ability of the antibodies to attach to bacteria is indicative of the species.

USES AND COMPLICATIONS

The use of Gram-staining methodology is arguably the single most important step in the identification of microorganisms; its applications are far-ranging. Most diseases of humans and other animals, as well as of plants, are caused by microorganisms. Isolation and identification of disease-causing bacteria are key aspects in understanding the etiology of such diseases. Many aspects of technology, from the discovery or development of new antibiotics to the development of new strains of microbes, utilize such methodologies as Gram's stain in the identification of fresh isolates.

Clinical methods for the identification of infectious agents follow a series of defined steps. The particular material involved depends on the type and site of infection and can include such fluids as blood, urine, pus, or saliva (sputum). The specific symptoms of the illness may also provide clues as to the particular agents involved.

For example, among the most common infections are those of the urinary tract. These are particularly common nosocomial, or hospital-acquired, infections. Samples are taken with a sterile swab, which is used to inoculate special types of selective or differential media. Generally speaking, such infections are usually associated with gram-negative bacteria. The majority of these infections, about 90 percent, are caused by *Escherichia coli* (*E. coli*), a common intestinal organism. To a lesser extent, such infections may be associated with other genera such as *Klebsiella*, *Pseudomonas*, *Proteus*, or *Streptococcus*. All but *Streptococcus* are gram-negative bacilli.

Confirmation of the Gram morphology follows growth on selective media. The media of choice in this example are those selective for gram-negative bacteria: either eosin-methylene blue or MacConkey agars. Both inhibit the replication of bacteria such as *Staphylococcus*, commonly found on the surface of the skin and a possible contaminant during the swabbing of the site of infection.

The presence of the sugar lactose in either MacConkey or EMB agar allows these media to be differential in addition to being selective. Lactose fermenters such as *Escherichia*, *Klebsiella*, or *Enterobacter* will produce pink colonies on MacConkey agar, while gram-negative organisms such as *Proteus*, *Pseudomonas*, or *Salmonella*, which do not ferment lactose, will produce colorless colonies on this medium. Analogous results can be seen with other differential enteric agars. More detailed types of analysis using other forms of media or utilizing immunological methods may be necessary to fine-tune the diagnosis, or antibiotic susceptibility tests may simply be conducted to determine the treatment of choice.

In some instances, Gram morphology may be sufficient for the identification of a microorganism. For example, the presence of gram-negative cocci in a cervical smear from a patient suspected of having contracted a sexually transmitted disease is indicative of a *Neisseria gonorrhea* infection. The identification can be confirmed using immunological methods or through growth on selective media such as Thayer-Martin agar, which contains antibiotics inhibitory to most other gram-negative bacteria.

If the clinical sample consists of blood or cerebrospinal fluid, both of which are normally sterile, either gram-negative or gram-positive organisms may be involved. The initial step toward identification is a Gram's stain of the material. Gram-negative bacteria can be identified using methods already described. Generally speaking, the bacterial content of blood during bacteremia will be too low for ready observation. For this reason, blood samples are inoculated into bottles of nonselective growth media, one of which is grown under aerobic conditions and one under anaerobic conditions. If and when growth becomes apparent, smears are prepared for Gram staining.

Gram-positive cocci will almost always be members of either of two genera: *Staphylococcus* or *Streptococcus*. The two can be differentiated on the basis of catalase production, an enzyme which degrades hydrogen peroxide; staphylococci produce the enzyme, while streptococci do not. A variety of commercial kits are available for rapid identification of species. These contain a battery of tests based on biochemical properties of the organisms, including tolerance of high salt, fermentation of unusual sugars, and growth characteristics on blood agar plates (nutrient agar containing sheep red blood cells).

The identification of gram-positive bacilli is more difficult, given their biochemical variation even within the genus. The major subdivisions of this group are based on their tolerance of oxygen. Obligate gram-positive anaerobes, organisms that cannot tolerate oxygen, include the genus *Clostridium*, members of which cause tetanus, gangrene, and food poisoning. Aerobes and facultative anaerobes, which are oxygen-tolerant, include the genera *Bacillus*, *Corynebacterium*, and *Listeria*. Further identification often requires immunological means.

The gram-negative bacillus *E. coli* is frequently used as a marker for sewage contamination of water supplies. Since it is a common intestinal organism and rarely found in soil, its presence in water samples is indicative of possible fecal contamination of that water. Testing for the presence and level of *E. coli* utilizes the biochemical properties of the microbe. Various quantities of the water sample are placed in tubes of lactose broth; growth is indicative of a lactose fermenter and is presumptive for the presence of *E. coli*. A sample of the lactose culture is then streaked on EMB agar. The development of metallic green-colored colonies of gram-negative bacilli confirms the presence of *E. coli*. The smaller the volume of the water sample that produced growth in lactose, the higher the level of *E. coli* in that sample. In a sense, *E. coli* serves as a surrogate marker in these tests. It may not itself be a pathogen (though some strains of *E. coli* may indeed cause severe intestinal infections), but other gram-negative intestinal pathogens such as *Salmonella*, *Shigella*, or *Vibrio*, even if present in water supplies, may be in a concentration too low for ready detection. Therefore, the presence of *E. coli* suggests possible fecal contamination, allowing for proper sewage treatment. Conversely, the absence of *E. coli* in the water sample indicates that fecal contamination, and therefore the presence of other intestinal pathogens, is unlikely.

PERSPECTIVE AND PROSPECTS

During the latter portion of the nineteenth century, the role of bacteria as etiological agents of disease became apparent. Eventually the experimental observations linking the presence of bacteria with various illnesses coalesced in the so-called germ theory of disease. During the early 1880's, the German physician Robert Koch, along with his colleagues and students, developed an experimental method that could be applied to associate a particular organism with a specific disease. These procedures eventually became known as Koch's postulates. Inherent in Koch's postulates was the necessity to observe the microbial agent, either in tissue or following growth in the laboratory. Staining methods, however, were often crude or imprecise. The best one might hope for was to be able to at least observe the organism.

Hans Christian Gram, a Danish physician working with C. Friedlander in Berlin during the early 1880's, was able to introduce a highly effective method of staining bacteria. Gram's method was a modification of that developed earlier by Paul Ehrlich. The procedure began by first staining the sample with Gentian Violet in aniline water, followed by treatment with iodine in a potassium iodide solution. Gram found that when tissue sections or smears treated in such a manner were washed with dilute alcohol, certain types of bacteria (or schizomycetes, as they were then known) became decolorized (gram-negative), while other forms of bacteria retained their violet appearance (gram-positive). The procedure, published in 1884, was shown to be applicable for most types of bacteria. As a result, a process for differentiation between various types of bacteria became available. In addition, the ability to detect smaller quantities of bacteria in tissue increased significantly.

—Richard Adler, Ph.D.

See also Bacterial infections; Bacteriology; Cells; Cytology; *E. coli* infection; Laboratory tests; Microbiology; Salmonella infection; Shigellosis; Staphylococcal infections; Streptococcal infections.

FOR FURTHER INFORMATION:

Alcamo, I. Edward. *Microbes and Society: An Introduction to Microbiology*. Sudbury, Mass.: Jones and

Bartlett, 2002. A nonscientific text for the liberal arts student that explores the importance of microbes to human life and their role in food production and agriculture, in biotechnology and industry, in ecology and the environment, and in disease and bioterrorism.

Alcamo, I. Edward, and Lawrence M. Elson. *Microbiology Coloring Book*. New York: HarperCollins, 1996. This volume is one in a series of "coloring books" that are excellent sources of information. Detailed instructions help the reader navigate the intricacies of the world of microbes through observation and reading. This book is jammed with useful facts about the biology of microorganisms and the methods used to study them.

Goodsell, David. *The Machinery of Life*. New York: Springer-Verlag, 1993. A short book on the biology of the cell for the general reader. The section on *Escherichia coli* as the prototype for bacteria is well written and easy to understand. Especially striking are the large number of computer graphics illustrating molecular structures.

Koneman, Elmer, Stephen Allen, V. R. Dowell, Jr., and Herbert Sommers. *Color Atlas and Textbook of Diagnostic Microbiology*. 5th ed. Philadelphia: J. B. Lippincott, 1997. Presents methods of identification for most organisms likely to appear in a clinical laboratory. Of particular interest are the large number of color photographs illustrating results for major staining methods and biochemical tests.

Madigan, Michael T., John M. Martinko, and Jack Parker. *Brock Biology of Microorganisms*. 10th ed. Upper Saddle River, N.J.: Prentice Hall, 2002. An outstanding microbiology text. The authors provide a thorough description of bacteria and the means by which they are studied. Relevant to this topic are chapters on methods of isolation and characterization.

Singleton, Paul. *Bacteria in Biology, Biotechnology, and Medicine*. 5th ed. New York: John Wiley & Sons, 1999. The author has written a concise description of bacteria and their roles in nature. Included are chapters on bacterial structure, staining, and methods of classification and identification. Portions of the book cover molecular aspects of cells.

Snyder, Larry, and Wendy Champness. *Molecular Genetics of Bacteria*. Rev. ed. Washington, D.C.: ASM Press, 2002. A text that introduces the field of bacterial molecular genetics and describes the mechanisms of mutations and gene exchange in bacteria and phages. Concentrates specifically on the bacterium *E. Coli* while using examples from other bacteria as appropriate.

Wilson, Michael, Brian Henderson, and Rod McNab. *Bacterial Virulence Mechanisms*. New York: Cambridge University Press, 2002. Basing their discussion on research advances in microbiology, molecular biology, and cell biology, the authors describe the interactions that exist between bacteria and human cells both in health and during infection.

GRAY HAIR

DISEASE/DISORDER

ANATOMY OR SYSTEM AFFECTED: Hair

SPECIALTIES AND RELATED FIELDS: Dermatology

DEFINITION: The reduction in hair pigmentation that is a natural by-product of aging.

CAUSES AND SYMPTOMS

Hair color is produced by tiny pigment cells in hair follicles called melanocytes. Each melanocyte has long, armlike extensions that carry the pigment granules known as melanin to the hair cells. In the course of a lifetime, the production of pigment-forming enzymes drops, and the activity of the melanocytes in each follicle begins to wane, resulting in gray hair. Each individual's melanocyte clock is different, but in Caucasians the reduction of melanocyte activity usually occurs earlier than in other ethnic groups. On the average, graying starts at age thirty-four in Caucasians, in the late thirties in Asians, and at age forty-four in African Americans.

Pigment loss starts at the root, with some strands of hair gradually fading in color, while others may grow in gray or white. Initial graying can be accelerated by

---

INFORMATION ON GRAY HAIR

CAUSES: Aging; also hyperthyroidism, anemia, autoimmune disease, severe stress, vitamin B_{12} deficiency, skin pigmentation disorders (vitiligo)

SYMPTOMS: Change in hair color; drier, coarser, more wiry hair

DURATION: Chronic

TREATMENTS: Masking via chemical and vegetable rinses and dyes

hyperthyroidism, anemia, autoimmune disease, severe stress, or vitamin B_{12} deficiency. Disorders of skin pigmentation, such as vitiligo, can also result in the loss of hair pigmentation.

Once gray hair begins to appear, the rate at which it progresses over the rest of the head depends entirely upon each individual. It does not appear to be a function of the original hair color or texture, ethnic background, or the condition of the scalp. By age fifty, 50 percent of Caucasians are significantly gray. As hair loses its pigment, it often gets drier, resulting in coarser, wirier hair.

TREATMENT AND THERAPY

For some individuals, gray hair is a symbol of maturity, while for others it is an embarrassing sign associated with the aging process. In most cases, graying can be readily masked if so desired. Effective chemical and vegetable rinses and dyes are available.

—*Alvin K. Benson, Ph.D.*

See also Aging; Hair; Hair loss and baldness; Hair transplantation; Pigmentation; Skin; Skin disorders.

FOR FURTHER INFORMATION:

Carper, Jean. *Stop Aging Now!* New York: Harper-Collins, 1995.

Feinberg, Herbert S. *All About Hair.* Alpine, N.J.: Wallingford Press, 1978.

Greenwood-Robinson, Maggie. *Hair Savers for Women: A Complete Guide to Preventing and Treating Hair Loss.* New York: Crown, 2000.

Levine, Norman. *Pigmentation and Pigmentary Disorders.* Boca Raton, Fla.: CRC Press, 1993.

Schneider, Edward L., and John W. Rowe. *Handbook of the Biology of Aging.* 5th ed. San Diego, Calif.: Academic Press, 2001.

Scott, Susan Craig, and Karen W. Pressler. *The Hair Bible.* New York: Simon & Schuster, 2003.

GRIEF AND GUILT

DISEASE/DISORDER

ANATOMY OR SYSTEM AFFECTED: Psychic-emotional system

SPECIALTIES AND RELATED FIELDS: Family practice, psychiatry, psychology

DEFINITION: Grief and accompanying guilt are common reactions to the fact or eventuality of serious losses of various kinds, especially death; every person eventually experiences grief, and while grief is normal, its effects can be incapacitating.

KEY TERMS:

abnormal grief: an unhealthy response to a loss, which may include anger, an inability to feel loss, withdrawal, and deterioration in health

grief: a multifaceted physical, emotional, psychological, spiritual, and social reaction to loss

guilt: a cognitive and emotional response often associated with the grief experience in which a person feels a sense of remorse, responsibility, and/or shame regarding the loss

loss: the sudden lack of a previously held possession, physical state, or social position or the death of a loved one

CAUSES AND SYMPTOMS

During life, people unavoidably experience a variety of losses. These may include the loss of loved ones, important possessions or status, or health and vitality, and ultimately the loss of self through death. "Grief" is the word commonly used to refer to an individual's or group's shared experience following a loss. The experience of grief is not a momentary or singular phenomenon. Instead, it is a variable, and somewhat predictable, process of life. Also, as with many phenomena within the range of human experience, it is a multidimensional process including biological, psychological, spiritual, and social components.

The biological level of the grief experience includes the neurological and physiological processes that take place in the various organ systems of the body in response to the recognition of loss. These processes, in turn, form the basis for emotional and psychological reactions. Various organs and organ systems interact with one another in response to the cognitive stimulation resulting from this recognition. Human beings are self-reflective creatures with the capacity for experiencing, reflecting upon, and giving meaning to sensations, both physical and emotional. Consequently, the physiological reactions of grief that take place in the body are given meaning by those experiencing them.

The cognitive and emotional meanings attributed to the experience of grief are shaped by and influence interactions within the social dimensions of life. In other words, how someone feels or thinks about grief influences and is influenced by interactions with family, friends, and helping professionals. In addition, the individual's religious or spiritual frame of reference may have a significant influence on the subjective experience and cognitive-emotional meaning attributed to grief.

INFORMATION ON GRIEF AND GUILT

CAUSES: Loss of loved ones, important possessions or status, health and vitality, and ultimately the loss of self through death

SYMPTOMS: Anxiety and/or depression; difficulty sleeping; feeling sad and/or that life has lost its meaning; feelings of loss, shock, shame, rage, numbness, relief, anger, and/or guilt; social isolation, withdrawal, or alienation

DURATION: Varies widely

TREATMENTS: Counseling, antidepressants

The grief reactions associated with a loss such as death vary widely. While it is very difficult and perhaps unfair to generalize about such an intensely personal experience, several predictors of the intensity of grief have become evident. The amount of grief experienced seems to depend on the significance of the loss, or the degree to which the individual subjectively experiences a sense of loss. This subjective experience is partially dependent on the meaning attributed to the loss by the survivors and others in the surrounding social context. This meaning is in turn shaped by underlying belief systems, such as religious faith. Clear cognitive, emotional, and/or spiritual frameworks are helpful in guiding people constructively through the grief process.

People in every culture around the world and throughout history have developed expectations about life, and these beliefs influence the grief process. Some questions are common to many cultures. Why do people die? Is death a part of life, or a sign of weakness or failure? Is death always a tragedy, or is it sometimes a welcome relief from suffering? Is there life after death, and if so, what is necessary to attain this afterlife? The answers to these and other questions help shape people's experience of the grief process. As Elisabeth Kübler-Ross states in *Death: The Final Stage of Growth* (1975), the way in which a society or subculture explains death will have a significant impact on the way in which its members view and experience life.

Another factor that influences the experience of grief is whether a loss was anticipated. Sudden and/or unanticipated losses are more traumatic and more difficult to explain because they tend to violate the meaning systems mentioned above. The cognitive and emotional shock of this violation exacerbates the grief process. For example, it is usually assumed that youngsters will not die before the older members of the family. Therefore, the shock of a child dying in an automobile crash may be more traumatic than the impact of the death of an older person following a long illness.

Death and grief are often distasteful to human beings, at least in Western Judeo-Christian cultures. These negative, fearful reactions are, in part, the result of an individual's difficulty accepting the inevitability of his or her own death. Nevertheless, in cultures which have less difficulty accepting death and loss as normal, people generally experience more complicated grief experiences. The Micronesian society of Truk is a death-affirming society. The members of the Truk society believe that a person is not really grown up until the age of forty. At that point, the individual begins to prepare for death. Similarly, some native Alaskan groups teach their members to approach death intentionally. The person about to die plans for death and makes provisions for the grief process of those left behind.

In every culture, however, the grief-stricken strive to make sense out of their experience of loss. Some attribute death to a malicious intervention from the outside by someone or something else; death becomes frightening. For others, death is in response to divine intervention or is simply the completion of "the circle of life" for that person. Yet for most people in Western societies, even those who come to believe that death is a part of life, grief may be an emotional mixture of loss, shock, shame, sadness, rage, numbness, relief, anger, and/or guilt.

Kübler-Ross points out in her timeless discourse "On the Fear of Dying" (*On Death and Dying*, 1969) that guilt is perhaps the most painful companion of death and grief. The grief process is often complicated by the individual's perception that he or she should have prevented the loss. This feeling of being responsible for the death or other loss is common among those connected to the deceased. For example, parents or health care providers may believe that they should have done something differently in order to detect the eventual cause of death sooner or to prevent it once the disease process was detected.

Guilt associated with grief is often partly or completely irrational. For example, there may be no way that a physician could have detected an aneurysm in her patient's brain prior to a sudden and fatal stroke. Similarly, a parent cannot monitor the minute-by-minute activities of his adolescent children to prevent lethal accidents. Kübler-Ross explains a related phenomenon among children who have lost a parent by pointing out the difficulty in separating wishes from deeds. A child whose wishes are not gratified by a parent may become angry. If the parent subsequently dies, the child may feel guilty, even if the death is some distance in time away from the event in question.

The guilt may also involve remorse over surviving someone else's loss. People who survive an ordeal in which others die often experience "survivor's guilt." Survivors may wonder why they survived and how the deceased person's family members feel about their survival, whether they blame the survivors or wish that they had died instead. As a result, survivors have difficulty integrating the experience with the rest of their lives in order to move on. The feelings of grief and guilt may be exacerbated further if survivors believe that they somehow benefited from someone else's death. A widow who is suddenly the beneficiary of a large sum of money attached to her husband's life insurance policy may feel guilty about doing some of the things that they had always planned but were unable to do precisely because of a lack of money.

Last, guilt may result when people believe that they did not pay enough attention to, care well enough for, or deserve the love of the person who died. These feelings and thoughts are prompted by loss—loss of an ongoing relationship with the one who died, as well as part of the empathetic response to what it might be like to die oneself.

Feelings of guilt are not always present, even if the reaction is extreme. If individuals experience guilt, however, they may "bargain" with themselves or a higher power, review their actions to find what they did wrong, take a moral inventory to see where they could have been more loving or understanding, or even begin to act self-destructively. Attempting to resolve guilt while grieving loss is doubly complicated and may contribute to the development of what is considered an abnormal grief reaction.

The distinctions between normal and abnormal grief processes are not clear-cut and are largely context-dependent; that is, what is normal depends on standards that vary among different social groups and historical periods. In addition, at any particular time the variety of manifestations of grief depend on the individual's personality and temperament; family, social, and cultural contexts; resources for coping with and resolving problems; and experiences with the successful resolution of grief.

Despite this diversity, the symptoms that are manifested by individuals experiencing grief are generally grouped into two different but related diagnostic categories: depression and anxiety. It is normal for the grieving individual to manifest symptoms related to anxiety and/or depression to some degree. For example, a surviving relative or close friend may temporarily have difficulty sleeping, or feel sad or that life has lost its meaning. Relative extremes of these symptoms, however, in either duration or intensity, signal the possibility of an abnormal grief reaction.

In *Families and Health* (1988), family therapist William Doherty and family physician Thomas Campbell identify the signs of abnormal grief reactions as including periods of compulsive overactivity without a sense of loss; identification with the deceased; acquisition of symptoms belonging to the last illness of the deceased; deterioration of health in the survivors; social isolation, withdrawal, or alienation; and severe depression. These signs may also include severe anxiety, abuse of substances, work or school problems, extreme or persistent anger, or an inability to feel loss.

TREATMENT AND THERAPY

There is no set time schedule for the grief process. While various ethnic, cultural, religious, and political groups define the limits of the period of mourning, they cannot prescribe the experience of grief. Yet established norms do influence the grief experience inasmuch as the grieving individuals have internalized these expectations and standards. For example, the typical benefit package of a professional working in the United States offers up to one week of paid "funeral" leave in the event of the death of a significant family member. On the surface, this policy begins to prescribe or define the limits of the grief process.

Such a policy suggests, for example, that a mother or father stricken with grief at the untimely death of a child ought to be able to return to work and function reasonably well once a week has passed. Most individuals will attempt to do so, even if they are harboring unresolved feelings about the child's death. Coworkers, uncomfortable with responding to such a situation and conditioned to believe that people need to "get on with life," may support the lack of expression of grief.

Helpful responses to grief are as multifaceted as is grief itself. Ultimately, several factors ease the grief process. These include validating responses from significant others, socially sanctioned expression of the experience, self-care, social or religious rituals, and possibly professional assistance. Each person responds to grief differently and requires or is able to use different forms of assistance.

Most reactions to loss run a natural, although varied, course. Since grief involves coming to grips with the reality of death, acceptance must eventually be both intellectual and emotional. Therefore, it is important to allow for the complete expression of both thoughts and feelings. Those attempting to assist grief-stricken individuals are more effective if they have come to terms with their own feelings, beliefs, and conflicts about death, and any losses they personally have experienced.

Much of what is helpful in working through grief involves accepting grief as a normal phenomenon. Grief-related feelings should not be judged or overly scrutinized. Supportive conversations include time for ventilation, empathic responses, and sharing of sympathetic experiences. Helpful responses may take the form of "To feel pain and sadness at this time is a normal, healthy response" or "I don't know what it is like to have a child die, but it looks like it really hurts" or "It is understandable if you find yourself thinking that life has lost its purpose." In short, people must be given permission to grieve. When it becomes clear that the person is struggling with an inordinate amount of feelings based on irrational beliefs, these underlying beliefs—not the feelings—may need to be challenged.

People tend to have difficulty concentrating and focusing in the aftermath of a significant loss. The symptoms of anxiety and depression associated with grief may be experienced, and many of the basic functions of life may be interrupted. Consequently, paying attention to healthy eating and sleeping schedules, establishing small goals, and being realistic about how long it may take before "life returns to normal" are important.

While the prescription of medication for the grief-stricken is fairly common, its use is recommended only in extreme situations. Antianxiety agents or antidepressants can interfere with the normal experiences of grief that involve feeling and coming to terms with loss. Sedatives can help bereaved family members and other loved ones feel better over the short term, with less overt distress and crying. Many experts believe, however, that they inhibit the normal grieving process and lead to unresolved grief reactions. In addition, studies suggest that those who start on psychotropic medication during periods of grief stay on them for at least two years.

The grief process is also eased by ritual practices that serve as milestones to mark progress along the way. Some cultures have very clearly defined and well-established rituals associated with grief. In the United States, the rituals practiced continue to be somewhat influenced by family, ethnic, and regional cultures. Very often, however, the rituals are confined to the procedures surrounding the preparation and burial of the body (for example, viewing the body at the mortuary, a memorial service, and interment). As limited as these experiences might be, they are designed to ease people's grief. Yet the grief process is often just beginning with the death and burial of the loved one. Consequently, survivors are often left without useful guidelines to help them on their way.

Another common, although unhelpful, phenomenon associated with the process is for the grief-stricken person initially to receive a considerable amount of empathy and support from family, friends, and possibly professionals (such as a minister or physician) only to have this attention drop off sharply after about a month. The resources available through family and other social support systems diminish with the increasing expectation that the bereaved should stop grieving and "get on with living." If this is the case, or if an individual never did experience a significantly supportive response from members of his or her social system, the role of psychotherapy and/or support groups should be explored. Many public and private agencies offer individual and family therapy. In addition, in many communities there are a variety of self-help support groups devoted to growth and healing in the aftermath of loss.

PERSPECTIVE AND PROSPECTS

The grief process, however it is shaped by particular religious, ethnic, or cultural contexts, is reflective of the human need to form attachments. Grief thus reflects the importance of relationships in one's life, and therefore it is likely that people will always experience grief (including occasional feelings of guilt). Processes such as the grief experience, with its cognitive, emotional, social, and spiritual dimensions, may affect an individual's psychological and physical well-being. Consequently, medical and other health care and human service professionals will probably always be called upon to investigate, interpret, diagnose, counsel, and otherwise respond to grief-stricken individuals and families.

In the effort to be helpful, however, medical science has frequently intervened too often and too invasively into death, dying, and the grief process—to the point of attempting to disallow them. For example, hospitals and other institutions such as nursing homes have become the primary places that people die. It is important to remember that it has not always been this way. Even now in some cultures around the world, people die more often in their own homes than in a "foreign" institution.

In the early phases of the development of the field of medicine, hospitals as institutions were primarily devoted to the care of the dying and the indigent. Managing the dying process was a primary focus. More recently, however, technological advances and specialty development have shifted the mission of the hospital to being an institution devoted to healing and curing. The focus on the recovery process has left dying in the shadows. Death has become equated with failure and associated with professional guilt.

It is more difficult for health care professionals to involve themselves or at least constructively support the grief process of individuals and families if it is happening as a result of the health care team's "failure." In a parallel fashion, society has become unduly fixated on avoiding death, or at least prolonging its inevitability to the greatest possible extent. The focus of the larger culture is on being young, staying young, and recoiling from the effects of age. As a result, healthy grief over the loss of youthful looks, stamina, health, and eventually life is not supported.

Medical science can make an important contribution in this area by continuing to define the appropriate limits of technology and intervention. The struggle to balance quantity of life with quality of life (and death) must continue. In addition, medical science professionals need to redouble their efforts toward embracing the patient, not simply the disease; the person, not simply the patient; and the complexities of grief in death and dying, not simply the joy in healing and living.

—Layne A. Prest, Ph.D.

See also Antidepressants; Death and dying; Depression; Emotions: Biomedical causes and effects; Midlife crisis; Neurosis; Phobias; Postpartum depression; Psychiatric disorders; Psychiatry; Psychiatry, child and adolescent; Psychiatry, geriatric; Psychoanalysis; Stress; Suicide.

FOR FURTHER INFORMATION:

Canfield, Jack L., and Mark Victor Hansen. *Chicken Soup for the Grieving Soul: Stories About Life, Death and Overcoming the Loss of a Loved One.* Deerfield Beach, Fla.: Health Communications, 2003. Part of a popular series. Offers personal stories of loss and grief and explores coping strategies and healing from the loss of a loved one.

Corr, Charles A., Clyde M. Nabe, and Donna M. Corr. *Death and Dying, Life and Living.* 4th ed. Belmont, Calif.: Wadsworth, 2002. This book provides perspective on common issues associated with death and dying for family members and others affected by life-threatening circumstances.

Doka, Kenneth J., ed. *Living with Grief After Sudden Loss: Suicide, Homicide, Accident, Heart Attack, Stroke.* Washington, D.C.: Taylor & Francis, Hospice Foundation of America, 1997. Provides information that will be useful for individuals dealing with the different kinds of adjustment related to the death of a loved one or the loss of functioning or abilities.

Greenspan, Miriam. *Healing Through the Dark Emotions: The Wisdom of Grief, Fear, and Despair.* Boston: Shambhala, 2003. Examines grief from a cultural perspective and argues that grief, fear, and despair are not pathologies to be medicated away but emotions that foster psychological and spiritual growth.

GriefNet. http://griefnet.org/. An Internet community of persons dealing with grief, death, and major loss. Offers more than forty e-mail support groups for adults and children.

James, John K. *When Children Grieve: For Adults to Help Children Deal with Death, Divorce, Pet Loss, Moving, and Other Losses.* New York: HarperCollins, 2002. Provides excellent guidelines for helping children develop a lifelong, healthy response to loss.

Klass, Dennis, Phyllis R. Silverman, and Steven L. Nickman, eds. *Continuing Bonds: New Understandings of Grief.* Washington, D.C.: Taylor & Francis, 1996. Examines cross-cultural manifestations of bereavement, particularly the psychological aspects. Includes a bibliography and an index.

Kübler-Ross, Elisabeth, ed. *On Death and Dying.* New York: Collier Books, 1970. This book is, and will remain, a classic in the field. Kübler-Ross shares the experience of many years working with dying patients and their families.

Staudacher, Carol. *Beyond Grief: A Guide for Recovering from the Death of a Loved One.* New York: Barnes & Noble Books, 2000. A clear and readable guide to the grief process. The author provides specific examples relevant for some of the most painful grief experiences: those following the death of a spouse, child, or parent at an early age.

GROWTH

BIOLOGY

ANATOMY OR SYSTEM AFFECTED: All

SPECIALTIES AND RELATED FIELDS: Embryology, endocrinology, obstetrics, orthopedics, pediatrics

DEFINITION: The development of the human body from conception to adulthood; growth occurs at different rates for different systems over this period, and varies by sex and individual as well.

KEY TERMS:

accretion: a type of growth in which new, nongrowing material is simply added to the surface

allometric growth: unequal rates of growth of different body parts, or in different directions

developmental biology: broadly, the study of ontogeny; narrowly, the study of how gene action is controlled

embryonic stage: that part of ontogeny during which organs are formed

fetal stage: that part of ontogeny after the organs are formed but before birth takes place

interstitial growth: growth throughout a structure, usually in all directions

isometric growth: equal rates of growth of all parts, or in all directions

ontogeny: the entire developmental sequence, from conception through the various embryonic stages, birth, childhood, maturity, senescence, and death; also, the study of this sequence

ossification: the formation of bone tissue

PROCESS AND EFFECTS

The human body grows from conception until adult size is reached. Adult size is reached in females around the age of eighteen and in males around twenty or twenty-one, but there is considerable variation in either direction. (Nearly all numerical measurements of growth and development are subject to much variation.) On the average, males end up with a somewhat larger body size than females because of these two or three extra years of growth.

Growth begins after conception. The first phase of growth, including approximately the first month after conception, is called embryonic growth, and the growing organism is called an embryo. During embryonic growth, the most important developmental process is differentiation, the formation of the various organs and tissues. After the organs and tissues are formed, the rest of prenatal growth is called fetal growth and the developing organism is called a fetus. Respiratory movements begin around the eighteenth week of gestation,

during the fetal stage; limb movements (such as kicking) begin to be felt by the mother around the twenty-fourth week, with a considerable range of variation. At birth, the average infant weighs about 3.4 kilograms (7.5 pounds) and measures about 50 centimeters (20 inches) in length.

Growth continues after birth and throughout childhood and adolescence. From the perspective of developmental biology, childhood is defined as the period from birth to puberty, which generally begins at twelve years of age, and adolescence continues from that point to the cessation of skeletal growth at around the age of eighteen in females and twenty or twenty-one in males. The long period of adulthood that follows is marked by a stable body size, with little or no growth except for the repair and maintenance of the body, including the healing of wounds. After about age sixty, there may be a slight decline in body height and in a few other dimensions.

By one year of age, the average baby is 75 centimeters (30 inches) long and weighs 10 kilograms (22 pounds). (There is actually a slight decline in weight in the first week of postnatal life, but this is usually regained by age three weeks.) For ages one to six, the average weight (in kilograms) can be approximated by the equation "weight = age × 2 + 8." For ages seven to twelve, growth takes place more rapidly: Average weight (in kilograms) can be approximated by "weight = age × 3.5 − 2.5," while average height (in centimeters) can be approximated for ages two to twelve by the equation "height = age × 6 + 77." Head circumference has a median value of about 34.5 centimeters at birth, 46.3 centimeters at an age of one year, 48.6 centimeters at age two, and 49.9 centimeters at age three. All these figures are about 1 centimeter larger in boys than in girls, with considerable individual variation. Median heights and weights, when differentiated by sex, reveal that boys and girls are generally similar until age fourteen, after which boys continue to gain in both dimensions.

Growth of the teeth takes place episodically. In most children, the first teeth erupt between five and nine months of age, beginning with the central incisors, the lower pair generally preceding the upper pair. The lateral incisors (with the upper pair first), the first premolars, the canines, and the second premolars follow, in that order. All these teeth are deciduous teeth ("baby teeth") that will eventually be shed, to be replaced during late childhood by the permanent teeth. At one year of age, most children have between six and eight teeth.

Growth from Infancy to Adulthood

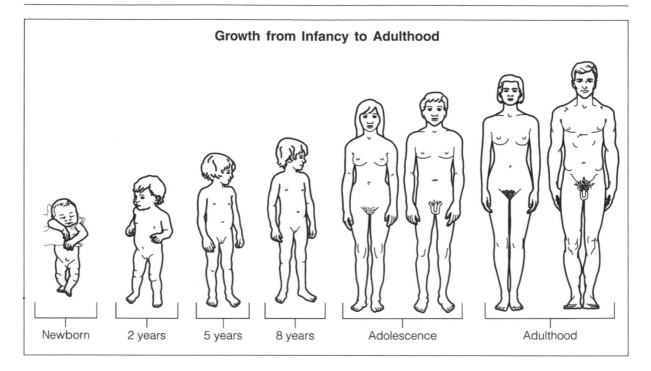

Newborn   2 years   5 years   8 years   Adolescence   Adulthood

Growth takes place in several directions. Growth at the same rate in all directions is called isometric growth, which maintains similar proportions throughout the growth process. Isometric growth occurs in nautilus shells and a variety of other invertebrates. Most of human growth, however, is allometric growth, which takes place at different rates in different directions. Allometric growth results in changes in shape as growth proceeds. Moreover, different parts of the body grow at different rates and in different directions. During fetal development, for example, the head develops in advance of the fore and hind limbs, and the fetus at about six months of age has a head which is about half its length. The head of a newborn baby is about one-third of its body length, compared to about one-seventh for an adult. In contrast, the legs make up only a small part of the body length in either the six-month-old fetus or the newborn baby, and their absolute length and proportionate length both increase throughout childhood and adolescence.

Growth of the skeleton sets the pace for growth of the majority of the body, except for the nervous system and reproductive organs. Most parts of the skeleton begin as fast-growing cartilage. The process in which cartilage tissue turns into bone tissue is called ossification, which begins at various centers in the bone. The first center of ossification within each bone is called the diaphysis; in long bones, this ossification usually takes place in the center of the bone, forming the shaft. Sec-

ondary centers of ossification form at the ends of long bones and at certain other specified places; each secondary center of ossification is called an epiphysis. In a typical long bone, two epiphyses form, one at either end. Capping the end of the bone, beyond the epiphysis, lies an articular cartilage. Between the epiphysis and the diaphysis, the cartilage that persists is called the epiphyseal cartilage; this becomes the most rapidly growing region of the bone. During most of the growth of a long bone, the increase in width occurs by accretion, a gradual process in which material is added at a slow rate only along a surface. In the case of a bone shaft, increase in width takes place only at the surface, beneath the surrounding membrane known as the periosteum. By contrast, the epiphyseal cartilage grows much more rapidly, and it also grows by interstitial growth, meaning that growth takes place throughout the growing tissue in all directions at once. As the epiphyseal cartilage grows, parts of it slowly become bony, and those bony portions grow more slowly.

During the first seven or eight years of postnatal life, the growth of the epiphyseal cartilage takes place faster than its replacement by bone tissue, causing the size of the epiphyseal cartilage to increase. Starting around age seven, the interstitial growth of the epiphyseal cartilage slows down, while the replacement of cartilage by bone speeds up, so that the epiphyseal cartilage is not growing as fast as it turns into bone tissue; the size of the epiphyseal cartilage therefore starts to decrease. At the time of puberty, the hormonal influences create an adolescent growth spurt during which the individual's bone growth increases for about a one-year period. In girls, the adolescent growth spurt takes place about two years earlier than it does in boys—the average age is around twelve in girls, versus about fifteen in boys—but there are tremendous individual variations both in the extent of the growth spurt and in its timing. At age fourteen, most girls have already experienced most of their adolescent growth spurt, while most boys are barely beginning theirs. Consequently, the average fourteen-year-old girl is a bit taller than the average fourteen-year-old boy.

At around eighteen years of age in females and twenty or twenty-one years of age in males, the replacement of the epiphyseal cartilage by bone is finally complete, and bone growth ceases. The age at which this occurs and the resulting adult size both vary considerably from one individual to another. For the rest of adult life, the skeleton remains more or less constant in size, diminishing only slightly in old age.

Most of the other organs of the body grow in harmonious proportion with the growth of the skeleton, reaching a maximum growth rate during the growth spurt of early adolescence and reaching a stable adult size at around age eighteen in women and age twenty or twenty-one in men. The nervous system and reproductive system, however, constitute major exceptions to this rule. The nervous system and brain grow faster at an earlier age, reaching about 90 to 95 percent of their adult size by one year of age. The shape of the head, including the shape of the skull, keeps pace with the development of the brain and nervous system. For this reason, babies and young children have heads that constitute a larger proportion of their body size than do the heads of adults.

The growth of the reproductive system also follows its own pattern. Most reproductive development is delayed until puberty. The reproductive organs of the embryo form slowly and remain small. The reproductive organs of children, though present, do not reach their mature size until adolescence. These organs, both the internal ones and the external ones, remain small throughout childhood. Their period of most rapid growth marks the time of puberty, which spans ages eleven through thirteen, with a wide range of variation. At this time, the pituitary gland begins secreting increased amounts of the follicle-stimulating hormone (FSH), which stimulates the growth and maturation of the gonads (the ovaries of females and the testes of males). The ovaries or testes then respond by producing increased amounts of the sex hormones testosterone (in males) or estrogen (in females), which stimulate the further development of both primary and secondary sexual characteristics. Primary sexual characteristics are those which are functionally necessary for reproduction, such as the presence of a uterus and ovaries in females or the presence of testes and sperm ducts in males. Secondary sexual characteristics are those which distinguish one sex from another, but which are not functionally necessary for reproduction. Examples of secondary sexual characteristics include the growth of breasts or the widening of the hips in females, the growth of the beard and deepening of the voice in males, and the growth of hair in the armpits and pubic regions of both sexes.

MEDIAN HEIGHTS AND WEIGHTS FROM CHILDHOOD TO ADULTHOOD

	Boys		Girls	
Age	Height (cm)	Weight (kg)	Height (cm)	Weight (kg)
2	87	12	87	12
3	95	15	94	14
4	103	17	102	16
5	110	19	108	18
6	117	21	115	20
7	122	23	121	22
8	127	25	127	25
9	132	28	132	28
10	138	31	138	33
11	143	35	145	37
12	150	40	152	42
13	157	45	157	46
14	163	51	160	50
15	169	57	162	54
16	174	62	162	56
17	176	66	163	57
18	177	69	164	57

Growth takes place psychologically and socially as well as physically. Newborn babies, though able to respond to changes in their environment, seem to pay attention to such stimuli only on occasion. At a few weeks of age, the baby will respond to social stimuli (such as the sound of the mother's voice) by smiling. Babies usually can grasp objects by five months of age, depending on the size and shape of the object. By six months, most babies will show definite signs of pleasure in response to social stimulation; this may include an open-mouth giggle or laugh. At seven months of age, most babies will respond to adult facial expressions and will show different responses to familiar adults as opposed to strangers. The age at which babies learn to crawl varies greatly, but most infants learn the technique by nine or ten months of age. Social imitation begins late in the first year of life. Also, by this time, children learn object permanence, meaning that they will search for a missing object if they have watched it being hidden. Walking generally develops around eighteen months of age, but the time of development varies greatly.

Jean Piaget (1896-1980) was a pioneer in the study of the social and cognitive development of children. Piaget identified four stages of cognitive and social growth, which he called sensorimotor, preoperational, concrete operational, and formal operational. In the sensorimotor stage, from birth to about two years of age, infants begin with reflexes such as sucking or finger curling (in response to touching their palms). Starting with these reflexes, they gradually learn to understand their senses and apply the resulting information in order to acquire important adaptive motor skills that can be used to manipulate the world (as in picking up things) or to navigate about and explore the world (as in walking). Socially, infants develop ways to make desirable stimuli last by such acts as smiling. In the preoperational stage, which lasts from about two to six years of age, children acquire a functional use of their native language. Their imagination flourishes, and pretending becomes an important and frequent activity. Most of the thinking at the preoperational stage is egocentric, however, which means that the child perceives the world only from his or her own point of view and has difficulty seeing other points of view.

The concrete operational stage spans the years from about seven to eleven years of age. This is the stage at which children learn to apply logic to concrete objects. For example, they realize that liquid does not change volume when poured into a taller glass, and they develop the ability to arrange objects in order (for example, by size) or to classify them into groups (for example, by color or shape). The final stage is called the formal operational stage, beginning around age twelve. This is the stage of adolescence and adulthood, when the person learns to manipulate abstract concepts in such areas as ethical, legal, or mathematical reasoning. This is also the stage at which people develop the ability to construct hypothetical situations and to use them in arguments.

COMPLICATIONS AND DISORDERS

Disorders of growth include dwarfism, gigantism, and several other disorders such as achondroplasia (chondrodystrophy). Dwarfism often results from an insufficiency of the pituitary growth hormone, also called somatostatin or somatotrophic hormone. Some short-statured individuals are normally proportioned, while others have proportions differing from those of most other people. An overabundance of growth hormone causes gigantism, a condition marked by unusually rapid growth, especially during adolescence. In some individuals, the amount of growth hormone remains normal during childhood but increases to excessive amounts during the teenage years; these individuals are marked by acromegaly, a greater than normal growth which affects primarily the hands, feet, and face.

Achondroplasia, also called chondrodystrophy, is a genetically controlled condition caused by a dominant gene. In people having this condition, the epiphyseal cartilages of the body's long bones turn bony too soon, so that growth ceases before it should. Those exhibiting chondrodystrophy therefore have short stature and childlike proportions but rugged faces that look older than they really are.

Inadequate growth can often result from childhood malnutrition, particularly from insufficient amounts of protein. If a child is considerably shorter or skinnier than those of the same age, that child's diet should be examined for the presence of malnutrition. Intentional malnutrition is one of the characteristic features of anorexia nervosa. The opposite problem, overeating, can lead to obesity, although obesity can also result from many other causes, including diabetes and other metabolic problems.

By the late twentieth century, human growth hormone, a drug used since the 1950's to help very short children grow, was being used for "off-label" purposes that included anti-aging and body-building. In 2002, researchers suggested an apparent link between the use of the hormone and cancer, specifically Hodgkin's disease and colorectal cancer.

PERSPECTIVE AND PROSPECTS

As a phenomenon, growth of both wild and domestic animals was well known to ancient peoples. Hippocrates (c. 460-c. 370 B.C.E.), considered the father of medicine, wrote a treatise on embryological growth, and Aristotle (384-322 B.C.E.) wrote a longer and more complete work on the subject. During the Renaissance, Galileo Galilei (1564-1642) studied growth mathematically and distinguished between isometric and allometric forms of growth, arguing that the bones of giants would be too weak to support their weight.

The most important era in the study of human embryonic development was ushered in by the Estonian naturalist Karl Ernst von Baer (1792-1876), who discovered the human ovum. From this point on, detailed studies of human embryonic and postnatal development proceeded at a rapid pace, especially in Germany. Much of the modern understanding of growth in more general or mathematical terms derives from the classic studies of the British anatomist D'Arcy Wentworth Thomson (1860-1948). In the twentieth century, Piaget became a leader in the study of childhood social and cognitive growth phases.

—*Eli C. Minkoff, Ph.D.*

See also Aging; Childbirth; Conception; Dwarfism; Embryology; Endocrine disorders; Endocrinology; Endocrinology, pediatric; Failure to thrive; Gigantism; Glands; Hormones; Hypertrophy; Malnutrition; Menopause; Menstruation; Nutrition; Prader-Willi syndrome; Pregnancy and gestation; Puberty and adolescence; Sexuality; Vitamins and minerals; Weight loss and gain.

FOR FURTHER INFORMATION:

Behrman, Richard E., et al. *Nelson Textbook of Pediatrics.* 17th ed. New York: Elsevier, 2003. Text covering all medical and surgical disorders in children with authoritative information on genetics, endocrinology, aetiology, epidemiology, pathology, pathophysiology, clinical manifestations, diagnosis, prevention, treatment, and prognosis.

Brooks, S. J., and Robert S. Bar. *Early Diagnosis and Treatment of Endocrine Disorders.* Totowa, N.J.: Humana Press, 2003. Reviews the early signs and symptoms of endocrine diseases, surveys the clinical testing needed for a diagnosis, and presents recommendations for therapy.

Goodman, H. Maurice. *Basic Medical Endocrinology.* 3d ed. San Diego, Calif.: Academic Press, 2003. Focuses on research advances in the understanding of hormones involved in regulating most aspects of bodily functions. Includes in-depth coverage of individual glands and regulatory principles.

Marieb, Elaine N. *Essentials of Human Anatomy and Physiology.* 6th ed. Redwood City, Calif.: Benjamin/Cummings, 2003. This introductory anatomy and physiology textbook, easily accessible to those with little science background, is richly illustrated with diagrams and photographs, which help to illuminate body systems and processes.

Moore, Keith L., and T. V. N. Persaud. *The Developing Human.* 7th ed. Philadelphia: W. B. Saunders, 2003. An outstanding textbook on human embryonic development, with specific information about the causes of congenital malformations and common defects occurring in each of the body's systems.

Oski, Frank A., ed. *Oski's Pediatrics: Principles and Practice.* 3d ed. Philadelphia: J. B. Lippincott, 1999. Contains many good descriptions and illustrations of different stages of development, various disorders common in children, and several treatments for these disorders.

Rosse, Cornelius, and Penelope Gaddum-Rosse, eds. *Hollinshead's Textbook of Anatomy.* 5th ed. Philadelphia: Lippincott-Raven, 1997. A very thorough, up-to-date, detailed reference work. Provides helpful descriptions and illustrations, including descriptions of the immature stages of growth.

Tsiaras, Alexander, and Barry Werth. *From Conception to Birth: A Life Unfolds.* New York: Doubleday, 2002. Using state-of-the-art medical imaging technology, traces the development of a human life from conception through birth in spectacular, highly detailed photographs.

Williams, Peter L., et al., eds. *Gray's Anatomy.* 38th ed. New York: Churchill Livingstone, 1995. The classic work on anatomy, containing the most thorough descriptions. The excellent color illustrations provide much realistic detail in most cases and well-selected highlights in a few. Developmental stages are covered in detail.

GUILLAIN-BARRÉ SYNDROME
DISEASE/DISORDER

ALSO KNOWN AS: Acute inflammatory demyelinating polyneuropathy

ANATOMY OR SYSTEM AFFECTED: Immune system, muscles, musculoskeletal system, nerves, nervous system

SPECIALTIES AND RELATED FIELDS: Internal medicine, neurology

DEFINITION: An acute degeneration of peripheral motor and sensory nerves, known to physicians as acute inflammatory demyelinating polyneuropathy, a common cause of acute generalized paralysis.

KEY TERMS:

antibody: a substance produced by plasma cells which usually binds to a foreign particle; in Guillain-Barré syndrome, antibodies bind to myelin protein

antigen: any substance that stimulates white blood cells to mount an immune response

areflexia: loss of reflex

autoimmune disorder: a condition in which the immune system attacks the body's own tissue instead of foreign tissue

B cell: a type of white blood cell that produces antibodies

CSF protein: a protein in the cerebrospinal fluid which is usually very low

demyelination: a loss of the myelin coating of nerves

electromyogram: the external recording of electrical impulses from muscles

macrophage: a white blood cell that engulfs foreign protein; in Guillain-Barré syndrome, it also attacks myelin

motor weakness: muscle weakness resulting from the failure of motor nerves

nerve conduction velocity: the speed at which a nerve impulse travels along a nerve

neurogenic atrophy: shrinkage of muscle caused by a loss of nervous stimulation

neuropathy: a condition in which nerves are diseased, are inflamed, or show abnormal degeneration

phagocytosis: the process of engulfing particles

polyneuropathy: neuropathy found in many areas

CAUSES AND SYMPTOMS

Guillain-Barré syndrome (GBS) is an acute disease of the peripheral nerves, especially those that connect to muscles. It causes weakness, areflexia (loss of reflex), ataxia (difficulty in maintaining balance), and sometimes ophthalmoplegia (eye muscle paralysis). GBS demonstrates a variable, multifocal pattern of inflammation and demyelination of the spinal roots and the cranial nerves, although the brain itself is not obviously affected. By the 1990's, it was the most common cause of generalized paralysis in the United States, averaging two cases per 100,000 people per year. The disease was first described in the early 1900's by Georges Guillain and Jean-Alexander Barré, two French neurologists. Little was known of the cause of GBS or the mecha-

nism for its symptoms, however, until the 1970's. Since then, symposia sponsored by the National Institute of Neurological and Communicative Disorders and Stroke have shed more light on this condition.

Most individuals with GBS have a rapidly progressing muscular weakness in more than one limb and also experience paresthesia (tingling) and numbness in the hands and feet. These sensations have the effect of reducing fine muscle control, balance, and one's awareness of limb location. The prevailing scientific opinion regarding GBS is that it is an autoimmune disorder involving white blood cells, which for some unknown reason attack nerves and/or produce antibodies against myelin, the insulating covering of nerves. The weakness is usually ascending in nature, beginning with numbness in the toes and fingers and progressing to total limb weakness. The demyelination is more prominent in the nerves of the trunk and occurs to a lesser extent in the more distal nerves. The brain and spinal cord are protected from GBS by the blood-brain barrier, although antibodies to myelin have been found in the cerebrospinal fluid of some patients.

With GBS, there is often a precipitating event such as surgery, pregnancy, upper respiratory infection, viral infection (such as cytomegalovirus), or vaccination. Preexisting debilitating illnesses such as systemic lupus erythematosus (SLE) or Hodgkin's disease also seem to predispose a person to GBS. GBS has been diagnosed in patients having heart transplants in spite of the fact that they are receiving immunosuppressive drugs. The increased risk with such surgery may be attributable to the stress associated with the procedure.

INFORMATION ON GUILLAIN-BARRÉ SYNDROME

CAUSES: Autoimmune disorder; often with precipitating event such as surgery, pregnancy, upper respiratory infection, viral infection (such as cytomegalovirus), vaccination

SYMPTOMS: Weakness; loss of reflex; difficulty maintaining balance; eye muscle paralysis; tingling and numbness in hands and feet; reduced fine motor control, balance, and awareness of limb location; paralysis of vocal cords

DURATION: Chronic with acute episodes

TREATMENTS: Plasmapheresis, administration of cyclosporine or corticosteroids

Most patients who come down with GBS have had some prior condition that placed stress on the immune system prior to the appearance of GBS.

The patient with GBS is frequently incapable of communicating as a result of paralysis of the vocal cords. Typically, motor paralysis will worsen rapidly and then plateau after four weeks, with the patient bedridden and often in need of respiratory support. Autonomic nerves can also be affected, causing gastrointestinal disturbances, adynamic ileus (loss of function in the ileum of the small intestine), and indigestion. Other, less common symptoms include pupillary disturbances, pooling of blood in limbs, heart rhythm disturbances, and a decrease in the heart muscle's strength. These patients are usually hypermetabolic because considerable caloric energy goes into an immune response that is self-destructive and into mechanisms that are attempting to repair the damage.

In addition to the loss of myelin, cell body damage to nerves may result and may be associated with permanent deficits. If the nerve cell itself is not severely damaged, regrowth and remyelination can occur. Antibodies to myelin proteins and to acidic glycolipids are seen in a majority of patients. Blood serum taken from patients with GBS has been shown to block calcium channels in muscle, and experiments in Germany have found that cerebrospinal fluid from GBS patients blocks sodium channels.

Like most autoimmune conditions, GBS is cyclic in nature; the patient will have "good" days and "bad" days because the immune system is sensitive to the levels of steroid hormones in the body, which are known to fluctuate. In addition to paralysis, there is significant pain with GBS. Many of the nerve fibers that register the pain response (nociceptors) are nonmyelinated and therefore are not interrupted in GBS. Pain management can be difficult, requiring the use of such drugs as fentanyl, codeine, morphine, and other narcotics. The course of the disease is variable and is a function of the level of reactivity of the patient's immune system. The autoimmune attack is augmented in those patients experiencing activation of serum complement protein induced by antibodies. Recovery usually takes months, and frequently the patient requires home health care. Complications can lead to death, but most patients recover fully, though some have residual weakness.

The physician must be careful to distinguish GBS from lead poisoning, chemical or toxin exposure, polio, botulism, and hysterical paralysis. Diagnosis can be confirmed using cerebrospinal fluid (CSF) analysis.

GBS patients have protein levels greater than 0.55 gram per deciliter of CSF. Macrophages are frequently found in the CSF, as well as some B cells. Nerve conduction velocity will be decreased in these patients to a value that is 50 percent of normal in those nerves that are still functioning. These changes can take several weeks to develop. With GBS, macrophages and T cells have been shown to be in contact with nerves, as evidenced in electron micrographs. T-cell and macrophage activation in these individuals point to an immune response gone awry, possibly precipitated by a virus or exposure to an antigen that is foreign but similar in appearance to one of the proteins in myelin. T cells, upon encountering an unrecognizable antigen, will produce interleukin 2, initiate attack, and recruit macrophages to participate. The use of an anti-T-cell drug theoretically should improve nerve function, but researchers at the University of Western Ontario failed to find any benefit from the infusion of an anti-T-cell monoclonal antibody. Unexpectedly, GBS has been found in patients testing positive for the human immunodeficiency virus (HIV) who are asymptomatic, in spite of the fact that their T cells are under attack from the HIV virus and are diminished in number. Although myelin proteins are thought to be the immunogens, other candidates include gangliosides in the myelin. Antiganglioside antibodies have been seen in a majority of the GBS patients. This trait may distinguish GBS from amyotrophic lateral sclerosis (Lou Gehrig's disease) and multiple sclerosis, which seem to involve different myelin proteins as antigens.

In GBS, the white blood cells attack peripheral motor nerves more often than other types of nerves, implying a biochemical difference between motor and sensory nerves that has yet to be discovered. One possible cause of this disease is a similarity between a protein or glycolipid that is present normally in myelin and coincidentally on an infectious agent, such as a virus. The immune system responds to the agent, resulting in a sensitization of the macrophages and T cells to that component of myelin. B cells are then stimulated to produce antibodies against this antigen, and they unfortunately cross-react with components of the myelin protein. The severity of the disease will depend on the number of macrophages and lymphocytes activated and whether serum complement-binding antibodies are being produced. Serum complement proteins are activated by a particular class of antibodies, resulting in the activation of enzymes in the blood that potentiate tissue destruction and neurogenic atrophy. Serum complement levels can be determined by a serum complement fixation test.

In severe cases of GBS, intercostal muscles are more severely compromised and respiratory function needs to be monitored closely. The immune response will subside when T-suppressor cells have reached their peak levels. Halting the autoimmune response will not reverse the symptoms immediately, since it takes time for antibody levels to decrease and for the nerves to regrow and remyelinate, which occurs at the rate of 1 to 2 millimeters per day. Some nerves will undergo retrograde degeneration and be lost from the neuronal pool. Other nerves will have more closely spaced nodes and conduct impulses at a lower velocity. Nerve sprouting will also occur, which will result in one nerve's being responsible for more muscle fibers or serving a larger sensory area and in decreased fine motor control.

TREATMENT AND THERAPY

In Guillain-Barré syndrome, the amount of muscle and nerve involvement can be assessed by performing an electromyogram, which can reveal the amount of motor nerve interruption and the conduction velocity of the nerves that continue to function. Based upon the assumption that an autoimmune response is in progress, corticosteroids such as prednisolone and methylprednisolone are sometimes administered in high doses. The benefits of such drugs have been shown to be marginal, while the side effects are considerable.

More recently, a procedure known as plasmapheresis has been tried with better results, especially when performed in the first two weeks. This procedure involves removing 250 milliliters (a little more than a pint) of plasma from the blood every other day and replacing this volume with a solution containing albumin, glucose, and appropriate salts. Six treatments are typical and usually result in a faster recovery of muscle control than for those not receiving plasmapheresis. Because relapses may occur if the patient produces new antibodies to myelin, immunosuppressants are given to the patient after plasmapheresis. Another procedure, intravenous immunoglobulin therapy, is in the clinical trial stage and is based on the strategy of blocking the binding of antibodies to nerves.

Cyclosporine, a T-cell inhibitor, is also being tried, with some promising results. Some researchers note, however, that transplant patients, who routinely take cyclosporine, have a higher-than-normal risk of developing GBS. Others emphasize that no one knows what their risk for GBS would be without the administration

of cyclosporine. Because of the variability of the body's immune response, the benefits of this drug will depend on whether, in a given individual, it is an antibody response or T-cell response. Cyclosporine will benefit those who have a strong T-cell response. T-cell reactivity can be tested with the mixed lymphocyte assay, and T-cell counts can be done.

Cerebrospinal fluid filtration is also being tried in order to remove reactive white blood cells and antibodies. Serum so filtered loses its nerve-inhibiting effect, as evidenced by its application to in vitro nerve and muscle cells. GBS has been mimicked in animal models, which show antibody and T-cell reactivity to myelin protein. Guillain-Barré syndrome has many of the characteristics of an autoimmune disease and could serve as a model for an acquired autoimmune condition.

PERSPECTIVE AND PROSPECTS

Guillain-Barré syndrome is an example of a delicate physiological balance gone awry. The immune system has the difficult task of distinguishing between self and enemy, and if it detects the latter it must either inactivate or eliminate the intruder. Mistakes in recognition or communication between immune cells can cause either an unintended attack or the failure to attack when appropriate. GBS probably represents an unnecessary attack on self tissue, in this case myelin, and may be considered a form of hyperimmunity. Many diseases fall into this category. They include rheumatoid arthritis, juvenile diabetes, Crohn's disease, ulcerative colitis, Graves' disease, multiple sclerosis, amyotrophic lateral sclerosis, ankylosing spondylitis (inflammation of the joints between the vertebrae), and systemic lupus erythematosus. The other type of response, hypoimmune, is seen in cancer and immunodeficiency diseases such as acquired immunodeficiency syndrome (AIDS).

Questions that arise with GBS are the same ones that arise in many other diseases. It must be determined why the immune system chose this time to initiate an attack against a self-antigen. The answer could be a mistake in recognition, an error in translating the deoxyribonucleic acid (DNA) code in the bone marrow cells, an alteration of the antigen by some environmental factor, or an alteration of an antigen-detector protein on a white blood cell. Researchers also try to discover if there is a genetic predisposition for GBS. Seeking answers about GBS may shed light on other conditions as well, and treatments beneficial to GBS patients have a high probability of benefiting patients with other immune disorders. GBS is a reminder that physiological stress can translate to immunological stress, and under stress the immune system can make mistakes. Failure to react can result in diseases such as cancer, and unnecessary action can lead to diseases such as GBS.

—*William D. Niemi, Ph.D.*

See also Ataxia; Autoimmune disorders; Immune system; Immunology; Motor neuron diseases; Nervous system; Neuralgia, neuritis, and neuropathy; Neurology; Neurology, pediatric; Numbness and tingling; Paralysis; Stress.

FOR FURTHER INFORMATION:

Abbas, Abdul K., and Andrew K. Lichtman. *Basic Immunology: Functions and Disorders of the Immune System.* New York: Elsevier, 2001. Provides introductory text on the basics of immunology and describes the primary disorders that impair immunological function. Illustrations, case studies, review questions, key point summaries, and a glossary are included.

Adelman, Daniel C., et al., eds. *Manual of Allergy and Immunology.* Philadelphia: Lippincott Williams & Wilkins, 2002. Examines research developments and the clinical diagnosis and treatment of allergies and immune disorders.

Baron-Faust, Rita. *The Autoimmune Connection.* New York: McGraw-Hill, 2003. Examines myriad health issues in women and investigates their possible environmental triggers. Each chapter includes signs, diagnosis and tests, current and future treatments, and looks at the role of female hormones, menstruation, pregnancy, and menopause in affecting the course of each disease.

Barr, Murray L., and John A. Kiernan. *The Human Nervous System.* 7th ed. Philadelphia: J. B. Lippincott, 1998. A softbound text designed for a medical school introductory course in the basic sciences. Provides a good foundation for understanding the nervous system, with some discussion of demyelination.

Guillain-Barré Syndrome Foundation International. http://www.guillain-barre.com/index.html. A Web site focused on providing informative support and increasing the opportunities for patients, family, and friends to network and communicate.

Lechtenberg, Richard. *Synopsis of Neurology.* Philadelphia: Lea & Febiger, 1991. A pocket-sized book with summary descriptions of the most common neurological syndromes. Covers diagnostic techniques and symptoms associated with neurological problems, including Guillain-Barré syndrome.

Nicholls, John G., A. Robert Martin, and Bruce G. Wallace. *From Neuron to Brain.* 4th ed. Sunderland, Mass.: Sinauer Associates, 2000. An excellent and detailed neurobiology text that can help the reader understand the basis and consequences of demyelinating conditions such as Guillain-Barré syndrome.

Noback, Charles R., Norman L. Strominger, and Robert J. Demarest. *The Human Nervous System: Structure and Function.* 6th ed. Totowa, N.J.: Humana Press, 2003. A concise, easy-to-read paperback that offers a good balance of physiology and anatomy. Well illustrated.

Parker, James N., and Philip M. Parker, eds. *The Official Patient's Sourcebook on Guillain-Barrè Syndrome.* San Diego, Calif.: Icon Health, 2002. Draws from public, academic, government, and peer-reviewed research to provide a wide-ranging handbook for patients with Guillain-Barré syndrome.

Pearlman, Alan L., and Robert C. Collins. *Neurobiology of Disease.* New York: Oxford University Press, 1990. An advanced text that provides detailed descriptions of most neurological abnormalities. Contains a good description of Guillain-Barré syndrome and a chapter devoted to demyelinating disease.

Sticherling, Michael, and Enno Christophers. *Treatment of Autoimmune Disorders.* New York: Springer-Verlag, 2002. Explores the basic mechanisms of autoimmune disorders; neurological, gastrointestinal, ophthalmological, and skin diseases; and current and future therapeutic options.

GULF WAR SYNDROME
DISEASE/DISORDER

ANATOMY OR SYSTEM AFFECTED: Blood, brain, cells, chest, eyes, gastrointestinal system, gums, hair, immune system, joints, muscles, psychic-emotional system, skin

SPECIALTIES AND RELATED FIELDS: Biochemistry, environmental health, epidemiology, ethics, occupational health, psychology, public health

DEFINITION: A popular term used to describe collectively a variety of symptoms, not a specific disease, suffered by veterans of the Persian Gulf War.

KEY TERMS:

cytokines: proteins which are used by white blood cells to communicate with similar cells

organophosphates: chemical pesticides

pyridostigmine bromide: a chemical that prevents damage from possible nerve gas exposure

sarin: a nerve gas that can cause convulsions and death

CAUSES AND SYMPTOMS

This condition is characterized by flulike symptoms, which sufferers complain of experiencing simultaneously but which do not indicate any specific known disease. Such physical symptoms include chronic fatigue, fever, muscle and joint pain and weakness, and intense headaches. Some patients report episodes of memory loss, insomnia, nightmares, and limited attention spans as well as neuropsychological disorders, such as depression, anxiety attacks, and mood swings. Respiratory problems, diarrhea and gastrointestinal distress, blurred vision, arthritis, bleeding gums, hair loss, and skin rashes sometimes accompany other symptoms.

Physicians disagree about the causal factors of Gulf War syndrome. While some medical professionals diagnose veterans' symptoms as resulting from exposure to wartime toxins, bacteria, or viruses, other doctors state that the symptoms are psychosomatic and due to posttraumatic stress disorder. Gulf War syndrome has not been attributed to any infectious disease that veterans might have contracted in the Persian Gulf. Significantly, it has been difficult for researchers to prove any laboratory abnormality or unique characteristic for this disorder or to isolate any organ system as the primary system affected by this condition. Most medical professionals say that Gulf War syndrome is a condition representing factors of several diseases but is not a separate disease.

Many Persian Gulf War veterans believe their ailments are service related. Approximately eight hundred thousand coalition forces were deployed to the Persian Gulf after Iraq invaded Kuwait in August, 1990. About 10 percent of these veterans have claimed to have Gulf War syndrome (statistics vary according to sources). Soldiers hypothesize that exposure to sarin caused the syndrome. Other possible causes include germ and chemical warfare (although no evidence of either has been verified), antianthrax and botulism vaccines, pyridostigmine bromide (PB) tablets, and exposure to radiation from depleted uranium, fumes from burning oil wells, and organophosphates.

TREATMENT AND THERAPY

Because they do not think their concerns are being seriously addressed, many veterans rely on self-diagnosis based on other veterans' accounts exchanged orally, in the press, or on the Internet. Self-medication with over-the-counter pain relievers is a common treatment on which veterans depend for the soothing of symptoms. Physicians prescribe more potent pharmaceuticals and physical therapy to alleviate symptoms and reinforce patients' immune systems. The American, Canadian, and British governments have established medical programs through publicly funded veterans' administrations and privately endowed medical institutions to research the syndrome's causes, ascertain its etiology, identify derivative presentations of the syndrome, develop effective treatment methods, and offer medical care for veterans exhibiting Gulf War syndrome symptoms.

Physicians recommend that some veterans suffering Gulf War syndrome undergo counseling to address neuropsychological symptoms and assist readjustment to peacetime or civilian life and frustration with enduring chronic sickness. Exercise, a nutritional diet, and support groups are also helpful to many veterans suffering Gulf War syndrome. Genetic testing of veterans and their spouses is also sometimes pursued to determine causation of birth defects in some veterans' children, which are often incorrectly attributed to Gulf War service. Complications associated with treatment of Gulf War syndrome include possible common side effects of pain relievers, such as drowsiness. Patients also risk becoming addicted to pain relievers that they use to numb the ever-present aches associated with chronic illnesses.

PERSPECTIVE AND PROSPECTS

Originally identified when some American, British, and Canadian Gulf War veterans complained of various

---

INFORMATION ON GULF WAR SYNDROME

CAUSES: Unclear; possibly exposure to wartime toxins, bacteria, or viruses; psychosomatic factors; post-traumatic stress disorder

SYMPTOMS: Varies widely; can include chronic fatigue, fever, muscle and joint pain and weakness, intense headaches, episodes of memory loss, insomnia, nightmares, anxiety attacks, mood swings, respiratory problems, blurred vision, rashes

DURATION: Chronic

TREATMENTS: Self-medication with over-the-counter pain relievers, prescribed drug and physical therapy, counseling

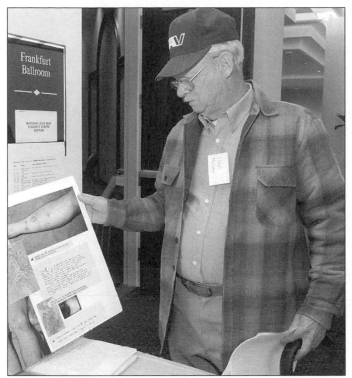

A Gulf War veteran examines a poster at a conference sponsored by the National Gulf War Resource Center. He returned from the conflict with headaches, dizziness, night sweats, memory loss, and numerous skin cancers and other lesions. (AP/Wide World Photos)

ailments after returning home in 1991, Gulf War syndrome was sensationalized in the press as a mystery illness. Physicians familiar with military medical history recognized similarities with symptoms documented in soldier populations as early as the American Civil War. This awareness suggested that the syndrome was indicative of a common wartime factor rather than a unique occurrence in the Gulf War.

Gulf War syndrome became politicized as government officials and veterans disagreed regarding description of and funding for treatment of the syndrome. After clinical investigations of twenty thousand Gulf War veterans, the Institute of Medicine declared that no Gulf War syndrome existed, although some soldiers did suffer nonchronic illnesses, such as malaria. Five independent panels confirmed the conclusion that no unique case of an illness had been proven.

Physicians and scientists representing the Departments of Defense, Veterans Affairs, and Health and Human Services stated that the rates of incidence of Gulf War veterans' symptoms, hospitalization, and mortality are not greater than those reported for the general population and that many veterans may have already been genetically predisposed to certain physiological conditions. They also questioned why veterans from other countries, especially Arab nations, did not report syndrome symptoms, nor were any similar reports issued after World War II soldiers returned from the Persian Gulf.

In 2002, in what veterans called a "stunning reversal," the U.S. Department of Defense admitted that there is increasing evidence that neural damage affects some veterans of the Gulf War and doubled research funding. The change in stance was partly in response to research emanating from the University of Texas Southwestern Medical Center in Dallas and the U.S. Department of Veterans Affairs. Using a statistical technique called factor analysis, researchers at these facilities identified unusual clusters of symptoms that could be divided into syndromes. Syndrome 1 involved sleep and memory disturbances, syndrome 3 involved joint and muscle pain, while syndrome 2, the most serious, involved confusion and dizziness. Using magnetic resonance spectroscopy (MRS), the research team found that veterans with syndrome 2 had lost nerve cells in the brain structures that are involved with the symptoms of the syndrome. Moreover, syndrome 2 veterans were also approximately eight times more likely as healthy veterans to have had a bad reaction to the PB tablets. Researchers surmise that chemical weapons, and the PB tablets that were designed to protect against them, affect the same physiological pathway. The increasing scientific evidence of real physiological damage among veterans has helped spur the U.S. government to begin more strenuous investigation into its causes. In 2002, the Department of Veterans Affairs appointed a Research Advisory Committee on Gulf War veterans.

Determined to understand Gulf War syndrome, some researchers hypothesize how variables possibly affected veterans' immune symptoms to cause physiochemical reponses, such as increased cytokine production and brain cell damage. Others claim that chemical exposure contaminated soldiers' bloodstreams and is to blame for renal failure and cancers. Unless additional research determines a singular illness, Gulf War syndrome will remain a puzzling, vague, controversial condition with no specific cure or prevention for future military forces. A Veterans Administration Persian Gulf Health Registry and Department of Defense Persian Gulf Health Surveillance System were also created to monitor veterans' health status and to detect patterns that might possibly provide further insights about the complexities of Gulf War syndrome.

—*Elizabeth D. Schafer, Ph.D.*

See also Biological and chemical weapons; Environmental diseases; Environmental health; Epidemiology; Poisoning; Toxicology.

FOR FURTHER INFORMATION:

Blanck, Ronald R., and members of the Persian Gulf Veterans Coordinating Board. "Unexplained Illnesses Among Desert Storm Veterans: A Search for Causes, Treatment, and Cooperation." *Archives of Internal Medicine* 155 (February 13, 1995): 262-268.

Bloom, Saul, et al. *Hidden Casualties: Environmental, Health, and Political Consequences of the Persian Gulf War.* Berkeley, Calif.: Arms Control Research Center, North Atlantic Books, 1994.

Eddington, Patrick G. *Gassed in the Gulf: The Inside Story of the Pentagon-CIA Cover-up of Gulf War Syndrome.* Washington, D.C: Insignia, 1997.

Gulf War Veteran Resource Pages. http://www.gulfweb.org/.

Hersh, Seymour M. *Against All Enemies: Gulf War Syndrome, the War Between America's Ailing Veterans and Their Government.* New York: Ballantine Books, 1998.

National Defense Research Institution. *A Review of the Scientific Literature as It Pertains to Gulf War Illnesses.* 7 vols. Santa Monica, Calif.: Rand, 1998.

Wheelwright, Jeff. *The Irritable Heart: The Medical Mystery of the Gulf War.* New York: W. W. Norton, 2000.

GUM DISEASE

DISEASE/DISORDER

ANATOMY OR SYSTEM AFFECTED: Gums, mouth, teeth

SPECIALTIES AND RELATED FIELDS: Dentistry

DEFINITION: Inflammation of the soft tissue that surrounds the teeth; in advanced disease, there is also loss of bone that holds the teeth in place.

CAUSES AND SYMPTOMS

Bacterial infection is the most common cause of gum disease. In early stages of the disease, only the soft tis-

---

> **INFORMATION ON GUM DISEASE**
>
> **CAUSES:** Bacterial infection
> **SYMPTOMS:** Red, swollen gums that bleed easily; may progress to bone loss. loose teeth, abscesses, and pain
> **DURATION:** Chronic and sometimes progressive
> **TREATMENTS:** Removal of plaque and tartar, antibiotics (oral and inserted into gum pockets), surgery

---

sues—the gums, or gingiva—are affected, but in later stages bacteria also attack the hard tissues underlying the gums.

The bacteria responsible for gum disease accumulate in plaque, which is a sticky biofilm of bacteria that forms on the teeth, both above and below the gum line. Plaque that remains on the teeth for more than about seventy-two hours may harden into tartar, which cannot be removed completely except by a professional. Plaque accumulation is usually the result of inadequate tooth brushing and flossing.

Plaque contains many different kinds of bacteria. Bacteria that live below the gum line, where oxygen is low or lacking, are the main culprits in gingivitis, an inflammation of the soft, gum tissues. Toxins produced by the bacteria destroy the collagen fibers that make up the connective tissue between the gum and the tooth, causing the gum to loosen and detach from the tooth. The widening and deepening of the space between tooth and gum produces a pocket. Whereas in healthy gums there is a crevice about 1 to 3 millimeters deep between the gum and tooth, in gingivitis there is a pocket up to 4 millimeters deep. The gum becomes movable instead of clinging to the tooth. The gum also swells, is red rather than a healthy pink, and bleeds when brushed or probed. At this early stage, there is little or no pain.

From a gum pocket, bacteria can advance to the bone and to the other hard tissues that support the tooth: the cementum, which covers the roots of the tooth, and the periodontal ligament, which anchors the tooth to the jawbone. Gum disease that has progressed to the bone is referred to as periodontitis. It usually results from a long-term accumulation of plaque and tartar.

In early periodontitis, the crests or peaks of the bone between the teeth have begun to erode. The patient may as yet be unaware of the problem because there is no pain. As the inflammation destroys the fibers of the periodontal ligament and further dissolves the bone, the pocket often deepens to between 4 and 8 millimeters. In advanced stages, most of the bone surrounding the tooth is destroyed and the tooth loosens. Abscesses and pain are common at this point. Advanced periodontitis can cause teeth to fall out or require extraction and is one of the main causes of tooth loss in adults.

In both gingivitis and periodontitis, the damage may be localized. Furthermore, the disease does not progress at a uniform rate but instead advances episodically, with periods of remission. Most adults have had gingivitis at one time or another, but some individuals are especially susceptible, including those who smoke, have certain medical conditions, or take particular medications.

Treatment and Therapy

Gum disease is treatable. To diagnose the disease, the dentist may use X rays to determine the extent of bone loss, and a dental probe to measure the depth of pockets. The dentist removes plaque and tartar by scaling the surfaces of the teeth and planing the surfaces of the roots. An ultrasonic scaler, which cleans the teeth with high-frequency vibrations, may also be used. Once the bacterial biofilm has been removed, the gums are able to heal and reattach to the teeth, thereby shrinking the pockets.

Oral antibiotics are also useful in fighting periodontitis, though they are not effective for gingivitis. In addition, antibiotic-impregnated materials inserted into deep gum pockets can deliver high concentrations of antibiotic directly to the infected area.

Surgery is performed on some patients, either by a general dentist or by a periodontist. Under local anesthesia, flaps of gum tissue are cut away from the underlying bone, thus allowing better access for scraping and cleaning the tooth roots and for correcting bone defects caused by the infection. Some of the infected gum tissue is also removed, and the remaining gum is sutured back in place.

An important tool in the fight against gum disease is good oral hygiene. The patient should brush and use dental floss daily to remove plaque. In addition to toothpastes, effective cleaning agents include baking soda, peroxide, and some mouth rinses. A regular schedule of teeth cleaning by a dental professional is also essential. Depending on how fast a patient accumulates tartar, professional cleaning may be required every three to six months.

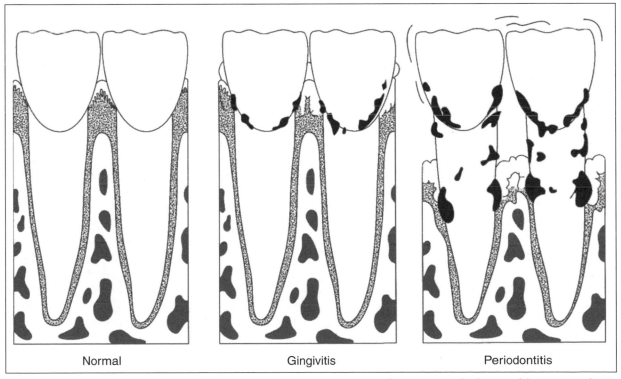

Normal   Gingivitis   Periodontitis

Gum disease begins with poor oral hygiene; if unchecked, it leads to gingivitis (inflammation and infection of the gums) and periodontitis (erosion of supporting bone and tooth loss).

PERSPECTIVE AND PROSPECTS

Humans have attempted to clean their teeth since prehistoric times. Early humans fashioned implements out of twigs and bone splinters to remove bits of food trapped between their teeth. Later, the toothpick became the main tooth-cleaning tool. The Chinese are credited with inventing the toothbrush around 1000 A.D. It was not until the late 1930's, however, that an inexpensive toothbrush became available.

Research on the causes, prevention, and treatment of gum disease is being conducted at dental schools and at the National Institute of Dental and Cranio-Facial Research. Research areas include attempts to regenerate periodontal tissues. Bone grafting can help restore lost bone, and guided tissue regeneration may help recreate periodontal ligament.

—Jane F. Hill, Ph.D.

See also Cavities; Dental diseases; Dentistry; Endodontic disease; Gingivitis; Periodontal surgery; Periodontitis; Root canal treatment; Teeth; Tooth extraction; Toothache.

FOR FURTHER INFORMATION:

Beers, Mark, ed. *The Merck Manual of Medical Information.* 2d ed. Rahway, N.J.: Merck Research Laboratories, 2003.

Christensen, Gordon J. *A Consumer's Guide to Dentistry.* 2d ed. St. Louis: Mosby, 2002.

Marsh, P. D. "Dental Plaque." In *Microbia Biofilms,* edited by Hilary Lappin-Scott and J. William Costerton. New York: Cambridge University Press, 1995.

Serio, Francis G. *Understanding Dental Health.* Jackson: University of Mississippi Press, 1998.

Smith, Rebecca W., and the Columbia University School of Dental and Oral Surgery. *The Columbia University School of Dental and Oral Surgery's Guide to Family Dental Care.* New York: W. W. Norton, 1997.

GYNECOLOGY

SPECIALTY

ANATOMY OR SYSTEM AFFECTED: Breasts, genitals, reproductive system, uterus

SPECIALTIES AND RELATED FIELDS: Endocrinology, family practice, obstetrics, oncology, psychiatry, psychology

DEFINITION: The branch of medicine concerned with the diseases and disorders that are specific to women, particularly those of the genital tract, as well as women's health, endocrinology, reproductive physiology, family planning, and contraceptive use.

KEY TERMS:

menarche: the onset of menstrual cycles in a woman

menopause: the permanent cessation of menstrual cycles, signifying the conclusion of a woman's reproductive life

menstruation: the cyclic bleeding that normally occurs, usually in the absence of pregnancy, during the reproductive period of the human female; typically occurs at twenty-eight-day intervals

Papanicolau (Pap) smear: a screening test for precancer and cancer of the cervix; it is performed by placing a sample of cervical cells on a microscope slide along with a preservative solution or by placing the cells into a small container filled with preservative solution

puberty: the physiological sequence of events by which a child acquires the reproductive capacities of an adult; the growth of secondary sexual characteristics occurs, reproductive functions begin, and the differences between males and females are accentuated

SCIENCE AND PROFESSION

Gynecology is the branch of medical science that treats the functions and diseases unique to women, particularly in the nonpregnant state. A gynecologist is a licensed medical doctor who has obtained specialty training. Unlike many fields in medicine which are clearly defined by surgical or nonsurgical practice, gynecology involves both. In the early 1800's, gynecology was closely tied to general surgery. In fact, one of the first reported cases of abdominal surgery in which the patient survived and was cured of a condition occurred in 1809, with the successful removal a massive ovarian tumor by Ephraim McDowell (without the benefit of anesthesia or antibiotics).

Today, gynecology is much more than just a surgical field. With the tremendous progress made in the basic sciences and medical sciences by the twenty-first century, gynecology now involves a broad spectrum of medical fields, including developmental and congenital disorders relating to puberty and adolescence, sexually transmitted diseases (STDs) and other infectious diseases, contraception, menstrual disturbances, endocrinology, early pregnancy issues, infertility, preventive health, menopausal problems, incontinence, and oncology, specifically dealing with cancers of the reproductive tract such as the ovaries, uterus, and breasts.

Many of the medical problems dealt with in gynecology have far-reaching social, ethical, and legal consequences. Among the most controversial issues in medicine today involve abortion and STDs (such as human immunodeficiency virus, or HIV), both of which are conditions commonly managed by gynecologists. Another example of a common problem managed by gynecologists with important social implications is contraception. Female steroid hormones were among the first biological substances to be purified in the laboratory in the twentieth century. These hormones were then intentionally fed to animals for their contraceptive effect and eventually given to human beings as well in the form of the birth control pill. The birth control pill is an invention that has been widely credited with providing women with a relatively easy means to control their own fertility. Many social scholars would argue that women's ability to harness their own fertility was key in enabling women to delay childbearing, pursue education and careers, and take roles in society that were formerly occupied almost exclusively by men.

To understand gynecology, it is first necessary to have a working knowledge of relevant female anatomy and physiology. Broadly, the female reproductive organs are divided into two groups, external and internal. Within each group are many specific components, most of which are analogous to structures in the male because they are derived from the same sources during embryological development. The external organs are the vulva (the fleshy "lips" covered with skin), vagina, and clitoris; the internal organs are the uterus (including the cervix), Fallopian tubes, and ovaries. These organs mature during puberty and communicate with regions of the brain, specifically the hypothalamus and pituitary, to coordinate function.

The vagina is a tube of tissue that connects the vulva with the uterus. In adult females, it is 9 to 10 centimeters in length. When a woman is standing upright, the vagina extends upward and backward from the opening to the uterus. There is a slight cuplike expansion near the uterus. It is here that the actual connection between the vagina and uterus is made through a muscular structure called the cervix. The muscles of the vagina are normally constricted, thus closing the tube. The vagina can stretch to accommodate a penis during intercourse and a fetus during birth.

The cervix is a ring of muscle; the central opening is called the cervical os. Throughout most of the month, the cervical os forms a tight barrier. When the lining of the uterus is sloughed during a menstrual period, the cervix relaxes slightly. During childbirth, the cervix dilates to 10 centimeters (about 4 inches).

The uterus is a hollow, thick-walled, muscular organ. It normally forms a right angle with the vagina, angling upward and anteriorly. The bladder is immediately anterior to the uterus. In a nonpregnant woman, the uterus is pear-shaped. In a woman who has never been pregnant, it is 8 centimeters in length, 6 centimeters wide, and 4 centimeters thick. It increases in size during pregnancy; after birth, it shrinks but does not quite return to its size prior to pregnancy. The lining of the uterus is shed approximately every twenty-eight days during a normal menstrual period.

The Fallopian tubes are two canals that transport eggs from the ovaries to the uterus. The Fallopian tube is the site where sperm meet the egg and fertilization occurs. The tubes are wide near the ovaries and become narrow toward the uterus. The ovaries are two almond-shaped bodies found in the pelvic cavity, and they brush up against the Fallopian tubes. The ovaries are about 3.5 by 2 by 1.5 centimeters in size, although there can be much variation. The ovaries contain eggs, which are released at monthly intervals between puberty and the menopause.

DIAGNOSTIC AND TREATMENT TECHNIQUES

As with all medical problems, a good history from the patient regarding the nature of the problem is crucial for diagnosis. The history is almost always followed by a physical examination. Probably the best known diagnostic technique in gynecology is the bimanual pelvic examination. Any woman who is sexually active or age eighteen should receive one from a physician. The purpose of the examination is to confirm normal anatomy, rule out pathological conditions, and prevent the development of cancers through screening tests such as the Pap smear.

The pelvic examination is typically performed with the woman on her back, knees apart, with feet and legs supported by stirrups. Visual inspection of the external genitalia is performed; this involves inspecting the pubic region to ensure normal secondary sexual development as well as to look for abnormalities such as unusual lesions on the labia, which may indicate infections (by fungi, bacteria, viruses, or parasites), skin conditions (such as eczema), or cancer. The next portion is a bimanual examination. The examiner places one hand on the patient's abdomen and gently inserts two fingers of the other hand into the patient's vagina; gloves are worn at all times. The examiner proceeds to feel the uterus and ovaries by gently pushing them toward the anterior abdomen. The external hand on the abdomen serves as a counterforce to enable the examiner to feel the contours of the uterus and ovaries and hence to assess their size.

The last portion of the examination is a visual inspection of the interior of the vagina and the surface of the cervix. Because the vagina is normally closed, a device called a speculum is carefully placed in the vaginal canal. The speculum has two "blades"; each blade is analogous to a tongue depressor which pushes the tongue out of the way to enable inspection of the throat. The blades are then slowly opened to part the vaginal tissues and enable visualization of the vaginal canal and cervix. The vaginal walls and cervix are inspected for abnormalities, and the consistency of vaginal fluid is noted. If any abnormalities are noted, cultures or biopsies may taken to facilitate diagnosis. When indicated, a Pap smear is performed by swabbing the exterior of the cervix as well as the cervical canal. The cells that are obtained from the swab can then be sent to the pathology laboratory for analysis to screen for precancer or cancer of the cervix.

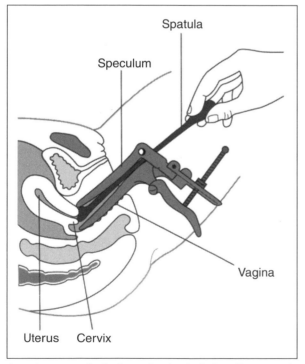

A routine gynecological examination includes a Pap smear, in which a spatula is used to perform a biopsy of the cervix for laboratory analysis.

Although the bimanual examination is the mainstay of office practice, this examination is but a small fraction of diagnostic modalities commonly employed by gynecologists. A complete physical examination, including breast examination, is often performed for a comprehensive survey to aid in diagnosis. When abnormalities are suspected, a vast array of imaging techniques and laboratory tests can be invaluable in diagnosis. For instance, when a pelvic mass is felt on bimanual examination, the gynecologist may order an ultrasound to better characterize the mass. Laboratory tests such as CA-125 levels may be indicated to help differentiate the pelvic mass from a benign growth versus a malignancy, such as of the ovary.

Other diagnostic tests commonly employed by gynecologists in office practice are blood and urine tests for pregnancy, blood or culture tests (for STDs such as HIV, syphilis, gonorrhea, chlamydia, and herpes), and biopsies of the external genitalia, which may assist in diagnosing skin conditions such as lichen sclerosus or precancers. If an endocrinologic abnormality is suspected, then blood tests to check the levels of various hormones (such as thyroid hormone, follicle-stimulating hormone, or prolactin) can help pinpoint the problem. In a patient with urinary incontinence, urodynamic testing, which records the pressures of the bladder and abdomen under different conditions, may help diagnose and characterize the type of incontinence.

A number of diagnostic tests commonly employed by gynecologists require going to an operating room, most often because of the need for patient sedation or anesthesia. One example is hysteroscopy, whereby a small camera mounted on a cannula is introduced through the cervix to visualize the cervical canal and uterine lining. Hysteroscopy can be useful in the diagnosis of polyps or fibroids (benign tumors of the uterus) which may be causing abnormal vaginal bleeding. Another example is diagnostic laparoscopy, whereby a small camera mounted on a cannula is introduced into the abdominal and pelvic cavity to inspect for abnormalities such as pelvic scarring, masses, or endometriosis, a condition in which cells resembling the uterine lining are found in the pelvic or abdominal cavities.

Gynecologists have a vast array of treatment options available to them. In the office setting, common treatment modalities include the use of antibiotics for uncomplicated pelvic infections, such as chlamydia, gonorrhea, or trichomoniasis. Another problem commonly treated in the office setting is undesired fertility. A number of contraceptive modalities exist, including the prescription of birth control pills, the placement of an intrauterine device (IUD), or the injection of sustained-release hormones. In women experiencing menopausal symptoms such as hot flashes, hormonal pills or other medications may be prescribed. Women with chronic pelvic pain may be treated with medications such as antidepressants. Urinary incontinence may respond to bladder training, pessaries, or medications.

In the operating room, procedures may be carried out in a controlled setting to treat disease. A woman with abnormal vaginal bleeding caused by fibroids who no longer desires childbearing may receive a hysterectomy, with or without removal of the ovaries. If a woman is interested in retaining her uterus, the fibroids can be isolated and removed surgically through a common surgical procedure called a myomectomy. In women who desire permanent sterilization, a common surgical procedure performed by gynecologists is tubal ligation. Another common surgical procedure is the removal of pelvic masses such as ovarian cysts. Endometriosis or pelvic scars can be removed or destroyed through laparotomy (also known as abdominal surgery) or laparoscopy (minimally invasive abdominal surgery). When a Pap smear or biopsy indicates non-invasive cancer of the cervix, treatment is possible through excision of the part of the cervix surrounding the cancer. In women with urinary incontinence not helped by medical management, surgery may be indicated to treat the problem. Women who are infertile as a result of blocked Fallopian tubes can be treated with in vitro fertilization. In this procedure, eggs are harvested from the woman in the operating room, and fertilization is performed in the laboratory. When the embryos are sufficiently developed, they are placed in the uterine cavity through an office procedure.

PERSPECTIVE AND PROSPECTS

The formation of a medical field specific to women's diseases largely began in the nineteenth century. At the time, the treatment of women's diseases was inextricably linked with the role of women in society. In the nineteenth century, women were often viewed as frail and limited by their cyclical physiology and childbearing role. Consequently, they were excluded from the male-dominated spheres of politics, professional careers, and education. For instance, influential psychiatrist Henry Maudsley (1835-1918) wrote about the harm that higher education would cause to the physiologic development of postpubescent girls. Edward

Clarke (1820-1877), a Harvard Medical School professor, wrote in 1873 that higher education might develop the intellect, but at the expense of the reproductive organs, leading to painful menstrual periods and abnormal uterine function.

The field has evolved dramatically since then, with much of the evolution tied to changes in the role of women in society as well as to technological and scientific advances. Today, one of the major forces changing gynecological practice (as well as many other fields of medicine) is the concept of evidence-based medicine. This movement is based on the idea that medical practice must be guided by scientific evidence as well as good intentions. Without objective evidence that a treatment is effective, even the best of intentions can result in patient harm. Although a physician may practice evidence-based medicine, this does not mean that clinical judgment and the tailoring of treatments to fit individual patients should be ignored. In fact, applying scientific evidence in an automatic way to all patients is not endorsed. Gynecologists today most often practice evidence-based medicine either by examining the available literature themselves, using evidence-based medical summaries developed by others, or using evidence-based protocols developed by others.

One example of evidence-based medicine guiding clinical practice involves Pap smear screening. Although the classical teaching had been that Pap smears were recommended on a yearly basis, this frequency was not based on any direct evidence that this protocol would lead to better outcomes than screening less frequently. Consequently, both the U.S. Preventative Services Task Force and the American Cancer Society have suggested lengthening the period between successive Pap smears in women thirty years of age or older who have had negative results on three or more consecutive Pap smears. In fact, the U.S. Preventative Services Task Force recommends Pap smears be performed "at least every three years" rather than every year.

Among the studies cited for this recommendation is one that followed more than 100,000 women at community-based clinics throughout the United States who had previously received three years of normal Pap smears. There was no statistically significant difference in the number of precancers or cancers of the cervix found on the new Pap smear based on the time interval since the last Pap smear (that is, one year versus three years). In an era where the optimum use of limited resources is of concern to patients, physicians, health maintenance organizations (HMOs), and insurance companies alike, the careful application of evidence-based medicine to appropriate situations in medical practice can result in the best overall benefit for all parties involved.

—*Anne Lynn S. Chang, M.D.*

See also Abortion; Amenorrhea; Assisted reproductive technologies; Biopsy; Breast biopsy; Breast cancer; Breast disorders; Breasts, female; Cervical, ovarian, and uterine cancers; Cervical procedures; Chlamydia; Circumcision, female, and genital mutilation; Conception; Contraception; Culdocentesis; Cyst removal; Cystectomy; Cystitis; Cysts; Dysmenorrhea; Electrocauterization; Endocrinology; Endometrial biopsy; Endometriosis; Endoscopy; Episiotomy; Gamete intrafallopian transfer (GIFT); Genital disorders, female; Glands; Gonorrhea; Herpes; Hormone replacement therapy (HRT); Hot flashes; Hysterectomy; In vitro fertilization; Incontinence; Infertility in females; Laparoscopy; Mammography; Mastectomy and lumpectomy; Mastitis; Menopause; Menorrhagia; Menstruation; Myomectomy; Nutrition; Obstetrics; Ovarian cysts; Pap smear; Pelvic inflammatory disease (PID); Placenta; Postpartum depression; Preeclampsia and eclampsia; Pregnancy and gestation; Premenstrual syndrome (PMS); Reproductive system; Sex change surgery; Sexual dysfunction; Sexuality; Sexually transmitted diseases (STDs); Sterilization; Syphilis; Toxic shock syndrome; Tubal ligation; Ultrasonography; Urethritis; Urinary disorders; Urology; Warts.

FOR FURTHER INFORMATION:

Boston Women's Health Book Collective. *Our Bodies, Ourselves for the New Century.* New York: Simon & Schuster, 1998. Contains in-depth discussions of topics related to gynecology. This book was written by women for women and is one of the best reference works available on this subject for the general reader.

Braunwald, Eugene, et al., eds. *Harrison's Principles of Internal Medicine.* 15th ed. New York: McGraw-Hill, 2001. Contains many good chapters on major women's health problems.

Novak, Emil, and Jonathan S. Berek. eds. *Novak's Gynecology.* 13th ed. Philadelphia: Lippincott Williams & Wilkins, 2002. A standard text covering all aspects of gynecology, with an emphasis on diagnosis and treatment. Topics include biology and physiology, family planning, sexuality, evaluation of pelvic infections, early pregnancy loss, benign breast disease, benign gynecologic conditions, malignant diseases of the reproductive tract, and breast cancer.

Rushing, Lynda, and Nancy Joste. *Abnormal Pap Smear: What Every Woman Needs to Know.* Amherst, N.Y.: Prometheus Books, 2001. Explains the causes of cervical neoplasia and the treatment procedures used. Numerous diagrams show the stages of cervical disease.

Scott, James R., et al., eds. *Danforth's Obstetrics and Gynecology.* 9th ed. Philadelphia: Lippincott Williams & Wilkins, 2003. A basic textbook that describes many common gynecological problems, along with their diagnosis, management, and treatment.

Speroff, Leon, Robert H. Glass, and Nathan G. Kase. *Clinical Gynecologic Endocrinology and Infertility.* 6th ed. Baltimore: Lippincott Williams & Wilkins, 1999. The authoritative textbook on the normal role of hormones in women, hormonal disturbances and the medical diseases to which they can lead, and the evaluation and treatment of infertility.

Stenchever, Morton A., et al. *Comprehensive Gynecology.* 4th ed. St. Louis: Mosby, 2001. The definitive textbook on gynecological problems.

Stewart, Elizabeth Gunther, and Paula Spencer. *V Book: A Doctor's Guide to Complete Vulvovaginal Health.* New York: Bantam Books, 2002. Covers a wealth of information related to vulvovaginal health, including picking a good gynecologist and asking the right questions, vulvovaginal hygiene, the safe use of tampons, common ailments and their symptoms, and which medical tests to insist upon from one's doctor.

Tierney, Lawrence M., Stephen J. McPhee, and Maxine Papadakis, eds. *Current Medical Diagnosis and Treatment 2004.* 43d ed. Stamford, Conn.: Appleton & Lange, 2003. An easy-to-read medical textbook with good chapters related to women's health.

Way, Lawrence W., and Gerard M. Doherty, eds. *Current Surgical Diagnosis and Treatment.* 11th ed. New York: Lange Medical Books/McGraw-Hill, 2003. Provides information on the surgical aspects of women's health and gynecology.

Weschler, Toni. *Taking Charge of Your Infertility.* Rev. ed. New York: HarperCollins, 2001. An excellent book that encourages women to become responsible for their own reproductive health. Includes discussions of infertility, natural birth control, and achieving pregnancy.

GYNECOMASTIA
DISEASE/DISORDER

ANATOMY OR SYSTEM AFFECTED: Breasts, chest, endocrine system, glands

SPECIALTIES AND RELATED FIELDS: Endocrinology
DEFINITION: An enlargement of the glandular part of the male breast that may affect one or both breasts and be painless or painful.

CAUSES AND SYMPTOMS

True gynecomastia must be distinguished from malignant or benign breast tumors and from enlargement of the fatty part of the breast because of obesity. Causes of gynecomastia include normal physiological changes, endocrine diseases, other diseases such as chronic liver or kidney disease, tumors, and many drugs.

Some newborn boys may have swollen breasts as a result of the maternal estrogen to which they are exposed during pregnancy. This enlargement may be accompanied by the secretion of milk, known as galactorrhea. Up to 70 percent of boys experience gynecomastia as they go through puberty, usually between the ages of twelve and fifteen. It is usually one-sided, but it may involve both breasts either at the same time or sequentially. This normally subsides within a year; the only treatment is reassurance that it will resolve on its own.

In athletes who take androgens and anabolic steroids, about half will develop gynecomastia. Other drugs that can cause this problem include alcohol, cimetidine, diazepam, diethylstilbestrol, digitalis, estrogens, some tranquilizers, many of the drugs used to treat schizophrenia, marijuana, methadone, synthetic narcotics, growth hormone, and tricyclic antidepressants.

Elderly men, particularly if they gain weight, may also develop gynecomastia because of the changes in the balance between male and female hormones that come with aging.

Types of cancer leading to gynecomastia include lung and testicular cancers. Likewise, tumors of the adrenal gland may cause this problem. Sometimes the enlargement of the breast tissue is the first sign of some serious underlying disease, but often it occurs for no apparent reason.

Men who develop gynecomastia where the cause is not obvious should have a radiographic study of the chest performed, along with blood studies to measure hormones such as prolactin, testosterone, luteinizing hormone, estradiol, and thyroid hormones. Some men may require genetic testing to determine the cause of their gynecomastia. Finally, a needle biopsy may be necessary.

INFORMATION ON GYNECOMASTIA

CAUSES: Normal physiological changes, endocrine diseases, diseases such as chronic liver or kidney disease, tumors, maternal estrogen during pregnancy, certain drugs (androgens, anabolic steroids, alcohol, cimetidine, diazepam, DES, digitalis, estrogens, some tranquilizers, schizophrenia drugs, marijuana, methadone, synthetic narcotics, growth hormone, tricyclic antidepressants)
SYMPTOMS: Enlargement of breasts in males, sometimes with milk secretion
DURATION: Within one year
TREATMENTS: None (self-resolving), cessation of drug use

TREATMENT AND THERAPY

The treatment of gynecomastia depends upon the cause. In the case of infant or pubertal boys, nothing is required but time for the problem to resolve on its own. When the condition is the result of a drug, it will usually resolve once the drug is stopped. Weight loss is indicated where the appearance of gynecomastia is attributable to obesity. Treating endocrine disorders, other illnesses, and tumors usually resolves the gynecomastia.

When the problem is painful, it may be treated with an antiestrogen drug. Severe or persistent gynecomastia may be treated by surgical means, although the results are not entirely satisfactory. In some cases, liposuction via the armpit and mastectomy performed under the skin may improve the situation.

—*Rebecca Lovell Scott, Ph.D., PA-C*

See also Breast cancer; Breast disorders; Breasts, female; Endocrine system; Endocrinology; Endocrinology, pediatric; Hormones, Neonatalogy; Pediatrics; Puberty and adolescence.

FOR FURTHER INFORMATION:

Beers, Mark, ed. *The Merck Manual of Medical Information*. 2d ed. Rahway, N.J.: Merck Research Laboratories, 2003.

Komaroff, Anthony, ed. *Harvard Medical School Family Health Guide*. New York: Simon & Schuster, 1999.

Masters, William H., Virginia E. Johnson, and Robert C. Kolodny. *Human Sexuality*. 5th ed. New York: HarperCollins College, 1995.

Hair

Anatomy

Anatomy or system affected: Hair, skin

Specialties and related fields: Dermatology

Definition: Threadlike outgrowths of nonliving, mostly proteinaceous material that cover much of the body of humans and other mammals.

Key terms:

alopecia: hair loss, especially if noticeable or significant

alopecia areata: loss of hair in patches

follicle: the structure in skin that manufactures hair

hirsutism: excessive hair growth

Structure and Functions

Humans grow three kinds of hair. The downy hair that covers the fetus is lanugo. Soon after birth, it is replaced by vellus (or villus) hair. Vellus hair covers the entire skin surface except for the palms of the hands and the soles of the feet. It is fine, short, nearly colorless, and slow-growing.

The thick, pigmented hair on the head, eyebrows, and eyelids is terminal hair. Somewhere between 65 and 95 percent (by weight) of terminal hair is protein. Other components include water, fats (lipids), trace elements (minerals), and pigment. Because proteins twist into complex three-dimensional shapes held together by chemical bonds, hair is both rigid and flexible. Terminal hair replaces villus hair on the genitals at puberty. Called pubic hair, it is coarse and curly. Also at puberty, terminal hair begins to grow in the armpits and on the faces of males.

The shaft of a single hair has three layers. The outer casing is the cuticle, made of overlapping layers of proteinaceous material. Inside the cuticle lies the cortex, a column of cells containing keratin, the same protein that hardens tooth enamel and fingernails. The central core of the hair is the medulla. Also called the pith, it is made of small, hardened cells snared in a web of fine filaments.

Hair grows from a tiny pouch below the skin's surface called a follicle. At the bottom of the follicle lies the papilla, an upward-growing finger of connective tissue. The papilla forms the root of the hair shaft. The actively growing part of the hair shaft is the hair bulb. The cells that generate the hair lie just above the hair bulb. As soon as hair cells are manufactured, they harden and die, forming the hair shaft.

Tiny blood vessels around each follicle supply nutrients. Sebaceous glands that open into the follicle produce the oily sebum that lubricates hair and skin. In the papilla of the follicle, melanocytes produce melanin, the same pigment that gives skin its color. There are two kinds of melanin: Eumelanin makes hair black or brown, while pheomelanin makes it red or blond. Melanin is deposited in the cortex of the hair shaft of terminal hair, giving it its color.

Hair helps insulate the body. Arrector muscles at the base of the follicle elevate hair in response to environmental stimuli, including cold. The high sulfur content of keratin gives it heat-retaining properties. Hair also retards water loss from the body. Body hair augments the sense of touch. Hair's movement facilitates the detection of light touches and slight temperature changes.

Terminal hair cushions the head against blows and protects the scalp from sunburn. Eyelashes keep dirt, insects, and foreign objects out of the eyes. Eyebrows keep sweat from running down into the eyes. The hair inside the ears is coated with the waxy substance cerumen that traps dirt and prevents infections. Hair in the nose filters dust and bacteria from the air.

Hair growth and replacement occur in three stages. Anagen is the active growth stage. It lasts from two to six years. During catagen, lasting about two weeks, the lower segment of the hair follicle breaks down. A "club hair" separates from the papilla and falls out. Then, during telogen, the follicle "rests." Telogen lasts several weeks or months. At any one time, about 80 to 90 percent of the hairs on the head are in anagen, 3 to 4 percent are in catagen, and the remainder are in telogen.

Disorders and Diseases

While a loss of fifty to one hundred scalp hairs per day is normal, alopecia, or noticeable hair loss, occurs in nearly one-third of women and two-thirds of men. Women typically notice a general thinning of the hair, while men usually experience male pattern baldness: loss at the hairline and crown first, followed by loss at top of the head. The cause is neither a loss of follicles nor a cessation of hair growth. Instead, follicles gradually shrink and become less active, producing shorter, finer vellus hairs. Three interacting factors—heredity, hormones, and aging—cause the change in follicles. Genetic programming controls the age when hair loss begins and how fast it progresses. Male hormones (even in women) must be present for balding to occur.

No drug can reverse baldness in its later stages. However, minoxidil (trade name Rogaine) slows the rate of hair loss or promotes regrowth in about 25 percent of men and 20 percent of women. It received the approval of the U.S. Food and Drug Administration (FDA) in

1988 and became available without a prescription in 1996. Another drug, finasteride (trade name Propecia), was approved in 1997 for use in men only.

Surgical alternatives are available for those bothered by baldness. To transplant or graft hair, surgeons remove segments of scalp from the sides and back of the head (where follicles are less sensitive to hormones) and transfer them to the top. To perform a scalp reduction, surgeons cut away a portion of hairless scalp, then stitch the remaining scalp together, reducing the total area of baldness. Another alternative is flap surgery. A flap of hair-bearing scalp is turned to cover the spot where bald scalp has been removed.

Alopecia areata is the loss of hair in round patches, usually on the scalp, beard, eyebrows, or pubic area. It is thought to be an autoimmune disease. The immune system "mistakes" the hair follicles for invading disease agents and attacks them, reducing their size and decreasing hair production. The disorder may result from fever, stress, surgery, allergies, crash diets, burns, scalds, and tumors. Other possible causes include radiation exposure, an overactive or underactive thyroid gland, liver or kidney disease, and illnesses ranging from influenza to scarlet fever. A deficiency of iron, zinc, or certain vitamins is the cause in some cases, as is chemotherapy for cancer. Hair loss is also a side effect of many drugs. Alopecia areata is seldom serious or permanent, but it can be disturbing. A doctor may prescribe drugs to combat it, but it generally resolves itself within a year.

Hirsutism, excessive hair growth on the face or body, can cause concern, especially for women. Although it can be triggered by tumors, diseases of the ovaries or adrenal glands, contraceptive pills, hormonal drugs, or anabolic steroids, the most common cause is menopause. As production of the female hormone estrogen declines, the relative concentration of male hormones (produced naturally by the adrenal glands) rises, causing dark hairs to appear on the upper lip, chin, and cheeks. Shaving, tweezing, waxing, sugaring, or using depilatory creams and lotions removes hair temporarily. Electrolysis, in which a needle inserted into the follicle delivers a current that destroys the follicle, removes hair permanently. In severe cases, doctors may prescribe drugs that block the action of male hormones to treat hirsutism in women.

PERSPECTIVE AND PROSPECTS

Since ancient times, people have sought to prevent or reverse the balding process. The Egyptians of the sixteenth century B.C.E. prescribed a blend of iron, red lead, onions, and alabaster, along with prayers to the sun god. In 420 B.C.E., the Greek Hippocrates, often called the founder of modern medicine, recommended a mixture of opium, horseradish, pigeon droppings, beetroot, and spices.

The concept of surgical hair transplantation arose in the early 1800's, and in the twentieth century reliable techniques were developed. Japanese physicians pioneered hair transplantation and grafting in the late 1930's and early 1940's, but it was not until the 1980's that procedures yielding cosmetically acceptable results were achieved in the United States. Drug treatments for baldness were discovered by chance as side effects. Minoxidil originally treated hypertension; finasteride ameliorated prostate enlargement.

Attempts to remove unwanted hair have roots in prehistory. Sharpened rocks and shells used for hair removal have been found in archaeological sites dating back twenty thousand years. The ancient Sumerians invented tweezers, and the Egyptians buried razors and arsenic-based depilatories with their dead. Native American men tweezed facial hair with clamshells, and North American colonists in the seventeenth century used caustic lye to burn hair away. In 1903, the American inventor King Gillette marketed the first razor with a disposable blade. Jacob Schick introduced the electric shaver in 1931.

In the 1960's, lasers were first used to heat and disable hair follicles over large areas, and hair removal entered the arena of medical practice. Early lasers emitted a continuous wave that risked overheating and skin damage. The invention of a switching device allowed light energy to enter the follicle in controlled pulses. In 1995, the FDA approved the first laser device for hair removal. Most developed since that time use water or gel to cool the skin and laser light to target the melanin in the hair. Other strategies are being investigated, and studies of such variables as beam width, pulse duration, and delivery rate may result in laser hair removal treatments that are safe, effective, and permanent.

Basic research on the nature and action of the immune system may lead to treatments for autoimmune disorders including alopecia areata. The cloning of individual hair follicles may facilitate hair transplantation. Gene therapy could, in theory, be used to alter the genetic control of follicles, preventing inherited baldness entirely.

—*Faith Hickman Brynie, Ph.D.*

See also Dermatology; Gray hair; Hair loss and baldness; Hair transplantation; Laser use in surgery; Plastic surgery; Skin; Skin disorders.

FOR FURTHER INFORMATION:

Anderson, Richard R. "Lasers in Dermatology: A Critical Update." *Journal of Dermatology* 27, no. 11 (November, 2000): 700-705.

Brynie, Faith Hickman. *101 Questions About Your Skin That Got Under Your Skin . . . Until Now.* Brookfield, Conn.: Twenty-first Century Books, 1999.

Champion, Robert H., et al., eds. *Rook/Wilkinson/ Ebling Textbook of Dermatology.* 5th ed. Malden, Mass.: Blackwell Science, 1998.

Freedburg, Irwin M. *Dermatology in General Medicine.* 6th ed. New York: McGraw-Hill, 2003.

Kuntzman, Gersh. *Hair: Mankind's Historic Quest to End Baldness.* New York: AtRandom, 2001.

HAIR LOSS AND BALDNESS
DISEASE/DISORDER

ANATOMY OR SYSTEM AFFECTED: Hair, head, skin

SPECIALTIES AND RELATED FIELDS: Dermatology, endocrinology, plastic surgery

DEFINITION: Symptoms of genetic factors, endocrine disorders, and aging which occur in both men and women, although more frequently in men, affecting more than one-half of the male population.

KEY TERMS:

alopecia: a condition in which all hair falls out, not only that on the scalp but also eyebrows, eyelashes, and even body hair

follicle: a small, saclike cavity for secretion or excretion

hair shaft: the hair itself, consisting of the central part (medulla), the middle part (cortex), and the outer part (cuticle)

psoriasis: a chronic skin disease characterized by scaly, reddish patches

seborrhea: a dermatologic condition characterized by an excessively dry skin (seborrhea oleosa) or oily skin (seborrhea sicca)

CAUSES AND SYMPTOMS

The major reason that hair on the scalp thrives more lavishly than on other parts of the body is that scalp hairs are produced by the largest follicles found in human skin. Throughout the early years of infancy, these follicles increase in size, shedding their hairs about every two to six years to clear a path for a new hair that grows thicker and longer than the one that it replaced. In the mid-teens, nearly every follicle in an individual's scalp is generating an actively growing hair, and by the late teens scalp hair reaches its adult size, populating the scalp in numbers that will never again be equaled.

For most adults entering their twenties, this situation reverses, and hair loss begins to occur—either permanently or temporarily. At this stage in their development, nearly every man and more than 80 percent of women find their hairlines receding. As the years progress, the shedding continues, and the density of scalp hair continues to diminish. Nearly all the permanent hair loss that affects the human scalp is produced by the natural aging process and/or common baldness.

Common, or male pattern, baldness (baldness is classified into various groups depending on its pattern on the scalp) affects at least 20 million Americans. The term "baldness" is often used when a definite hairline recession, a bald spot on the crown, thinning over the top of the scalp, or a combination of the three is detected. The sides and rear scalp fringe areas are usually spared, except for the inevitable thinning that accompanies age. These regions appear to be capable of generating enough two-to-six-year hair cycles to keep them well covered for most, if not all, of a male's average life span.

The less frequent causes of permanent hair loss can be categorized into three groups. The first involves injury to follicles created by constant tension or pulling of scalp hair. Tight ponytails or chignons, worn over a number of years, often result in permanent bald patches on the sides of the head. In addition, tight rollers and the process of hair weaving kill follicles. The second infrequent cause of permanent hair loss is physical injury, such as a laceration or burn. If hair is ironed as a method of straightening over a period of years, hair follicles will become damaged. The third cause involves various inflammatory skin disorders and growths that occasionally affect the scalp. For example, a scalp wen, or cyst, tends to occur in families and requires no treatment unless it appears to be growing. Removal involves a simple office procedure and eliminates the bald spot that results from pressure of the enlarging cyst upon adjacent scalp follicles.

Nearly all humans lose some scalp hair every day. The number of falling hairs, however, often varies considerably from day to day. This daily variation in hair loss is not an indication of abnormality. An average of thirty to sixty hairs may be shed from the scalp each day. While days, weeks, and months may pass with little to no hair loss, large numbers of hairs may be lost over similar time periods. The yearly average, however, remains fairly constant.

This daily variation in hair loss merely reflects the fact that hair follicles act independently of one another. Their three-year growth and three-month rest cycles occur randomly. Aside from the tendency to lose more hair in the autumn, chance dictates the periods when the scalp will contain more resting hairs (hairs having small whitish roots).

Dandruff and its two related conditions of seborrhea and psoriasis, both scaly scalp conditions, may create a significant diffuse hair loss. Because these conditions are so common, they account for most of the shedding that requires medical treatment. In most cases, these problems can be controlled without medical assistance.

Temporary hair loss can result from alopecia areata, pregnancy, severe illness, surgery, certain medications, hormonal disorders, or dieting. Alopecia areata is a condition that usually produces temporary shedding of scalp—and occasionally body—hair. In most cases, the hair regrows spontaneously or after medical therapy has ended. Occasionally, if this problem begins during childhood, all the scalp and body hair may be lost permanently. Extensive shedding may follow pregnancy or the discontinuation of birth control pills. After several months, however, the hair usually begins to regrow. Hair loss may also result from a severe illness associated with high fever (usually influenza) or an extensive surgical procedure. In the case of surgery, the cause is related to changes in body chemistry. Various medications can also create hair loss. The main offenders are the amphetamines, blood thinners, antithyroid drugs, anticancer drugs (as well as radiation treatments), and birth control pills. Hormonal disorders, particularly thyroid dysfunction, can create a thinning problem, but this condition is rarely an isolated symptom. In rare instances, improper nutrition can result in hair loss, such as in the case of dieters who eliminate protein from their daily food intake.

The conditions responsible for temporary shedding usually create a thinning problem quite rapidly. Aside from hair breakage or forcible extraction (hair pulling), the problem is usually one of increased numbers of resting hairs, resulting in massive hair loss. (The two conditions primarily responsible for creating permanent hair loss—aging and common baldness—usually develop slowly, over many years. Thinning occurs simply because the scalp follicles are no longer capable of producing new hairs.)

If something occurs to double the number of resting hairs from their normal 15 to 30 percent, then hundreds of hairs may fall each day. If this lasts for several months, about one-third of the scalp's hair may be lost. A loss of about 30 to 40 percent is required before thinning becomes obvious. After the shedding abates, it may take years for the scalp hair to return to its original density, since the new hairs can grow only about an inch every two months.

Treatment and Therapy

Scientific research in the area of hair loss has produced a drug that has been relatively effective in some individuals. The drug minoxidil was originally used as an antihypertensive medication; however, 70 percent of patients taking it reported unexpected hair growth, occasionally in such undesirable places as the forehead. A 0.2 percent minoxidil solution for external use was devised by a major drug company in the United States and marketed under the name Rogaine. The Food and Drug Administration approved Rogaine as the only prescription drug that effectively combats baldness.

Although it is uncertain how the drug works, it is believed that minoxidil enables shrunken follicles to grow back to a size capable of producing sturdy, visible hairs. Minoxidil has been shown to have promising, though limited, results. It is best at filling in those patchy gaps that herald the beginnings of baldness. Between one-third and one-half of men in some studies exhibited "significant" or "cosmetically acceptable" hair growth. Minoxidil is not a cure, however, and it requires a lifetime commitment. When the drug is stopped, hair thins out within months.

Another nonsurgical method for achieving permanent hair is hair weaving, a process that originated in the African American culture in the nineteenth century. Weaving hair involves braiding it tightly so that a toupee or smaller weft (section of hair) can be attached permanently. All that is required is a sufficient amount of hair remaining on the scalp to serve as an anchor for a hairpiece.

The braids are usually formed from the thicker hair found on the sides and back of the scalp. A semicircular ridge is created that holds a hairpiece firmly in place. If enough hair is still growing on top of the scalp, it can be twisted into smaller braids to anchor individual wefts. This type of weave permits better aeration and easier cleansing of the scalp.

A hair "fusion," "bonding," or "linking" is exactly like a weave except that the hairpiece or wefts are glued, instead of tied, onto the braided hair. This so-called chemical bond is insoluble in water and quite caustic. Frequent hair breakage has limited the usefulness of this method.

While weaved or fused hair does not grow, it still requires regular care and maintenance to keep it looking acceptable. The scalp hair used to anchor the weave naturally continues to grow. As it grows, the attached hair starts to ride above the scalp. Thus the weave or fusion must be reanchored frequently (as often as every three weeks). In addition, the tension placed on the anchoring scalp hair creates accelerated shedding, and this hair loss is often irreversible.

Hair implants, also known as medical or suture implants, have become the principal method for fixing a hairpiece securely to the scalp. Implants are usually not permanent, are only quasi medical, and are to be distinguished from transplants, with which they share a resemblance in name only. Implants are stitches made from either stainless steel or nylon-type materials that are sewn into the scalp and tied into rings. Like the weave hair braids, the knotted stitches act as anchors, holding a hairpiece or several wefts against the barren scalp. If the implants secure a hairpiece, only two or perhaps six stitches are needed. If the implants anchor many smaller wefts of hair, however, more than a dozen stitches must be sewn into the scalp. A physician must perform this procedure, since only someone with a medical license can inject a local anesthetic and sew stitches into the scalp. The problems generated by sewing and leaving stitches in the scalp, however, are pain, infection, and scarring.

In the 1970's, a surgical procedure known as tunnel grafting was developed. This procedure is not available in implant clinics. A small rectangle of skin is removed from behind each ear. The two pieces are immediately grafted to the front and back of the scalp to form two loops that serve as anchors for a hairpiece. While the operation is relatively simple to perform, extreme care must be taken to ensure proper graft acceptance and healing. Although this method avoids the pitfalls of implanted stitches, it still retains two of the problems common to any kind of artificial anchoring device. Since only two loops are available to fix a hairpiece, the

hairpiece can still lift off the scalp. In addition, the skin loops are as vulnerable to injury as suture loops. Scalp lacerations resulting from forcible removal of the hairpiece have occurred.

From the discovery of hair transplants in the 1960's to the late 1970's, it has been estimated that approximately one million people—both men and women—underwent such transplants. As with the implant procedure, a medical license is mandatory in order to inject a local anesthetic into the scalp and make the surgical incisions required for a hair transplant. Doctors who specialize in hair transplants are usually dermatologists; some are plastic surgeons.

Even the baldest scalp contains thousands of transplantable hair follicles. To move them where they are most needed, three surgical methods have been developed, employing scalp grafts known variously as "flaps," "strips," and "plugs." While all three methods are used, most hair transplants are performed with plug grafts because they are the simplest and safest to work with and yield the most satisfying results. The transplant

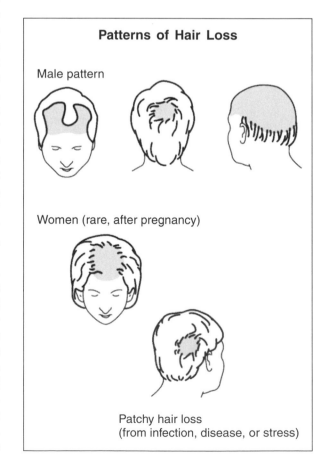

Patterns of Hair Loss

Male pattern

Women (rare, after pregnancy)

Patchy hair loss
(from infection, disease, or stress)

candidate need only be bald enough to justify undergoing the procedure and be endowed with enough side and rear fringe scalp hair to make the procedure worthwhile.

To create a flap or "full thickness" graft, a surgeon cuts out three sides of a rectangular patch of scalp from above the ears and swings it over to the bald area to create a new hairline. This is a major hospital procedure requiring considerable surgical expertise. Although a fairly large portion of bald scalp can be provided with instant hair density, this method is fraught with problems. To ensure a proper take, or graft survival, the blood vessels feeding the transplant must remain intact while they are moved along with it. Because the vessels are quite fragile, they are frequently damaged, resulting in poor graft survival and catastrophic hair loss.

To alleviate this problem, a variation of this type of transplant, known as a free flap procedure, was developed by a team of Japanese surgeons. The free flap is cut out on all four sides, completely severing the blood supply. After setting the graft into its new location, the surgeons meticulously reestablish its blood supply to the recipient blood vessels using a delicate microsurgical technique.

Even if this technical obstacle is surmounted, however, other aesthetic problems remain. The first problem involves the surgical scar that delineates the border between the forehead and the transplanted hairline. Little can be done to minimize this scar. The other problem concerns the unnatural direction in which the newly transplanted hair grows. A flap graft cannot provide hair that will grow in the direction of the hair that has been lost. Hairs growing from the sides of the scalp exit much closer to the surface than in other areas. When transplanted to the frontal area, these hairs lie much too flat against the scalp. Thus, while a flap may provide a faster way to achieve a high-density transplant, the problems of graft survival and poor aesthetic results have limited its usefulness.

A surgical strip graft is a narrow rectangular patch of scalp, cut out on all four sides, that is usually transplanted to create a hairline. Unlike the larger flap, its blood supply need not be moved along with it or be laboriously reestablished. After the strip is placed into its new location, the adjacent bald scalp sends new blood vessels directly into it. Like a flap graft, however, it must be sewn into place. If it is used to create a hairline, an unsightly scar will mark its border with the forehead as well. While this procedure can be performed in an office rather than at a hospital, extreme care must be taken to avoid damaging this delicate graft. Despite the most

painstaking precautions, poor takes result quite often. Areas of nongrowth are common, and not infrequently the entire graft becomes almost completely devoid of hair.

A "hair transplant" usually refers to a procedure in which a small cylinder of hair-bearing scalp, or plug, is taken from the rear or side fringe areas and transferred to either the bald crown or the scalp's frontal region. While this transplant method requires several sessions to approach the density of hair acquired with a flap graft, the ease with which it can be performed, coupled with its superior aesthetic results, make it the logical choice for surgically replacing hair.

The surgeon uses a trephine, or "punch," to remove the cylindrical section of scalp, properly called a donor graft rather than a plug. The graft is quite small, measuring about 0.8 centimeter deep by 0.5 centimeter in diameter. The hair follicle is intimately related to all three skin layers. The bulb—or hair-producing portion of the follicle—lies within and is cushioned by the fat, or adipose, layer. The entire follicle is supported by and receives its nourishment from the fibrous portion of skin, or dermis, which is about 0.6 centimeter thick in the scalp. The skin mantle, or epidermis, provides the opening, or "pore," through which the hair exits to the surface of the scalp.

When a donor graft is removed, all three skin layers must be included. The hair is actually superfluous to the procedure: The hair follicle is all that is essential. After removing the hair-bearing donor grafts, the physician next punches out identical sections of bald scalp. The term "plug" actually refers to the hairless cylinder of scalp that is taken from the bald area. The donor graft is placed into the void left by the removal of the bald plug. Light pressure is applied for several seconds to allow the blood to clot and hold the graft in place. Because these grafts are so small and clotting occurs so rapidly, stitches are not required to fix them in place.

Within hours, new blood vessels move into the graft from the surrounding skin to feed the new section. Within several days, as healing continues, the graft and its adjacent host skin become one. Keeping the grafts small facilitates easy penetration by these vital blood vessels. When larger grafts, or strips, are used, the blood supply may not reach all the hair follicles, and they die.

Because of the small size, the grafts' rounded edges blend into the host skin quite evenly, creating an acceptable hairline. While they might appear obvious on close inspection, they are always less noticeable than the borders left by flaps and strips. Because the grafts are small and are taken from the rear half of the scalp, where the hairs grow out in the same manner as the front and crown hairs, they can be directed to duplicate exactly the original pattern of growth in the bald host areas. This method is a minor office procedure that, in the hands of an experienced physician, is considered safe, with little discomfort experienced by the patient.

PERSPECTIVE AND PROSPECTS

The observation that eunuchs are not subject to gout or baldness was made by Hippocrates in the year 400 B.C.E. and is contained in the *Hippocratic Corpus* as a short medical truth or aphorism. Aristotle, himself balding, was interested in the fact that eunuchs did not become bald and were unable to grow hair on their chests. These observations were either forgotten or overlooked for the next twenty-five centuries, and medical science remained baffled by male pattern baldness until James B. Hamilton, an anatomist, in 1949 again made the observation that eunuchs did not become bald. His suggestion that androgens are a prerequisite and incitant in male pattern baldness and his later classification of the patterns and grades of baldness are landmarks in the study of male pattern baldness. Subsequent investigations of hair loss confirmed the significance of androgens in male pattern baldness, and Hamilton's classification remains in use.

Hamilton demonstrated conclusively that the extent and development of male pattern baldness were dependent on the interaction of three factors: androgens, genetic predisposition, and age. In summary, he found that genetic, endocrine, and aging factors are interdependent. No matter how strong the inherited predisposition, male pattern alopecia will not result if androgens are missing. Neither are the androgens able to induce baldness in individuals not genetically predisposed to baldness. The action of aging is demonstrated by the immediate loss of hair upon exposure to androgens in the sixth decade of life, whereas hair in young men exposed to androgens tends to remain much longer.

Over the centuries, men have tried every imaginable approach to retain hair. They have shampooed their scalps with tar, petroleum, goose dung, and cow urine. They have stuck their heads into rubber caps connected to vacuum pumps to suck recalcitrant hairs to the surface. In the 1960's, hair transplants became the most efficient and aesthetically pleasing method of retaining scalp hair. Research in the area of drug treatment continues.

—*Genevieve Slomski, Ph.D.*

See also Aging; Dermatology; Gray hair; Hair; Hair transplantation; Plastic surgery; Pregnancy and gestation; Psoriasis; Skin; Skin disorders.

FOR FURTHER INFORMATION:

"Bothered by Baldness? Here Are Your Options." *Health News* 18, no. 3 (June/July, 2000): 3. The vast majority of men with thinning hair have "male pattern baldness." Some of the treatments available to men to prevent baldness are discussed, including medication and hair transplants.

Greenwood-Robinson, Maggie. *Hair Savers for Women: A Complete Guide to Preventing and Treating Hair Loss.* New York: Crown, 2000. Provides guidelines for dealing with hair loss that stems from stress, hormonal imbalance, illness, chemotherapy, or medical side effects. Medical and natural approaches are covered as baldness remedies.

Marritt, Emanuel. *Hair Replacement Revolution: A Consumer's Guide to Effective Hair Replacement Techniques.* Garden City Park, N.Y.: Square One, 2000. An easy-to-understand guide that explores the three basic approaches to hair replacement—drug therapies, artificial hair systems, and surgical procedures—and the strengths, weaknesses, and breakthroughs of each.

Regrowth.com. http://www.hairloss.org. Site dedicated to researching treatments for hair loss and verifying product claims for hair growth.

Scott, Susan Craig, and Karen W. Pressler. *The Hair Bible.* New York: Simon & Schuster, 2003. Covers a wide range of hair-related topics, including basics of hair care, remedies for scalp troubles, female pattern baldness, the emotional effects of hair loss, and hair grafts or scalp reductions that can mitigate hair loss.

Setterberg, Fred. "The Naked Truth About Baldness." *In Health* 3 (September/October, 1989): 112-118. This article summarizes for the general reader the main causes of permanent hair loss and discusses treatment options such as transplants and the drug minoxidil.

Stough, Dow B., and Robert S. Haber, eds. *Hair Replacement: Surgical and Medical.* St. Louis: C. V. Mosby, 1996. This book discusses hair loss and its various treatments, such as stimulants and transplantation.

Thompson, Wendy, and Jerry Shapiro. *Alopecia Areata: Understanding and Coping with Hair Loss.* Baltimore: Johns Hopkins University Press, 2000. Details current research, diagnosis, treatment options, and practical strategies for living with the condition.

HAIR TRANSPLANTATION

PROCEDURE

ANATOMY OR SYSTEM AFFECTED: Hair, head, skin

SPECIALTIES AND RELATED FIELDS: Dermatology, general surgery, plastic surgery

DEFINITION: The surgical relocation of healthy hair follicles to a part of the scalp where shrunken follicles are producing short, thin hair or no hair.

INDICATIONS AND PROCEDURES

There are several types of balding that may cause a patient to seek out a hair transplantation procedure. Androgenetic alopecia (common baldness) is a condition that can affect both men and women who are genetically predisposed to it. Usually beginning in late adolescence or early adulthood, androgenetic hormones cause hair follicles gradually to grow smaller and eventually to yield hair that can be detected only by a microscope, or no hair at all.

Different patterns of balding have been observed. Frontal recession is a gradual process during which the frontal hairline retreats from the forehead. In vertex thinning, the hair on the crown of the head gradually disappears, exposing the scalp; the denuded area grows slowly in a concentric pattern. With complete balding, progressive frontal recession combines with vertex balding to create a condition in which hair is present only in a rim at the sides and back of the scalp.

Several surgical styles have been developed to perform hair transplantation, and techniques continue to evolve to improve the appearance of the scalp and hair. In one common procedure, small grafts of scalp containing one or two healthy hair follicles, called micrografts, are removed surgically and set into the frontal scalp to create a natural-looking hairline. The area behind the frontal hairline is filled in with large grafts, and the gaps between the large grafts are filled in with minigrafts, which contain three or four hairs. This process can involve several sessions over a long time, sometimes as long as ten years, depending on the patient's natural hair thickness and degree of balding. The freshly grafted hair falls out but is replaced with new growth in a few weeks.

More than fifty thousand hair transplantation procedures are performed each year in the United States, and the number is expected to increase as more practitioners are trained and the cost, which often amounts to several thousand dollars, is reduced.

—*Russell Williams, M.S.W.*

See also Dermatology; Grafts and grafting; Hair; Hair loss and baldness; Plastic surgery; Skin; Transplantation.

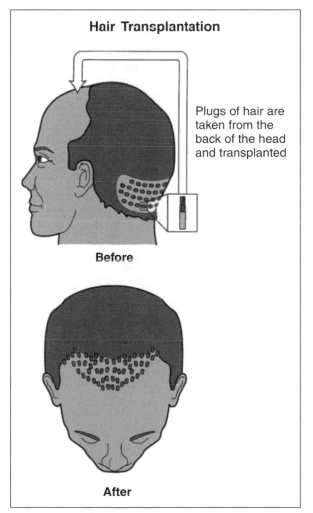

Hair Transplantation

Plugs of hair are taken from the back of the head and transplanted

Before

After

In the punch graft method of hair transplantation, tiny plugs of hair are taken from areas of the scalp where hair growth is still abundant and are inserted into areas where growth has stopped, usually the forehead or the crown.

FOR FURTHER INFORMATION:

Hannapel, Coriene E. "Hair Transplant Advances Add Up to Better Results." *Dermatology Times* 21, no. 6 (June, 2000): 35. Dr. Walter P. Unger, codirector of dermatologic surgery at the University of Toronto, discusses the shift to using only follicular units for transplanting, as opposed to using both follicular units and minigrafts.

Regrowth.com. http://www.hairloss.org. Site dedicated to researching treatments for hair loss and verifying product claims for hair growth.

Sams, W. Mitchell, Jr., and Peter J. Lynch, eds. *Principles and Practice of Dermatology*. 2d ed. New York: Churchill Livingstone, 1996. A dermatology reference guide and text emphasizing accurate diagnosis by succinct discussions in eighty-five presentations featuring color photographs. The contributing dermatologists detail all major topics in the field of dermatology.

Scott, Susan Craig, and Karen W. Pressler. *The Hair Bible*. New York: Simon & Schuster, 2003. Covers a wide range of hair-related topics, including basics of hair care, remedies for scalp troubles, female pattern baldness, the emotional effects of hair loss, and hair transplantations or scalp reductions that can mitigate hair loss.

Segell, Michael. "The Bald Truth About Hair." *Esquire* 121, no. 5 (May 1, 1994): 111-117. A guide to avoiding baldness is offered. Baldness can occur in three ways: vertex baldness (the top of the head), frontal recession, or a combination of both.

Thompson, Wendy, and Jerry Shapiro. *Alopecia Areata: Understanding and Coping with Hair Loss*. Baltimore: Johns Hopkins University Press, 2000. Details current research, diagnosis, treatment options, and practical strategies for living with the condition.

HALITOSIS

DISEASE/DISORDER

ANATOMY OR SYSTEM AFFECTED: Gums, lungs, mouth, nose, stomach, teeth, throat

SPECIALTIES AND RELATED FIELDS: Dentistry, gastroenterology, microbiology, otorhinolaryngology

DEFINITION: Bad breath that is often caused by bacterial activity in the mouth.

CAUSES AND SYMPTOMS

The primary cause of halitosis stems from anaerobic bacteria that reside in the back of the mouth, particularly on the back of the tongue. These bacteria break down proteins and generate smelly gases, especially hydrogen sulfide and methyl mercaptan. More than twenty-two different bacteria have been identified as producing bad odors in the mouth. Periodontal disease, decayed teeth, and infected tonsils are also sources of bad breath. Dry mouth caused by a decreased flow of saliva can produce halitosis. Foods such as onions, garlic, and hot peppers produce chemical odors that are expelled in the breath. In general, particles of food that remain in the mouth on the tongue or between teeth collect bacteria and can cause bad breath. Tobacco

---

INFORMATION ON HALITOSIS

CAUSES: Anaerobic bacteria; also periodontal disease, decayed teeth, infected tonsils, certain foods (onions, garlic, hot peppers), tobacco products

SYMPTOMS: Foul-smelling breath, bad taste in mouth, white-to-yellow coating on tongue, bleeding gums

DURATION: Chronic

TREATMENTS: Brushing of the teeth, tongue, and gums after each meal; flossing; mouthwash; regular dentist visits; adequate fluids; fresh fruits and vegetables

---

products cause halitosis, stain teeth, and irritate gum tissues.

Outside the mouth, chronic infections of the sinuses or lungs can also cause halitosis. Kidney failure has been associated with ammonia-smelling breath, while inadequate diabetic control results in sweet-smelling breath. Halitosis originating from the stomach is very rare, since the esophagus is a closed tube that connects the stomach with the mouth.

Symptoms associated with halitosis include foul-smelling breath, a bad taste in the mouth, a white-to-yellow coating on the tongue, and bleeding gums. For many people, the problem of bad breath is manifest only when they begin to talk. To detect bad breath, one should ask a family member, close friend, or dentist how one's breath smells.

TREATMENT AND THERAPY

The basic treatment for halitosis includes brushing the teeth, tongue, and gums properly after each meal; flossing the teeth at least once a day; visiting the dentist regularly; drinking adequate fluids; and eating fresh, fibrous fruits and vegetables. Although it may take time and patience to overcome the gagging reflex, it is important periodically to clean the back of the tongue thoroughly and gently with a toothbrush or a scraper.

Some mouthwashes have been clinically proven to reduce bad breath effectively, as have some toothpastes. Chewing sugarfree gum, mint, cloves, or fennel seeds for a short time can likewise reduce the odor. Dentures should be cleaned properly every day and should not be kept in the mouth overnight. Nose and throat infections resulting in halitosis may need medical treatment.

PERSPECTIVE AND PROSPECTS

More than fifty million people in the United States suffer some degree of halitosis. It originates in the mouth in more than 90 percent of the cases. Although Islamic and Jewish teachings implicate the stomach as a source of bad breath, it almost never originates there. In almost all cases, halitosis is treatable. Rarely is it an indication of a significant general health problem.

—*Alvin K. Benson, Ph.D.*

See also Alcoholism; Bacterial infections; Cavities; Dental diseases; Dentistry; Dentures; Endodontic disease; Food biochemistry; Gastroenterology; Gastroenterology, pediatric; Gastrointestinal disorders; Gastrointestinal system; Gum disease; Nasopharyngeal disorders; Otorhinolaryngology; Pharyngitis; Sense organs; Sinusitis; Smell; Smoking; Sore throat; Taste; Tonsillitis.

FOR FURTHER INFORMATION:

Conrad, David. *Burps, Boogers, and Bad Breath*. Minneapolis: Compass Point Books, 2002.

Miller, Richard A. *Beating Bad Breath: Your Complete Guide to Eliminating and Preventing Halitosis*. Baltimore: Noble House, 1995.

Rosenberg, Mel, and Daniel van Steenberghe, eds. *Bad Breath: A Multidisciplinary Approach*. Leuven, Belgium: Leuven University Press, 1996.

HALLUCINATIONS

DISEASE/DISORDER

ANATOMY OR SYSTEM AFFECTED: Brain, nervous system, psychic-emotional system

SPECIALTIES AND RELATED FIELDS: Neurology, psychiatry, psychology

DEFINITION: The perception of sensations without relevant external stimuli.

Society often associates hallucinations with psychotic behavior, because schizophrenia and other forms of mental illness frequently involve hallucinations. Another widely publicized example of these symptoms is the use of hallucinogenic drugs, for example, LSD (lysergic acid diethylamide) or marijuana. One must also consider the role of hallucinations in religious experiences and megalomania; such perceptions occur when ordinary people are subjected to extraordinary stimuli.

Medical science has resisted the study of hallucinations and treated them as symptoms of mental illness. Increasing evidence shows, however, that they arise

---

INFORMATION ON HALLUCINATIONS

CAUSES: Psychological disorders, various diseases, use of hallucinogenic drugs

SYMPTOMS: Varies; can include depression, insomnia, maniclike mood swings

DURATION: Short-term to chronic

TREATMENTS: Counseling, drug therapy

---

from specific brain and nervous system structures involving specific biological experiences and common reactions to stimuli. Consequently, people suffering from drug abuse, alcoholism, and disorders similar to Alzheimer's disease, in which severe loss of memory can provoke illusions, are subject to hallucinations.

Since a hallucination can be the result of physical causes as well as the traditional mental unbalance of schizophrenia or manic depression, it is difficult to categorize its symptoms. An individual experiencing hallucinations at times other than waking or falling asleep should see his or her doctor. If the incidents are attributable to a serious illness, early detection is possible. If they are an effect of a particular medication, the prescription should be changed immediately.

—*K. Thomas Finley, Ph.D.*

See also Addiction; Alcoholism; Alzheimer's disease; Bipolar disorder; Brain; Brain disorders; Delusions; Dementias; Intoxication; Narcolepsy; Neurology; Neurology, pediatric; Paranoia; Poisonous plants; Psychiatric disorders; Psychiatry; Psychiatry, child and adolescent; Psychiatry, geriatric; Psychosis; Schizophrenia; Sleep disorders; Stress.

FOR FURTHER INFORMATION:

Asaad, Ghazi. *Hallucinations in Clinical Psychiatry: A Guide for Mental Health Professionals*. New York: Brunner/Mazel, 1990. Discusses the diagnosis and treatment of hallucinations. Includes bibliographical references and an index.

Bloom, Floyd E., et al., eds. *The Dana Guide to Brain Health*. New York: Simon and Schuster, 2003. An easy-to-understand health guide to the brain from neuroscience, neurology, and psychiatry perspectives. More than seventy psychiatric and neurological disorders, their diagnoses, and their treatments are covered.

Lennox, Belinda R., et al. "Spatial and Temporal Mapping of Neural Activity Associated with Auditory Hallucinations." *The Lancet* 353, no. 9153 (February

20, 1999): 644. Results show the strong association of the right middle temporal gyrus with the experience of auditory hallucination in the patient studied, supporting the hypothesis that auditory hallucinations reflect abnormal activation of the auditory cortex.

Nolte, John. *Human Brain: An Introduction to Its Functional Anatomy.* 5th ed. New York: Elsevier, 2001. Text covering major concepts and structure-function relationships in the human neurological system.

Sadock, Benjamin James, and Virginia A. Sadock. *Kaplan and Sadock's Synopsis of Psychiatry: Behavioral Sciences/Clinical Psychiatry.* 9th ed. Philadelphia: Lippincott Williams & Wilkins, 2002. Integrates biological, psychological, and sociological perspectives to provide a comprehensive overview of the field of psychiatry.

Siegel, Ronald K. *Fire in the Brain: Clinical Tales of Hallucination.* New York: E. P. Dutton, 1992. This textbook describes clinical case studies of patients suffering from hallucinations. Includes bibliographical references.

Slade, P. D., and R. P. Bentall. *Sensory Deception: A Scientific Analysis of Hallucinations.* Baltimore: Johns Hopkins University Press, 1988. Discusses the mechanisms of hallucination. Includes bibliographical references and an index.

Stephens, G. Lynn, and George Graham. *When Self-Consciousness Breaks: Alien Voices and Inserted Thoughts.* Cambridge, Mass.: MIT Press, 2003. Utilizes a number of case studies to explain alienated self-consciousness. Includes bibliographical references and an index.

HAMMERTOE CORRECTION
PROCEDURE

ANATOMY OR SYSTEM AFFECTED: Blood vessels, bones, feet, musculoskeletal system, nervous system, tendons

SPECIALTIES AND RELATED FIELDS: General surgery, orthopedics, podiatry

DEFINITION: The surgical removal of ligaments and joining of the middle joints in the toes to correct hammertoe, a deformity in which the toes bend downward abnormally.

INDICATIONS AND PROCEDURES

A hammertoe is a painful deformity which usually affects the second toe. The clawlike appearance of the toe results from malignancy of the joint surface or shortening and weakening of the foot and toe muscle. People with diabetes mellitus are prone to hammertoe development because of the nerve and muscle damage frequently associated with the disease. In other cases, hammertoe results from the wearing of shoes that are too short and do not fit properly. High-heeled shoes, which place pressure on the front of the foot and compress the smaller toes tightly together, can contribute to hammertoe formation. Painful calluses form on the tops of toes when the deformed toe rubs against the top of the shoe. Special orthotics and pads are often used to redistribute pressure and relieve pain. In severe cases, surgery may be required.

Before the operation, blood and urine studies are conducted and X rays are taken of both feet. Hammertoe correction surgery begins with the injection of a local anesthetic. To prevent bleeding in the surgical area, a tourniquet is applied above the ankle. An incision is made through the skin above the affected joint. The tendons that attach to the toes are located and cut free of the connective tissue to the foot bone. The tendons are then divided, enabling the toe to straighten. To keep the toe from bending, the middle joints are permanently connected together with fine pins and wires. Fine sutures are used to close the skin, and the tourniquet is removed. After the surgery, additional blood studies are taken. Sutures are usually removed seven to ten days after the procedure.

USES AND COMPLICATIONS

The correction of hammertoe usually arises out of a need to correct severe deformity or relieve persistent pain. During recovery, flat, comfortable shoes should be worn. After recovery, shoes should be worn that fit well and do not cramp the toes or put undue stress on the front of the foot. Though full recovery from surgery is expected in four weeks, vigorous exercise should be avoided for six weeks after surgery. Once the time for healing has passed, the affected toe will appear in a normal position, and pain will be relieved. Because of the connecting of joints in the toe, however, movement of the toes will be limited.

Possible complications associated with hammertoe correction include excessive bleeding and surgical wound infection.

—Jason Georges

See also Bone disorders; Bones and the skeleton; Feet; Foot disorders; Hammertoes; Lower extremities; Orthopedic surgery; Orthopedics; Podiatry.

FOR FURTHER INFORMATION:

Copeland, Glenn, and Stan Solomon. *The Foot Doctor.* Emmaus, Pa.: Rodale Press, 1986.

Currey, John D. *Bones: Structures and Mechanics.* Princeton, N.J.: Princeton University Press, 2002.

Lippert, Frederick G., and Sigvard T. Hansen. *Foot and Ankle Disorders: Tricks of the Trade.* New York: Thieme, 2003.

Lorimer, Donald L., ed. *Neal's Common Foot Disorders: Diagnosis and Management.* 6th ed. New York: Churchill Livingstone, 2001.

Van De Graaff, Kent M., and Stuart I. Fox. *Concepts of Human Anatomy and Physiology.* 5th ed. Dubuque, Iowa: Wm. C. Brown, 2000.

HAMMERTOES

DISEASE/DISORDER

ANATOMY OR SYSTEM AFFECTED: Feet

SPECIALTIES AND RELATED FIELDS: Orthopedics, podiatry

DEFINITION: Toes that are bent permanently at the joint nearest to the foot; the closely related term "clawtoe" denotes a toe that is bent at both joints.

CAUSES AND SYMPTOMS

Hammertoes and clawtoes can occur in one or more of the four smaller toes on each foot, with the second toe being the most common site for these deformities. Hammertoes and clawtoes are thought to be caused by muscle imbalance, contraction of the tendons, and enlargement of the toe joints. Although anyone can develop these conditions, they are felt to be caused primarily by wearing high heels or shoes that are too tight. It is common for people to develop painful corns and calluses in association with these conditions, particularly on the top or on the tip of the toe where it is most likely to rub against the shoe. Furthermore, people with hammertoes or clawtoes may experience considerable pain if the toe gets inflamed and may also develop skin ulcers from the rubbing of their shoes against the bent toe. These ulcers can become infected and develop abnormal channels to the skin surface called sinus tracts. These conditions may also cause significant problems with walking for the affected individual.

TREATMENT AND THERAPY

Treatment of hammertoes or clawtoes depends on the severity of the condition and whether there are secondary complications such as corns or ulcers. The simplest treatment is to change to shoes with broad toes and soft soles that cushion the foot and to avoid wearing high heels and shoes that pinch the toes. Accompanied by excellent foot care such as callus and corn removal, this may be all that is required to prevent pain and irritation of the toes. In cases that are more advanced, various inserts can be added to the shoes. These include metatarsal bars, orthotics, and other devices. A metatarsal bar supports the ball of the foot, spreading the pressure normally put on this area over a greater part of the foot. Orthotics are specially molded plastic devices that serve much the same purpose. In some cases, podiatrists (foot doctors) or orthopedists recommend toe caps, padded sleeves that help prevent friction between the toe and the shoe. In a few cases, it may be necessary to cut the tendons in the toe or to perform arthroplasty (repair of the joint itself) to provide relief.

—*Rebecca Lovell Scott, Ph.D., PA-C*

See also Bone disorders; Bones and the skeleton; Corns and calluses; Foot disorders; Hammertoe correction; Lower extremities; Skin; Skin disorders.

INFORMATION ON HAMMERTOES

CAUSES: Muscle imbalance, tendon contraction, enlargement of toe joints, improper footwear

SYMPTOMS: Pain, inflammation, corns and calluses, skin ulcers

DURATION: Typically short-term

TREATMENTS: Change of footwear, use of corrective inserts or devices, sometimes arthroplasty or cutting of affected tendon

---

FOR FURTHER INFORMATION:

Copeland, Glenn, and Stan Solomon. *The Foot Doctor.* Emmaus, Pa.: Rodale Press, 1986.

Lippert, Frederick G., and Sigvard T. Hansen. *Foot and Ankle Disorders: Tricks of the Trade.* New York: Thieme, 2003.

Lorimer, Donald L., ed. *Neale's Common Foot Disorders: Diagnosis and Management.* Rev. 6th ed. New York: Churchill Livingstone, 2001.

Shangold, Jules, and Frank Greenberg. *Opportunities in Podiatric Medicine.* Skokie, Ill.: VGM Career Horizons, 1982.

HAND-FOOT-AND-MOUTH DISEASE
DISEASE/DISORDER

ANATOMY OR SYSTEM AFFECTED: Gastrointestinal system, mouth, skin

SPECIALTIES AND RELATED FIELDS: Dermatology, pediatrics, virology

DEFINITION: An enteroviral disease which usually affects children, causing vesicular eruptions on the hands, feet, oral mucosa, and tongue.

CAUSES AND SYMPTOMS

Hand-foot-and-mouth disease is usually caused by Coxsackievirus A16, but it may also be associated with a number of other coxsackieviruses and enterovirus 71. Young children, ages one to five, are most commonly infected in the summer or early fall. They often become infected through contact with the oral secretions of infected children, and nursery school outbreaks may occur. Skin lesions and fecal material may also contribute to the spread of the virus. The incubation period is three to six days.

The illness commences with a low-grade fever (100 to 101 degrees Fahrenheit) and a sore mouth. Oral lesions begin as small, red macules and evolve rapidly into fragile vesicles that rupture, leaving painful ulcers. Any part of the mouth may be involved, but the hard palate buccal mucosa and tongue are mainly affected with an average of five to ten lesions. Similar lesions develop on the skin over the next one to two days; they usually number twenty to thirty, but there may be as many as one hundred. Discrete macular lesions, about 4 millimeters in diameter, appear on the hands and feet and sometimes the buttocks. These lesions often occur along skin lines and progress to become papules and white or gray flaccid vesicles containing infective virus. The lesions may be painful or tender. The fever occurs during the first one to two days of the illness, which resolves in seven to ten days. Rarely, the viral infection is complicated by meningoencephalitis, carditis, or pneumonia.

TREATMENT AND THERAPY

There is no specific treatment for hand-foot-and-mouth disease. The infection usually resolves without complications in about one week. Topical anesthetic agents, such as viscous lidocaine, may be used to soothe the discomfort of the mouth lesions.

PERSPECTIVE AND PROSPECTS

The first described outbreak of this disease occurred in Toronto, Canada, in 1957. British authors first coined

---

INFORMATION ON HAND-FOOT-AND-MOUTH DISEASE

CAUSES: Viral infection

SYMPTOMS: Low-grade fever, sore mouth, oral lesions that rupture into painful ulcers, skin lesions on hands and feet

DURATION: Seven to ten days

TREATMENTS: None (self-resolving); topical anesthetic agents for mouth lesions

---

the term "hand-foot-and-mouth disease" when they reported an outbreak in Birmingham, England, in 1959. While there currently are no medications available for treating enteroviral infections, a number of antiviral agents are being studied and might be useful for complicated forms of this disease, such as meningoencephalitis.

—*H. Bradford Hawley, M.D.*

See also Childhood infectious diseases; Dermatology, pediatric; Encephalitis; Fever; Meningitis; Rashes; Skin; Skin disorders; Viral infections.

FOR FURTHER INFORMATION:

Belshe, Robert B., ed. *Textbook of Human Virology*. 2d ed. St. Louis: Mosby Year Book, 1991.

Freedberg, Irwin M., et al., eds. *Fitzpatrick's Dermatology in General Medicine*. 6th ed. New York: McGraw-Hill, 2003.

Mandell, Gerald L., John E. Bennett, and Raphael Dolin, eds. *Mandell, Douglas, and Bennett's Principles and Practice of Infectious Diseases*. 5th ed. New York: Churchill Livingstone, 2000.

HANTA VIRUS
DISEASE/DISORDER

ANATOMY OR SYSTEM AFFECTED: Kidneys, lungs, respiratory system

SPECIALTIES AND RELATED FIELDS: Critical care, environmental health, epidemiology, internal medicine, public health, pulmonary medicine, virology

DEFINITION: An often-fatal viral infection carried by rodents that causes influenza-like symptoms and respiratory failure.

CAUSES AND SYMPTOMS

Hanta virus, which is distantly related to Ebola virus, is transmitted through contact with the urine and droppings of wild rodents, such as the deer mouse and cotton rat. Contact usually involves the inhalation of contaminated particles in dust. Hanta virus is not transmissible between humans.

Infection takes two major forms. In South America, one strain causes hemorrhagic fever with renal syndrome, involving kidney failure, hemorrhaging, and shock. In the United States, another strain results in hantavirus pulmonary syndrome. Early symptoms mimic influenza; they include fever, chills, muscle aches, nausea and vomiting, malaise, and a dry cough. After initial improvement, increasing shortness of breath follows and may progress to pulmonary edema, internal bleeding, respiratory failure, and death.

TREATMENT AND THERAPY

Diagnosis of hantavirus pulmonary syndrome involves physical examination for hypoxia, hypotension, and adult respiratory distress syndrome. Laboratory tests show an elevated white blood cell count and a decreasing platelet count, and chest X rays may reveal edema. The presence of hanta virus is confirmed through serological testing.

There is no cure for hantavirus pulmonary syndrome; treatment is focused on alleviating the symptoms. This condition must be treated in the intensive care unit (ICU) of a hospital, as careful monitoring of respiratory function and blood gases is essential. In severe cases, the use of an endotracheal tube and a ventilator becomes necessary. Experiments have been performed with intravenous ribavirin therapy; the efficacy of this treatment is being evaluated. Unfortunately, even with aggressive measures, the death rate ranges from 50 to 80 percent.

PERSPECTIVE AND PROSPECTS

The incidence of hantavirus pulmonary syndrome seemed to rise sharply in the 1990's. Epidemiologists were uncertain whether the number of cases increased or more cases were reported following identification of the virus in the United States in 1993.

Because much remains to be learned about the transmission, development, and treatment of hanta virus infection, public health efforts have been in education and prevention. Hikers and campers are thought to be at a greater risk; they are urged to avoid exposure to rodent droppings and questionable water sources. People entering cabins, sheds, or other buildings that have not been used recently should air out the building first and use disinfectant on all surfaces.

—*Tracy Irons-Georges*

> ### INFORMATION ON HANTA VIRUS
>
> **CAUSES:** Viral infection spread through contact with urine and droppings of wild rodents
> **SYMPTOMS:** Fever, chills, muscle aches, nausea and vomiting, malaise, dry cough, kidney failure, hemorrhaging, shock
> **DURATION:** Acute
> **TREATMENTS:** None; alleviation of symptoms

See also Edema; Environmental diseases; Environmental health; Epidemiology; Lungs; Pulmonary diseases; Pulmonary medicine; Respiration; Viral infections; Zoonoses.

FOR FURTHER INFORMATION:

Cockrum, E. Lendell. *Rabies, Lyme Disease, Hanta Virus, and Other Animal-Borne Human Diseases in the United States and Canada*. Tucson, Ariz.: Fisher Books, 1997.

Meyer, Andrea S., and David R. Harper. *Of Mice, Men, and Microbes: Hantavirus*. New York: Academic Press, 1999.

Murray, P. R., et al. *Medical Microbiology*. 4th ed. New York: Elsevier, 2001.

Pan American Health Organization. *Hantavirus in the Americas: Guidelines for Diagnosis, Treatment, Prevention, and Control*. Washington, D.C.: Author, 1999.

Robbins, Stanley L., Ramzi S. Cotran, and Vinay Kumar, eds. *Robbins' Pathologic Basis of Disease*. 6th ed. Philadelphia: W. B. Saunders, 1999.

Sompayrac, Lauren. *How Pathogenic Viruses Work*. 5th ed. Sudbury, Mass.: Jones and Bartlett, 2002.

Strauss, James, and Ellen Strauss. *Viruses and Human Disease*. New York: Elsevier, 2001.

HARE LIP. *See* CLEFT LIP AND PALATE.

HASHIMOTO'S THYROIDITIS
DISEASE/DISORDER

ALSO KNOWN AS: Struma lymphomatosa, lymphadenoid goiter, chronic lymphocytic thyroiditis, autoimmune thyroiditis

ANATOMY OR SYSTEM AFFECTED: Endocrine system, glands, immune system, neck

SPECIALTIES AND RELATED FIELDS: Endocrinology

DEFINITION: An inflammation of the thyroid gland caused when abnormal blood antibodies and white blood cells infiltrate and attack thyroidal cells.

INFORMATION ON HASHIMOTO'S THYROIDITIS

CAUSES: Unknown; possibly autoimmune in origin
SYMPTOMS: Mild pressure on thyroid gland, goiter, fatigue, weight gain, cold intolerance, constipation, hair loss
DURATION: Chronic
TREATMENTS: Hormonal therapy with thyroxine, surgery if required

CAUSES AND SYMPTOMS

Hashimoto's thyroiditis is a common type of hypothyroidism. The cause and etiology of this disorder is not fully understood; however, it is thought to have an autoimmune origin, in which abnormal blood antibodies and white blood cells, called lymphocytes, infiltrate and attack thyroid cells. The combative interplay between the lymphocytes and the thyroid may lead to a complete absence of thyroid cells.

The highest incidence of the disease is observed in young or middle-aged women, but it may occur at any age. The onset is very slow, and the disease may progress for many months or years before it is fully detected. The symptoms may vary, but the condition is usually characterized by a mild pressure on the thyroid gland. In some cases, a firm, slightly irregular, and sometime tender goiter (enlarged thyroid gland) may develop in the neck region. In more severe cases, the disease may cause symptoms related to low thyroid function (hypothyroidism), such as fatigue, weight gain, intolerance to cold, constipation, and hair loss.

The symptomology of Hashimoto's thyroiditis may resemble other medical conditions. Therefore, in addition to a full medical examination, the diagnostic procedure must also include blood tests to determine the levels of thyroid hormone and thyroid antibodies. If a patient has developed the classic symptoms that accompany Hashimoto's thyroiditis but has a normal blood test, then a biopsy in which a needle is inserted into the thyroid and some cells are removed may be performed to confirm the diagnosis.

TREATMENT AND THERAPY

Though a specific treatment is not yet available, the hypothyroidism resulting from Hashimoto's thyroiditis can be treated with hormones. Medical practitioners opt to commence hormone therapy, in the form of thy-roxine, as soon as a diagnosis is made, even if thyroid function is normal at the time. The hormone therapy is expected to shrink any goiter that has developed. If there is no response, then surgery may be required.

The prognosis for a full recovery is usually very good because the disease remains dormant or stable for many years.

—Nicholas Lanzieri

See also Endocrine disorders; Endocrinology; Glands; Goiter; Hormones; Hyperparathyroidism and hypoparathyroidism; Metabolism; Parathyroidectomy; Thyroid disorders; Thyroid gland; Thyroidectomy.

FOR FURTHER INFORMATION:

Bayliss, R. I. S., and W. M. Tunbridge. *Thyroid Disease: The Facts*. 3d ed. New York: Oxford University Press, 1999.

Burrow, Gerard N., Jack H. Oppenheimer, and Robert Volpé. *Thyroid Function and Disease*. Philadelphia: W. B. Saunders, 1990.

Wood, Lawrence C., David S. Cooper, and E. Chester Ridgway. *Your Thyroid: A Home Reference*. 3d ed. New York: Ballantine Books, 1995.

HAY FEVER

DISEASE/DISORDER

ALSO KNOWN AS: Seasonal allergic rhinitis
ANATOMY OR SYSTEM AFFECTED: Eyes, immune system, lungs, lymphatic system, nose, respiratory system, throat
SPECIALTIES AND RELATED FIELDS: Immunology, otorhinolaryngology
DEFINITION: A damaging immune response to otherwise harmless foreign substances such as pollen grains and mold spores.

CAUSES AND SYMPTOMS

The most common cause of hay fever is wind-dispersed pollen. These tiny grains are produced in phenomenal numbers to ensure transfer of the pollen (which contains the plant's sperm) to other flowers of the same plant species. Trees, grasses, and certain forbs (especially the ragweeds) are the most common culprits. The first time that a susceptible person is exposed, the pollen acts to sensitize the immune system. On second and subsequent exposures, the pollen triggers an allergic response called hay fever.

This response is triggered by the formation of a specific antibody against the proteins on the pollen grains (generally called antigens and in this case called allergens). Antibodies identified as immunoglobulin E (IgE) are produced in large amounts. IgE attaches to tissue cells called mast cells by one end and to the pollen grains at the other end. This attachment causes the mast cells to release defensive substances, the best known of which is histamine. These substances cause increased permeability of capillaries and the production and release of mucous and watery substances from the nasal passages and eyes. Itching and sneezing accompany the release. The tendency to produce IgE, and thus the tendency to develop allergies, appears to be inherited.

TREATMENT AND THERAPY

It is generally agreed that avoidance of the allergen is the most effective therapy for hay fever. Staying inside a building with air conditioning or well-filtered air during the worst allergy season helps. However, avoiding an allergen completely, such as ragweed pollen during ragweed's flowering season, is essentially impossible.

The most common treatments employed are desensitization and drugs. Desensitization involves a series of injections of slowly increasing concentrations of the allergen, in the hope of turning the patient's immune system from the production of IgE to the production of immunoglobulin G, which does not trigger the mast cells. Drugs such as antihistamines, which block the action or the release of histamine and the other substances released by mast cells, are commonly recommended, either in prescription strength or over the counter. Drugs that block the action or production of IgE are also being explored. All such drugs have side effects, which should be carefully monitored.

PERSPECTIVE AND PROSPECTS

IgE was discovered early in the twentieth century, although it was some time before its role in allergies was understood. The pathway from exposure to the allergen to the allergic response is complex, involving many substances and many steps. The prospect that one or more of those substances can be targeted to exert more effective control over the allergic response is the subject of ongoing research.

—*Carl W. Hoagstrom, Ph.D.*

See also Allergies; Antihistamines; Autoimmune disorders; Decongestants; Immune system; Nasopharyngeal disorders; Otorhinolaryngology; Sense organs; Sinusitis; Smell; Sneezing.

FOR FURTHER INFORMATION:

Abbas, Abul K., and Andrew H. Lichtman. *Basic Immunology: Functions and Disorders of the Immune System.* 2d ed. Philadelphia: W. B. Saunders, 2004.

Janeway, Charles, Paul Travers, Mark Walport, and Mark Shlomchik. *Immunobiology: The Immune System in Health and Disease.* 5th ed. New York: Garland, 2001.

Nairn, Roderick, and Matthew Helbert. *Immunology for Medical Students.* New York: Mosby International, 2002.

Roitt, Ivan, and Arthur Rabson. *Really Essential Medical Immunology.* Malden, Mass.: Blackwell Science, 2000.

HEAD AND NECK DISORDERS
DISEASE/DISORDER

ANATOMY OR SYSTEM AFFECTED: Bones, brain, head, muscles, musculoskeletal system, neck, nervous system, respiratory system, spine, throat

SPECIALTIES AND RELATED FIELDS: Dentistry, emergency medicine, neurology, otolaryngology, sports medicine

DEFINITION: Physical trauma or neurological problems affecting the head and neck, including the spinal cord.

The head and neck region of the human body houses a sophisticated collection of structures including the special sense organs (structures for breathing, speaking, and eating) and the brain, brain stem, and cervical (neck) portion of the spinal cord. A multitude of disorders or injuries can occur in this complex region.

Trauma to the head and neck. Head or neck trauma can result from a harsh blow on the head, as can occur in a fall or with a strike from an object. These injuries are commonly seen in young, basically healthy persons who come to emergency rooms during evenings or weekends as a result of sports accidents, automobile accidents, or domestic or street violence. In the older age group, strokes and aneurysms are more common problems. Some of these accidents or events can cause permanent nerve and brain damage to the injured person.

Concussions and contusions of the head are common results of head trauma, which induces an internal neurological response. A concussion is a loss of consciousness or awareness of one's surroundings that may last a few minutes or days. Sometimes a concussion appears only as a moderately decreased level of awareness and not a total loss of consciousness. There is no evidence of a change in the brain's structure but, oddly, there is a change in the way in which the brain operates so that alertness is altered. Concussion is presumably a temporary change in brain chemistry, and the damage is reversible unless repeated head blows, such as a professional boxer may experience, are endured. Concussions may occur from other trauma, such as loss of blood flow to the brain, but such trauma is more closely associated with the more urgent threat of permanent brain damage. A contusion is popularly referred to as a bruise. The color associated with a fresh bruise is attributable to an aggregation of blood in an area that was damaged, causing many small blood vessels to rupture and release blood into the surrounding tissue. A bruise around the eye, temple, or forehead causes a black eye.

Automobile accidents rank as one of the common causes of head and neck injury. One of the more familiar complaints after a car accident is the condition called whiplash. Whiplash is the layperson's term for hyperextension of the neck, whereby the head is thrust backward (posteriorly) abruptly and beyond the normal range of neck motion. Hyperflexion occurs when the head is abruptly thrust in the forward (anterior) direction—sometimes as a recoil from hyperextension. The pain of whiplash originates from the damage to the anterior longitudinal ligament along the neck region of the spinal cord. This ligament can be overly stretched or even torn as a result of a sudden snap or jerk of the neck. Furthermore, the bony vertebrae may also grind

against one another after the trauma, causing additional irritation, swelling, and pain in the neck area.

One of the common troubles of a gun or knife wound to the head and neck region is superficial and deep lacerations (cuts). If left unsutured, a deep scalp wound can cause death by hemorrhage. Superficial lacerations to the face may also cause considerable bleeding; such wounds generally are not life-threatening, but they often require stitches in order to heal.

Trauma to the head and neck area can arise from spontaneous internal events such as a stroke, an embolus, or an aneurysm. Each of these conditions is serious and potentially life-threatening because of the risk of losing blood flow to the brain and other vital tissues of the head and neck region.

Neurological problems of the head and neck. Although the bony cranium offers some protection to the head, the neck is, in some regards, more vulnerable to intrusion. Breathing can be interrupted by severing the left or right phrenic nerve, each of which innervates its corresponding half of the most important muscle of breathing, the diaphragm.

The left or right vagus nerve may also be severed. The vagus nerves supply the sympathetic system of the thorax and abdomen, and they also innervate the vocal cords. Severance of one of the vagus nerves causes a hoarseness of the voice as a result of the loss of function of one-half of the vocal cords. If both vagus nerves are damaged—a rare event—then the ability to speak is forever lost.

The sympathetic trunk is another nerve at risk in the neck. Severance of this nerve leads to Horner's syndrome, which consists of a group of signs including ptosis (drooping eyelids), constricted pupils, a flushed face as a result of vasodilation, and dry skin on the face and neck because of the inability to sweat.

Transection (the complete severance) of the lower cervical spinal cord causes upper and lower limb paralysis and trouble with urination, and damage to the upper cervical cord can cause death because of loss of innervation to the muscles of respiration. Hemisection (partial severance) of the cervical spinal cord can also cause Horner's syndrome. Damage to the spinal cord can occur from a knife or gun wound or from crushing or snapping the cord by sudden impact, as with an injury from an earthquake or an automobile accident.

—*Mary C. Fields, M.D.*

See also Amnesia; Aneurysmectomy; Aneurysms; Ataxia; Botox; Brain; Brain disorders; Cluster headaches; Coma; Computed tomography (CT) scanning;

INFORMATION ON HEAD AND NECK DISORDERS

CAUSES: Injury, neurological problems
SYMPTOMS: Pain, bruising, whiplash, alignment problems, inflammation
DURATION: Short-term to chronic
TREATMENTS: Surgery, drug therapy, corrective devices

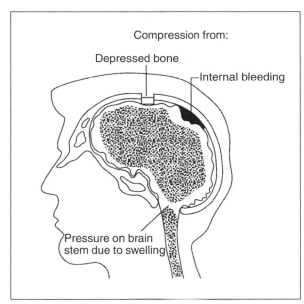

Head trauma may result in compression of the brain, consequent distortions, and severe neurological reactions.

Concussion; Craniosynostosis; Craniotomy; Dementias; Dizziness and fainting; Electroencephalography (EEG); Embolism; Encephalitis; Epilepsy; Hallucinations; Headaches; Hemiplegia; Hydrocephalus; Laryngitis; Memory loss; Meningitis; Migraine headaches; Nasal polyp removal; Nasopharyngeal disorders; Neuralgia, neuritis, and neuropathy; Neurology; Neurology, pediatric; Neurosurgery; Numbness and tingling; Palsy; Paralysis; Paraplegia; Pharyngitis; Quadriplegia; Seizures; Shunts; Sinusitis; Spinal cord disorders; Sports medicine; Strokes; Thrombosis and thrombus; Torticollis; Transient ischemic attacks (TIAs); Unconsciousness; Voice and vocal cord disorders; Whiplash.

FOR FURTHER INFORMATION:

Clayman, Charles B., ed. *The American Medical Association Family Medical Guide.* New York: Random House, 1994. The perfect beginner's guide, not only to head and neck medicine but to any common medical topic as well.

Larson, David E., ed. *Mayo Clinic Family Health Book.* 3d ed. New York: HarperResource, 2003. Perhaps the best general medical text for the layperson, this book covers the entire medical field. While the information is derived from a wide variety of highly technical sources, the articles are written to be easily understood by a general audience.

Marieb, Elaine N. *Essentials of Human Anatomy and Physiology.* 6th ed. Redwood City, Calif.: Benjamin/

Cummings, 2003. This introductory anatomy and physiology textbook, easily accessible to those with little science background, is richly illustrated with diagrams and photographs, which help to illuminate body systems and processes.

Moore, Keith L. *Clinically Oriented Anatomy.* 4th ed. Baltimore: Williams & Wilkins, 1999. Moore addresses the normal human anatomy and offers clinical commentary for the sake of relevance. Enhanced by multicolored, detailed sketches. Expertly written.

Nicholls, John G., A. Robert Martin, and Bruce G. Wallace. *From Neuron to Brain.* 4th ed. Sunderland, Mass.: Sinauer Associates, 2000. An excellent and detailed neurobiology text that can help the reader understand the basis and consequences of conditions arising from head injuries.

Noback, Charles R., Norman L. Strominger, and Robert J. Demarest. *The Human Nervous System: Structure and Function.* 6th ed. Totowa, N.J.: Humana Press, 2003. A concise, easy-to-read paperback that offers a good balance of physiology and anatomy. Well illustrated.

Scanlon, Valerie, et al. *Essentials of Anatomy and Physiology.* 4th ed. Philadelphia: F. A. Davis, 2002. A text designed around three themes: the relationship between physiology and anatomy, the interrelations among the organ systems, and the relationship of each organ system to homeostasis.

HEADACHES

DISEASE/DISORDER

ANATOMY OR SYSTEM AFFECTED: Brain, head, nervous system, psychic-emotional system

SPECIALTIES AND RELATED FIELDS: Family practice, internal medicine, neurology

DEFINITION: A general term referring to pain localized in the head and/or neck, which may signal mere tension or serious disorders.

KEY TERMS:

cluster headache: a severe type of headache, characterized by excruciating pain; attacks occur in groups, or clusters

migraine headache: a type of headache characterized by pain on one side of the head, often accompanied by disordered vision and gastrointestinal disturbances

prophylactic treatment: a treatment focusing on preventing disease, illness, or their symptoms from occurring

symptomatic treatment: a treatment focusing on aborting disease, illness, or their symptoms once they have occurred

tension-type headache: a type of headache characterized by bandlike or caplike pain over the head

CAUSES AND SYMPTOMS

In 1988, an ad hoc committee of the International Headache Society developed the current classification system for headaches. This system includes fourteen exhaustive categories of headache with the purpose of developing comparability in the management and study of headaches. Headaches most commonly seen by health care providers can be classified into four main types: migraine, tension-type, cluster, and "other" acute headaches.

Migraine headaches have been estimated to affect approximately 12 percent of the population. The headaches are more common in women, and they tend to run in families; they are usually first noticed in the teen years or young adulthood. For the diagnosis of migraine without aura ("aura" refers to visual disturbances or hallucinations, numbness and tingling on one side of the face, dizziness, or impairment of speech or hearing—symptoms that occur twenty to thirty minutes prior to the onset of the headache), the person must experience at least ten headache attacks, each lasting between four and seventy-two hours with at least two of the following characteristics: The headache is unilateral (occurs on one side), has a pulsating quality, is moderate to severe in intensity, or is aggravated by routine physical activity. Additionally, one of the following symptoms must accompany the headache: nausea and/or vomiting, or sensitivity to light or sounds. The person's medical history, a physical examination, and (where appropriate) diagnostic tests must exclude other organic causes of the headache, such as brain tumor or infection. Migraine with aura is far less common.

Migraines may be triggered or aggravated by physical activity, by menstruation, by relaxation after emotional stress, by ingestion of alcohol (red wine in particular) or certain foods or food additives (chocolate, hard cheeses, nuts, fatty foods, monosodium glutamate, or nitrates used in processed meats), by prescription medications (including birth control pills and hypertension medications), and by changes in the weather. Yet the precise pathophysiology of migraines is unknown. It had been posited that spasms in the blood vessels of the brain, followed by the dilation of these same blood vessels, cause the aura and head pain; however, studies us-

ing sophisticated brain and cerebral blood-flow scanning techniques indicate that this is likely not the case and that some type of inflammatory process may be involved related to the permeability of cerebral blood vessels and the resultant release of certain neurochemicals.

Tension-type headaches are the most common type of headache; its prevalence is approximately 79 percent. Tension-type headaches are not hereditary, are found more frequently in females, and are first noticed in the teen years of young adulthood, although they can appear at any time of life. For the diagnosis of tension-type headaches, the person must experience at least ten headache attacks lasting from thirty minutes to seven days each, with at least two of the following characteristics: The headache has a pressing or tightening (nonpulsating) quality, is mild or moderate in intensity (may inhibit but does not prohibit activities), is bilateral or variable in location, and is not aggravated by physical activity. Additionally, nausea, vomiting, and light or sound sensitivity are absent or mild. Furthermore, the patient's medical history and physical or neurological examination exclude other organic causes for the headache apart from the following: oral or jaw dysfunction, muscular stress, or drug overuse. Tension-type headache sufferers describe these headaches as a bandlike or caplike tightness around the head, and/or muscle tension in the back of the head, neck, or shoulders. The pain is described as slow in onset with a dull or steady aching.

Tension-type headaches are believed to be precipitated primarily by emotional factors but can also be stimulated by muscular and spinal disorders, jaw dysfunction, paranasal sinus disease, and traumatic head injuries. The pathophysiology of tension-type headaches is controversial. Historically, tension-type headaches were attributed to sustained muscle contractions of the pericranial muscles. Studies indicate, however, that most patients do not manifest increased pericranial muscle activity and that pericranial muscle blood flow and/or central pain mechanisms might be involved in the pathophysiology of tension-type headaches. It is also believed that muscle contraction and scalp muscle ischemia play some role in tension-type headache pain.

Cluster headaches are the least frequent of the headache types and are thought to be the most severe and painful. Cluster headaches are more common in males, with estimates of 0.4 to 1.0 percent of males being affected. Traditionally, these headaches first appear at about thirty years of age, although they can start later in life. There is no genetic predisposition to these headaches. For the diagnosis of cluster headaches, the person must experience at least ten severely painful headache attacks, typically on one side of the face and lasting from fifteen minutes to three hours. One of the following symptoms must accompany the headache on the painful side of the face: a bloodshot eye, tearing, nasal congestion, nasal discharge, forehead and facial sweating, contraction of the pupils, or drooping eyelids. Physical and neurological examination and imaging must exclude organic causes for the headaches, such as tumor or infection. Cluster headaches often occur once or twice daily, or every other day, but can be as frequent as ten attacks in one day, recurring on the same side of the head during the cluster period. The temporal "clusters" of these headaches give them their descriptive name.

A cluster headache is described as a severe, excruciating, boring, sharp, and burning pain through the eye. The pain is occasionally throbbing but always unilateral. Radiation of the pain to the teeth has been reported. Duration of a headache can range from ten minutes to three hours, with the next headache in the cluster occurring sometime the same day. Cluster headache sufferers are often unable to sit or lie still and are in such pain that they have been known, in desperation, to hit their heads with their fists or to smash their heads against walls or floors.

Cluster headaches can be triggered in susceptible patients by alcohol consumption, subcutaneous injections of histamine, and sublingual use of nitroglycerine. Because these agents all cause the dilation of blood vessels, these attacks are believed to be associated with dilation of the temporal and ophthalmic arteries and other extracranial vessels. There is no evidence that intracranial blood flow is involved. Cluster headaches have been shown to occur more frequently during the weeks before and after the longest and shortest days of the year, lending support for the hypothesis of a link to seasonal changes. Additionally, cluster headaches often occur at about the same time of day in a given sufferer, suggesting a relationship to the circadian rhythms of the body. Vascular changes, hormonal changes, neurochemical excesses or deficits, histamine levels, and autonomic nervous system changes are all being studied for their possible role in the pathophysiology of cluster headaches.

Acute headaches, using the International Headache Society's classification scheme, constitute many of the headaches not mentioned above. Distinct from the other headache types, which are often considered to be chronic in nature, acute headaches often signify underlying disease or a life-threatening medical condition. These headaches can display pain distribution and quality similar to those seen in chronic headaches. The temporal nature of acute headaches, however, often points to their seriousness. Acute headaches of concern are usually the first or worst headache the patient has had or are headaches with recent onset that are persistent or recurrent. Other signs that cause a high index of suspicion include an unremitting headache that steadily increases without relief, accompanying weakness or numbness in the hands or feet, an atypical change in the quality or intensity of the headache, headache upon exertion, recent head trauma, or a family history of cardiovascular problems. Such headaches can point to hemorrhage, meningitis, stroke, tumor, brain abscess, hematoma, and infection, which are all potentially life-threatening conditions. A thorough evaluation is necessary for all patients exhibiting the danger signs of acute headache.

INFORMATION ON HEADACHES

CAUSES: Genetic factors, physical activity, hormones, stress, dietary irritants or food additives, certain medications, environmental factors, muscular and spinal disorders, head trauma

SYMPTOMS: Numbness and tingling, dizziness, speech or hearing impairment, nausea and vomiting, sensitivity to light or sounds

DURATION: Acute, chronic, or episodic

TREATMENTS: Surgery, drug therapy, stress management, relaxation training, biofeedback, psychotherapy, dietary and lifestyle modification

TREATMENT AND THERAPY

Because there are several hundred causes of headaches, the evaluation of headache complaints is crucial. Medical science offers myriad evaluation techniques for headaches. The initial evaluation includes a complete history and physical examination to determine the factors involved in the headache complaint, such as the general physical condition of the patient, neurological functioning, cardiovascular condition, metabolic status, and psychiatric condition. Based on this initial evaluation, the health care professional may elect to perform a number of diagnostic tests to confirm or reject a diagnosis. These tests might include blood studies, X rays, computed tomography (CT) scans, psychological evaluation, electroencephalograms (EEGs), magnetic resonance imaging (MRI), or studies of spinal fluid.

Once a headache diagnosis is made, a treatment plan is developed. In the case of acute headaches, treatment may take varying forms, from surgery to the use of prescription medications. For migraine, tension-type, and cluster headaches, there are several common treatment options. Headache treatment can be categorized into two types: abortive (symptomatic) treatment or prophylactic (preventive) treatment. Treatment is tailored to the type of headache and the type of patient.

A headache is often a highly distressing occurrence for patients, sometimes causing a high level of anxiety, relief-seeking behavior, and a dependency on the health care system. The health care provider must consider not only biological elements of the illness but also possible resultant psychological and sociological elements as well. An open, communicative relationship with the patient is paramount, and treatment routinely begins with soliciting patient collaboration and providing patient education. Patient education takes the form of normalizing (or "decatastrophizing") the headache experience for patients, thereby reducing their fears concerning the etiology of the headache or about being unable to cope with the pain. Supportiveness, understanding, and collaboration are all necessary components of any headache treatment.

There are a number of abortive pharmacological treatments for migraine headaches. Ergotamine tartrate (an alkaloid or salt) is effective in terminating migraine symptoms by either reducing the dilation of extracranial arteries or in some way stimulating certain parts of the brain. Isomethaptine, another effective treatment for migraine, is a combination of chemicals that stimulates the sympathetic nervous system, provides analgesia, and is mildly tranquilizing. Another class of medications for migraines are nonsteroidal anti-inflammatory drugs (NSAIDs); these drugs, as the name implies, work on the principle that inflammation is involved in migraine. Both narcotic and nonnarcotic pain medications are often used for migraines, primarily for their analgesic properties; the concern in prescribing potent narcotic pain medications is the potential for their overuse. Antiemetic medications prevent or arrest vomiting and have been used in the treatment of migraines. Sumatriptan, a vasoactive agent that in-creases the amount of the neurochemical serotonin in the brain, shows promise in treating migraines that do not respond to other treatments.

Prophylactic treatments for migraines include beta-blockers, methysergide, and calcium channel blockers, which are believed to interfere with the dilation or contraction of extracranial arteries by acting on the sympathetic nervous system or on the central nervous system itself. Antidepressants, medications used typically for the treatment of depression, have also been found to prevent migraine attacks; there appears to be an analgesic effect from certain antidepressants that is effective for chronic migraines. Antiseizure medications have been found to be useful for some migraine patients, although the mechanism of action is unknown. NSAIDs have also been used as a preventive measure for migraines.

There are several nonpharmacological treatment options for migraine headaches. These include stress management, relaxation training, biofeedback (a variant of relaxation training), psychotherapy (both individual and family), and the modification of headache-precipitating factors (such as avoiding certain dietary precipitants). Each of these treatments has been found to be effective for certain patients, particularly those with chronic migraine complaints. For some patients, they can be as effective as pharmacological treatments. The exact mechanism of action for their effect on migraines has not been established. Other self-management techniques include lying quietly in a dark room, applying pressure to the side of the head or face on which the pain is experienced, and applying cold compresses to the head.

The abortive treatment options for tension-type headaches include narcotic and nonnarcotic analgesics, because of their pain-reducing properties. More often with tension-type headaches, the milder over-the-counter pain medications (such as aspirin or acetaminophen) are used. NSAIDs, simple muscle relaxants, or antianxiety drugs can also be used. Muscle relaxants and antianxiety drugs are believed to relax smooth muscles, reducing scalp muscle ischemia and therefore head pain.

Prophylactic treatments for tension-type headaches include antidepressants, narcotic and nonnarcotic analgesics, muscle relaxants, and antianxiety drugs. Occasionally, "trigger-point injections" are used to relieve tension-type headaches. Trigger points are areas within muscles, primarily in the upper back and neck, that are hypersensitive; when stimulated, they can cause headaches. These trigger points can be injected with a local anesthetic or steroid to decrease their sensitivity or to eliminate possible inflammation in the area.

Nonpharmacological treatment of tension-type headaches is similar to that for migraines and includes stress management, relaxation training, biofeedback, and psychotherapy. Psychotherapy has been found to be a very important adjunct to any treatment of tension-type headaches because the illness, particularly when chronic, can lead to a pain syndrome characterized by family dysfunction, medication overuse, and vocational disruptions. Other self-management techniques include taking a hot shower or bath, placing a hot water bottle or ice pack on the head or back of the neck, exercising, and sleeping.

For cluster headaches, one of the most excruciating types of headache, the most common abortive treatment is administering pure oxygen to the patient for ten minutes. The exact mechanism of action is unknown, but it might be related to the constriction of dilated cerebral arteries. Ergotamine tartrate or similar alkaloids given orally, intramuscularly, or intravenously can also abort the attack in some patients. Nasal drops of a local anesthetic (lidocaine hydrochloride) or cocaine have been used to interrupt the activity of the trigeminal nerve that is believed to be involved in cluster attacks. The efficacy of these treatments is inconclusive.

Prophylactic treatment of this headache type is crucial. Ergotamine, methysergide, calcium channel blockers, antiseizure medications, and steroidal anti-inflammatory medications have been used with some success in the prevention of cluster attacks. The mechanism of action for these medications is unknown. Lithium carbonate, a drug commonly prescribed for bipolar disorder, has been found to be effective for some cluster patients. This medication is believed to affect certain regions of the brain, possibly the hypothalamus.

While no nonpharmacological treatment strategies are routinely offered to cluster headache patients, surgery is an option in severe cases, particularly if the headaches are resistant to all other available treatments. Percutaneous radio frequency thermocoagulation of the trigeminal ganglion is a surgical procedure that destroys the trigeminal nerve pathway, the chief nerve pathway to the face. Modest successes have been found with this extreme treatment option.

PERSPECTIVE AND PROSPECTS
Headaches are among the most common complaints to physicians and quite likely have been a problem since the beginning of humankind. Accounts of headaches can be found in the clinical notes of Arateus of Cappadocia, a first century physician. Descriptions of specific headache subtypes can be traced to the second century in the writings of the Greek physician Galen. Headaches are a prevalent health problem that affects all ages and sexes and those from various cultural, social, and educational backgrounds.

The lifetime prevalence estimates of headaches is 93 percent for males and 99 percent of females. Studies in the United States estimate that 65 to 85 percent of the population will experience a headache within a year. Data from cross-cultural studies echo the significance of this public health problem: Frequent, severe headaches are reported by 10.4 percent of men and 35.3 percent of women in Thailand; 17.6 percent of men and 20.2 percent of women in urban Africa report a history of recurrent headaches; 57 percent of men and 73 percent of women in Finland report at least one headache in the previous year; and 39 percent of men and 60 percent of women in New Zealand also report an annual headache frequency.

As these data indicate, the prevalence of headaches is greater in women, although the reason is unknown. Age seems to be a mediating factor as well, with significantly fewer people sixty-five years of age or older reporting headache problems. There are no socioeconomic differences in prevalence rates, with persons in high-income and low-income brackets having similar rates. There are data to suggest that people with college educations or higher report headaches more often than those with only some high school education. The only vocational area that has been tied to increased rates of headaches are people who work at computer terminals.

The total economic costs of headaches are staggering. Headaches constitute approximately 1.7 percent of all visits to physician offices. Of visits to hospital emergency rooms, 2.5 percent are for headaches. The expenses associated with advances in assessment techniques and routine health care have risen rapidly. The cost in lost workdays adds to this economic picture. Thirty-six percent of headache sufferers in one study reported missing one or more days of work in the previous year because of headaches. The scientific study of headaches is necessary to understand this prevalent illness. Efforts, such as those by the International Headache Society, to develop accepted definitions of headaches will greatly assist efforts to identify and treat headaches.

—Oliver Oyama, Ph.D.

See also Anxiety; Brain; Brain disorders; Caffeine; Cluster headaches; Head and neck disorders; Migraine headaches; Multiple chemical sensitivity syndrome; Neuralgia, neuritis, and neuropathy; Neurology; Neurology, pediatric; Sinusitis; Stress; Stress reduction; Tumor removal; Tumors.

FOR FURTHER INFORMATION:

Blanchard, Edward B., and Frank Andrasik. *Management of Chronic Headaches: A Psychological Approach.* New York: Pergamon Press, 1985. The authors review the evaluation and treatment of headaches from a psychological perspective. Alternative, nonpharmacological treatments for headaches are described in detail.

Diamond, Seymour. "Migraine Headaches." *The Medical Clinics of North America* 75, no. 3 (May 1, 1991): 545-566. Diamond is one of the world's authorities on headaches. His article is well organized and comprehensively addresses the subject of migraines in a readable and interesting format. A practical guide to treating the headache patient.

Ivker, Robert S. *Headache Survival: The Holistic Medical Treatment Program for Migraine, Tension, and Cluster Headaches.* New York: Putnam, 2002. A guide that surveys nutritional and holistic remedies that aim to treat the cause, as well as the symptoms, of headaches.

Lang, Susan, and Lawrence Robbins. *Headache Help: A Complete Guide to Understanding Headaches and the Medications That Relieve Them.* Boston: Houghton Mifflin, 2000. Discusses a wide range of topics related to headaches including treatment options for migraines, cluster headaches, and tension headaches; the actions and side effects of over-the-counter and prescription medications; how hormones affect migraines; and alternative treatments, including herbs and acupuncture.

National Headache Foundation. http://www.headaches .org/. Operates local support groups and provides information for headache sufferers, their families, and physicians.

Paulino, Joel, and Ceabert J. Griffith. *The Headache Sourcebook.* New York: McGraw-Hill, 2001. Reviews types of headaches, provides information on diagnosis and treatment, and offers advice on effectively communicating one's symptoms to doctors to expedite correct care.

Rapoport, Alan M., and Fred D. Sheftell. *Headache Relief.* New York: Simon & Schuster, 1991. The book takes the often-complicated theory, evaluation, and treatment of headaches and explains each area in very understandable terms for the layperson. The authors describe a "how-to" approach to treating headaches.

Saper, Joel R., et al., eds. *Handbook of Headache Management: A Practical Guide to Diagnosis and Treatment of Head, Neck, and Facial Pain.* 2d ed. Baltimore: Williams & Wilkins, 1999. A manual for doctors with patients complaining of headache pain.

HEALING

BIOLOGY

ANATOMY OR SYSTEM AFFECTED: All

SPECIALTIES AND RELATED FIELDS: Alternative medicine, cytology, dermatology, family practice, hematology, histology, immunology, plastic surgery, vascular medicine

DEFINITION: The process of mending damaged tissue by which an organism restores itself to health.

KEY TERMS:

collagen: a white fibrous protein produced by the body to fill in areas destroyed by injury; the healing component more commonly thought of as scar tissue

delayed primary closure: a procedure in which the wound is left open four to six days and then sewn closed; used for infected or contaminated wounds

healing by primary intention: the most desirable healing in the least amount of time, with minimal scar tissue formation; the edges of the wound close together

healing by secondary intention: less desirable healing of a wound, with replacement of damaged area by granulation tissue; delayed healing and excessive scar formation occur

regeneration: the renewal, regrowth, or restoration of destroyed or missing tissue; the production of new tissue

tensile strength: the greatest stress that can be placed on a tissue without tearing it apart; relative to the strength of a tissue

wounds: injuries classified as open or closed depending on whether the skin is broken; types of open wounds include abrasions, lacerations, avulsions, punctures, and incisions

THE HEALING PROCESS

The human body is not able to reproduce injured parts during the healing process. Most injured tissue in the body is replaced with collagen, a white protein known as scar tissue. Body areas capable of reproducing, or regenerating, include the outer layer of skin and the inner layers of the intestines.

The human body is involved in a continuous process of self-healing every day. The outer layer of the skin is constantly rubbed off, yet the body is able to replace (regenerate) new skin to take its place. Another body area capable of regeneration is the innermost layer of the intestine. All other types of tissue, however, such as muscle, fat, blood vessels, or even bones, must rely on other ways to heal when injured. How quickly the body heals depends on many factors, but the process is a predictable one. The healing process includes three phases: the acute inflammatory phase, the repair or regeneration phase, and the remodeling phase.

The first phase of healing, the immediate inflammatory phase, includes the first three or four days after the injury. This process, carried out by vascular, chemical, and cellular events, leads to the repair of tissue, to regeneration, or to scar tissue formation. If the hand is sliced open by a piece of broken glass, the first healing response would be a temporary decrease in blood flow, known as vasoconstriction, that lasts from a few seconds up to several minutes. This narrowing of the blood vessel occurs because of a decrease in the diameter of the blood vessels at the injury site and prevents the person from bleeding to death. With extensive vessel damage, however, the body is unable to close off enough vessels, and life-threatening hemorrhaging may occur.

When only a small amount of tissue is cut, the blood begins to seal the broken vessels by coagulation, also known as blood clot formation. The next step is activation of the chemicals needed in the healing process, which is possible only after the blood vessel diameter increases in a process called vasodilation. During vasodilation, the blood flow is slowed and the blood becomes thicker, resulting in swelling. At this point, a buildup or accumulation of fluid results from the seeping of plasma, the fluid portion of the blood, through the vessel walls. This seeping or leakage results from the difference in pressure within the vessel and outside its walls. The amount of swelling at the injury site depends on the amount of seeping, which in turn depends on how much tissue damage has occurred.

Because the blood flow is slower, the concentration of red blood cells and white blood cells is increased. The white blood cells line up and adhere to the inside walls of small blood vessels, known as venules. These white blood cells then pass through the venule walls and are chemically attracted to the injury site over the next several hours. A specialized connective tissue cell,

known as a mast cell, is also sent to the injury site. Mast cells contain heparin and histamine. Heparin prolongs the clotting time of blood by temporarily preventing coagulation, while histamine causes dilation of the capillaries. During this earliest phase, both heparin and histamine are important factors, since their actions allow other specialized cells to move into the injured area. The amount of bleeding and fluid buildup at the injury site depends on the extent of damage and how easily materials can cross the walls of intact vessels. Both of these conditions influence the healing process.

The second phase of healing can be called the repair or regeneration phase. For tissue capable of regeneration, this phase involves the restoration of destroyed or missing tissue. For other types of tissue, this second phase would entail the repair process. The healing of a deep cut in the hand would not be considered regeneration, since the body is not able to remake all the different layers of skin and muscle injured. This healing phase would extend forward from the previously described inflammatory phase. During this phase, the cut is naturally cleaned through the body's ability to remove cellular waste, the help of the red blood cells, and the formation of a blood clot.

Two types of healing can occur. Primary healing, or healing by primary intention, could take place in the hand laceration example, since the edges are even and close together. If this injury resulted in a large piece of tissue being removed, then the body would fill the gap with scar tissue. The replacement of tissue with scar tissue is an example of secondary healing, or healing by secondary intention. A torn muscle would be an example of secondary healing if it is allowed to heal on its own by the formation of scar tissue within the muscle.

No matter which type of healing occurs, several factors regulate how quickly and how completely this process takes place. Because blood vessels and cells are deprived of oxygen and die from the injury, this new cellular waste or debris must be cleaned from the area before repair or regeneration can take place. This tissue death promotes the formation of new capillary buds on the walls of the intact vessels. As these mature, the injury site is newly supplied with oxygenated blood and the healing process continues into the third phase.

The third phase of healing, known as the remodeling phase, includes the laying down of young scar tissue that increases in strength over the next year. Although the healing process has no distinct time frame, it is believed that three to six weeks are needed for the production of scar tissue. There must be a balance between the toughness and the elasticity of the scar. The amount of stress placed on a newly formed scar will determine the tensile strength of the collagen content. If stress or strain is placed on this forming scar tissue too early, the healing process will take longer. A desirable outcome would be a scar of adequate collagen content through the development of sufficient mature collagen fibers of proper tensile strength. Adequate tensile strength is also affected by how long inflammation is present.

If an injury site has inflammation that lasts up to one month, it is considered a subacute inflammation. When it lasts for months or years, it is then called chronic inflammation. Chronic inflammation is a condition where small traumas happen repeatedly; it is often seen in overuse injuries. Because this type of injury lasts longer, different types of chemicals try to initiate com-

plete healing. The role of some of these special chemicals is not completely understood.

The healing of a broken bone, similar in many ways to the healing of the skin, is somewhat easier to understand. The first phase shows the same acute inflammation that lasts about four days, involving clotting blood, dead bone cells, and soft tissue damage around the injury site. The second phase, the repair and regeneration phase, differs slightly when a bone is broken, since the blood clot (hematoma) becomes granulated and builds between the two bone ends. The bone produces a specialized cell that turns into a soft or hard fibrous callus, matures into cartilage, and finally becomes bone with a firmly woven network of cells.

The beginning soft callus is a network of unorganized bone that forms at the two broken edges and is later absorbed and replaced by a hard callus. With appropri-

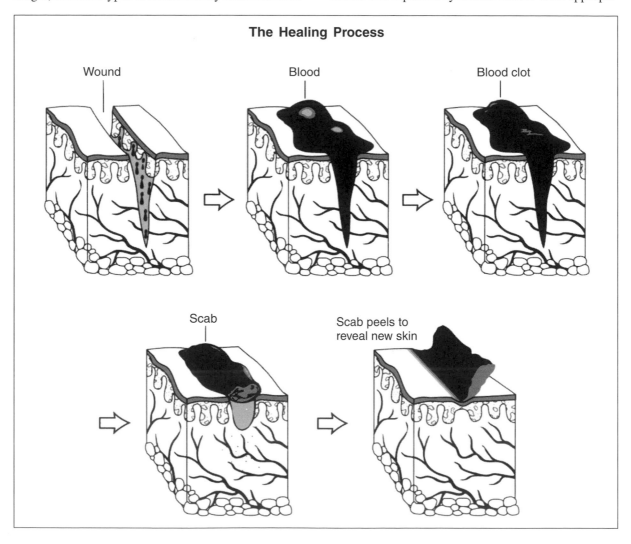

The Healing Process

Wound

Blood

Blood clot

Scab

Scab peels to reveal new skin

ate care, a broken bone will develop a new network in the center and eventually become primary bone. The amount of oxygen available in the area determines this development. It is important to keep in mind that when the injury is severe enough to break a bone, then the blood supply is interrupted, lowering the amount of oxygen that is available. Low oxygen could result in the formation of only fibrous tissue or cartilage. Strong, healthy bone results when oxygen and the correct amount of compression are available. The third phase, the remodeling phase, describes the time when the callus has been reabsorbed and special intersecting bone fibers cover the broken area. It may take many years for this entire process to be completed, until the bone has regained its normal shape and ability to withstand stresses.

DISORDERS AND TREATMENT

Any of the three stages of healing can be delayed or prevented. The three main causes for failed healing are poor blood supply, poor immobilization, or infection.

The healing process within the body can be seriously hampered if the blood supply is poor, since the delivery of nutrients, chemicals, hormones, and specialized building materials to the injury site is hampered. It is extremely important that oxygen levels are adequate for proper healing. If the blood supply is not sufficient, then the tissue may die, especially in broken bone fragments. Fortunately, most tissues of the body have a good blood supply, as demonstrated by the amount of bleeding that takes place when the skin and underlying tissues are injured.

The second condition that interferes with healing is excessive movement because the body part was not immobilized. In order for the scar tissue or even new bone to become well organized, the two edges of the injured tissue must be kept close together.

The third reason for poor healing is infection. Although the body has many defenses against infection, foreign material can slow healing. If this infectious material invades the space between the two bone ends of a fracture, the necessary building materials may not reach the site. Infection invading the hand tissue cut by the glass could prevent the edges from healing together because of pus, scab formation, or the interference of germs.

There are many different types of injuries, and several steps must be taken in caring for each type. Soft tissues, the first line of defense against injuries, can be used to describe all tissues other than bone. Soft tissue injuries are classified as either closed or open. In a closed wound, the damage lies below the surface of the skin and the skin remains intact. A sprained ankle or a bruised knee are classified as closed wounds. In an open wound, the skin or mucous membranes such as the lining of the mouth are broken or torn.

There are four types of open soft tissue injuries; each has specific characteristics and heals differently. The first type is an abrasion, in which part of the outer layer of the skin and some underlying tissue is rubbed or scraped off. A common injury of this type is a scraped knee resulting from a fall on the sidewalk. The second type, the laceration, results from a sharp object cutting the skin, such as the previous example of a piece of glass cutting the skin either superficially or very deeply. The third type, an avulsion, results when a piece of skin or even an entire fingertip is torn off or left loosely hanging by a small flap of skin. It is important that this flap not be removed since a physician can sometimes reattach the part. The last type of soft tissue injury is the puncture wound, which results when a sharp object penetrates the skin and into a body part. Such an injury could be a stab from a knife or an ice pick, a splinter stuck in the foot, or even a bullet shot into the leg. The initial management is the same for all four types of injury.

Management of open wounds must include control of bleeding, infection prevention, and immobilization. Two of the above injuries, an avulsion and a puncture wound, require additional special care. In the case of an avulsed body part, the amputated part should be saved; wrapped in a dry, sterile piece of gauze; and placed in a plastic bag. If this bag is kept in something cool, such as a bucket of ice, the possibility of reattachment is increased. An impaled object remaining in a puncture wound should never be removed but held in place and all movement restricted until medical care can be given.

Several medical treatments can aid in promoting the healing process, as can commonsense first aid measures taken immediately after an injury occurs. For example, with a glass cut to the hand one should immediately stop the bleeding by placing a sterile piece of gauze, or a very clean cloth, directly over the laceration. By adding direct pressure over the gauze, the circulation is reduced. If the cut is deep, if the bleeding cannot be controlled, or if a piece of glass remains in the wound, then it is advisable to seek medical attention. A physician would then thoroughly clean the injury site and stitch the two edges together. Immobilizing the two flaps of skin together by sewing them will allow the first two phases of healing to progress. By having the wound inspected and cleaned by medical personnel, the risk of infection is reduced. A small injury can be cared for at home, but infection must be prevented through proper cleansing. Even soap and water, along with a bandage or dressing, will help to ward off infections.

PERSPECTIVE AND PROSPECTS

Many strategies to improve the healing of human tissue have evolved over time—from ancient times, when healers packed mud on the top of sores to draw out the infection, to modern alternative medicines. Every person, at one time or another, receives a cut, scrape, bump, or bruise. Therefore, there is much interest in speeding up the healing process.

Renewed interests in nontraditional approaches to medicine explore the healing powers locked within the human body. The use of homeopathy, acupuncture, and acupressure are examples of alternatives to antibiotics and standard first aid measures to help an injury heal. Holistic health care, hypnosis, and osteopathic medicine offer other areas of exploration. The practice of Chinese medicine includes the use of herbs, crystals, massage, and meditation to allow healing to proceed quickly but through natural means. Even the use of aromatherapy—treatment through the inhalation of specific smells—has gained a foothold in the medical world. The manipulations done by chiropractic doctors offer other possibilities. Some seek cures in nature, from sources below the sea or deep in the forest. Yet, many untapped resources remain. The continuing research in genetics offers vast possibilities, and the link between mental attitude and the immune system presents a rich area for further exploration. Even innovations as simple as a special glue, used to replace sutures or staples for closing wounds, would have an important influence on the future of the healing process.

—*Maxine M. Urton, Ph.D.*

See also Antibiotics; Aromatherapy; Bleeding; Blood and blood disorders; Chiropractic; Circulation; Dermatology; Grafts and grafting; Histology; Host-defense mechanisms; Immune system; Immunology; Infection; Inflammation; Laceration repair; Meditation; Skin; Surgery, general; Vascular system; Wounds.

FOR FURTHER INFORMATION:

Browner, Bruce, Lenworth M. Jacobs, and Andrew N. Pollack, eds. *Emergency Care and Transportation of the Sick and Injured.* Rev. 7th ed. Rosemont, Ill.: American Academy of Orthopaedic Surgeons, 1999. Covers soft tissue injuries. Offers graphic photo-graphs of actual injuries and discusses care and management. This text is often used in the training of emergency medical technicians, yet chapters are easily understood by the nonmedical layperson.

DiPietro, Luisa A., and Aime L. Burns, eds. *Wound Healing: Methods and Protocols.* Totowa, N.J.: Humana Press, 2003. A clinical text that describes classic and contemporary laboratory methods for studying tissue repair and examines systemic and genetic conditions that influence the healing process.

Eisenberg, David. *Encounters with Qi.* New York: W. W. Norton, 1995. Extensive explanations of the Chinese principles in medicine are covered, from ancient practices through current uses. Examines the uses of herbs, acupuncture, and psychic healing to restore the body's inner balance.

Gach, Michael R. *Acupressure's Potent Points: A Guide to Self-Care for Common Ailments.* New York: Bantam Books, 1990. An extensively illustrated book showing the self-use of acupressure to relieve physical problems by activating the body's natural self-healing processes.

Goldberg, Linn, and Diane L. Elliot. *The Healing Power of Exercise: Your Guide to Preventing and Treating Diabetes, Depression, Heart Disease, High Blood Pressure, Arthritis, and More.* New York: Wiley, 2000. This book explains how exercise can reduce your risk of certain diseases as well as alleviate symptoms.

Handal, Kathleen A. *The American Red Cross First Aid and Safety Handbook.* Boston: Little, Brown, 1992. A comprehensive, fully illustrated guide outlining basic first aid and emergency care steps to be taken until medical assistance can be obtained. Updated materials can also be obtained directly from local Red Cross Association chapters listed in telephone books.

Hill, James A., ed. *AMA Handbook of First Aid and Emergency Care.* 3d rev. ed. New York: Random House, 2000. Provides a listing of injuries, illnesses, and medical emergencies accompanied by easy-to-follow instructions and illustrations.

Kemper, Kathi J. *The Holistic Pediatrician: A Pediatrician's Comprehensive Guide to Safe and Effective Therapies for the Twenty-five Most Common Ailments of Infants, Children, and Adolescents.* New York: HarperCollins, 2002. Integrates mainstream and alternative medicine to aid parents in dealing with the most common childhood health problems and injuries.

Woodham, Anne, and David Peters. *The Encyclopedia of Healing Therapies.* New York: Dorling Kindersley, 1997. This book explains holistic and complementary medicine and offers a guide to well-being. Also contains information on finding practitioners, a directory of associations, a glossary, and a bibliography.

HEALTH MAINTENANCE ORGANIZATIONS (HMOs)

ORGANIZATION

ALSO KNOWN AS: Competitive medical plans

DEFINITION: A business competitor within a free market economy that provides health care insurance and services to group and individual clients for an established, prepaid monthly premium and that generally attempts to provide care at a lower cost than traditional fee-for-service insurance programs by transferring financial risk to physicians through capitation and other incentives.

KEY TERMS:

disability insurance: a health coverage policy that protects against loss of income resulting from sickness or accident, whereby benefits are structured to pay approximately 40 to 60 percent of earnings up to a maximum total amount

group model HMO: an HMO organized by physicians whereby a private professional corporation is established which then individually contracts with an HMO to provide services exclusively for its subscribers

independent practice association model HMO: a flexible arrangement whereby several office physicians in a community form a networked professional corporation that seeks group contracts among local employers and provides all medical care for a capitated rate per client per month to subscribers, who often choose a personal primary care physician

managed care: the techniques by which an HMO, a health insurance carrier, or a self-insuring employer makes certain that the health care services it is endorsing are cost-effective and of a high quality

point-of-service model HMO: also called an open-ended HMO; a model that includes an option which allows subscribers to seek medical care outside the established network and receive partial reimbursement, with all remaining expenses paid out-of-pocket

preferred providers: physicians and other health care providers and hospitals who choose to provide health care at a reduced cost for subscribers to an HMO

staff model HMO: an HMO that is directly controlled at its headquarters, with all physicians and other health care workers being full-time, salaried employees

ROLE IN THE HEALTH CARE INDUSTRY

A health maintenance organization (HMO) in a free market economy functions in a dual role as both a health insurance company and a provider of health services, roles that were previously separated within the U.S. health care system. HMOs—also known as competitive medical plans, managed care plans, or alternative delivery systems—are generally organized by an employer, physician group, union, consumer group, insurance company, or for-profit health care agency. They were originally formed from one, or a mixture, of the following models: point of service, staff, group, and independent practice association.

The role of an HMO as an insurer is to seek group contracts with employers and individual clients and to negotiate premiums to be prepaid in exchange for covering preagreed benefits. Its role in service delivery is to affiliate with or hire directly physicians to provide the expected volume of care that is required for all subscribers under contract. An HMO owns or contracts with one or more health centers for ambulatory care and with hospitals for inpatient care. Within its private health center or in contracts with freestanding providers, an HMO will furnish services from other health care providers such as physical and occupational therapy, pharmacy, and mental health care, which are rapidly increasing in their level of responsibility.

HMOs are attractive to employers because the annual medical bill for the average subscriber-patient consistently has proved to be approximately 30 percent less than that of conventional insurers. One advantage of HMO membership is that all medical expenses, from routine and emergency care to hospitalization, are covered within a single, fixed monthly premium. In addition, presenting an HMO membership card at time of services with a small copayment means no forms to fill out, no deductibles to pay, and no bills to submit. Disadvantages include that new subscribers often cannot keep a trusted physician they have had for years, providers become extremely busy when they are assigned hundreds of patients in exchange for a fixed fee, and subscribers often must accept fewer choices in treatment options.

PRACTICES AND PROCEDURES

The term "managed care" describes the techniques by

which an HMO, a health insurance carrier, or a self-insuring employer makes certain that the health care services that it endorses are high in quality and cost-effective. This system was once used in many countries. Workers joined a mutual aid association and paid premiums, and the association was responsible for hiring enough quality full-time or part-time physicians to provide the required services. These restrictive arrangements could not survive within a country that has a national health insurance law because every covered citizen would then have the right to choose any provider and subsequently bill the system. Managed care is able to survive in the United States only because a compulsory national health insurance law has not been enacted, as has been done in other industrialized countries.

The headquarters of an HMO competitively markets its services to employer groups and individuals and administers the revenue and payments. An HMO generally contracts or directly hires a limited number of physicians in addition to building, staffing, and equipping the necessary number of health centers and hospitals. Its marketing claim is to provide good quality care within the employer's group premium, without seeking further supplements from the employer. Because an HMO and its providers are at personal financial risk, the organization directly imposes financial discipline upon its physicians, hospitals, and other health care providers. The HMO retains a percentage of the premiums paid from employers for its administrative and facility costs and pays a monthly "capitated rate" per client to the providers. HMOs have historically had persistent difficulty in recruiting and retaining physicians, and patients have consistently informed the HMOs that they prefer private offices to health centers.

Managed care procedures generally involve the HMO establishing a network of physicians with superior reputations in each region, with these physicians agreeing to bill the carriers according to limited reimbursement rules. Each client is assigned to a "primary care gatekeeper" who is expected to provide most care in his or her private office for limited fees. When a referral to a specialist, laboratory, or hospital is necessary, authorization is required from the headquarters of the managed care organization. Hospitals contract with these organizations to limit their charges and follow established rules about economical care and prompt discharge. The managed care organization reviews utilization by physicians and hospitals, attempts to correct wasteful practices, and subsequently drops health care providers with expensive and/or poor practice styles.

In contrast to more traditional HMOs, point-of-service plans have more recently emerged. These plans enable clients to have freedom of choice with respect to providers and some treatment options but requires them personally to pay the balance for their chosen higher-priced services. If the patient goes to physicians, hospitals, and other providers within the network and follows rules about utilization and authorization, the out-of-pocket financial costs are minimal. The patient retains the option to go to an out-of-plan provider, pay the bill in full, and then be reimbursed for the limited amount established in the individual plan. The employer's group contract with the managed care organization provides for limited and predictable premiums. The considerable costs of out-of-plan services thus are shifted from the group contract to the individual patient.

Managed care plans will continue to monitor closely the treatment patterns of physicians and encourage them to prescribe cheaper medications, to develop standards that physicians are expected to follow in treatment of various diseases, and to hold utilization review panels that review patient records and decide which treatments a patient's health plan will cover and which it will not. Because of the numerous consumer complaints that arose from actions resulting from the decisions of case managers, who often do not have any medical training, nineteen states had passed comprehensive managed care laws by 1997. In the year 1997 alone, states passed a record 182 laws related to managed care, up from 100 in 1996. Legislation during the late 1990's and into the twenty-first century focused on issues such as adopting measures to ban physician gag clauses, establishing consumer grievance procedures, requiring disclosure of financial incentives for physicians to withhold care, holding external reviews of internal decisions to deny care, and ensuring the ability to sue an HMO for malpractice. In 2001, many of these issues were addressed via a legislative "Bill of Rights" for patients. The bill led to a contentious debate over whether and how to regulate managed care plans. The bill was passed, but critics claim its provisions do not apply to all of the more than 160 million people enrolled in health insurance plans and fail to give unhappy patients the right to sue their health plans for punitive damages. Several states have also attempted—with some, like Washington State, succeeding—to implement their own managed care reforms.

PERSPECTIVE AND PROSPECTS

The first HMOs in the United States were established in the 1930's with the pioneering efforts of the Ross-Loos Medical Group in California, but most experienced only minimal growth until the 1970's. Beginning in the early 1970's, HMOs proliferated rapidly, primarily as a result of escalating costs for health care services and increasing competition among a growing number of physicians. The Health Maintenance Organizations Act of 1973 provided federal grants and loans for the establishment of HMOs and required many employers to offer HMO membership to employees as a health insurance alternative. The federal government began to promote the HMO concept as a means by which to control costs by discouraging physicians from performing unnecessary and costly procedures, to meet the increased demand for health insurance particularly in underserved areas, and to foster preventive medicine. Monetary incentives, which are strongly supported by numerous politicians, are in theory the major forces behind personal freedom of choice, containment of costs, and assurance of quality. Innovated by the Kaiser Foundation Health Plan in California, the Health Insurance Plan of Greater New York, and the Group Health Cooperative of Puget Sound, greater numbers of preferred provider organizations began to appear in the 1980's and 1990's as a more flexible alternative to standard HMOs. Many major health insurers such as Blue Cross and Blue Shield then began exerting control over the daily operations of both HMOs and preferred provider organizations. Managed care was spread rapidly across the United States by the large health insurance companies, largely stimulated by the ongoing difficulties experienced by national policy in containing medical costs. In 1970, there were approximately thirty different managed care plans; by 1997, this number had grown to more than fifteen hundred. In 1997, more than 80 percent of HMOs were for-profit organizations. The significance of this figure is that an increasing amount of money that could be spent on medical care is now being spent on marketing costs and stockholder dividends.

The largest looming question regarding the future of HMOs is whether physicians and other health care workers, as well as client subscribers, will continue to enroll in and thus support the system. Managed care necessarily adds substantial administrative overhead, with the ongoing question of whether the final result is greater efficiency for the entire system or simply for subscribing employers. Another controversial topic of discussion involves the responsibility of an HMO to provide disability insurance, which becomes necessary when a client incurs loss of income resulting from sickness or an accident that is not covered by workers' compensation. An organization that will exert considerable influence in future HMO developments is the American Association of Retired Persons (AARP), a large, nonprofit advocacy group for Americans over the age of fifty with more than 30 million members. It has begun giving endorsements to HMOs that meet its standards of quality and price.

In other industrialized nations, both the services covered and the extent of coverage equal or exceed the coverage of a standard HMO within the United States. Several countries have universal health care insurance coverage, although in many industrialized nations certain categories of residents may be exempt. Notable examples include Germany, which requires the purchase of private health insurance by law; Canada and Sweden, which have public insurance coverage for essentially any citizen; and Great Britain, which has a majority of medical services located within the public sector.

—*Daniel G. Graetzer, Ph.D.*

See also Allied health; Ethics; Law and medicine; Malpractice.

FOR FURTHER INFORMATION:

Birenbaum, Aaron. *Wounded Profession: American Medicine Enters the Age of Managed Care.* Westport, Conn.: Greenwood Press, 2002. Traces the evolution of health care in the United States during the 1990's and examines the rising costs, consumer backlash, and new legislation.

Brink, Susan, and Nancy Shute. "Are HMOs the Right Prescription?" *U.S. News and World Report* 123, no. 4 (October 13, 1997): 60-65. Covered in this well-researched article is the growing dissatisfaction of subscribers with the quality of health care received, with a rating of the best HMOs in the United States.

Dranove, David. *The Economic Evolution of American Health Care: From Marcus Welby to Managed Care.* Princeton, N.J.: Princeton University Press, 2002. Traces the economic, technological, and historical forces that have transformed the health care field.

Freeborn, D. K., and C. R. Pope. *The Promise and Performance of Managed Care: The Prepaid Practice Model.* Rev. ed. Baltimore: Johns Hopkins University Press, 1999. This excellent text highlights the evolution of several common promises of HMOs that employ the prepaid practice model and evaluates their performance based on relevant criteria.

Johnsson, Julie. "HMOs Dominate, Shape the Market." *American Medical News* 39, no. 4 (1996): 1-3. A well-written article that outlines the competition among HMOs and how they attempt to obtain lower prices from providers as premiums continue to drop.

Kongstvedt, Peter R., and Wendy Knight. *Managed Care: What It Is and How It Works.* 2d ed. Sudbury, Mass.: Jones and Bartlett, 2002. Provides a historical overview of managed care and covers organizational structures, concepts, and practices of the managed care industry.

Lairson, D. R., et al. "Managed Care and Community-Oriented Care: Conflict or Complement?" *Journal of Health Care for the Poor and Underserved* 8, no. 1 (1997): 36-55. This informative article evaluates models for community health planning and health care reform designed for the medically indigent, including programs that receive support from the U.S. government and programs that do not.

Ludmerer, Kenneth M. *Time to Heal: American Medical Education from the Turn of the Century to the Managed Care Era.* New York: Oxford University Press, 2001. Ludmerer looks at the future of medicine in America and reveals some very disturbing trends in managed care, education, and research funding. Contains a wealth of factual details and insightful questions.

Zelman, W. A. *The Changing Health Care Market Place.* San Francisco: Jossey-Bass, 1996. An excellent evaluation of past trends in HMOs and predictions of what the future might hold.

HEARING AIDS

TREATMENT

ANATOMY OR SYSTEM AFFECTED: Ears

SPECIALTIES AND RELATED FIELDS: Audiology, otorhinolaryngology

DEFINITION: Electromechanical devices meant to improve ease of communication and minimize listening fatigue. Patients with profound sensorineural hearing loss receive little or no benefit from conventional hearing aids but may use a cochlear implant, an electronic prosthetic device surgically placed in the inner ear to deliver electrical signals to the brain, where they are interpreted as sounds.

KEY TERMS:

assistive listening devices: earphones or a headset with amplification to supplement or substitute for traditional hearing aids

audiogram: a graph used to display one's hearing ability for average speech sounds, in which decibels have been converted from sound pressure levels to hearing levels

audiologist: a diagnostician who administers hearing tests and dispenses hearing aids

cochlea: an inner ear cavity shaped like a snail surrounded by fluid; when set in motion, this fluid displaces rows of thousands of microscopic hair cells, each of which functions to receive electrical activity and transfer it to the central auditory system

presbycusis: a hearing loss of unknown cause, often attributed to aging

INDICATIONS AND PROCEDURES

Hearing loss is one of the most common conditions affecting older adults, but it is not limited to that age group. In the early twenty-first century, it was estimated that about one in ten individuals in the United States had a significant hearing loss and that 120 million people worldwide had hearing loss significant enough to interfere with communication. In the United States, approximately one million people each year purchase hearing aids. These devices were developed to help those people affected by hearing loss ranging from mild to severe and resulting from a number of causes. The most common type of hearing loss, sensorineural, is linked to a variety of physical and psychosocial dysfunctions (isolation, depression, hypertension, and stress), as well as illnesses such as ischemic heart disease and arrhythmias.

Over the years, hearing aids have evolved in several ways. Two major trends have been in signal processing and size. In the 1960's, the best available hearing aids were limited to help in quiet only; in loud situations, they made things worse. Therefore, it was common practice to remove them around noise. They produced sound like cheap transistor radios. Starting in the 1980's and 1990's, advanced circuitry has offered consumers improved quality of hearing in quiet as well as some increased ability to hear in noise; sound distortion is now minimal. Certain hearing aids can be electronically adjusted for individual users; for example, they can be reprogrammed to accommodate increased hearing loss. Certain hearing aids have volume controls; others adjust automatically. Research has shown that consumers report greater satisfaction with sound quality than they did in the past, and people with hearing loss in both ears tend to be more satisfied with two hearing aids, enabling them to determine the direction of sounds.

Prior to the 1940's, hearing aids were large and required carrying a battery pack strapped to one's body. In the 1940's, vacuum tubes reduced the size of hearing aids to that of a transistor radio. Hearing aids in the ear or on the head were not available until the 1960's. Because of the size reduction of hearing aids, they have become more comfortable and less noticeable.

For patients with bilateral profound sensorineural hearing loss, which does not respond to traditional hearing aids, a cochlear implant is now possible. A cochlear implant is an electronic prosthesis surgically implanted in the inner ear. It has external parts that are worn outside the ear, including a microphone, speech processor, headpiece antenna, and cable. It is not a hearing aid. A cochlear implant delivers electrical signals to the brain, where they are interpreted as sounds. Potential candidates for these implants include both children and adults in a wide age range. Generally, children should be at least eighteen months old, and many successful implant recipients are in their eighties. Adults who become deaf later in life, and who have fully developed speech and language before their hearing loss, have better results with the implant than do those who were born deaf or who lost their hearing early in life. It has been shown, however, that the child who is born deaf who is given a cochlear implant early in life can receive great benefit from it. In adults, the memory of sound appears to be one of the most important factors for success. For children, early implantation and placement in an educational program that emphasizes the development of auditory skills appear to be important factors for success.

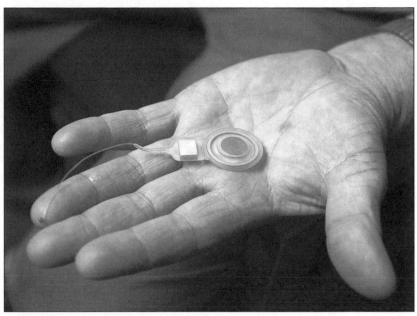

This hearing aid is implanted in the patient. When used with an external component, it enhances middle-ear function and provides a better signal to the cochlea. (AP/Wide World Photos)

USES AND COMPLICATIONS

One of the biggest impediments to hearing aid use is patient reactions to hearing loss. Many people try to cover up the fact that they have hearing difficulties, and when hearing loss is confirmed, they experience a wide range of emotions, from horror, denial, disbelief, and withdrawal to embarrassment, sadness, resentment, and gradual acceptance and coping. People's coping skills and behavior patterns vary, in part because hearing loss generally occurs gradually and may take a long time to be recognized.

For those who embrace hearing aids, a variety of technological and cosmetic choices are available. A number of options exist regarding hearing aid style: behind-the-ear, custom in-the-ear, in-the-canal, and the smallest, the completely in-canal hearing aid. In addition to aesthetic considerations and sound fidelity, one's anatomy and manual dexterity may dictate the style that is most effective and efficient. The degree of hearing loss and other medical conditions are also important factors when evaluating the best hearing aid.

PERSPECTIVE AND PROSPECTS

Hearing aid technology has improved such that patients with mild to moderate hearing loss will be candidates for hearing aids and those with severe loss will be candidates for hearing aids or cochlear implants, depending upon how well they function with a particular device. Patients with profound hearing loss will benefit best from cochlear implants.

Initially, only those patients who were completely deaf in both ears were considered candidates for cochlear implants. With significant improvements in implant technology, however, the benefits gained by implanted patients, both children and adults, have markedly improved. This, in turn, has led to a broadening of criteria for implant patients. Select patients with severe hearing loss who receive some benefit from hearing aids are considered possible implant candidates.

—*Marcia J. Weiss, J.D.*

See also Aging; Audiology; Ear surgery; Ears; Hearing loss; Hearing tests; Otorhinolaryngology; Sense organs.

FOR FURTHER INFORMATION:

Biderman, Beverly. *Wired for Sound: A Journey into Hearing.* Toronto: Trifolium Books, 1998.

Carmen, Richard, ed. *The Consumer Handbook on Hearing Loss and Hearing Aids: A Bridge to Healing.* Sedona, Ariz.: Auricle Ink, 1998.

Romoff, Arlene. *Hear Again: Back to Life with a Cochlear Implant.* New York: League for the Hard of Hearing, 1999.

HEARING LOSS

DISEASE/DISORDER

ANATOMY OR SYSTEM AFFECTED: Ears, nervous system

SPECIALTIES AND RELATED FIELDS: Audiology, geriatrics and gerontology, neurology, occupational health, otorhinolaryngology

DEFINITION: Loss of sensitivity to sound pressure changes as a result of congenital factors, disease, traumatic injury, noise exposure, or aging.

KEY TERMS:

aging process: the process in which physiological, neurological, and biological changes affect behavior and function

auditory: referring to the ear and to the sense of hearing

auditory cortex: that portion of the temporal lobe in the human brain where the ascending auditory pathway terminates

auditory nerve: the cochlear branch of the eighth cranial nerve

neural hearing loss: hearing impairment caused by a loss of the neural tissue that constitutes the ascending pathway of the auditory system

ossicles: three small bones located in the middle ear that convey sound pressure changes from the tympanic membrane (eardrum) to the oval window of the cochlea; the bones are commonly referred to as the hammer (malleus), anvil (incus), and stirrup (stapes)

phonology: the study of the sounds that make up any verbal language system

sensory hearing loss: hearing impairment caused by a loss of sensory cells (nerve cells) in the cochlea

THE PHYSIOLOGY OF THE EAR

The normal, young ear is capable of detecting frequencies (tones) from as low as 20 hertz to as high as 20,000 hertz. (Hertz is the current notation for cycles per second.) Actually, in terms of frequency, humans can hear as low as 2 hertz, but about 20 hertz is required for a perception of "tonality." This is an amazing range. At the very low end of the frequency scale, one is not certain whether a tone is being "heard" or whether the sensation is a "tactile" one. (There is some neuroanatomical speculation that the organ of hearing is a very specialized tactile sensor.) At the very high end of the frequency scale, one can detect the highest strings of the violin, the rustle of leaves as they are disturbed by the wind, and the distinctive cry of birds and animals. A host of other sounds in between the lowest and highest frequencies can also be perceived. The subjective, psychological correlate of frequency is pitch. In general, the higher the frequency of a sound, the higher is the perceived pitch.

The ear performs an amazing feat in dealing with the broad range of intensities. Intensity is directly proportional to the magnitude of sound pressure change. The ear is so sensitive to small changes in sound pressure that the normal ear is capable of detecting pressure changes no greater than the diameter of a hydrogen molecule. At the other end of this continuum, the human ear can withstand great amplitude changes in sound pressure without damage. In terms of sound pressure units, the range from the weakest sound detected to the loudest sound tolerated represents a ratio of 10,000,000:1. In other words, the most intense sound pressure that is bearable is on the order of 10,000,000 times as great as the softest one that is perceptible under optimum listening conditions.

Intensity is expressed in decibels. Essentially, the higher the decibel value, the more intense or louder the sound. The ear is sensitive to a range of intensities from about 0 decibels to about 135 decibels. At the very extreme of this range, pain is experienced and permanent damage can occur if the sound intensity is prolonged. The psychological correlate of intensity is loudness. Under ideal conditions, if the intensity is increased by 9 decibels, the signal is perceived as being twice as loud.

The ability to process acoustic information correctly depends on the critical relationship between frequency and intensity. The critical frequency range needed to understand the English phonological system extends from about 300 hertz to 4,000 hertz. Theoretically, if one heard no other sounds above 4,000 hertz and below 300 hertz, one would experience no difficulty in understanding the intended message. Relative to intensity, a listener would have no difficulty in information processing if speech were presented at 65 decibels at a distance of one meter. In addition to the listener's distance from the speech source, speech understanding is also influenced by ambient background noise. For adequate processing to occur, speech must be louder than the ambient noise.

Sound is produced by a generating source such as a musical instrument, sounds of nature, or the vibrations of the human vocal cords that create a voice. The resulting series of sound pressure changes represents all the frequency and intensity characteristics generated at the source. These sound pressure changes travel through the atmosphere at a constant speed (approximately 335 meters per second at sea level). They are channeled through the external ear canal and strike the eardrum (tympanic membrane). The eardrum is sensitive to negative and positive changes in sound pressure and moves in concert with these changes. The greater the sound pressure, the greater is the magnitude of movement. Similarly, the higher the frequency, the more rapid are the movements of the eardrum. In the middle ear of the hearing system are three small bones, called ossicles. The first of these, the hammer (malleus), is attached to the eardrum. The second, the anvil (incus), is attached by ligaments to the malleus and to the third ossicle, the stirrup (stapes), which in turn attaches to the oval window membrane of the cochlea. As the eardrum is displaced in a negative or positive direction by sound pressure changes in the external ear canal, there is an absolute and corresponding movement of the ossicles.

In the cochlea, there are three anatomical divisions: the scala vestibuli, the scala tympani, and the scala media. Each of these spaces is filled with a fluid. The fluid of the scala media is chemically different from the fluid in the other two spaces. Housed in the scala media are all the specialized nervous tissues that respond to the movement of the fluid. These specialized nerve cells are situated on top of an anatomical structure called the basilar membrane. The wave forms generated within the fluid are caused by the movement of the stapes bones, as the oval window membrane communicates directly with the fluid of the cochlear space. The rate at which the stapes moves will cause the basilar membrane to be displaced at a site-specific location along its length. High-frequency sounds generate amplitude changes of the membrane at the apical portion. The movement of the membrane causes the small nerve cells (hair cells) to "fire," creating a neural discharge that travels from the cochlea to the temporal cortex of the brain. The neural events generated by sound pressure changes are interpreted by the brain.

CAUSES, SYMPTOMS, AND TREATMENTS

In the truest sense, hearing loss is any reduction in threshold sensitivity for any frequency, including those below or above the range for the normal hearing of speech. The real issue, however, is whether minor changes in sensitivity create significant problems in understanding speech and other information-bearing acoustic signals. For example, it is known that loss of threshold sensitivity below 300 hertz and above 4,000 hertz has a minimal effect on understanding speech information. It is when hearing loss exists within this critical frequency range that an individual may experience appreciable difficulty in understanding intended messages. The question becomes, then, "What conditions may cause a permanent or temporary loss of hearing, and how is such a loss managed by medical, surgical, or rehabilitative intervention?"

Conductive Hearing Loss. Any barrier or impedance that keeps sound from reaching the cochlea of the human auditory system at its intended loudness is termed "conductive hearing loss." A very common cause of conduction loss is a buildup of earwax (cerumen) in the external ear canal. The production of earwax in the ear canal is essential. It prevents the skin of the ear canal from drying and sloughing off, and it may serve to trap minute foreign particles and keep them from causing damage to the external canal. Normally, earwax will migrate out of the ear and create no conduction prob-

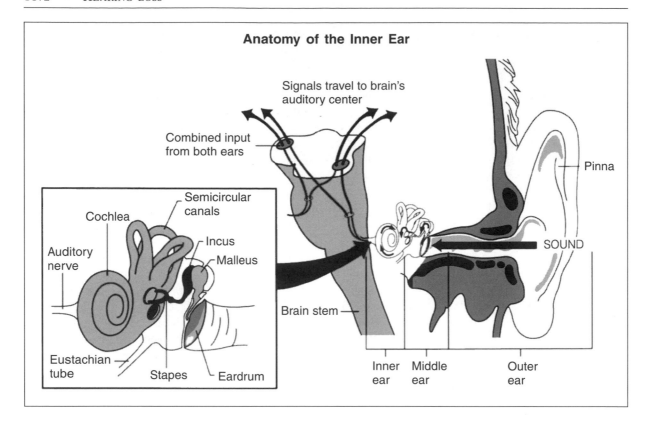

Anatomy of the Inner Ear

Signals travel to brain's auditory center

Combined input from both ears

Pinna

SOUND

Semicircular canals

Cochlea

Incus

Auditory nerve

Malleus

Brain stem

Eustachian tube

Stapes

Eardrum

Inner ear   Middle ear   Outer ear

lem. It is when the earwax accumulates to an amount sufficient to block sound from entering the ear that something needs to be done. In most cases, earwax can be removed by irrigation. A physician washes out the earwax using a special liquid solution that does not damage the tissue of the ear canal or the eardrum itself.

Another cause of conductive hearing loss is a hole (perforation) in the eardrum, which can be created by a number of conditions, including injury. Depending on the size and location of the hole, surgery (tympanoplasty) is often successful in restoring normal hearing function. For some persons, otosclerosis (a disease causing hardening and fixing of the three small bones in the middle-ear space) results in significant conductive hearing impairment. Otosclerosis prevents these tiny bones from moving efficiently as the eardrum moves, and hearing sensitivity is reduced. Fortunately, advances in surgical procedures have allowed the surgeon to replace the stapes bone with a suitable prosthesis, reinstating relatively normal activity of the ossicles and greatly improving hearing ability.

Congenital malformation of the pinna or the ear canal, known as atresia, is an infrequent cause of conductive hearing loss. Often, when the pinna is malformed, there is no opening into the ear canal. In some cases, the ear canal has failed to develop. Depending on the severity of the malformation, of either the pinna or the ear canal, surgery may be successful in restoring function. Other causes of conductive hearing loss include Eustachian tube malfunction, disruption of the ossicular chain (the three tiny bones in the middle ear), and swelling (edema) of the external ear canal.

A frequently occurring cause of conductive pathology is otitis media. Otitis media may refer to inflammation involving the middle-ear space or to a disorder in which the middle ear is filled with a watery fluid. In some cases, the fluid may harbor bacteria, creating significant medical problems if this condition is not treated early. Such middle-ear effusions are more common in children than in adults. If fluid is present in the middle ear, its mass will restrict the movement of the ossicles and create hearing impairment. Generally, patients with otitis media can be successfully treated through medical or surgical intervention.

It must be noted that conductive pathology does not affect the behavior of inner-ear structures; that is, the inner ear is capable of normal auditory performance. If the conductive pathology is eliminated by appropriate treatment, normal hearing will be restored. Severity of the condition may prevent the restoration of hearing, however, even if an aggressive treatment program is followed.

Sensorineural Hearing Loss. As a major classification of hearing loss, this term is somewhat misleading. Actually, there are two types of hearing loss within this classification. One is a sensory loss which involves the destruction of nerve cells (hair cells) in the cochlea. The other is a neural loss which involves neural cells in the ascending auditory pathway from the cochlea to the brain. It is possible to experience one type of loss without the other. Some examples of sensory loss include the following: loss of nerve cells resulting from traumatic injury to the cochlea, such as from whiplash, sharp blows to the head, or sudden, brief, and intense noises; loss of sensory cells from viral infections such as measles; loss of sensory cells caused by ototoxic drugs such as those in the mycin group (such as streptomycin or kanamycin); congenital problems associated with a lack of embryonic development; and exposure to loud and continuous (long-term) noise, a very common cause of hearing loss in adults. This last type of impairment is different from traumatic injury resulting from sudden, intense noise because it may take months or years for hearing loss caused by long-term noise to manifest itself. Research has also established a clear correlation between the normal aging process and sensory hearing impairment.

When sensory hearing impairment occurs, it is permanent. At the moment, there is no way of regenerating sensory tissue after the cell body has died. The only exception to this rule is found in those patients suffering from Ménière's disease. This disorder is often characterized by vertigo, dizziness, vomiting, and hearing loss. In the initial stages, however, the loss of sensitivity to sound is the result of changes in cellular physiology rather than of necrosis (death) of the nerve cells.

Examples of neural hearing loss are found among those hearing-impaired individuals with tumors, acoustic neuromas (benign tumors), cysts, and other anomalous conditions affecting the transmission of nerve impulses from the cochlea to the brain. Depending on the magnitude of the disorder, neural hearing loss has a much more devastating effect on speech understanding and signal processing than does sensory loss. As with sensory hearing impairment, neural hearing loss is a rather frequent occurrence associated with the aging process. For a sizable portion of those who experience hearing impairment, components of both sensory and neural loss are present. If the cause of the hearing deficit is entirely neural in nature, then the impairment is referred to as a retrocochlear loss.

For some types of neural pathology, medical or surgical intervention can be undertaken successfully. Acoustic neuromas are often removed after they have

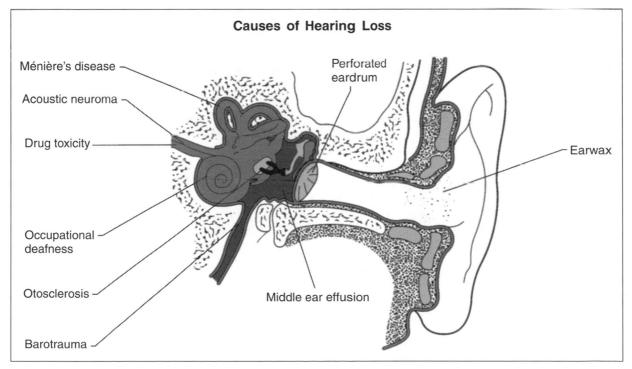

Causes of Hearing Loss

Ménière's disease

Acoustic neuroma

Drug toxicity

Occupational deafness

Otosclerosis

Barotrauma

Perforated eardrum

Earwax

Middle ear effusion

been confirmed by audiologic, otologic, radiologic, and other diagnostic modalities. The size and location of the neuroma or tumorous growth will often dictate whether hearing can be preserved following surgery.

For those millions suffering from hearing impairment, it is the loss of speech discrimination ability that is of greatest concern. Thousands of studies have been undertaken to investigate the correlation between the magnitude, type, and length of hearing loss and the degree of speech recognition difficulty. One of the essential findings of these studies indicates that, in general, hearing loss is more pronounced for the high frequencies (above 1,000 hertz), whether the loss is caused by disease, drugs, noise, or the aging process. Another major finding is that one's ability to identify vowel and consonant information is frequency-dependent. Vowel identification is dependent on frequencies from about 200 hertz to 1,000 hertz, while consonant identification is dependent on frequencies above 1,000 hertz. A listener understands about 68 percent of speech sounds if nothing above 1,500 hertz is heard and about 68 percent of speech if nothing below 1,500 hertz is heard.

PERSPECTIVE AND PROSPECTS

Hearing loss is quite common and affects some twenty million Americans, ranging from infants to the elderly. The primary reason for preserving hearing is to maintain social adequacy in communication skills. Hearing conservation programs have been instituted by public and private schools, industry, military installations, construction organizations, and more recently, the U.S. government. In 1970, the Occupational Safety and Health Act (OSHA) was passed, making it mandatory for employers to provide safe work areas for workers exposed to noise levels exceeding government standards.

For the hearing impaired, understanding of speech is related to the degree of loss and the type of impairment. Because medical or surgical care cannot always ameliorate the loss, rehabilitation programs may take the form of speech or lipreading to improve communication skills. These rehabilitative programs constituted the treatment of choice until the introduction of wearable electric hearing aids.

Before the advent of electric hearing aids, however, the early ear trumpets were very effective for some in restoring speech recognition ability. Through ingenious design, some of the ear trumpets were "acoustically tuned" to provide more amplification in the higher frequencies than in the lower, but the volume of sound was determined by the person talking—often a major problem for the hearing impaired.

With the development of the vacuum tube in the early part of the twentieth century, electric hearing aids became the treatment of choice when medical or surgical intervention was not indicated in resolving the hearing loss. It was possible not only to control the loudness of the hearing aid sound (volume) but also to shape the frequency response of the instrument to match the acoustic needs of the patient. In the second half of the twentieth century, there were significant advances in hearing aid technology. Transistor technology makes it possible to reduce the size of the hearing aid device without sacrificing performance. Computer science has also been used in the design of hearing aids. With digital technology, it is now possible to program electroacoustic characteristics into the hearing aid, which extends its utility.

Recently, major emphasis has been given to hearing conservation. Such continuing efforts have been instrumental in conserving the hearing of tens of thousands who might otherwise suffer from hearing losses sufficient to create problems in speech understanding. Although such programs are too late for millions of hearing-impaired individuals, advances in rehabilitative practices and the scientific application and use of hearing aids have provided them with a quality of life that was not possible only a generation ago.

—*Robert Sandlin, Ph.D.*

See also Aging; Audiology; Ear infections and disorders; Ear surgery; Ears; Hearing aids; Hearing tests; Ménière's disease; Nasopharyngeal disorders; Neuralgia, neuritis, and neuropathy; Otorhinolaryngology; Sense organs; Speech disorders.

FOR FURTHER INFORMATION:

Dugan, Marcia B. *Living with Hearing Loss*. Washington, D.C.: Gallaudet University Press, 2003. Offers a range of practical advice for those with hearing loss, including strategies for dealing with everyday situations and emergencies, speech reading, oral interpreters, and assertive communication.

Ferrari, Mario. *Ear, Nose, and Throat Disorders*. New York: Elsevier, 2002. A clinical yet accessible reference text that provides a comprehensive list of disorders, with a summary of the condition, background, diagnosis, treatment, outcomes, prevention, and resources.

Gelfand, Stanley A. *Essentials of Audiology*. 2d ed. New York: Thieme, 2001. Undergraduate text covering a wide range of relevant topics, including acoustics, anatomy and physiology, sound perception, auditory disorders, and the nature of hearing impairment.

Hearing Exchange. http://www.hearingexchange.com/ An online community designed to foster the exchange of information and the provision of support for the hearing impaired.

Katz, Jack, ed. *Handbook of Clinical Audiology*. 5th ed. Philadelphia: Lippincott Williams & Wilkins, 2002. Text that examines advances in the scientific, clinical, and philosophical understanding of audiology. Sections of the book cover behavioral tests, physiologic tests, special populations, and the management of hearing disorders.

Pascoe, David. *Hearing Aids: Who Needs Them?* St. Louis: Big Bend Books, 1991. This easy-to-read text presents an abundance of data relative to hearing, hearing aid devices, and their use. Answers many questions that may arise concerning hearing aid use in direct and simple terms. One of the most significant aspects of this book is that it explains, in reasonable detail, how to use and evaluate hearing aids.

Yost, William. *Fundamentals of Hearing*. 4th ed. San Diego, Calif.: Academic Press, 2000. This text describes, in easy-to-understand terms, the organ of hearing and its contribution to an individual's behavior. Simple auditory theory is examined, as is the nature of the ear's response to acoustic energy.

HEARING TESTS

PROCEDURE

ANATOMY OR SYSTEM AFFECTED: Ears, nervous system

SPECIALTIES AND RELATED FIELDS: Audiology, neurology, otorhinolaryngology, speech pathology

DEFINITION: Evaluation techniques for determining the type and severity of hearing loss in children.

KEY TERMS:

auditory brainstem response: measurement of the nervous discharge produced by the central auditory system as a response to sound stimulation; also known as brainstem auditory evoked response (BAER) or auditory brainstem potentials (ABR)

auditory nerve: the nerve that conducts sound stimuli to the brain for interpretation

behavioral audiometry: a technique that the audiologist employs to evaluate hearing in infants, toddlers, or uncooperative patients (both children and adults) with developmental deficits

cochlea: the organ localized in the inner portion of the auditory system that detects sound

mastoid: referring to the bone behind the ear

middle ear: the part of the auditory system, consisting of the ossicular chain and the auditory tube, that serves as a conductor of and transducer of sound

otoacoustic emissions: sound produced in the middle ear as a response to the vibration produced by the cochlea when it is stimulated by external sounds

INDICATIONS AND PROCEDURES

Hearing tests are done to establish the presence, type, and severity of hearing impairment in children and adults. Such tests are conducted by an audiologist, although screening tests can also be done by a technician under the supervision of an audiologist. The severity of hearing loss is classified as mild, moderate, moderately severe, severe, and profound. It is also classified according to the anatomic region affected: conductive, sensorineural, or mixed hearing loss.

The selection of tests to evaluate hearing will depend on the patient's age and ability to follow directions and the ability of the audiologist to elicit responses from the patient. When a patient cannot follow instructions such as lifting a hand or pressing a button, a test that does not require the patient's cooperation is used. Two tests that do not require the patient's cooperation are the auditory brainstem potential (ABR) test and the evoked otoacoustic emissions (EOAE) test. Both tests require only that the patient be quiet. For this purpose, the patient may need sedation if normal sleep cannot be induced.

The ABR test requires the placement of four electrodes in the child's head: in both mastoid regions and in the mid forehead and upper center of the head. A stimulus is sent through a small microphone placed in the patient's external ear canal or via headphones. The instrument records the average of the electrical discharges generated by the auditory nerve in response to sound stimuli and produces a tracing of waves that correspond to the different electrical potentials generated in response to the stimuli. Analysis of the waves can determine the presence of hearing loss and measure its severity. The ABR test may be used for screening, to determine whether the subject can hear, or for the clinical evaluation of hearing loss. It can be done at any age. An automated method of ABR testing is available for screening newborn infants for hearing loss; it automatically determines if the patient has passed or failed. The clinical ABR test requires specially trained personnel and takes from forty-five to fifty minutes to perform. The automated method can be applied by a technician.

The EOAE test involves recording the sound produced by hair cells within the cochlea by way of a microphone placed in the outer ear canal. Normally, when sound enters the cochlea, the hair cells produce a sound that bounces backward and can be recorded. This sound correlates with the sound sent to the auditory nerve. If there is damage to the hair cells in the cochlea, then no sound is elicited. The EOAE test can be performed without sedation if the patient cooperates by staying quiet. It can be done by a technician and takes approximately ten minutes or less. The EOAE test is used for universal screening of newborn infants. It can be done at all ages to help determine the integrity of the cochlea and thus whether an observed hearing defect is within the cochlea.

Behavioral techniques are the most practical, cost-effective, and time-efficient methods for the accurate assessment of hearing. They give more complete information on the child's hearing as well as functional information about how the child uses his or her hearing. The simplest test is behavioral observation audiometry, in which the audiologist records the behavioral response to an applied sound stimuli of a known frequency. This test can be done with infants up to six months of age, toddlers, and uncooperative patients, such as children or adults with developmental delays. Visual reinforcement audiometry is done with infants and toddlers from six months to twenty-four months of age. It is also used with uncooperative patients. In this test, the patient is submitted to sounds of different intensity and trained to respond to the sound stimuli by means of an attractive stimulus. Every time that the sound appears, the stimulus illuminates. When the patient hears the sound, he or she will look for the reinforcement. Play audiometry is a test that can be used in children over two years of age. The child is taught to move a block or place a puzzle piece every time he or she hears a sound.

Perspective and Prospects

Early detection of hearing loss has become a priority among intervention services because it has devastating effects on language development and consequently on social adaptation. It has been found that the mean age at which deafness is diagnosed is around three, which is after speech development should have occurred. Thus, children with hearing loss are placed at a disadvantage with their peers.

In 1993, the National Institutes of Health (NIH) developed a consensus statement by which all newborn infants in the United States were to be screened for hearing loss. The aim was that by the year 2000, all newborns would have been screened before being discharged from the hospital.

The role of otitis media (middle-ear infections) in producing hearing impairment is an area of great concern and controversy. Special attention to the hearing evaluation of children with recurrent and chronic otitis media is indicated.

—*Gloria Reyes Báez, M.D.,*
and Hilda Velez Rodriguez, M.S.

See also Ear infections and disorders; Ears; Hearing loss; Neonatology; Physical examination; Screening; Sense organs.

For Further Information:

Elder, Nina. "Now Hear This—Check Your Baby's Hearing." *Better Homes and Gardens* 78, no. 5 (May, 2000): 264. One out of every three hundred U.S. babies is born with a hearing problem, yet only 25 percent of newborns get hearing tests. If a hearing problem is detected within the first six months of life, a child has a good chance of catching up with his or her peers.

Glaser, Gabrielle. "Pediatricians Urge Hearing Tests at Birth." *The New York Times*, April 6, 1999, p. 7. Hearing impairment in infants can cause delays in speech, language, and cognitive development, according to Dr. Philip Ziring. Often, hearing loss is not diagnosed in children until they are two or three years old and are not speaking properly.

Hall, James A. *Handbook of Auditory Evoked Response*. Boston: Allyn & Bacon, 1992. An exhaustive study of auditory evoked response aimed at the medical professional. Includes bibliographical references and an index.

Hearing Exchange. http://www.hearingexchange.com/ An online community designed to foster the exchange of information and the provision of support for the hearing impaired.

McCormick, Barry, ed. *The Medical Practitioner's Guide to Paediatric Audiology*. New York: Cambridge University Press, 1995. A handbook of hearing disorders in infancy and childhood. Includes discussion of the various hearing tests and aids available.

Martin, Frederick N., and John Greer Clark. *Introduction to Audiology*. 8th ed. Englewood Cliffs, N.J.: Prentice Hall, 2002. In addition to providing thorough coverage of the physics of sound, anatomy, and physiology of the auditory system, covers the causes and treatment of hearing disorders and the relevant diagnostic and therapeutic techniques.

Northern, Jerry L., and Marion P. Downs. *Hearing in Children*. 5th ed. Baltimore: Williams & Wilkins, 2001. Topics covered include hearing and hearing loss, auditory mechanics, medical aspects of hearing loss, deviation of auditory behavior, and amplification.

Roush, Jackson. *Screening for Hearing Loss and Otitis Media in Children*. San Diego: Singular, 2001. Although clinical in nature, describes myriad hearing tests in great detail.

HEART

ANATOMY

ANATOMY OR SYSTEM AFFECTED: Blood, blood vessels, chest, circulatory system

SPECIALTIES AND RELATED FIELDS: Cardiology, exercise physiology

DEFINITION: The muscle that pumps blood through the body by means of rhythmic contractions.

KEY TERMS:

arteries: vessels that take blood away from the heart and toward the tissues

atria: the upper receiving chambers of the heart that lie above the ventricles

atrioventricular (A-V) node: a small region of specialized heart muscle cells that receives the electrical impulse from the atria and begins its transmission to the ventricles

coronary arteries: the arteries that supply blood to the heart muscle

diastole: the period of relaxation of the heart between beats

sinoatrial (S-A) node: a small region of specialized heart muscle cells that spontaneously generates and sends an electrical signal which gives the heart an automatic rhythm for contraction

systole: the period of contraction of the heart when blood moves out of the heart chambers and into the arteries

veins: vessels that take blood to the heart and from the tissues

ventricles: the lower pumping chambers of the heart located below the atria; they force blood into the arteries

STRUCTURE AND FUNCTIONS

All the cells in the human body are dependent on the blood in the cardiovascular system (the heart and blood vessels) for the transport of gases, nutrients, hormones, and other factors. Likewise, the tissues must have a way to dispose of waste products so that they do not build to harmful levels. All these substances are dissolved in the blood, but something must provide the force to transport the blood to all parts of the body at all times—the heart. This organ must beat continuously from early in development to death. It beats without conscious control and can vary how quickly it moves blood throughout the body depending on the needs and activities of the tissues.

In humans, an individual's heart is about the size of his or her fist and is enclosed in the center of the chest cavity between the lungs. The heart contains specialized muscle cells known as cardiac muscle. These cardiac cells make up most of the thickness of the walls of the heart; they are responsible for moving blood out of the heart and are also involved in maintaining the rhythm of the heartbeat. This heavily muscled layer is referred to as the myocardium. The inner lining of the heart is called the endocardium; it is continuous with the lining of all the blood vessels in the body. The outermost layer of the heart is the epicardium, which covers the myocardium. The heart moves as it beats and is contained within a fluid-filled bag called the pericardial sac. The rhythmically beating heart has the potential to rub against adjacent structures (such as the lungs), harming itself and those structures. Therefore, it is important that the heart be encased in the pericardial sac, with its lubricating fluid.

The human heart has four separate chambers. These internal cavities can be identified by their location and function. The upper pair of smaller chambers are known as atria, and the lower larger chambers are called ventricles. Because the atria and ventricles have a muscular wall which separates them into right and left halves, one can refer to the individual chambers as the right atrium and left atrium, and the right ventricle and left ventricle. The wall that separates the right and left halves of the heart is called the septum. The septum prevents any mixing of blood from the right and left sides of the heart. The atria and ventricles on the same side, however, must allow blood to pass between them in a single direction. This action is accomplished by one-way valves between the atria and ventricles. The valve that allows blood to pass from the right atrium to the right ventricle is called the tricuspid valve because it is made of three flaps. On the left side of the heart is the bicuspid valve (with two flaps), which is also known as the mitral valve. The bicuspid valve allows blood from the left atrium to flow only into the left ventricle. This rather complex anatomy is necessary because the heart must pump blood in one direction and into two separate systems.

The anatomy of the heart often makes more sense if one understands its function or physiology. As an example, one may consider an active cell in the body, perhaps a muscle cell which moves the foot. This cell utilizes oxygen to help metabolize food for energy. During this process, carbon dioxide is produced as a waste product, and high levels of carbon dioxide can be harmful to cells. Therefore, one of the jobs of the cardiovascular system is to deliver oxygen and take away carbon dioxide. Once the carbon dioxide is picked up by the blood, it travels back to the heart via veins and enters the right atrium. From the right atrium, the blood passes the tricuspid valve and enters the right ventricle. The right ventricle then sends the blood past a one-way valve called the semilunar valve into blood vessels that transport it to the lungs. At the lungs, the blood loses carbon dioxide and picks up oxygen. This oxygenated blood must now be delivered to the tissues. First, the blood returns to the heart and enters the left atrium. From the left atrium, blood is pushed past the bicuspid valve into the left ventricle. The blood is then pumped from the powerful left ventricle through another set of semilunar valves into the blood vessels that will carry the blood to all the tissues of the body, including the heart itself. The blood vessels that feed the heart directly are known as coronary vessels.

The orderly pattern by which blood flows through the heart, lungs, and body requires the chambers of the

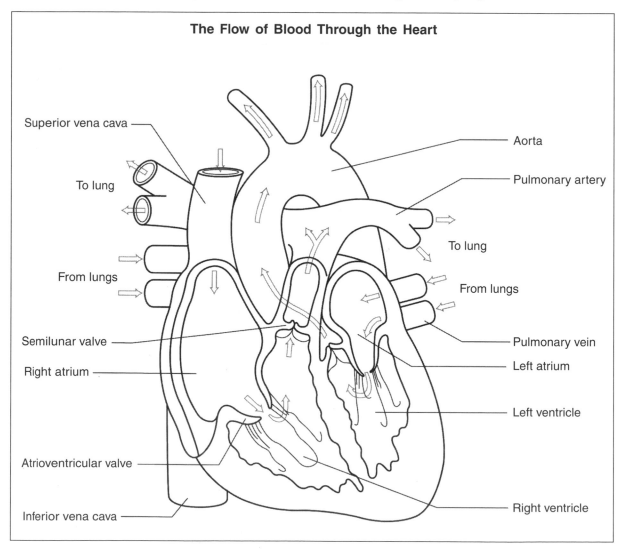

The Flow of Blood Through the Heart

Superior vena cava

To lung

From lungs

Semilunar valve

Right atrium

Atrioventricular valve

Inferior vena cava

Aorta

Pulmonary artery

To lung

From lungs

Pulmonary vein

Left atrium

Left ventricle

Right ventricle

heart to work in a coordinated fashion. The atria contract together to help send blood into the ventricles. The ventricles then contract together so that blood flows through the lungs from the right ventricle and through the tissues of the body from the left ventricle. The tricuspid and bicuspid valves prevent a backflow of blood into the atria when the ventricles contract, and the semilunar valves prevent blood from returning to the ventricles after they have contracted.

Something must coordinate the contraction of the heart so that the atria contract together before the ventricles do so. Highly specialized cells of the myocardium have the ability to conduct electrical impulses rapidly and to discharge spontaneously at a certain rate. These properties allow the heart to be stimulated in a synchronous way and for it to generate its own rate and rhythm. One region of the right atrium is known as the sinoatrial (S-A) node; it functions as the heart's pacemaker. The S-A node has the ability to generate spontaneously an electrical signal with a relatively rapid rhythm. Therefore, it serves to "pace" the heart rate. When the S-A node sends its electrical impulse throughout the atria, the atria contract. There is a slight delay before the impulse reaches the ventricles, which allows the atria to contract fully before the ventricles. The atrioventricular (A-V) node will then pick up the electrical signal and send it through both ventricles via specialized conductive heart muscle fibers known as Purkinje's fibers. Purkinje's fibers transmit the electrical signal ensuring that all the ventricular muscle cells contract at nearly the same time. The ventricles contract in such a way that the bottom tip of the heart (apex) contracts slightly before the region of the ventricles next to the atria (base). Additionally, the ventricles contract in a somewhat twisting motion that causes the heart to "wring out" the blood.

This rather complex system allows the heart to contract at its own rate and in a highly synchronous fashion. Nevertheless, one's heart rate varies depending on one's physical activity or emotional state. For example, during exercise or when an individual is under stress, the heart rate goes up. When one is relaxed, the heart does not beat as rapidly. Therefore, the body must have a way to regulate the rate at which the S-A node signals the heart to contract.

The autonomic nervous system, which functions without one's conscious control, regulates the heart rate. It is divided into two systems: parasympathetic and sympathetic. The parasympathetic nervous system is active during periods of rest and has the ability to slow the heart. During periods of physical or emotional stress, the sympathetic nervous system stimulates the heart to contract more forcefully and at a more rapid rate. The parasympathetic and sympathetic systems communicate with the heart via chemical messengers known as neurotransmitters. The parasympathetic nervous system uses the neurotransmitter acetylcholine to slow the heart, while norepinephrine and epinephrine are the chemicals used by the sympathetic nervous system to increase the heart rate.

DISORDERS AND DISEASES

Even though the heart seems to be adaptable to a variety of situations throughout one's life, it can malfunction. In fact, diseases of the heart and blood vessels are the number one killer in the United States. One common disease that affects the heart directly is coronary artery disease, which can lead to life-threatening heart attacks. Although medical researchers are still investigating the causes of coronary artery disease, most of the evidence points to hypertension (high blood pressure) and atherosclerosis (a buildup of fatty plaque in the walls of arteries).

Hypertension is usually defined as a blood pressure greater than 140/90 millimeters of mercury (mmHg) at rest. A typical blood pressure for a young, healthy adult is 120/80 mmHg. The top number measures the force of blood against an artery wall during the contraction of the heart; this is referred to as the systolic pressure. The bottom number, the diastolic pressure, is a measurement of force when the heart is relaxed. If either systolic or diastolic pressure exceeds 140/90 mmHg, the patient is considered hypertensive. The cause of hypertension has not been determined, but it is known that with hypertension the heart must work harder to push the blood through the arteries, including the coronary arteries. Physicians treat hypertension by prescribing drugs that block the effect of the sympathetic nervous system on the heart, such as metoprolol (Lopressor). They may also prescribe drugs such as prazosin (Minipress) that prevent the arteries from becoming too narrow.

Hypertension is also seen in patients who have atherosclerosis. This buildup of fatty materials such as cholesterol under the lining of the artery causes the plaque to protrude, narrowing the diameter of the vessel. This can lead to blood clot formation on artery walls which are irregular. This clot, also known as a thrombus, may dislodge and travel in the bloodstream. Eventually, it may block a small artery, thereby preventing the flow of blood to the tissue. If this happens in a coronary artery, a myocardial infarction (heart attack) will result.

A heart attack occurs when a portion of the heart dies because of a lack of oxygen or a buildup of waste products. Heart muscle has no way of repairing itself, and the resulting damage is permanent. If the patient is transported to the hospital immediately, the emergency room physician may give drugs to prevent further blood clot formation (aspirin and heparin) and to help dissolve the already formed clot (streptokinase and tissue plasminogen activator, or TPA). If the coronary artery is only partially blocked, the patient may suffer from angina pectoris, a chest pain which radiates down the left arm. These patients usually take drugs such as nitroglycerin which help dilate (widen) blood vessels, reestablishing adequate flow to the heart.

Another devastating disease of the heart is congestive heart failure, a condition in which the heart fails to pump enough blood to meet the demands of the body's tissues. The heart becomes enlarged because of the resulting excessive increase in blood volume. There are several causes of heart failure, most of which stem from the fact that the heart loses its ability to pump efficiently. For example, a patient who has had a heart attack may have lost significant function as a result of heart damage. Even without a heart attack, some individuals may have malfunctioning heart valves or other problems that cause an inefficient ejection of blood and thus heart failure.

The cardiovascular system attempts to compensate for heart failure in several ways. The sympathetic nervous system increases the heart rate, and the kidneys retain more fluid to increase blood volume. These compensatory mechanisms help to reestablish adequate blood flow for a while. Because of the increase in blood volume, however, more blood enters the chambers of the heart and causes them to stretch. At some point, the ventricles can no longer force out the increased amount of blood entering them, and they enlarge. This increase in the size of the heart chamber further enlarges the heart and strains the heart muscle. The heart will continue to weaken, unable to keep up with the body's demands. Compensatory mechanisms attempt to meet the body's need for continuous blood flow but in doing so further overload the heart. This vicious circle may lead to complete heart failure and death.

Congestive heart failure may involve only one side of the heart, perhaps because of a heart attack which affected that side. If the heart failure occurs on the left side, the right ventricle is pumping blood to the lungs in an efficient manner but the left ventricle cannot pump all the blood returning from the lungs. Therefore, blood backs up and pools in the lung tissues. Similarly, if the right ventricle begins to fail and the left ventricle is normal, blood begins to pool throughout the body since the right side of the heart cannot keep up in its pumping.

Physicians are able to slow the progression of congestive heart failure by prescribing drugs such as digoxin that increase the force of heart muscle contraction and thereby the amount of blood ejected with each beat. Therapeutic agents such as captopril (Capoten) help to reduce the fluid retention in the kidneys.

Coronary artery disease and heart failure are related to the inability of the heart to contract. In addition, the specialized heart muscle cells that provide the heart's rhythm and conduct the electrical signals necessary for a coordinated heartbeat may be affected by disease. In the resting adult, the heart normally beats about seventy to eighty times per minute. Several conditions exist whereby the heart loses control of its normal rate and rhythm, a serious condition.

For example, if the heart begins to beat too rapidly, the ventricles do not have enough time to fill and the movement of blood to the heart muscle and the rest of the body is impaired. The atria or ventricles may contract at a high rate and lose their coordinated sequence of contraction; this is referred to as atrial or ventricular fibrillation. If immediate action is not taken to reestablish the normal rate and conduction sequence, the patient will die. Emergency measures such as electrical defibrillation may shock the heart into reestablishing its normal rhythm and conduction pathways. It is easy to understand how these abnormal patterns of heart activity occur if one imagines more than one pacemaker attempting to control heart function. The cause of these and other, less severe heart rhythms may be heart damage affecting the conductive pathway, drugs, or even psychological distress.

Heart disease is a major cause of death, but most experts agree that many heart problems are preventable. High blood pressure and high blood levels of fat and cholesterol are associated with an increased incidence of coronary artery disease. Cigarette smoking and excessive weight are also correlated with heart disease. Additionally, exercise seems to be critical in maintaining a healthy heart, as sedentary individuals have a twofold increase in their risk of heart disease when compared to active people.

It is likely that individuals who are at risk can lessen the probability of having heart problems by adopting a more healthful lifestyle, including eating a low-fat diet, stopping smoking, reducing excessive weight and mental stress, and engaging in enjoyable physical activities (with their physicians' permission).

PERSPECTIVE AND PROSPECTS

The role of the heart in the functioning of the human body was questioned by the ancient Egyptians, who attributed breathing to the heart. It was the Chinese who first documented that the heart is responsible for the pulse and movement of blood. They also believed that the heart was the seat of happiness. The ancient Greeks had a different idea about the function of the heart, believing that it was the region where thinking originated.

It was not until William Harvey (1578-1657), an English physiologist, published his experiments on the heart and circulation that scientists believed blood was pumped continuously by the heart. He observed that both ventricles of the heart contracted and expanded at the same time. Harvey also noted that when the heart was removed from an animal, it continued to contract and relax; that is, it had an automatic rhythm.

More than one hundred years after Harvey published his work, Stephen Hales made the first blood pressure measurements. He did so by inserting a tube into the neck artery of a horse and watching the blood rise 3 meters above the animal. Then early in the twentieth century Willem Einthoven invented an instrument to measure electrical currents. This instrument was used by Thomas Lewis to measure the electrical activity in the heart, the first electrocardiograph (ECG).

By the mid-nineteenth century, heart surgeries were being performed to correct heart defects. These early surgeries had to be done with the heart still beating. In 1953, the heart-lung machine was used to take over the pumping function of the heart during surgery so that the surgeon could stop the heart. In 1967, Christiaan Barnard performed the first heart transplantation in a human. Heart transplants were performed during the next ten years with no long-term survivors, usually because of tissue rejection. In 1982, a completely artificial heart was implanted into a patient. This patient died in the spring of 1983.

Heart transplants have become much more successful, however, mainly because of the use of immunosuppressive drugs which help to prevent rejection of the transplanted heart. Similarly, newer drugs and procedures such as coronary bypass surgery, angioplasty, and atherectomy are becoming more effective in treating heart disease. Nevertheless, perhaps the best approach to maintaining a healthy heart is to practice preventive medicine. Scientists are making comparable strides in finding ways to prevent heart disease as they are in treating already existing conditions.

—*Matthew Berria, Ph.D.*

See also Anatomy; Aneurysmectomy; Aneurysms; Angina; Angiography; Angioplasty; Anxiety; Arrhythmias; Arteriosclerosis; Biofeedback; Blue baby syndrome; Bypass surgery; Cardiac rehabilitation; Cardiology; Cardiology, pediatric; Cardiopulmonary resuscitation (CPR); Catheterization; Circulation; Congenital heart disease; Electrical shock; Electrocardiography (ECG or EKG); Embolism; Endocarditis; Exercise physiology; Heart attack; Heart disease; Heart failure; Heart transplantation; Heart valve replacement; Hypertension; Internal medicine; Mitral valve prolapse; Pacemaker implantation; Palpitations; Resuscitation; Reye's syndrome; Rheumatic fever; Shock; Sports medicine; Strokes; Systems and organs; Thoracic surgery; Thrombolytic therapy and TPA; Thrombosis and thrombus; Transplantation; Vascular medicine; Vascular system.

FOR FURTHER INFORMATION:

Hales, Dianne. *An Invitation to Health.* 10th ed. Belmont, Calif.: Wadsworth Thomson Learning, 2003. This text should be read by anyone who wishes an overview of health topics. Several chapters deal with the function of the heart and how lifestyle influences its health.

The Incredible Machine. Washington, D.C.: National Geographic Society, 1994. A colorful book which describes in layperson's terms how the body works and how one alters one's own health. The chapter on the cardiovascular system is well written and contains exciting photographs and drawings of the heart.

McGoon, M. *The Mayo Clinic Heart Book.* 2d ed. New York: William Morrow, 2000. One of the most respected texts for laypeople on heart disease. Covers all aspects of anatomy, physiology, diagnosis, treatment, and prevention.

Mackenna, B. R., and R. Callander. *Illustrated Physiology.* 6th ed. New York: Churchill Livingstone, 1996. Provides the reader with a visual explanation of physiology on a basic level. Chapter 5 contains many excellent diagrams, illustrations, and explanations of cardiovascular anatomy and physiology.

Marieb, Elaine N. *Human Anatomy and Physiology.* 6th ed. Redwood City, Calif.: Benjamin/Cummings, 2003. Nonscientists at the advanced high school level or above will be able to understand this fine textbook. It includes a complete glossary, index, pronunciation guide, and other helpful features.

Park, Myung K. *Pediatric Cardiology Handbook.* 3d ed. New York: Elsevier, 2002. A text for the medical specialist with discussion of all congenital heart defects, including atrial septal defects, ventricular septal defects, cushion defects, coarctation, and interrupted aortic arch.

Tortora, Gerard J., and Sandra R. Grabowski. *Principles of Anatomy and Physiology.* 10th ed. New York: John Wiley & Sons, 2003. An outstanding textbook of human anatomy and physiology, covering the heart and circulatory system in depth.

HEART ATTACK
DISEASE/DISORDER

ALSO KNOWN AS: Myocardial infarction

ANATOMY OR SYSTEM AFFECTED: Circulatory system, heart

SPECIALTIES AND RELATED FIELDS: Cardiology, critical care, emergency medicine, internal medicine

DEFINITION: Myocardial infarction; the sudden death of heart muscle characterized by intense chest pain, sweating, shortness of breath, or sometimes none of these symptoms.

KEY TERMS:

atherosclerosis: narrowing of the internal passageways of essential arteries caused by the buildup of fatty deposits

atria: the chambers in the right and left top portions of the heart that receive blood from the veins and pump it to the ventricles

fibrillation: wild beating of the heart, which may occur when the regular rate of the heartbeat is interrupted

myocardium: the muscle tissue that forms the walls of the heart, varying in thickness in the upper and lower regions

sinoatrial node: the section of the right atrium that determines the appropriate rate of the heartbeat

ventricles: the chambers in the right and left bottom portions of the heart that receive blood from the atria and pump it to the arteries

CAUSES AND SYMPTOMS

Although varied in origin and effect on the body, heart attacks (or myocardial infarctions) occur when there are interruptions in the delicately synchronized system either supplying blood to the heart or pumping blood from the heart to other vital organs. The heart is a highly specialized muscle whose function is to pump life-sustaining blood to all parts of the body. The heart's action involves the development of pressure to propel blood through arriving and departing channels—veins and arteries—that must maintain that pressure within their walls at critical levels throughout the system.

The highest level of pressure in the total cardiovascular system is to be found closest to the two "pumping" chambers on the right and left lower sections of the heart, called ventricles. Dark, bluish-colored blood, emptied of its oxygen content and laden with carbon dioxide waste instead of the oxygen in fresh blood, flows into the upper portion of the heart via the superior and inferior venae cavae. It then passes from the right atrium chamber into the right ventricle. Once in the ventricle, this blood cannot flow back because of one-way valves separating the "receiving" from the "pumping" sections of the total heart organ.

After this valve closes following a vitally synchronized timing system, constriction of the right ventricle by the myocardium muscle in the surrounding walls of the heart forces the blood from the heart, propelling it toward the oxygen-filled tissue of the lungs. Following reoxygenation, bright red blood that is still under pressure from the thrust of the right ventricle flows into the left atrium. Once channeled into the left ventricle, the pumping process that began in the right ventricle is then repeated on the left by muscular constriction, and oxygenated blood flows out of the aortic valve under pressure throughout the cardiovascular system to nourish the body's cells. Because the force needed to supply blood under pressure from the left ventricle for the entire body is greater than the first-phase pumping force needed to move blood into the lungs, the myocardium surrounding the left ventricle constitutes the thickest muscular layer in the heart's wall.

The efficiency of this process, as well as the origins of problems of fatigue in the heart that can lead to heart attacks and eventual heart failure, is tied to the maintenance of a reasonably constant level of blood pressure. If pulmonary problems (blockage caused by the effects of smoking or environmental pollution, for example) make it harder for the right ventricle to push blood through the lungs, the heart must expend more energy in the first stage of the cardiovascular process. Similarly, and often in addition to the added work for the heart because of pulmonary complications, the efficiency of the left ventricle in handling blood flow may be reduced by the presence of excessive fat in the body,

INFORMATION ON HEART ATTACK

CAUSES: Pulmonary problems, atherosclerosis, smoking, high blood pressure, diabetes mellitus
SYMPTOMS: Varies but often includes intense chest pain, sweating, shortness of breath
DURATION: Acute
TREATMENTS: Drug therapy, surgery, preventive medication, exercise, dietary change, medical devices

causing this ventricle to expend more energy to propel oxygenated blood into vital tissues.

Although factors such as these may be responsible for overworking the heart and thus contributing to eventual heart failure, other causes of heart attacks are to be found much closer to the working apparatus of the heart, particularly in the coronary arteries. The coronary arteries begin at the top of the heart and fan out along its sides. They are responsible for providing large quantities of blood to the myocardium muscle, which needs continual nourishment to carry out the pumping that forces blood forward from the ventricles. The passageways inside these and other key arteries are vulnerable to the process known as atherosclerosis, which can affect the blood supply to other organs as well as to the heart. In the heart, atherosclerosis involves the accumulation, inside the coronary arteries, of fatty deposits called atheromas. If these deposits continue to collect, less blood can flow through the arteries. A narrowed artery also increases the possibility of a variant form of heart attack, in which a sudden and total blockage of blood flow follows the lodging of a blood clot in one of these vital passageways.

A symptomatic condition called angina pectoris, characterized by intermittent chest pains, may develop if atherosclerosis reduces blood (and therefore oxygen) supply to the heart. These danger signs can continue over a number of years. If diagnosis reveals a problem that might be resolved by preventive medication, exercise, or recommendations for heart surgery, then this condition, known as myocardial ischemia, may not necessarily end in a full heart attack.

A full heart attack occurs when, for one of several possible reasons including a vascular spasm suddenly constricting an already clogged artery or a blockage caused by a clot, the heart suddenly ceases to receive the necessary supply of blood. This brings almost immediate deterioration in some of the heart's tissue and causes the organ's consequent inability to perform its vital functions effectively.

Another form of attack and disruption of the heart's ability to deliver blood can come either independently of or in conjunction with an arterially induced heart attack. This form of attack involves a sustained interruption in the rate of heartbeats. The necessary pace or rate of myocardial contractions, which can vary depending on the organism's rate of physical exertion or age, is regulated in the sinoatrial node in the right atrium, which generates its own electrical impulses. The ultimate sources for the commands to the sinoatrial node are to be found in the network of nerves coming directly from the brain. There are, however, other so-called local pacemakers located in the atria and ventricles. If these sources of electrical charges begin giving commands to the myocardium that are not in rhythm with those coming from the sinoatrial node, then dysrhythmic or premature beats may confuse the heart muscle, causing it to beat wildly. In fact, the concentrated pattern of muscle contractions will not be coordinated and instead will be dispersed in different areas of the heart. The result is fibrillation, a series of uncoordinated contractions that cannot combine to propel blood out of the ventricles. This condition may occur either as the aftershock of an arterially induced heart attack or suddenly and on its own, caused by the deterioration of the electrical impulse system commanding the heart rate. In patients whose potential vulnerability to this form of heart attack has been diagnosed in advance, a heart physician may decide to surgically implant a mechanical pacemaker to ensure coordination of the necessary electrical commands to the myocardium.

TREATMENT AND THERAPY

Extraordinary medical advances have helped reduce the high death rates formerly associated with heart attacks. Many of these advances have been in the field of preventive medicine. The most widely recognized medical findings are related to diet, smoking, and exercise. Although controversy remains, there is general agreement that cholesterol absorbed by the body from the ingestion of animal fats plays a key role in the dangerous buildup of platelets inside arterial passageways. It has been accepted that regular, although not necessarily strenuous, exercise is an essential long-term preventive strategy that can reduce the risk of heart attacks. Exercise also plays a role in therapy after a heart attack.

IN THE NEWS:
LOW-GRADE INFLAMMATION AS A TRIGGER

Researchers have suspected for some time that the body's inflammatory response may play a critical role in heart attacks and strokes. It is well known that risk factors for heart attack and stroke include obesity, high cholesterol levels, high blood pressure, and smoking. Blood tests in a 1988 study in Finland, however, showed the presence of a bacterium called *Chlamydia pneumoniae* inside the cells of people with coronary artery disease. It seemed apparent, however, that *C. pneumoniae* alone was not a risk factor or cause of heart disease.

Researchers in the Helsinki Heart Study also looked for the presence of human heat-shock protein 60 (hHsp60), indicating an immune response which could possibly lead to atherosclerosis, and of C-reactive protein (CRP), which sends white blood cells to the site of injury or infection but can cause harm if prolonged or excessive. An eight-year follow-up of this study showed that the risk for heart disease increased when levels of *C. pneumoniae* or hHsp60 antibodies were high. However, the risk was greatest when all three factors were elevated, indicating a possible synergistic effect. It was concluded that chronic infection, autoimmunity, and inflammation in combination contributed to coronary events in the study population.

The research of Dr. Paul Ridker of Boston's Brigham and Women's Hospital further showed that levels of CRP over 3 milligrams per liter of blood more than doubled the risk of heart attack and stroke. A test for CRP levels is available, but there are questions of who should be tested and when.

High CRP levels have also been associated with being overweight, a known risk factor for heart disease. Adjusting for age, smoking, and other chronic diseases, the association was especially strong for obese women, who were six times as likely to have elevated CRP levels, while obese men were twice as likely. One theory to explain this outcome would be that many overweight or obese persons have persistent low-grade inflammation. This may be the result of another protein, interleukin 6, produced by fat tissue, which in turn stimulates the production of CRP by the liver.

Scientific research continues to establish definitive links between heart disease and chronic infections, inflammation, and autoimmune conditions. These links could lead to attacking the basic processes of atherosclerosis, to treatment with anti-inflammatory drugs, and to the prevention of heart attacks and stroke.

—Martha Loustaunau, Ph.D.

The actual application of medical scientific knowledge to assist in the campaign against the deadly effects of heart disease involves multiple fields of specialization. These may range from the sophisticated use of electrocardiograms (ECGs) to monitor the regularity of heartbeats, to specialized drug therapies aimed at preventing heart attacks in people who have been diagnosed as high-risk cases, to coronary bypass surgery or even heart transplants. In the 1980's, highly specialized surgeons at several university and private hospitals began performing operations to implant artificial hearts in human patients.

In the case of ECGs, it has become possible, thanks to the use of portable units that record the heartbeat patterns of persons over an extended period of time, to gain a much more accurate impression of the actual functioning of the heart. Previous dependence on electrocardiographic data gathered during an appointed and limited examination provided only minimal information to doctors.

In 2003, the Food and Drug Administration (FDA) approved a simple blood test that, when used with ECGs, could greatly improve the ability of doctors to confirm or rule out a heart attack in patients visiting emergency rooms (ERs). Nearly five million Americans visit ERs each year with possible heart attack symptoms but only about one in five actually is experiencing a heart attack. The test, which uses the metal cobalt to hunt changes in a blood protein that occur during an attack, helped rule out a heart attack 70 percent of the time when used with standard heart attack tests during initial studies.

The domains of preventive surgery and specialized drug treatment to prevent dangerous blood clotting are

In both preventive and postattack contexts, it has been medically proven that the entire cardiovascular system profits from the natural muscle-strengthening process (in the heart's case) and general cleansing effects (in the case of oxygen intake and stimulated blood flow) that result from controlled regular exercise.

vast. Statistically, the most important and widely practiced operations that were developed in the later decades of the twentieth century were replacement of the aortic valve, the coronary bypass operation, and, with greater or lesser degrees of success, the actual transplantation of voluntary donors' hearts in the place of those belonging to heart disease patients. Coronary bypass operations involve the attachment to the myocardium of healthy arteries to carry the blood that can no longer pass through the patient's clogged arterial passageways; these healthy arteries are taken by the heart surgeon from other areas of the patient's own body.

Another sphere of medical technology, that of balloon angioplasty, held out a major nonsurgical promise of preventing deterioration of the arteries leading to the heart. This sophisticated form of treatment involves the careful, temporary introduction of inflatable devices inside clogged arteries, which are then stretched to increase the space within the arterial passageway for blood to flow. By the 1990's, however, doctors recognized one disadvantage of balloon angioplasty. By stretching the essential blood vessels being treated, this procedure either stretches the plaque with the artery or breaks loose debris that remains behind, creating a danger of renewed clogging. Thus another technique, called atherectomy, was developed to clear certain coronary arteries, as well as arteries elsewhere in the body.

Atherectomy involves a motorized catheter device resembling a miniature drill that is inserted into clogged arteries. As the drill turns, material that is literally shaved off the interior walls of arteries is retrieved through a tiny collection receptacle. Early experimentation, especially to treat the large anterior descending coronary artery on the left side of the heart, showed that atherectomy was 87 percent effective, whereas, on the average, angioplasty removed only 63 percent of the blockage. In addition, similar efforts to provide internal, nonsurgical treatment of clogged arteries using laser beams were being made by the early 1990's.

PERSPECTIVE AND PROSPECTS

The modern conception of cardiology dates from William Harvey's seventeenth century discovery of the relationship between the heart's function as a pump and the circulatory "restoration" of blood. Harvey's much more scientific views replaced centuries-old conceptions of the heart as a blood-warming device only.

Although substantial anatomical advances were made over the next two centuries that helped explain most of the vital functions of the heart, it was not until the early decades of the twentieth century that science developed therapeutic methods to deal with problems that frequently cause heart attacks. Drugs that affect the liver's production of substances necessary for normal coagulation of blood, for example, were discovered in the 1930's. A large variety of such anticoagulants have since been developed to help thin the blood of patients vulnerable to blood clotting. Other drugs, including certain antibiotics, are used to treat persons whose susceptiblitity to infection is known to be high. In these cases, the simple action of dislodging bacteria from the teeth when brushing can cause an invasion of the vital parts of the heart by an infection. This bacterial endocarditis, the result of the actual destruction of heart tissue or the sudden release of clots of infectious residue, could lead to a heart attack in such individuals although they have no other symptoms of identifiable heart disease.

Pain Associated with Heart Attack

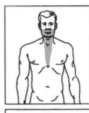

Pain radiating up into jaw and through to back

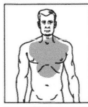

Pain felt in upper abdomen

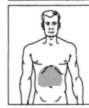

Pressure in the central chest area, from mild to severe

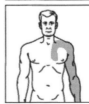

Pain radiating down left arm; may cause sensation of weakness in the arm

The most spectacular advance in the scientific treatment of potential heart attack victims, however, has been in the field of cardiac surgery. Many advances in open heart surgery date from the late 1950's, when the development of heart and lung replacement machines made it safe enough to substitute electronic monitors for some of the organism's normal body functions. Before the 1950's, operations had been limited to surgical treatment of the major blood vessels surrounding the heart.

Various technical methods have also been developed that help identify problems early enough for drug therapy to be attempted before the decision to perform surgery is made. The use of catheters, which are threaded into the coronary organ using the same vessels that transport blood, became the most effective way of locating problematic areas. The process known as angiography, which uses X rays to trace the course of radiopaque dyes injected through a catheter into local heart areas under study, can actually tell doctors if drug therapy is having the desired effects. In cases where such tests show that preventive drug therapy is not effective, an early decision to perform surgery can be made, preventing the source of coronary trouble from multiplying the patient's chances of suffering a heart attack.

—*Byron D. Cannon, Ph.D.*

See also Angina; Arrhythmias; Arteriosclerosis; Bypass surgery; Cardiac rehabilitation; Cardiology; Cardiopulmonary resuscitation (CPR); Cholesterol; Circulation; Critical care; Electrocardiography (ECG or EKG); Embolism; Emergency medicine; Heart; Heart disease; Heart failure; Heart transplantation; Heart valve replacement; Hypercholesterolemia; Hyperlipidemia; Hypertension; Ischemia; Mitral valve prolapse; Pacemaker implantation; Palpitations; Phlebitis; Resuscitation; Thrombolytic therapy and TPA; Thrombosis and thrombus.

FOR FURTHER INFORMATION:

American Heart Association. http://www.american heart.org/. Site provides comprehensive information on heart disease and conditions, healthy lifestyles, and resources, and provides interactive health tools.

Baum, Seth J. *The Total Guide to a Healthy Heart: Integrative Strategies for Preventing and Reversing Heart Disease.* New York: Kensington, 2000. This book brings together the practices of both conventional and alternative approaches to reversing heart disease and maintaining heart health. Offers great insight into why the integrative approach to maintaining a healthy heart will be the medicine of the new millennium.

Berra, Kathleen, et al. *Heart Attack: Advice for Patients by Patients.* New Haven, Conn.: Yale University Press, 2001. After an introductory chapter detailing diagnosis, treatment, and rehabilitation, offers eleven other chapters authored by heart attack survivors—including several medical professionals—and their lessons learned. Diet and nutrition, advances in treatment, and cardiac rehabilitation programs are covered.

Crawford, Michael, ed. *Diagnosis and Treatment in Cardiology.* New York: McGraw-Hill, 2002. Discusses advances in cardiac diagnostics, treatments, and prognostic indicators and includes extensive information on prevention techniques.

Eagle, Kim A., and Ragavendra R. Baliga. *Practical Cardiology: Evaluation and Treatment of Common Cardiovascular Disorders.* Philadelphia: Lippincott Williams & Wilkins, 2003. Details advances in cardiac medicine.

Gersh, Bernard J., ed. *The Mayo Clinic Heart Book.* 2d ed. New York: William Morrow, 2000. One of the most respected texts for laypeople on heart disease. Covers all aspects of anatomy, physiology, diagnosis, treatment, and prevention.

Gillis, Jack. *The Heart Attack Prevention and Recovery Handbook.* Point Roberts, Wash.: Hartley & Marks, 1995. Using simple, brief explanations, Gillis's text covers essential information that heart attack victims and families need immediately for reassurance and recovery. Presents excellent discussions of emotional effects on patients, medications, and treatments.

Kligfield, Paul. *Cardiac Recovery Handbook: The Complete Guide to Life After Heart Attack or Heart Surgery for Patients and Their Families.* Long Island City, N.Y.: Hatherleigh Press, 2003. A clearly written book that details all aspects of cardiac recovery, including the initial diagnosis of heart disease, medications and surgical options, hospitalization, rehabilitation, diet and exercise, and financial planning.

Yannios, Thomas A. *The Heart Disease Breakthrough: What Even Your Doctor Doesn't Know About Preventing a Heart Attack.* New York: Wiley, 1999. Yannios, associate director of critical care and nutritional support at Ellis Hospital in Schenectady, New York, describes the smallest components of cholesterol, which can do more damage to the heart than the overall LDL levels that concern so many people.

Zaret, Barry L., Marvin Moser, and Lawrence S. Cohen, eds. *Yale University School of Medicine Heart Book*. New York: William Morrow, 1992. Discusses the prevention and control of heart disease. Illustrated, with a bibliography and an index.

HEART DISEASE

DISEASE/DISORDER

ANATOMY OR SYSTEM AFFECTED: Blood vessels, circulatory system, heart

SPECIALTIES AND RELATED FIELDS: Cardiology, family practice, internal medicine

DEFINITION: One of the leading causes of death in many industrialized nations; heart diseases include atherosclerotic disease, coronary artery disease, cardiac arrhythmias, and stenosis, among others.

KEY TERMS:

cardiac arrhythmia: a disturbance in the heartbeat

coronary arteries: blood vessels surrounding the heart that provide nourishment and oxygen to heart tissue

nodes: areas of electrochemical transmission within the heart that regulate the heartbeat

plaque: an accumulation of matter within artery walls that can impede blood flow

CAUSES AND SYMPTOMS

The heart is a fist-sized organ located in the upper left quarter of the chest. It consists of four chambers: the right and left atria on top and the right and left ventricles at the bottom. The chambers are enclosed in three layers of tissue: the outer layer (epicardium), the middle layer (myocardium), and the inner layer (endocardium). Surrounding the entire organ is the pericardium, a thin layer of tissue that forms a protective covering for the heart. The heart also contains various nodes that transmit electrochemical signals, causing heart muscle tissue to contract and relax in the pumping action that carries blood to organs and cells throughout the body.

Signals from the brain cause the heart to contract rhythmically in a sequence of motions that move the blood from the right atrium down through the tricuspid valve into the right ventricle. From here, blood is pushed through the pulmonary valve into the lungs, where it fulfills one of its major functions: to pick up oxygen in exchange for carbon dioxide. From the lungs, the blood is pumped back into the heart, entering the left atrium from which it is pumped down through the mitral valve into the left ventricle. Blood is then pushed through the aortic valve into the main artery of the body, the aorta, from which it starts its journey to the organs and cells. As it passes through the arteries of the gastrointestinal system, the blood picks up nutrients which, along with the oxygen that it has taken from the lungs, are brought to the cells and exchanged for waste products and carbon dioxide. The blood then enters the veins, through which it is eventually returned to the heart. The heart nourishes and supplies itself with oxygen through the coronary arteries, so called because they sit on top of the heart like a crown and extend down the sides.

The heart diseases collectively include all the disorders that can befall every part of the heart muscle: the pericardium, epicardium, myocardium, endocardium, atria, ventricles, valves, coronary arteries, and nodes. The most significant sites of heart diseases are the coronary arteries and the nodes; their malfunction can cause coronary artery disease and cardiac arrhythmias, respectively. These two disorders are responsible for the majority of heart disease cases.

Coronary artery disease occurs when matter such as cholesterol and fibrous material collects and stiffens on the inner walls of the coronary arteries. This plaque that forms may narrow the passage through which blood flows, reducing the amount of blood delivered to the heart, or may build up and clog the artery entirely, shutting off the flow of blood to the heart. In the former case, when the coronary artery is narrowed, the condition is called ischemic heart disease. Because the most common cause of ischemia is narrowing of the coronary arteries to the myocardium, another designation of the condition is myocardial ischemia, referring to the fact that blood flow to the myocardium is impeded. Accumulation of plaque within the coronary arteries is referred to as coronary atherosclerosis.

INFORMATION ON HEART DISEASE

CAUSES: Pulmonary problems, atherosclerosis, smoking, diabetes, hypertension, infection, high-fat diet and obesity, stress

SYMPTOMS: Varies; can include pain, sweating, shortness of breath, inability to exercise, irregular heartbeat, dizziness, loss of consciousness

DURATION: Acute or chronic

TREATMENTS: Drug therapy, surgery, preventive medication, exercise, dietary change, medical devices

As the coronary arteries become clogged and then narrow, they can fail to deliver the required oxygen to the heart muscle, particularly during stress or physical effort. The heart's need for oxygen exceeds the arteries' ability to supply it. The patient usually feels a sharp, choking pain, called angina pectoris. Not all people who have coronary ischemia, however, experience anginal pain; these people are said to have silent ischemia.

The danger in coronary artery disease is that the accumulation of plaque will progress to the point where the coronary artery is clogged completely and no blood is delivered to the part of the heart serviced by that artery. The result is a myocardial infarction (commonly called a heart attack), in which some myocardial cells die when they fail to receive blood. The rough, uneven texture of the plaque instead may cause the formation of a blood clot, or thrombus, which closes the artery in a condition called coronary thrombosis.

Although coronary ischemia is usually thought of as a disease of middle and old age, in fact it starts much earlier. Autopsies of accident victims in their teens and twenties, as well as young soldiers killed in battle, show that coronary atherosclerosis is often well advanced in young persons. Some reasons for these findings and for why the rates of coronary artery disease and death began to rise in the twentieth century have been proposed. While antibiotics and vaccines reduced the mortality of some bacterial and some viral infections, Western societies underwent significant changes in lifestyle and eating habits that contributed to the rise of coronary heart disease: high-fat diets, obesity, and the stressful pace of life in a modern industrial society. Further, cigarette smoking, once almost a universal habit, has been shown to be highly pathogenic (disease-causing), contributing significantly to the development of heart disease, as well as lung cancer, emphysema, bronchitis, and other disorders. In the early and middle decades of the twentieth century, coronary heart disease was considered primarily an ailment of middle-aged and older men. As women began smoking, however, the incidence shifted so that coronary artery disease became almost equally prevalent, and equally lethal, among men and women.

Other conditions such as hypertension or diabetes mellitus are considered precursors of coronary artery disease. Hypertension, or high blood pressure, is an extremely common condition that, if unchecked, can contribute to both the development and the progression of coronary artery disease. Over the years, high blood pressure subjects arterial walls to constant stress. In response, the walls thicken and stiffen. This "hardening" of the arteries encourages the accumulation of fatty and fibrous plaque on inner artery walls. In patients with diabetes mellitus, blood sugar (glucose) levels rise either because the patient is deficient in insulin or because the insulin that the patient produces is inefficient at removing glucose from the blood. High glucose levels favor high fat levels in the blood, which can cause atherosclerosis.

Cardiac arrhythmias are the next major cause of morbidity and mortality among the heart diseases. Inside the heart, an electrochemical network regulates the contractions and relaxations that form the heartbeat. In the excitation or contraction phase, a chain of electrochemical impulses starts in the upper part of the right atrium in the heart's pacemaker, the sinoatrial or sinus node. The impulses travel through internodal tracts (pathways from one node to another) to an area between the atrium and the right ventricle called the atrioventricular node. The impulses then enter the bundle of His, which carries them to the left atrium and left ventricle. After the series of contractions is complete, the heart relaxes for a brief moment before another cycle is begun. On the average, the process is repeated sixty to eighty times a minute.

This is normal rhythm, the regular, healthy heartbeat. Dysfunction at any point along the electrochemical pathway, however, can cause an arrhythmia. Arrhythmias range greatly in their effects and their potential for bodily damage. They can be completely unnoticeable, merely annoying, debilitating, or frightening. They can cause blood clots to form in the heart, and they can cause sudden death.

The arrhythmic heart can beat too quickly (tachycardia) or too slowly (bradycardia). The contractions of the various chambers can become unsynchronized, or out of step with one another. For example, in atrial flutter or atrial fibrillation, the upper chambers of the heart beat faster, out of synchronization with the ventricles. In ventricular tachycardia, ventricular contractions increase, out of synchronization with the atria. In ventricular fibrillation, ventricular contractions lose all rhythmicity and become uncoordinated to the point at which the heart is no longer able to pump blood. Cardiac death can then occur unless the patient receives immediate treatment.

An arrhythmic disorder called heart block occurs when the impulse from the pacemaker is "blocked." Its progress through the atrioventricular node and the bundle of His may be slow or irregular, or the impulse may fail to reach its target tissues. The disorder is rated in three degrees. First-degree heart block is detectable only on an electrocardiogram (ECG), in which the movement of the impulse from the atria to the ventricles is seen to be slowed. In second-degree heart block, only some of the impulses generated reach from the atria to the ventricles; the pulse becomes irregular. Third-degree heart block is the most serious manifestation of this disorder: No impulses from the atria reach the ventricles. The heart rate may slow dramatically, and the blood flow to the brain can be reduced, causing dizziness or loss of consciousness.

Disorders that affect the heart valves usually involve stenosis (narrowing), which reduces the size of the valve opening; physical malfunction of the valve; or both. These disorders can be attributable to infection (such as rheumatic fever) or to tissue damage, or they can be congenital. If a valve has narrowed, the passage of blood from one heart chamber to another is impeded. In the case of mitral stenosis, the mitral valve between the left atrium and the left ventricle is narrowed. Blood flow to the left ventricle is reduced, and blood is retained in the left atrium, causing the atrium to enlarge as pressure builds in the chamber. This pressure forces blood back into the lungs, creating a condition called pulmonary edema in which fluid collects in the air sacs of the lungs. Similarly, malfunctions of the heart valves that cause them to open and close inefficiently can interfere with the flow of blood into the heart, through it, and out of it. This impairment may cause structural changes in the heart that can be life-threatening.

Heart failure may be a consequence of many disease conditions. It occurs primarily in the elderly. In this condition, the heart becomes inefficient at pumping blood. If the failure is on the right side of the heart, blood is forced back into the body, causing edema in the lower legs. If the failure is on the left side of the heart, blood is forced back into the lungs, causing pulmonary edema. There are many manifestations of heart failure, including shortness of breath, fatigue, and weakness.

Numerous diseases afflict the tissues of the heart wall—the epicardium, myocardium, and endocardium, as well as the pericardium. They are often caused by bacterial or viral infection, but they may also result from tissue trauma or a variety of toxic agents.

TREATMENT AND THERAPY

The main tools for diagnosing heart disease are the stethoscope, the electrocardiograph (ECG), and the X ray. With the stethoscope the doctor listens to heart sounds, which provide information about many heart functions such as rhythm and the status of the valves. The doctor can determine whether the heart is functioning normally in pumping blood from one chamber into the other, into the lungs, and into the aorta. The ECG gives the doctor a graph representation of heart function. Twelve to fifteen electrodes are placed on various parts of the body, including the head, chest, legs, and arms. The activities of the heart are printed on a strip of paper as waves or tracings. The doctor analyzes the printout for evidence of heart abnormalities, changes in heart function, signs of a heart attack, or other problems. Generally, the electrocardiographic examination is conducted with the patient at rest. In some situations, however, the doctor wishes to view heart action during physical stress. In this case, the electrodes are attached to the patient and the patient is required to exercise on a treadmill or stationary bicycle. The physician can see what changes in heart function occur when the cardiac workload is increased. The X ray gives the doctor a visual picture of the heart. Any enlargements or abnormalities can be seen, as well as the status of the aorta, pulmonary arteries, and other structures.

Another standard diagnostic tool is the echocardiograph. High-frequency sound waves are pointed at the heart from outside the body. The sound waves bounce against heart tissue and are shown on a monitor. The general configuration of the heart can be seen, as well as the shape and thickness of the chamber walls, the valves, and the large blood vessels leading to and from the heart. Velocity and direction of blood flow through the valves can be determined.

Various procedures can help the doctor assess the degree of ischemia within the heart. In one test, a radioactive isotope is injected into a vein and its dispersion in the heart is read by a scanner. This procedure can show which parts of the heart are being deprived of oxygen. In another test using a radioactive isotope, the reading is made while the patient exercises, in order to detect any changes in expansion and contraction of the heart wall that would indicate impaired circulation. The coronary angiogram gives a picture of the blockage within the coronary arteries. A thin tube called a catheter is threaded into a coronary artery, and a dye that is opaque to X rays is released. The X-ray picture will reveal narrowings in the artery resulting from plaque buildup.

The main goals of therapy in treating heart diseases are to cure the condition, if possible, and otherwise help the patient live a normal life and prevent the condition from becoming worse. In coronary artery disease, the physician seeks to maintain blood flow to the heart and to prevent heart attack. Hundreds of medications are available for this purpose, including vasodilators (agents that relax blood vessel walls and increase their capacity to carry blood). Chief among the coronary vasodilators are nitroglycerin and other drugs in the nitrate family. Also, calcium channel blockers are often used to dilate blood vessels. Beta-blocking agents are used because they reduce the heart's need for oxygen and alleviate the symptoms of angina. In addition, various support measures are recommended by physicians to stop plaque buildup and halt the progress of the disease. These include losing weight, reducing fats in the diet, and stopping smoking. The physician also treats concomitant illnesses that can contribute to the progress of coronary artery disease, such as hypertension and diabetes.

Sometimes medications and diet are not fully successful, and the ischemia continues. In a relatively new procedure, the cardiologist can unblock a clogged artery by a procedure called angioplasty. The physician threads a catheter containing a tiny balloon to the point of the blockage. The balloon is inflated to widen the inner diameter of the artery, and blood flow is increased. This procedure is often successful, although it may have to be repeated. When it is not successful, coronary bypass surgery may be indicated. In this procedure, clogged coronary arteries are replaced with healthy blood vessels from other parts of the body.

When coronary artery disease progresses to a heart attack, the patient should be treated in the hospital or similar facility. The possibility of sudden death is high during the attack and remains high until the patient is stabilized. Emergency measures are undertaken to minimize the extent of heart damage, reduce heart work, keep oxygen flowing to all parts of the body, and regulate blood pressure and heartbeat.

Cardiac arrhythmias can be managed by a variety of medications and procedures. Digitalis, guanidine, procainamide, tocanamide, and atropine are widely used to restore normal heart rhythm. In acute situations, the patient's heart rhythm can be restored by electrical cardioversion, in which an electrical stimulus is applied from outside the body to regulate the heartbeat. When a slowed heartbeat cannot be controlled by medication, a pacemaker may be implanted to regulate heart rhythm.

Treatment of heart valve disorders and disorders of the heart wall is directed at alleviating the individual condition. Antibiotics and/or valve replacement surgery may be required. In many cases, valve disorders can be completely corrected. Cardiac transplantation remains a possible treatment for some heart patients. This is an option for comparatively few patients because there are ten times as many candidates for heart transplants as there are available donor hearts.

Perspective and Prospects

Heart disease became a major killer in the United States in the twentieth century. In the early decades, the best that the medical community could do was to treat symptoms. Since then, the emphasis has shifted to prevention. Hundreds of investigative studies have been undertaken to determine the causes of the most prevalent heart dysfunction, coronary artery disease. Many of these studies have involved tens of thousands of subjects, and they point to a general consensus that coronary artery disease is a multifactorial disorder, the primary elements of which are cholesterol and other fatty substances circulating in the bloodstream, smoking, diabetes, high blood pressure, stress, and obesity.

The reasons that mortality from heart disease is declining include improved medications and treatment modalities, and much credit has to be given to the success of preventive measures. Millions of Americans have stopped smoking and have begun watching their diets. Entire industries are devoted to helping Americans eat more intelligently. While fast-food outlets continued to offer high-fat standards, such as hot dogs and hamburgers, they have also added salads and leaner selections.

Perhaps most important, medical and sociological authorities have turned their attention to children. Because advanced atherosclerosis has been detected in young men and women, cholesterol-watching has become a major preoccupation with parents and school dieticians. In addition, national programs have been instituted to discourage smoking among the young. Whether the rates of coronary heart disease will be lower in these individuals than in their parents remains to be seen, but the success of these measures in the older populations indicates that the prognosis is good.

The prognosis is also good for other heart diseases. New drugs continue to be licensed for the treatment of arrhythmias, and more versatile and reliable pacemakers increase the prospects of a normal life for many patients. Improvements in heart surgery have been particularly impressive, especially those for managing congenital heart defects in neonates and infants. Heart transplants have been successfully performed on these patients, and numerous other procedures promise significant improvement in the prospects of young people with heart disease.

Rheumatic fever, however, one of the major causes of heart disease in children, remains a threat. No vaccine is available for immunization against the streptococcus strains that cause rheumatic fever, but fortunately there are effective antibiotics to control infection in these patients. Rheumatic fever usually develops subsequent to a throat infection. Careful monitoring of the child with a sore throat can avoid progression of the infection to rheumatic fever.

—*C. Richard Falcon*

See also Aneurysms; Angina; Arrhythmias; Arteriosclerosis; Blue baby syndrome; Bypass surgery; Cardiac rehabilitation; Cardiology; Cardiology, pediatric; Cholesterol; Circulation; Claudication; Congenital heart disease; Diabetes mellitus; Electrocardiography (ECG or EKG); Embolism; Endocarditis; Heart; Heart attack; Heart failure; Heart transplantation; Heart valve replacement; Hypercholesterolemia; Hyperlipidemia; Hypertension; Ischemia; Mitral valve prolapse; Obesity; Pacemaker implantation; Palpitations; Phlebitis; Pulmonary hypertension; Thrombolytic therapy and TPA; Thrombosis and thrombus; Varicose veins; Venous insufficiency.

FOR FURTHER INFORMATION:

American Heart Association. http://www.american heart.org/. Site provides comprehensive information on heart disease and conditions, healthy lifestyles, and resources, and provides interactive health tools.

Baum, Seth J. *The Total Guide to a Healthy Heart: Integrative Strategies for Preventing and Reversing Heart Disease.* New York: Kensington, 2000. This book brings together the practices of both conventional and alternative approaches to reversing heart disease and maintaining heart health. Offers great insight into why the integrative approach to maintaining a healthy heart will be the medicine of the new millennium.

Dranov, Paula. *Heart Disease.* New York: Random House, 1990. Devoted to helping the reader become knowledgeable about heart disease and how it is being treated.

Gersh, Bernard J., ed. *The Mayo Clinic Heart Book.* 2d ed. New York: William Morrow, 2000. One of the most respected texts for laypeople on heart disease. Covers all aspects of anatomy, physiology, diagnosis, treatment, and prevention.

Goldberg, Nieca. *Women Are Not Small Men: Life-Saving Strategies for Preventing and Healing Heart Disease in Women.* New York: Random House, 2002. Written by the founder and chief of the Women's Heart Program at New York's Lenox Hill Hospital, details the way in which women experience heart disease and recovery in fundamentally different ways than men do. Physiology, symptoms, and treatment and medications are scrutinized.

Kramer, Gerri Freid, and Shari Mauer. *Parent's Guide to Children's Congenital Heart Defects: What They Are, How to Treat Them, How to Cope with Them.* New York: Crown, 2001. Experts in pediatric cardiology provide easy-to-understand answers to help parents coping with a child's heart disease. Includes the latest information on diagnosis, treatment options, surgery, aftercare, and growing up with heart defects, as well as stories from parents who have lived through the ordeal.

Larson, David E., ed. *Mayo Clinic Family Health Book.* 3d ed. New York: HarperResource, 2003. Perhaps the best general medical text for the layperson, this book covers the entire medical field. The sections on the heart diseases are exemplary for clarity and thoroughness.

Piscatella, Joseph, and Barry Franklin. *Take a Load Off Your Heart: 109 Things You Can Do to Prevent or Reverse Heart Disease.* New York: Workman, 2002. Easy-to-follow guide that details such preventive measures as managing stress, improving diet, and exercising and offers more than one hundred practical tips for preventing, stabilizing, and reversing heart disease.

Taylor, George J. *Primary Care Management of Heart Disease.* St. Louis: Mosby, 2000. A resource on the therapy and diagnosis of heart disease. Includes bibliographical references and an index.

Yannios, Thomas A. *The Heart Disease Breakthrough: What Even Your Doctor Doesn't Know About Preventing a Heart Attack.* New York: Wiley, 1999. Yannios, associate director of critical care and nutritional support at Ellis Hospital in Schenectady, New York, describes the smallest components of cholesterol, which can do more damage to the heart than the overall LDL levels that concern so many people.

Zaret, Barry L., Marvin Moser, and Lawrence S. Cohen, eds. *Yale University School of Medicine Heart Book.* New York: William Morrow, 1992. This text will give the reader a clear understanding of the various heart diseases, as well as of methods of treating and preventing them.

HEART FAILURE

DISEASE/DISORDER

ANATOMY OR SYSTEM AFFECTED: Circulatory system, heart

SPECIALTIES AND RELATED FIELDS: Cardiology, internal medicine, vascular medicine

DEFINITION: A condition in which the heart cannot pump enough blood to meet the needs of the body because its ability to contract is impaired.

KEY TERMS:

congestive heart failure: the stage of heart failure that occurs when a backup of pressure results in accumulation of fluid in the veins and tissues

coronary arteries: the arteries that supply blood to the heart muscle

diuretic: a drug that stimulates the kidneys to eliminate more salt and water from the body

edema: the accumulation of fluid around the cells in tissue

ejection fraction: the ratio of the stroke volume to the residual volume, expressed as a percentage

hormone: a chemical messenger released by a gland which is carried by the blood to its target

inotropic agent: a drug that improves the ability of the heart muscle to contract

optimal length: the length of a heart muscle cell at which stimulation can elicit the maximum possible force development

residual volume: the blood volume left in the heart chamber at the end of a heartbeat

stroke volume: the blood volume leaving either the right or the left side of the heart with each beat; each side usually ejects the same volume per beat

vasodilator: a drug that relaxes blood vessels

CAUSES AND SYMPTOMS

The circulation of the blood has many functions. It is essential for the delivery of oxygen, nutrients, and elements of the immune system to tissues. It also contributes to regulation and communication between different parts of the body by moving chemical messengers from where they are produced to where they have a biological effect. The delivery of warm blood to the surface of the skin is one essential element in temperature control. The blood pressure determines how much water can move across the exchange surfaces in the kidneys, thus affecting water balance in the body. The movement of blood through the kidneys, the lungs, and all tissues is important for waste removal.

All these functions depend on the ability of the heart to contract and eject blood. Blood is pumped, in two serial circuits, from the right heart through the lungs into the left heart and from the left heart around the body back to the right heart. In each circuit, the blood travels through large arteries, then to smaller arterioles, to capillaries (where exchange takes place), and back via small venules and veins to the heart. Heart failure describes the situation in which heart function is reduced. While still able to beat, the heart is unable to meet the circulatory needs of the body. That is, the heart muscle is unable to contract enough to pump the blood adequately.

The severity of the heart failure can be gauged by the ejection fraction, a measure of the pumping capacity of the heart. It is the percentage calculated from the stroke volume (the volume of blood leaving a heart chamber with each beat) divided by the residual volume (the volume left in the heart chamber at the end of a heartbeat). Thus the ejection fraction measures how much blood in the heart chamber can actually leave when the heartbeat occurs. In normal, healthy hearts, this value is 100 percent: The amount that stays in the heart is approximately equal to the amount that leaves it. In mild or moderate heart failure, it ranges approximately between 15 and 40 percent: Less blood leaves the heart with each beat, and more blood remains behind.

The pressure inside the heart at the end of a heartbeat is another index of heart performance. If the heart is failing and more blood is left behind in the heart at the end of a beat, the pressure inside the heart at the end of the beat will be increased. In cases of severe failure, the pressure in the arteries outside the heart will fall.

In failure, the heart cannot supply enough blood for all the functions of the circulation. This fact accounts for the variety of symptoms that accompany heart failure: labored breathing; light-headedness; generalized weakness; cold, pale, or even bluish skin tone; and accumulation of fluid in the extremities and/or lungs. Other possible symptoms include distended neck veins, accumulation of fluid in the abdomen, abnormal heart rate and rhythm, and chest pain.

The specific symptoms of the condition depend on the type of failure, its severity, its underlying causes, and the ways in which the body attempts to compensate. There are several ways to categorize types of heart failure: acute or chronic, forward or backward, and right-sided or left-sided.

Acute heart failure refers to a sudden decrease in heart function. It can be caused by toxic quantities of drugs, anesthetics, or metals or by certain disease states, such as infections. Most often, however, it is

INFORMATION ON HEART FAILURE

CAUSES: Varies; can include inherited or acquired diseases, allergic reactions, connective tissue or metabolic abnormalities, high blood pressure, anatomical defects, toxic quantities of drugs, sudden blockage of coronary arteries

SYMPTOMS: Labored breathing; light-headedness; generalized weakness; cold, pale, or even bluish skin tone; accumulation of fluid in extremities and/or lungs; distended neck veins; abnormal heart rate and rhythm; chest pain

DURATION: Acute or chronic

TREATMENTS: Drug therapy, surgery, preventive medication, exercise, dietary change, medical devices

caused by a sudden blockage of the coronary arteries supplying the heart muscle. A sudden blockage caused by a blood clot can induce a heart attack and subsequent heart failure, causing chest pain and often abnormal heart rate or rhythm. These effects are sometimes so rapid that there is little time for the body to attempt compensation.

Chronic heart failure is a progressive reduction in heart function that develops over time. It can be caused by inherited or acquired diseases, allergic reactions, connective tissue or metabolic abnormalities, high blood pressure, and anatomical defects. The most common cause, however, is coronary artery disease. This disease narrows blood vessels and leads to a reduction in the amount of blood reaching the heart muscle. It causes reduced oxygen availability and, eventually, a reduction in the ability of the heart muscle to contract.

In the early stages of chronic failure, the hormone and nervous systems promote compensation in the heart, blood vessels, and kidneys to help the heart continue to pump enough blood. These systems stimulate the heart muscle directly to make it beat harder. They also take advantage of the fact that modest stretching of the heart muscle increases its ability to contract. By stimulating the blood vessels to contract, more blood moves back toward the heart, causing a cold, pale, or even bluish skin tone. Stimulation of the kidney to retain water and sodium results in an increase in blood volume, which also moves more blood back to the heart. In each case, the heart muscle is stretched by these increases and, therefore, can contract harder.

Yet these reactions do not constitute a long-term solution. The heart muscle can become fatigued from overwork and can become overstretched. A resulting accumulation of fluid in the heart reduces its ability to contract. Compensation fails, and the additional fluid in the blood starts to back up in the circulation. This condition is called backward heart failure. At the same time, the heart is unable to pump hard enough to move the blood forward against the higher resistance caused by the contraction of the blood vessels. This condition is termed forward heart failure. Congestive heart failure is the stage that occurs when the backup of pressure is worsened by fluid retention and blood vessel contraction. The congestion, or accumulation of fluid, occurs in the veins and tissues.

Left-sided or right-sided heart failure can occur alone or together. The right side of the heart pumps blood to the lungs to be oxygenated, and the left side of the heart pumps oxygenated blood to the organs of the body. Normally, these two sides are well matched so that the same volume moves through each side. When the right heart cannot contract properly, however, blood accumulates upstream in the veins and somewhat less blood reaches the lungs to pick up oxygen, resulting in distended veins and shortness of breath. It is primarily a backward heart failure. Fluid can back up in the veins and increase pressure in the capillaries so that it starts to leak out of the circulation into the surrounding tissues. This leads to an accumulation of fluid (called edema), especially in the liver and lower extremities. In isolated right-sided heart failure, this pressure rarely backs up to such an extent that it causes problems through the rest of the circulation to the left side of the heart.

In contrast, when the left side of the heart cannot contract properly, it can back up pressure so badly that it creates a pressure overload against which the right side of the heart must pump. This increase in the workload on the right side of the heart frequently leads to two-sided heart failure. This outcome is especially common since the disease conditions that exist in the left side are likely to exist on the right as well. In left-sided heart failure, blood accumulates upstream in the lungs, increasing pressure enough to cause a leakage of fluid into the lungs (pulmonary edema). This leakage interferes with oxygen uptake and therefore causes shortness of breath. It also results in inadequate blood flow to the body's tissues, including the muscles and brain, resulting in generalized weakness and light-headedness. Left-sided heart failure is thus both a backward and a forward failure.

TREATMENT AND THERAPY

Treatments for cardiac failure, like its symptoms, depend on a variety of factors. The first goal of treatment is to avoid any obvious precipitating causes of the failure, such as alcohol, drugs, the cessation of necessary essential medications, acute stress, a salt-loaded diet, overexercise, infection, illness, or surgery. The next approach is to take the simplest measures to reduce distension of the heart by controlling salt and water retention and to decrease the workload of the heart by altering the circulatory needs of the tissues. The former can be achieved by dietary salt restriction, restriction of fluid consumption, or mechanical removal of fluid accumulating around the lungs or abdomen. The latter can be accomplished with bed rest and weight loss.

Typically, drug therapy is also required in order to treat heart failure. No single agent meets all the requirements for optimal treatment, which includes rapid relief of labored breathing and edema, enhanced heart performance, reduced mortality, reduced progression of the underlying disease, safety, and minimal side effects. Therefore, drugs are used in combination to achieve control over sodium and water retention, improve heart contraction, reduce heart work, and protect against blood clots.

The purpose of therapy with diuretic drugs (drugs that increase salt and water loss through the kidneys) is threefold: to reduce the pooling of fluid that can take place in the lungs, abdomen, and lower extremities; to minimize the buildup of back pressure from the accumulation of blood in the veins; and to reduce the circulating blood volume. All these things will lessen the overstretch of the heart muscle and bring it to a level of stretch that is closer to its optimum. Care must be taken, however, not to reduce severely the water content of the blood, which could reduce the stretch on the heart muscle to below the optimum and consequently impair heart contraction. One way to monitor how much water

IN THE NEWS:
HOMOCYSTEINE LEVELS AND CONGESTIVE HEART FAILURE

In the January, 2003, issue of the *Journal of the American Medical Association* (JAMA), a team of researchers from the National Heart, Lung, and Blood Institute's Framingham Heart Study, the U.S. Department of Agriculture Human Nutrition Research Center on Aging, and Boston University reported that elevated levels of total homocysteine in the blood are associated with an increased risk for congestive heart failure, a condition in which the heart is unable to maintain adequate blood circulation to the tissues.

The correlation between elevated homocysteine levels and increased risk of cardiovascular disease in general—and specifically myocardial infarction (heart attack), arteriosclerosis, coronary heart disease, and stroke—has been well established, but this was the first study to pinpoint congestive heart failure.

Homocysteine is an amino acid, but unlike most amino acids, it is not a component of proteins. Its primary role seems to be to act as an intermediate in the formation and breakdown of other molecules. Excess levels of homocysteine probably result from its accumulation when its conversion to the next intermediate occurs too slowly, a process often thought to be caused by folic acid deficiency. This conversion can be accelerated by the administration of folic acid.

The subjects of this eight-year study were 2,491 participants of the Framingham Heart Study, who at the start of the study had no histories of myocardial infarction or congestive heart failure. Their average age was seventy-two years. Patients were examined at various times after the initial measurement of plasma homocysteine, and the examinations included plasma homocysteine measurement, blood pressure measurement, electrocardiogram evaluation, systematic assessment of cardiovascular risk factors, and a review of cardiovascular events in each patient's medical record. There were 156 patients who developed congestive heart failure, and the association between plasma homocysteine levels and the incidence of congestive heart failure was examined. Patients with higher-than-average homocysteine levels were more likely to develop congestive heart failure. Women with higher-than-average homocysteine levels had twice the risk for congestive heart failure when compared to the total female population of the study. Researchers noted, however, that additional studies to evaluate the effect of folic acid supplementation on the risk of congestive heart failure are needed.

—*Lorraine Lica, Ph.D.*

is lost or retained is for patients to empty their bladders and then weigh themselves each day before breakfast. If weight changes steadily or suddenly, then sodium and water loss may be too great or too little. In either case, an adjustment is in order. Some generic diuretic drugs used to treat heart failure include furosemide, ethacrynic acid, the thiazides, and spironolactone.

The purpose of therapy with inotropic drugs (drugs that increase the contractile ability of heart muscle) is to improve the pumping action of the heart. This effect causes an increase in stroke volume (more blood moves out of the heart per beat) and helps compensate for forward failure. The increased output also reduces the backup of blood returning to the heart and thus also compensates for backward failure.

Digitalis, a derivative of the foxglove plant which originated as a Welsh folk remedy, is still the most frequently used inotropic drug for the treatment of chronic heart failure. Because it improves heart muscle contraction, it reverses to some extent all the symptoms of heart failure. Digitalis exerts its effects by increasing the accumulation of calcium inside the heart muscle cells. Calcium interacts with the structure of the shortening apparatus inside the cell to make more contractile interactions within the cell possible. Its disadvantages are that it becomes toxic in high doses and that it can severely damage performance of an already healthy heart.

Other inotropic agents also act to improve contraction by increasing calcium levels within the heart muscle cells. Some of them mimic the naturally produced hormones and neurotransmitters that are released and depleted in early stages of heart failure. These are called the sympathomimetic drugs. They include drugs such as dopamine, terbutaline, and levodopa. While these drugs improve heart performance, they can have serious side effects: increased heart rate, palpitations, and nervousness. One group of inotropic agents improves cardiac contraction while relaxing blood vessels. These drugs, called phosphodiesterase inhibitors, stop the breakdown of an essential cellular messenger molecule which helps to manage calcium levels and other events inside both heart cells and blood vessel cells. Examples of these drugs include amrinone and milrinone. Their use is not common because they can cause stomach upset and fatigue and because they are not clearly superior to other treatments.

The purpose of therapy with vasodilator drugs (drugs that relax the blood vessels) is to decrease the work of the heart. The resulting expansion of the blood vessels makes it easier for blood to be pumped through them. It also leaves room for pooling some of the blood in the veins, decreasing the amount of blood returning to the heart and so reducing overstretching as well. Some of the vasodilators, such as hydralazine, pinacidil, dipyridamole, and the nitrates, act directly on the blood vessels. Other vasodilators, such as angiotensin-converting enzyme (ACE) inhibitors and adrenergic inhibitors, inhibit the release of naturally produced substances that would make the blood vessels contract. Sometimes it is hard to predict the effects of vasodilators because they may act differently in different blood vessels and the body may attempt to offset the effects of the drug by releasing substances that contract blood vessels. Vasodilator drug therapy is usually added to other treatments when the symptoms of heart failure persist after digitalis and diuretic therapy are used.

The purpose of therapy with antithrombotics (blood clot inhibitors) is to prevent any further obstruction of the circulation with blood clots. Because heart failure changes the mechanics of blood flow and is the result of damaged heart muscle, it can increase the formation of blood clots. When blood clots form an obstruction in the large blood vessels of the lungs, it is often fatal. Clots can also lodge in the heart, causing further damage to heart muscle, or in the brain, where they could cause a stroke. Both the short-acting clot inhibitor heparin and oral agents such as aspirin are used to prevent these effects.

The combination of all these drug therapies, while unable to reverse the permanent damage of heart failure, makes it possible to treat the condition. Individuals treated for heart failure can lead comfortable, productive lives.

If the heart failure progresses to acutely life-threatening proportions and the patient is in all other ways healthy, the next alternative is surgical replacement of the heart. Artificial hearts are sometimes used as a transition to heart transplant while a donor is sought. Yet transplantation is not a perfect solution. Transplanted hearts do not have the nervous system input of a normal heart and so their control from moment to moment is different. They are also subject to rejection. Nevertheless, they provide an enormous improvement in quality of life for severe heart failure patients.

PERSPECTIVE AND PROSPECTS

The vital significance of the pulse and heartbeat have been part of human knowledge since long before recorded history. Pulse taking and herbal treatments for poor heartbeat have been recorded in ancient Chinese,

Egyptian, and Greek histories. Digitalis has been used in treatment for at least two hundred years. It was first formally introduced to the medical community in 1785 by the English botanist and physician William Withering. He learned of it from a female folk healer named Hutton, who used it with other extracts to treat more than one kind of swelling. Withering identified the foxglove plant as the source of its active ingredient and characterized it as having effects on the pulse as well as on fluid retention. The plant is indigenous to both the United Kingdom and Europe and may well have been employed as a folk remedy for far longer. It is still the most widely used agent for the treatment of heart failure.

The developments in physiology and medicine during the nineteenth century set the stage for greater understanding and further treatments of heart failure. It was then that the stethoscope and blood pressure cuff were created for diagnostic purposes. In basic science, cell theory, hormone theory, and kidney physiology led to a better understanding of how heart muscle contraction and fluid balance might be coordinated in the body. The concepts and techniques required to keep organs and tissues alive outside the body with an artificial circulation system were conceived and introduced. Anesthesia and sterile techniques essential for cardiac surgery were developed.

These ideas and accomplishments contributed to important discoveries in the early twentieth century that greatly enhanced the understanding of the early compensatory responses to heart failure. For example, it was found that when heart muscle is stretched, it will contract with greater force on the next beat and that heart muscle usually operates at a muscle length that is less than optimal. Thus, when the amount of blood returning to the heart increases and stretches the muscle in the walls of the heart, the heart will contract with greater force, ejecting a greater volume of blood. This phenomenon, called the Frank-Starling mechanism, was first demonstrated in isolated heart muscle by the German physiologist Otto Frank and in functional hearts by the British physiologist Ernest Henry Starling in 1914.

Subsequent developments in the second half of the twentieth century, such as more specific vasodilator and diuretic drugs as well as the heart-lung machine, have led to the options of more complete drug therapy, artificial hearts (first introduced to replace a human heart by William DeVries in 1982), and heart transplant (first performed by Christiaan Barnard in 1967) as options for the treatment of heart failure.

—*Laura Gray Malloy, Ph.D.*

See also Arrhythmias; Arteriosclerosis; Cardiology; Cardiology, pediatric; Cholesterol; Circulation; Congenital heart disease; Edema; Endocarditis; Heart; Heart attack; Heart disease; Heart transplantation; Hypercholesterolemia; Hyperlipidemia; Hypertension; Ischemia; Mitral valve prolapse; Obesity; Palpitations; Vascular medicine; Vascular system.

FOR FURTHER INFORMATION:

Campbell, Neil A. *Biology: Concepts and Connections.* 6th ed. San Francisco: Benjamin/Cummings, 2002. This classic introductory textbook provides an excellent discussion of essential biological structures and mechanisms, including a chapter on cardiovascular function and disease.

Crawford, Michael, ed. *Diagnosis and Treatment in Cardiology.* New York: McGraw-Hill, 2002. Discusses advances in cardiac diagnostics, treatments, and prognostic indicators and includes extensive information on prevention techniques.

Dox, Ida G., B. John Melloni, and Gilbert M. Eisner. *The HarperCollins Illustrated Medical Dictionary.* 4th ed. New York: HarperCollins, 2001. A home medical dictionary with more than 26,000 medical terms and 2,500 illustrations, including all those of most concern to cardiovascular patients. Defines relevant anatomical structures, functional terminology, and some widely used chemical compounds and drugs under generic names. An excellent resource for high school or college students.

Gersh, Bernard J., ed. *The Mayo Clinic Heart Book.* 2d ed. New York: William Morrow, 2000. One of the most respected texts for laypeople on heart disease. Covers all aspects of anatomy, physiology, diagnosis, treatment, and prevention.

Sherwood, Lauralee. *Human Physiology: From Cells to Systems.* 5th ed. Belmont, Calif.: Wadsworth, 2003. A basic physiology textbook oriented toward an understanding of human function and disease. Superbly well written and offers excellent illustrations. Includes chapters that address cardiovascular function, with specific reference to heart failure and the cardiovascular abnormalities that precipitate it.

HEART TRANSPLANTATION
PROCEDURE

ANATOMY OR SYSTEM AFFECTED: Chest, circulatory system, heart, lungs, nervous system, respiratory system

SPECIALTIES AND RELATED FIELDS: Cardiology, critical care, emergency medicine, general surgery

DEFINITION: The removal of a diseased heart and its replacement with a healthy donor heart.

KEY TERMS:

cardiomyopathy: a serious acute or chronic disease in which the heart becomes inflamed; it may result from multiple causes, including viral infection

congenital: present at birth

congestive heart failure: abnormal heart function characterized by circulatory congestion caused by cardiac disorders, especially myocardial infarction of the ventricles

coronary atherosclerosis: the accumulation of cholesterol, lipids, and other cellular debris in the coronary arteries, thereby limiting circulation in the heart

immunity: a defense function of the body that produces antibodies to destroy invading antigens and other disease-causing organisms

leukocytes: white blood cells that are important in the development of immunity

primary cardiomyopathy: cardiomyopathy that cannot be attributed to a specific cause

secondary cardiomyopathy: cardiomyopathy that is attributable to a specific cause (such as hypertension) and that is often associated with diseases involving other organs

INDICATIONS AND PROCEDURES

Heart transplantation is performed when congestive heart failure or heart injury cannot be treated by other conventional medical or surgical means. It is reserved for patients with a high risk of dying within two years. The procedure involves removal of a diseased heart and its replacement with a healthy human heart or possibly an animal heart. In special cases, the surgeon may place the donor heart next to the diseased heart without removing it; this is called a piggyback transplant.

Patients who are candidates for heart transplantation include those with valvular disease, congenital heart disease, or rare conditions such as tumors. The selection of recipients is based on which patients are likely to exhibit the most pronounced improvement, functional capacity, and life expectancy after surgery. In the United States, the limited availability of donor hearts has necessitated the creation of a national organ procurement and distribution network called the United Network for Organ Sharing (UNOS), which distributes organs based on severity of illness, waiting time, donor and recipient blood types, and body size match.

USES AND COMPLICATIONS

The first human heart transplantation was performed on December 3, 1967, by Christiaan Barnard in Capetown, South Africa. The heart transplantation procedures that were tried soon afterward usually had a low success rate because the patient's body often rejected the new heart when leukocytes and other cells of the immune system recognized the new heart as foreign material and attacked it. With an improved understanding of immune system functioning and drug intervention, however, survival rates have gradually improved. Currently in the United States, approximately two thousand patients undergo heart transplantation annually in more than 230 heart transplantation centers. The one-year survival rate is 80 percent, the five-year survival rate is 70 percent, the ten-year survival rate is nearly

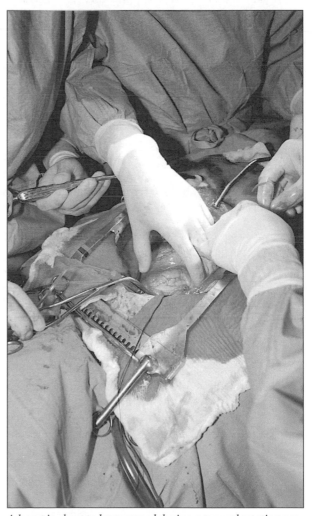

A heart is about to be removed during a transplantation procedure. (PhotoDisc)

50 percent, and some patients have lived longer than twenty years, according to statistics from the American Heart Association. About fifteen thousand Americans aged fifty-five or younger (and forty thousand aged sixty-five or younger) would benefit from heart trans- plantation. Transplantation has been conducted with newborn babies, and adult patients have run marathons and even played professional sports. The average age at which the procedure is performed is forty-seven years for men and thirty-nine years for women.

The complications immediately following this type of surgery in- clude irreversible damage to the heart, because of coronary athero- sclerosis or multiple heart attacks, and primary or secondary cardio- myopathy, because the cardiac muscle cells cannot contract nor- mally. Heart transplant recipients must take immunosuppressive (antirejection) medications for the remainder of their lives to pre- vent rejection; thus they must also cope with the numerous side ef- fects of these drugs. For at least one year after transplantation, the heart is denervated (cut away from the body's nervous system), causing a resting pulse rate of up to 130 beats per minute, as com- pared to 60 to 80 beats per minute in a normal heart. The chances for long-term success depend in part on the amount of damage or dis- ease in other organs as a result of stroke, chronic obstructive lung disease, and liver or kidney dis- ease. Transplant recipients must also deal with the psychological and emotional strain of the opera- tion and its aftermath. Patients with a history of alcohol and drug abuse or mental illness, and those who lack a social support net- work of family and friends, are not considered good candidates for heart transplantation.

IN THE NEWS: THE ABIOCOR ARTIFICIAL HEART

Scientific efforts at developing an artificial heart have been impor- tant because only about two thousand human donor hearts are available in the United States per year, despite many thousands of patients re- quiring a heart transplant. The initial experimental model, the Jarvik-7 in 1982, required a large pump outside the body and tethered the recipi- ent to its 375-pound machine. Technological advances in miniaturiza- tion and energy transfer permitted the creation of the AbioCor, the first implantable artificial heart affording full mobility to the patient.

The AbioCor is made of titanium and a unique plastic designed to withstand being flexed forty million times a year. Before receiving Food and Drug Administration (FDA) approval for a clinical trial with fifteen patients, the makers of the AbioCor heart had to demonstrate that it could beat two hundred million times, enough beats to last five years. The device uses a wireless power transfer system. An external battery worn on the waist connects with an external coil on the chest, which transfers energy via radio waves to a coil inside the chest. No wires break the skin or provide a route for infection. A computer chip inside the chest controls the pumping action, and the external battery can operate four or five hours without recharging. An internal battery, kept continually charged by the external battery, provides thirty min- utes of emergency power, permitting the user to disconnect the external power when showering.

Only patients likely to die within thirty days and unable to receive a live heart transplant were eligible to take part in the clinical trial. Suc- cess was defined as survival for 60 days with clear improvement in quality of life. On July 2, 2001, the first person to receive an implant lived for 151 days. Five more pumps were implanted in 2001, followed by an additional pump in 2002. Two patients died on the operating ta- ble, but the others lived more than 60 days. The longest surviving re- cipient lived 512 days and spent several months at home with his fam- ily before dying on February 7, 2003. The company temporarily suspended implants in 2002 and modified the AbioCor after two pa- tients died of strokes. Clinical trials resumed in 2003, with three pa- tients receiving artificial hearts in January and March of that year.

The dimensions of the AbioCor heart limit its usability. The human heart is about the size of a fist and weighs about 10 ounces. The AbioCor, the size of a grapefruit, weighs 2 pounds, too large for 50 per- cent of men and 80 percent of women. The developers hope to over- come this problem in future models.

—*Milton Berman, Ph.D.*

PERSPECTIVE AND PROSPECTS

The rapid increase in the num- ber of heart transplantations per- formed worldwide is attributable to specialized medical care and to numerous advances in knowl- edge regarding surgery, tissue preservation, immunology, and infectious disease. The extraordinary degree of success since the 1970's has enabled many patients who have undergone heart transplantation to live longer and more independent lives. Tremendous strides have been made in diagnosing rejection and developing immunosuppressive medications, and the development of several new antirejection drugs is anticipated soon. New techniques for diagnosing rejection candidates without the performance of a heart biopsy will be a major focus of future research, as will increasing access to donor organs. A better understanding of the immune system may give doctors greater success in transplanting organs from other species (a procedure called a xenograft) instead of human organs. Ongoing research will continue to focus on identifying risk factors for heart disease—such as high blood cholesterol and abnormal lipid subfractions, high blood pressure, diabetes mellitus, family history, and cigarette smoking—as early as possible in order to delay reaching the point at which heart transplantation is necessary.

—*Daniel G. Graetzer, Ph.D.*

See also Cardiac rehabilitation; Cardiology; Cardiology, pediatric; Circulation; Electrocardiography (ECG or EKG); Grafts and grafting; Heart; Heart disease; Heart failure; Heart valve replacement; Immune system; Immunology; Transplantation; Xenotransplantation.

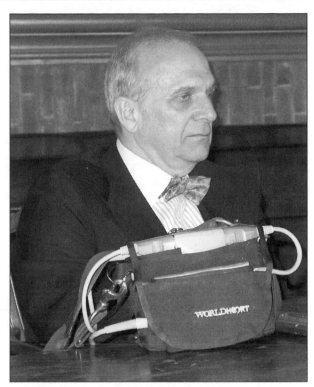

Pete Kenyon survived with an artificial heart for three years until he could receive a donor organ. The pump mechanism is carried in a pouch. (AP/Wide World Photos)

For Further Information:

American College of Sports Medicine. *ACSM's Guidelines for Exercise Testing and Prescription.* 6th ed. Baltimore: Williams & Wilkins, 2000. Covers the standards of exercise testing and therapy, including instruction for patients suffering from heart disease.

American Heart Association. *Heart and Stroke Facts.* Dallas: Author, 1994. Contains information for the layperson on cardiovascular and cerebrovascular disease. Includes an index.

Crawford, Michael, ed. *Diagnosis and Treatment in Cardiology.* New York: McGraw-Hill, 2002. Discusses advances in cardiac diagnostics, treatments, and prognostic indicators and includes extensive information on prevention techniques.

Deng, Mario C., et al. "Effect of Receiving a Heart Transplant: Analysis of a National Cohort Entered on to a Waiting List, Stratified by Heart Failure Severity." *British Medical Journal* 321, no. 7260 (September 2, 2000): 540-545. A study of cardiac transplantation in Germany reveals that patients with a predicted low or medium risk of mortality have no reduction in mortality risk as a result of transplantation.

Eagle, Kim A., and Ragavendra R. Baliga. *Practical Cardiology: Evaluation and Treatment of Common Cardiovascular Disorders.* Philadelphia: Lippincott Williams & Wilkins, 2003. Details advances in cardiac medicine.

Ewert, Ralf, et al. "Relationship Between Impaired Pulmonary Diffusion and Cardiopulmonary Exercise Capacity After Heart Transplantation." *Chest* 117, no. 4 (April, 2000): 968. Diffusion impairment and reduced performance in cardiopulmonary exercise testing have been found in patients after heart transplantation.

Krau, Stephen D., ed. *Heart Transplantation.* Philadelphia: W. B. Saunders, 2000. Discusses organ procurement, evaluation criteria for the pretransplant patient, and the long-term management of heart transplantation patients, including immunosuppression, complications, and psychological adjustments.

HEART VALVE REPLACEMENT

PROCEDURE

ANATOMY OR SYSTEM AFFECTED: Chest, circulatory system, heart

SPECIALTIES AND RELATED FIELDS: Cardiology, general surgery

DEFINITION: A surgical procedure that involves removing a defective heart valve and replacing it with another tissue valve or with a mechanical valve.

KEY TERMS:

anticoagulants: a class of drugs that slow the clotting time of blood

bacterial endocarditis: bacterial infection of the heart, which may scar or destroy a valve

murmur: the sound made by blood flowing backward through a heart valve

regurgitation: the leakage of blood backward through a valve

stenosis: a condition in which valve tissue has hardened and thickened, interfering with blood flow through the valve

INDICATIONS AND PROCEDURES

Valve replacement surgery is a procedure used when a heart valve no longer functions properly. There are several reasons that a heart valve may fail. Sometimes, a major defect present at birth must be repaired immediately. Minor defects present at birth may go undetected for years. When and if these minor defects become worse as a result of aging, valve replacement surgery may be necessary. Another cause of heart valve damage is infection. Rheumatic fever can cause the scarring of a valve. These scars can become more of a problem with age, and surgery may eventually be necessary. Bacterial endocarditis is another type of infection that can damage the heart very quickly. Valve replacement surgery is often needed as a result of this type of infection.

When a heart valve is damaged, the result is usually stenosis or regurgitation. Stenosis occurs when the valve becomes thick and hard. As a result, normal blood flow through the valve is obstructed. A valve that becomes stretched or weak may not close properly, resulting in blood flowing backward through the valve; this is called regurgitation. When the blood flows backward through the valve, a sound is made. This sound, called a murmur, generally can be heard with a stethoscope.

When a heart valve fails to function properly, the ability of the heart to do work is impaired. In an attempt to maintain normal work levels, the heart begins to enlarge, or experience hypertrophy. When further hypertrophy is no longer possible, the heart fails. This condition will result in permanent damage to the heart muscle and eventually death. Some of the symptoms of valve problems include chest pain or tightness, shortness of breath, temporary blindness, slurred speech, weakness, numbness, lack of coordination, unusually rapid weight gain, fatigue, and loss of consciousness. These symptoms are typically the result of inadequate blood flow, particularly to the brain.

In some cases, surgery can be used to repair the valve. Many times, however, the damage is too extensive for this type of surgery, and the valve must be replaced. The replacement valve may come from a deceased person's heart or from an animal's heart (usually that of a pig), or it may be a mechanical (prosthetic) valve. Prosthetic valves are made from metal, plastic, or carbon ceramic.

During valve replacement surgery, the chest is opened to expose the heart. Blood flow through the heart is diverted through an oxygenator and a pump that maintains the flow of oxygenated blood throughout the body. The surgeon removes the damaged valve and sutures a replacement valve to the heart. Upon completion of the surgery, if the replaced valve functions effectively, normal blood flow is restored through the heart.

USES AND COMPLICATIONS

Heart valve replacement is a very reliable procedure. Although problems with the new valve are possible, the majority of these surgeries are 100 percent effective. Nevertheless, there are two long-term concerns for the patient. Blood thinners or anticoagulants—drugs that slow the clotting process and may prevent blood clots—are usually required with prosthetic valves. These drugs help prevent blood from coagulating in and around the new valve. Some patients must also take antibiotics to prevent additional infections in the heart. Antibiotics are needed especially when patients visit the dentist, when bleeding is likely. If bleeding occurs, bacteria may enter the blood and become lodged in the replacement valve. The ensuing infection can cause further damage to the heart.

When one compares the use of tissue versus mechanical (prosthetic) valves for replacement, some differences emerge. In general, tissue valves work better. In addition, they are less likely to require drugs to increase blood-clotting time. On the other hand, they are harder to obtain. With more people acting as donors and with better preservation techniques becoming available, tissue replacements are preferred.

PERSPECTIVE AND PROSPECTS

Mechanical valves were first used as replacements for damaged valves in the early 1960's. In 1962, the initial clinical use of tissue valves was described. Tissue valve replacements were conducted simultaneously by Donald Ross in England and Sir Brian Barratt-Boyes in New Zealand. The acceptance of tissue valve use was slow because the number of donors was small and the methods for preserving valves for later use were poor. The result was shorter survival times for the replacement valves used in the 1960's and early 1970's.

By the 1980's, better preservation techniques were developed, which allowed surgeons to use living human tissue. These replacements have been found to be superior to nonliving tissues and mechanical valves. In

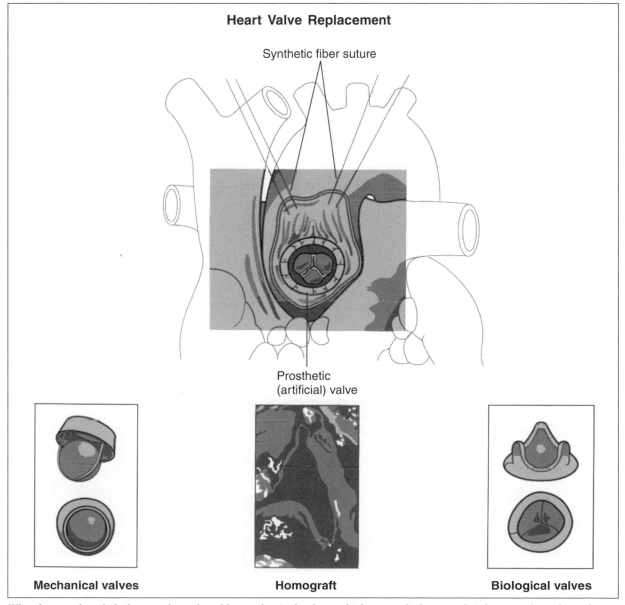

Heart Valve Replacement

Synthetic fiber suture

Prosthetic (artificial) valve

Mechanical valves   **Homograft**   **Biological valves**

When heart valves fail, they can be replaced by mechanical valves, which are made from artificial materials such as plastic, metal, and carbon fibers; by homografts, which are taken from cadavers; or by biological valves, which are either taken from pigs or constructed from the tissues of the patient or of a cow.

the future, both mechanical and tissue replacements will continue to be used, based on availability and the specific needs of the patient.

—*Bradley R. A. Wilson, Ph.D.*

See also Angiography; Angioplasty; Bleeding; Blood and blood disorders; Bypass surgery; Cardiac rehabilitation; Cardiology; Cardiology, pediatric; Circulation; Electrocardiography (ECG or EKG); Endocarditis; Heart; Heart attack; Heart disease; Heart failure; Heart transplantation; Pacemaker implantation; Rheumatic fever; Thrombolytic therapy and TPA.

FOR FURTHER INFORMATION:

Bonhoeffer, Philipp, et al. "Percutaneous Replacement of Pulmonary Valve in a Right-Ventricle to Pulmonary-Artery Prosthetic Conduit with Valve Dysfunction." *The Lancet* 356, no. 9239 (October 21, 2000): 1403-1405. The authors show that percutaneous valve replacement in the pulmonary position is possible. With further technical improvements, this new technique might be used for valve replacement in other cardiac and noncardiac positions.

Crawford, Michael, ed. *Diagnosis and Treatment in Cardiology.* New York: McGraw-Hill, 2002. Discusses advances in cardiac diagnostics, treatments, and prognostic indicators and includes extensive information on prevention techniques.

Eagle, Kim A., and Ragavendra R. Baliga. *Practical Cardiology: Evaluation and Treatment of Common Cardiovascular Disorders.* Philadelphia: Lippincott Williams & Wilkins, 2003. Details advances in cardiac medicine.

Kramer, Gerri Freid, and Shari Mauer. *Parent's Guide to Children's Congenital Heart Defects: What They Are, How to Treat Them, How to Cope with Them.* New York: Crown, 2001. Experts in pediatric cardiology provide easy-to-understand answers to help parents coping with a child's heart disease. Includes the latest information on diagnosis, treatment options, surgery, aftercare, and growing up with heart defects, as well as stories from parents who have lived through the ordeal.

Mitka, Mike. "Final Report on Mechanical vs. Bioprosthetic Heart Valves." *The Journal of the American Medical Association* 283, no. 15 (April 19, 2000): 1947-1948. A long-term follow-up study presented at the annual meeting of the American College of Cardiology has given surgeons a clear answer to the question of whether to perform heart valve replacement with a mechanical or a bioprosthetic device.

Nauer, Kathleen A., Barbara Schouchoff, and Kathleen Demitras. "Minimally Invasive Aortic Valve Surgery." *Critical Care Nursing Quarterly* 23, no. 1 (May, 2000): 66-71. Heart surgery has seen the emergence of minimally invasive techniques in the quest for less traumatic and less painful surgery. This procedure can be provided without the increased cost of endoscopic instrumentation by use of standard instrumentation, cannulation, and prostheses.

Otto, Catherine M. "Timing of Aortic Valve Surgery." *Heart* 84, no. 2 (August, 2000): 211. The timing of aortic valve surgery is described for patients complaining of two conditions: aortic stenosis and chronic aortic regurgitation.

Rahimtoola, Shahbudin H., ed. *Valvular Heart Disease.* 3d ed. Philadelphia: Lippincott, Williams & Wilkins, 2000. Discusses diseases of the heart valve and their treatments. Includes bibliographical references and an index.

HEARTBURN

DISEASE/DISORDER

ALSO KNOWN AS: Acid indigestion

ANATOMY OR SYSTEM AFFECTED: Chest, gastrointestinal system, throat

SPECIALTIES AND RELATED FIELDS: Family medicine, gastroenterology, internal medicine

DEFINITION: A feeling of warmth or discomfort in the chest.

CAUSES AND SYMPTOMS

Heartburn occurs when acid travels backward from the stomach to the esophagus. Acid is normally present at

---

INFORMATION ON HEARTBURN

CAUSES: Malfunction of lower esophageal sphincter, allowing stomach acid to rise into esophagus

SYMPTOMS: Hot, burning feeling in chest thirty minutes to one hour after eating, sour taste in mouth, sore throat, hoarseness

DURATION: Several minutes

TREATMENTS: Avoidance of dietary and lifestyle factors (tobacco, excessive alcohol, fatty foods, chocolate, caffeine), medications (*e.g.*, antacids), surgery

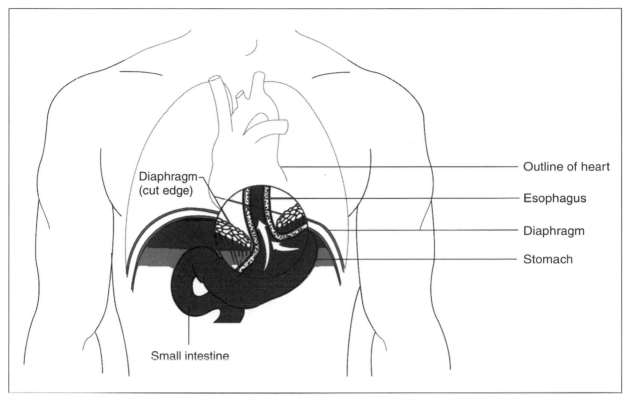

Diaphragm (cut edge)

Outline of heart

Esophagus

Diaphragm

Stomach

Small intestine

Heartburn is caused by a reflux of stomach acid into the esophagus shortly after eating.

very high concentrations in the stomach, where it aids digestion. Contrary to popular belief, most people who suffer from heartburn do not produce too much acid. Rather, they have a malfunction of the lower esophageal sphincter (LES), a ring of muscle between the stomach and the esophagus. Except when food is being swallowed, the LES stays closed. This keeps acid confined to the stomach. If the LES remains open, or if it is weakened, then stomach acid can travel freely to the esophagus and irritate its inner lining, resulting in heartburn.

Heartburn is described as a hot, burning feeling in the chest. It usually occurs thirty minutes to one hour after eating and lasts for several minutes. It is often worsened by lying down or bending over and is improved by standing up. Other associated symptoms may include a sour taste in the mouth, sore throat, or hoarseness. Some patients develop a dry cough as a result of acid irritating the throat. Heartburn must be distinguished from more ominous causes of chest pain, including a heart attack or other heart-related chest pain. Usually, chest pain attributable to such causes becomes worse with exertion, while heartburn should not.

TREATMENT AND THERAPY

The initial therapy for heartburn includes elimination of dietary and lifestyle factors that weaken the LES: tobacco, excessive alcohol, fatty foods, chocolate, and caffeine. Medications such as calcium-channel blockers and nitrates can also worsen heartburn, but they should not be discontinued without consulting a physician. It has been suggested that avoiding late-night meals and elevating the head of the bed with blocks underneath the headboard can improve heartburn, especially if symptoms occur mostly at nighttime. Occasional heartburn can be treated with over-the-counter antacids or medications such as ranitidine, which reduces acid production. If symptoms do not improve, then prescription medications are also available.

Surgery to reinforce the LES, called a Nissen fundoplication, is another option. Although results are excellent, patients often must take acid-suppressive medications after the procedure. Heartburn that is persistent or accompanied by trouble swallowing, weight loss, or bleeding requires more thorough investigation, as with endoscopy, to exclude the possibility of cancer or other serious medical conditions.

—Ahmad Kamal, M.D.

See also Acid reflux disease; Caffeine; Chest; Digestion; Gastroenterology; Gastroenterology, pediatric; Gastrointestinal disorders; Gastrointestinal system; Indigestion; Nausea and vomiting; Pain; Stress; Stress reduction; Ulcer surgery; Ulcers; Vagotomy.

FOR FURTHER INFORMATION:

Braunwald, Eugene, et al., eds. *Harrison's Principles of Internal Medicine.* 15th ed. New York: McGraw-Hill, 2001.

Cheskin, Lawrence J., and Brian E. Lacy. *Healing Heartburn.* Baltimore: Johns Hopkins University Press, 2002.

Minocha, Anil, and Christine Adamec. *How to Stop Heartburn: Simple Ways to Heal Heartburn and Acid Reflux.* New York: John Wiley & Sons, 2001.

HEAT EXHAUSTION AND HEAT STROKE
DISEASE/DISORDER

ANATOMY OR SYSTEM AFFECTED: Blood vessels, circulatory system, skin

SPECIALTIES AND RELATED FIELDS: Critical care, emergency medicine, family practice, internal medicine, sports medicine

DEFINITION: Heat-related illnesses in which the body temperature rises to dangerous levels and cannot be controlled through normal mechanisms, such as sweating.

CAUSES AND SYMPTOMS

The human body is well equipped to maintain a nearly constant internal body temperature. In fact, the body temperature of human beings is usually controlled so closely that it rarely leaves a very narrow range of 36.1 to 37.8 degrees Celsius (97 to 100 degrees Fahrenheit) regardless of how much heat the body is producing or what the environmental temperature may be. Humans maintain a constant temperature so that the millions of biochemical reactions in the body remain at an optimal rate. An increase in body temperature of only 1 degree Celsius will cause these reactions to move about 10 percent faster. As internal temperatures rise, however, brain function becomes slower because important proteins and enzymes lose their ability to operate effectively. Most adults will go into convulsions when their temperature reaches 41 degrees Celsius (106 degrees Fahrenheit), and 43 degrees Celsius (110 degrees Fahrenheit) is usually fatal.

A special region of the brain known as the hypothalamus regulates body temperature. The hypothalamus

detects the temperature of the blood much like a thermostat detects room temperature. When the body (and hence the blood) becomes too warm, the hypothalamus activates heat-loss mechanisms. Most excess heat is lost through the skin by the radiation of heat and the evaporation of sweat. To promote this heat loss, blood vessels in the skin dilate (open up) to carry more blood to the skin. Heat from the warm blood is then lost to the cooler air. If the increase in blood flow to the skin is not enough, then sweat glands are stimulated to produce and secrete large amounts of sweat. The process, called perspiration, is an efficient means of ridding the body of excess heat as long as the humidity is not too high. In fact, at 60 percent humidity, evaporation of sweat from the skin stops. When the body cannot dissipate enough heat, heat exhaustion and heat stroke may occur.

Heat exhaustion is the most prevalent heat-related illness. It commonly occurs in individuals who have exercised or worked in high temperatures for long periods of time. These people have usually not ingested adequate amounts of fluid. Over time, the patient loses fluid through sweating and respiration, which decreases the amount of fluid in the blood. Because the body is trying to reduce its temperature, blood has been shunted to the skin and away from vital internal organs. This reaction, in combination with a reduced blood volume, causes the patient to go into mild shock. Common signs and symptoms of heat exhaustion include cool, moist skin that may appear either red or pale; headache; nausea; dizziness; and exhaustion. If heat exhaustion is not recognized and treated, it can lead to life-threatening heat stroke.

Heat stroke occurs when the body is unable to eradicate the excess heat as rapidly as it develops. Thus, body temperature begins to rise. Sweating stops because the water content of the blood decreases. The loss of evaporative cooling causes the body temperature to continue rising rapidly, soon reaching a level that can cause organ damage. In particular, the brain, heart, and kidneys may begin to fail until the patient experiences convulsions, coma, and even death. Therefore, heat stroke is a serious medical emergency which must be recognized and treated immediately. The signs and symptoms of heat stroke include high body temperature (41 degrees Celsius or 106 degrees Fahrenheit); loss of consciousness; hot, dry skin; rapid pulse; and quick, shallow breathing.

TREATMENT AND THERAPY

As with most illnesses, prevention is the best medicine

INFORMATION ON HEAT EXHAUSTION AND HEAT STROKE

CAUSES: Dehydration
SYMPTOMS: For heat exhaustion, cool and moist skin that appears either red or pale, headache, nausea, dizziness, exhaustion; for heat stroke, cessation of perspiration, hot and dry skin, rapid pulse, quick and shallow breathing
DURATION: Acute
TREATMENTS: Cooling of body, replacement of body fluids, treatment of shock, emergency resuscitation

ministration because the patient is usually unable to drink as a result of convulsions or confusion and may even be unconscious. Once the body temperature has been brought back to normal, the patient is usually hospitalized and watched for complications. With early diagnosis and treatment, 80 to 90 percent of previously healthy people will survive.

—*Matthew Berria, Ph.D.*

See also Critical care; Critical care, pediatric; Dehydration; Emergency medicine; Fever; Hyperthermia and hypothermia; Resuscitation; Shock; Unconsciousness.

FOR FURTHER INFORMATION:

Browner, Bruce, Lenworth M. Jacobs, and Andrew N. Pollack, eds. *Emergency Care and Transportation of the Sick and Injured.* Rev. 7th ed. Rosemont, Ill.: American Academy of Orthopaedic Surgeons, 1999. Covers soft tissue injuries. Offers graphic photographs of actual injuries and discusses care and management. This text is often used in the training of emergency medical technicians, yet chapters are easily understood by the nonmedical layperson.

Clayman, Charles B., ed. *The American Medical Association Encyclopedia of Medicine.* New York: Random House, 1994. A concise presentation of numerous medical terms and illnesses. A good general reference.

Hales, Dianne. *An Invitation to Health.* 10th ed. Belmont, Calif.: Wadsworth Thomson Learning, 2003. This text should be read by anyone who wishes an overview of health topics.

Hill, James A., ed. *AMA Handbook of First Aid and Emergency Care.* 3d rev. ed. New York: Random House, 2000. Provides a listing of injuries, illnesses, and medical emergencies accompanied by easy-to-follow instructions and illustrations.

McArdle, William, Frank I. Katch, and Victor L. Katch. *Exercise Physiology: Energy, Nutrition, and Human Performance.* 5th ed. Philadelphia: Lippincott Williams & Wilkins, 2001. A wide ranging text on exercise and the human body, covering topics such as nutrition, energy transfer, exercise training, systems of energy delivery and utilization, enhancement of energy capacity, the effect of environmental stress, and the effect of exercise on successful aging and disease prevention.

Marieb, Elaine N. *Human Anatomy and Physiology.* 6th ed. Redwood City, Calif.: Benjamin/Cummings, 2003. Nonscientists at the advanced high school

for heat exhaustion and heat stroke. When exercising in hot weather, people should wear loose-fitting, lightweight clothing and drink plenty of fluids. When individuals are not prepared to avoid heat-related illness, however, rapid treatment may save their lives. When emergency medical personnel detect signs and symptoms of sudden heat-induced illness, they attempt to do three major things: cool the body, replace body fluids, and minimize shock.

For heat exhaustion, the initial treatment should be to place the patient in a cool place, such as a bathtub filled with cool (not cold) water. The conscious patient is given water or fruit drinks, sometimes containing salt, to replace body fluids. Occasionally, intravenous fluids must be given to return blood volume to normal in a more direct way. Hospitalization of the patient may be necessary to be sure that the body is able to regulate body heat appropriately. Almost all patients treated quickly and effectively will not advance to heat stroke. The activity that placed the patient in danger should be discontinued until one is sure all symptoms have disappeared and steps have been taken to prevent a future episode of heat exhaustion.

Heat stroke requires urgent medical attention, or the high body temperature will cause irreparable damage and often death. Body temperature must be reduced rapidly. With the patient in a cool environment, the clothing is removed and the skin sprinkled with water and cooled by fanning. Contrary to popular belief, rubbing alcohol should not be used, as it can cause closure of the skin's pores. Ice packs are often placed behind the neck and under the armpits and groin. At these sites, large blood vessels come close to the skin and are capable of carrying cooled blood to the internal organs. Body fluid must be replaced quickly by intravenous ad-level or above will be able to understand this fine textbook. It includes a complete glossary, index, pronunciation guide, and other helpful features.

HEEL SPUR REMOVAL
PROCEDURE

ANATOMY OR SYSTEM AFFECTED: Bones, feet, musculoskeletal system

SPECIALTIES AND RELATED FIELDS: General surgery, orthopedics, podiatry

DEFINITION: The surgical removal of a heel spur, a hard, bony growth on the heel.

INDICATIONS AND PROCEDURES

Heel spurs, also known as calcaneal spurs, are hard, bony growths on the heel bone. Pain and tenderness in the sole of the foot under the heel bone are common first indicators of this condition. Painful heel spurs can cause difficulty in walking and standing. Running, jogging, and prolonged standing often contribute to their development, especially when unpadded shoes are worn. When efforts to alleviate pain, such as activity modification and the use of shoes with cushioned heels, have been exhausted, it may be necessary for the spur to be surgically removed.

Most heel spur removal operations are performed at outpatient surgical facilities. Before the operation, blood and urine studies are conducted, and X rays are taken of both feet. Local or spinal anesthetics are administered. The surgeon, orthopedist, or podiatrist conducting the operation will choose a convenient site to make an incision, usually over the spur. Using special instruments, the heel spur is carved free and removed. The opening in the skin is closed with sutures. Barring complications, the sutures can be removed ten to fourteen days later. After the surgery, additional blood studies are taken, and laboratory examination of the removed tissue is performed.

USES AND COMPLICATIONS

Heel spurs form as a result of hard pounding or prolonged stress on the heel of the foot. Shock-absorbing soles in shoes and orthopedic inserts that cushion hard blows to the heel during vigorous exercise can help prevent and aid in recovery from heel spur operations. Following a removal operation, vigorous exercise can be resumed in approximately three months.

Clean cloths or tissues can be pressed against the wound for ten minutes if bleeding occurs within the first twenty-four hours after the surgery. The scar from the incision will recede gradually. Although it is important to keep the foot clean, the wound must be kept dry between baths. For the first two or three days after surgery, the wound should be covered with a dry bandage. Complications associated with heel spur removal surgery can include excessive bleeding and surgical wound infection, which should be examined by a doctor.

—*Jason Georges*

See also Bone disorders; Bones and the skeleton; Feet; Foot disorders; Lower extremities; Orthopedic surgery; Orthopedics; Podiatry.

FOR FURTHER INFORMATION:

Copeland, Glenn, and Stan Solomon. *The Foot Doctor.* Emmaus, Pa.: Rodale Press, 1986.

Currey, John D. *Bones: Structures and Mechanics.* Princeton, N.J.: Princeton University Press, 2002.

Lippert, Frederick G., and Sigvard T. Hansen. *Foot and Ankle Disorders: Tricks of the Trade.* New York: Thieme, 2003.

Lorimer, Donald L., ed. *Neale's Common Foot Disorders: Diagnosis and Management.* Rev. 6th ed. New York: Churchill Livingstone, 2001.

Shangold, Jules, and Frank Greenberg. *Opportunities in Podiatric Medicine.* Skokie, Ill.: VGM Career Horizons, 1982.

Van De Graaff, Kent M., and Stuart I. Fox. *Concepts of Human Anatomy and Physiology.* 5th ed. Dubuque, Iowa: Wm. C. Brown, 2000.

HEIMLICH MANEUVER
PROCEDURE

ANATOMY OR SYSTEM AFFECTED: Chest, lungs, mouth, neck, respiratory system, throat

SPECIALTIES AND RELATED FIELDS: Emergency medicine

DEFINITION: An emergency technique used to prevent suffocation when the airway becomes blocked.

INDICATIONS AND PROCEDURES

The Heimlich maneuver is an emergency technique, introduced in 1974 by Dr. Henry J. Heimlich, that guides a rescuer through a set of manipulative procedures to prevent suffocation when a victim's airway (windpipe) becomes blocked by food, water, or other foreign material. The maneuver lifts the diaphragm and forces enough air from the lungs to create an artificial cough. This cough intends to move the obstructive foreign body from the windpipe in order to resume normal and functional breathing (ventilation).

The Heimlich maneuver should be performed only if a choking victim cannot speak, cough, or breathe. Several indications may signal such a situation: frantic gestures to the throat, a face that turns blue in color because of lack of oxygen, and the production of loud noises in an attempt to take in breaths of air.

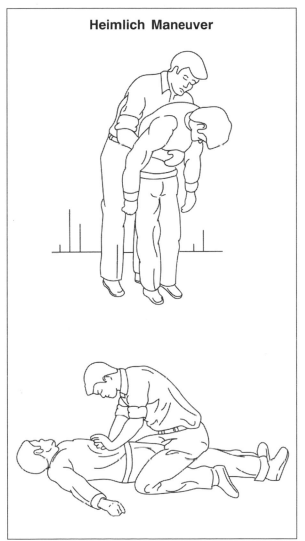

Heimlich Maneuver

The Heimlich maneuver is ideally performed on a standing or seated victim who has indicated consent that this maneuver be performed by nodding or another gesture of affirmation; if unconscious, the victim may be lying on his or her back, and abdominal thrusts are administered using the heel of the hand. Note: The illustration depicts only part of the procedure, which is not fully detailed above; for full information on the protocols for first aid for persons with obstructed airways, such as CPR, refer to the American Heart Association's Heartsaver Manual, *which is periodically updated.*

Before attempting the Heimlich maneuver, permission in the form of an affirmative nod or gesture should be given by a conscious victim to the intended administrator of the maneuver. When performing the technique, the rescuer is usually positioned behind the sitting or standing victim, with his or her arms around the victim's waist. The rescuer makes a fist with one hand and places that hand, with the thumb toward the victim, just above the victim's navel or below the rib cage and above the waist. The free hand should clasp the fisted hand tightly. Then, in a series of sharp thrusts upward and inward, the rescuer attempts to develop enough air pressure in the airway to force the lodged foreign object back up the trachea. The procedure may have to be repeated several times before the foreign object is expelled. Once the airway is cleared, the victim should start coughing and/or regain normal breathing. In cases when breathing is not resumed, then cardiopulmonary resuscitation (CPR) may have to be administered. In more serious choking cases in which the airway is not cleared of the obstruction, a small incision to the windpipe called a tracheostomy may have to be completed.

USES AND COMPLICATIONS

In addition to choking victims, the Heimlich maneuver may be administered to asthmatics and drowning victims. While it can be performed on all people, modifications should be adapted when executed upon infants (it is not recommended for infants less than one year old), children, and very obese, pregnant, or unconscious adults. The Heimlich maneuver may also be self-administered.

The Heimlich maneuver is one of the best courses to follow for the prevention of asphyxiation during a choking episode, but it does come with several precautions. In addition to modifications depending on the age and situation of the victim, incorrect administration of the Heimlich maneuver by incorporating techniques such as chest thrusts, back slaps, and abdominal thrusts can cause bruised ribs, broken bones, damage to internal organs, and even death. If all the guidelines are effectively followed by the administrator, however, then the victim should feel little or no bodily discomfort and should recover quickly.

—*Nicholas Lanzieri*

See also Asphyxiation; Asthma; Cardiopulmonary resuscitation (CPR); Choking; Emergency medicine; Emergency medicine, pediatric; Lungs; Pulmonary medicine; Pulmonary medicine, pediatric; Respiration; Resuscitation.

FOR FURTHER INFORMATION:

"Heimlich Maneuver." In *Everything You Need to Know About Medical Treatments*. Springhouse, Pa.: Springhouse, 1996.

Tintinalli, Judith E., Gabor D. Kelen, and J. Stephan Stapczynski, eds. *Emergency Medicine: A Comprehensive Study Guide*. 6th ed. New York: McGraw Hill, 2004.

White, R. D. "Foreign Body Airway Obstruction: Considerations in 1985." *Circulation* 74, no. 6, pt. 2 (1986): IV60-62.

HEMATOLOGY

SPECIALTY

ANATOMY OR SYSTEM AFFECTED: Blood, circulatory system, immune system, liver, musculoskeletal system, spleen

SPECIALTIES AND RELATED FIELDS: Cardiology, cytology, forensic medicine, genetics, immunology, oncology, pathology, serology, vascular medicine

DEFINITION: The study of the blood, including its normal constituents, and such blood disorders as anemia, leukemia, and hemophilia.

KEY TERMS:

anemia: a condition characterized by a deficiency of red blood cells or hemoglobin

bone marrow: the soft substance that fills the cavities within bones and that is the site of blood cell production

clotting factors: chemicals circulating in the blood which are necessary for the process of blood clotting

hematologist: one who specializes in the study of blood, its components and disorders

hemoglobin: the iron-containing molecule within red blood cells responsible for oxygen and carbon dioxide transport

leukemia: a condition characterized by the presence of numerous immature white blood cells in the circulating blood

plasma: the fluid portion of blood, containing water, proteins, minerals, nutrients, hormones, and wastes

platelets: specialized cell fragments that initiate blood clotting

red blood cell: a flexible, biconcave blood cell that contains hemoglobin

white blood cell: one of several types of colorless, large blood cells that work together to combat infections

SCIENCE AND PROFESSION

Most branches of medical science study a particular organ that is made of specific tissues and is located in a definite part of the body. Hematology is unique because its subject, the blood, is a liquid tissue constantly in motion and therefore in constant contact with every other tissue and organ of the body.

It has been estimated that blood travels about 16 kilometers (10 miles) an hour. It takes six seconds for blood to travel from the heart to the lungs, about eight seconds from the heart to the brain, and only fourteen seconds from the heart all the way to the toes. Hematologists studying these shifting currents of the blood are able to detect patterns that allow the early discovery of many disorders of the blood itself and of the organs that it supplies.

Blood is a complex material composed of approximately 55 percent plasma and 45 percent cells, which are also called formed elements. The plasma, or liquid portion of the blood, is about 90 percent water and 10 percent substances dissolved or suspended in that water. Part of that 10 percent consists of a remarkable array of substances, including nutrients, gases, salts, wastes, and hormones being transported around the body. The other, larger part of the 10 percent is another remarkable array—plasma proteins such as fibrinogen, albumin, and globulins with a great diversity of functions to accomplish. The modern hematologist's ability to measure and monitor all these plasma components precisely has greatly aided physicians in the treatment of innumerable diseases.

Beyond an analysis of the ingredients of the plasma, hematologists focus on the normal and abnormal conditions of the blood's cells. An individual has 25 trillion red blood cells; 10 million of these cells die or are destroyed each second, and 200 billion new ones need to be made each day. Hematologists discovered that these tiny, biconcave discs packed with hemoglobin transport the vast majority of the oxygen needed constantly by every cell of every organ for energy production.

Before each red blood cell is released from the bone marrow where it is produced, the bulk of its living nucleus is expelled. A small amount of nuclear material remains, as a fine network, in these young cells called reticulocytes. The number of reticulocytes released into the blood is an indication of the activity of the bone marrow. Hematologists use this number in both the diagnosis and the assessment of the response to treatment, in conditions such as the various forms of anemia.

Not only the total number and maturity but also the shape, diameter, and flexibility of red blood cells can give the hematologist important information. For years, such information was gathered by laborious manual methods. Electronic counters can now obtain this information with great speed and even greater accuracy.

Hematologists can also gauge the effectiveness of red blood cells by seeing how much hemoglobin they contain. The amount of this red pigment present—and therefore functioning—was once estimated by being matched against progressively darker-colored glass "standards." Now this figure too is accurately perceived using a precise, photoelectric technique.

Another useful test is called the packed cell volume (PCV) test. It not only reveals the proportion of the red blood cells to the plasma but also allows the calculation of their average size and their hemoglobin content.

An equally common blood investigation is the erythrocyte sedimentation rate (ESR). The erythrocytes, the term that hematologists use to describe red blood cells, normally fall slowly down through the plasma in a standard tube. A very rapid sedimentation rate demonstrates a disturbance in the plasma proteins that may be very dangerous. Usually, the faster they settle out, the sicker the patient, with a wide variety of inflammations as possible causes.

Beginning in the middle of the twentieth century, an increasing number of radioactive tests were developed by which hematologists can assess more accurately total blood volume and the survival time of red blood cells or platelets in circulation. Assessing total volume is important. A loss of more than 1 liter (2 pints) is quite dangerous because it can cause a total collapse of the blood vessels.

This reaction gives a clue about the importance of a second kind of blood cell, the platelet, and its work in stopping bleeding. When a blood vessel is first cut, platelets (or thrombocytes) rush to the site. They swell into irregular shapes, become sticky, clog the cut, and create a plug. The smallest blood vessels rupture hundreds of times a day, and platelets alone are able to make the necessary repairs. If the cut is too large, platelets—which are like sponges filled with diverse and biologically active compounds—disintegrate. Their ingredients react with numerous clotting factors in the plasma to initiate clot formation.

Hematologists check blood samples carefully to ascertain whether their patients possess the normal number of platelets—more than a trillion for the average adult. Since platelets only live about ten days, it is necessary to monitor those patients who exhibit significantly low amounts of these cells. If their bone marrow is not constantly replacing these platelets, these pa-

tients might bleed to death from a small cut. On the other hand, doctors must monitor any tendency toward the formation of too many platelets because of the danger of thrombophlebitis, the blockage of a vein by a blood clot.

As with red blood cells, the widespread use of electronic counters has made the measurement of the numbers of platelets and of white blood cells (the third type of blood cell) rapid, efficient, and extremely accurate.

White blood cells are hardest to count because they are the least numerous, making up only 0.1 percent of the total blood. Their number also varies dramatically from 4,000 to 11,000 per cubic centimeter of blood, according to the individual, the time of day, the outside temperature, and many other ordinary factors.

Hematologists can deduce the degree of maturity of circulating white blood cells from the appearance of their nuclei. There are five kinds of white blood cells (or leukocytes), whose normal proportions in the blood are quite specific and change drastically if an infection is present. The number of monocytes, for example, is normally 5 percent. If typhus, tuberculosis, or Rocky Mountain spotted fever organisms are present, the number will rise to 20 or 30 percent. The normal 60 percentage of neutrophils will increase to 75 percent or more in the presence of pneumonia or appendicitis.

DIAGNOSTIC AND TREATMENT TECHNIQUES

Blood to be tested by a hematologist is withdrawn from a vein. A thin smear or film of the blood is placed on a glass slide and stained to bring out identifying features more prominently. The microscope then reveals the proportion of different cell types and any variation from the normally expected amount. This examination alone may give an immediate diagnosis of a particular blood disorder. For example, a red blood cell count that is less than 4 million or more than 6 million per cubic centimeter of blood is considered unusual and is probably an indication of disease.

It often becomes necessary to study not only the circulating blood cells but also the original cells within the bone marrow which produce the erythrocytes, thrombocytes, and leukocytes. The hematologist must then use a long, thin needle to remove a sample of the marrow from within the tibia (shinbone) of a child or the pelvis (hipbone) or sternum (breastbone) of an adult. This test can provide a reliable diagnosis of a specific blood disorder.

The blood disorders that hematologists are routinely called on to diagnose and treat include diseases of the red blood cells, white blood cells, platelets, and clotting factors and failures of correct blood formation.

The disorders involving a deficiency of red blood cells or their hemoglobin are called anemias. There are many types of anemia, which are named, distinguished, and treated according to their causes. Some anemias exist because of a lack of the materials needed to build red blood cells: iron, vitamin B$_{12}$, and folic acid. Other anemias are caused by a shortening of the life span of red blood cells or by inherited abnormalities in hemoglobin. Still others are attributable to chronic infections or cancer.

Iron-deficiency anemia is by far the most common; it is particularly prevalent in women of childbearing age and in children. In young children who are growing rapidly, constant increase in muscle mass and blood volume will cause anemia unless a high enough level of iron is present in the diet. All women between puberty and the menopause lose iron with the menstrual flow of blood and, therefore, are always prone to iron-deficiency anemia. A pregnant woman is even more likely to develop this condition; iron is literally removed from her body and transferred through the placenta to the developing fetus.

The symptoms of iron-deficiency anemia may include a reduced capacity for physical work, paleness, breathlessness, increased pulse and, possibly, a sore tongue. The hematologist witnessing small, misshapen red blood cells deficient in hemoglobin will recommend an increase in iron in the diet. The hematologist will also send this patient for various gastrointestinal tests because of the possibility of internal bleeding or failure of the intestine to absorb iron properly.

Another class of anemias involves a lack of vitamin B$_{12}$ or of folic acid. Without the help of these two substances, the bone marrow cannot build red blood cells correctly. These anemias are diagnosed when the hematologist finds bizarre cells called megaloblasts in the patient's bone marrow. Both vitamin B$_{12}$ and folic acid can be added to the diet or given by injection. The problem may stem, however, not from an insufficient amount of vitamin B$_{12}$ in the diet but from the inability of the stomach lining to produce a substance called intrinsic factor. In this case, the patient will never be able to absorb this vitamin properly and is said to suffer from pernicious anemia.

Those anemias characterized by the early and too frequent destruction of red blood cells are grouped together as hemolytic anemias. Some of these disorders are acquired, while others are inherited. In both types,

hemoglobin from the destroyed red blood cells can be detected by the hematologist in the plasma, the urine, or the skin, where it causes the yellowing called jaundice.

Because the many types of anemia are so common, hematologists find that the diagnosis and treatment of these diseases form a large part of their everyday practice. All types of leukemia, on the other hand, are quite rare. They are caused by a change in one kind of primitive blood cell in the bone marrow. The result is uncontrolled growth of these cells, which do not mature but which invade the blood as badly functioning cells. Leukemia is often thought of as cancer of the blood.

Although it is not known what causes leukemia in a particular person, the disease seems to be associated with certain factors, including injury by chemicals or radiation, viruses, and genetic predisposition. Many cases of acute leukemia occur either in children who are under fourteen or in adults who are between fifty-five and seventy-five years of age. In children, it is almost always a disorder in the bone marrow cells that produce the white blood cells, called lymphocytes. This disorder is called acute lymphoblastic leukemia, or ALL. Adult leukemia usually occurs in the bone marrow that forms some other type of white blood cell and is called acute nonlymphoblastic leukemia, or ANLL.

Hematologists diagnose both conditions by their shared symptoms: abnormal bone marrow tissue and a lack of normal white blood cells and platelets in the circulating blood. The patient will often have been referred to the hematologist because of an uncontrollable infection (from a lack of normal white blood cells) or uncontrollable bleeding (from a lack of normal platelets). In both children and adults, anemia usually accompanies acute leukemia because defective bone marrow is not able to produce red blood cells properly either.

Less rare than acute leukemia are the various chronic types. One type called chronic granulocytic leukemia (CGL) occurs most often after the age of fifty. Unfortunately, its early symptoms are few and vague, so that the disease may have progressed greatly before its presence would even be suspected. By such time, an enormous enlargement of the spleen, along with elevations in both white blood cell and platelet counts, can be noted.

Two stages are usually seen in chronic granulocytic leukemia. Early treatment can relieve all symptoms, shrink the spleen, and return all blood cells to normal values. Eventually, however, the leukemic condition recurs, and the patient usually lives an average of only three years. Bone marrow transplantation from a suitable donor or a more recent process by which one's own marrow is removed, irradiated, and returned to the bones have become the increasingly common recommendations of the hematologist confronted with this condition.

A second type of chronic leukemia is known as chronic lymphatic leukemia (CLL). Unlike most of the other leukemias, CLL has no known cause, but it is most often found in male patients over the age of forty. Often quite symptomless, it is only discovered by chance. The hematologist is able to diagnose CLL by an increased proportion of abnormal white blood cells present in the blood. Surprisingly, this form of leukemia can vary from a case that remains symptomless, with the patient surviving twenty years or more, to a rapidly progressing case with increasing anemia and constant infections.

The third major class of disorders diagnosed and treated by hematologists consists of those involving abnormal bleeding. The diagnosis is quite simple. The hematologist notes whether bleeding from a tiny puncture in the ear lobe stops within three minutes, as it should. If the bleeding does not stop, the determination of the cause may be difficult: It may involve too few platelets or abnormal or missing clotting factors.

Very precise tests of an increasingly sophisticated nature are now used by hematologists to determine whether a bleeding disorder is attributable to inheritance (as with hemophilia), a vitamin K deficiency, or a side effect of medication or is secondary to a type of leukemia.

PERSPECTIVE AND PROSPECTS

That blood and the vessels that carry it are important to life and health was evident even to ancient peoples. Around 500 B.C.E., Alcmaeon, a Greek, was the first to discover that arteries and veins are different types of vessels. A century later, Hippocrates observed that blood, left to stand, settles into three distinct layers. The top or largest layer is a clear, straw-colored liquid that is now called plasma. The middle layer is a narrow white band that is now known to contain white blood cells. The bottom, quite large layer, he observed to be red; it contains the cells that are now called red blood cells.

Very little else of value seems to have been learned about the blood until the seventeenth century, which witnessed many discoveries in medical science. In 1628, William Harvey, an English doctor, demonstrated scientific evidence of circulation. He found proof of a circular route and of the purpose of circulation. By 1661, the Italian scientist Marcello Malpighi

reported seeing the tiny vessels called capillaries in the lungs of the frog.

Another giant step toward modern hematology occurred in the 1660's because of the efforts of Richard Lower of England and Jean-Baptiste Denis of France. Almost simultaneously, they accomplished blood transfusions from dog to dog and, soon after, from animal to human. Some transfusions were very successful; others were fatal to the patient. Almost 250 years would pass before the reason for success or failure would be learned.

In 1688, the Dutch scientist Antoni van Leeuwenhoek was able to describe and measure red blood cells accurately. He also observed that they changed shape to squeeze through tiny blood vessels. It was almost a hundred years later, in the 1770's, that Joseph Priestley, in England, found that the oxygen in the air changed dark blood from the veins into a bright red color. Only in the 1850's did the German researcher Otto Funke find within those red blood cells the compound hemoglobin, which is affected by the presence or absence of oxygen.

Although the first research on blood clotting, by William Hewson, occurred in 1768, the disease called hemophilia, or the failure of the blood to clot, was not described until 1803, by John Otto.

In the United States in the early 1900's, Karl Landsteiner discovered why certain blood can be safely transfused: the existence of the ABO blood types. This renowned hematologist was still advancing his science forty years later when he discovered the Rh system of blood types.

Another renowned hematologist, Max Perutz, worked steadily from 1939 to 1978 to understand fully the structure and function of the hemoglobin molecule. The 1940's had seen another breakthrough when Edwin Cohn, another American, discovered how to separate and purify the various plasma proteins. His work gave fellow hematologists the tools to study individual plasma components in order to learn the exact role of each in the blood. Since that time, scores of hematologists have so advanced this medical science that blood seems to have yielded most of its secrets. The ability of hematologists to treat so many types of anemia, leukemia, and other blood disorders successfully is the fruit of their tireless work.

—*Grace D. Matzen*

See also Acquired immunodeficiency syndrome (AIDS); Anemia; Bleeding; Blood and blood disorders; Blood testing; Bone marrow transplantation; Cholesterol; Circulation; Cytology; Cytopathology; Dialysis; Disseminated intravascular coagulation (DIC); Fluids and electrolytes; Forensic pathology; Hematology, pediatric; Hemolytic disease of the newborn; Hemophilia; Histiocytosis; Histology; Hodgkin's disease; Host-defense mechanisms; Hypercholesterolemia; Hyperlipidemia; Immune system; Immunology; Infection; Ischemia; Jaundice; Kidney disorders; Kidneys; Laboratory tests; Leukemia; Liver; Lymphadenopathy and lymphoma; Lymphatic system; Nephrology; Nephrology, pediatric; Rh factor; Septicemia; Serology; Sickle cell disease; Thalassemia; Thrombocytopenia; Thrombolytic therapy and TPA; Thrombosis and thrombus; Transfusion; Vascular medicine; Vascular system; Von Willebrand's disease; Wiskott-Aldrich syndrome.

FOR FURTHER INFORMATION:

Avraham, Regina. *The Circulatory System.* Philadelphia: Chelsea House, 2000. Contains a brief but excellent description of the blood: its many components and their diverse functions. Includes a useful glossary and a lengthy appendix listing other sources of information about blood and circulatory disorders.

Bick, Roger L. *Disorders of Thrombosis and Hemostasis: Clinical and Laboratory Practice.* 3d ed. Philadelphia: Lippincott Williams & Wilkins, 2002. An excellent introduction to the diagnosis and management of clotting and bleeding disorders.

Hackett, Earle. *Blood: The Biology, Pathology, and Mythology of the Body's Most Important Fluid.* New York: Saturday Review Press, 1973. This old but classic and, therefore, still relevant volume contains an entertaining but nevertheless factual history of the study of blood from the viewpoint of many peoples in many cultures, from ancient to modern times.

Lichtman, Marshall L., et al. *Williams Manual of Hematology.* 6th ed. New York: McGraw-Hill, 2002. An accessible handbook that covers the pathogenetic, diagnostic, and therapeutic essentials of blood cell and coagulation protein disorders.

Rodak, Bernadette. *Hematology.* 2d ed. New York: Elsevier Science, 2002. A comprehensive textbook covering all aspects of hematology and hemostasis.

Tortora, Gerard J. *Introduction to the Human Body: The Essentials of Anatomy and Physiology.* 6th ed. New York: Wiley, 2003. A general textbook of anatomy and physiology. Contains comprehensive information about the blood, the vessels in which it travels, the heart that pumps it, and the relationship of blood to immunity.

HEMATOLOGY, PEDIATRIC
SPECIALTY

ANATOMY OR SYSTEM AFFECTED: Blood, bones, circulatory system, immune system, liver, musculoskeletal system, spleen

SPECIALTIES AND RELATED FIELDS: Cytology, genetics, immunology, neonatology, pathology, pediatrics, perinatology, serology, vascular medicine

DEFINITION: The diagnosis and treatment of blood disorders in infants and children.

KEY TERMS:

anemia: a red blood cell deficiency caused by a decrease in hemoglobin or red cell production, an increase in cell destruction, or blood loss

erythrocytes: red blood cells

hematology: the scientific, medical study of blood and blood-forming tissues

hematopoiesis: the production of red and white cells and platelets, which occurs mainly in bone marrow

hemorrhage: the loss of a large amount of blood in a short period of time

leukemia: the presence of an increased number of leukocytes in the blood, with the specific disorder classified according to the predominant proliferating cells, the clinical course, and the duration of the disease

leukocytes: white blood cells

leukopenia: an abnormal decrease in white blood cells

neonate: a newborn infant

pediatric: pertaining to neonates, infants, and children up to the age of twelve

polycythemia: an abnormal increase in red blood cells

thrombocytes: platelets

venipuncture: a method of obtaining blood from a vein using a tourniquet, needle, and syringe

SCIENCE AND PROFESSION

Blood, the body's life-sustaining fluid, is composed of red and white cells and platelets floating in plasma. Blood transports oxygen from the lungs to the tissues; removes waste products such as carbon dioxide, urea, and lactic acid; transports hormones and nutrients; removes body heat from central to peripheral parts of the body; clots in order to seal hemorrhages; transports leukocytes and antibodies to fight injury and infection; and stores and circulates elements such as calcium and iron. The diagnosis of hematologic disorders requires the comparison of blood and bone marrow values to established reference ranges. These ranges can vary considerably during a child's growing years, with such important changes as polycythemia in the neonatal period followed by physiologic anemia of infancy, which is maximal at two and a half to three months.

Pediatric hematology involves the ongoing assessment of an infant's or child's blood and bone marrow. This specialty requires such skills as the identification of problems, the setting of goals, the use of appropriate interventions (including diet, teaching, and medication), and an evaluation of the outcome of this care. Routine blood screening involves the removal of blood by a medical laboratory phlebotomist using venipuncture in children and heel or finger stick in infants to assess the following: a complete coronary risk profile with lipid fractionation, a complete blood count (CBC), a chemistry 27 profile, an iron-deficiency profile, and diabetes mellitus screening.

A complete coronary risk profile with lipid fractionation is an assessment of total serum cholesterol, high-density lipoprotein cholesterol, low-density lipoprotein cholesterol, very-low-density lipoprotein cholesterol, total cholesterol/high-density lipoprotein cholesterol ratio, triglycerides, chylomicrons, and possibly apolipoproteins. A CBC involves an analysis of hemoglobin, hematocrit, and red and white blood cell counts with white blood cell differential, including granulocytes (neutrophils, eosinophils, and basophils) and agranulocytes (lymphocytes and monocytes). A chemistry 27 profile assesses important blood constituents such as iron and protein storage, uric acid, several electrolytes, and enzymes. An iron-deficiency profile includes measurements of total iron-binding capacity, percentage of transferrin saturation, and serum ferritin. Diabetes mellitus screening, an assessment of glucose and protein-bound glucose (indicative of the previous seven to fifteen days), is important because only an estimated one-half of all diabetics are diagnosed.

Some of the major manifestations of hematologic disease in infants and children are disorders in the function of red blood cells, white blood cells, or hemostasis. Red blood cell disorders include anemia caused by the inadequate production of erythrocytes and/or hemoglobin as a result of genetic disease or iron deficiency, anemia caused by excessive loss of erythrocytes as a result of hemorrhage or hemolytic problems, polycythemia, erythrocytosis, erythremia, and blood transfusion. Disorders of white blood cells include leukopenia, agranulocytosis, periodic neutropenia, Chediak-Higashi syndrome, and leukemias. Blood diseases associated with defects in hemostasis include disturbances in the mechanism for clotting, such as hemophilia, Von Willebrand's syndrome, deficiencies in factor II (prothrombin), factor XII deficiency, and disorders involving fibrinogen and fibrin; and defects in hemostasis in small vessels, such as thrombocytopenia, Aldrich's syndrome, and thrombopoietin deficiency.

DIAGNOSTIC AND TREATMENT TECHNIQUES

The diagnosis of pediatric hematological disorders begins with a routine blood chemistry analysis, leading to more specific tests and a medical history of the infant or child and family members to determine if the problem is congenital or acquired, chronic or episodic, and static or progressive. Iron deficiency (also called anemia) is probably the most common nutritional problem in the world today. Anemia decreases work capacity by restricting oxygen and carbon dioxide transport and reducing aerobic energy production via the inhibition of iron-dependent muscle enzymes. Therapy for anemia generally involves diet manipulation and medication but is highly variable and depends on the specific causative factors. Since the prevalence of anemia correlates strongly with socioeconomic status, screening intervals and therapy must be planned individually for each child. Up to 20 percent of children from poor homes may be anemic at one year of age, while only 4 percent of children from higher-income homes will be anemic. Anemia becomes less common between three and five years of age, thus diminishing the need for regular screening.

PERSPECTIVE AND PROSPECTS

Future research in pediatric hematology will probably include further investigation of reticulocytes, immature red blood cells that are larger than mature erythrocytes yet nonnucleated, that circulate in the blood for one to two days while maturing. Research into the causes of and prevention techniques for the development of anemia will continue to be a major focus.

Public health authorities have recommended routine screening of the entire newborn population for a variety of hereditary diseases, including acquired immunodeficiency syndrome (AIDS). This recommendation is likely to generate considerable controversy. Many states have recently required screening for phenylketonuria (PKU), a condition which can be toxic to brain tissue, even though it occurs in fewer than 1 in 16,000 neonates.

—*Daniel G. Graetzer, Ph.D.*

See also Acquired immunodeficiency syndrome (AIDS); Anemia; Bleeding; Blood and blood disorders; Blood testing; Bone marrow transplantation; Circulation; Cytology; Cytopathology; Dialysis; Disseminated intravascular coagulation (DIC); Fluids and electrolytes; Hematology; Hemolytic disease of the newborn; Hemophilia; Histiocytosis; Histology; Host-defense mechanisms; Immune system; Immunology; Infection; Ischemia; Jaundice; Kidney disorders; Kidneys; Laboratory tests; Leukemia; Liver; Lymphadenopathy and lymphoma; Lymphatic system; Nephrology, pediatric; Pediatrics; Rh factor; Septicemia; Serology; Sickle cell disease; Thalassemia; Thrombocytopenia; Transfusion; Vascular medicine; Vascular system; Von Willebrand's disease; Wiskott-Aldrich syndrome.

FOR FURTHER INFORMATION:

Keene, Nancy. *Childhood Leukemia: A Guide for Families, Friends and Caregivers*. 3d ed. Cambridge, Mass.: O'Reilly and Associates, 2002. Keene uses the story of her daughter's battle with leukemia as a vehicle to explore the physical and emotional impacts of the disease. Offers guidance on coping with procedures, hospitalizations, school, and associated social, emotional, and financial problems.

Kimball, Chad T. *Childhood Diseases and Disorders Sourcebook: Basic Consumer Health Information About Medical Problems Often Encountered in Pre-Adolescent Children*. Detroit: Omnigraphics, 2002. Offers basic facts about cancer, sickle cell disease, diabetes, and other chronic conditions in children and discusses frequently used diagnostic tests, surgeries, and medications. Long-term care for seriously ill children is also presented.

Nathan, David G., and Stuart H. Orkin, eds. *Nathan and Oski's Hematology of Infancy and Childhood*. Rev. 6th ed. Philadelphia: W. B. Saunders, 2003. This textbook will undoubtedly be useful to many readers not directly involved in clinical or research pediatric hematology. First, it provides basic scientists with a clinical perspective. Second, pediatric and adult subspecialists will occasionally need it to read about rare conditions, and it should be included in the reference collection of every library on adult hematology or general pediatrics.

Smith, C. H. *Smith's Blood Diseases of Infancy and Childhood*. Edited by Denis R. Miller et al. St. Louis: C. V. Mosby, 1978. A thorough text on all aspects of pediatric hematology. Includes bibliographical references and an index.

Wintrobe, M. M., et al. *Wintrobe's Clinical Hematology*. 11th ed. Philadelphia: Lea & Febiger, 2003. In-

cludes good information on laboratory hematology, with emphasis on interpretation, immunodiagnosis, flow cytometry, clusters of differentiation, cytogenetics, and molecular genetics.

HEMIPLEGIA

DISEASE/DISORDER

ANATOMY OR SYSTEM AFFECTED: Arms, brain, head, joints, legs, muscles, musculoskeletal system, nervous system, tendons

SPECIALTIES AND RELATED FIELDS: Exercise physiology, family practice, neurology, orthopedics, physical therapy

DEFINITION: Paralysis of one side of the body, usually caused by brain damage.

CAUSES AND SYMPTOMS

Hemiplegia is paralysis or partial paralysis of one side of the body, typically involving the leg, arm, and trunk. It is caused by damage or disease of the part of the brain that controls the motor nervous system. The damage may occur prior to birth, during birth, or after birth as a result of an accident, illness, or stroke. The most common cause is a cerebrovascular disease that leads to clotting of the cerebral arteries or bleeding from the diseased arterial wall, eventually producing a stroke. The site most often affected is the internal capsule, where packed nerve fibers descend from the cortex of the brain into the spinal cord.

Immediately after a stroke, the affected body parts are initially limp. In a few days or weeks, the limbs become stiff and spastic. Symptoms of hemiplegia can in-

---

INFORMATION ON HEMIPLEGIA

CAUSES: Brain damage or disease as a result of accident, illness, or stroke

SYMPTOMS: Paralysis on one side of body, muscle weakness and spasticity, poor balance, speech difficulties, epileptic seizures, visual field defects, emotional and behavioral problems, gait problems

DURATION: Long-term

TREATMENTS: Depends on severity; may include physical therapy, speech therapy, occupational therapy, braces or orthotics, electrical stimulation, drugs, Botox injections, surgery, acupuncture

clude paralysis on one side of the body, muscle weakness and spasticity, poor balance, speech difficulties, epileptic seizures, visual field defects, emotional and behavioral problems, and gait problems, including limping and toe drop. Increased energy expenditure results from compensatory adjustments during walking that produce abnormal movements of the body's center of gravity.

TREATMENT AND THERAPY

Treatments for hemiplegia are designed to improve strength and range of motion, increase bodily functions, and reduce or prevent spasticity. Long-term care is very important. Depending on the severity of the disorder, physical therapy, speech therapy, occupational therapy, braces or orthotics, electrical stimulation, drugs, Botox injections, and surgery may be used as corrective procedures. Acupuncture and electroacupuncture procedures may be promising treatments for hemiplegia. Children who suffer from hemiplegia may also receive special educational services to help improve specific learning difficulties caused by the disorder. Affected children should involve the weaker side of the body in everyday activities so that they become as two-sided as possible.

PERSPECTIVE AND PROSPECTS

The side of the body affected by hemiplegia depends on which side of the brain has been damaged. The left side of the brain controls the right side of the body, while the right side controls the left side of the body. Depending on which side of the body is affected, the disease is often referred to as right hemiplegia or left hemiplegia.

Childhood hemiplegia affects up to one child per one thousand. An associated rare neurological disorder, alternating hemiplegia of childhood (AHC), produces periodic transient attacks of hemiplegia that affect one side of the body or the other. An attack of AHC may last from a few minutes up to days. The attacks may alternate from one side of the body to the other. The symptoms are usually relieved with bed rest and proper sleep.

—*Alvin K. Benson, Ph.D.*

See also Brain; Brain disorders; Nervous system; Neurology; Neurology, pediatric; Paralysis; Paraplegia; Physical rehabilitation; Quadriplegia; Strokes.

FOR FURTHER INFORMATION:

Bobath, Berta. *Adult Hemiplegia: Evaluation and Treatment.* 3d ed. London: Heinemann Medical Books, 1999.

Davies, Patricia M. *Steps to Follow: The Comprehensive Treatment of Patients with Hemiplegia.* 2d ed. New York: Springer Verlag, 2000.

Spivak, Barney S., ed. *Evaluation and Management of Gait Disorders.* New York: Marcel Dekker, 1995.

HEMOCHROMATOSIS

DISEASE/DISORDER

ALSO KNOWN AS: Bronze diabetes

ANATOMY OR SYSTEM AFFECTED: Genitals, heart, liver, pancreas

SPECIALTIES AND RELATED FIELDS: Cardiology, endocrinology, gastroenterology, internal medicine

DEFINITION: A multisystem disease characterized by increased iron absorption and storage.

CAUSES AND SYMPTOMS

Iron is used by the body for various processes, such as making hemoglobin, the oxygen-carrying molecule in blood. Hemochromatosis is an inherited disorder characterized by the excessive absorption and accumulation of iron from the diet. This excess iron is deposited in various organs. Damage to these organs from years of iron accumulation results in the symptoms of hemochromatosis. The most commonly affected organs are the pancreas (causing diabetes), the skin (causing bronzelike skin pigmentation), the testes (causing loss of libido and erectile dysfunction), and the heart (causing abnormal heart rhythms or heart failure). The pituitary gland, which regulates sex hormones and metabolism, can also be affected. Although the liver is commonly involved as well, this usually results in mild abnormalities in blood tests of liver enzymes rather than liver failure. However, cirrhosis of the liver can occur, and these patients are at risk for developing liver

---

INFORMATION ON HEMOCHROMATOSIS

CAUSES: Genetic defect in iron production

SYMPTOMS: Damage to pancreas, skin, testes, and heart, causing diabetes mellitus, bronzelike skin pigmentation, loss of libido and erectile dysfunction, and abnormal heart rhythms or heart failure

DURATION: Chronic

TREATMENTS: Phlebotomy (blood removal) to create mild anemia

cancer. Unfortunately, most of the above warning symptoms occur late in the disease, after decades of iron accumulation and organ damage have already taken place.

TREATMENT AND THERAPY

Ideally, hemochromatosis should be detected and treated before the onset of symptoms. Screening for patients with a family history of this disease can be performed via blood tests, such as the iron saturation index. More recently, a genetic test for a common mutation that causes hemochromatosis has been developed. Liver biopsy is sometimes needed to confirm the diagnosis. Treatment consists of repeated phlebotomy, or the removal of blood. Typically one unit of blood is removed per week until the patient becomes mildly anemic. Hemochromatosis may require the removal of up to 150 units of blood over several years. Subsequently, phlebotomy is repeated every three to four months, and the patient's iron stores (ferritin) are monitored. If phlebotomy is started before liver cirrhosis develops, then many complications can be avoided.

PERSPECTIVE AND PROSPECTS

Hemochromatosis was initially described in 1865 as a triad of glucose in the urine, dark pigmentation of the skin, and liver cirrhosis. Research into the disease has resulted in tremendous advances in the understanding of iron metabolism. The gene responsible for hemochromatosis has been mapped to chromosome 6. Although the genetic defect is present in both men and women, men develop the disease much more often, since menstruation removes excess iron in women. A test to screen for one common mutation in this gene is available, but its usefulness is limited since several other mutations may cause the disease, especially in non-Caucasian ethnic groups.

—*Ahmad Kamal, M.D.*

See also Hematology; Hematology, pediatric; Liver disorders; Metabolism; Nephrology; Nephrology, pediatric.

FOR FURTHER INFORMATION:

Barton, James C., and Corwin Q. Edwards, eds. *Hemochromatosis: Genetics, Pathophysiology, Diagnosis, and Treatment*. New York: Cambridge University Press, 2000.

Burke, W., and P. D. Phatak. *Iron Disorders Institute Guide to Hemochromatosis*. Nashville: Cumberland House, 2001.

Parker, James N., and Philip M. Parker, eds. *The Official Patient's Sourcebook on Hemochromatosis*. San Diego, Calif.: Icon Health, 2002.

HEMOLYTIC DISEASE OF THE NEWBORN
DISEASE/DISORDER

ALSO KNOWN AS: Erythroblastosis fetalis, Rh incompatibility, ABO incompatibility

ANATOMY OR SYSTEM AFFECTED: Blood, brain, liver, skin

SPECIALTIES AND RELATED FIELDS: Hematology, neonatology, neurology

DEFINITION: The destruction of red blood cells in a fetus by antibodies transferred from the mother.

KEY TERMS:

antibodies: proteins produced by the immune system to destroy invading organisms or those perceived as foreign to the body

bilirubin: a pigment derived from the breakdown of red blood cells

Coombs' test: a test used to determine whether sensitization has occurred

exchange transfusion: the exchange of all or most of a patient's blood for donor blood; in a baby with hemolytic disease, usually performed through the umbilical vein

hemolysis: the rapid destruction of red blood cells

jaundice: yellow pigmentation resulting from the deposition of bilirubin in the skin

kernicterus: brain damage produced by the deposition of bilirubin in the brain

Rhogam: a protein that destroys Rh-positive cells

sensitization: the development of antibodies to a substance

CAUSES AND SYMPTOMS

Hemolytic disease of the newborn is a disorder in which maternal antibodies induce hemolysis of the red blood cells of the fetus or newborn, producing jaundice. The most common causes are ABO or Rh incompatibilities. ABO incompatibility occurs when the mother's blood is type O and the baby's blood is either type A or type B. The newborn develops jaundice within the first forty-eight hours of birth as a result of increasing bilirubin levels in the blood. Rh incompatibility can arise when an Rh-negative woman is carrying a second Rh-positive fetus. During the delivery of the first Rh-positive baby, blood from the newborn may pass into the mother's circulation. If no treatment is given, the woman may develop anti-Rh antibodies,

INFORMATION ON HEMOLYTIC DISEASE OF THE NEWBORN

CAUSES: Blood incompatibilities between mother and fetus
SYMPTOMS: Pale skin, enlarged liver and spleen, progressive jaundice and anemia within twenty-four hours of birth, deafness
DURATION: Varies
TREATMENTS: Light therapy, drug therapy, blood transfusions, iron and folic acid supplementation

which will remain in her circulation. If the fetus in her next pregnancy is also Rh-positive, the anti-Rh antibodies will cross over into the baby's blood, causing hemolysis of the red blood cells. In severe cases, the hemolysis starts in utero and the fetus will develop anemia, progressing to generalized edema with heart failure (hydrops fetalis) and death if the anemia is not corrected.

During the pregnancy, a positive Coombs' test indicates that the woman has been exposed and thus sensitized to Rh factor. A woman who is Rh-negative can become sensitized in three ways: by having delivered an Rh-positive baby following a previous pregnancy and not having received the protein Rhogam; by receiving an erroneous infusion of Rh-positive blood; and by having a spontaneous or induced abortion of an Rh-positive embryo or fetus. A rising concentration of antibodies during the course of the pregnancy indicates that hemolysis is occurring in the fetus. A small amount of amniotic fluid is obtained through a needle inserted through the mother's abdomen to determine the severity of the disease in the fetus. At birth, the baby may have pale skin and an enlarged liver and spleen. Progressive jaundice and anemia develop within the first twenty-four hours. High levels may cause the bilirubin to enter the brain and produce kernicterus. The baby with kernicterus shows little activity (hypoactivity), refuses to suck milk, and experiences seizures that can progress to permanent neurologic damage or to coma and death. Deafness may be a consequence of high bilirubin levels during the newborn period.

TREATMENT AND THERAPY
There is no preventive treatment for ABO incompatibility. Phototherapy, or light therapy, is used to decrease the level of bilirubin. Phototherapy acts on the bilirubin deposited in the skin and makes it water soluble, so that the pigment can be excreted through the gastrointestinal tract. An exchange transfusion may be required to decrease the concentration of bilirubin if it rises to dangerous levels. These levels will depend on the baby's maturation and clinical condition.

Preventive treatment for Rh incompatibility consists of giving Rhogam to all Rh-negative pregnant women at twenty-eight weeks of gestation and within the first seventy-two hours after the delivery of an Rh-positive baby. All Rh-negative women who have experienced an abortion or who have erroneously received a transfusion of Rh-positive blood should also receive Rhogam.

An Rh-negative pregnant woman with a positive Coombs' test needs to have periodic Coombs titers, or antibody concentration measurements, to determine what type of intervention, if any, is required. This test should first be done between sixteen and eighteen weeks of gestation. Rising Coombs titers indicate that hemolysis is occurring in the fetus. Prenatal interventions may include correcting fetal anemia by giving red blood cells directly to the fetus, either into the abdomen or into the umbilical vein. The fetus must be observed with sonography for the development of fetal edema, an ominous sign. At birth, the baby may have severe anemia requiring immediate correction. Phototherapy and an exchange transfusion may be needed if bilirubin rises above acceptable levels. Other modes of therapy such as phenobarbital, agar gel, and rectal suppositories are of limited value in reducing bilirubin in infants with hemolytic disease.

Before discharge from the hospital nursery, a hearing test must be done for all infants who have had jaundice during the neonatal period. Anemia may develop during the first six weeks of life as a result of the persistence of antibodies in the baby's blood. Close follow-up of hemoglobin levels must be done after discharge from the hospital. Blood transfusions may be indicated, as well as iron and folic acid supplementation.

PERSPECTIVE AND PROSPECTS
The incidence of Rh incompatibility has decreased remarkably since the advent of Rhogam. Nevertheless, it still occurs, particularly when unidentified miscarriages have occurred. Rh-negative fetuses can be identified early using special techniques available only in large medical centers. Therapy for hydrops fetalis has improved with the use of cordocentesis. This therapy, which consists of obtaining and transfusing blood directly into the umbilical cord while the fetus is in utero,

is available in specialized medical centers and has helped many sensitized babies to survive. Immunoglobulin has been used to block hemolysis, but it cannot be used for treatment. Agents that can metabolize bilirubin are currently under investigation.

—*Gloria Reyes Báez, M.D.*

See also Anemia; Blood and blood disorders; Critical care, pediatric; Emergency medicine, pediatric; Hearing loss; Immune system; Jaundice; Neonatology; Umbilical cord.

FOR FURTHER INFORMATION:

Behrman, Richard E., et al. *Nelson Textbook of Pediatrics.* 17th ed. New York: Elsevier, 2003. Text covering all medical and surgical disorders in children with authoritative information on genetics, endocrinology, aetiology, epidemiology, pathology, pathophysiology, clinical manifestations, diagnosis, prevention, treatment, and prognosis.

Gruslin-Giroux, Andrée, and Thomas R. Moore. "Erythroblastosis Fetalis." In *Neonatal-Perinatal Medicine: Diseases of the Fetus and Infant,* edited by Avroy A. Fanaroff and Richard J. Martin. 7th ed. St. Louis: C. V. Mosby, 2001. A chapter in an exhaustive resource covering all the major diseases of the infant and fetus. Includes bibliographical references and an index.

Kemper, Kathi J. *The Holistic Pediatrician: A Pediatrician's Comprehensive Guide to Safe and Effective Therapies for the Twenty-five Most Common Ailments of Infants, Children, and Adolescents.* New York: HarperCollins, 2002. Integrates mainstream and alternative medicine to aid parents in dealing with the most common childhood health problems such as fever, diaper rash, ear infections, and allergies.

Levy, Joseph. "Newborn Jaundice." *Parents Magazine* 69, no. 7 (July, 1994): 59-60. Jaundice is a fairly common condition in newborns because many do not have mature enough livers to process and excrete bilirubin, which causes the yellow color of jaundiced babies. The different types of jaundice, symptoms, and treatments for the disease are discussed.

Nathanson, Laura Walther. *The Portable Pediatrician: A Practicing Pediatrician's Guide to Your Child's Growth, Development, Health, and Behavior from Birth to Age Five.* 2d ed. New York: HarperCollins, 2002. An engaging, easy-to-read guide for parents to assess their child's development, medical symptoms, and behavioral problems.

HEMOPHILIA

DISEASE/DISORDER

ANATOMY OR SYSTEM AFFECTED: Blood

SPECIALTIES AND RELATED FIELDS: Genetics, hematology, serology

DEFINITION: A genetic disorder characterized by the blood's inability to form clots as a result of the lack or alteration of certain trace plasma proteins.

KEY TERMS:

clotting factors: substances present in plasma that are needed for the coagulation of blood

hemophilia A: a genetic blood disease characterized by a deficiency of clotting factor VIII

hemophilia B: a genetic blood disease characterized by a deficiency of clotting factor IX

hemostasis: the process of stopping the flow of blood at an injury site

von Willebrand's disease: a genetic blood disease characterized by a deficiency of the von Willebrand clotting factor

CAUSES AND SYMPTOMS

The circulatory system must be self-healing; otherwise, continued blood loss from even the smallest injury would be life-threatening. Normally, all except the most catastrophic bleeding is rapidly stopped in a process known as hemostasis. Hemostasis takes place through several sequential steps or processes. First, an injury stimulates platelets (unpigmented blood cells) to adhere to the damaged blood vessels and then to one another, forming a plug that can stop minor bleeding. This association is mediated by what is called the von Willebrand factor, a protein that binds to the platelets. As the platelets aggregate, they release several substances that stimulate vasoconstriction, or a reduction in size of the blood vessels. This reduces the blood flow at the injury site. Finally, the aggregating platelets and damaged tissue initiate blood clotting, or coagulation. Once bleeding has stopped, the firmly adhering clot slowly contracts, drawing the edge of the wounds together so that tough scar tissue can form a permanent repair on the site.

Formation of a blood clot involves the participation of nearly twenty different substances, most of which are proteins synthesized by plasma. All but two of these substances, or factors, are designated by a roman numeral and a common name. A blood clot will be defective if one of the clotting factors is absent or deficient in the blood, and clotting time will be longer. The clotting factors, with some of their alternative names, are factor

I (fibrinogen), factor II (prothrombin), factor III (tissue factor or thromboplastin), factor IV (calcium), factor V (proaccelerin), factor VII (proconvertin), factor VIII (antihemophilic factor), factor IX (Christmas factor), factor X (Stuart factor), factor XI (plasma thromboplastin antecedent), factor XII (Hageman factor), and factor XIII (fibrin stabilizing factor).

Several of the clotting factors have been discovered by the diagnosis of their deficiencies in various clotting disorders. The inherited coagulation disorders are uncommon conditions with an overall incidence of probably no more than 10 to 20 per 100,000 of the population. Hemophilia A, the most common or classic type of coagulation disorder, is caused by factor VIII deficiency. Hemophilia B (or Christmas disease) is the result of factor IX deficiency. It is quite common for severe hemophilia to manifest itself during the first year of life. Hazardous bleeding occurs in areas such as the central nervous system, the retropharyngeal area, and the retroperitoneal area. Bleeding in these areas requires admission to the hospital for observation and therapy. Joint lesions are very common in hemophilia because of acute spontaneous hemorrhage in the area, specially in weight-bearing joints such as ankles and knees. Urinary bleeding is often present at some time. The appearance of pseudotumors, caused by swelling involving muscle and bone produced by recurrent bleeding, is also common.

Hemophilia is transmitted entirely by unaffected females (carriers) to their sons in a sex-linked inheritance deficiency. Congenital deficiencies of the other coagulation factors are well recognized, even though bleeding episodes in these cases are uncommon. Deficiency of more than one factor is also possible, although documentation of such cases is very rare, perhaps because only patients with milder variations of the disease survive.

Von Willebrand's disease, unlike the hemophilias that mainly involve bleeding in joints and muscles, involves mainly bleeding of mucocutaneous tissues or skin. It affects both men and women. This disease shares clinical characteristics with hemophilia A, or classic hemophilia, including decreased levels of clotting factor VIII. This similarity made the differentiation between the two diseases very difficult for a long time. It has now been established that there are two different factors involved in von Willebrand's disease, each with a different function. The von Willebrand factor is involved in the adhesion of platelets to the injured blood vessel wall and to one another and, together with

---

INFORMATION ON HEMOPHILIA

CAUSES: Genetic blood defect
SYMPTOMS: Loss of large amounts of blood from even small injuries, hemorrhaging without apparent cause, bruising, pain, swelling, joint lesions, urinary bleeding, pseudotumors
DURATION: Chronic
TREATMENTS: Fresh frozen plasma, clotting factor concentrates, drug therapy

---

factor VIII, circulates in plasma as a complex held by electrostatic and hydrophobic forces. The von Willebrand factor is a very large molecule, consisting of a series of possible multimeric structures. The bigger and heavier the multimer, the better it works against bleeding. Von Willebrand's disease is one of the least understood clotting disorders. Three types have been identified, with at least twenty-seven variations. With type I, all the multimers needed for successful clotting are present in the blood, but in lesser amounts than in healthy individuals. In type II, the larger multimers, which are more active in hemostasis, are lacking, and type III patients exhibit a severe lack of all multimers.

TREATMENT AND THERAPY

The normal body is continually producing clotting factors in order to keep up with natural loss. Sometimes the production is stepped up to cover a real or anticipated increase in the need for these factors, such as in childbirth. Hemophiliacs, lacking some of these clotting factors, may lose large amounts of blood from even the smallest injury and sometimes hemorrhage without any apparent cause. The symptoms of their diseases may be alleviated by the intravenous administration of the deficient clotting factor. How this is done depends on the specific factor deficiency and the magnitude of the bleeding episode, the age and size of the patient, convenience, acceptability, cost of product, and method and place of delivery of care.

There are many sources for clotting factors. Fresh frozen plasma contains all the clotting factors, but since the concentration of the factors in plasma is relatively low, a large volume is required for treatment. Therefore, it can be used only when small amounts of clotting factor must be delivered. Its use is the only therapy for deficiencies of factors V, XI, and XII. Plasma is commonly harvested from single donor units to minimize the risk of infection by the hepatitis virus or human immunodeficiency virus (HIV), thus eliminating the risk involved in using pooled concentrates from many donors. Cryoprecipitates are the proteins that precipitate in fresh frozen plasma thawed at 4 degrees Celsius. The precipitate is rich in factors VIII and XIII and in fibrinogen, and carries less chance of infection with hepatitis. Its standardization is difficult, however, and is not required by the Food and Drug Administration. As a result, dosage calculation can be a problem. In addition, there is no method for the control of viral contamination. Therefore, cryoprecipitates are not commonly used unless harvested from a special known and tested donor pool. Clotting factor concentrates present many advantages. They are made from pooled plasma obtained from plasmapheresis or a program of total donor unit fractionation and are widely available. Factors VIII and IX can also be produced from plasma using monoclonal methods. Porcine factor VIII presents an alternative to patients with a naturally occurring antibody to human factor VIII.

Other substances can replace missing clotting factors as well. The synthetic hormone desmopressin acetate (also known by the letters DDAVP) has been used to stimulate the release of factor VIII and von Willebrand factor from the endothelial cells lining blood vessels. It is commonly used for patients with mild hemophilia and von Willebrand's disease. DDAVP has no effect on the concentration of the other factors, and aside from the common side effect of water retention, it is a safe drug. Antifibrinolytic drugs prevent the natural breakdown of blood clots that have already been formed. Although such drugs are not useful for the primary care of hemophiliacs, they are useful for use after dental extractions and in the treatment of other open wounds, after a clot has formed.

Between 10 and 15 percent of the patients affected with severe hemophilia develop factor VIII inhibitors (antibodies), which prevents their treatment with the usual methods. Newer therapeutic approaches have provided additional options for the management and control of bleeding episodes. The use of prothrombin complex concentrates or porcine factor VIII concentrates is indicated for low responders (those with a low amount of antibodies present in their system). An option for high responders is to try to eradicate the inhibitor present in their systems. One way to do this is with a regimen of immunosuppressive drugs. These are very limited in value, however, and cannot be used with HIV-positive hemophiliacs. The drugs used in this approach include substances such as cyclophosphamide,

vincristine, azathioprine, and corticosteroids. Another approach utilizes intravenous doses of gamma globulin to suppress, but not eradicate, the inhibitors. Yet another strategy is an immune tolerance regimen, in which factor VIII is administered daily in small amounts. This method causes the inhibitors to decrease and, in some cases, disappear. The regimen can also involve the prophylactic use of factor VIII (or factor VIII in combination with immunosuppressive drugs).

The introduction of plasma clotting factor concentrates has changed the treatment of patients with clotting factor deficiencies. It has brought about a remarkable change in the longevity of these patients and their quality of life. The availability of cryoprecipitates and concentrates of factors II, VII, VIII, IX, X, and XIII has made outpatient treatment for bleeding episodes routine and home infusion or self-infusion a possibility for many patients. Hospitalization for inpatient treatment is rare, and early outpatient therapy of bleeding episodes has decreased the severity of joint deformities.

Nevertheless, other problems are apparent in hemophiliac patients. Viral contamination of the factor concentrates has allowed the development of chronic illnesses, infection with HIV, immunologic diseases, liver and renal diseases, joint disorders, and cardiovascular diseases. While the use of heat for virus inactivation, beginning in 1983, resulted in a reduction in HIV infections, the majority of patients exposed to the virus had already been infected. The strategies to prevent contraction of hepatitis from these concentrates include vaccination against the contaminating viruses and the elimination of viruses from the factor replacement product. The non-A, non-B hepatitis virus is very difficult to remove, however, and the use of monoclonal factors seems to be the only solution to this problem. In general, difficulties associated with treatment have been largely eliminated through the production of the required clotting factors using recombinant DNA techniques, a process performed independent of human blood.

Treatment of von Willebrand's disease also includes pressure dressing, suturing, and oral contraceptives. A pasteurized antihemophiliac concentrate that contains substantial amounts of von Willebrand factor is used in severe cases.

Hematomas, or hemorrhages under the skin and within muscles, can frequently be controlled by application of elastic bandage pressure and ice. The ones that cannot be controlled easily within a few hours may cause muscle contraction and require factor replacement therapy. Exercise is recommended for joints after bleeding, as it helps protect joints by increasing muscle bulk and power and can also help relieve stress. Devices to protect joints, such as elastic bandages and splints, are commonly used. In extreme cases, orthopedic surgical procedures are readily available.

Analgesics, or painkillers, play an important part in the alleviation of chronic pain. Because patients cannot use products with aspirin and/or antihistamines, which inhibit platelet aggregation and prolong bleeding time, substances such as acetaminophen, codeine, and morphine are used. Chronic joint inflammation is reduced by the use of anti-inflammatory agents such as ibuprofen and of drugs used in rheumatoid arthritis patients.

The need for so many specialties and disciplines in the management of hemophilia has led to the development of multidisciplinary hemophilia centers. Genetic education (information on how the disease is transmitted), genetic counseling (the discussion of an individual's genetic risks and reproductive options), and genetic testing have provided great help to patients and affected families. Early and prenatal diagnosis and carrier detection have provided options for family planning.

PERSPECTIVE AND PROSPECTS

Descriptions of hemophilia are among the oldest known accounts of genetic disease. References to a bleeding condition highly suggestive of hemophilia go back to the fifth century, in the Babylonian Talmud. The first significant report in medical literature appeared in 1803 when John C. Otto, a Philadelphia physician, described several bleeder families with only males affected and with transmission through the mothers. The literature of the nineteenth century contains many descriptions of the disease, particularly the clinical characteristics of the hemorrhages and family histories. The disease was originally called haemorrhaphilia, or "tendency toward hemorrhages," but the name was later contracted through usage to hemophilia ("tendency toward blood"), the accepted name since around 1828.

Transfusion therapy was proposed as early as 1832, and the first successful transfusion for the treatment of a hemophiliac patient was reported in 1840 by Samuel Armstrong Lane. The use of blood from cows and pigs in the transfusions was explored but abandoned because of the numerous side effects. It was not until the beginning of the twentieth century that serious studies on clotting in hemophilia were started. Attention was directed to the use of normal human serum for treat-

ment of bleeding episodes. Some of the patients responded well, while others did not. This result is probably attributable to the fact that some had hemophilia A—these patients did not respond because factor VIII, in which they are deficient, is not present in serum— while some others had hemophilia B, for which the therapy worked. In 1923, harvested blood plasma was used in transfusion, and it was shown to work as well as whole blood. With blood banking becoming a reality in the 1930's, transfusions were performed more frequently as a treatment for hemophilia.

The history of the fractionation of plasma began around 1911 with Dr. Addis, who prepared a very crude fraction by acidification of plasma. In 1937, Drs. Patek and Taylor produced a crude fraction which, on injection, lowered the blood-clotting time in hemophiliacs. In the period from 1945 to 1960, a number of plasma fractions with antihemophiliac activity were developed. The use of fresh frozen plasma increased as a result of advances in the purification of the fractions. Some milestones can be identified in the production of the plasma fractions: the development of quantitative assays for antihemophiliac factors, the discovery of cryoprecipitation, and the development of glycine and polyethylene precipitation.

In 1952, four significant and independent publications indicated that there is a plasma-clotting activity separate from that concerned with classic hemophilia—in other words, that there are two types of hemophilia. One (hemophilia A) is characterized by a deficiency in factor VIII, while the other (hemophilia B) is characterized by deficiency in factor IX. Carriers of hemophilia A can have a mean factor VIII level that is 50 percent lower than that of normal females, while carriers of hemophilia B show levels of factor IX that are 60 percent below normal. The two diseases have the same pattern of inheritance, are similar in clinical appearance, and can be distinguished only by laboratory tests.

Hemophilias are caused by a disordered and complex biological mechanism that continues to be explored. Recombinant DNA techniques have now revealed the molecular defect in factor VIII or factor IX deficiencies in some families, demonstrating that a variety of gene defects can produce the classic phenotype of hemophilia. These techniques have also provided new tools for carrier detection and prenatal diagnosis.

Current treatment of hemophilia has converted the hemophiliac from an in-hospital patient to an individual with more independent status. Crucial in this development has been the creation of comprehensive care centers and of the National Hemophilia Foundation, which provide comprehensive treatment for the hemophilia patient. With the advancement of recombinant DNA technology, the future looks brighter for the sufferers of this disease.

—*Maria Pacheco, Ph.D.*

See also Acquired immunodeficiency syndrome (AIDS); Bleeding; Blood and blood disorders; Genetic diseases; Genetics and inheritance; Transfusion; Von Willebrand's disease.

FOR FURTHER INFORMATION:

Bloom, Arthur L., ed. *The Hemophilias*. Methods in Hematology 5. New York: Churchill Livingstone, 1982. The series presents accounts of methods for the study of blood and its disorders. This book concentrates on hemophilia, presenting a description of available assay methods, purification methods, and prenatal diagnosis.

Hilgartner, Margaret W., and Carl Pochedly, eds. *Hemophilia in the Child and Adult*. 3d ed. New York: Raven Press, 1989. A compilation of the thoughts and experiences of clinicians who deal with hemophilia, as well as some practical approaches to patient care. A well-organized and informative book.

Jones, Peter. *Living with Haemophilia*. 5th ed. New York: Oxford University Press, 2002. An excellent book for the layperson, it was written specifically for patients and their families. In an easy-to-read, understandable format, explains the transmission of bleeding disorders through families, their manifestations, and their management.

King, Richard A., et al., eds. *Genetic Basis of Common Diseases*. 2d ed. New York: Oxford University Press, 2002. Covers advances in the understanding of molecular processes involved in genetic susceptibility and disease mechanisms. Examines a range of diseases in detail and includes a chapter on genetic counseling.

Massimini, Kathy, ed. *Genetic Disorders Sourcebook: Basic Consumer Information About Hereditary Diseases and Disorders, Including Cystic Fibrosis, Down Syndrome, Hemophilia, Huntington's Disease, Sickle Cell Anemia, and More*. 2d ed. Detroit: Omnigraphics, 2000. This nontechnical sourcebook offers basic information about lifestyle expectations, disease management techniques, and current research initiatives for the most common types of genetic disorders, including a resource list of three hundred genetic disorders and related topics.

National Hemophilia Foundation. http://www.hemophilia.org/. A Web site that promotes education, research and advocacy on behalf of people with bleeding disorders.

Parker, James N., and Philip M. Parker, eds. *The 2002 Official Patient's Sourcebook on Hemophilia*. San Diego, Calif.: Icon Health, 2002. Draws from public, academic, government, and peer-reviewed research to provide a wide-ranging handbook for patients with hemophilia.

Rodak, Bernadette. *Hematology*. 2d ed. New York: Elsevier Science, 2002. A comprehensive textbook covering all aspects of hematology and hemostasis.

Voet, Donald, and Judith G. Voet. *Biochemistry*. Rev. ed. New York: John Wiley & Sons, 2002. A comprehensive biochemistry textbook with an excellent section on blood and blood-clotting mechanisms.

HEMORRHOID BANDING AND REMOVAL

PROCEDURE

ANATOMY OR SYSTEM AFFECTED: Anus, blood vessels, circulatory system, gastrointestinal system, intestines

SPECIALTIES AND RELATED FIELDS: Family practice, gastroenterology, general surgery, proctology

DEFINITION: The surgical ligation and removal of protruding veins from the lower rectum.

INDICATIONS AND PROCEDURES

Hemorrhoids, or piles, result from the protrusion or varicosity of veins found within the mucous membranes of the rectum. Hemorrhoids may develop either inside or outside the rectum, and they are among the more common of human afflictions.

Hemorrhoids generally develop as a result of increased pressure placed on veins within the rectum. The pressure may be attributable to straining as a result of constipation or to prolonged sitting. In women, they often develop during pregnancy and following childbirth. Treatment depends on the severity of discomfort and location of the hemorrhoid.

External hemorrhoids are often not painful, and they may respond to the application of cool compresses or over-the-counter astringent creams. Creams and suppositories containing steroids may be prescribed by a physician. Internal hemorrhoids may not be noticeable unless a vein ruptures, causing some bleeding, pain, and itching. Since bacteria regularly pass through the rectal area, infection may increase the itching and pain, eventually requiring treatment. If discomfort continues and is not relieved through simple medication, the hemorrhoids may require surgical removal. Several methods exist for removal. Often, the vein is stretched and cut off at its base. Local anesthetics may be necessary, and there may be bleeding and discomfort. Internal hemorrhoids may also be eliminated through cryosurgery, the application of subfreezing temperatures to eliminate tissue. The complete surgical removal of the hemorrhoid, hemorrhoidectomy, may be warranted under certain circumstances.

Hemorrhoid banding, also referred to as rubber band ligation and Barron ligation, involves the placement of a tight rubber band at the base of the hemorrhoid. Over the next few days, the vein will degenerate and slough off. The procedure is relatively simple and can be performed on an outpatient basis. Aside from some discomfort for several days, there are few side effects associated with the banding procedure. Warm sitz baths and local astringents may be helpful in reducing any swelling or pain, and the patient should eat a diet conducive to a soft stool.

—*Richard Adler, Ph.D.*

See also Colon and rectal surgery; Colonoscopy and sigmoidoscopy; Constipation; Cryosurgery; Hemorrhoids; Pregnancy and gestation; Proctology; Varicose veins; Vascular medicine; Vascular system.

FOR FURTHER INFORMATION:

Becker, Barbara. *Relief from Chronic Hemorrhoids.* New York: Dell, 1992.

The Hemorrhoid Book: A Look at Hemorrhoids—How They're Treated and How You Can Prevent Them from Coming Back. San Bruno, Calif.: Krames Communications, 1991.

Parker, James N., and Philip M. Parker, eds. *The Official Patient's Sourcebook on Hemorrhoids.* San Diego, Calif.: Icon Health, 2002.

Pcikin, Steven R. *Gastrointestinal Health.* Rev. ed. New York: HarperCollins, 1999.

Sachar, David B., Jerome D. Waye, and Blair S. Lewis, eds. *Pocket Guide to Gastroenterology.* Rev. ed. Baltimore: Williams & Wilkins, 1991.

Wanderman, Sidney E., with Betty Rothbart. *Hemorrhoids.* Yonkers, N.Y.: Consumer Reports Books, 1991.

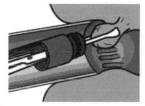
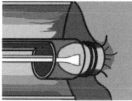

The Removal of Hemorrhoids

A proctoscope applying
a band to a hemorrhoid

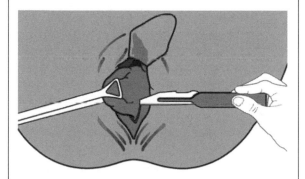

A hemorrhoid being withdrawn
by a clamp and cut off with a scalpel

Severe and distended hemorrhoids may be removed in one of two ways: through the placement of a rubber band around the base of the hemorrhoid, which constricts its blood supply and causes it to wither and drop off; or through surgical excision.

HEMORRHOIDS
DISEASE/DISORDER

ANATOMY OR SYSTEM AFFECTED: Anus, blood vessels, circulatory system, gastrointestinal system, intestines

SPECIALTIES AND RELATED FIELDS: Family practice, gastroenterology, proctology

DEFINITION: Blood-swollen enlargements of specialized tissues that help close the anus, as a result of intravenous pressure in the hemorrhoidal plexus; sometimes called piles.

KEY TERMS:

anus: the valve at the end of the rectum that prevents waste matter from leaking out until a person is ready to defecate

cauterize: to sear tissue with heat or a corrosive substance

dentate line: the junction in the anus where the external skin meets the internal mucosa

gastroenterologist: a physician who specializes in the gastrointestinal tract and related organs

mucosa: the mucus-secreting membrane that lines the surface of internal organs directly exposed to elements from outside the body, such as the lungs and intestines

proctologist: a physician who specializes in diseases of the rectum

rectum: the storage compartment at the end of the colon where wastes collect before defecation

stool: the excreted waste products of digestion

thrombosis: the condition of having a clot in a blood vessel

Causes and Symptoms

Hemorrhoids, some physiologists suggest, are one of the prices that humans pay for walking upright. The vascular system—the veins and arteries that circulate blood—evolved in an animal that walked on all fours. Now that humans spend most of their time standing, gravity puts awkward pressure on the system, and at the bottom of major parts of the system, as in the tissue around the anus, the column of blood above weighs heavily on the network of small blood vessels there. It does not take much additional pressure to cause a vessel's wall to balloon out. When it does, the result is a hemorrhoid, a little pouch protruding on the surface of the anus, similar to a hernia or varicose vein. Most people have hemorrhoids, even if they do not realize it, and the major symptoms are rarely dangerous, although they can be extremely annoying. Sometimes, however, hemorrhoids develop into or mask life-threatening diseases.

The term "hemorrhoid" derives from Greek words meaning "blood flowing," an apt description of the circulatory activity in the anal walls and an inadvertently apt warning of what most alarms people—hemorrhoids

---

Information on Hemorrhoids

Causes: Increased pressure in lower abdomen resulting from constipation, diarrhea, long periods of sitting, pregnancy and childbirth

Symptoms: Burning, itching, bleeding around anus

Duration: Often short-term but can be chronic

Treatments: Change in dietary and/or lifestyle habits; use of ointments, creams, medicated pads, and suppositories; surgery if needed

---

occasionally bleed. (The alternative, and now obsolescent, term "piles" comes from Latin *pila*, a ball, apparently a metaphor for the appearance of hemorrhoids.) Specifically, the "blood flowing" refers to the supple blood vessels of the internal rectal plexus, a series of pouches that act as cushions to help seal the anus shut. When these pouches become enlarged, they turn into hemorrhoids, which jut from the anus wall and swell up to 3 centimeters in length.

Because of the sphincter that controls defecation, not all hemorrhoids are visible without the aid of special instruments. The anus, an oval opening about 3 centimeters in front of the spine, is the valve ending the digestive tract. Like the mouth's lips, which begin the tract, the anus can purse shut, a state made possible by two concentric, circular sphincter muscles which act like drawstrings on a cloth bag. When sensors in the rectum signal the time to defecate, these muscles relax to pass stool and then immediately contract to close the anus again. As in the mouth, external skin meets the internal mucosal membrane in the anus; the meeting place is a corrugated joint called the dentate line (or, alternatively, the anorectal juncture or pectinase line). It is in this area—between the skin covering the external (or lower) sphincter and the mucosa over the internal (or upper) sphincter—that hemorrhoids form. Those that bulge out from the dentate line or above are hidden from sight by the closed anus and are called internal hemorrhoids; those that protrude below the closed anus, and so can be seen or felt, are called external hemorrhoids.

External hemorrhoids are the ones famed for vexing people. When the skin is stretched over swelled hemorrhoids, its sense receptors are activated, making the hemorrhoids burn and itch, sometimes so intolerably that the urge to scratch them is uncontrollable. Scratching, especially with abrasive materials such as toilet paper, often scrapes and tears the tissue. The bright red blood from these lesions is easily noticeable on the toilet paper and may even drip into the toilet bowl or onto underclothes. Likewise, the passage of a hard, dry stool often abrades hemorrhoids to the point of bleeding.

Internal hemorrhoids do not itch or burn and rarely cause pain because the mucosal tissue over them has no nerve endings, but they can also bleed when a passing stool damages them. (Pain may be "referred," however, from a damaged internal hemorrhoid to the sciatic nerve, bladder, lower back, or genitals; that is, a person feels little or no pain in the anorectal area, but suddenly pain flares in one of these other areas.) An especially

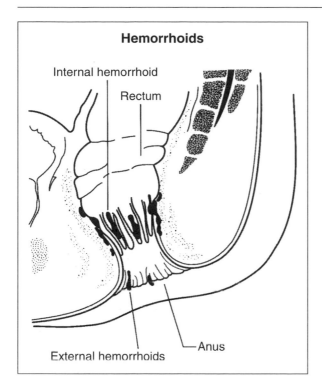

Hemorrhoids

Internal hemorrhoid

Rectum

External hemorrhoids

Anus

elongated internal hemorrhoid at times can protrude through the anus, a condition called prolapse. Usually, it spontaneously recedes or can be pushed back inside with a finger, but upon rare occasion a group of internal hemorrhoids prolapse, swelling and sending the internal sphincter into painful spasms. A doctor's help may then be required to reduce the pain and fit the hemorrhoids inside.

The blood vessels in the internal rectal plexus swell so easily because they lack valves. Without valves to regulate the local flow of blood, the walls are vulnerable to any sudden increase in pressure. Even a small, transient increase above the normal pressure of blood circulation can cause the vessels to bulge. Often, these bulges disappear when the excess pressure disappears or remain swollen only briefly afterward. If the increased pressure is high enough, however, a permanent protrusion results, drooping from the anal wall like lumps of melted wax on a candle. Even then, if the hemorrhoid is internal, the patient may feel no discomfort and may not realize that a hemorrhoid has formed.

Some people are more susceptible to chronic hemorrhoids than others because of a hereditary lack of elasticity in the blood vessels. In such people, standing for long periods of time can add enough pressure to make hemorrhoids swell. Nevertheless, anyone can get hemorrhoids; all that is needed is enough pressure in the

lower abdomen. Straining on the toilet to pass stool is the most common cause. People strain when they are constipated or have diarrhea, and since a poor diet can lead to these conditions, hemorrhoids can be a secondary effect of poor eating habits. Those who like to sit on the toilet a long time, reading or watching television while waiting for a bowel movement, also increase pressure on the anus because of the posture and the compressing effect of the toilet ring; they are likely to develop hemorrhoids. People who regularly lift heavy weights as part of their jobs or for recreation are especially susceptible if they hold their breath while lifting: This action pushes the diaphragm downward on organs below it, including the anus, putting pressure on them. Similarly, during pregnancy women can develop hemorrhoids as the expanding womb crowds and increases pressure on nearby organs; these hemorrhoids are exacerbated by delivery, but they usually go away afterward. Psychologists add to these causes the guilt that some people feel about eating and excreting, guilt spawned by overindulgence in food or bad toilet training; they bear down on their bowels to defecate as quickly as possible and by doing so stress the hemorrhoidal vessels. Finally, hemorrhoids occasionally develop because of some serious diseases, such as heart failure and cirrhosis of the liver, which elevate pressure in the veins, and rectal cancer, which can create a false sense of fullness so that the person strains to pass a stool that is not really there.

Although they seldom do more than itch, external hemorrhoids can thrombose—develop clots of coagulated blood from a burst or swollen vessel under the skin—and grow as large as a grape. A doctor can relieve the pain by slicing open the hemorrhoid and squeezing out the clot. Left alone, a thrombosed hemorrhoid may rupture, causing a painful and bloody mess that is ripe for infection. Yet the greatest threat of hemorrhoids lies not in the symptoms themselves but in how they might be confused with those of other, deadly diseases. Colorectal cancer, inflammatory bowel disease, and sexually transmitted diseases such as syphilis, gonorrhea, and herpes can lead to discharges of blood, as can anal fissures (cracks in the anal canal), fistulas (tunnel-like passages between an infected gland and mucosa or skin), and abscesses (pus-filled sacs under the mucosa). A person who dismisses the bloody discharge as simply a flare-up of hemorrhoids may be delaying treatment for the real cause. In the case of colorectal cancer, one of the most common cancers in the United States, such a delay can be fatal. Only a doctor has the tools and vantage point to distinguish between the relatively benign hemorrhoids and a dangerous disorder.

Treatment and Therapy

Since hemorrhoid-like symptoms can be produced by deadly diseases, a thorough checkup at the doctor's office includes an examination of the anus and rectum, especially if the patient has noticed bleeding. In addition to the visual inspection and "digital" examination, during which the doctor inserts a finger and feels around for enlarged hemorrhoids or other masses, patients provide clues by describing the color, amount, and time of bleeding. If the blood is bright red and occurs in small quantities during or just after defecation, hemorrhoids are most likely to blame. If dark red blood or clots appear in the stool or seep out randomly, however, the doctor will look for other causes, inspecting the anus, rectum, and colon with various types of endoscopes, fiber-optic-filled flexible tubes that can also collect tissue samples. Once the doctor rules out other diseases, the patient has three basic choices: change habits, rely on therapy, or have the hemorrhoids removed.

If a person's hemorrhoids do not cause severe discomfort, the doctor will likely recommend a diet with high fiber and water intake. Fiber and water together make stools bulky and soft. They pass more easily during defecation than small, hard, dry stools. The patient does not have to strain, and so no further pressure is put on existing hemorrhoids. Furthermore, soft stools do not scrape hemorrhoids and cause them to bleed. The doctor will also suggest regular exercise, since this helps the bowels work more efficiently and reduces the chance of constipation. Finally, the patient may receive instructions on the proper way to breathe during heavy exertion so as to lessen the stress on the hemorrhoids. With a better diet, more exercise, and less physical straining, patients may find that hemorrhoids have disappeared completely.

Until hemorrhoids shrink, they plague the patient, and to reduce the itching and burning a number of therapies prove effective, if only temporarily. An ice compress eases the discomfort, as does a sitz bath (sitting for at least fifteen minutes in shallow warm water), which also cleanses the site of potentially infecting wastes and promotes healing in damaged tissue. Should these relatively simple and cheap measures be impracticable, a variety of ointments, creams, medicated pads, and suppositories, either prescription or nonprescription, may provide relief. Some are inert, such as petroleum jelly, and coat and lubricate the hem-

orrhoids, protecting them from irritation. Some have an astringent effect, tightening and sealing tissue and thereby protecting it. Others have anesthetic ingredients, numbing the tissue, or anti-inflammatory effects, decreasing swelling. None of these medications has a proven capacity to make swelling go away entirely, and those with active ingredients may cause an allergic response. For patients with constipation, doctors may prescribe stool softeners to eliminate straining during defecation. Laxatives are usually to be avoided because the chemicals in them irritate hemorrhoids, and the resulting diarrhea often causes urgency and pressure in the rectal area.

When hemorrhoids become chronically and unusually swollen or the patient can no longer endure the discomfort, removing them is the last resort. This cure is certain, although not necessarily permanent, but it has its cost in pain and recovery time. There are seven basic methods, six that cause the target hemorrhoid to shrivel, to drop off on its own, or both, and one, surgery, that removes it directly.

The surgical removal of hemorrhoids, called hemorrhoidectomy, is a relatively simple operation; nevertheless, it is usually reserved for those patients who for one reason or another cannot undergo one of the other methods. The patient is given a local anesthetic to deaden the tissue in the anus, although some patients are rendered unconscious with a general anesthetic; the surgeon cuts off the hemorrhoid at its base and then sews the wound closed with absorbable sutures. The recovery period may require hospitalization for up to a week, during which pain medication, stool softeners, and anal pads are necessary until the tissues heal. Bed rest after hospitalization and sitz baths may also be necessary. Because of this recovery time—as much as a month all together—hemorrhoidectomies are not widely popular among patients or physicians. Moreover, urine retention, infection, and hemorrhaging after the operation are possible complications.

The remaining methods avoid the trauma of cutting, and the first of them, ligation, is the oldest of all the methods, referred to in the writings of Hippocrates (c. 460-c. 370 B.C.E.). Ancient Greek physicians tied a thread around a hemorrhoid to strangle its blood supply; modern gastroenterologists or proctologists use special rubber bands. The effect is the same: The hemorrhoid dries up, shrivels, and falls off. Little pain accompanies the procedure, which is done in the doctor's office. Ligation, however, can only be used for internal hemorrhoids.

Likewise, sclerotherapy, cryosurgery, and infrared coagulation are only for internal hemorrhoids because the pain would be too intense on external hemorrhoids. In sclerotherapy, the doctor injects a liquid—usually phenol in oil or quinine in urea—that seals closed the blood vessels at the base of the hemorrhoid. With no blood in them, the vessels eventually shrink to normal dimensions and, if stressing pressure on them is not resumed, the hemorrhoid disappears. In cryosurgery, super cold liquid nitrogen or nitrous oxide is applied to the hemorrhoid, freezing it and killing the tissue. The hemorrhoid slowly melts and, as it does, shrinks and finally sloughs off. Popular in the 1970's and early 1980's, cryosurgery lost favor because of the messy and extended recovery time. Useful for mild, small hemorrhoids, infrared coagulation involves a beam of infrared light that, aimed at the hemorrhoid, shrinks it by cauterizing the tissue. The heat of the beam can cause pain in other parts of the anus during the procedure.

The remaining methods, laser surgery and electric current coagulation, can be used on external hemorrhoids. Like infrared coagulation, laser surgery trains a beam of light—in this case intense visible light—that burns and shrinks the hemorrhoid to a stub. Since the laser cauterizes as it destroys tissue and therefore seals off blood vessels, its main advantage over regular surgery lies in reduced bleeding. Recovery time is shorter, about a week, and hospitalization is usually not necessary. This procedure is much more expensive than a hemorrhoidectomy or ligation, however, because of the cost of laser technology. In electric current coagulation, electrodes pass either direct or alternating current through the hemorrhoids. Because tissue is a poor conductor, the resistance to the current creates heat, which cooks the hemorrhoid, coagulating and shrinking it.

Which method the surgeon, gastroenterologist, or proctologist uses depends partly upon the physician's and patient's preferences and partly upon the size and location of the hemorrhoid. Ligation remains the most frequently used method because it is relatively cheap and fast.

PERSPECTIVE AND PROSPECTS

According to Napoleon's personal physician, piles cost the emperor the Battle of Waterloo, which ended his reign. His hemorrhoids were so inflamed and painful on the morning of the battle that he could not get out of bed, much less sit on his horse. Without his personal direction, the French lost. Popular writers often cite this dramatic example, sometimes with humorous overtones, to demonstrate how seriously hemorrhoids can interfere with the lives of even the great.

Certainly, hemorrhoids are no laughing matter. Yet the long-standing taboo in the United States about excretion and the anus has prompted many Americans either to laugh nervously about their hemorrhoids or to keep silent, preferring to suffer stoically rather than to risk becoming the target of jokes. For this reason, it is nearly impossible to say how many sufferers there are in the United States. Estimates vary from several million people to the entire population over the age of thirty.

Whatever the exact statistic, clearly many people share a problem that embarrasses them too much to discuss openly or that they believe is too trivial for medical attention. If they need relief from the itching and pain, they treat themselves. A large industry in home remedies and over-the-counter medications serves them: Rectal medications alone earned drug companies $178 million in 1999, according to the Consumer Healthcare Products Association. The benefits of such medications are difficult to assess, and some authorities claim that petroleum jelly eases the itching and burning as much as any preparation specifically intended for hemorrhoids. Folk remedies, such as suppositories made of tobacco or compresses soaked in papaya juice, can damage tissue outright, making the problem worse. Moreover, throughout the United States specialized clinics offer surgical cures for hemorrhoids, promising patients quick relief on an outpatient basis and using expensive methods, particularly laser surgery.

Therefore, many people spend a considerable amount of money and time, often wasting both, to tend a chronic discomfort that can as readily be prevented or palliated by a change in habits, doctors claim. Like colon cancer and many other intestinal ailments, hemorrhoids are most common in populations whose diet includes a high number of processed foods, which are low in fiber. While fiber is no panacea, people in cultures whose diet contains significant fiber have larger stools and fewer intestinal complaints in general.

Because hemorrhoids are in most cases preventable or controllable without treatment, they have been cited, along with deadly maladies such as colon cancer and inflammatory bowel disease, in criticisms of both the American diet and Americans' eagerness to rely on medical intervention to save them from their own unhealthy habits. In the case of hemorrhoids—while they are not exclusively a malady of Western civilization—the fast pace and pressures of life, the attitudes about defecation, and the eating habits of industrial cultures help give them a distracting prominence.

—*Roger Smith, Ph.D.*

See also Colon and rectal polyp removal; Colon and rectal surgery; Colon cancer; Colon therapy; Colonoscopy and sigmoidoscopy; Cryosurgery; Endoscopy; Hemorrhoid banding and removal; Intestinal disorders; Intestines; Pregnancy and gestation; Thrombosis and thrombus.

FOR FURTHER INFORMATION:

Becker, Barbara. *Relief from Chronic Hemorrhoids.* New York: Dell, 1992. An excellent book for general readers, it gives advice on every aspect of diagnosis, treatment, removal procedures, and alternative therapies. Special attention is given to improving the patient's diet, and extensive, very specific tables on proper foods accompany the argument for this self-help approach.

"Help for Hemorrhoids Includes Fiber, Fluids, and Fitness." *Environmental Nutrition* 23, no. 4 (April, 2000): 7. Hemorrhoids are a common medical problem, especially for people over age fifty. The best way to prevent hemorrhoids is to avoid constipation by combining a high-fiber diet with plenty of fluids and regular physical activity.

Larson, David E., ed. *Mayo Clinic Family Health Book.* 3d ed. New York: HarperResource, 2003. Perhaps the best general medical text for the layperson, this book covers the entire medical field. While the information is derived from a wide variety of highly technical sources, the articles are written to be easily understood by a general audience.

Minkin, Mary Jane. "Prevent Hemorrhoids." *Prevention* 50, no. 6 (June, 1998): 76. Pushing or straining too hard due to constipation is a major reason hemorrhoids develop. Tips on how to prevent constipation are offered.

Okie, Susan. "Colon Susceptible to Other Woes Besides Cancer; The Basics on Everything from Crohn's Disease to Hemorrhoids." *The Washington Post*, February 10, 1998, p. Z19. Between 10 and 20 percent of American adults suffer from irritable bowel syndrome, a set of symptoms that can be painful, inconvenient, and at times disabling.

Peikin, Steven. *Gastrointestinal Health.* Rev. ed. New York: HarperCollins, 1999. Concerned almost wholly with the effect of nutrition on GI maladies, the author offers a self-help guide for the afflicted. After explaining the GI tract's workings and describing common symptoms, Peikin specifies diets that he argues will relieve symptoms.

Sachar, David B., Jerome D. Waye, and Blair S. Lewis, eds. *Pocket Guide to Gastroenterology.* Rev. ed. Baltimore: Williams & Wilkins, 1991. This diagnosis-oriented handbook gives information on all gastroenterological ailments in outline form, making it valuable for quick studies on major problems. The section on hemorrhoids, though superficial, lays out the basic symptoms and treatments.

Wanderman, Sidney E., with Betty Rothbart. *Hemorrhoids.* Yonkers, N.Y.: Consumer Reports Books, 1991. Providing a simple but thorough overview of anatomical problems, causes, medications, therapies, and removal methods, this short book also discusses related complaints, such as fissures and fistulas, and dangerous diseases whose symptoms can be mistaken for those of hemorrhoids.

HEPATITIS

DISEASE/DISORDER

ANATOMY OR SYSTEM AFFECTED: Liver

SPECIALTIES AND RELATED FIELDS: Epidemiology, internal medicine, toxicology, virology

DEFINITION: An inflammatory condition of the liver, characterized by discomfort, jaundice, and enlargement of the organ and bacterial, viral, or immunological in origin; may also result from use of alcohol and other toxic drugs.

KEY TERMS:

alanine aminotransferase: a liver enzyme associated with the metabolism of the amino acid alanine; elevated levels are an indication of liver damage

aspartate aminotransferase: a liver enzyme associated with metabolism of the amino acid aspartate; elevated levels are an indication of liver damage

cirrhosis: chronic degeneration of the liver, in which normal tissue is replaced with fibroid tissue and fat; commonly associated with alcohol abuse but can also result from hepatitis

hepatitis A virus: the virus associated with certain forms of hepatitis; generally contracted through fecal contamination of food and water

hepatitis B virus: the agent associated with severe forms of viral hepatitis; contracted through contaminated blood or hypodermic needles or through contaminated body fluids, and sometimes found in association with hepatitis D virus

hepatitis C virus: formerly referred to as the etiological agent for non-A, non-B viral hepatitis; most often passed in contaminated blood

hepato: a prefix denoting anything associated with the liver—for example, a hepatocyte is a liver cell

jaundice: a symptom of a variety of liver disorders which manifests as yellowish discoloration of the skin, the whites of the eyes, and other tissues; hepatocellular jaundice results from hepatitis

CAUSES AND SYMPTOMS

Hepatitis, a pathology referring to inflammation of the liver, may result from any of a variety of causes but commonly follows bacterial or viral infection. Hepatitis may be associated with an autoimmune phenomenon in which the body produces antibodies against liver tissue. Liver inflammation may also be an aftereffect of the use of alcohol or various hepatotoxic chemicals, either through the taking of illegal drugs or as a side effect of the legal use of pharmacological agents. Among the pharmaceuticals that can cause liver damage are antibiotics such as isoniazid and rifampin and the painkiller acetaminophen.

Symptoms associated with hepatitis are a reflection of the function of the liver. The liver is arguably the most complex organ in the body. More than five hundred different functions have been associated with the organ, including the production of bile for emulsification of fats and the secretion of glucose, proteins, or vitamins for use elsewhere in the body. The liver plays a major role in the detoxification of the blood, removing alcohol, nicotine, and other potentially poisonous substances. The Kupffer cells in the liver function in the removal of infectious agents or foreign material from the blood. More than 10 percent of the blood supply in the body is found within the liver at any time.

Among the functions of the liver is the removal of hemoglobin in the blood, released as a result of the lysis (disintegration) of red blood cells. A breakdown product of hemoglobin is the yellowish compound bilirubin. It is the buildup of bilirubin in blood that results in the appearance of jaundice in cases of inadequate liver function, such as during hepatitis.

Although hepatitis may develop from a variety of causes, it most commonly results from infection of the liver. Nearly any infectious agent may potentially damage the liver, but generally these involve one of several types of viruses, bacteria, fungi, or amoebas. Liver disease may also be significantly exacerbated by alcohol abuse, as is seen in patients with cirrhosis. Regardless of the specific cause, symptoms of liver disease remain similar in most cases. The liver is often enlarged and tender to physical examination. The person may feel tired and run a low-grade fever. It is not unusual for the person to feel nauseous and lose weight. Jaundice is common in most patients; the concentrations of the enzymes alanine aminotransferase (ALT) and aspartate aminotransferase (AST) may rise. Levels of these enzymes, however, are not necessarily indications of the severity of liver disease; in any event, their levels often fall over the course of the disease.

Three particular viruses have been associated with most forms of viral hepatitis (types A, B, and C), while a fourth (type D) appears as a passenger during some cases of hepatitis B. Several additional viruses, designated hepatitis E (HEV) through hepatitis G (HGV), have also been linked to forms of the disease. Hepatitis A results from infection with hepatitis A virus (HAV), a virus classified in the same group as the poliovirus and rhinoviruses (cold viruses). The disease is transmitted through a fecal-to-oral method and is self-limited (running a definite and limited course). Often the disease is subclinical (undetectable), particularly as seen in children. Replication of the virus occurs in hepatocytes (liver cells); the virus then passes into the intestine and is eliminated with the feces. A long incubation period following ingestion may occur, sometimes as long as a month, and during much of this period the person is capable of transmitting the disease. In otherwise healthy individuals, recovery is complete and occurs over several weeks. Anti-HAV antibodies are present in the blood of about 30 to 40 percent of the general population, reflecting the widespread nature of the disease.

Hepatitis B (HBV), formerly called serum hepatitis, is a potentially much more severe form of the disease. The disease in young children is frequently asymptomatic, with appearance of symptoms in older individuals

---

INFORMATION ON HEPATITIS

CAUSES: Bacterial or viral infection, immunological disorder, abuse of alcohol and other toxic drugs

SYMPTOMS: Jaundice, liver enlargement, discomfort, fatigue, low-grade fever, nausea, weight loss

DURATION: Ranges from short-term to chronic

TREATMENTS: Antibiotics, hospitalization

being more common. In general, however, the most frequent result of primary infection with HBV is a mild or subclinical course of infection. The disease is most commonly seen in the fifteen-to-thirty-five age group, in part reflecting its method of transmission (through blood or body fluids).

Persistent infection with HBV, occurring in approximately 1 to 3 percent of patients, can be associated with either an asymptomatic carrier state or chronic hepatitis. The chronic state may be severe, with progression to cirrhosis and cellular degeneration or inflammation. In fact, it is the immune response to the presence of HBV that may contribute to liver degeneration. HBV infection results in the expression of viral antigens, which stimulate an immune response, on the surface of liver cells. Among the inflammatory cells present at the sites of infection are a large proportion of lymphocytes. These include cytotoxic T cells, lymphocytes associated with the killing of virally infected cells. Because immunologically impaired individuals infected with HBV often suffer a mild form of the disease, the possibility exists that it is the immune response itself that contributes to the ensuing liver damage.

Hepatitis B transmission occurs through blood or bodily fluids, including semen and vaginal secretions. Because HBV is also found in saliva, the disease may be transmitted among family members through nonsexual contact. Maternal-neonatal transmission may occur, occasionally while the fetus is in the uterus but more likely during the labor or birth process. There is, however, no evidence for transmission through food or water or by an airborne means.

Clinical features of HBV infections are similar to those associated with other forms of hepatitis. In the asymptomatic form of type B disease, AST or ALT levels may be elevated, but jaundice is absent. Adults with symptomatic hepatitis B may suffer jaundice (icteric hepatitis), or they may not (nonicteric hepatitis). There is generally a mild fever, fatigue, and weakness.

Accompanying an indeterminant number of HBV infections is a second virus, designated the hepatitis D virus (HDV). HDV is a defective virus, capable of replication only in the presence of HBV. Not surprisingly, its geographic distribution and mode of transmission are similar to those of HBV. The prevalence of HDV has been found to be as high as 70 percent in some outbreaks of HBV and nonexistent in others. In most cases, HDV infection results in subclinical or mild hepatitis. In about 15 percent of cases, the disease may progress to a more severe form. HDV may itself be cytopathic

(causing pathological changes) for hepatocytes, but this remains to be established firmly.

Based on the exclusion of other types of etiologic agents, including HAV, HBV, Epstein-Barr virus, and cytomegalovirus, non-A, non-B (NANB) hepatitis was considered a clinical entity. During the late 1980's, NANB hepatitis was determined to be caused by a newly isolated infectious agent, designated hepatitis C virus (HCV). The study of HCV was hampered by the inability to grow the virus in cell culture. Ironically, the virus was cloned and characterized before it was even physically observed, allowing for the development of a screening assay used for the detection of contaminated serum. In the United States, approximately 25 percent of hepatitis is associated with HCV. Before screening procedures were put into place in 1992, HCV infection was the major complication of blood transfusions or transfusions of blood products. Infection now occurs through sexual intercourse, the sharing of intravenous needles, and accidental needle punctures among health care workers. HCV has been increasingly recognized as a major health threat. It creates serious liver damage and is the leading cause of liver transplants. It is all the more dangerous because patients are often asymptomatic and learn of the infection when the blood is screened for other reasons. As a result, many people are unknowing carriers of the virus.

Outbreaks of an enterically transmitted NANB hepatitis (NANB hepatitis transmitted through the intestines), designated hepatitis E, have also been found in some parts of the world. Though hepatitis E has been around at least since 1955 (and no doubt earlier, but undocumented), it was only in the late 1980's that it was determined to be a unique form of the disease. Trans-

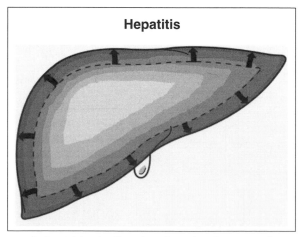

Hepatitis

In hepatitis, the liver is enlarged and congested.

mission occurs through eating or drinking contaminated food or water, though there is evidence that household contact with infected persons may also transmit the disease. Hepatitis E is most common in the poor countries of Asia, with sporadic outbreaks elsewhere. The few cases found in the United States have involved travelers to these areas.

Acute hepatitis is less commonly associated with infection by other viruses. These include the herpes family of viruses, such as herpes simplex, cytomegalovirus, and Epstein-Barr virus. Because the prevalence of these viruses is quite high, immunosuppressed or immunodeficient patients may be at particular risk.

Certain forms of hepatitis are associated with an autoimmune response. In these cases, the cause is not an infectious agent but rather a form of rejection by the body of its own liver tissue. Autoimmune hepatitis is suspected in individuals in which the disease persists for at least six months with no evidence of exposure to an infectious agent or hepatotoxin. In nearly one-third of these individuals, other immunological diseases such as lupus or arthritis may be present. The clinical manifestations of autoimmune hepatitis are similar to those of other forms of the disease. Most patients exhibit jaundice, a mild fever, weakness, and weight loss. The liver is often enlarged and tender. Unlike other forms of hepatitis, found equally in men and women, autoimmune hepatitis is most commonly found in women. Prognosis of the disease is unclear, as an unknown percentage of cases are subclinical. Severe forms have a high fatality rate.

TREATMENT AND THERAPY

Treatment for the various forms of viral hepatitis is, for the most part, symptomatic and supportive. Hospitalization may be required in severe cases, but, in general, any restriction of activity is left up to the patient. This is particularly convenient, since recovery often involves a long convalescence. As long as a healthy diet is maintained, no special dietary requirements exist, but a high-calorie diet is often preferable. Drugs or chemicals that are potentially damaging to the liver, including alcohol and certain antibiotics or painkillers, should be avoided.

Hepatitis induced by other forms of infectious agents such as bacteria or fungi may be treated using an appropriate course of antibiotic therapy. In cases of drug-induced disease, avoidance of the chemical is a key to recovery. Bacterial infections of the liver are often associated with patients who are malnourished, such as

the elderly or alcoholics, or who may be immunosuppressed. These problems must also be addressed during the course of treatment.

Prevention of the disease is preferable, however, and because the means of viral spread has been well established in most cases, appropriate measures can often be taken. For the most part, the viruses associated with hepatitis have little in common with one another aside from their predilection for hepatocytes. Thus, preventing their spread involves different strategies.

HAV is almost always spread through a fecal-oral means of transmission. Often the source is an infected person involved in the preparation of uncooked foods. Common sense dictates that the person should wash after every use of a toilet, but this is often not the case. Not surprisingly, children attending day care centers frequently become infected. Contaminated groundwater is also a potential source of outbreaks in areas in which proper sewage treatment does not take place. Less commonly, HAV is spread directly from person to person through sexual contact. A method called immunoprophylaxis can prevent the development of symptoms in individuals exposed to hepatitis A by utilizing a form of passive immunity. Developed during World War II, the procedure involves the pooling of serum from immune individuals. Inoculation of the serum into exposed persons is effective in prevention of the disease in most cases.

In 1994, SmithKline Beecham Pharmaceuticals developed and received Food and Drug Administration (FDA) approval for the first vaccine shown to be safe and effective in preventing HAV infection. Manufactured under the trade name Havrix, the vaccine consists of a formalin-inactivated strain of HAV, to be administered in three doses to children. In 1996, a similar vaccine was developed by Merck and Co., to be sold under the trade name Vagta.

The transmission of HBV generally involves passage via contaminated blood or body secretions. In the period prior to the screening of blood, transfusions were the most common means of spreading the disease—hence the designation "serum hepatitis." Since the 1980's, the most common means of documented spread has been through either sexual contact or the sharing of contaminated hypodermic needles. Semen, vaginal secretions, and saliva from infected individuals all contain the active virus, and limiting exchange of these fluids is key to prevention of transmission. Even so, the means of infection in nearly one-third of symptomatic cases remains unknown.

An effective vaccine for prevention of HBV infection was first developed during the 1970's and early 1980's. The vaccination procedure was later modified to create an effective combined active-passive vaccine. Passive immunization utilizes antibodies purified from the blood of donors who have recovered from HBV infection. This hepatitis B immune globulin (HBIG) is combined with a recombinant yeast vaccine that contains hepatitis virus proteins but lacks the genetic material necessary for the virus to replicate. Because HBIG already contains a high level of anti-HBV antibody, it is effective as a postexposure preventive for an individual who has come in contact with the disease. For example, a person exposed to the virus through an accidental needle stick, such as an unimmunized health care worker, may not have time to proceed through the regimen of treatment. The use of HBIG provides a short-term means of protection. The combined vaccine is used as a method of pre-exposure immunization. In the early 1990's, vaccination was recommended to only those persons at high risk for exposure to HBV. This group is composed of homosexual or bisexual men, health care workers (including physicians and dentists), and persons dealing with individuals in whom the disease is commonly found.

Because hepatitis D virus is defective in replication, requiring the presence of HBV, no specific measures of prevention are necessary. Immunization against HBV is sufficient to prevent the spread of HDV.

The deadly HCV is treated with antiviral agents, such as ribavirin and shots of interferon. A longer-acting form called pegylated interferon (Pegasys) is still in the experimental stage but is showing some promise against this liver-destroying infection.

The transmission of the hepatitis E virus is also through a fecal-oral route. The drinking of water contaminated by sewage has been the most common source of transmission. Because no active means of prevention has been developed, prevention of exposure requires that the individual avoid any food or water potentially contaminated with sewage. This is particularly true in areas of the world in which hepatitis E is found. Though the precaution may seem obvious, the safety of the water, as well as any object washed in the water, is not always readily apparent.

Autoimmune hepatitis results from an aberrant immune system rather than from an infectious agent. Treatment generally involves the use of immunosuppressive drugs to limit the immune response. Corticosteroids such as prednisone, sometimes in combination with azathioprine, have proven effective in the therapy of many patients. Still, in some cases the disease progresses to cirrhosis and results in death. Treatment generally is carried out over a long period of time, at least a year, and relapses are common. Often, the patient requires lifetime therapy. The immunosuppressive activity of the therapy may also leave the patient more susceptible to infection. In some cases, liver transplantation has proven effective, at least in the short term. Because the liver rejection was caused by an autoimmune response in the first place, the transplant may also be subject to the same phenomenon.

Perspective and Prospects

Inflammation of the liver resulting in hepatitis can develop from a variety of mechanisms. Most often, these mechanisms are associated with either a chemical injury or infection by a microbiological agent.

Infections of the liver generally involve one of several viral agents. The association of liver disease, or at least jaundice, with an infectious agent was suspected as early as the time of Hippocrates (the fifth century B.C.E.). Hippocrates described a syndrome which was undoubtedly viral hepatitis. The disease was also described in the Babylonian Talmud about eight hundred years later. Epidemics of the disease have been reported since the Middle Ages; these most likely involved outbreaks of hepatitis A. The spread of this disease through personal contact was confirmed in the 1930's.

Type B, or serum hepatitis, was described as a clinical entity by A. Lurman in 1855. Lurman observed that 15 percent of shipyard workers in Bremen, Germany, who received a smallpox vaccine containing human lymph developed jaundice within the following six months. In the early years of the twentieth century, jaundice frequently developed among patients who received vaccines prepared from convalescent serums or who underwent procedures such as venipuncture using instruments which had not been properly sterilized. By 1926, the blood-borne nature of the disease had been confirmed. In 1942, more than twenty-eight thousand American soldiers developed jaundice after vaccination with a yellow fever vaccine prepared from pooled human serums. By then it had become obvious that at least two forms of infectious agents were associated with viral hepatitis.

The isolation of HBV occurred as a result of studies initiated by Baruch Blumberg in 1963. Blumberg was actually attempting to correlate the development of diseases such as cancer with particular patterns of proteins found in the serum of individuals. His approach was to collect blood from persons in various parts of the world and then analyze their serum proteins. Blumberg found an antigen, a protein, in the blood of Australian aborigines which reacted with antibodies in the blood of an American hemophiliac. Blumberg called the protein the Australia (Au) antigen. It later became apparent that the Au antigen could be isolated from the blood of patients with serum hepatitis. By 1970, it was established that what Blumberg had referred to as the Au antigen was in fact the HBV particle.

HBV is associated with more than simply viral hepatitis. Chronic hepatitis associated with HBV can often develop into hepatocellular carcinoma, or cancer of the liver. The precise reason is unclear; the cancer may result from the chronic damage to liver tissue associated with long-term infection by HBV.

An effective vaccine for the prevention of HBV infection was licensed in 1982. By the late 1990's, the effectiveness of a worldwide vaccination program, under the auspices of the World Health Organization, had led to the possibility that hepatitis resulting from HBV infection, as well as hepatocelluar carcinoma, could be controlled within another decade.

Cases of HCV continue to climb because of the high numbers of asymptomatic carriers. In 2003, it was estimated that four million Americans were infected with HCV and that approximately ten thousand would die from it each year, with that number expected to triple by 2010. About 170 million people were infected worldwide. As a result, HCV may prove to be one of the next important threats to global health.

—Richard Adler, Ph.D.;
updated by Tracy Irons-Georges

See also Addiction; Alcoholism; Autoimmune disorders; Cirrhosis; Immunization and vaccination; Jaundice; Liver; Liver cancer; Liver disorders; Liver transplantation; Viral infections.

FOR FURTHER INFORMATION:

Everson, Gregory T., and Hedy Weinberg. *Living with Hepatitis C: A Survivor's Guide.* 3d ed. Long Island City, N.Y.: Hatherleigh Press, 2002. An invaluable resource that reviews the latest clinical trials; updates all of the organizations, resources, and information that has changed since the last edition; and offers chapters on research trends, liver transplants, children, coinfection with HIV/AIDS or hepatitis B, and the nutritional, emotional, and financial challenges that accompany infection with hepatitis C.

Frank, Steven A. *Immunology and Evolution of Infectious Disease.* Princeton, N.J.: Princeton University Press, 2002. Blends research from molecular biology, immunology, pathogen biology, and population dynamics to discuss how and why parasites vary to escape recognition by the immune system, vaccine design, and the control of epidemics.

Gorbach, Sherwood L., John G. Bartlett, and Neil R. Blacklow, eds. *Infectious Diseases.* 3d ed. Philadelphia: W. B. Saunders, 2003. A thorough discussion of infectious diseases. Included is a brief history, an account of the mechanisms of disease and immunity, and a concise discussion of a broad range of infectious agents. The section on hepatitis viruses is well written and not particularly detailed.

Hepatitis Foundation International. http://www.hepfi .org/. A foundation that teaches the public and hepatitis patients how to prevent, diagnose, and treat viral hepatitis and supports research into prevention, treatment, and cures for the disease.

Kelley, William, et al., eds. *Textbook of Internal Medicine.* 4th ed. Philadelphia: Lippincott Williams & Wilkins, 2000. A medical textbook on the subject. The book contains an extensive section on liver diseases, including a concise description of viral hepatitis. The discussion of hepatitis viruses is thorough, clear, but not overly detailed.

Levine, Arnold. *Viruses.* New York: W. H. Freeman, 1992. A well-written outline of viruses and their history. Some basic knowledge of biology is helpful in certain areas of the book, but overall the format and style should reach nearly all general readers. The book is profusely and colorfully illustrated. Several sections deal specifically with viral hepatitis.

Palmer, Melissa. *Dr. Melissa Palmer's Guide to Hepatitis and Liver Disease.* Garden City Park, N.Y.: Avery, 2000. Palmer, a nationally recognized hepatologist, provides plainly written medical information explaining how the liver is integral to every aspect of daily functioning and well-being. Includes "The Basics," "Understanding and Treating Viral Hepatitis," "Understanding and Treating Other Liver Diseases," and "Treatment Options and Lifestyle Changes."

Shaw, Michael, ed. *Everything You Need to Know About Diseases.* Springhouse, Pa.: Springhouse Press, 1996. This well-illustrated consumer reference, compiled by more than one hundred doctors and medical experts, describes five hundred illnesses and conditions, their causes, symptoms, diagnosis, treatment, and prevention. Of particular interest is chapter 6, "Liver and Gallbladder."

Spector, Steven. *Viral Hepatitis: Diagnosis, Therapy, and Prevention.* Totowa, N.J.: Humana Press, 1999. This clearly written and readable review of viral hepatitis provides useful information for family physicians interested in this protean disorder. Each chapter is divided into sections, allowing the reader to quickly access desired information.

Zakim, David, and Thomas Boyer, eds. *Hepatology: A Textbook of Liver Disease.* 4th ed. Philadelphia: W. B. Saunders, 2002. A thorough compendium on most aspects of liver disease. The section on hepatitis contains a complete clinical description of the disease and of the biology of the hepatitis viruses.

HERBAL MEDICINE

TREATMENT

ALSO KNOWN AS: Plant medicine

ANATOMY OR SYSTEM AFFECTED: All

SPECIALTIES AND RELATED FIELDS: All

DEFINITION: The traditional and scientific application of chemicals directly derived from any part of plants for medicinal purposes. The medicinal uses of plants are for both preventive and curative purposes.

KEY TERMS:

alkaloid: a large group of compounds that contain nitrogen and usually have a basic reaction (for example, cocaine, caffeine, nicotine, quinine, and morphine)

antiseptic: a chemical substance that inhibits the growth of bacteria

glycoside: a compound containing a carbohydrate molecule (sugar) that yields glucose on hydrolysis and a nonsugar component called aglycone

hormone: chemical messengers produced by the tissues of an organism to act as signaling compounds for the regulation of functions

hypertension: persistent high blood pressure

hypotension: low blood pressure

leukemia: a cancer of the blood-forming organs, marked by the abnormal multiplication and development of leukocytes

pathogen: any agent or microorganism capable of producing disease

pharmaceutical: a medicinal drug

purgative: referring to substances that promote the rapid elimination of material from the digestive tract

THE CHEMICALS OF PLANT-DERIVED MEDICINES

Plants synthesize a wide array of secondary compounds that play a role in the physiology of plants but do not usually constitute an important part of the basic metabolism of plants. Secondary compounds enable plants to attract animals and also help plants to avoid or overcome their natural enemies of infection, parasitism, and predation. These secondary compounds are the main chemicals in plants that humans use as medicinal herbs. Fatty acids, essential oils, gums, resins, alkaloids, and steroids are the most common secondary compounds in plants.

Humans use oils and gums as purgatives and as carriers or emulsifiers in many drug preparations. Volatile oils and resins are often used to help processes that seek to penetrate tissues of the body and are also used as antiseptics. Alkaloids and steroids are the two major classes of plant-derived compounds used in human medicine today. These chemical compounds can occur in different forms that have one or more sugar molecules attached. Such forms, called glycosides, are often the medicinally active form of a compound.

All forms of steroids are complex chemical compounds that have the same fundamental structure of four carbon rings, called the backbone. When different chemical groups are added at different places on the backbone, a variety of steroidal compounds are produced as a result. For example, when sugar molecules are added to the carbon rings, steroidal glycosides are produced. Various cardiac glycosides and steroid hormones are produced by the addition of specific side chains or extra rings to the steroid backbone.

The second major group of medicinally important chemicals synthesized in plants is the alkaloids. They contain nitrogen and usually exhibit an alkaline reaction. Alkaloids were formerly considered secondary products, but unlike steroids, they have recently been shown occasionally to enter into the primary metabolism of plants. Many alkaloids are extremely poisonous to humans, and many have been used as poisons in many cultures around the world. Several of these plant chemicals possess antimicrobial properties and are used to kill harmful microorganisms that are pathogenic. A number of them are used as dietary supplements for balanced human nutrition and good health.

MEDICINAL PLANTS OF IMPORTANCE

In the past, some natural chemicals and oils were of tremendous medicinal use in treating diseases. Quinine was used for the treatment of malaria, cocaine was used as a calming agent and a local anesthetic, and chaulmoogra oil was employed for the treatment of leprosy.

Although these herbal medicines are rarely used today, many plants are still of great importance as sources of medicinal compounds. Both steroids and glycosides occur in many angiosperms.

To cite a few examples, certain members of the yam genus *Dioscorea* contain particular kinds of steroids in their tubers called saponins that are similar to human sex hormones. The chemical diosgenin can be extracted from the tubers, which is a good starting point for the chemical synthesis of saponins. The majority of the hormones synthesized from diosgenin are used in birth control pills, for the production of hormones that regulate the menstrual cycle, or as a component of fertility drugs. Cortisone and hydrocortisone are two other important hormones that are synthesized from diosgenin. They are used for the treatment of severe allergic reactions, arthritis, and Addison's disease, which is caused by malfunctioning of the adrenal glands.

Opium poppy, *Papaver somniferum*, is one of the oldest and still predominant sources of analgesics, which relieve pain. More than twenty-six different alkaloids have been isolated from opium, but only three of them—morphine, codeine, and papaverine—are used extensively. Morphine and codeine are used as painkillers, and papaverine is used primarily in drugs for the treatment of internal spasms, particularly those of the intestinal tract.

Another group of alkaloids is obtained from members of the potato family. They are considered analgesics and are used for controlling a variety of muscle spasms and in psychiatry. Alkaloids from *Atropa belladonna* are prescribed for stomach and bladder cramps and to prevent nausea and vomiting caused by motion sickness. They are prescribed for victims of Parkinson's disease to decrease stiffness and tremors and are often given to patients before surgery as a relaxant and to reduce salivation. These alkaloids, especially atropine, are helpful in cases of nerve gas (organophosphate insecticides) or mushroom poisoning. Alkaloids of the North American lily such as American false hellebore, *Veratrum viride*, have hypotensive properties and are used to treat high blood pressure.

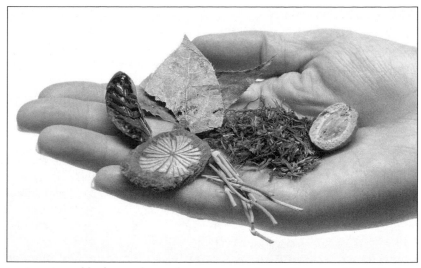

A variety of herbs can be used to prevent and treat illnesses. (PhotoDisc)

Cinchona, the genus known primarily as a source of quinine, produces about thirty other alkaloids, including the compound quinidine, which is useful in treating heart disease. Quinidine inhibits abnormal rapid contractions of the upper right chamber of the heart and corrects improper heart rhythms.

Rauwolfia serpentina was used in the past for treating snakebites. It was later found to be useful in the treatment of hypertension by relaxing the heart muscle and thus lowering blood pressure, but it produced the side effects of depression and tremors, and its use was therefore discontinued. In 1952, the important alkaloid reserpine was isolated in Switzerland from the root where it is concentrated, although it occurs everywhere in the plant. The dramatic effects of reserpine completely altered practices in mental institutions because of its pronounced calming effect on schizophrenics without producing undesirable side effects. A relatively New World species, *R. tetraphylla*, is also a source of the alkaloid.

The few known substances that are able to arrest cancer cells are plant alkaloids. The common periwinkle, *Catharanthus reseus*, has been used in its native range in Europe for hundreds of years as a folk treatment for diabetes. It is now used effectively to treat some leukemias, especially those that commonly afflict children. The two active alkaloids are vinblastine and vincristine. Mayapple, *Podophylum peltatum*, contains antitumor alkaloids. Today mayapple alkaloids are used as the basis of VM-26 (teniposide), a drug used to treat testicular tumors and, with other agents, breast and lung cancer. The alkaloid colchicine is extracted from the corms of the autumn crocus, *Colchicum autumnale*. Colchicine is primarily used for the reduction of inflammation and pain caused by gout but is also used in the treatment of cancer. Taxol, a compound most abundant in the bark of the Pacific yew, *Taxus brevifolia*, has been a major success in the treatment of breast and uterine cancer.

Several mucilaginous compounds of plant origin are used in soothing ointments and as carriers for other medicines. Species of *Aloe*, primarily *A. barbadensis*, have been used for their soothing gels. Chymopapain, an enzyme that exhibits specificity in its dissolution of proteins, is obtained from papaya, *Carica papaya*. It is injected by doctors into the soft central area of a deformed disk in humans to dissolve a large part of it and relieve the pressure on adjacent nerves.

PERSPECTIVE AND PROSPECTS

The medicinal uses of plants by humans have been known since ancient times and can be said to predate written history. Every culture on earth has used plants to cure disease, ease pain, and heal the ills and discomforts of the human body. People first started to keep records of herbal medicine about five thousand to seven thousand years ago in China and Mesopotamia. Sumerian drawings of opium poppy capsules from 2500 B.C.E. suggest that considerable knowledge of medicinal plants was in place. A substantial record of the use of herbs in medicine comes from the Code of Hammurabi, a series of tablets carved under the direction of the king of Babylon in about 1770 B.C.E. These tablets mention plants, such as henbane, licorice, and mint, that are still used in medicines at the present time. The Egyptians later recorded their knowledge of illnesses and cures on temple walls and in the Ebers papyrus (1550 B.C.E.), which contains more than seven hundred medicinal formulas.

In Greece, Hippocrates (c. 460-c. 370 B.C.E.) prescribed sound nutrition, purgatives, and botanical drugs for humans. He consequently earned the reputation as the father of medicine by being the first person to document illnesses and their treatment in a rational and orderly fashion. The most significant contribution made by Greeks toward the documentation of plants with healing properties was made by Dioscorides in his five-volume work entitled *De Materia Medica*. His encyclopedia described the preparation of about one thousand simple drugs. For several centuries afterward, it was the foundation text for practitioners of herbal medicine throughout Europe.

A stronger link was established between the studies of botany and medicine during the Middle Ages, and printed herbals became more available with the invention of the printing press in 1439. More herbs were added to the list from the New World when Europeans arrived in North America and learned Native American herbal uses. In the fourteenth century, the Renaissance led Europe into the determination of the medicinal uses of plants.

In the seventeenth and eighteenth centuries, science and philosophy advanced to the stage of experiments and hypothesis testing. It was not until the early 1800's, however, that scientists first began to isolate and extract healing compounds from plants. This experimental approach to medicine led to an improved understanding of physiology and provided a framework for the careful testing of medical treatments, including medicinal herbs.

The first half of the twentieth century saw tremendous advancements in medicine as more causes of diseases were discovered and new effective drugs were produced. Several modern medicines were produced as isolated and purified products of traditional plant-derived extracts, including morphine, quinine, and ephedrine. Medical chemists then began to determine the structures of these compounds and the possibility of their synthesis. In addition, they explored the chances of using the knowledge of the active ingredients of a natural healing herb to synthesize chemically related compounds that were potentially better medicines than the original one.

In the latter part of the twentieth century and the beginning of the twenty-first century, the prevalence of some diseases in some parts of the world and the emergence of diseases such as acquired immunodeficiency syndrome (AIDS) and severe acute respiratory syndrome (SARS) have challenged scientists, botanists, and doctors to explore plant sources for drugs that will offer possible or better cures.

Medicinal herbs are central to alternative therapies, which are gaining popularity in the twenty-first century. This trend is partly attributable to modern research into plant medicine and the remarkable healing results of herbal application to some diseases. For example, years of studies have shown that garlic can help control blood pressure and cholesterol. Yet few mainstream doctors recommend it, even though garlic is cheaper than pharmaceuticals and causes fewer side effects. This situation is beginning to change, however, because of a growing interest in natural sources of medicine. An estimated 80 percent of the world's population still rely on herbs for treating and preventing disease. In the United States, an estimated 25 percent of pharmaceuticals are still derived from plant sources. Native American herbs are still used by North American doctors in the twenty-first century. Many people do not realize that medical herbs are a key link between alternative therapies and mainstream medicine. Scientists around the world depend on herbs to develop new, more potent medications, and the search continues for plants with healing properties.

—*Samuel V. A. Kisseadoo, Ph.D.*

See also Alternative medicine; Antioxidants; Food biochemistry; Homeopathy; Marijuana; Nutrition; Pharmacology; Pharmacy; Self-medication; Supplements; Toxicology.

FOR FURTHER INFORMATION:

Castleman, Michael. *Blended Medicine: The Best Choices in Healing.* Emmaus, Pa.: Rodale Press, 2000. Provides comprehensive knowledge on the use of medicinal plants as the center of alternative medicine. Discusses how different forms of treatment can be "blended" for different diseases.

Maleskey, Gale, and the editors of Prevention Health Books. *Nature's Medicines.* Emmaus, Pa.: Rodale Press, 1999. Contains a detailed account of health supplements and the use of natural herbs to prevent and cure several common ailments. Includes an index, charts, and elaborate information of the names of many plants and natural supplements, plus steps that one can follow in order to use them effectively.

Simpson, Beryl Brintnall, and Molly Conner Ogorzaly. *Economic Botany.* 3d ed. Boston: McGraw-Hill, 2001. Gives an excellent account of the history and use of medicinal plants in different cultures over the centuries. Highlights modern utility and research into herbal medicine. Contains good illustrations, photographs, references, the scientific and common names of plants, a glossary, and an index.

White, B. Linda, and Steven Foster. *The Herbal Drugstore.* Emmaus, Pa.: Rodale Press, 2000. Provides one of the best natural alternatives to over-the-counter and prescription medicines. Contains charts, illustrations, scientific names, and an index.

Yeager, Selene. *The Doctors Book of Food Remedies.* Emmaus, Pa.: Rodale Press, 1998. Gives a very detailed account of the healing properties of most common food items and herbs. Contains outlines of various preparations, charts, illustrations, and an index.

HERMAPHRODITISM AND PSEUDOHERMAPHRODITISM

DISEASE/DISORDER

ANATOMY OR SYSTEM AFFECTED: Genitals, reproductive system, urinary system

SPECIALTIES AND RELATED FIELDS: Embryology, endocrinology, genetics, gynecology, urology

DEFINITION: Abnormal primary sexual characteristics caused by developmental defects.

CAUSES AND SYMPTOMS

Hermaphroditism is a condition in which testicular and ovarian tissues are found in the same person and their urogenital development is ambiguous. A baby with an enlarged clitoris resembling a penis and fused labial-scrotal folds is often designated a male, whereas a baby with a normal clitoris and open labial folds might be considered a female. Generally, inappropriate levels of male and female hormones during fetal development are responsible for ambiguous genitals at birth.

Pseudohermaphroditism is a condition in which either testicular tissues or ovarian tissues, but not both, are found in an individual with ambiguous urogenital development. XY pseudohermaphrodites develop internal testes, but their external genitals and appearance at birth are female. They lack ovaries, Fallopian tubes, and a uterus, but they have a blind (dead-end) vagina. There are two types of XY pseudohermaphrodites, those with testicular feminization syndrome (TFS) and those with *huevodoce* (or *guevedoces*) syndrome (HDS).

As individuals with TFS enter puberty, they begin to grow genital hair and breasts and have the appearance of normal females because they are unable to respond to any form of testosterone. When individuals with HDS begin puberty, the clitoris enlarges into a penis-like structure without a urethra. The urethral opening is at the base of the enlarged clitoris. One or both of the internal testes descend into scrotal sacs, and the teenager

---

INFORMATION ON HERMAPHRODITISM AND PSEUDOHERMAPHRODITISM

CAUSES: Genetic defect of sex organs

SYMPTOMS: Abnormal appearance of primary sexual characteristics

DURATION: Chronic unless corrected

TREATMENTS: Hormonal therapy, surgery

begins to develop masculine body and facial hair, but there is no breast development. In some cases, the voice deepens, and muscle mass and body shape become more masculine. Individuals with *huevodoce* syndrome develop as they do because they are unable to convert testosterone to 5-alpha-dihydrotestosterone (DHT), the inducer necessary for the early development of male tissues. At puberty, the testes produce very large amounts of testosterone, which is able to make up for the lack of DHT and to stimulate some tissues to develop further.

TREATMENT AND THERAPY

Hormone therapy or even operations to remove vestigial testes at birth might be of value in promoting the development of normal external genitals in hermaphroditic babies. In children with HDS, hormone therapy helps to resolve the ambiguous development of external genitalia at puberty. There are no treatments or therapies for individuals with TFS because these individuals are not responsive to testosterone.

PERSPECTIVE AND PROSPECTS

In general, persons with TFS think of themselves as females. They are sexually attracted to men and usually marry. No treatment should be considered for these individuals. Many individuals with HDS remain in a female role, but some take on the male role as they change at puberty. Hormone therapy might be of value in helping to establish the roles they desire in their culture.

—*Jaime S. Colomé, Ph.D.*

See also Genetic diseases; Genetics and inheritance; Puberty and adolescence; Reproductive system; Sexual differentiation.

FOR FURTHER INFORMATION:

Dreger, Alice Domurat. *Hermaphrodites and the Medical Invention of Sex.* Cambridge, Mass.: Harvard University Press, 2000.

Fausto-Sterling, Anne. *Sexing the Body: Gender Politics and the Construction of Sexuality.* New York: Basic Books, 2000.

Hellinga, Gerhardus. *Clinical Andrology: A Systematic Approach, with a Chapter on Intersexuality.* London: Heinemann, 1976.

Hunter, R. H. F. *Sex Determination, Differentiation, and Intersexuality in Placental Mammals.* New York: Cambridge University Press, 1995.

Kessler, Suzanne. *Lessons from the Intersexed.* New Brunswick, N.J.: Rutgers University Press, 1998.

Moore, Keith L., and T. V. N. Persaud. *The Developing Human.* 7th ed. Philadelphia: W. B. Saunders, 2003.

HERNIA

DISEASE/DISORDER

ANATOMY OR SYSTEM AFFECTED: Abdomen, gastrointestinal system, intestines, reproductive system, stomach

SPECIALTIES AND RELATED FIELDS: Gastrointestinal system, internal medicine

DEFINITION: A pouchlike mass consisting of visceral material encased in properitoneal tissue (the hernial sac) protruding through an aperture in the abdomen—a result of a weakening in the abdominal wall.

KEY TERMS:

Bassini technique: the most widely accepted surgical method for treating hernias; named after the Italian surgeon Edoardo Bassini

hernioplasty: the surgery performed to treat hernia patients

incarceration: an advanced and dangerous hernial stage which occurs when the hernial sac protrudes well beyond the abdominal aperture and is constricted at the neck

inguinal hernia: the most common form of hernia, in which the hernial sac protrudes into the lower groin area

reducible hernia: a hernia that has not advanced significantly beyond the weakened aperture in the abdomen; such hernias were formerly treated by means of the externally applied pressure of a truss

CAUSES AND SYMPTOMS

A hernia condition exists when either tissues from, or actual portions of, vital internal organs protrude beyond the enclosure of the abdomen as a result of an abnormal opening in several possible areas of the abdominal wall. In most hernias, the protruding material remains encased in the tissue of the peritoneum. This saclike extension forces itself into whatever space can be ceded by neighboring tissues outside the abdomen. Because of the swelling effect produced, the hernia is usually visible as a lump on the surface of the body. As there are several types of hernias that may occur in different areas of the abdomen, the place of noticeable swelling and the internal organs affected may vary. With the single exception of the pancreas, hernia cases have been recorded involving all other organs contained in the abdomen. The most common hernial protrusions, however, involve the small intestine and/or the omenta, folds of the peritoneum. Another category of hernia, referred to as hernia adipose, consists of a protrusion of peritoneal fat beyond the abdominal wall.

Generally speaking, the cause of hernial conditions involves not only an internal pressure pushing portions of the viscera against the abdominal wall (hence the danger of bringing on a hernia through heavy physical exertion in work or athletics) but also a point of weakness in the abdominal wall itself. Two such points of potential weakness exist in all normal, healthy individuals: the original umbilical ring, which should normally "heal" over after the umbilical cord is severed; and the groin tissues in the lower portion of the abdomen—the region where the most common hernia, the inguinal hernia, occurs. Another possible source of vulnerability to hernia protrusions is connected to the individual's prior surgical history: Scar tissue may prove to be the weakest point of resistance to pressures originating anywhere in the abdominal region.

It should be noted that, because the abdominal tissues of infants and young children are particularly delicate, there is a proportionately higher occurrence of hernial conditions among babies and toddlers. If the hernia is diagnosed and treated early enough, complete healing is almost certain in such cases, most of which do not develop beyond the preliminary, or reducible, stage.

The several stages, or degrees, of hernial development usually begin with what doctors call a reducible hernia condition. At this stage, a patient suffering from hernia, sensing the onset of the disorder, may be able to obtain temporary relief from a developing protrusion by changing posture angle when upright or by lying down. Until the late twentieth century, some physicians preferred to treat reducible hernias by means of an externally attached pressure device, or truss, rather than resorting to surgical intervention. This form of treatment was gradually dropped in favor of increasingly effective hernioplasty operations.

When a hernial condition enters what is called the stage of incarceration, the advanced protrusion of the sac containing portions of viscera through the opening, or ring, in the abdominal wall can cause very severe complications. If, as is frequently the case, the protruding hernia sac passes through the ring as a fingerlike tube and then assumes a globular form outside the abdominal wall, a state of incarceration exists. As this state advances, the patient runs the risk of hernial strangulation. The constricting pressure of the ring's edges on the hernial sac interferes with circulatory functions in the herniated organ, causing destruction of tissues and, unless surgical intervention occurs, rapid spread of gangrene throughout the affected organ. It was the sixteenth century French surgeon Pierre Franco who carried out the first operation to release a strangulated hernia by inserting a thin instrument between the incarcerated bowel and the herniated sac, then incising the latter without touching the extruded vital organ.

A surprisingly wide range of hernial conditions have been noted and studied. These include hernias in the umbilical, epigastric (upper abdominal), spigelian (transversus abdominal muscle), interparietal, and groin regions. Hernias in the groin can be either femoral or inguinal. Inguinal hernias affecting the groin area have always been by far the most common, accounting for more than three-quarters of hernial cases, particularly among males.

Inguinal hernias share a number of common characteristics with one another and with the other closely associated form of groin hernia, the femoral hernia. Inguinal hernias are all caused by the abnormal introduction of a hernial sac into one of the four-centimeter-long inguinal canals located on the sides of the abdomen. These canals originate in the lower portion of the abdomen at an aperture called the inguinal ring. They have an external exit point in the rectus abdominal tissue. Located inside each inguinal canal are the ilioinguinal nerve, the genital branch of the genitofemoral nerve, and the spermatic cord. A comparable passageway from the abdomen into the groin area is found at the femoral ring, through which both the femoral artery and the femoral vein pass.

It may take a long period, sometimes years, for the sac to engage itself fully in the inguinal or femoral ring. Once the ring is passed, however, pressures from inside the abdomen help it descend through the canal rather quickly. If the external inguinal ring is firm in structure,

---

INFORMATION ON HERNIA

CAUSES: Presence of scar tissue, heavy physical exertion in work or athletics, obesity, aging, congenital abnormality

SYMPTOMS: Heartburn, swallowing difficulty, chest pain, belching

DURATION: Acute or chronic

TREATMENTS: Surgery

and particularly if the narrow passageway is largely filled with the thickness of the spermatic cord, the inguinal hernia may be partially arrested at this point. In men, once it passes beyond the external inguinal ring, however, it quickly descends into the scrotum. In women, the inguinal canal contains the round ligament, which may also temporarily impede the further descent of the hernial sac beyond the external inguinal opening.

TREATMENT AND THERAPY

Given the widespread occurrence of hernia conditions at all age levels in most societies, physicians receive extensive training in the diagnosis and, among those with surgical training, the treatment of hernia patients. Near-total consensus among doctors now demands surgery (external trusses having been largely abandoned), but different schools support different surgical methods. With the exception of operations involving the insertion of prosthetic devices to block the extension of hernia damage, most recent inguinal hernioplasty methods derive from the model finalized by the Italian Edoardo Bassini in the late nineteenth century.

Bassini believed that the surgical methods of his time fell short of the goal of complete hernial repair, since most postoperational patients were required to wear a truss to guard against recurring problems. In the simplest of surgical terms, his solution involved the physiological reconstruction of the inguinal canal. The operation provided for a new internal passageway to an external opening, as well as strengthened anterior and posterior inguinal walls. After initial incisions and ligation of the hernial sac, Bassini's method involved a separation of tissues between the internal inguinal ring and the pubis. A tissue section referred to as the "triple layer" (containing the internal oblique, the transversus abdominal, and the transversalis fascia tissue layers) was then attached by a line of sutures to the Poupart ligament, with a lowermost suture at the edge of the rectus abdominal muscle. Such local reconstruction of the inguinal canal proved to strengthen the entire zone against the recurrence of ruptures.

Physicians operating on indirect, as opposed to direct, inguinal hernias confront a relatively uncomplicated set of procedures. In the former case, a high ligation of the peritoneal sac (a circular incision of the peritoneum at a point well inside the abdominal inguinal ring) usually makes it possible to remove the sac entirely. Complications can occur if the patient is obese, since a large mass of peritoneal fatty material may be joined to the sac, obstructing access to the inguinal

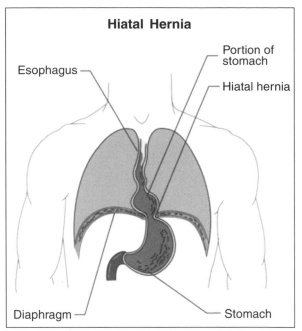

Hiatal Hernia

Esophagus

Portion of stomach

Hiatal hernia

Diaphragm

Stomach

A portion of the stomach has pushed through the weakened abdominal wall.

ring. For normal indirect inguinal hernias, the next basic step, after ensuring that no damage has occurred to the viscera either during formation of the hernia or in the process of relocating the contents of the hernial sac inside the abdomen, is to use one of several surgical methods to reduce the opening of the inguinal ring to its normal size. The physician must also ensure that no damage to the posterior inguinal wall has occurred and that its essential attachment to Cooper's ligament does not require additional surgical attention.

One must contrast the relative simplicity of indirect inguinal hernia surgery to treatment of direct inguinal hernias. In these cases, the hernia does not protrude through the existing inguinal aperture, but, as a result of a weakening of local tissues, passes directly through the posterior inguinal wall. The direct inguinal hernia is usually characterized by a broad base at the point of protrusion and a relatively short hernial sac. When a physician recommends surgical treatment of such hernias, the surgeon must be prepared for the extensive task of surgical reconstruction of the posterior inguinal wall as part of the operation.

Two additional reasons tend to discourage an immediate decision to operate on direct inguinal hernias. First, this form of hernia rarely strangulates the affected viscera, since the aperture stretches to allow protrusion of the hernial sac. Second, once physicians find obvious symptoms of a direct inguinal hernia (a ceding of the weakened posterior inguinal wall to pressures originating in the abdomen), they may decide to examine the patient more thoroughly to determine whether the cause behind the symptoms demands an entirely different prognosis. Such causes of abdominal pressures may range from the effects of a chronic cough to much more serious problems, including inflammation of the prostate gland or other forms of obstruction in the colon itself.

PERSPECTIVE AND PROSPECTS

Because the phenomenon of hernias has been the subject of scientific observation since the onset of formal medical writing itself, a stage-by-stage development of prognoses has been associated with this condition. A main dividing line appears between the mid-eighteenth and mid-nineteenth centuries, however, between the extremely rudimentary surgical treatments of the late Middle Ages and Renaissance and what can be called modern prognoses.

Without doubt the surgical contribution of the sixteenth century Frenchman Pierre Franco, who performed the first operation to release an incarcerated hernia, must be considered a landmark. The major general cause for advancement in knowledge of hernias, however, is tied to the birth of a new era in medical science, characterized by the use, from about 1750 onward, of anatomical dissection to investigate the essential characteristics of a number of common diseases.

Before the relatively long line of contributions that led to general adoption of the Bassini technique of operating on hernias, surgeons tended to follow the so-called Langenbeck method, named after the German physician who pioneered modern hernioplasty. This method held that simple removal of a hernial sac at the point of its protrusion from the abdomen and closing the external aperture would lead to a closing of the sac by "adhesive inflammation." Such spontaneous closing occurs when a severed artery "recedes" to the first branching-off point.

It took contributions by at least two lesser-known late nineteenth century forerunners to Edoardo Bassini to convince the surgical world that hernia operations must involve a high incision of the hernial sac. Both the American H. O. Marcy (1837-1924) and the Frenchman Just Marie Marcellin Lucas-Championnière (1843-1913) have been recognized for their insistence on the necessity of high-incision operations. Their hernia operations, by incising the external oblique fascia,

were the first to penetrate well beyond the external ring to expose the entire hernial sac. Following removal of the sac, it was then possible for surgeons to close the transversalis fascia and to repair the higher interior tissues that might have been damaged by the swollen hernia.

Following initial acceptance of the technique of high-incision hernial operations, a number of physicians recommended a variety of methods that might be used to repair internal tissue damage. These methods ranged from simple ligation of the sac at the internal ring, without more extensive surgery involving either the abdominal wall or the spermatic cord, to the much more extensive method practiced by Bassini. Even after the Bassini method succeeded in gaining almost universal recognition, other adaptations (but nothing that represented a full innovation) would be added during the middle decades of the twentieth century. One such method, which borrowed from the German physician Georg Lotheissen's use of Cooper's ligament to serve as a foundation for suturing damaged layers of lower abdominal tissues, earned its proponent, the American Chester McVay, the honor of having the operation named after him.

Finally, one should note that, although few significant changes have occurred in most doctors' view of what must be done surgically to treat hernia patients, surgical use of laser beams in the 1990's began to affect the techniques of hernioplasty, particularly in terms of recovery time.

—*Byron D. Cannon, Ph.D.*

See also Abdomen; Abdominal disorders; Gastroenterology; Gastroenterology, pediatric; Gastrointestinal disorders; Gastrointestinal system; Hemorrhoids; Hernia repair; Intestinal disorders; Intestines.

FOR FURTHER INFORMATION:

Bendavid, Robert. *Abdominal Wall Hernias: Principles and Management*. New York: Springer-Verlag, 2000. A comprehensive examination of advances in hernia repair surgery.

Hernia Resource Center. http://www.herniainfo.com/. Provides FAQs about hernias, latest medical news and research, information on surgical treatment options, and tools to help find a doctor specializing in hernias.

Kurzer, Martin, Allan E. Kark, and George W. Wantz. *Surgical Management of Abdominal Wall Hernias*. London: Martin Dunitz, 1999. Although surgeons generally agree that hernias should be treated surgically, which surgical approach is the most appropriate for hernia repair is a much-debated issue. This book examines the various approaches.

Nyhus, Lloyd M., and Robert E. Condon, eds. *Hernia.* 5th ed. Philadelphia: J. B. Lippincott, 2001. Widely recognized and updated joint contribution by a large number of specialized physicians. Examines such topics as the etiology, history, and anatomy of hernias; conventional, laparoscopic, and endoscopic groin hernia repairs; complications of groin hernia; and pediatric hernias.

Ponka, Joseph L. *Hernias of the Abdominal Wall.* Philadelphia: W. B. Saunders, 1980. A general medical textbook containing excellent illustrative plates.

HERNIA REPAIR

PROCEDURE

ANATOMY OR SYSTEM AFFECTED: Abdomen, gastrointestinal system, intestines, stomach

SPECIALTIES AND RELATED FIELDS: Gastroenterology, general surgery

DEFINITION: Surgery to correct organ or tissue protrusions.

KEY TERMS:

congenital: referring to a disorder which is present at birth

diaphragm: the muscular partition that separates the abdominal and thoracic cavities

esophagus: the muscular tube through which food passes from the throat to the stomach

gangrene: death and decay of a body part as a result of injury, disease, or inadequate blood supply

peritonitis: potentially fatal abdominal inflammation and infection

INDICATIONS AND PROCEDURES

A hernia is an abnormal protrusion of an organ or organ part from its normal body cavity, most often tissue protruding through the abdominal wall. Abdominal hernias may occur in the groin (inguinal hernia), upper thigh (femoral hernia), navel (umbilical hernia), and diaphragm (hiatal hernia). They may be congenital or acquired in later life. Herniated tissue is most often part of the small or large intestine. It can also be part of the bladder or the stomach in femoral and hiatal hernias, respectively. Most hernias occur as a result of strain to the abdominal wall or its injury. For example, they are often caused by athletic overexertion or hard labor. Consequently, men are more subject to acquired hernias than women.

Congenital inguinal hernias in male infants can occur when the testicles of a developing fetus work their way down the inguinal canal to the scrotum. If the tissue sac accompanying them does not close off correctly, congenital hernia occurs. In men, acquired inguinal hernias occur when excess abdominal strain ruptures the intestinal wall and releases a loop of intestine. Inguinal hernias are less common in women and are associated with the canal that holds the round ligament of the uterus. Femoral hernias in both sexes lie on the inner sides of the blood vessels of the thighs and are always acquired, often by overexertion. Umbilical hernias, which may be congenital or acquired, protrude from the navel.

Incisional hernia is caused by the incomplete healing of surgical wounds of the abdomen. A fifth hernia type is hiatal hernia, which occurs at the opening where the esophagus passes through the diaphragm (the hiatus). Such hernias, in which part or all of the stomach passes through the diaphragm, may cause no external symptoms and be diagnosed only when chest X rays are taken for other reasons. If symptoms do occur, they usually include heartburn and chest pain.

Hernias are classified according to severity. Reducible hernias are those which can be resolved by pushing herniated tissue back into its proper position. Irreducible hernias are more serious. They cannot be pushed back manually because of their position, or because of the presence of adhesions that bind them in place. Such hernias can only be corrected with surgery. Strangulated hernias are those whose size and location pinch herniated tissue, cutting off blood flow. They require immediate surgical treatment to prevent the development of gangrene or peritonitis, both of which can be fatal.

Surgical repair is the suggested treatment for most hernias. If the patient is temporarily too ill for surgery, a truss may be used to diminish pain and swelling for inguinal, femoral, umbilical, and incisional hernias. Trusses, however, provide only temporary, symptomatic relief, except perhaps in umbilical hernias of very young children. Extreme caution is necessary: Reducible hernias treated with trusses can become irreducible or strangulated.

Standard hernia surgery can be accomplished in several ways. For the correction of inguinal or umbilical hernias, first the muscle wall is opened. Then, after the herniated loop is moved into an appropriate position, the muscle wall is closed as normally as possible. In more severe types of hernia repair involving visible protrusions, the abdominal wall is opened, adhesions are cut away, and the tissue is returned to a normal position. Then, the muscle wall is closed to restore normal muscle layers. When strangulation occurs, damaged tissue is cut away, normal sections are joined together, and viable tissue is returned to the abdomen, followed

Hernia Repair

Abdominal wall

Intestine

Muscle   Fascia

Abdominal wall hernia

Femoral hernia

A hernia is the protrusion of a tissue or organ (usually a loop of intestine) into another area of the body. With abdominal wall hernias, which include inguinal and umbilical hernias, the intestine protrudes through a weakness in the abdomen; with femoral hernias, the intestine passes down the canal containing the major blood vessels to the thigh and appears as a bulge in the groin area. When a hernia presents a danger to the patient, the intestine must be surgically returned to its proper position.

by abdominal closure. Incisional hernias are treated similarly, in a fashion dependent on the extent of the external damage and the degree of herniation.

Hiatal hernias are treated medically, whenever possible, because they tend to recur after surgery. Medical treatment includes restriction of activity, weight loss, and diet modification. Surgery is carried out when these efforts fail or if severe adhesions and/or strangulation occurs. The goal of this surgery is to strengthen the closure at the junction between the diaphragm and the esophagus.

USES AND COMPLICATIONS

The surgeries to correct inguinal, femoral, umbilical, and incisional hernias are straightforward. In all cases, but especially in strangulation, patients are checked before release to ensure that normal bowel movement occurs, that incisions have not become infected, and that fever has not developed. At this time, patients are also shown how to protect their incisions before coughing, are advised to maintain a high fluid intake to engender normal bowel function, are warned against overexertion, and are made aware of signs of incision infection. Furthermore, they are advised to resume work or physical activity only after consulting the physician involved.

Patients who have undergone surgery to correct a hiatal hernia are given much the same advice. Their surgery, however, is more extensive and prone to more complications. Therefore, they are provided with recommendations concerning which foods and activities to avoid. Furthermore, they are advised of the extended time period required before they can return to normal function and are told that without careful compliance, the problem will recur.

PERSPECTIVE AND PROSPECTS

Major advances in the treatment of hernias have included better diagnosis of their extent and the necessary means of their correction. Computed tomography (CT) scanning and other imaging techniques can make possible very accurate diagnoses. Progress in the surgical techniques used in hernia repair includes laparoscopy, in which a fiber-optic tube is used to visualize the chest cavity and thus to minimize incision size in the correction of hiatal hernias. All these methodologies are expected to improve in the future.

—*Sanford S. Singer, Ph.D.*

See also Abdomen; Abdominal disorders; Gangrene; Gastroenterology; Gastroenterology, pediatric;

Gastrointestinal disorders; Gastrointestinal system; Hernia; Internal medicine; Intestinal disorders; Intestines; Pediatrics; Peritonitis.

FOR FURTHER INFORMATION:

Berkow, Robert, and Andrew J. Fletcher, eds. *The Merck Manual of Diagnosis and Therapy.* 17th ed. Rahway, N.J.: Merck Sharp & Dohme Research Laboratories, 1999. Contains a useful exposition of the characteristics, etiology, diagnosis, and treatment of hernia. Designed for physicians, the material is also useful for less specialized readers. Information on related topics is also included.

Greenfield, Lazar J., et al. *Surgery: Scientific Principles and Practice.* 3d ed. Philadelphia: Lippincott Williams & Wilkins, 2001. Covers the scope and practice of surgery and includes reviews of wound biology, immunology, the management of trauma and transplantation, surgical practice according to anatomic region and specialty, and musculoskeletal, neurologic, genitourinary, and reconstructive surgery.

Maingot, Rodney. *Maingot's Abdominal Operations.* Edited by Michael J. Zinner et al. 10th ed. Stamford, Conn.: Appleton and Lange, 1997. This textbook has long been considered the classic work on all surgical disciplines.

Nyhus, Lloyd M., and Robert E. Condon, eds. *Hernia.* 5th ed. Philadelphia: J. B. Lippincott, 2001. Widely recognized and updated joint contribution by a large number of specialized physicians. Examines such topics as the etiology, history, and anatomy of hernias; conventional, laparoscopic, and endoscopic groin hernia repairs; complications of groin hernia; and pediatric hernias.

Tierney, Lawrence M., Stephen J. McPhee, and Maxine Papadakis, eds. *Current Medical Diagnosis and Treatment 2004.* 43d ed. Stamford, Conn.: Appleton & Lange, 2003. This text, updated yearly, is the point of reference for physicians and other health care practitioners. It incorporates each year's biomedical research discoveries that have immediate, relevant, and applicable use for the patient.

HERNIATED DISK. *See* SLIPPED DISK.

HERPES
DISEASE/DISORDER
ANATOMY OR SYSTEM AFFECTED: Genitals, mouth, reproductive system

SPECIALTIES AND RELATED FIELDS: Family practice, gynecology, internal medicine, virology

DEFINITION: A family of viruses that cause several diseases, including infectious mononucleosis, cold sores, genital herpes, and chickenpox; for most individuals, these widespread diseases are mild and of brief duration, but they may be fatal to those with impaired immune systems.

KEY TERMS:

antibody: a protein found in the blood and produced by the immune system in response to bodily contact with a foreign substance, such as a virus

congenital disease: a disease resulting from heredity or acquired while in the womb

disseminated: spread throughout the body

immune system: the body system that is responsible for fighting off infectious disease

immunocompromised: a condition in which the immune system is impaired in some way, such as being not fully developed, deficient, or suppressed

latent: lying hidden or concealed

primary infection: a person's first infection with a particular virus

recurrent infection: an infection caused by the reactivation of a latent virus

vaccine: a substance given in order to prevent or ameliorate the effect of some disease

virus: the simplest entity that can reproduce; viruses are essentially made of some genetic material in a protective coating; viruses can reproduce only inside a living cell

TYPES OF HERPESVIRUS
Herpesviruses that affect humans include herpes simplex virus types 1 and 2, Epstein-Barr virus, varicella-zoster virus, and cytomegalovirus. Herpesviruses cause three types of infections: primary, latent, and recurrent. Most first-time, or primary, infections with herpesviruses cause few or no symptoms in the victim. Following the primary infection, herpesviruses have the unique ability to become latent, or hidden, in the body. Latent infections may persist for the life of the individual with no further symptoms, or the virus may reactivate (come out of hiding) and cause a recurrent infection. Although herpesvirus infections are often mild in healthy persons, they can cause potentially fatal infections in immunocompromised patients. Persons in this group include infants, whose immune systems are not fully developed; immunodeficient persons, whose immune systems are lacking some important component;

and immunosuppressed patients, such as cancer or transplant patients, whose immune systems are being suppressed by immunosuppressive drugs or radiation. Herpesviruses have also been implicated in causing certain types of cancer.

Herpes simplex viruses exist in two forms: type 1 (HSV1) and type 2 (HSV2). HSV1 and HSV2 infections cause the formation of painful or itchy vesicular (blisterlike) lesions, which ulcerate, crust over, and heal within a few weeks. The virus is transmitted from one person to another by direct contact with infected lesions, and the virus enters the recipient through broken skin or mucous membranes. HSV1 usually causes infections above the waist—for example, in the mouth, throat, eye, skin, and brain. Gingivostomatitis, the most common form of primary HSV1 infection, is seen mostly in small children and is characterized by ulcerative lesions inside the mouth. Herpes labialis, or cold sores, the most common recurrent disease caused by HSV1, is characterized by blisters on the outer portion of the lips. HSV1 can also cause infection in any area of the skin where trauma (for example, a burn, scrape, or eczema) gives the virus an opening to get in. HSV1 infection of the eye can lead to scarring and blindness, and HSV1 infection of the brain can lead to death. Genital herpes, a disease transmitted by sexual contact, is most often caused by HSV2. The virus infects the penis in males and the cervix, vulva, vagina, or perineum in females. Two to seven days after infection, painful blisters appear in the genital area; they ulcerate, crust over, and disappear in a few weeks. Fever, stress, sunlight, or local trauma may trigger the virus to come out of hiding and cause a recurrent infection, and about 88 percent of persons with an HSV2 genital infection will have recurrences at a frequency of up to five to eight times per year. A severe form of HSV2 infection, neonatal herpes, occurs when a mother suffering from genital herpes passes the virus to her baby as it travels through the birth canal during delivery. This type of infection is usually disseminated, its death rate is high, and its survivors suffer from severe neurological damage.

Varicella-zoster virus (VZV) causes two diseases: chickenpox (varicella) and shingles (zoster). Chickenpox is a highly contagious common childhood disease caused by a primary infection with VZV. The virus is transmitted during close personal contact with an infected patient via airborne droplets that enter the respiratory tract or via direct contact with skin lesions. Once inside a person, the virus travels from the respiratory tract to the blood, and then to the skin. Ten to twenty-one days after infection, a typical rash appears on the skin and mucous membranes. On skin, the rash begins as red spots that develop into clear, fluid-filled vesicles that become cloudy, ulcerate, scab over, and fall off in a few days. Mucous membrane lesions in the mouth, eyelid, rectum, and vagina rupture easily and appear as ulcers. Fever, headache, tiredness, and itching may accompany the rash. Recovery from chickenpox confers lifelong immunity to reinfection but not latency. Reye's syndrome, an occasional severe complication of chickenpox, is associated with the use of aspirin. A few days after the initial infection has receded, the patient persistently vomits and exhibits signs of brain dysfunction. Coma and death can follow if the syndrome is not treated. Chickenpox infection in adults is often more severe than in children, and adults run the risk of developing a fatal lung or brain infection.

Individuals with prior varicella infection may later develop shingles, which is caused by the reactivation of latent VZV. More than 65 percent of cases of shingles appear in adults older than forty-five years of age. The mechanism of reactivation is unknown, but recurrence is often associated with physical and emotional stress or a suppressed immune system. Shingles is usually localized to one area of the skin; it begins with pain in the nerves, and then a chickenpox-like rash appears on the skin over the nerves. The pain may be severe for one to four weeks, and recovery occurs in two to five weeks, with pain persisting longer in some elderly patients.

Epstein-Barr virus (EBV) causes infectious mononucleosis, an infection of the lymphatic system. In infected persons, the virus is present in saliva and blood, and thus it is transmitted by intimate oral contact (for example, kissing), sharing food or drinks, or by blood transfusions. Primary infection early in life usually causes no symptoms of disease, whereas primary infection later in life usually causes symptoms of infectious mononucleosis. In countries where sanitation is poor, most people have been infected by the age of five, without symptoms. In contrast, in countries where sanitation is good, primary infection is delayed until adolescence or young adulthood, and thus more than half the people in this age group develop symptoms. Once the infection begins, the virus grows in the throat and spreads to blood and lymph, invading white blood cells called B lymphocytes. The typical symptoms of infectious mononucleosis are extreme exhaustion, sore throat, fever, swollen lymph nodes, and sometimes an enlarged liver and spleen. The disease is self-limiting, and recovery takes place in four to eight weeks. The virus remains latent in the blood, lymphoid tissue, and throat and can continue to be transmitted to others even when no signs of active infection are present. EBV infection has also been associated with chronic fatigue syndrome and several types of cancer.

The widespread cytomegalovirus (CMV) is responsible for a broad spectrum of diseases. As is the case with EBV infection, primary infection by CMV early in life usually results in no symptoms, while primary infection as an adult yields mononucleosis-like symptoms. CMV also causes congenital cytomegalic inclusion disease and is a significant danger to bone marrow transplant patients. The virus is found in body secretions such as saliva, urine, semen, cervical secretions, and breast milk. Babies may acquire the virus from infected mothers congenitally, during birth while passing through the birth canal, or through breast milk. Children in day care may acquire CMV from other children who orally excrete the virus, and parents may get it from their children. CMV may be acquired through sexual transmission and blood transfusions. Patients undergoing transplants, especially bone marrow transplants, are at higher risk for CMV infection, since the virus may be present in the transplanted organs. The mononucleosis-like disease caused by CMV has the same symptoms as EBV-induced mononucleosis except the sore throat, swollen lymph nodes, and enlarged spleen. Congenital cytomegalic inclusion disease causes severe neurological damage, mental retardation, and death in infants; it is a result of primary CMV infection of the mother during pregnancy.

CAUSES, SYMPTOMS, AND TREATMENTS

A physician can often tell whether a person has an HSV infection based on the presence of the characteristic lesions and a history of exposure or previous lesions. For more severe HSV infections, the virus can

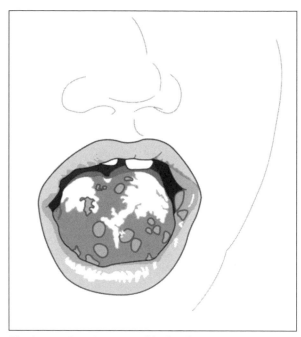

The herpesvirus is responsible for the common cold sore.

be isolated and identified from infected tissue to confirm HSV as the causative agent. The major treatment procedure for most mild HSV infections is supportive care. These measures, such as bed rest and medication to relieve itching or pain, treat the symptoms but not the infection. For most infections, the symptoms eventually go away by themselves. For more severe HSV infections, several antiviral drugs have been used. Idoxuridine and trifluridine have been used to treat eye infections. Vidarabine and acyclovir are used to treat encephalitis and disseminated disease; both reduce the severity of the infection but do not reverse any neurological damage or prevent recurrent infections. Acyclovir has also been useful in reducing the duration of primary genital herpes, but not recurrent infection. The use of oral acyclovir to suppress recurrent infection may cause more severe and more frequent infections once the therapy has stopped. The best way to prevent infection with HSV is to avoid contact with a person with active lesions. Victims of genital herpes should avoid all sexual contact during episodes of lesions, to avoid transmitting the virus to someone else. Using condoms may be somewhat helpful in preventing the sexual transmission of HSV2. Newborns, children with eczema or other skin problems, burn patients, and immunocompromised patients should avoid persons with active HSV lesions. Pregnant females with active genital lesions must be delivered by cesarean section, in order to prevent the infection of their infants.

A diagnosis of chickenpox or shingles is based mainly on the symptoms of the patient, since they are so characteristic. It is possible to grow the virus from tissue samples or test the person for antibodies to VZV if necessary. Chickenpox takes care of itself and disappears after a few weeks; therefore, the only treatment needed is supportive care for the patient during that time. Often, drying lotions such as calamine help relieve the itching. It is important to cut the fingernails of especially young children so that they cannot scratch hard enough to break through the skin and leave themselves susceptible to secondary bacterial infection. It is extremely important not to give a child aspirin for the fever, because of the association between the use of aspirin during chickenpox and the development of Reye's syndrome. A child may be given acetaminophen if necessary. Zoster is treated mostly with pain medication to control the pain. Steroids given early in the infection help reduce the severity of the infection, and acyclovir increases the rate of recovery. Antiviral drugs such as acyclovir, interferon, and vidarabine have been used in the treatment of immunocompromised patients with chickenpox to help reduce the potential severe complications of the disease. For most healthy persons, it is not necessary to prevent chickenpox, since it is a mild disease. It is important for newborns and immunocompromised patients to avoid exposure to persons with chickenpox because of threats such as pneumonia, encephalitis, and death. Since 1981, varicella-zoster immune globin (VZIG) has been available for the prevention and treatment of chickenpox in these patients. VZIG provides a short time of immunity, can lessen symptoms, and is recommended for immunocompromised children exposed to chickenpox, but it has no value once chickenpox has started. A VZV vaccine has been developed and shown to provide temporary protection from severe infection in immunocompromised children.

Unlike diagnoses of most VZV or HSV infections, the diagnosis of an EBV infection cannot be made based on the symptoms alone, because the virus causes a wide range of symptoms that could be caused by many other disease-causing agents. The diagnosis of EBV infection is made, therefore, based on laboratory tests. One test is a blood test in which technicians count the number of and kinds of white blood cells present in a patient. Persons with infectious mononucleosis have an abnormally large number of lymphocytes (one type of white blood cell) in their blood, and many of these lymphocytes have an odd appearance. A second test involves mixing patients' blood serum (the fluid portion from their blood) with the red blood cells of sheep. The serum from 90 percent of persons with infectious mononucleosis will cause the sheep cells to clump. It is unknown why serum from infectious mononucleosis patients has this odd property (referred to as heterophil-positive). Persons suspected of having EBV but who give a heterophil-negative test are tested more rigorously for antibodies in their blood that are specific for EBV. The isolation of EBV from patients is not routinely performed to confirm a diagnosis of EBV infection, because the techniques needed are too complex for most laboratories. Infectious mononucleosis is a self-limiting disease, which means that it will eventually run its course and go away. Therefore, treatment involves mostly supportive care, such as bed rest and aspirin or acetaminophen for the fever and sore throat. It is also recommended that mononucleosis patients avoid contact sports, to prevent possible rupture of an enlarged spleen. In some severe cases, steroids are administered, and antiviral drugs are in the process of being tested to determine whether they are of any therapeutic value. The best way to prevent an EBV infection is to avoid intimate contact (for example, kissing) with an infected individual. Unfortunately, many persons shed the virus in their saliva without exhibiting any symptoms, so one cannot always tell who is infected and who is not.

Like EBV infection, CMV infection causes vague symptoms, and therefore diagnosis depends on laboratory tests. The virus can be grown from tissue samples, tissue can be examined to look for typical infected cells or the presence of virus, or the blood can be tested to look for antibodies to CMV. Mild cases of CMV need no treatment except supportive measures. Antiviral drugs such as interferon, vidarabine, idoxuridine, and cytosine arabinoside as well as CMV immune globin have all been tested for their benefit in severe cases of CMV infections, but none has been successful. The drug ganciclovir has been shown to have some therapeutic value. Most preventive measures have been aimed at developing a vaccine to prevent congenital CMV and CMV infection in immunosuppressed patients. A CMV vaccine has been developed, but further work is needed. Until better measures are available, it is important to try to avoid infection in immunocompromised patients, especially transplant recipients. The screening of organ donors for the presence of CMV may be helpful in accomplishing this goal. In addition, to prevent congenital CMV, pregnant females need to avoid primary CMV infection during their pregnancies. All pregnant females should be tested for CMV antibodies to determine whether they have already been infected; if not, they should avoid contact with small children who might carry CMV.

PERSPECTIVE AND PROSPECTS

Between 20 and 40 percent of the people in the United States suffer from cold sores, and more than 20 million persons suffer from genital herpes. In addition, HSV1 infection of the eye is the most common cause of corneal blindness in the United States. Two hundred babies in the United States die each year, and 200 more suffer physical or mental impairment caused by HSV infection.

Chickenpox is the second most reported disease in the United States, with more than 200,000 cases per year. This number is probably too low, since many cases go unreported. About 100 deaths per year are attributed to chickenpox.

EBV infection is worldwide, and EBV antibodies can be found in more than 90 percent of most adult populations. EBV infection has been shown to be an important factor in the development of Burkitt's lymphoma (a cancer of the jaw) in Africa and nasopharyngeal carcinoma (a fatal cancer of the nose) in China. EBV has also been linked to chronic fatigue syndrome, but the relationship is not conclusive.

CMV infection is worldwide, with 40 to 100 percent of a population possessing antibodies to CMV. Almost all kidney transplant recipients and half of bone marrow recipients get CMV infection. Congenital CMV infection is the cause of severe neurological damage in more than 5,000 children born each year in the United States.

It is clear from these facts that infections with herpesviruses are a very important public health problem. The infections are widespread, and they cause a significant amount of distress, sickness, and death. The development of vaccines and other drugs to treat these diseases is important for infants and other immunocompromised persons whose lives can be threatened by acquiring a herpesvirus infection. The viruses' ability to become latent and the lack of drugs to destroy the latent viruses, however, make it virtually impossible to eradicate these diseases from the human population. Persons are infected for life, and they may continue to transmit the infection to other persons. Many other viral diseases, such as smallpox, measles, and polio, have been controlled by the use of vaccines that prevent a person from getting the disease, but the development of vaccines for herpesviruses is a complex problem. First, most of the diseases they cause are mild and self-limiting, so there is no pressing need to develop a vaccine quickly. Second, the association of the viruses with cancer causes scientists to proceed with caution in the development of a vaccine. Third, even if a vaccine does become available, it will be a long time before the viruses will be gone from the human population. Since herpesviruses can remain hidden in a person and stay there for life, they will not disappear until all currently infected persons die.

—*Vicki J. Isola, Ph.D.*

See also Canker sores; Cervical, ovarian, and uterine cancers; Chickenpox; Chronic fatigue syndrome; Cold sores; Genital disorders, female; Genital disorders, male; Gynecology; Mononucleosis; Reye's syndrome; Sexually transmitted diseases (STDs); Shingles; Viral infections; Warts.

FOR FURTHER INFORMATION:

Biddle, Wayne. *Field Guide to Germs.* 2d ed. New York: Henry Holt, 2002. This comprehensive book is easily accessible to the nonspecialist and includes a discussion of nearly every virus, bacterium, and fungus known to cause human and nonhuman animal disease. The history of the microbe and the treatment of diseases are included.

Ebel, Charles. *Managing Herpes: How to Live and Love with a Chronic STD.* Rev. ed. Research Triangle Park, N.C.: American Social Health, 2002. Easy-to-read guide to living with herpes. Provides information on the diagnosis and treatment of genital herpes as well as a bibliography, glossary, and resource list.

Gorbach, Sherwood L., John G. Bartlett, and Neil R. Blacklow, eds. *Infectious Diseases.* 3d ed. Philadelphia: W. B. Saunders, 2003. A thorough discussion of infectious diseases. Included is a brief history, an account of the mechanisms of disease and immunity, and a concise discussion of a broad range of infectious agents.

Herpes Resource Center. http://www.ashastd.org/hrc/. A group that focuses on increasing education, public awareness, and support to anyone concerned about herpes.

Parker, James N., and Philip M. Parker, eds. *The Official Patient's Sourcebook on Genital Herpes.* San Diego, Calif.: Icon Health, 2002. Draws from public, academic, government, and peer-reviewed research to provide a wide-ranging handbook for patients with genital herpes.

Radetsky, Peter. *The Invisible Invaders: The Story of the Emerging Age of Viruses*. Boston: Little, Brown, 1995. Discusses viruses in general, how they were discovered, and the diseases they cause. Chapter 10 gives an interesting account of the discovery of the links between EBV infection and chronic fatigue syndrome, infectious mononucleosis, and Burkitt's lymphoma.

Sompayrac, Lauren. *How Pathogenic Viruses Work*. 5th ed. Sudbury, Mass.: Jones and Bartlett, 2002. An engaging exploration of the basics of virology. The author uses twelve of the most common viral infections to demonstrate how viruses "devise" various solutions to stay alive.

Strauss, James, and Ellen Strauss. *Viruses and Human Disease*. New York: Elsevier, 2001. An undergraduate text that examines virology from a human disease perspective.

Wagner, Edward K., and Martin Hewlett. *Basic Virology*. 2d ed. Boston: Blackwell, 2003. A very readable undergraduate text covering issues of virology and viral disease, properties of viruses and virus-cell interaction, working with viruses, and replication patterns of specific viruses.

Zinsser, Hans. *Zinsser Microbiology*. Edited by Wolfgang K. Joklik et al. 20th ed. Norwalk, Conn.: Appleton and Lange, 1992. The information presented in this textbook is thorough, logical, and supplemented by interesting diagrams, photographs, and charts. Chapter 66, "Herpesviruses," gives a complete description of infections with HSV, VZV, EBV, and CMV.

HICCUPS

DISEASE/DISORDER

ALSO KNOWN AS: Hiccoughs

ANATOMY OR SYSTEM AFFECTED: Chest, lungs, muscles, respiratory system, throat

SPECIALTIES AND RELATED FIELDS: Family practice, gastroenterology, neurology

DEFINITION: Involuntary, spasmodic contractions of the diaphragm and the simultaneous closure of the glottis.

CAUSES AND SYMPTOMS

A hiccup is caused by an involuntary, spasmodic contraction of the diaphragm, the large partition of muscles

---

INFORMATION ON HICCUPS

CAUSES: Overdistension of stomach, gastric irritation from spicy or rich foods, nerve spasms

SYMPTOMS: Involuntary, spasmodic contractions of diaphragm and simultaneous closure of glottis; stomach upset

DURATION: Ranges from short-term to chronic

TREATMENTS: Varies; can include holding one's breath, drinking a glass of water, breathing deeply or into paper bag

---

and tendons that separates the chest from the abdomen. The diaphragm draws air into the lungs through rhythmic contractions. When it contracts suddenly, an opening located toward the top of the trachea (windpipe) between the vocal cords in the larynx (voice box) called the glottis snaps shut abruptly. The combination of air being forced through the vocal cords in the larynx and the abrupt closure of the glottis causes the sound associated with hiccups.

There are a number of causes of hiccups, the most common being overdistension of the stomach. Other causes include gastric irritation from spicy or rich foods and nerve spasms. There is some indication that hiccups are controlled by the central nervous system.

Hiccups generally last for a very short time, usually stopping within minutes. People who suffer from hiccups for more than twenty-four hours or who have repetitive attacks are said to suffer from chronic hiccups. This condition is very rare.

People of all ages can suffer from hiccups. Pregnant women report that fetuses sometimes have hiccups in the womb.

TREATMENT AND THERAPY

An attack of hiccups is not serious and is generally self-limiting. A number of techniques to stop are practiced, including holding one's breath, drinking a glass of water, breathing deeply, or breathing into a paper bag.

Babies often suffer from hiccups, particularly during nursing. Some mothers report that feeding the baby a quarter of a teaspoon of sugar mixed in 4 ounces of water calms the hiccups. Doctors suggest that hiccup-prone babies be fed before they are overly hungry and when they are calm.

—*Diane Andrews Henningfeld, Ph.D.*

See also Abdomen; Breast-feeding; Coughing; Respiration.

FOR FURTHER INFORMATION:

Gluck, Michael, and Charles E. Pope II. "Hiccups and Gastrointestinal Reflux Disease: The Acid Perfusion Test as a Provocative Maneuver." *Annals of Internal Medicine* 105 (1996): 219-220.

Heuman, Douglas M., A. Scott Mills, and Hunter H. McGuire, Jr. *Gastroenterology.* Philadelphia: W. B. Saunders, 1997.

Launois, J. L., W. A. Bizec, J. C. Whitelaw et al. "Hiccup in Adults: An Overview." *European Respiratory Journal* 6 (1993): 563-575.

Shay, Steven D. S., Robert L. Myers, and Lawrence F. Johnson. "Hiccups Associated with Reflux Esophagitis." *Gastroenterology* 87 (1984): 204-207.

HIP FRACTURE REPAIR

PROCEDURE

ANATOMY OR SYSTEM AFFECTED: Bones, hips, joints, legs, musculoskeletal system

SPECIALTIES AND RELATED FIELDS: Geriatrics and gerontology, orthopedics

DEFINITION: The repair or replacement of a broken hip joint.

KEY TERMS:

arthroplasty: joint replacement

osteoporosis: a loss of bone mass accompanied by increasing fragility and brittleness

INDICATIONS AND PROCEDURES

Hip fracture repair constitutes one of the most common procedures performed by orthopedic surgeons. The human hip consists of two bones, the hipbone and the thighbone (femur), and their point of intersection, a cup-shaped cavity called the acetabulum. This hip joint forms a ball-and-socket mechanism that allows the leg to move in different directions. As a major weight-bearing joint, the hip is vulnerable both to sudden trauma, such as sports injuries, and to degenerative disorders of aging, such as osteoporosis. If the loss of bone mass associated with osteoporosis is sufficiently advanced, a simple fall from a standing position can shatter the hip joint. The most common fracture involves the femur snapping or cracking just below the rounded end that fits into the acetabulum.

PERSPECTIVE AND PROSPECTS

The repair of hip fractures involves the realignment of the bone fragments and the insertion of a long nail into the bone to hold them together. A plate is attached to the nail and to the healthy bone surrounding the fracture in order to give support.

Because broken bones heal slowly in the elderly, in the past a broken hip almost inevitably resulted in these patients becoming permanent invalids restricted to wheelchairs or, at best, forced to rely on walkers and enjoying only limited mobility. This bleak prognosis changed in the 1960's when orthopedic specialists working with biomedical engineers developed artificial hip joints. The combination of prosthetic devices and surgical techniques known as total hip arthroplasty (THA) allows physicians to return patients to active, independent lives. In THA, the weakened end of the femur is removed and an artificial replacement installed. The replacement can consist of any of a variety of materials, but typically it is constructed of a chromium steel alloy coated with a ceramic polymer that helps resist corrosion as well as providing a surface with which the patient's bone can bond. The end of the prothesis and the surface of the acetabulum are coated with plastic polymers to reduce friction. Research indicates that artificial hip joints last fifteen years or longer before wear and tear on the lining of the ball-and-socket joint creates problems.

—*Nancy Farm Mannikko, Ph.D.*

See also Aging: Extended care; Arthroplasty; Arthroscopy; Bone disorders; Bone grafting; Bones and the skeleton; Emergency medicine; Fracture and dislocation; Fracture repair; Geriatrics and gerontology; Hip replacement; Orthopedic surgery; Orthopedics; Osteoporosis; Physical rehabilitation.

FOR FURTHER INFORMATION:

Currey, John D. *Bones: Structures and Mechanics.* Princeton, N.J.: Princeton University Press, 2002.

Morrey, Bernard. *Joint Replacement Arthroplasty.* 3d ed. New York: Elsevier, 2003.

Nelson, Miriam, and Sarah Wernick. *Strong Women, Strong Bones: Everything You Need to Know to Prevent, Treat and Beat Osteoporosis.* New York: Berkley, 2001.

Sabiston, David C., Jr., ed. *Textbook of Surgery.* 16th ed. Philadelphia: W. B. Saunders, 2001.

Schwartz, Seymour I., ed. *Principles of Surgery.* 7th ed. New York: McGraw-Hill, 1999.

Way, Lawrence W., and Gerard M. Doherty, eds. *Current Surgical Diagnosis and Treatment.* 11th ed. Norwalk, Conn.: Appleton & Lange, 2003.

Wilmore, Douglas W., et al., eds. *Care of the Surgical Patient.* New York: Scientific American, 1992.

HIP REPLACEMENT

PROCEDURE

ANATOMY OR SYSTEM AFFECTED: Bones, hips
SPECIALTIES AND RELATED FIELDS: Orthopedics, rheumatology
DEFINITION: The removal of diseased bone tissue in the hip and its replacement with an artificial device.

INDICATIONS AND PROCEDURES

The most common reason for hip replacement surgery is the decline in efficiency of the hip joint that often results from osteoarthritis. Osteoarthritis is a common form of arthritis that causes joint and bone deterioration, which may lead to the wearing down of cartilage and cause the underlying bones to rub against each other. This may result in severe pain and stiffness in the affected areas. Other conditions that may lead to the need for hip replacement include rheumatoid arthritis (a chronic inflammation of the joints), avascular necrosis (loss of bone caused by insufficient blood supply), and injury.

Generally, physicians may be more inclined to choose less invasive techniques such as physical therapy, medication, or walking aids before resorting to surgery. In some cases, exercise programs may help reduce hip pain. In addition, if preliminary treatment does not improve the patient's condition, doctors may use corrective surgery that is not as invasive as hip replacement. However, when these efforts do not reduce pain or increase mobility, hip replacement may be the best option. In addition, the age of the patient may be an important factor in the decision to replace the hip. The majority of hip replacements are performed on individuals over the age of sixty-five. One of the reasons for this is that the activity level of older adults is lower than that of younger adults, therefore reducing the concern that the new hip will wear out or fail. However, technological advances have improved the quality of the artificial hip, making hip replacement surgery a more likely intervention for younger adults as well.

Generally, a candidate for total hip replacement surgery (THR) possesses a hip that has worn out from arthritis, falls, or other conditions. The hip consists of a ball-and-socket joint where the head of the femur (thigh bone) fits into the hip socket, or acetabulum. In a normal hip, this arrangement provides for a relatively wide range of motion. For some older adults, however, deterioration caused by arthritis and other conditions reduces the effectiveness of this arrangement, compromising the integrity of the hip socket or the femoral head. This state can lead to extreme discomfort.

Total hip replacement may provide the best long-term relief for these symptoms. Total hip replacement involves the removal of diseased bone tissue and the replacement of that tissue with prostheses (artificial devices used to replace missing body parts). Usually, both the femoral head and hip socket are replaced. The femoral head is replaced with a metal ball that is attached to a metal stem and placed into the hollow marrow space of the femur. The hip socket is lined with a plastic socket. Other materials have been used effectively as hip replacements.

In some cases, the surgeon will use cement to bond the artificial parts of the new hip to the bone tissue. This approach has been the traditional method of ensuring that the artificial parts hold. One problem with this method is that over time, cemented hip replacements may lose their bond with the bone tissue. This may result in the need for an additional surgery. However, a cementless hip replacement has been developed. This approach includes a prosthesis that is porous so that bone tissue may grow into the metal pores and keep the prosthesis in place.

Both procedures have strengths and weaknesses. In general, recovery time may be shorter with cemented prostheses since one does not have to wait for bone growth to attach to the artificial prostheses. However, the potential for long-term deterioration of the replaced hip must be considered. A cemented hip generally lasts about fifteen years. With this in mind, physicians may be more likely to use a cemented prosthesis for patients over the age of seventy. Cementless hip replacement may be more advisable for younger and more active patients. Some physicians have used a combination of approaches, known as a "hybrid" or "mixed" hip. This combination relies on an uncemented socket and a cemented femoral head.

USES AND COMPLICATIONS

Total hip replacements are generally quite successful, with about 96 percent of surgeries proceeding without complications. In rare instances, however, complications occur, including blood clots and infections during surgery, and hip dislocation or bone fracture after surgery. In addition, in some cases, bone grafts may be used to assist in the restoration of bone defects. In these instances, bone may be obtained from the pelvis or the discarded head of the femur. Other postoperative complications may include some pain and stiffness.

Patients recovering from total hip replacement usually remain in the hospital up to ten days if there are no complications. However, physical therapists may initiate therapy as soon as the day after surgery. Physical therapy involves the use of exercises that will improve recovery. Many patients are able to sit on the edge of their bed, stand, and even walk with assistance as early as two days after surgery. Patients must remember that their artificial hip may not provide the same full range of motion as an undiseased hip. Physical therapists teach patients how to perform daily activities without placing an undue burden on their new hips. This may require learning a new method of sitting, standing, and performing other activities.

While many factors may affect recovery time, full recovery from surgery may take up to six months. At that point, many patients enjoy such activities as walking and swimming. Doctors and physical therapists may discourage patients from participating in such high-impact activities as jogging or playing tennis, which may burden the new hip. Despite these restrictions, many patients are able to perform normal activities without pain and discomfort. Nonetheless, people who have undergone hip replacement surgery are advised to consult with their doctor about proper exercise and activity levels.

Pᴇʀsᴘᴇᴄᴛɪᴠᴇ ᴀɴᴅ Pʀᴏsᴘᴇᴄᴛs

Total hip replacement is one of the most common surgical interventions that older adults face. The American Academy of Orthopedic Surgeons estimates that more than 120,000 hip replacement surgeries are performed in the United States each year. The average age of the patient who undergoes hip replacement surgery is sixty-seven years, while 67 percent of total hip replacements are performed on individuals age sixty-five or older. Approximately 60 percent of hip replacement surgeries are performed on women.

—*H. David Smith, Ph.D.*

See also Arthritis; Bone disorders; Bones and the skeleton; Hip fracture repair; Orthopedics.

Fᴏʀ Fᴜʀᴛʜᴇʀ Iɴғᴏʀᴍᴀᴛɪᴏɴ:

Bucholz, Robert, and Joseph A. Buckwalter. "Orthopedic Surgery." *Journal of the American Medical Association* 275, no. 23 (June 19, 1996). The research focus of orthopedic surgery is discussed, including research on the use of recombinant growth factors to induce bone repair and the regeneration of cartilaginous surfaces.

Duffey, Timothy P., Elliott Hershman, Richard A. Sanders, and Lori D. Talarico. "Investigating the Subtle and Obvious Causes of Hip Pain." *Patient Care* 31, no. 18 (November 15, 1997). A delay in diagnosing the cause of a patient's acute hip pain could lead to significant impairment of the hip. Talarico explains how to maximize one's investigative effort and make the most of treatment.

Dunkin, Mary Anne. "Hip Replacement Surgery." *Arthritis Today* 12, no. 2 (March/April, 1998). Two types of joint prostheses are discussed. Illustrations by Kevin A. Somerville show the difference between a healthy hip joint and cartilage that is damaged.

Finerman, Gerald A. M. *Total Hip Arthroplasty Outcomes.* New York: Churchill Livingstone, 1998. Discusses topics such as the anatomic medullary looking prosthesis, the porous-coated anatomic prosthesis, the anatomic porous replacement system, long-term results of hybrid prostheses, and the hybrid total hip replacement.

Horosko, Marian. "Connected to the Hip Bone." *Dance Magazine*, February, 1999, 89. This article includes a description of metal-metal hip replacement surgery.

Lane, Nancy E., and Daniel J. Wallace. *All About Osteoarthritis: The Definitive Resource for Arthritis Patients and Their Families.* New York: Oxford University Press, 2001. A comprehensive look at the degeneration of bones and joints accompanied by detailed illustrations of key joints—knees, hips, fingers, backs, hands, and necks. Covers the steps of diagnosis, how the body is affected, and ways to manage the disease, including new medications and surgical options.

MacWilliam, Cynthia H., Marianne U. Yood, James J. Verner, Bruce D. McCarthy, and Richard E. Ward. "Patient-Related Risk Factors That Predict Poor Outcome After Total Hip Replacement." *Health Services Research* 31, no. 5 (December, 1996). A study identifies factors associated with poor outcome after total hip replacement (THR) surgery. It is the first to present results from the American Medical Group Association (AMGA) THR consortium.

Morrey, Bernard. *Joint Replacement Arthroplasty.* 3d ed. New York: Elsevier, 2003. Reviews arthroplasty of all joints. Each section concludes with chapters on alternatives and future directions of research and practice.

Silber, Irwin. *Patient's Guide to Knee and Hip Replacement: Everything You Need to Know.* New York: Simon & Schuster, 1999. Written by a hip-replacement patient, guides readers through the complete joint-replacement process, from the initial diagnosis and the decision whether to have surgery, the hospital stay, and the full recovery period.

Trahair, Richard C. S. *All About Hip Replacement: A Patient's Guide*. Oxford, England: Oxford University Press, 1999. Includes bibliographical references and an index.

Van De Graaff, Kent M., and Stuart Ira Fox. *Concepts of Human Anatomy and Physiology*. 5th ed. Dubuque: Iowa: Wm. C. Brown, 2000. Chapters 8 through 11 present a first-rate introduction to bones, the skeleton, and joints. The many clear illustrations, photographs, clinical commentaries, and X rays, as well as a pronunciation guide, a complete index, and a glossary, make this a very accessible book for the nonspecialist reader.

HIPPOCRATIC OATH

ETHICS

DEFINITION: A document, written in the fifth century B.C.E., to offer guidelines for the emerging medical profession, which continues to be the subject of debate in modern practice because of the ethical issues that it addresses.

KEY TERMS:

euthanasia: the practice (particularly in cases involving patients of advanced age) of withholding medical treatments that might sustain life that would otherwise expire "naturally"; in a more controversial form, it is associated with the administration of drugs by physicians in order to avert prolonged suffering

living will: a legally binding document instructing a physician not to prolong life by externally administered life support systems if the patient is unable to express his or her decision concerning forms of medical treatment recommended by a physician

malpractice insurance: insurance policies held by physicians in order to protect them financially in the event of a patient-initiated lawsuit alleging incidents of improper medical decisions or incompetence

MEDICAL CODES OF ETHICS

Western civilization has long held the writings of the fifth century B.C.E. Greek physician Hippocrates, and in particular the Hippocratic oath, as a model of ethical values to be followed in the medical profession. As the nature of Western civilization itself has changed over the centuries, interpretations of the ethical values behind the Hippocratic oath have also changed. The circumstances of modern medical practice and ethical values, however, have ironically made certain elements of

the classical Hippocratic tradition even more relevant than they may have appeared in previous eras.

In fact, the Hippocratic oath is only the introductory section of the *Corpus Hippocraticum* (Hippocratic Collection) traditionally attributed to Hippocrates. (There is debate about whether he is the author of all the books or only some.) The actual medical observations of Hippocrates were studied and applied for many centuries, until scientific research rendered many of them recognizably obsolete. A number of sections of the corpus, however, reflect the Greek physician's recurring concern for rules to guide the medical profession. Hippocrates' chapters on "The Art," "Decorum," and "The Law" complement the more famous ethical precepts contained in the oath.

The first part of the oath itself covers the physician's lifelong commitment to his or her teachers. This commitment extends not only to the symbolic bonds of respect but also to obligation to share one's medical practice and even to provide financial assistance to one's teachers, if requested. Additionally, the physician is committed to train, free of charge, the families of his or her teachers in the art of medicine.

The second part of the Hippocratic oath contains the more general pledges that would contribute to its value as an ethical guide for the medical profession. The physician is bound, in a very general way, to help the sick according to his or her ability and judgment in a manner that can never be interpreted as involving injury or wrongdoing. The physician is bound both to confidentiality concerning direct experiences in the patient-doctor relationship and to extreme discretion to avoid the circulation of professional knowledge that is not appropriate for publication abroad.

In addition to these general precepts, all of which have an ethical timelessness that would survive the centuries, there were two points in the oath that refer to specific issues that cannot be separated from the modern debate over medical ethics. Addressing the questions of euthanasia ("mercy killing") and abortion, Hippocrates stated: "I will give no deadly drug to any, though it be asked of me, nor will I counsel such, and especially I will not aid a woman to procure abortion."

Anyone searching for wider guidelines can glean many items of timeless wisdom from other sections of Hippocrates' writings. In the pieces titled "The Physician" and "Decorum," for example, the personal behavior of doctors is discussed. In all cases, Hippocrates exhorted physicians to maintain even levels of dignity and patience, to practice exemplary personal hygiene, and to avoid excesses in living habits that could introduce an element of distance between themselves and the patients who depend on them. Many centuries later, as in the eighteenth century English essay by Samuel Bard titled "A Discourse upon the Duties of a Physician," one can see similar concerns for behavioral propriety toward the defenseless: for example, "Never affect to despise a man for the want of a regular education, and treat even harmless ignorance with delicacy and compassion" and protect against the effects of "foolhardiness and presumption." These admonitions are indicative of the defining boundaries of the views of Hippocrates and those of the later, Christian era on the practice of medicine. The main attention of commentators on the Hippocratic corpus in recent generations has been directed to two broad divisions in the main ethical issues that he formulated: the physician's role in abortion and in the decision to end life by either withholding or administering certain treatments. It took many centuries, however, for degrees of emphasis in analyzing the Hippocratic oath to take form. In the interim, and after a delay that separated the classical world from the late medieval world, different interpretations of the Hippocratic oath would appear, each reflecting the cultural environment to which it was meant to apply.

Several factors may explain why centuries passed before systematic attention was given to the rules of medicine first broached in the classical Greek and Roman worlds. The first of these was the general decline of political and economic conditions after the fall of Rome (fifth century C.E.), which had repercussions in a variety of cultural areas. Medical practices tended to revert to quite crude levels until the rediscovery of early medical texts, including those of Hippocrates, sparked interest in improving conditions of medical treatment in the late Middle Ages.

One can say that, in addition to editing elements of Hippocratic teachings to Christianize the pagan references that they contained, a second important redirection occurred in setting down medieval rules for the practice of medicine. It was Holy Roman Emperor Frederick II, around 1241, who specified for the first time that the higher authority of the state alone should define institutional procedures for certifying physicians. This was to be done through formal training and examinations in the universities of Naples or Salerno, and later in universities throughout the Western world.

In addition to rules leading to physicians' certification, Frederick II stipulated that doctors must take an oath binding them to obligations that, in comparison to the Hippocratic oath or modern codes of medical ethics, covered very specific issues. One of these was an obligation to report any irregularities in an apothecary's preparation of drugs that were to be dispensed to patients. Another enjoined doctors to provide free medical services to the poor.

If one looks at more modern standards for the regulation of relations between physician and patient, it is possible to suggest that—until some very major changes took place in society's views on delicate questions previously reserved for ecclesiastical law—similar operatives continued to govern the guidelines for medical ethics. In the "Code of Medical Ethics" (1846-1847) by the American Medical Association (AMA), for example, primary focus is still visibly on the physician's obligation to place the patient's interest before his or her own, particularly in terms of prospects for material or other forms of personal gain. Defense of the public's interest against quackery or the distribution of drugs that are either dangerous or illegally prepared follows, as well as avoidance of "crude hypotheses" or "magnification of the importance of services" sought, merely for the purpose of "temporary effect and popularity." Although there are enormous time spans between the classical Hippocratic model, the medieval variant offered by Frederick II, and the mid-nineteenth century AMA code, all are comparable in their focus on what, in the terminology of the 1847 code, would be called "Duties for Support of Professional Character" (part 1, article 1) or "Duties of the Profession to the Public" (part 2, article 1).

One hundred years later, however, different societal attitudes toward medical ethics would establish themselves in most Western nations, including the United States. Generally stated, the basic changes reflected in ethical debates emphasized (or questioned the rising emphasis on) the protection of individual rights and privacy in matters relating to human life and the intervention of physicians. On one hand, changing directions in the expression of ethical orientations stemmed from advances made in key areas of medical science in the twentieth century, such as technologies for combating terminal disease, saving the lives of severely preterm infants, and prolonging life in old age. On the other hand, and in an even broader context, extraordinary scientific discoveries concerning the genetic keys behind life itself introduced an entirely different dimension to medical ethics, that of responsibility for monitoring or "engineering" life that has not yet been conceived.

MODERN APPLICATIONS

Although neither the original nor edited versions of the Hippocratic oath are applied today as a condition for becoming a doctor, the medical profession in the United States has definitely formalized publication of what it considers to be a necessary code of medical ethics. Evolving versions of this "Code of Medical Ethics" date from the original (1847) text of the AMA as revised by specific decisions in 1903, 1912, and 1947.

When the AMA adopted a statement under the title "Guide to Responsible Professional Behavior" in 1980, it assigned to a formal body within its organization, the Council on Ethical and Judicial Affairs, the task of publishing, on a yearly basis, updated paragraphs that reflect ethical guidelines for the profession as a whole. These evolving guidelines are organized under such subheadings as "Social Policy Issues," "Interprofessional Relations," "Hospital Relations," "Confidentiality," and "Fees and Charges."

At the turn of the twenty-first century, the public's growing uncertainty about a doctor's role in a market-oriented health care delivery system and increasing mistrust in the face of malpractice suits prompted physicians to question their professional responsibilities and roles within modern medicine. In 2002, a joint effort between the American Board of Internal Medicine (ABIM), the American College of Physicians-American Society of Internal Medicine (ACP-ASIM), and the European Federation of Internal Medicine (EFIM) introduced a new professional code of conduct designed to address these issues and help physicians meet the needs of patients in the twenty-first century. The charter incorporated traditional understanding of professional norms into the unique circumstances of modern medicine by addressing issues such as patient autonomy and choice, working in physician teams and respecting other professionals, managing conflicts of interest, social justice and equality in health care access, and market forces—issues not relevant during the time of Hippocrates. The American-British team noted that they hoped their efforts reaffirmed to a wary public the profession's commitment to putting the needs of the patient first and offered guidelines to physicians for coping with the ethical problems in the modern world.

Along with such modern-day charters, physicians are bound to respect the ethical guidelines provided to them by their professional association. Failure to respect these guidelines is tantamount to breaking one's binding ethical obligations and can lead to expulsion from the medical profession.

Several major changes, both in levels of medical technology and in social attitudes toward issues relating to medical practice, have played key roles in several spheres of an ongoing debate concerning medical ethics. In two cases, those of abortion and euthanasia, debate has focused on the ethics of deciding to end life; in the third, referred to generally as genetic engineering, the central question involves both the living and those yet to be born. In all these spheres, the legal and ethical debates have revolved around potential conflicts between physicians and patients but also in the context of wider social values.

Movement from the historical domain of idealized codes or oaths to the more practical and contemporary realm of changing societal reactions to what constitutes injury or breach of professional ethics in several areas of modern medicine is facilitated by reference to landmark legal decisions that have given a modern and quite different meaning to Hippocratic concepts.

Probably the most widely recognized issue reflecting such ethical conflicts, and one that received specific attention in the Hippocratic oath itself, involves abortion. In the United States, the climate of public opinion toward doctor-assisted pregnancy terminations was altered considerably by the landmark 1973 Supreme Court decision *Roe v. Wade*. In this decision, the Court judged that state laws defining abortion as a criminal offense were unconstitutional. The main thrust of the argument in *Roe v. Wade* was that, although the Constitution does not provide a specific guarantee of a civil right of privacy that could be applied to questions of life and death in medical care, parallels exist in Supreme Court decisions on other matters of individual rights with respect to procreation. These rights tend to fall under the Fourteenth Amendment's concept of personal liberty and restrictions on state action. These rights, in the Court's words, are "broad enough to encompass a woman's decision whether or not to terminate her pregnancy."

Reference to the fundamental right of "personal privacy" in *Roe v. Wade* granted individual women and their physicians recourse against specific state laws criminalizing abortion. It did not, however, consider the right to have an abortion to be unqualified. Nor did it extend beyond the domain of pregnancy termination to cover a general assumption that constitutional protection of the right of privacy included the individual's right to "do with one's body as one pleases." In fact, there was an explicit suggestion that the legal definition of protection of an individual's right to privacy where critical medical decisions affecting vital life processes are concerned is "not unqualified and must be considered against important state interests in regulation."

As time passed in the evolving debate over abortion, definitions of what this could mean became colored by the inevitable introduction of religious conceptions of defense of the unborn individual—the fetus—as a possessor of life separate from that of the pregnant woman. This was a precursor to the "right to life" versus "right to choice" debate that would place physicians between two poles of opinion as to where their final obligations should lie.

What seemed most important in the beginnings of the abortion debate (and then, a few years later, the euthanasia debate) was the Supreme Court's inclusion of commentary on Hippocratic ethical precepts as part of its argument justifying recognition of individual rights to final responsibility for the disposition of someone else's "future" life or the disposition of one's own life. The *Roe v. Wade* brief actually argued that the strict Hippocratic injunction against abortion must be recognized as a reflection of only one segment of opinion and values (specifically Pythagorean) at a particular time in history. By underlining the fact that other views and practices were known to be current throughout antiquity, and that later Christian ethics chose to ignore diversity of interpretations of medical ethics in such matters, *Roe v. Wade* implied that diversity of ethical opinion within a social environment must be recognized in order to avoid too narrow a definition of what standards should be followed by physicians in dealing with their patients.

The implications of these two directions in interpreting the ethical bonds between patient and physician—the right to privacy in reaching individual decisions and recognition of a degree of social relativity in defining guidelines for medical ethics—are equally visible in the debate concerning the ultimate source of authority for deciding when to terminate life and the presumed authority of the Hippocratic oath in this process.

Two issues, one involving the ethics of sustaining life by means of advanced medical technology and the other involving the "engineering" of lives according to genetic predictions, fall under the provisions of the Hippocratic oath. As one approaches more contemporary statements of professional obligations of medical doctors, such as the "Principles of Medical Ethics" (1957) of the American Medical Association, one finds that, as certain areas of specificity in classical Hippo-

cratic or Christian medical ethics (the illegality of abortions or the administration of deadly potions) tend to decline in visibility, another area begins to come to the forefront—namely, striving continually to improve medical knowledge and skills to be made available to patients and colleagues.

This more modern concern for the application of advancements in medical knowledge, especially in the technology of medical lifesaving therapy, has introduced a new focus for ethical debate: not "lifesaving" but "life-sustaining" techniques, particularly in cases judged to be otherwise terminal or hopeless. As with the issue of abortion, the question of a doctor's responsibility to use every means within his or her reach to sustain life, even when there is no hope of a meaningful future for the patient, reflects a dilemma regarding Hippocratic injunctions. This debate is more important now than in any earlier era because advanced medical technology has made it possible either to extend the lives of aged patients who would die without life-sustaining machines or—in the case of younger persons afflicted by brain damage, for example—to sustain life although the patient remains in a comatose state.

A prototype in the latter case was a 1976 Supreme Court decision that allowed the parents of New Jersey car accident victim Karen Quinlan to instruct her physician to remove life support systems so that their comatose daughter would die. At issue in this complicated case, which also rested on legal discussions of the constitutional right of privacy, was the question of who should decide that inevitable natural death is preferable to prolongation of life by externally administered means. When the Court took this decision away from an appointed court guardian and gave it to those closest to the patient, the question became whose privacy was being protected. This dilemma is not unlike that inherent in the abortion debate, where the privacy of the pregnant woman is weighed against that of the as-yet-unconscious, unborn child. To whom does the physician's oath to avoid doing injury actually apply?

Legal solutions to subareas of the euthanasia debate were attained in stages, especially in cases of the very aged or patients afflicted with known terminal diseases. A living will, for example, allows individuals to instruct their physicians not to sustain their lives by artificial means if, beyond a certain point, they are unable to express their own will to die. In some cases, this discretion is assigned to the next of kin. In both cases, the objective is to remove ultimate responsibility for inevitable natural death from the physician's shoulders and to place it as closely as possible to within the private sphere of the patient.

A final area of contemporary debate over medical ethics illustrates how far conceptions of ultimate responsibility for the protection of life have gone beyond frames of reference that might have been familiar not only in Hippocrates' time but also as recently as the generation of doctors trained before the 1980's. Impressive advances in the research field of human genetics by the mid-1980's began to make it possible to predict, through analysis of deoxyribonucleic acid (DNA) structures, the likelihood that certain genetic traits (specifically debilitating chronic diseases) might be transmitted to the offspring of couples under study. Inherent in the rising debate over the ethics of such studies, which range from the prediction of reproductive combinations (genetic counseling) through actual attempts to detach and splice DNA chains (genetic engineering), was the delicate question of who, if anyone, should hold the responsibility of determining if individuals have ultimate control over their genes. In the most extreme hypothetical argument, a notion of scientific exclusion of certain gene combinations, or planning of desirable gene pools in future generations, began to appear in the 1980's and 1990's. These notions represent potential problems for medical ethics that, because of exponential changes in technological possibilities, surpass the entire realm of Hippocratic principles.

PERSPECTIVE AND PROSPECTS

Despite the introduction of certain legal precedents that tried to protect both physicians and their patients against dilemmas stemming from the assumed immutable ethical principles of the Hippocratic oath, society continues to witness practical shortcomings in modern understanding of who needs to be protected and how such protection should be institutionalized.

Malpractice insurance offers legal protection to physicians against personal damage claims levied by aggrieved patients or those surviving deceased patients; by the late twentieth century in the United States, these rates had soared. The larger debate regarding whether what physicians have done in individual cases was right or wrong rests on the assumption that his or her judgment can be put to the test by private parties defending their rights against professional incompetence. Therefore, the issue, as well as the institutional and/or legal devices pursued to resolve it, lies beyond the strict realm of a patient's privacy vis-à-vis a physician's responsibilities.

More characteristic examples of the contemporary social-ethical dilemma of whether doctors are fulfilling their appropriate professional responsibilities in recognizing patients' rights to certain types of treatment continue to fall into legally unresolved categories. The most obvious appears to be the ongoing debate concerning the legality of physician-assisted abortions. The considerations that have been introduced clearly go beyond the black-or-white principles that simple comparison with the content of the Hippocratic oath might involve. Courts and legislators involved in the ethics of abortion have had to devote extensive attention to the considerations of how pregnancies were induced (with attention to the anomalies of incest or rape, for example) or to questions of whether tax-appropriated funds gathered from an ethically divided public body can be dispensed to pay for medically approved abortions.

Still other dimensions of contemporary physician-patient relationships reveal that new forms of legislation will be needed before debates over the applicability of Hippocratic principles to modern society will recede from front-page prominence. With living wills having more or less resolved the question of individuals' right to instruct physicians or families to make decisions for them when personal capacities decline to incoherence, signs of new legal dilemmas began to emerge in the 1990's concerning fully coherent, terminally ill patients. Despairing of future suffering that can come well before any question of life support devices arises, some patients contracted their physicians—initially one physician in particular, Jack Kevorkian of Detroit, Michigan—to perform "mercy killing" by the administration of lethal poisons. Thus, one of the specific negative injunctions of the original Hippocratic oath returned the question of individual physicians' ethical and legal obligations to the forefront of public attention and court proceedings more than two millennia after its initial statement.

—*Byron D. Cannon, Ph.D.*

See also Abortion; American Medical Association (AMA); Cloning; Education, medical; Ethics; Euthanasia; Genetic engineering; Law and medicine; Malpractice.

FOR FURTHER INFORMATION:

Cambell, Alistair V., Gareth Jones, and Grant Gillett. *Medical Ethics.* 3d ed. New York: Oxford University

Press, 2002. A text that takes an interdisciplinary approach in examining major ethical questions in medical practice, including issues in genetics, prenatal and neonatal care, AIDS, mental health, geriatrics, and end-of-life care.

Casarett, David J., Frona Daskal, and John Lantos. "Experts in Ethics? The Authority of the Clinical Ethicist." *The Hastings Center Report* 28, no. 6 (November/December, 1998): 6-11. This article examines the work of Jurgen Habermas, which provides a basis for a model of clinical ethics consultation in which consensus, grounded in moral theory, assumes a central theoretical role.

Devine, Richard J. *Good Care, Painful Choices: Medical Ethics of Ordinary People.* 2d ed. Mahwah, N.J.: Paulist Press, 2000. An accessible survey of medical ethics for the layperson. Covers moral concepts such as personhood and conscience, abortion, genetics, organ transplants, end-of-life issues, and social health issues, including informed consent and health care access and reform.

Fletcher, John C., et al., eds. *Introduction to Clinical Ethics.* 2d ed. Frederick, Md.: University, 1997. This group of essays by contributing authors addresses the topic of ethics in contemporary medicine. Includes a bibliography.

Harron, Frank, John Burnside, and Tom Beauchamp. *Biomedical-Ethical Issues.* New Haven, Conn.: Yale University Press, 1983. A collection of key contemporary documents, including court decisions, state and federal laws, and policy statements by a number of professional associations regarding the most-debated ethical issues in medicine.

Jonsen, Albert R., Mark Siegler, and William J. Winslade. *Clinical Ethics: A Practical Approach to Ethical Decisions in Clinical Medicine.* 5th ed. New York: McGraw-Hill, 2002. Discusses the whole range of medical ethics, including legal issues, confidentiality, care of the dying patient, and euthanasia and assisted suicide.

Munson, Ronald. *Intervention and Reflection: Basic Issues in Medical Ethics.* 7th ed. New York: Wadsworth, 2003. An undergraduate text that combines social context, case studies, readings, and decision scenarios for topics that include abortion, advances in gene therapy, genetic discrimination, and health care rights.

Pence, Gregory. *Classic Cases in Medical Ethics: Accounts of Cases That Have Shaped Medical Ethics, with Philosophical, Legal, and Historical Backgrounds.* 4th ed. New York: McGraw-Hill, 2003. Surveys important cases that have defined and shaped the field of medical ethics. Each case is accompanied by careful discussion of pertinent philosophical theories and legal and ethical issues.

HIRSCHSPRUNG'S DISEASE
DISEASE/DISORDER

ALSO KNOWN AS: Congenital megacolon

ANATOMY OR SYSTEM AFFECTED: Anus, intestines, nerves

SPECIALTIES AND RELATED FIELDS: Cytology, family practice, obstetrics, pediatrics, proctology

DEFINITION: A disease of the large intestine that makes bowel movements difficult or impossible.

CAUSES AND SYMPTOMS

Hirschsprung's disease is caused when the lower part of the large intestine (colon), including the rectum, does not have the ganglion nerve cells to control the muscles that produce the contractions necessary for a bowel movement. Occasionally, the whole large intestine and even portions of the small intestine may be missing these nerve cells. The disease develops prior to birth. In the normal development of a fetus, the ganglion nerve cells grow from the top of the intestine down to the anus. For some unknown reason, the nerve cells stop growing at some distance down the intestine in children who experience Hirschsprung's disease.

The disease manifests itself most often in young children, although it can appear when an individual is a teenager or an adult. In an individual with Hirschsprung's disease, the healthy upper portion of the colon pushes stool down until it reaches the affected part. The stool then stops. New stool backs up behind it. Severe constipation results. In some cases, the victim may not be able to have any bowel movements at all. Babies

---

INFORMATION ON HIRSCHSPRUNG'S DISEASE

CAUSES: Lack of ganglion nerve cells for muscle control in lower colon

SYMPTOMS: Severe constipation, vomiting of bile, swollen abdomen, enterocolitis

DURATION: Acute

TREATMENTS: Surgery to remove affected area of colon

with Hirschsprung's disease often vomit up bile and experience swollen abdomens after eating. Infections, particularly enterocolitis, may develop in the intestines, which could even burst the colon.

TREATMENT AND THERAPY

Diagnosis of the disorder is confirmed by a barium enema X ray and a biopsy of the rectum. Barium makes the intestine show up better on an X ray. Manometry is also often used by the doctor to diagnose the disease. In this procedure, a small balloon is inflated inside of the rectum. If the anal muscle does not relax, the patient may have Hirschsprung's disease.

A pull-through operation removes the affected area of the intestine. The remaining ends are joined together. After this surgery, 85 to 90 percent of the patients pass feces normally, although some may experience diarrhea or constipation for a period of time. Eating high-fiber foods can help reduce diarrhea and constipation. Since the intestine is shortened by the surgery, not as much fluid is absorbed by the body. Consequently, the patient will need to drink plenty of fluids.

PERSPECTIVE AND PROSPECTS

Hirschsprung's disease occurs in approximately 1 out of every 5,000 births. About 80 percent of patients are boys. Children with Down syndrome are at a high risk for developing the disorder.

Hirschsprung's disease has been found to be hereditary, with the risk greater if the mother has the condition. Even if the parents have not had the disorder develop in their own lives, they may pass it on to their children. If one child in a family has the disease, other children are at greater risk to be born with it.

—*Alvin K. Benson, Ph.D.*

See also Constipation; Gastroenterology; Gastroenterology, pediatric; Gastrointestinal system; Genetic diseases; Intestinal disorders; Intestines; Neonatology; Peristalsis; Surgery, pediatric.

FOR FURTHER INFORMATION:

Eichenwald, Heinz F., Josef Ströder, and Charles M. Ginsburg, eds. *Pediatric Therapy*. 3d ed. St. Louis: Mosby Year Book, 1993.

Holschneider, Alexander M., and Prem Puri, eds. *Hirschsprung's Disease and Allied Disorders*. 2d ed. Philadelphia: Dunitz Martin, 2000.

Wester, Tomas. *Aspects of the Human Enteric Nervous System*. Uppsala, Sweden: University of Uppsala, 1999.

HISTIOCYTOSIS

DISEASE/DISORDER

ALSO KNOWN AS: Langerhans cell histiocytosis (LCH), histiocytosis X, eosinophilic granuloma, Hand-Schüller-Christian disease, Letterer-Siwe disease

ANATOMY OR SYSTEM AFFECTED: Blood, bones, ears, gastrointestinal system, immune system, liver, lungs, nervous system, skin, throat

SPECIALTIES AND RELATED FIELDS: Hematology, immunology

DEFINITION: A group of relatively rare blood disorders characterized by the abnormal accumulation of white blood cells called histiocytes, leading to a wide range of adverse bodily responses.

CAUSES AND SYMPTOMS

There is no clear understanding of the exact etiology of histiocytoses, blood disorders characterized by an accumulation of white blood cells called histiocytes, including monocytes and macrophages. Langerhans cell histiocytosis (LCH) is the most common type. At least four or five people per million are affected, with more males affected than females. The disorder affects both children and adults.

LCH may develop in response to underlying immunodeficiency or as a secondary effect from a viral infection. Symptoms vary based on the severity of the disease, and patients may be relatively symptom-free. LCH may be localized to one area or organ, or it may be more diffuse, involving multiple organs. It can cause lesions on bone, especially skull bones, or it may manifest itself as a skin rash. Respiratory symptoms such as cough or shortness of breath may signify that LCH has

---

INFORMATION ON HISTIOCYTOSIS

CAUSES: Response to underlying immunodeficiency or secondary effect from viral infection

SYMPTOMS: Depends on severity; may include bone lesions (especially skull), rashes, respiratory problems (cough, shortness of breath), gastrointestinal problems (bleeding, elevated liver enzymes)

DURATION: Short-term or long-term

TREATMENTS: Depends on the severity; may include chemotherapy

affected the lungs. Gastrointestinal manifestations of the disease include bleeding within the gastrointestinal tract or elevated liver enzymes. LCH can also affect the lymph nodes or the central nervous system and may contribute to the development of diabetes insipidus, growth hormone deficiency, and hypopituitarism (underactive pituitary gland).

Definitive diagnosis requires a biopsy, and the differential diagnosis (other diseases similar to it) is broad. Making the diagnosis requires a high index of suspicion because it is rare and easily missed. Helpful radiologic tests might include a chest X ray or a skeletal survey.

TREATMENT AND THERAPY

Treatment options vary widely based on the severity of the disease. On one hand, minimal treatment may be needed for symptom-free, single-system involvement, especially as LCH affecting only one system often remits completely. On the other hand, more severe disease affecting many systems may warrant chemotherapy, with characteristic remissions and relapses.

PERSPECTIVE AND PROSPECTS

The histiocytoses are classified into three types: LCH, hemophagocytic lymphohistiocytosis (HLH), and malignant histiocytosis. The impacts of LCH can be many, some with short-term and others with long-term consequences: stunted growth, dental problems, hearing loss, and hepatic fibrosis, to name a few. Though caregivers from a variety of medical specialties are often involved in caring for LCH patients and tremendous strides in diagnosis and treatment have been made, many patients still suffer from problematic, recurrent disease.

—Leonard Berkowitz, D.O.,
and Paul Moglia, Ph.D.

See also Blood and blood disorders; Hematology; Hematology, pediatric; Immune system; Immunology; Immunopathology.

FOR FURTHER INFORMATION:

Arceci, Robert J., B. Jack Longley, and Peter D. Emanuel. "Atypical Cellular Disorders." *Hematology*, 2002, 297-314.

Histiocytosis Association of America. www.histio.org.

Tebbi, Cameron K. "Histiocytosis." *Medline: Instant Access to the Minds of Medicine.* www.emedicine .com (May, 2002): 1-36.

HISTOLOGY

SPECIALTY

ANATOMY OR SYSTEM AFFECTED: All

SPECIALTIES AND RELATED FIELDS: Biochemistry, cytology, dermatology, hematology, internal medicine, oncology, pathology, vascular medicine

DEFINITION: The study of the body's tissues—epithelial, connective, muscle, and nerve tissues—to find the changes in structure that can be induced by disease.

KEY TERMS:

collagen: a fibrous protein occurring in many types of connective tissue

connective tissues: tissues containing large amounts of matrix outside the cells

epithelia: tissues that originate in broad, flat surfaces

matrix: organic or inorganic material occurring in connective tissues but located outside the cells

muscle tissues: tissues specialized in such a manner that they respond to stimulation by contracting along their long axes

nerve tissues: tissues specialized in such a manner that they respond to stimulation by conducting nerve impulses along their surfaces

tissues: groups of similar cells that are closely interrelated in function and organized together spatially

TYPES OF TISSUES

Histology is the study of tissues, which are groups of similar cells that are closely interrelated in their function and are organized together by location and structure. The four major types of tissues are epithelial tissue, connective tissue, muscle tissue, and nervous tissue.

Epithelial tissue (or epithelia) includes those tissues that originate in broad, flat surfaces. Their functions include protection, absorption, and secretion. Epithelia can be one-layered (simple) or multilayered (stratified). Their cells can be flat (squamous), tall and thin (columnar), or equal in height and width (cuboidal). Some simple epithelia have nuclei at two different levels, giving the false appearance of different layers; these tissues are called pseudostratified. Some simple squamous epithelia have special names: The inner lining of most blood vessels is called an endothelium, while the lining of a body cavity is called a mesothelium. Kidney tubules and most small ducts are also lined with simple squamous epithelia. The pigmented layer of the retina and the front surface of the lens of the eye are examples of simple cuboidal epithelia. Simple columnar epithelia form the inner lining of most digestive organs and the linings of the small bronchi and gallbladder. The epithelia lining the Fallopian tube, nasal cavity, and bronchi are ciliated, meaning that the cells have small hairlike extensions called cilia.

The outer layer of skin is a stratified squamous epithelium; other stratified squamous epithelia line the inside of the mouth, esophagus, and vagina. Sweat glands and other glands in the skin are lined with stratified cuboidal epithelia. Most of the urinary tract is lined with a special kind of stratified cuboidal epithelium called a transitional epithelium, which allows a large amount of stretching. Parts of the pharynx, larynx, urethra, and the ducts of the mammary glands are lined with stratified columnar epithelia.

Glands are composed of epithelial tissues that are highly modified for secretion. They may be either exocrine glands (in which the secretions exit by ducts that lead to targets nearby) or endocrine glands (in which the secretions are carried by the bloodstream to targets some distance away). The salivary glands in the mouth, the glandular lining of the stomach, and the sebaceous glands of the skin are exocrine glands. The thyroid gland, the adrenal gland, and the pituitary gland are endocrine glands. The pancreas has both exocrine and endocrine portions; the exocrine parts secrete digestive enzymes, while the endocrine parts, called the islets of Langerhans, secrete the hormones insulin and glucagon.

Connective tissues are tissues containing large amounts of a material called extracellular matrix, located outside the cells. The matrix may be a liquid (such as blood plasma), a solid containing fibers of collagen and related proteins, or an inorganic solid containing calcium salts (as in bone).

Blood and lymph are connective tissues with a liquid matrix (plasma) that can solidify when the blood clots. In addition to plasma, blood contains red cells (erythrocytes), white cells (leukocytes), and the tiny platelets that help to form clots. The many kinds of leukocytes include the so-called granular types (basophils, neutrophils, and eosinophils, all named according to the staining properties of their granules), the monocytes, and the several types of lymphocytes. Lymph contains lymphocytes and plasma only.

Most connective tissues have a solid matrix that includes fibrous proteins such as collagen and also elastic fibers, in some cases. If all the fibers are arranged in the same direction, as in ligaments and tendons, the tissue is called regular connective tissue. The dermis of the skin, however, is an example of an irregular connective

tissue in which the fibers are arranged in all directions. Loose connective tissue and adipose (fat) tissue both have very few fibers. The simplest type of loose connective tissue, with the fewest fibers, is sometimes called areolar connective tissue. Adipose tissue is a connective tissue in which the cells are filled with fat deposits. Hemopoietic (blood-forming) tissue, which occurs in the bone marrow and the thymus, contains the immature cell types that develop into most connective tissue cells, including blood cells. Cartilage tissue matrix contains a shock-resistant complex of protein and sugarlike (polysaccharide) molecules. Cartilage cells usually become trapped in this matrix and eventually die, except for those closest to the surface. Bone tissue gains its supporting ability and strength from a matrix containing calcium salts. Its typical cells, called osteocytes, contain many long strands by means of which they exchange nutrients and waste products with other osteocytes, and ultimately with the bloodstream. Bone also contains osteoclasts, large cells responsible for bone resorption and the release of calcium into the bloodstream.

Mesenchyme is an embryonic connective tissue made of wandering amoebalike cells. During embryological development, the mesenchyme cells develop into many different cell types, including hemocytoblasts, which give rise to most blood cells, and fibroblasts, which secrete protein fibers and then usually differentiate into other cell types.

Muscle tissues are tissues that are specially modified for contraction. When a nerve impulse is received, the overlapping fibers of the proteins actin and myosin slide against one another to produce the contraction. The three types of muscle tissue are smooth muscle, cardiac muscle, and skeletal muscle.

Smooth muscle contains cells that have tapering ends and centrally located nuclei. Muscular contractions are smooth, rhythmic, and involuntary, and they are usually not subject to fatigue. The cells are not cross-banded. Smooth muscle occurs in many digestive organs, reproductive organs, skin, and many other organs.

The term "striated muscle" is sometimes used to refer to cardiac and skeletal muscle, both of which have cylindrical fibers marked by cross-bands, which are also called cross-striations. The striations are caused by the lining up of the contractile proteins actin and myosin.

Cardiac muscle occurs only in the heart. Its crossstriated fibers branch and come together repeatedly. Contractions of these fibers are involuntary and rhythmic, and they occur without fatigue. Nuclei are located in the center of each cell; the cell boundaries are marked by dark-staining structures called intercalated disks.

Skeletal muscle occurs in the voluntary muscles of the body. Its cylindrical, cross-striated fibers contain many nuclei but no internal cell boundaries; a multinucleated fiber of this type is called a syncytium. Skeletal muscle is capable of producing rapid, forceful contractions, but it fatigues easily. Skeletal muscle tissue always attaches to connective tissue structures.

Nervous tissues contain specialized nerve cells (neurons) that respond rapidly to stimulation by conducting nerve impulses. All neurons contain RNA-rich granules, called Nissl granules, in the cytoplasm. Neurons with a single long extension of the cell body are called unipolar, those with two long extensions are called bipolar, and those with more than two long extensions are called multipolar. There are two types of extensions: Dendrites conduct impulses toward the cell body, while axons generally conduct impulses away from the cell body. Many axons are surrounded by a multilayered fatty substance called the myelin sheath, which is actually made of many layers of cell membrane wrapped around the axon.

Nervous tissues also contain several types of neuroglia, which are cells that hold nervous tissue together. Many neuroglia have processes (projections) that wrap around the neurons and help nourish them. Among the many types of neuroglia are the tiny microglia and the larger protoplasmic astrocytes, fibrous astrocytes, and oligodendroglia.

Two major tissue types make up most of the brain and spinal cord, or central nervous system. The first type, gray matter, contains the cell bodies of many neurons, along with smaller amounts of axons, dendrites, and neuroglia cells. The second type, white matter, contains mostly the axons, and sometimes also the dendrites, of neurons whose cell bodies lie elsewhere, along with the myelin sheaths that surround many of the axons. Clumps of cell bodies are called nuclei within the brain and ganglia elsewhere. Bundles of axons are called tracts within the central nervous system and nerves in the peripheral nervous system.

Histology as a Diagnostic Tool

Many diseases produce changes in one or more body tissues; these changes are so characteristic that the diagnosis of a disease often depends on the microscopic observation of changes in tissues. In order for such a diagnosis to be made, the tissue must be sliced very thin on a machine called a microtome. Some tissues are sliced while frozen; others must be hardened (or "fixed") in chemical solutions. After being sliced, the tissue is usually stained with chemical dyes that make viewing easier. Some tissues are viewed under the light microscope; others are sliced even thinner for viewing by electron microscopy.

Most hospitals have a pathology department that is responsible for these operations. After the tissues are sliced and examined, the pathologist makes a report that usually includes a diagnosis of the disease shown by the tissue samples.

Many diseases result in marked changes in the tissue at the microscopic level. Adaptively altered changes, which are usually reversible, include an increase in cell size (hypertrophy), increase in cell numbers (hyperplasia), a change from one cell or tissue type to another (metaplasia), and a decrease in size by withering (atrophy). Prolonged or repeated insults to the tissue may result in altered or atypical growth patterns (dysplasia). Overwhelming or sustained injury results in irreversible changes such as tissue degeneration or death. Tissue degeneration often includes the accumulation of abnormal amounts of fatty, fibrous, or pigmented tissue. Tissue death in a body that goes on living is called necrosis, and it may be of several types. If tissue death exceeds a certain limit, then the death of the organism results. Once this occurs, the tissues usually release protein-digesting enzymes that digest their own cell contents, a process known as autolysis.

Changes to cellular organelles can often be seen with an electron microscope before they become apparent at the light microscope level. Disturbances of the cell membrane may alter the flow of fluids (especially water) and cause changes to occur in the fluid composition of the cytoplasm. Too much fluid may result in swelling and eventually in bursting of the cells; too little fluid results either in shrinkage or in the coagulation of proteins. Swelling may also be induced by the lack of oxygen flow to the mitochondria, which can also result in the deposition of fats or calcium. The increase in the water content of the cells can also cause swelling in the endoplasmic reticulum and the detachment of ribosomes from the surfaces of the rough endoplasmic reticulum. Most damaging of all are the disturbances of the lysosomes, which can release their protein-digesting enzymes and cause autolysis.

At the light microscope level, other changes that may result from disease processes include the coalescence of numerous dropletlike vacuoles into a single, large, fluid-filled space. Other changes that may indicate disease are abnormal cell shapes, changes in the proportion of blood cells, and the rupture of cell membranes or other structures. Substances that may accumulate in diseased cells include glycogen (a sugar storage product), fibrous deposits of collagen and other proteins, and mineral deposits such as calcium salts. Abnormalities of the nucleus may include nuclear fragmentation, loss of the staining properties of the nucleus, or pyknosis, a shrinkage of the nucleus that also includes the clumping of its chromosomal material.

Edema, or tissue swelling, is a condition that can easily be confirmed by microscopic examination of histological sections. The swelling is marked by an increase in the amount of extracellular fluid. In the case of pulmonary edema, the fluid stains pink and fills the usually empty lung spaces (alveoli).

A different type of change is seen in Barrett's esophagus, a condition caused by the repeated backflow (or reflux) of gastric fluids into the esophagus. The inner lining of the esophagus is usually a stratified squamous epithelium, but in Barrett's esophagus the surface cells become taller, and the lining is changed into a columnar epithelium resembling that of the stomach.

Most cancers are recognized by abnormalities of the affected tissues, usually including more cells in the process of cell division (mitosis). The most dangerous cancers are marked by large tumors with ill-defined, irregular margins. If the cancer tumor is well-defined, small, and has a smooth, circular margin, the cancer is much less of a threat.

In juvenile diabetes, histological examination of the pancreas reveals a greatly reduced number of pancreatic islets, and those that remain are smaller and more fibrous. Herpes simplex infection causes the epidermal cells of the skin to undergo a buildup of fluid and a consequent balloonlike swelling. Warts of the skin are marked by a thickening of the outermost layer (stratum corneum) of the epidermis. Pernicious anemia, or vitamin B_{12} deficiency, results in a deterioration of the glands in the stomach lining. Crohn's disease produces swelling of the affected parts of the intestine, deposition of fat and lymphoid tissue, and ultimately tissue loss and deposition of fibrous scar tissue; the affected parts typically alternate with healthy regions. Cirrhosis of the liver, which is most commonly the result of chronic alcohol abuse, proceeds through a fatty stage (marked by deposition of fatty tissue), a fibrotic stage (marked by small nodules and scars), and an end stage

marked by abnormal shrinkage (atrophy) of liver tissue, scars, and larger nodules up to 1 centimeter in diameter. Emphysema, a lung disease found in many smokers, is recognizable histologically by an enlargement of the air spaces and by the presence of black, tarlike deposits within the lung tissue. Fibrocystic changes of the breast may be marked by the deposition of fibrous tissue, by increasing cell numbers, and by the enlargement of the glandular ducts.

Lupus erythematosus, a connective tissue disease, often produces red skin lesions marked by degeneration and flattening of the lower layers of the epidermis, drying and flaking of the outermost layer, dilation of the blood vessels under the skin, and the leakage of red blood cells out of these vessels, adding to the red color. (The word "erythematosus" means "red.")

Muscular dystrophy has several forms; the most common form is marked in its advanced stages by enlarged muscles in which the muscle tissue is replaced by a fatty substance. Another muscular disease, myasthenia gravis, is often marked by overall enlargement of the thymus and an increase in the number of thymus cells. Myocardial infarction (heart attack), a form of heart disease marked by damage to the heart muscle, is indicated in histological section by dead, fibrous scar tissue replacing the muscle tissue in the heart wall. In patients with arteriosclerosis, the usually elastic walls of the arteries become thicker and more fibrous and rigid. Many of the same patients also suffer from atherosclerosis, a buildup of deposits on the inside of the blood vessels that partially or completely blocks the flow of blood.

In nervous tissue, damage to peripheral nerves often results in a process called chromatolysis in the cell bodies of the neurons from which these axons arise. The nuclei of these cells enlarge and are displaced to one side, while the Nissl granules disperse and the cell body as a whole undergoes swelling. Increased deposits of fibrous tissue characterize multiple sclerosis and certain other disorders of the nervous system. Some of these diseases are also marked by a degeneration of the myelin sheath around nerve fibers. In the case of a cerebrovascular stroke, impaired blood supply to the brain causes degeneration of the neuroglia, followed by general tissue death and the replacement of the neuroglia by fibrous tissue. Cranial hematoma (abnormal bleeding in any of several possible locations) results in the presence of blood clots (complete with blood cells and connective tissue fibers) in abnormal locations. Alzheimer's disease is marked by granules of a proteinlike substance called amyloid, often containing aluminum, surrounded by additional concentric layers of similar composition. Advanced stages of alcoholism are marked in brain tissue by the destruction of certain neurons and neuroglia. Poliomyelitis, or polio, is marked by the destruction of nervous tissue in the anterior horn of the spinal cord.

PERSPECTIVE AND PROSPECTS

The microscopic study of tissues began historically with Robert Hooke's *Micrographia* (1665) and the studies of Marcello Malpighi (1628-1694), but early microscopes were low in quality by today's standards. As microscopes improved, so did their use in studying tissues. During the 1830's, the Scottish botanist Robert Brown (1773-1858) discovered the cell nucleus. Soon, German biologists Matthias Jakob Schleiden (1804-1881) and Theodor Schwann (1810-1882) developed the so-called cell theory, a theory which proclaimed that all living things are constructed of cells and that all biological processes are rooted in processes occurring at the level of cells and tissues. The greatest advances in microscopic optics were made between 1870 and 1900, mostly in Germany, and the study of histology benefited greatly.

The great pathologist Rudolph Virchow (1821-1902) was the first to emphasize the structural changes in cells caused by the disease process; he showed that many diseases could be detected at the cellular level under the microscope. This claim, coupled with the enthusiasm for the cell theory, aroused great interest in the study of cells throughout Europe and later in America. Advances in tissue-staining techniques in microanatomy were made in various countries over a long period; the Czech histologist and physiologist Jan Evangelista Purkinje (1787-1869) was one of the leaders of this early period. Early in the twentieth century, histologists Santiago Ramón y Cajal (1852-1934) of Spain and Camillo Golgi (1844-1926) of Italy shared the 1906 Nobel Prize in Physiology or Medicine for their detailed work on the tissue structure of the nervous system. In the decades after World War II, the electron microscope became a standard instrument for the ultrafine study of tissue details at and even below the cellular level. Today, pathology laboratories routinely use the microscopic examination of tissues as an important tool in diagnosis.

—*Eli C. Minkoff, Ph.D.*

See also Alzheimer's disease; Arteriosclerosis; Biopsy; Bleeding; Blood and blood disorders; Bones and the skeleton; Cells; Cirrhosis; Crohn's disease; Cytology; Dermatology; Emphysema; Glands; Herpes; Lupus erythematosus; Lymphatic system; Multiple sclerosis; Muscles; Muscular dystrophy; Nervous system; Neurology; Orthopedics; Pathology; Poliomyelitis; Skin; Strokes.

FOR FURTHER INFORMATION:

Fawcett, D. W. *A Textbook of Histology.* 12th ed. New York: Chapman & Hall, 1994. A classic standard, well illustrated with a variety of light micrographs (often in color) and electron micrographs. Most thorough in its descriptions of physiological functions.

Junqueira, Louis Carlos, and Jose Carneiro. *Basic Histology.* 10th ed. New York: McGraw-Hill, 2002. A leading text that describes the structure and function of cells and the function and specialization of the four tissue groups: epithelial, connective, adipose, and nerve. Also includes chapters on the cytoplasm and cell nucleus that review recent discoveries in cell biology.

Kerr, Jeffrey B. *Atlas of Functional Histology.* St. Louis: Mosby, 1999. This volume includes discussion of histology as it applies to the major biological systems, such as the endocrine, respiratory, reproductive, gastrointestinal, nervous, and circulatory systems.

Kessel, Richard G. *Basic Medical Histology.* Oxford, England: Oxford University Press, 1998. This textbook is derived from Kessel's notes, figures, and references accumulated over thirty-five years of teaching histology at the University of Iowa. Suitable for advanced undergraduate students in biology or possibly first-year medical students.

Lewin, Benjamin. *Genes: VIII.* New York: Oxford University Press, 2003. A college textbook that discusses the entire field of molecular biology and genetics, with many references to the structure and activity of the cell nucleus. Although written at the college level, it is readable and accessible to a general audience. Many highly informative illustrations and diagrams are included.

Ross, Michael H., et al. *Histology: A Text and Atlas.* 4th ed. Philadelphia: Lippincott Williams & Wilkins, 2002. Introductory text on histology that covers vast array of topics, including methods, the cell, the classification of tissues, epithelial tissue, connective tissue, cartilage, bone, blood, muscle, nerves, cardiovascular tissue, lymphatic tissue, and the esophagus and gastrointestinal tract.

HIV. *See* Human immunodeficiency virus (HIV).

Hives

Disease/disorder

Also known as: Urticaria

Anatomy or system affected: Immune system, skin

Specialties and related fields: Dermatology, family practice, immunology, internal medicine, pediatrics

Definition: Pink swellings called wheals that may occur in groups on any part of the skin.

> ### Information on Hives
>
> **Causes:** Allergic reactions, foods, drugs, environmental toxins, infections, insect bites, internal diseases, physical stimuli (*e.g.*, heat, cold)
> **Symptoms:** Inflammation, itchiness
> **Duration:** Acute or chronic
> **Treatments:** Antihistamines

Causes and Symptoms

Hives are produced by blood plasma leaking through tiny gaps between the cells lining small vessels in the skin. A natural chemical called histamine is released from mast cells, which lie along the blood vessels in the skin. Allergic reactions, foods, drugs, or other chemicals can cause histamine release.

Hives can vary in size from as small as a pencil eraser to as large as a dinner plate, and they may join together to form larger swellings. When hives are forming, they are usually very itchy; they may also burn or sting. Nearly 20 percent of the general population will have at least one episode of hives in their lifetime. Acute hives may last for a few days to weeks. If they last for more than six weeks, they are called chronic hives.

The most common causes of acute hives are foods, drugs, infections, insect bites, and internal diseases. Other causes are physical stimuli, including pressure, cold, and sunlight.

Treatment and Therapy

The best treatment for hives is to find the cause and then eliminate it. Unfortunately, this is not always an easy task. Even if a cause cannot be found, antihistamines are usually prescribed to provide some relief. Antihistamines work best if taken on a regular schedule. It may be necessary to try more than one or use different combinations of antihistamines to find out what works best. In severe cases of hives, an injection of epinephrine (adrenalin) or a cortisone preparation can bring dramatic relief.

Perspective and Prospects

In 1927, Sir Thomas Lewis reported the association between wheals and small blood vessel dilation, which later confirmed the importance of histamine as a cause of hives. Years of research showed that apart from allergy, nonimmunological stimuli can cause hives as well. A recent report that some patients with chronic hives may have formed antibodies against the immunoglobulin IgE receptor suggests that the cause of hives could be multifactorial.

—*Shih-Wen Huang, M.D.*

See also Allergies; Antihistamines; Bites and stings; Dermatology, pediatric; Immune system; Itching; Rashes; Skin; Skin disorders.

For Further Information:

Adelman, Daniel C., et al., eds. *Manual of Allergy and Immunology.* Philadelphia: Lippincott Williams & Wilkins, 2002.

Joneja, Janice M. V., and Leonard Bielory. *Understanding Allergy, Sensitivity, and Immunity.* New Brunswick, N.J.: Rutgers University Press, 1990.

Kuby, Janis. *Immunology.* 4th ed. New York: W. H. Freeman, 2000.

Middlemiss, Prisca. *What's That Rash? How to Identify and Treat Childhood Rashes.* London: Hamlyn, 2002.

Roitt, Ivan. *Essential Immunology.* 10th ed. Boston: Blackwell Scientific, 2001.

Young, Stuart, Bruce Dobozin, and Margaret Miner. *Allergies.* Rev. ed. New York: Plume, 1999.

Hodgkin's disease

Disease/disorder

Anatomy or system affected: Lymphatic system

Specialties and related fields: Hematology, internal medicine, oncology, serology

Definition: A neoplastic disorder originating in the tissues of the lymphatic system, recognized by distinctive histologic changes and defined by the presence of Reed-Sternberg cells.

Key terms:

chemotherapy: a modality of cancer treatment consisting of the administration of cytotoxic drugs *combination chemotherapy:* the use of multiple chemical agents in the treatment of cancer, each in a lower dosage so that the overall toxicity, but not the effectiveness, is reduced

neoplastic: pertaining to cancerous growths

prognosis: a prediction of the outcome of treatment for a disease on the basis of clinical and pathologic parameters, such as pathology, clinical stage, and presence or absence of symptoms such as fever, night sweats, and unexplained weight loss

radiotherapy: the use of radiation to kill cancer cells or shrink cancerous growth; when high and full doses of radiation (measured in units called rads) are used, the patient is said to be given a "megavoltage"

CAUSES AND SYMPTOMS

Malignant lymphomas are neoplasms of lymphoid tissues and are of two general categories: those related to Hodgkin's disease and others that are collectively called non-Hodgkin's lymphomas. The lymphoid tissues represent the structural expressions of the immune system, which defends the body against microbes. This system is widely spread throughout the body, is highly complex, and interacts closely with other physiologic systems of the body—especially the mucosa that lines the airways and digestive tract, where there is direct exposure to environmental microbes and other foreign substances. The components of this system are aggregations of lymphocytes in the mucosal linings (such as tonsils and adenoids), lymph nodes, and the spleen. The components of the lymphatic system connect with one another via small lymphatic vessels. The lymph nodes, which are situated in anatomical regions all over the body, interconnect and drain centrally toward the great veins of the body. The cellular components of

the immune system are the lymphocytes, also called immunocytes. These account for about 20 percent of blood cells; lymphocytes make up the bulk of the lymphoid tissue that makes up the lymphatic system. The blood cells have a finite life and are disposed of in the spleen, which is the largest lymphoid organ in the body.

There are two major functional immunologic classes of lymphocytes and several other subclasses. Nevertheless, all share similar morphologic appearance, being small round cells almost completely occupied by a round nucleus. The B lymphocyte (the B refers to its bone marrow derivation) can, under proper antigenic stimulation, transform and mature into a plasma cell, which is the cell in charge of producing antibodies. Antibodies are the protein products of the immune system that act by capturing and removing foreign substances, called antigens. The other major class of lymphocytes is the T lymphocyte (the T refers to its thymus derivation). T lymphocytes are of at least two major functional subclasses, which either help or suppress the B lymphocytes in their transformation into plasma cells; thus they are termed helper and suppressor T cells, respectively. Other cellular components of the immune system, cellular monocytes and macrophages, play an important role in carrying and transferring specific immunologic information between the various cellular components of the immune-lymphatic system. This, then, is a highly organized and complex system, with positive and negative biofeedback that maintains optimal, balanced proportions of all the cellular components that make up the system.

Hodgkin's disease is a neoplasm of the lymphoid tissues that usually arises in lymph nodes, often in the neck, and has a varied histologic appearance characterized by the presence of Reed-Sternberg cells. The Reed-Sternberg cell is a giant cell having two nuclei that are situated in a mirror-image fashion. Treatment and prognosis in Hodgkin's disease are determined by two parameters: the histopathologic classification, whereby the morphologic appearance is evaluated by the pathologist, and the clinical staging classification, whereby the extent of spread of the disease and its localization are determined by clinical studies. The pathology is studied by reviewing thinly cut sections of diseased lymph nodes removed from the patient. This study is most important for establishing a diagnosis of Hodgkin's disease and ruling out other conditions that may closely simulate its clinical and/or pathologic features. At times, peer consultations are used to confirm the diagnosis.

INFORMATION ON HODGKIN'S DISEASE

CAUSES: Unknown

SYMPTOMS: Persistent fever and fatigue; chills and night sweats; painless swelling of lymph nodes in neck, armpits, or groin; unexplained weight loss and loss of appetite; eventual tumors

DURATION: Possibly recurrent

TREATMENTS: Radiation therapy, chemotherapy, bone marrow transplantation

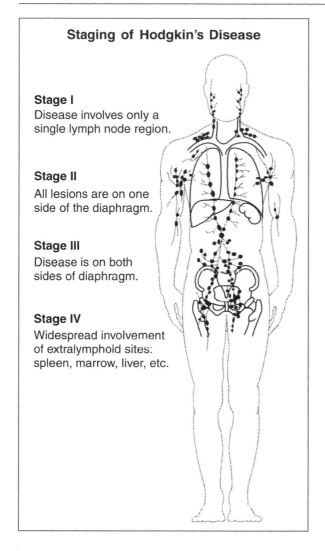

Staging of Hodgkin's Disease

Stage I
Disease involves only a single lymph node region.

Stage II
All lesions are on one side of the diaphragm.

Stage III
Disease is on both sides of diaphragm.

Stage IV
Widespread involvement of extralymphoid sites: spleen, marrow, liver, etc.

Reed-Sternberg cells have a characteristic appearance and must be identified to make a diagnosis of Hodgkin's disease. The pathologic classification of this disease, based on microscopic study, recognizes four different types, each with its own clinical implications regarding survival and prognosis. The classification is based on the relative dominance of lymphocytes when compared to the number of the neoplastic Reed-Sternberg cells. In the most favorable type, the lymphocytes predominate and Reed-Sternberg cells are sparse; this type is called lymphocyte predominance. In the worst type, the lymphocytes are very sparse and there are many more Reed-Sternberg cells and their variants; this type is called lymphocyte depletion. In between these two extremes are the mixed-cellularity type, in which there is an even mixture of lymphocytes and Reed-Sternberg cells, and nodular sclerosis, which forms

nodules of fibrous scar tissue that surround the mixture of lymphocytes and Reed-Sternberg cells.

This classification has important prognostic implications. It correctly presumes that the neoplastic cells are the Reed-Sternberg cells and their variants, and that the lymphocytes are induced by the immune system to multiply and to fight the spread of the neoplastic cells. It follows that the more the process is successful, the better is the prognosis. Hence lymphocyte predominance carries a more favorable outlook than lymphocyte depletion, with mixed-cellularity types somewhere in between. Nodular sclerosis also carries a good prognosis. Other inflammatory cells are invariably mixed with the lymphocytes and Reed-Sternberg cells; these cells are also part of the body's immune response against cancer cells.

The clinical staging classification of Hodgkin's disease was formulated by a group of experts who met at a workshop in Ann Arbor, Michigan, in 1971. It is based on the proposition that the disease begins in a single group of lymph nodes (usually in the neck) and then spreads to the next adjacent group of lymph nodes, on the same side, before it crosses over to the other side of the body. The disease then advances further across the diaphragm muscle, which separates the thorax from the abdominal cavity, and finally disseminates into the blood to involve the bone marrow and other distant sites. In this schema, stage I represents early stage, with involvement of only a single lymph node region, and stage II is the condition in which two or more such regions are involved on the same side of the diaphragm (that is, either above or below the diaphragm).

In the United States, Hodgkin's disease is an uncommon neoplasm accounting for an estimated 7,600 cases, or fewer than 1 percent of all new cases of cancer, a year. In 2002, the disease resulted in approximately 1,300 deaths according to American Cancer Society statistics. The incidence in the United States is slightly higher in males than females, and in whites than blacks. Incidence trends show a mild rise for the nodular sclerosis type in young adults and a mild decrease of Hodgkin's disease over the age of forty.

Hodgkin's disease can occur at any age, although the highest peak incidence occurs in adolescents and young adults, and smaller peaks occur in the fifth and sixth decades of life. Most patients come to clinical attention because of painless, nontender, enlarged lymph nodes in the neck or armpits (above the diaphragm) or, less commonly, in the groin. In the young adult or adolescent, a mass in the chest may press against the airways to produce a dry, hacking cough and shortness of breath, which may be the patient's first symptoms. Some patients may have anemia or severe itching. At times, especially when the disease is aggressive and extensive, the patient may have a fever, which may run for a few days and then disappear, only to recur after a week or two; there can also be night sweats and weight loss. These symptoms—fever, night sweats, and weight loss—indicate a less favorable prognosis. Younger patients and those with lymphocyte predominance and nodular sclerosis histologic types (favorable histologic types) tend to have limited disease—that is, stages I and II—found primarily above the diaphragm. Older patients and those with mixed-cellularity or lymphocyte depletion types are more likely to have extensive disease involving lymph nodes on both sides of the diaphragm (stage III) or even involving the liver, spleen, and bone marrow (stage IV).

When a patient with persistent lymph node enlargement seeks medical attention, a lymph node biopsy is usually made to make sure of the diagnosis. Other cancers that may simulate Hodgkin's disease must be excluded, as well as a long list of benign conditions such as infectious mononucleosis and tuberculosis. A series of blood tests, X-ray and other imaging studies, and a bone marrow biopsy are done in order to evaluate the spread of disease and to assign the proper clinical stage. At times, even surgical exploration of the abdomen, with biopsies of abdominal lymph nodes, the liver, and the spleen, is done to assign an accurate stage of Hodgkin's disease; this procedure is called staging laparotomy.

TREATMENT AND THERAPY

Modern cancer therapy has achieved its greatest triumph in the treatment of Hodgkin's disease. The advent of a generally acceptable histopathologic classification, accurate staging, improved radiotherapy, effective chemotherapy, and supportive care, such as antibiotics and the transfusion of platelets, have contributed to the impressive 80 percent overall cure rate. The therapy is enhanced by an effective teamwork of medical experts in oncology, radiation therapy, surgery, pathology, and diagnostic radiology.

Because Hodgkin's disease spreads in an orderly fashion through adjacent lymph node groups, effective high-dose radiation can be directed at affected lymph nodes and at their neighboring, uninvolved nodes. Irradiation, with a full dose of 3,500 to 4,000 rads in three

to four weeks, can eradicate Hodgkin's disease in involved nodes within the treatment field more than 95 percent of the time. In addition, extended-field irradiation of the adjacent uninvolved nodes is a standard practice used to eradicate minimal or early disease in these lymph nodes.

Stages I and II can be treated with radiotherapy alone by an extended field to include all areas above the diaphragm bearing lymph nodes (the axilla, neck, and chest), and in most cases the lymph nodes in the abdomen. Such treatment cures about 90 percent of patients. For patients in which the disease is found extensively in the chest, chemotherapy is added to the radiotherapy and results in prolonged, relapse-free survival in 85 percent of patients.

A variety of cytotoxic drugs (those that kill cells) are available to treat Hodgkin's disease. Such drugs are similar to nitrogen mustard (which was once used in war) and are toxic to the body. It has been found that when more than one drug is used, each in a smaller dose, the toxicity can be reduced without diminishing effectiveness. Thus combination chemotherapy has

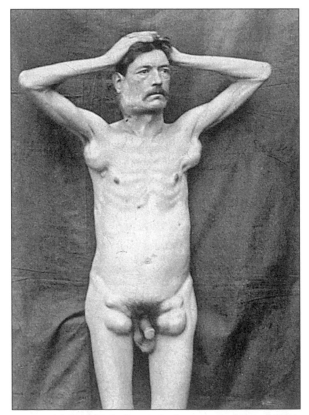

A man with Hodgkin's disease is shown in the Atlas of Clinical Medicine *(1892).* (National Library of Medicine)

evolved. There are many effective regimens of combination chemotherapy that are called by the initials of the individual components; the most widely used is MOPP (mechlorethamine, Oncovin, procarbazine, and prednisone). In stage III, chemotherapy with or without radiotherapy is used, depending upon specific variations within the stage, with cure rates achieved in 75 to 80 percent of patients. Even in stage IV disease, combination chemotherapy (particularly with MOPP) has produced a complete remission in about 75 percent of patients, with a cure rate of more than 50 percent.

Bone marrow transplantation, which is the intravenous infusion of normal marrow cells into the patient shortly after treatment in order to protect the patient from toxicity, has permitted the use of much higher doses of certain drugs. It allows the therapist to irradiate all the patient's bone marrow, eradicating both "good" and "bad" cells, with the hope that the normal marrow cells that are infused will populate the bone marrow and grow there. Bone marrow transplantation has been successfully used mainly in young patients who were resistent to conventional chemotherapy.

PERSPECTIVE AND PROSPECTS

Thomas Hodgkin of Guy's Hospital in London was the first to recognize the disease that would bear his name. In 1832, he described the gross autopsy findings and clinical features of seven patients who had simultaneous enlargement of grossly diseased lymph nodes and spleens, and he considered the condition to be a primary affliction of these organs. This condition, he himself records, was vaguely outlined by Marcello Malpighi in 1665. Four years earlier than Hodgkin, David Craige had described the autopsy findings of a similar case. Subsequent histologic examination of tissues from Hodgkin's original cases confirmed the disease in three of them. In 1865, Sir Samuel Wilks elaborated on the autopsy studies of similar cases and published the findings on fifteen patients, calling the condition Hodgkin's disease.

Important histopathologic observations were contributed by William Greenfield in 1878 and E. Goldman in 1892. George Sternberg described the giant cells but believed the condition to be a peculiar form of tuberculosis. The recognition that these cells were an integral part of the disease awaited the careful pathologic observation of Dorothy Reed of The Johns Hopkins Hospital in Baltimore. These cells, appropriately named Reed-Sternberg cells, are the hallmark of Hodgkin's disease.

Controversy as to the nature of this disease led early investigators to study infectious agents as possible etiologic causes, especially the tuberculosis bacillus, but to no avail. More recent studies have examined the roles of other viral infectious agents, especially the agent of infectious mononucleosis, but with no consistent results. At present, the condition is accepted as neoplastic, probably triggered by some unknown environmental agent or agents.

Between 1930 and 1950, major advances included the recognition of meaningful histologic subtypes of Hodgkin's disease correlating with prognosis, and the development by Vera Peters of a clinical staging system. Impressive responses to X-ray therapy were reported at the beginning of the twentieth century, and treatment with megavoltage therapy was further developed. By World War II, it became realistic to speak of curing some patients with early Hodgkin's disease. The potential for a cure meant that accurate histologic diagnosis and estimation of the extent and localization of disease were imperative in planning treatment; a multidisciplinary approach to diagnosis and treatment was developed. Modern concepts of histologic classification became codified at a conference held in Rye, New York, in 1965, and the clinical staging system was refined into its present form at a workshop held at Ann Arbor, Michigan, in 1971.

Modern effective chemotherapy was developed concurrently with these advances in classification, staging, and radiotherapy. The alkylating agents, created as an outgrowth of studies on nitrogen mustard gas during World War II, provided the first drugs to produce impressive shrinkage of the tumor and significant palliation of the disease. The subsequent developments in modern pharmacology and therapeutics enabled Vince DeVita and his coworkers, in 1970, to design the first effective combination chemotherapy regimen, MOPP.

Today, many more such regimens are being tested; the possibility for cure has become a realistic hope for every patient with Hodgkin's disease. This is the case because of the refinement of ancillary therapies with antibiotics (for infections that may occur during the necessary phases of suppression of the immune system by these powerful toxic drugs) and platelet transfusion technology. Bone marrow transplantation technology also offers strong hope of curing patients with advanced cases who are resistant. The bone marrow is harvested and then reintroduced into a patient whose marrow has been effectively disabled. Immunotherapy is also being investigated. It can boost the patient's ability to combat disease by modulating the body's responses. The drawback to aggressive combinations of chemotherapy and radiotherapy, however, is the emergence of therapy-related leukemia and leukemia-like malignancies several years after the completion of successful therapy for Hodgkin's disease.

—*Victor H. Nassar, M.D.*

See also Bone marrow transplantation; Cancer; Chemotherapy; Lymphadenopathy and lymphoma; Lymphatic system; Malignancy and metastasis; Oncology; Radiation therapy.

FOR FURTHER INFORMATION:

CA: A Cancer Journal for Clinicians 43, no. 1. January/February, 1993. A journal published by the American Cancer Society. This special issue is devoted to a discussion of cancer statistics, including those regarding Hodgkin's disease.

Dollinger, Malin, Ernest H. Rosenbaum, and Greg Cable. *Everyone's Guide to Cancer Therapy.* 4th rev. ed. Kansas City, Mo.: Andrews & McMeel, 2002. An excellent source of medical information about cancer, written for the general public. A helpful glossary of medical terminology is provided.

Lee, G. Richard, et al., eds. *Wintrobe's Clinical Hematology.* 11th ed. Philadelphia: Lea & Febiger, 2003. A textbook of hematologic disorders, with an excellent review of Hodgkin's disease. Written for clinicians and students of medicine.

Lymphoma Information Network. http://www.lymphomainfo.net/hodgkins/. Offers information on the diagnosis and treatment options for adult and childhood Hodgkin's disease and resources for further research.

Murphy, G., L. Morris, and D. Lange. *Informed Decisions: The Complete Book of Cancer Diagnosis, Treatment, and Recovery.* 2d ed. New York: Viking Press, 2001. This text from the American Cancer Society is intended for the layperson. It is exemplary in its discussion of cancer.

Parker, James N., and Philip M. Parker, eds. *The Official Parent's Sourcebook on Childhood Hodgkin's Disease.* San Diego, Calif.: Icon Health, 2002. Draws from public, academic, government, and peer-reviewed research to provide a wide-ranging handbook for families of children with Hodgkin's disease.

_____. *Official Patient's Sourcebook on Adult Hodgkin's Disease.* San Diego, Calif.: Icon Health, 2002. Draws from public, academic, government, and peer-reviewed research to provide a wide-ranging handbook for adult patients with Hodgkin's disease.

Williams, Stephanie F., Ramez Farah, and Harvey M. Golomb, eds. *Hodgkin's Disease.* Philadelphia: W. B. Saunders, 1989. A volume in the series Hematology/Oncology Clinics of North America. A thorough review of this disease—its diagnosis, pathology, and treatment. Includes bibliographical references and an index.

Williams, W. J., E. Beuter, A. J. Erslev, and M. A. Lichtman, eds. *Williams Hematology.* 6th ed. New York: McGraw-Hill, 2002. An up-to-date textbook that offers an authoritative review of all aspects of Hodgkin's disease.

HOLISTIC MEDICINE

SPECIALTY

ANATOMY OR SYSTEM AFFECTED: All

SPECIALTIES AND RELATED FIELDS: Alternative medicine, environmental health, nursing, osteopathic medicine, preventive medicine, psychology

DEFINITION: The practice of medicine to maintain both physical and psychological health as a natural deterrent to disease and as a way of realizing one's highest potential.

KEY TERMS:

hospice care: an alternative to hospitalization for the terminally ill or aged that allows for the dignified acceptance of impending death

stress management: the alleviation of stress, a form of preventive medicine borrowed from holistic approaches to common emotional disorders

SCIENCE AND PROFESSION

Although the phenomenon of holistic medicine gained increased attention in the latter half of the twentieth century, most of the principles associated with it have appeared in various forms and in various cultures over the centuries. Ironically, it may have been the progress of medical science generally and the widespread use by doctors of new drugs to treat disease that sparked what some would call holistic medicine's call for a return to basics. For example, some proponents of holism oppose automatic reliance on surgical methods of treating some ailments for not recognizing either their causes or more beneficial modes of treatment. In addition, holists oppose a reliance on drugs not only because they hold certain maladies to be curable (or indeed totally avoidable) without them but also because of possible negative side effects.

A number of quite sophisticated principles could fall under the presumed "basics" of the holistic approach to health. Primary among these is a conviction that—short of obvious conditions involving attacks by virus, bacteria, or chronic debilitation of certain organs of the body, including the nervous system—increased awareness of the nature of bodily functions can help maintain a healthy level of balance within the total organism. Essential to the principle of balance is recognition of the importance of the mind in influencing one's reactions, both psychological and physical, to circumstances in the surrounding environment. Some holists adhere to the Abraham Maslow school of psychology, which places strong emphasis on questions of drive toward "need fulfillment" in both the physical and psychological domains. Certain bodily states can easily be linked to biologically stimulated drives, including hunger and sexuality. Less apparent psychological drives, however, may also trigger physical reactions. Imbalances in fulfilling the natural drives for love or success are held responsible for many forms of physical disorder that could be averted, such as anorexia nervosa, ulcers, and stress.

Several approaches to holistic medicine consider the end goal of good physical health to be not only the avoidance of disease but also the realization of a positive, life-enhancing experience. In some cases, the inspiration for such theories comes from long traditions in Asian philosophies and religions that assume close links between the psychic and the physical realms of life. An assumption that may or may not be shared between such philosophies and holists is that a "true" state of health leads to superior levels of awareness in both spheres.

Physicians interested in holistic medicine need not, however, be tied solely to disease-specific or "consciousness-heightening" aspects of what can be a very general field. Some specialists in geriatrics, for example, adopt holistic approaches to counseling the elderly about natural stages of aging, preparing them to accept, with a minimum of anxiety, the gradual decline that accompanies the end of life. Growing emphasis on hospice care for the terminally ill or aged, as opposed to hospitalization, is connected with this aspect of holistic medicine.

DIAGNOSTIC AND TREATMENT TECHNIQUES
Although individual physicians may espouse holistic approaches, many persons without formal medical training choose to practice it themselves to maintain their bodies and minds in the healthiest state possible. Such practices may be individual and personal, ranging from exercise and dietary habits to meditation. They may also involve group associations supported by the participation of trained physicians or laypersons. It has become possible to find method-specific holistic centers specializing in a range of techniques. These range from, for example, very general holistic health and nutrition institutes to highly specialized centers that strive to treat those suffering from chronic pain through localized electrical nerve stimulation.

Essential to almost all holistic approaches to treatment is an emphasis on the physician's role as a facilitator—someone who is able to help the patient recognize what he or she should do to adopt various attitudes and actions that can alleviate all or part of the observed disorder. In this connection, a number of general practitioners maintain auxiliary personnel to provide various therapies (massages, controlled breathing, and so on) to supplement, or sometimes to replace, such standard treatments as drug prescriptions or minor surgery.

PERSPECTIVE AND PROSPECTS
It was the South African political figure Jan Smuts who, in 1926, first used the specific word "holism" to describe, not holistic medicine per se, but the philosophical principle which holds that whole systems (and therefore whole organisms) involve entities that are greater than, and different from, the sum of their component parts. In medicine, the idea that external factors intervene to affect the way that an organism functions is almost as old as medicine itself. Hippocrates, for example, is known to have been concerned about environmental causes for certain disorders and to have included emotional and nutritional considerations in diagnosing patients.

Two aspects of holistic approaches to health and daily life in the postindustrial world are likely to increase in importance in coming generations: concern over improving dietary habits and exercise patterns. The discovery of the possible long-term harm that can come from poorly balanced diets (particularly those with a high fat content or excessive chemical additives) has made such specialized practices of holists as vegetarianism and fasting more familiar and at least partly attractive to the wider public. Likewise, the holistic emphasis on regular physical exercise for people of all ages has increasingly become part of many general practitioners' standard advice to their patients.

—*Byron D. Cannon, Ph.D.*

See also Aging; Aging: Extended care; Alternative medicine; Death and dying; Environmental diseases; Environmental health; Exercise physiology; Family practice; Meditation; Nutrition; Osteopathic medicine; Preventive medicine; Psychiatry; Psychiatry, child and adolescent; Psychiatry, geriatric; Terminally ill: Extended care.

FOR FURTHER INFORMATION:

American Holistic Health Association. http://www .ahha.org/. A Web site dedicated to honoring the whole person and encouraging people to actively participate in their own health and health care.

Goldberg, Burton Allan, and Max Allan Goldberg. *Alternative Medicine: The Definitive Guide*. 2d ed. Berkeley, Calif.: Ten Speed Press, 2002. An encyclopedic volume with contributions from four hundred alternative physicians who review safe, affordable, and effective remedies for more than two hundred medical conditions.

Kemper, Kathi J. *The Holistic Pediatrician: A Pediatrician's Comprehensive Guide to Safe and Effective Therapies for the Twenty-five Most Common Ailments of Infants, Children, and Adolescents*. New York: HarperCollins, 2002. Integrates mainstream and alternative medicine to aid parents in dealing with the most common childhood health problems such as fever, diaper rash, ear infections, and allergies.

Nordenfelt, Lennart. *On the Nature of Health*. Rev. 2d ed. Boston: Kluwer, 1995. Deals with the relationship between good health and the welfare of individuals and society as they interact.

Pelletier, Kenneth R. *The Best Alternative Medicine: Sorting Fact from Fiction in Complementary and Alternative Medicine*. New York: Simon & Schuster, 2000. Surveys alternative therapies such as homeopathy, Western herbal medicine, traditional Chinese medicine, acupuncture, and naturopathy and provides definitions, background, and examples of specific treatments.

_____. *Holistic Medicine*. New York: Delacorte Press, 1979. A general text that seeks to strengthen the public image of holistic medicine, both for the prevention and for the treatment of disease, while discounting some popular myths.

Salmon, J. Warren, ed. *Alternative Medicines*. New York: Tavistock, 1984. Offers comparative views of Western and Chinese approaches to holistic medicine but also includes other, less widely recognized alternatives, ranging from chiropractic to psychic healing.

Woodham, Anne, and David Peters. *The Encyclopedia of Healing Therapies*. New York: Dorling Kindersley, 1997. This book explains holistic and complementary medicine and offers a guide to well-being. Also contains information on finding practitioners, a directory of associations, a glossary, and a bibliography.

HOMEOPATHY
SPECIALTY

ANATOMY OR SYSTEM AFFECTED: All

SPECIALTIES AND RELATED FIELDS: Immunology, pathology, pharmacology

DEFINITION: A system of medicine based on the principle that an ill patient can be provided effective and nontoxic treatment through the use of weak or very small doses of a substance that would cause similar symptoms in a healthy individual.

KEY TERMS:

antidote: anything that counteracts the effect of a substance, such as a homeopathic remedy

Materia Medica: the homeopathic pharmacopoeia, a list of remedies with their associated symptoms and uses

potency: the strength of a homeopathic remedy, according to the number of times it has been diluted and succussed

proving: the testing of a substance or remedy on healthy volunteers (provers), who take repeated doses and record in detail any symptoms produced by it

Repertory: an index of symptoms, each heading listing the drugs known to cause the symptom

succussion: violent shaking at each stage of dilution in the preparation of a remedy

tincture: a remedy in liquid form, normally with alcohol and water as a solvent; the most concentrated form is called the mother tincture, from which all dilutions are made

SCIENCE AND PROFESSION

In conventional medicine, diseases, or changes from the normal physiological state, are diagnosed on the basis of symptoms and physical signs. This enables the physician to find a cause for which there is a specific treatment, or to treat the patient's symptoms. There are few treatments, however, that cure the patient as a whole. Sometimes, symptoms are assumed to be the disease, and the method of action is to try to fix the symptoms and not the disease. Suppressing or removing symptoms does not necessarily constitute a cure. Curing patients means restoring them to a sense of well-being that is physical, emotional, and mental. Homeopathic medicine is a form of treatment that studies the person as a whole, with particular interest in the patient as an individual. Homeopathy is a therapeutic method that consists of prescribing for a patient weak or infinitesimal doses of a substance which, when administered to a healthy person, causes symptoms similar to those exhibited by the ill patient. Homeopathic remedies stimulate the defense mechanisms of the body, causing them to work more effectively and making them capable of curing the individual. While controversial and not accepted by most physicians, homeopathy is not intended to substitute for conventional medicine. Rather, it is a system of therapeutics which is meant to enlarge and broaden the physician's outlook, and in some cases, it might bring about a cure not possible with the usual drugs.

The word "homeopathy" is derived from the Greek words *homoios*, meaning "like" or "similar," and *pathos*, meaning "suffering." A symptom is defined as the changes felt by the patient or observed by another individual that may be associated with a particular disease. When a homeopathic drug or remedy is administered in repeated doses to a group of healthy persons, certain symptoms and signs of toxicity are produced. These symptoms are carefully annotated in what is called the proving of a remedy. In some cases, there are accidental provings—cases in which the symptoms produced by a drug in a healthy person are observed because of an accident, such as being bitten by a snake. Other sources for the proving of a remedy are the cases in which, after a remedy has been successfully prescribed, symptoms cured by it that were not present in the provings are noted. Some of these symptoms are common to many drugs, and a few are characteristic of particular ones. It is then possible to build a symptom-complex picture which is unique to each drug or remedy. In many cases, when the symptom-complex presented by the patient is compared to the symptom-complex produced by a certain remedy, there will be a resemblance—often a close one—between the patient's symptom picture and the effects of a given drug on healthy persons.

The first and fundamental principle of homeopathy is the selection and use of the similar remedy, based on the patient's symptoms and characteristics and the drug's toxicology and provings. A second principle is the use of remedies in extremely small quantities. The most successful remedy for any given occasion will be the one whose symptomatology presents the clearest and closest resemblance to the symptom-complex of the sick person in question. This concept is formally presented as the Law of Similars, which expresses the similarity between the toxicological action of a substance and its therapeutic action; in other words, the same things that cause the disease can cure it. For example, the effects of peeling an onion are very similar to the symptoms of acute coryza (the common cold). The remedy prepared from *Allium cepa* (red onion) is used to treat the type of cold in which the symptoms resemble those caused by peeling onions. In the same way, the herb white hellebore, which toxicologically produces cholera-like diarrhea, is used to treat cholera.

The homeopathic principle is being applied whenever a sick person is treated using a method or drug that can cause similar symptoms in healthy persons. For example, conventional medicine uses radiation therapy, which causes cancer, to treat this disease. Orthodox medicine, however, does not follow other fundamental principles of homeopathy, such as the use of infinitesimal doses.

Homeopathy stimulates the defense mechanism to make it work more effectively and works on the concept of healing instead of simply treating a disease, combating illness, or suppressing symptoms. Individualization plays a crucial role in homeopathic treatment. Even when two individuals have the same ailment, their symptoms can be different. Remedies are therefore selected on an individual basis, depending on the specific, complete symptom picture of the individual. Homeopathic physicians must develop a different approach to their patients, which involves a diagnosis as well as a study of the whole individual. The way in which some homeopathic remedies work is still unknown, but the persistence of homeopathy since the mid-nineteenth century would seem to suggest its effectiveness in helping sick people.

Some conditions do not respond well to homeopathy, such as those requiring surgery, immediately life-threatening situations such as severe asthma attacks, or situations for which an improvement requires a change in diet (such as iron deficiency) or reduced exposure to environmental stress (a change in lifestyle). Nevertheless, homeopathy appears to help in these cases. For example, it can be useful for faster, complete healing after surgery or after the necessary change in lifestyle has been made. In the United States, both the Food and Drug Administration (FDA) and traditional homeopaths have been concerned about the use of homeo-

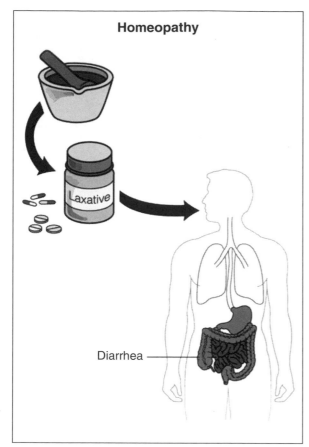

Homeopathy

Laxative

Diarrhea

The principle underlying homeopathy is that taking small amounts of a substance that normally produces a certain symptom will stimulate the immune system to counteract that very symptom. For example, a patient suffering from diarrhea may be given an infinitesimally small dose of a laxative which has been ground into a fine powder with a mortar and pestle.

pathic remedies to treat serious problems, such as cancer, and their use by unlicensed practitioners. In some cases, the ability to prescribe homeopathic remedies has been restricted to osteopaths, naturopaths, and medical doctors. In some cases, homeopathy does not work; the reason is unknown.

Individuals who have benefited from these remedies may not care whether homeopathy can be scientifically explained or whether research has proven its effectiveness. Nevertheless, some facts suggest that homeopathic medicines are not placebos and that the infinitesimal doses produce true biological action. For example, homeopathic medicines work on animals and are also commonly and successfully used on infants; it is doubtful that psychological suggestion can explain their success in these cases. Moreover, homeopathic micro-

doses have the capacity to cause symptoms in healthy individuals, and the experience of what is called a healing crisis—temporary exacerbation of symptoms that is sometimes observed during the healing process—cannot be produced by placebos or psychological suggestion. The major drawback to most homeopathic research, however, is that it is rarely published in respected scientific journals, and whatever little has been published has been received with much skepticism from the medical community.

The action of homeopathic medicines supports the theory that each organism expresses symptoms in an effort to heal itself. This homeopathic action can augment, complement, and sometimes replace present medical technologies. For example, abuse of strong medications can lead to resistance to the drugs themselves, allergies, and other unpleasant side effects. In homeopathy, small drug doses have been shown to be more effective than larger ones, which in itself can reduce the undesired side effects associated with the use of common medications.

DIAGNOSTIC AND TREATMENT TECHNIQUES

The first step in treating an illness using homeopathy is taking the case history or symptom picture (the detailed account of what is wrong with the patient as a whole). This is carried out in a similar way by classical doctors and homeopathic practitioners, since most homeopaths are doctors or have some conventional medical training. The symptoms are divided into three categories: general, mental/emotional, and physical.

The homeopath then consults the *Materia Medica* (the encyclopedia of drug effects) and/or the *Repertory* (an index of symptoms from the *Materia Medica* listed in alphabetical order, used as a cross-reference between symptoms and remedies) to decide on the remedy to be used. The professional homeopath works with a number of *Materia Medica* texts compiled by different homeopaths.

The classical homeopath will give only one remedy at a time in order to gauge its effect more efficiently. The best-known unconventional usage of homeopathic medicines is of combination medicines or complexes, normally a mixture of between three and eight low-potency remedies. This approach is useful when the correct remedy is not available or when the practitioner is unsure as to which one to use. These mixtures are commonly sold in health food stores and are named for the disease or symptom that they are supposed to cure. Another unconventional use is what is called pluralism, which is the application of two or more medicines at a time, each of which is taken at a different time of day. This approach is most commonly used in Europe.

Homeopathy is a natural pharmaceutical system that utilizes microdoses of substances to arouse a healing response by stimulating the patient's immune system. Homeopathic remedies are always nontoxic because of the small concentrations used. They do not act chemically but rather according to a particular physical state linked to the way in which they are prepared. They have the capacity of making the ill subject react to his or her disease, and in this way they are considered specific stimulants.

Homeopathic remedies come from the plant, mineral, and animal kingdoms. Plants are the source of more than half of the remedies. They are harvested in their natural state according to strict norms by qualified specialists and are used fresh after thorough botanical inspection. Mineral remedies include natural salts and metals, always in their purest state. Animal remedies may contain venoms, poisonous insects, hormones, or physiological secretions such as musk or squid ink.

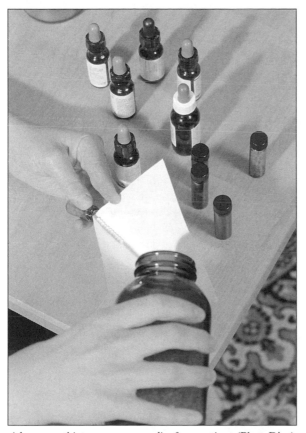

A homeopathist prepares remedies for a patient. (PhotoDisc)

In all cases, the starting remedy is made from a mixture of the substance itself, which has been steeped in alcohol for a period of time and then strained. This starting liquid is called a tincture or mother tincture. In the decimal scale, a mixture of one-tenth tincture and nine-tenths alcohol is shaken vigorously, a process known as succussion; this first dilution is called a 1X. (The number in the remedy reveals the number of times that it has been diluted and succussed; thus, 6X means diluted and succussed six times.) In the centesimal scale, the remedy is diluted using one part tincture in a hundred, and the letter *C* is used after the number. The number indicates the degree of the dilution, while the letter indicates the technique of preparation (decimal or centesimal). Insoluble substances are diluted by grinding them in a mortar with lactose to the desired dilution. The greater the dilution of a remedy, the greater its potency, the longer it acts, the deeper it heals, and the fewer doses are needed.

A medicine is chosen for its similarity to the person's symptoms, so that the person's bioenergetic processes are hypersensitive to the substance. One theory used to explain the success of homeopathic remedies, even when they are used in such small concentrations, is that they work through some kind of resonance within the individual's system. There are other examples of high sensitivity to small amounts of substances in the animal kingdom, such as in the case of pheromones, sex attractants that affect only animals of the same species in very small amounts and at a very long distance.

Constantine Hering (1800-1880), the founder of American homeopathy, was the first to make note of the specific features of the healing process to create a holistic assessment tool that can be used to evaluate a patient's progress. His observations are summarized in Hering's Law of Cure. First, the human body seeks to externalize disease, to dislodge it from more serious, internal levels to more superficial ones; for example, in the healing of asthma the patient may exhibit an external skin rash before complete cure is achieved. Second, the healing progresses from the top of the body to the bottom; someone with arthritis will feel better in the upper part of the body earlier than in the lower part. Third, the healing proceeds in the reverse order of the appearance of the symptoms; that is, the more recent symptoms will heal first, and old symptoms may reappear before complete healing.

Homeopathic remedies are most commonly available in tablet form, combined with sugar from cow's milk. The tablets can be soft (so that they dissolve easily under the tongue and are easy to crush) or hard (so that they must be chewed and held in the mouth for a few seconds before being swallowed), or they can be prepared as globules (tiny round pills). The liquid remedies are dissolved in alcohol. Also available are powders that are wrapped individually in small squares of paper (convenient if the remedy is needed for only a few doses or is to be sent by mail), wafers, suppositories, and liniments. Homeopathic tablets will keep their strength for years without deteriorating, but they must be stored in a cool, dark, and dry place with their bottle tops screwed on tightly, away from strong-smelling substances.

The prescribed quantities are the same for babies, children, adults, and older people. The size of a dose is immaterial; it is how often it is taken that counts. The strength (potency) that is needed changes with the circumstances. The greater the similarity between the symptoms and the remedy, the greater the potency to be used (that is, the more dilute the remedy).

The following substances all counteract the effects of a homeopathic remedy to some extent (and as such are considered antidotes): camphor, coffee, menthol/eucalyptus, peppermint, recreational drugs, and any strong-smelling or strong-acting substance.

As with all treatments, there are some dangers associated with homeopathic cures, such as unintentional provings. These take place when, after an initial improvement, the symptoms characteristic of the remedy appear, creating a worse situation for the patient. Sometimes, this reaction takes place because the individual has been taking the remedy for too long, and it can be stopped by discontinuing the remedy or by using an antidote. In other cases, there is a confused symptom picture, the effect being that the remedy is working in a limited way or curing a restricted number of symptoms.

Homeopathy is important in the treatment of bacterial infections (where resistance to antibiotics can develop) and viral conditions. Homeopathic remedies stimulate the person's resistance to infection without the side effects of antibiotics, and they help the body without suppressing the organism's self-protective responses. The remedies used are safer than regular medicines because they exhibit minimal side effects, and counterreactions between medicines can be prevented.

Homeopathic remedies are exempt from federal review in the United States. In 1938, any drug listed in the *Homeopathic Pharmacopoeia of the United States* was accepted by the FDA. Consequently, prescribed homeopathics do not have to undergo the rigorous safety and effectiveness testing the regulating agency requires of drugs used in orthodox medicine. Nonprescription homeopathics are also exempt and can be purchased in pharmacies, greengroceries, and health food stores throughout the country. The FDA requires that, as with any over-the-counter drug, a remedy be sold only for a self-limiting condition (such as headaches, menstrual cramps, or insomnia) and that the indications be printed on the label. The ingredients and their dilution must also be listed. Nonhomeopathic active ingredients cannot be included in the preparation.

PERSPECTIVE AND PROSPECTS

The Law of Similars was observed twenty-five centuries ago by Hippocrates and was utilized by people of many cultures, including the Mayans, Chinese, Greeks, and American Indians. In the following centuries, other doctors made similar observations, but they did not come to any practical conclusions. It was not until the end of the eighteenth century that a German physician, Christian Friedrich Samuel Hahnemann, studied the matter further, developed it, and gave it a scientific basis.

Hahnemann recruited a group of healthy subjects to take the remedies and report in a diary the symptoms that they caused, a process called proving the substance. He and his subjects proved more than a hundred remedies and produced a very accurate collection for use by other homeopathy practitioners. He also found that the remedies worked better in very small doses. Homeopathy was initially rejected by the medical profession, but its methods became more accepted when Hahnemann obtained astonishing results with his patients. In 1810, he published a book called *Organon der rationellen Heilkunde* (*The Organon of Homœopathic Medicine*, 1836), in which he presented the philosophy of homeopathy. He also published *Materia Medica pura* in six volumes between 1811 and 1821. These volumes contain the compilations of his provings. As new remedies are discovered, they are added to the compilation. By the time of Hahnemann's death in 1843, homeopathy was established around the world.

In the 1820's, homeopathy arrived in the United States at a time when the state of orthodox medicine was worse than in Europe. Many ordinary people consulted herbalists and bonesetters, so homeopathy was easily accepted and soon flourished. In 1844, the American Institute of Homeopathy was founded. In 1846, however, the American Medical Association (AMA) was founded, and it adopted a code of ethics which forbade its members to consult homeopaths. Nevertheless, public demand continued. The 1860's through the 1880's saw the heyday of homeopathy in the United States, with the institution of training programs, hospitals, and asylums and the training of thousands of homeopaths in the country.

Developments in orthodox medicine around the end of the nineteenth century strengthened this camp, however, while the homeopathic establishment was weakened by internal division. In 1911, the AMA moved to close many homeopathic teaching institutions because they were considered to provide a poor standard of education. By 1950, all the homeopathic colleges in the United States were either closed or no longer teaching homeopathy. By the 1990's, it was roughly estimated that only five hundred to one thousand medical doctors used homeopathics in their practices, though the number of homeopaths and osteopaths prescribing them had probably increased. Although the AMA has no official statement on homeopathy, it is no longer part of the medical school curriculum.

Homeopathy has exhibited a renaissance, and it is popular throughout the world, especially in France. Perhaps the reasons for this revived popularity include both skepticism surrounding conventional medicine and a need for alternatives in the face of challenging health problems: Homeopathy offers a safe alternative as it seeks to improve the general level of health of the whole person, emotionally as well as physically. It must not be forgotten, however, that this brand of medicine has a long way to go before its curative powers are proven.

—*Maria Pacheco, Ph.D.*

See also Alternative medicine; Disease; Herbal medicine; Immune system; Immunology; Pathology; Pharmacology; Toxicology.

FOR FURTHER INFORMATION:

Aubin, Michel, and Philippe Picard. *Homeopathy: A Different Way of Treating Common Ailments.* Translated by Pat Campbell and Robin Campbell. Bath, England: Ashgrove Press, 1989. An easy-to-read book which includes a critical analysis of orthodox medicine from the perspective of an orthodox doctor turned homeopath, a description of homeopathy, and a section on self-treatment with homeopathy.

Castro, Miranda. *The Complete Homeopathy Handbook: A Guide to Everyday Health Care.* New York: St. Martin's Press, 1991. Examines the principles underlying the theory of homeopathy, as well as how to prescribe and learn the best use of homeopathic medicines that are available over the counter.

Josephson, Laura. *Homeopathic Handbook of Natural Remedies: Safe and Effective Treatment of Common Ailments and Injuries.* New York: Random House, 2002. Gives an overview of the healing principles and history of homeopathy, guidelines for identifying and treating symptoms, and instructions for preparing and stocking your home kit. Includes an entire section on childhood conditions, an extensive directory of homeopathic pharmacies, and a list of articles and other publications that provide further information.

McCabe, Vinton. *Practical Homeopathy: A Comprehensive Guide to Homeopathic Remedies and Their Acute Uses.* New York: St. Martin's Press, 2000. McCabe, president of the Connecticut Homeopathic Association and a member of the faculty and board of the Hudson Valley School of Classical Homeopathy, joins philosophy and pharmacy in a practical way in this resource. Includes homeopathic remedies.

National Center for Homeopathy. http://www.homeopathic.org/. Offers resources on research, training, and how to find a homeopath.

Ullman, Dana. *Discovering Homeopathy: Medicine for the Twenty-first Century.* Rev. ed. Berkeley, Calif.: North Atlantic Books, 1991. Includes sections on the history and research methods of homeopathy and an excellent section on sources (books, computer programs, tapes) and general information on homeopathy. Lists pharmacies, organizations, schools, and training programs in the United States.

_____. *Essential Homeopathy: What It Is and What It Can Do for You.* Novato, Calif.: New World Library, 2002. Provides answers to frequently asked questions, introduces readers to the practice, and explains which conditions respond best to homeopathic treatment. Surveys treatments for common ailments including digestive troubles, colds, flus, allergies, and headaches.

HORMONE REPLACEMENT THERAPY (HRT)

TREATMENT

ANATOMY OR SYSTEM AFFECTED: Blood vessels, bones, brain, breasts, circulatory system, genitals, heart, psychic-emotional system, reproductive system, skin, urinary system, uterus

Specialties and related fields: Cardiology, endocrinology, family practice, geriatrics and gerontology, gynecology, hematology, internal medicine, oncology, orthopedics, preventive medicine, vascular medicine

Definition: Estrogens, with or without progestogens, given to women in the perimenopause to treat or prevent a variety of conditions.

Key terms:

hypothalamus: a part of the brain that controls many body functions; its releasing hormones stimulate the pituitary to secrete hormones of its own

incontinence: inability to control the bladder or bowel

menopause: the last menstrual period that a woman experiences

osteoporosis: thinning of the bones, which occurs in all people as they age

perimenopause: a period of years around the menopause, during which changes occur in the balance among the reproductive hormones, leading to the cessation of menses and the end of fertility; this time of transition from reproductive to postreproductive life is also known as the climacteric

pituitary gland: the body's master gland that produces various hormones which in turn stimulate other glands in the body to produce their own hormones; in women, the pituitary produces follicle-stimulating hormone and luteinizing hormone, which stimulate the ovary to produce estrogens and progesterone

progestogen: any of a number of substances (natural or synthetic) that have a progesterone-like effect

prolapse: the slipping out of place of an internal organ, such as the uterus

transdermal: through the skin; transdermal medications are those which are applied as creams, gels, or patches and are then absorbed through the skin

Indications and Procedures

During a woman's reproductive years, a complex feedback loop among the hypothalamus, pituitary gland, and ovaries causes the ovaries to produce various sex hormones, the major ones being estrogens and progesterone. These hormones are responsible for developing the secondary sexual characteristics such as breasts and pubic hair, for governing the menstrual cycle, and for maintaining a pregnancy should one occur. They also have profound effects on a woman's skin, heart, blood vessels, lipids (blood fats, such as cholesterol), bones, blood, and other systems.

As women approach the menopause, changes begin to occur in the hormone feedback loop. The menstrual cycle typically becomes shorter and more irregular, and then menses cease altogether. As hormone levels decline and the ratio between the estrogens and progesterone changes, the woman's body undergoes other changes such as thinning of the mucous membranes in the reproductive and urinary tract, drying of the skin, thinning of the bones, and alterations in cholesterol levels. Perimenopausal women may also experience hot flashes, night sweats, insomnia, mood swings, and other uncomfortable symptoms. Postmenopausal women do continue to produce sex hormones, although in smaller amounts. The adrenal glands are responsible for much of the postmenopausal hormone production, and some production occurs by conversion of other hormones in the body tissues.

The menopause normally occurs between the ages of forty-five and fifty-five. If a woman undergoes the menopause before age forty, it is called premature menopause. A woman who stops menstruating because of a total hysterectomy, in which not only the uterus but also the Fallopian tubes and ovaries are removed, undergoes what is called a surgical menopause. Women who undergo radiation of the ovaries will also experience an artificial menopause. The discomforts associated with the menopause may be exaggerated in these women.

Health care providers have used hormone replacement therapy (HRT) to treat uncomfortable perimenopausal symptoms and to prevent or treat a number of conditions associated with the postmenopausal state. HRT may include estrogen alone or a combination of estrogen and progesterone. At times, other hormones such as testosterone may be used to treat symptoms, but it is the estrogen-progesterone combination that comprises what is commonly thought of as HRT. Estrogen replacement therapy by itself is known as ERT.

Uses and Complications

A variety of estrogens and progestogens are available for the treatment of menopausal symptoms and for the prevention of health problems that accelerate after the menopause. They include oral estrogens and progestins, transdermal estrogens, injectable estrogens and progestins, and topical estrogens. Available oral estrogens for HRT include conjugated estrogens, micronized estradiol, piperazine estrone, ethinyl estradiol, quinestrol, and chlorotrianisene. Of these, the conjugated equine estrogens have been most extensively studied over a long period of time. They are usually well tolerated by patients. Various estrogens are also available as transdermal patches or vaginal creams. The oral progestogens used for HRT include medroxy-progesterone acetate and micronized progesterone.

At various periods throughout the twentieth century, health care providers and researchers have recommended that all women in the perimenopause begin hormone replacement. However, important questions about the safety and effectiveness of HRT have subsequently limited its use. In the first decade of the twenty-first century, recommendations from major medical organizations were generally that the decision whether to use HRT and for how long should be individualized. It should be used only to provide relief for severe symptoms and to prevent or treat specific conditions in women at high risk for problems.

Serious potential side effects and contraindications must be considered before making the decision to begin HRT. First, women who take estrogen supplementation without a progestogen are at increased risk for developing excessive thickening of the lining of the uterus. This situation can ultimately result in carcinoma (cancer) of the uterus. For this reason, women who have not had a hysterectomy are advised to take combination estrogen-progestogen HRT. If the combination is given on a cyclical basis, however, the woman will most likely experience monthly withdrawal bleeding. This is not always acceptable to postmenopausal women. About 90 percent of women who take a continuous dose of a lower-dose progestogen will not bleed at all after a year of its continuous use; the remainder will bleed occasionally.

Another risk to be considered is the possible development of breast cancer. Scientific studies have produced conflicting results about this risk. Some studies have shown a small increased risk of breast cancer with postmenopausal estrogen replacement used for extended periods of time. Adding a progestogen does not appear to change this risk.

Women who take oral estrogen supplements have an increased tendency to develop blood clots. This is not the case, however, for women who used transdermal formulations. Estrogen replacement therapy is also associated with an increased risk of gallbladder disease.

Women who should not take estrogen-containing hormone replacement at all include those with unexplained vaginal bleeding, a history of uterine or breast cancer, liver disease, or a history of blood clots in the veins. HRT should be used with caution in women with seizure disorders, high blood pressure, diabetes melli-

tus, migraines, gallbladder disease, and certain other conditions.

Minor adverse effects of hormone treatment include swelling, breast tenderness, bloating, headaches, and increased cervical mucus.

Some specific changes associated with the menopausal state that may be altered or prevented through the use of HRT are reproductive tract changes, urinary tract changes, vasomotor instability, osteoporosis, cardiovascular changes, skin and hair changes, and psychological changes, including dementia.

As the supply of estrogen decreases, women experience thinning and drying of the vaginal tissues. The cervix, uterus, and ovaries become smaller in size, and the cervix stops producing mucus. In addition, the ligaments that support the reproductive organs become more relaxed. These changes may lead to painful sexual intercourse, bleeding with minor trauma, itching, vaginal discharge, and prolapse of the uterus. The Food and Drug Administration (FDA) recommends vaginal cream formulations if vaginal thinning and dryness are the woman's only problem, rather than oral medications which affect the entire body.

The tissues of the bladder and urethra also become thinner, which may lead to urinary urgency, painful urination, or increased frequency. Some women even become incontinent. The evidence is not entirely clear about the usefulness of estrogen replacement therapy in this setting.

Vasomotor instability refers to the changes that lead to hot flashes and increased sweating. These flushes may be accompanied by heart palpitations, weakness, fatigue, dizziness, or lightheadedness. The episodes may cause nighttime awakening or insomnia, which in turn may lead to memory problems or irritability. The major treatment for vasomotor instability is the administration of estrogen, although progestogens have been used in women who cannot take estrogen. Some women find relief from a different type of drug called clonidine. Other treatments, which have not been studied as thoroughly as estrogen and progesterone, include various vitamin and mineral supplements, tranquilizers, and antidepressants.

All people gradually lose bone mass as they age, but in the years following the menopause this process accelerates in women, particularly in the type of bone known as trabecular bone. Postmenopausal women's risk for hip fracture becomes two to three times that of men. For this reason, estrogen has been recommended for prevention of osteoporosis, particularly in women who are thin, smoke cigarettes, have a strong family history of osteoporosis, drink large amounts of alcohol, or have some other risk factor. Studies have shown that women who take postmenopausal estrogen decrease their risk of hip fracture by up to 50 percent. The risk for fracture of the vertebrae in the spine decreases by about half as well.

With concerns about the safety of estrogens, however, other drugs are increasingly used to prevent or treat osteoporosis, including drugs from the classes known as bisphosphonates and selective estrogen receptor modulators (SERMs). Calcitonin and progestogens may also be used but do not seem to be as effective as the estrogens, bisphosphonates, or SERMs. All menopausal women should probably take supplemental calcium and vitamin D, exercise regularly, stop smoking if needed, and limit alcohol, caffeine, salt, and animal proteins in order to minimize their risk of developing osteoporosis.

Before the menopause, very few women have heart attacks. This state changes rapidly after the menopause, and by age seventy women have the same risk of heart attack as men. The conclusion has been that the higher levels of estrogen in premenopausal women must have a beneficial effect on the heart. Medical studies, however, have provided contradictory evidence about the effect of postmenopausal HRT on cardiovascular disease, with some studies indicating that HRT protects women and others indicating no effect or even an increased risk for heart disease with HRT.

From a theoretical standpoint, postmenopausal estrogen could affect cardiovascular health in two ways. First, estrogen supplementation increases the type of cholesterol that protects the heart (high-density lipoprotein, or HDL) and decreases the amount of harmful cholesterol (low-density lipoprotein, or LDL). Second, estrogen seems to have a direct effect on the blood vessels, helping to prevent atherosclerotic plaques from building up and narrowing the arteries.

In actual practice, however, no studies have clearly shown a benefit in terms of reduced heart attack or cardiac death rates in women who take HRT. One section of a long-term study funded by the National Institutes of Health (NIH), called the Women's Health Initiative, compared thousands of women who took combination HRT to women who received a placebo (sugar pill). Those on the combination treatment had an increased risk for heart disease, stroke, and blood clots in the lung. Major medical organizations, including the American Heart Association (AHA), the American

College of Obstetricians and Gynecologists (ACOG), and the North American Menopause Society (NAMS), have recommended that combination therapy not be used for the prevention of cardiac disease.

As people age, they experience changes in the skin and hair. The skin becomes thinner and less elastic, particularly in sun-exposed areas. There is some loss of pubic hair and hair in the armpits. Some women experience balding, and some develop coarse facial hair. Body hair may either increase or decrease. The skin has estrogen receptors, so those changes are thought to be caused by decreased estrogen. Hair changes are more likely to result from a change in the ratio of estrogen to testosterone in the body after the menopause. Testosterone levels remain nearly the same before and after the menopause, while estrogen levels drop drastically. HRT does seem to improve or prevent skin changes.

Some studies have found that women in the early menopause experience more irritability, depression, and feelings of anxiety. It is not clear if these changes are attributable to some change in brain chemistry as a result of decreased estrogen, societal expectations about aging, or some other factor. Some researchers have suggested that the lack of sleep caused by hot flashes and night sweats is the source of mood changes, rather than being a function of the menopause itself. Furthermore, many perimenopausal women have multiple stressors, such as caring for aging parents, that may contribute to depression and anxiety. On the other hand, some researchers found that women who did not have hot flashes but did experience depression improved with the administration of estrogen. Some evidence exists that the areas of the brain responsible for memory are affected by estrogen, leading to the suggestion that Alzheimer's disease and other dementias may be prevented or treated by HRT.

In summary, the clearest indications for HRT are severe menopausal symptoms and the prevention of osteoporosis in women at high risk. For women with severe vasomotor symptoms, a fairly high dose of estrogen is probably indicated at first but this amount should be reduced as soon and as rapidly as possible. If the primary problem is vaginal dryness or discomfort, then estrogen cream may be helpful and have fewer side effects than oral estrogen. Other treatment modalities may limit further the use of estrogen in the prevention of osteoporosis.

PERSPECTIVE AND PROSPECTS

Feminist thinkers and researchers have periodically raised important questions about the use of sex hormones in women. They point out that many of the conditions that are treated with hormones are a part of women's normal life experience. By declaring such events as pregnancy and the menopause as "problems" and treating them with hormones, normal life events become "medicalized"—a condition to be treated at great expense and some risk to health and well-being. A second important issue raised by feminists is that hormones have been administered to women for various conditions without adequate testing and with serious consequences. For example, in the mid-twentieth century, physicians encouraged perimenopausal women to take estrogen to remain "forever young." Because these women were given estrogen without the progesterone needed to protect against the development of uterine cancer, cancer rates rose dramatically and estrogen alone was withdrawn as a treatment for the menopause.

—*Rebecca Lovell Scott, Ph.D., PA-C*

See also Aging; Arteriosclerosis; Breast cancer; Cervical, ovarian, and uterine cancers; Endocrinology; Endometrial cancer; Gynecology; Heart disease; Herbal medicine; Hormones; Hot flashes; Hysterectomy; Infertility in females; Menopause; Menstruation; Midlife crisis; Osteoporosis.

FOR FURTHER INFORMATION:

Love, Susan, and Karen Lindsey. *Dr. Susan Love's Menopause and Hormone Book: Making Informed Choices*. New York: Random House, 2003. An excellent overview of the menopause and the pros and cons of hormone replacement therapy with alternative treatments.

National Women's Health Network. *The Truth About Hormone Replacement Therapy: How to Break Free from the Medical Myths of Menopause*. Roseville, Calif.: Prima, 2002. A feminist, strongly anti-HRT argument.

Seaman, Barbara. *The Greatest Experiment Ever Performed on Women: Exploding the Estrogen Myth*. New York: Hyperion, 2003. A history of the medicalization of the menopause and other normal stages of a woman's life and the use of estrogen. Offers a strong critique and details about the dangers of estrogen.

HORMONES
BIOLOGY

ANATOMY OR SYSTEM AFFECTED: Circulatory system, endocrine system, glands, psychic-emotional system

SPECIALTIES AND RELATED FIELDS: Biochemistry, endocrinology, pharmacology

DEFINITION: Chemical substances that are secreted by endocrine glands or specialized secretory cells into the blood or nearby tissues to act on those tissues and affect its function.

KEY TERMS:

adrenal glands: endocrine organs located on top of the kidneys; their function is to produce steroid hormones such as cortisol and sex hormones

deoxyribonucleic acid (DNA): the basic building block of life, which bears encoded genetic information; it is found mainly in chromosomes and can reproduce

messenger ribonucleic acid (mRNA): a single-stranded RNA that arises from and is complementary to double-stranded DNA; it passes from the nucleus to the cytoplasm, where its information is translated into proteins

prohormone: a hormone that must be cut or modified in a specific way in order to achieve full activity

receptor: a molecular structure at the cell surface or inside the cell that is capable of combining with hormones and causing a change in cell metabolism or function

STRUCTURE AND FUNCTIONS

The definition of the term "hormone" has continued to change over the years. The classic definition is that of an endocrine hormone—that is, one secreted by ductless glands directly into the blood and acting at a distant site. The definition can be expanded to include any chemical substance secreted by any cell of the body that has a specific effect on another cell. A hormone can affect a nearby cell (paracrine action) or the cell that secretes it (autocrine action). Certain hormones are produced by the brain and kidneys, which are not thought of as classic endocrine glands. In fact, the largest producer of hormones is the gastrointestinal tract, which is not usually thought of as an endocrine gland.

Hormones fall into two major categories: peptide hormones, which are derived from amino acids, and steroid hormones, which are derived from cholesterol. The different classes of hormones have different mechanisms of action. Peptide hormones work by interacting with a specific receptor located in the plasma membrane of the target cell. Receptors have different regions, or domains, that perform specialized functions. One part of the receptor has a specific three-dimensional structure similar to a keyhole into which a certain hormone can fit. This design allows a specific action of a hormone despite the fact that the hormone is often circulating in minute quantities in the bloodstream along with myriad other hormones.

There are different classes of plasma membrane receptors. One class is that of the receptor kinases. The insulin receptor is an example. In this case, the part of the receptor molecule that faces the cytoplasm, or inside of the cell, is able to perform a specific function. When insulin interacts with its receptor, a chemical change occurs on the receptor that allows it to activate proteins within the cell. Many hormones use a similar cascade of chemical reactions to control and amplify signals from outside the cell and effect change within the cell itself.

Another class of membrane receptors includes the G-protein coupled receptor. An example is the beta-2 adrenergic receptor. Epinephrine interacts with this receptor, causing the activation of a signal transducer or G protein. This activated G protein then leads to the modification of a specific protein, which leads to a cascade of biochemical events within the cell. This is another example of an amplification mechanism.

Steroid hormones exert their effects by means of a different mechanism. For example, glucocorticoids exert their effects by entering the cell and binding to specific glucocorticoid receptors in the cell nucleus. The glucocorticoid-receptor complex is able to bind specific regulatory DNA sequences, called glucocorticoid response elements. This binding is able to activate gene transcription, which causes an increase in mRNA and, ultimately, the translation of the mRNA to deliver a newly secreted protein. The protein can then act to change the cell's metabolism in some way. Cortisol, a type of glucocorticoid, is produced by the adrenal glands when a person is under stress. It can lead to changes in blood sugar levels, affect immune system function, and, at high levels, increase fat deposition in characteristic areas of the body.

Most hormones that circulate in the blood are attached to binding proteins. The general binding proteins in the body are albumin and transthyreitin. These two proteins bind many different hormones. There are also specific binding proteins, such as thyroid-binding globulin, which binds thyroid hormone, and insulin-like growth factor-binding proteins, which bind to the family of insulin-like growth factors. The bound hormone is considered the inactive hormone, and the free hormone is the active hormone. Therefore, binding proteins make it possible to control an active hormone precisely, without having to synthesize a new hormone.

Hormones can be secreted in a variety of time frames. Some hormones, such as testosterone, are secreted in a pulsatile fashion that changes over minutes or hours. Other hormones, such as cortisol, are secreted in a diurnal pattern, with levels varying depending on the time of day. Cortisol levels are highest at about 8 A.M. and fall throughout the day, with the lowest levels occurring between midnight and 2 A.M. The menstrual cycle is an example of the weekly to monthly variation of hormone production. For instance, progesterone (a steroid hormone) levels rise throughout the menstrual cycle and fall prior to the onset of menses. The exact control mechanisms that determine the rhythmicity of hormone production are unknown.

The ability to study and utilize hormones in treating human disease has been revolutionized by molecular biology. The first hormone to be synthesized for clinical use was insulin. The need for a secure and steady supply of insulin prompted scientists to look for alternative sources of this hormone in the 1970's. At that time, insulin was isolated and purified from animal pancreas glands, mostly those of cows and pigs. It was suspected, however, that insulin could be made in the laboratory via genetic engineering. Native insulin is produced from a prohormone, proinsulin. Recombinant DNA human insulin is currently made by encoding for the proinsulin molecule and then using enzymes to cut the molecule in the proper places, yielding insulin and a piece of protein called C peptide. This process, which is very similar to the process that the body uses to create insulin, produces high yields of active hormone.

Modern molecular biology techniques were used to identify a hormone and receptor involved in weight regulation. Originally discovered in mice, a gene called *ob* was identified in human beings which produced a hormone called leptin. Leptin and its receptor are believed to play a role in signaling satiety to the brain. If the leptin signal does not reach the brain as the result of a faulty receptor, the brain will not produce the satiety signal. Appetite will remain high. Thus, a defective leptin system may contribute to obesity in human beings. The functioning of leptin may also be responsible for cycles of weight loss and gain in dieters. As obese individuals lose adipose tissue, less leptin is synthesized and the brain may not send out sufficient signals to indicate satiety, thus increasing appetite and food consumption. The leptin-obesity connection is under intensive study.

THE MEDICAL USE OF HORMONES

The biological roles of hormones are numerous and critical to the normal function of important organ systems in human beings, and there are many examples of medical uses for hormones. In general, any derangements in the amount of hormones made, or in the timing of their production, can result in significant human disease or discomfort. For example, in women who reach the menopause, declining levels of estrogen and progesterone from the ovaries can lead to undesirable consequences such as hot flushes, vaginal dryness, and bone mineral density loss. Taking exogenous estrogen and progesterone, in the form of hormone replacement therapy, can reduce or stop these consequences. Another example of exogenous hormone use in human disease is thyroid hormone. People with thyroid disease, such as Hashimoto's thyroiditis, do not produce adequate levels of thyroid hormone. This condition can lead to intense fatigue and weight gain. These symptoms may be relieved by taking a synthetic thyroid hormone called levothyroxine.

Another example of the medical use of hormones is the role of synthetic erythropoietin in treating and preventing anemia. Normally, erythropoietin is made by the kidneys. It is essential for the differentiation and development of stem cells from the bone marrow into red blood cells. Most patients who develop kidney failure also suffer from severe anemia because the ability to synthesize erythropoietin is lost as the kidneys are destroyed by disease. Giving this hormone to a patient with kidney disease can lead to the restoration of that patient's red blood cell mass. Correcting the anemia that accompanies chronic renal disease can improve the exercise tolerance and overall quality of life of kidney disease patients. The hormone must be given by injection several times per week. It has been made available to the almost 50,000 Americans with chronic renal failure who require dialysis. Erythropoietin can also be given to renal failure patients who do not yet require dialysis but who do have anemia.

Another example of a hormone that has been synthesized for treatment of human disease is calcitonin. Calcitonin is a polypeptide hormone secreted by specialized C cells of the thyroid gland (also called parafollicular cells). The parafollicular cells make up about 0.1 percent of the total mass of the thyroid gland, and the cells are dispersed within the thyroid follicles. Calcitonin has been isolated from several different animal species, including the salmon, eel, rat, pig, sheep, and chicken. The main physiologic function of the hormone is to lower the serum calcium level. It does this by inhibiting calcium resorption from bone. Calcitonin has been used to treat patients with Paget's disease, a disorder of abnormal bone remodeling that can lead to deformities, bone pain, fractures, and neurological problems. Calcitonin has also been used in the past to treat patients with osteoporosis, a condition of bone density depletion associated with aging which can lead to bone fractures.

The first and most commonly used form of the hormone in the United States is salmon calcitonin. This form is a more potent inhibitor of bone resorption than the human form. A small number of patients given the drug will develop a resistance to it. The etiology of this resistance may be the development of antibodies to the salmon calcitonin. Subsequently, calcitonin was synthesized via recombinant DNA technology. Although the human form is somewhat less potent, the fact that its amino acid structure is identical to that of the native hormone makes it much less immunogenic than salmon calcitonin, and theoretically less likely to produce resistance. In fact, patients who were resistant to salmon calcitonin may be switched to human calcitonin and achieve a therapeutic effect.

An example of a hormone with multiple medical uses is vasopressin, also known as antidiuretic hormone. Normally, vasopressin is produced in the posterior pituitary gland (located in the brain); it is responsible for water conservation. An increase in plasma osmolality or a decrease in circulating blood volume will normally cause its release. Central diabetes insipidus, a disorder involving an absence or abnormal decrease of vasopressin, is characterized by an inappropriately dilute urine. Central diabetes insipidus can be caused by a variety of factors, including trauma, neurosurgery, brain tumors, brain infections, and autoimmune disorder. The clinical symptoms of the disease are polyuria and polydipsia. The patient may put out up to 18 liters of urine per day. If such large volume deficits are not remedied, more serious symptoms will ensue, including dangerously low blood pressure and coma. The acute treatment of any patient with central diabetes insipidus involves the replacement of body water with intravenous fluids. The chronic therapy involves replacement of the hormone vasopressin.

Several different forms of the hormone may be used, depending on the clinical situation. Aqueous vasopressin is useful for diagnostic testing and for acute management following trauma or neurosurgery. For diagnostic testing, it is often given subcutaneously at the end of the water deprivation test to determine whether the patient will respond to the hormone with a decrease in urine output and an increase in urine osmolality greater than 50 percent. After surgery, vasopressin can be given either intramuscularly, with a duration of action of about four to six hours, or by continuous intravenous infusion to ensure a steady level of the hormone.

In obstetrics, vasopressin is also known as pitocin, a hormone that can cause powerful uterine contractions. It is commonly used to augment labor, as when the mother's own uterine contractions are not adequate to expel the baby. It is given intravenously and titrated up until regular contractions of the uterus occur. Another use of vasopressin is in the acute setting of advanced cardiac life support, also known as a code situation. A patient noted to have a cardiac arrhythmia such as ventricular fibrillation may receive vasopressin as well as shocks from a defibrillator in an attempt to restore a perfusing cardiac rhythm.

One of the most important uses of hormones in medicine is for contraception, specifically in the form of birth control pills. In the early 1900's, the observation was made that mice that were fed extracts from ovaries could be rendered infertile. In the 1920's, the critical substance responsible for this infertility was discovered to be sex steroid hormones. The production of birth control pills dates back to the 1920's and 1930's, when steroid hormones such as progesterone were isolated from animal sources, such as pigs. By the 1940's, progesterone could be isolated in large quantities from Mexican yams, which caused the prices for progesterone to fall dramatically. With the fall in prices, the idea that progesterone could be sold in the mass market as a birth control pill became more feasible. The first clinical trial of the birth control pill in human beings occurred in 1956. Since then, several generations of progesterones have been mass produced for the purposes of birth control. Each successive generation of progesterone has caused fewer undesirable side effects, and the dosage necessary to achieve a contraceptive effect has been found to be much lower than those found in the original birth control pills.

Birth control pills and the progesterone contained within them have other medical uses besides contraception. Birth control pills can be used to regulate menstrual cycles in women who suffer from irregular menstrual cycles or abnormal vaginal bleeding. They can be used to decrease heavy menstrual periods. They can even be useful in decreasing acne, which can lead to permanent scarring when it is severe.

PERSPECTIVE AND PROSPECTS

The study of hormones has been instrumental in understanding how human beings adapt to and live in their environment. Hormones are involved in the regulation of body homeostasis and all critical aspects of the life cycle. The study of hormones has expanded as scientists have produced large amounts of synthetic hormones in the laboratory for use in research.

The history of insulin discovery and production is an example of the rapid scientific progress made in the field of hormone research. In 1889, Joseph von Mering and Oskar Minkowski demonstrated that dogs whose pancreases had been removed exhibited abnormalities in glucose metabolism that were similar to those seen in human diabetes mellitus patients. This fact suggested that some factor made by the pancreas lowered the blood glucose. The search for this factor led to the discovery of insulin in 1921 by Frederick C. Banting and Charles H. Best. They were able to extract the active substance from the pancreas and to demonstrate its therapeutic effects in dogs and humans. The chemistry of insulin progressed with the establishment of the amino acid sequence and three-dimensional structure in the 1960's. In 1960, insulin became the first hormone to be measured by radioimmunoassay. With advances in laboratory techniques in the 1970's, it became the first hormone to be commercially available via recombinant DNA technology, thus ensuring the availability of pure hormone without the need for animal sources.

The ability to synthesize hormones and their receptors has increased greatly. In fact, scientists can clone genes, or parts of genes, and synthesize the associated protein in order to make hormones that are encoded by the body. This method involves amplifying small amounts of DNA isolated from the cell using the technique of polymerase chain reaction (PCR). This allows large amounts of the same piece of DNA to be made in a matter of hours, which can then be transcribed into RNA and translated to yield the hormone. These powerful techniques, developed in the research laboratory, have been applied on a commercial basis and have provided enormous benefits to people. One such example is the production of growth hormone.

—RoseMarie Pasmantier, M.D.;
Karen E. Kalumuck, Ph.D.;
updated by Anne Lynn S. Chang, M.D.

See also Addison's disease; Corticosteroids; Cushing's syndrome; Diabetes mellitus; Dwarfism; Endocrine disorders; Endocrinology; Endocrinology, pediatric; Genetic engineering; Gigantism; Glands; Goiter;

Growth; Hormone replacement therapy (HRT); Hyper-parathyroidism and hypoparathyroidism; Hypoglyce-mia; Insulin resistance syndrome; Leptin; Melatonin; Menopause; Metabolism; Obesity; Paget's disease; Pancreas; Pancreatitis; Pregnancy and gestation; Puberty and adolescence; Steroid abuse; Steroids; Thyroid disorders; Weight loss and gain.

For Further Information:

Barinaga, Marcia. "Obesity: Leptin Receptor Weighs In." *Science* 271 (January 5, 1996): 29. This article presents a summary of leptin receptor research accessible to the nonspecialist, as well as a discussion of the prospects for obesity drug research.

Bliss, Michael. *The Discovery of Insulin.* Edinburgh, Scotland: Paul Harris, 1987. Very stimulating reading that re-creates the excitement surrounding the discovery of insulin. This novel gives the reader a feeling for the circumstances leading up to that momentous event.

Griffin, James E., and Sergio R. Ojeda, eds. *Textbook of Endocrine Physiology.* 5th ed. New York: Oxford University Press, 2004. A well-written book that presents an excellent summary of how hormones work and affect the body.

Larsen, P. Reed, et al., eds. *Williams Textbook of Endocrinology.* 10th ed. Philadelphia: W. B. Saunders, 2003. This extensive book on endocrinology covers all different aspects of the field. It is written by recognized experts in endocrinology in a very readable style.

Marieb, Elaine N. *Essentials of Human Anatomy and Physiology.* 7th ed. San Francisco: Benjamin/Cummings, 2003. This introductory anatomy and physiology textbook, easily accessible to those with little science background, is richly illustrated with diagrams and photographs that help to illuminate body systems and processes.

Tierney, Lawrence M., Stephen J. McPhee, and Maxine Papadakis, eds. *Current Medical Diagnosis and Treatment 2004.* 43d ed. Stamford, Conn.: Appleton & Lange, 2003. Contains a good chapter on endocrinology that describes common diseases which are a result of hormone abnormalities. Concisely and clearly written, with a medical focus.

Hospice

Health care system

Definition: Hospice care is a holistic approach to caring for the dying and their families by addressing their physical, emotional, and spiritual needs.

Hospice is a philosophy of care directed toward persons who are dying. Hospice care uses a family-oriented holistic approach to assist these individuals in making the transition from life to death in a manner that preserves their dignity and comfort. This approach, as Elisabeth Kübler-Ross would say, allows dying patients "to live until they die." Hospice care encourages patients to participate fully in determining the type of care that is most appropriate for their comfort. By creating a secure and caring community sensitive to the needs of the dying and their families and by providing palliative care that relieves patients of the distressing symptoms of their disease, hospice care can aid the dying in preparing mentally as well as spiritually for their impending death.

Unlike traditional health care, where the patient is viewed as the client, hospice care, with its holistic emphasis, treats the family unit as the client. There are usually specific areas of stress for the families of the dying. In addition to the stress of caring for the physical needs of the dying, family members often feel tremendous pressure maintaining their own roles and responsibilities within the family itself. The conflict of caring for their own nuclear families while caring for dying relatives places a huge strain on everyone involved and can be a source of anxiety and guilt for the patient as well. Another area of stress experienced by family members involves concern for themselves, that is, having to put their own lives on hold, keeping from getting physically run down, dealing with their newly acquired time constraints, and viewing themselves as isolated from friends and family. Compounding this is the guilt that many caregivers feel over not caring for the dying relative as well or as patiently as they might, or secretly wishing for the caregiving experience to reach an end.

Due to the holistic nature of the care provided, the hospice team is actually an interdisciplinary team composed of physicians, nurses, psychological and social workers, pastoral counselors, and trained volunteers. This medically supervised team meets weekly to decide on how best to provide physical, emotional, and spiritual support for dying patients and to assist the surviving family members in the subsequent grieving process.

This type of care can be administered in three different ways. It can be home-health-agency based, delivered in the patient's own home. It can be dispensed in an institution devoted solely to hospice care. It can even be administered in traditional medical facilities (such as hospitals) that allot a certain amount of space (perhaps a wing or floor, or even a certain number of beds) to this type of care. Fewer than 20 percent of hospices are totally independent and unaffiliated with any hospitals.

PRINCIPLES

Hospice care attempts to enhance the quality of dying patients' final days by providing them with as much comfort as possible. It is predicated on the belief that death is a natural process with which humans should not interfere. The principles of hospice care, therefore, revolve around alleviating the anxieties and physical suffering that can be associated with the dying process, and not prolonging the dying process by using invasive medical techniques. Hospice care is also based on the assertion that dying patients have certain rights that must be respected. These rights include a right to absent themselves from social responsibilities and commitments, a right to be cared for, and the right to continued respect and status. The following seven principles are basic components of hospice care.

The first principle is highly personalized and holistic care of the dying, which includes treating dying patients emotionally and spiritually as well as physically. This interpersonal support, known as bonding, helps patients in their final days to live as fully and as comfortably as possible, while retaining their dignity, autonomy, and individual self-worth in a safe and secure environment. This one-on-one attention involves what can be called therapeutic communication. Knowing that someone has heard, that someone understands and is concerned, can be profoundly healing.

Another principle is treating pain aggressively. To this end, hospice care advocates the use of narcotics at dosages that will alleviate suffering while, at the same time, enabling patients to maintain a desired level of alertness. Efforts are made to employ the least invasive routes to administer these drugs (usually orally, if possible). In addition, pain medication is administered before the pain begins, thus alleviating the anxiety of patients waiting for pain to return. Since it has been shown that fear of pain often increases the pain itself, this type of aggressive pain management gives dying patients more time and energy to respond to family members and friends and to work through the emotional and spiritual stages of dying. This dispensation of pain medication before the pain actually occurs, however, has proven to be perhaps the most controversial element in hospice care, with some critics charging that the dying are being turned into drug addicts.

A third principle is the participation of families in caring for the dying. Family members are trained by hospice nurses to care for the dying patients and even to dispense pain medication. The aim is to prevent the patients from suffering isolation or feeling as if they are surrounded by strangers. Participation in care also helps to sustain the patients' and the families' sense of autonomy.

The fourth principle is familiarity of surroundings. Whenever possible, it is the goal of hospice care to keep dying patients at home. This eliminates the necessity of the dying to spend their final days in an institutionalized setting, isolated from family and friends when they need them the most. It is estimated that close to 90 percent of all hospice care days are spent in patients' own homes. When this is not possible and patients must enter institutional settings, rules are relaxed so that their rooms can be decorated or arranged in such a way as to replicate the patients' home surroundings. Visiting rules are suspended when possible, and visits by family members, children, and sometimes even pets are encouraged.

The fifth principle is emotional and spiritual support for the family caregivers. Hospice volunteers are specially trained to use listening and communicative techniques with family members and to provide them with emotional support both during and after the patient's death. In addition, because the care is holistic, the caregivers' physical needs are attended to (for example, respite is provided for exhausted caregivers), as are their emotional and spiritual needs. This spiritual support applies to people of all faith backgrounds, as impending death tends to put faith into a perspective where particular creeds and denominational structures assume less significance. In attending to this spiritual dimension, the hospice team is respectful of all religious traditions while realizing that death and bereavement have the ability to both strengthen and weaken faith.

The sixth principle is having hospice services available twenty-four hours a day, seven days a week. Because of its reliance on the assistance of trained volunteers, round-the-clock support is available to patients and their families.

The seventh principle is bereavement counseling for the survivors. At the time of death, the hospice team is available to help families take care of tasks such as planning the funeral and probating the will. In the weeks after the death, hospice volunteers offer their support to surviving family members in dealing with their loss and grief and the various phases of the bereavement process, always aware of the fact that not all bereaved need or want formal interventions.

HISTORY

The term "hospice" comes from the Latin *hospitia*, meaning "places of welcome." The earliest documented example of hospice care dates to the fourth century, when a Roman woman named Fabiola apparently used her own wealth to care for the sick and dying. In medieval times, the Catholic Church established inns for poor wayfarers and pilgrims traveling to religious shrines in search of miraculous cures for their illnesses. Such "rest homes," usually run by religious orders, provided both lodging and nursing care, since the medieval view was that the sick, dying, and needy were all travelers on a journey. This attitude also reflects the medieval notion that true hospitality included care of the mind and spirit as well as of the body. During the Protestant Reformation, when monasteries were forcibly closed, the concepts of hospice and hospital became distinct. Care of the sick and dying was now considered a public duty rather than a religious or private one, and many former hospices were turned into state-run hospitals.

The first in-patient hospice establishment of modern times (specifically called "hospice") was founded by Mary Aitkenhead and the Irish Sisters of Charity under her leadership in the 1870's in Dublin, Ireland. Cicely Saunders, a physician at St. Joseph's Hospice in London, which was founded by the English Sisters of Charity in 1908, began to adapt the ancient concept of hospice to modern palliative techniques. While there, Saunders became extremely close to a Holocaust survivor who was dying of cancer. She found that she shared his dream of establishing a place that would meet the needs of the dying. Using the money he bequeathed her at his death as a starting point, Saunders raised additional funds and opened St. Christopher's Hospice in Sydenham, outside London, in 1967. Originally it housed only cancer patients, but with the financial support of contracts with the National Health Service in England and private donations, it later expanded to meet the needs of all the dying. In fact, no patient has ever been refused because of inability to pay. St. Christopher's has served as a model for the hospices to be built later in other parts of the world.

Even though hospice care did not originate with Cicely Saunders, she is usually credited with founding the first modern hospice, since she introduced the concept of dispensing narcotics at regular intervals in order to preempt the pain of the dying. She was also the first to identify the need to address other, nonphysical sources of pain for dying patients.

Two years after St. Christopher's Hospice was opened, Kübler-Ross wrote *On Death and Dying*, which validated the hospice movement by relating stories of the dying and their wishes as to how they would be treated. In 1974, the United States opened its first hospice, Hospice, Inc. (later called the Connecticut Hospice), in New Haven, Connecticut. Within the next twenty-five years, over three thousand hospice programs would be implemented in the United States. In Canada, the first "palliative care" unit (as hospices are referred to in Canada) was opened in 1975 by Dr. Balfour M. Mount at the Royal Victoria Hospital in Montreal. This is considered to be the first hospital-based hospice in North America.

COST

Because of hospice care's reliance on heavily trained volunteers and contributions, and because death is seen as a natural process that should not be prolonged by invasive and expensive medical techniques, hospice care is much less costly than traditional acute care facilities. Because hospice care is a philosophy of care rather than a specific facility, though, legislation to provide monetary support for hospice patients took a great deal of time to be approved. In 1982, the U.S. Congress finally added hospice care as a Medicare benefit. In 1986, it was made a permanent benefit. Medicare requires, however, that there be a prognosis of six months or less for the patient to live. Hospice care is also reimbursable by many private insurance companies.

The National Hospice Organization (NHO) originated in 1977 in the United States as a resource for the many groups across the country who needed assistance in establishing hospice programs in their own communities. The purpose of this organization is to provide information about hospice care to the public, to establish conduits so that information may be exchanged between hospice groups, and to maintain agreed-upon standards for developing hospices around the country. The NHO publishes *Guide to the Nation's Hospices* on an annual basis.

—Mara Kelly-Zukowski, Ph.D.

See also Death and dying; Euthanasia; Grief and guilt; Hospitals; Medicare; Terminally ill: Extended care.

FOR FURTHER INFORMATION:

Buckingham, Robert W. *The Handbook of Hospice Care.* New York: Prometheus Books, 1996. Covers the history and philosophy of hospice care while providing practical information as to its cost, how to find hospice programs in your own community, and how to manage grief. Focuses on two target populations for hospice care: children and AIDS victims.

Byock, Ira. *Dying Well: The Prospect for Growth at the End of Life*. New York: Riverhead Books, 1997. President of the American Academy of Hospice and Palliative Medicine at the time he wrote this book, Dr. Byock uses the personal stories of his patients to show the best ways to die. Provides information for the families of the dying who wish to make their loved ones' final days as comfortable and meaningful as possible.

Connor, Stephen R. *Hospice: Practice, Pitfalls, and Promise*. Washington, D.C.: Taylor & Francis, 1998. This book provides a useful outline of the history, structure, and function of hospice programs in the United States, with understandably less emphasis on medical issues. There is clear evidence of wide experience and consideration of the real world of hospice care, not second-hand distillation from the literature.

Corr, Charles A., Clyde M. Nabe, and Donna M. Corr. *Death and Dying, Life and Living*. 4th ed. Belmont, Calif.: Wadsworth, 2002. This book provides perspective on common issues associated with death and dying for family members and others affected by life-threatening circumstances.

Lattanzi-Licht, Marcia, John J. Mahoney, and Galen W. Miller. *The Hospice Choice: In Pursuit of a Peaceful Death*. New York: Simon & Schuster, 1998. Definitive resource from the National Hospice Organization. Provides practical information such as range of hospice services, methods of payment, and so on. Intersperses stories of families who have received hospice care with a thorough explanation of its history, principles, and benefits.

Meyer, Maria M., and Paula Derr. *Comfort of Home: An Illustrated Step-by-Step Guide for Caregivers*. 2d ed. Portland, Oreg.: CareTrust, 2002. A very useful guide to caregiving in the home. Provides a chronological structure to define preparation for caregiving and the day-to-day expectations, and gives a listing of numerous research resources.

National Hospice and Palliative Care Organization. http://www.nhpco.org/templates/1/homepage.cfm. A group that advocates for the terminally ill and their families, develops public and professional educational programs and materials to enhance understanding and availability of hospice and palliative care, and conducts research, among other activities.

Sendor, Virginia F., and Patrice M. O'Connor. *Hospice and Palliative Care: Questions and Answers*. Lanham, Md.: Scarecrow, 1997. The user-friendly question-and-answer style of this volume allows for use as a quick reference. The purpose is to address the questions often asked by individuals faced with a terminal illness and those involved in the care of the terminally ill.

Sheehan, Denice C., and Walter B. Forman. *Hospice and Palliative Care: Concepts and Practice*. 2d ed. Sudbury, Mass.: Jones and Bartlett, 2002. A text that examines the theoretical perspectives and practical information about hospice care. Other topics include community medical care, geriatric care, nursing care, pain management, research, counseling, and hospice management.

HOSPITALS

HEALTH CARE SYSTEM

DEFINITION: Institutions focused on the management, prevention, and treatment of illness; utilizing a staff of medical and allied health professionals, hospitals provide medical, surgical, and psychiatric treatment along with emergency care and evaluation.

KEY TERMS:

emergency room: a place where rapid evaluation and treatment of sudden illnesses, accidents, and traumas occur

intensive care: continuous medical treatment involving vigilant monitoring of the vital signs of patients with grave physical conditions

outpatient care: evaluation and treatment services not requiring an overnight stay

triage: a process in which patient needs are evaluated by a health care team and preliminary treatment plans are made

ORGANIZATION AND FUNCTIONS

Hospitals are run both privately and under public auspices, such as a local, state, or federal government. In general, they can be classified in three ways: nonprofit versus for-profit, general versus specialty, and short-term versus long-term care. Typically, they are organized in a hierarchical fashion: A governing body, such as a board of directors and its committees, oversees an administrator who, in turn, oversees a variety of departmental managers. While the governing body is responsible for defining and fostering the hospital's mission, the administrator guides the implementation of the mission, and the managers enact it. As such, hospitals have feedback mechanisms from the departments and chief administrator back to the board to ensure quality and progress.

STAFF AND SERVICES

Most hospitals have five primary departments for service management: financial, support, nursing, medical, and ancillary. The first two, financial and support, provide nonmedical services, while the remainder provide direct and indirect medical services. The financial department relies on office personnel and manages business functions, such as admissions, data management, accounting, and collections. In contrast, the support department manages administrative functions (such as volunteer services, medical records, purchasing, personnel), environmental concerns (such as maintenance and housekeeping), and nonmedical patient services (such as dietary needs and social services). This department hosts a diverse service staff, ranging from janitors to dietitians to social workers.

As patients, individuals typically enter hospitals through admissions, the emergency room, or a hospital clinic, or via referral from a private doctor. Thus, depending on a patient's route of admission, his or her interaction with different departmental service staff may vary considerably. In any hospital, however, the nursing service has perhaps the greatest visibility, as it fulfills functions in the emergency and operating rooms, outpatient clinics, and inpatient units. In fact, nurses may perform any of the following duties, depending on their level of training and where they work within a hospital: triage, charting, medical room preparation, medication administration, vital signs monitoring, assistance of patients with meals and hygiene, and staff training. In addition, the nursing service typically dominates short-term special care units, such as intensive care and the emergency room, and nonacute care units, such as renal dialysis centers, psychiatric and substance abuse units, and long-term care centers for chronic illnesses.

Equally well known is the medical service, consisting of physicians, osteopathic physicians, podiatrists, dentists, and psychologists. Typically, this service manages the delivery of care for general medicine, surgery, obstetrics and gynecology, pediatrics, and psychiatry. While the nursing service historically has dominated the emergency room, more recently medical staff are leading in this service area. Many different classes of emergency rooms exist, however, ranging from highly

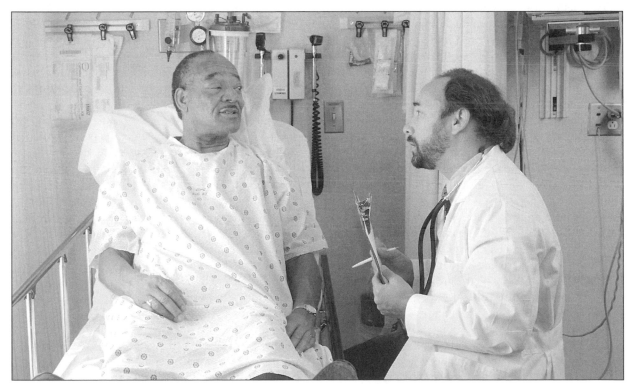

Older adults may find themselves hospitalized for acute illnesses, chronic illnesses, or injuries—all of which present higher risks for the elderly than for younger adults. (Digital Stock)

staffed by physicians and specialists (twenty-four-hours on site) to minimally staffed (an on-call emergency nurse or technician who transfers patients to hospitals with life support equipment). Consequently, this balance between nursing and medical services may vary considerably among hospital emergency rooms.

Finally, ancillary service professionals assist the medical service staff in rendering diagnoses and treating patients. These staff members are highly trained and commonly use sophisticated equipment and methods. Subdepartments composing this service include the laboratory, pharmacy, anesthesiology, physical therapy, electrocardiography (ECG or EKG), electroencephalography (EEG), magnetic resonance imaging (MRI), and inhalation therapy departments. Radiology is also included and has three divisions: diagnostic radiology, therapeutic radiology, and nuclear medicine.

PERSPECTIVE AND PROSPECTS

The word "hospital" was derived from the Greek word *hospitum*, meaning a place for the reception of pilgrims, and the Latin word *hospes*, meaning "guest" or "host." Originally, hospitals existed as temples or churches in ancient Greece and Rome, where priest-physicians performed healing miracles on the mind, body, and spirit. Later, hospitals were run by Christians and church bishops in Europe and served primarily as places of refuge and service for travelers. It was not until 600 C.E. that European hospitals specifically began caring for the sick. Similarly, in America, hospitals were not established until the eighteenth century—and then, only in larger cities. At that time, they primarily functioned as places where the urban poor could receive care and where individuals with contagious diseases could be confined during epidemics. With the advent of modern medicine and developments such as anesthesia and antibiotic drugs, hospitals were seen less as places to be sick and more as places to get well. As a result, they began to take in patients from all sectors of society and with a broader diversity of medical needs.

Today, hospitals are large, financially driven institutions that focus not only on the provision of emergency medical services and healing the very sick but also on the prevention of illness. Increasingly, specialty hospitals are addressing specific groups of patients, such as children, women, elders, and individuals with particular illnesses, such as cancer. In addition, specialty hospitals are taking on identities as centers for research and teaching as they improve treatment methods and strategies. With improved drug therapies and medical procedures, there is also a trend in general hospitals toward outpatient and day care for chronic illnesses replacing a long history of inpatient services. In the future, these trends toward service specialization and outpatient service are expected to continue, with hospitals increasing their use of illness prevention strategies, as well as continuing to improve their delivery of critical care and emergency services for diverse groups of patients.

—*Nancy A. Piotrowski, Ph.D.*

See also Anesthesiology; Critical care; Critical care, pediatric; Emergency care; Geriatrics and gerontology; Malpractice; Nursing; Obstetrics; Oncology; Paramedics; Pediatrics; Physician assistants; Psychiatry; Psychiatry, child and adolescent; Psychiatry, geriatric; Surgery, general; Surgery, pediatric; Terminally ill: Extended care.

FOR FURTHER INFORMATION:

Birenbaum, Aaron. *Wounded Profession: American Medicine Enters the Age of Managed Care*. Westport, Conn.: Greenwood Press, 2002. Traces the evolution of health care in the United States during the 1990's and examines the rising costs, consumer backlash, and new legislation.

Christman, Luther, and Michael A. Counte. *Hospital Organization and Healthcare Delivery*. Boulder, Colo.: Westview Press, 1981. Details guidelines and rationale for health care risk management, looking beyond conventional hospital-based, clinical initiatives to encompass a variety of health care settings.

Clifford, Joyce C. *Restructuring: The Impact of Hospital Organization on Nursing Leadership*. Chicago: AHA Press, 1998. An examination of the evolution of the role of the chief nursing officer in hospitals responding to a dramatically changing health care environment. Clifford examines the impact of change on the management and administration of clinical nursing services and considers the opportunities and ramifications of how present actions can affect the future of nursing.

Dranove, David. *The Economic Evolution of American Health Care: From Marcus Welby to Managed Care*. Princeton, N.J.: Princeton University Press, 2002. Traces the economic, technological, and historical forces that have transformed the health care field.

Melnick, Glenn, Emmett Keeler, and Jack Zwanziger. "Market Power and Hospital Pricing: Are Nonprofits Different?" *Health Affairs* 18, no. 3 (June, 1999): 167-173. This study shows that nonprofit and government hospitals have steadily become more willing to raise prices to exploit market power and discusses the implications for antitrust regulators and agencies that must approve nonprofit conversions.

Sloane, Robert M., and Beverly LeBov Sloane. *A Guide to Health Facilities: Personnel and Management*. 3d ed. Ann Arbor, Mich.: Health Administration Press, 1992. Offers an overview of health facilities, with a look at hospital administration. Includes bibliographical references and an index.

HOST-DEFENSE MECHANISMS
BIOLOGY

ANATOMY OR SYSTEM AFFECTED: Blood, cells, gastrointestinal system, immune system, skin, urinary system

SPECIALTIES AND RELATED FIELDS: Hematology, immunology, preventive medicine, serology

DEFINITION: Immunological methods that the body uses to protect against external infectious agents and to maintain internal homeostasis, such as those rooted in the skin, sweat, urine, tears, phagocytes, and "helpful" bacteria.

KEY TERMS:

antibodies: proteins produced by immune cells called lymphocytes; antibodies bind to targets called antigens in a highly specific manner

antigen: any substance that causes the formation of a specific antibody; generally a protein

complement: a series of serum proteins that, when activated, carry out a variety of immune functions; the most notable complement function is the lysis of a target

granulocyte: a white blood cell characterized by large numbers of cytoplasmic granules, including neutrophils, eosinophils, and basophils

innate immunity: nonspecific immunity in the sense that prior contact with an infectious agent is not required for proper innate immune response

interferons: a family of proteins; some of these proteins induce an antiviral state within a cell, while others serve to regulate aspects of the immune response

lymphocyte: either of two kinds of small white blood cells; B lymphocytes function to secrete antibodies, while T lymphocytes function to destroy virus-infected cells

macrophage: any of several forms of either circulating or fixed phagocytic cells of the immune system

neutrophil: a circulating white blood cell that serves as one of the principal phagocytes for the immune system

phagocyte: any cell capable of surrounding, ingesting, and digesting microbes or cell debris; in a certain sense, phagocytes function as scavengers

STRUCTURE AND FUNCTIONS

Humans exist in an environment that contains a wide variety of potentially infectious agents. These agents range in size from microscopic viruses—such as rhinoviruses, which cause the common cold—to a wide variety of bacteria and even macroscopic agents such as parasitic worms. In the absence of a functioning immune system, as is observed in persons with acquired immunodeficiency syndrome (AIDS) or congenital immune deficiencies, a person will eventually succumb to overwhelming infections.

Host-defense mechanisms consist of two major components: an innate system that is not dependent on prior exposure to an infectious agent and an acquired immunity that is stimulated by exposure to an agent. In general, the innate system functions in a nonspecific manner, while the acquired immune responses are highly specific.

The first major lines of host defense are the physical barriers to infection. These include the intact skin and the mechanical or physical barriers that serve to protect body openings. Few infectious agents are capable of penetrating intact skin. Numerous sweat glands and follicles are also associated with skin, and their secretion of fatty acids or lactic acid serves to produce an acid environment that inhibits the growth of bacteria. In addition, the high salt content found on the surface of the body also serves to inhibit growth. Bacteria that can resist the high levels of salt and acid, such as *Staphylococcus* or *Streptococcus*, tend to cause skin-related problems such as acne or boils.

Openings of the body, such as the mouth, anus, and vagina, exhibit both the physical barrier of skin and a variety of other defense strategies. Secreted mucus serves to trap foreign particles, which can then be expelled, depending on the tissue, by the ciliary action of the cells, coughing or sneezing, or the washing action of saliva, urine, or tears. Many of these secretions also contain antibacterial or antiviral agents. Gastric juices contain hydrochloric acid, while the enzyme lysozyme, found in tears and saliva, serves to cause the breakdown of certain bacteria.

The normal flora of organisms found within the body also plays an important role in defense. Bacteria in the mouth and gut serve to suppress any external agents that may find their way to those regions. Removal of the innate flora with antibiotics may result in yeast infections of the mouth or vaginal tract, or ulceration by "opportunistic" organisms of the gut.

Penetration of the host by infectious agents initially brings into action other aspects of the innate immune system. This can take the form of a series of "professional" phagocytes, cells that literally eat foreign particles such as bacteria; also included are chemical agents found in tissue and blood.

Two major forms of phagocytes are found in blood and tissues: neutrophils and monocytes/macrophages. Neutrophils represent the most numerous white cells in blood, approximately 60 to 70 percent of the total. They can be recognized by their multilobed nuclei, which confer the ability to pass between the endothelial cells of capillaries into sites of tissue infections. When neutrophils locate a target, such as an infectious agent or a dead cell, they surround that target with membranous arms called pseudopods and ingest it. Once the particle is incorporated within this "phagosome," it is ready for killing and digestion.

The killing of ingested organisms such as bacteria involves a series of complicated reactions, the major products of which are highly reactive oxidizing agents such as peroxides or metabolic by-products such as acid. At the same time, digestive organelles within the phagocyte, called lysosomes, fuse with the phagosome. Lysosomes contain numerous digestive enzymes, and these function to digest the engulfed particle. In effect, the particle now ceases to exist.

Monocytes, which are most often observed in their differentiated macrophage stage, function in a similar manner. Unlike circulating cells such as neutrophils, however, macrophages constitute the mononuclear phagocytic system that is associated with many tissues in the body. Examples of tissue-associated macrophages are the Kupffer cells of the liver, the microglia of the brain, and certain alveolar cells of the lungs. In addition to serving a nonspecific phagocytic function, macrophages serve as antigen-presenting cells (APCs) for specific immune responses.

A variety of blood chemicals also can be associated with innate immunity. Complement represents a series of some twenty blood proteins, activated in a cascade fashion, which exhibit a variety of pharmacologic activities. The complement pathway can be initiated upon exposure to certain bacteria. Components of the pathway can serve as chemoattractants for neutrophils. They can increase the efficiency of phagocytosis (opsonization), and they can form a mem-

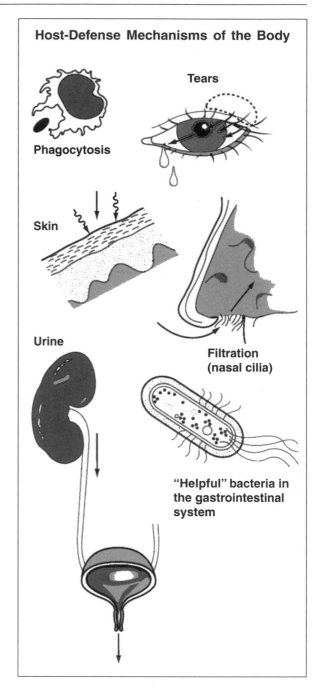

Host-Defense Mechanisms of the Body

Phagocytosis

Tears

Skin

Urine

Filtration (nasal cilia)

"Helpful" bacteria in the gastrointestinal system

brane attack complex on the surface of a target, resulting in lysis.

Another type of blood cell may play a role in certain types of parasitic infections: the eosinophil. Granulocytes like the neutrophils, eosinophils contain within their granules digestive enzymes capable of being released against targets such as parasitic worms. The binding of these enzymes on the surface of a target damages the parasite's membrane, resulting ultimately in death of the parasite.

Acquired host defenses, while involving mechanisms similar to those of the innate systems, differ in one important way: They require prior exposure to the antigen. Acquired immunity consists of two major arms: humoral immunity, which represents substances soluble in the blood; and cellular immunity, which utilizes cells targeted against agents in a specific manner.

Humoral immunity centers primarily on proteins called antibodies. Exposure to foreign antigens triggers a series of reactions among three separate types of blood cells: antigen-presenting cells, T lymphocytes, and B lymphocytes. It is the B cell that actually secretes the antibodies.

The process starts when an APC encounters and phagocytizes an antigen. The antigen is digested, and pieces, or determinants, of the antigen are expressed on the surface of the cell. The most common APC is the macrophage, but antigen presentation can also be carried out by dendritic cells found in the dermis of the skin. This portion of the process is analogous to the series of events associated with innate immunity. At this point, however, the determinant is "presented" to appropriate T and B lymphocytes. Only those lymphocytes that possess specific receptors for that antigenic determinant can interact with the APC; it is this aspect that represents the specificity of the reaction. In association with a subclass of T lymphocytes called T helper cells (also known as CD4+ cells), the B cell is stimulated to begin the secretion of large quantities of antibodies. The antibodies recognize and bind only those antigens against which they were produced.

The formation of antigen-antibody complexes is the key to the humoral response. The result of the reaction depends upon the form taken by the antigen. The binding of antibodies to a bacterium or virus results in opsonization, a significantly enhanced ability of phagocytes to engulf the target. Antibody binding to a virus may also inhibit the agent's binding to a target cell, rendering the virus inactive. If the antigen is a toxin, antibody binding will neutralize the molecule.

The other arm of acquired immunity directly utilizes cellular defenses. The key cell here is the T lymphocyte. T lymphocytes mature in an organ called the thymus, which is located in humans near the thyroid in the neck and which provides the basis for the cells' name. T cells are often referred to as "killer cells" (or CD8+ cells), because of their function. They possess receptors on their surfaces that bind to specific target cells, which are generally cells infected with viruses, though T cells are also associated with rejection of foreign grafts. Once the T cell binds to the target, pharmacologically active granules are released that bind to and disrupt the membrane of the target. Thus, the humoral response is directed primarily against extracellular agents such as bacteria, while the cellular response is directed primarily against internal parasites.

DISORDERS AND DISEASES

In their most obvious form, the mechanisms of host defense protect against disease. Humans exist in an environment that is a sea of microorganisms. Most infections, while often uncomfortable, are not life-threatening. It is only when the immune system fails to function properly or is overwhelmed that illness results in the death of the individual. Ironically, the study of these circumstances has provided much knowledge of the functioning of the immune system.

Throughout history, diseases have periodically plagued humanity. Epidemics of viral diseases such as polio and bacterial infections such as bubonic plague or cholera have killed untold millions of persons. Among the most important advances in medicine since the eighteenth century has been the development of vaccination as a means of preventing disease. In the case of passive immunity, host defenses are temporarily augmented, while active immunity, mimicking an actual infection, often provides lifelong protection.

Passive immunity involves the acquisition of preformed antibodies by an individual. Since colostrum, or milk from a nursing mother, contains a form of antibody, this is the most common form of passive immunization. Preformed antibodies may also be given to a person exposed to potentially lethal toxins under circumstances in which there may be insufficient time for a proper immune response. These can include persons exposed to snake venom or tetanus toxin. While temporarily providing protection, passively acquired antibodies survive in the individual only for a short period.

More commonly, vaccines are utilized to provide active immunization by stimulating the acquired host defenses. These vaccines generally utilize inactivated or attenuated parasites that stimulate specific cellular or humoral responses. The prototypes of active immunization are the polio vaccines developed by Jonas Salk and Albert Sabin in the 1950's. Salk's vaccine utilizes a formalin-inactivated poliovirus, while Sabin's consists of attenuated virus. While controversy exists regarding which is superior, both vaccines act in basically the same manner. Exposure to either vaccine results in the production of protective antibodies in the circulation of the individual. In the event of actual infection by poliovirus, the agent would be neutralized before it could reach its target in the central nervous system. Analogous vaccines have been developed against previously common viral diseases such as smallpox, measles, and mumps, and against bacterial diseases such as pertussis (whooping cough) and diphtheria.

The process by which the acquired immune process functions is in part defined by the nature of the antigen. It is also important to remember that the humoral and cellular defense systems are not self-exclusive; each functions in conjunction with the other. If the antigen in question is a bacterium, it is primarily the role of the humoral system to deal with the infection. This can take several forms. The antibody may bind to the surface of the cell, inactivating the cell wall or membrane enzymes, resulting in the death of the cell. The antibody-antigen (bacterium) complex may also activate the complement pathway, resulting in either opsonization or the formation of a membrane attack complex by complement components. Indeed, antibody binding by itself may result in opsonization.

If the antigen is a virus-infected cell, the cellular portion of the response comes into play. Cytotoxic T cells can bind to the target through specific receptors, causing the death of the virus-infected cell. If an antibody binds to viral receptors on the infected cell, cytotoxic cells with receptors for the antibody may show increased affinity for the target in a process called antibody-dependent cell-mediated cytotoxicity (ADCC). The result is the death of the target. The antibody may also serve to neutralize a cell-free virus before the particle can even infect the target cell. Certain bacteria, however, such as the mycobacteria associated with tuberculosis and leprosy, are actually found as intracellular parasites. In such cases, it is the cellular immune system that plays a major role in defense. In this manner, the humoral and cellular defense mechanisms complement each other.

Failure of the immune system to function is clearly illustrated in persons infected with the human immunodeficiency virus (HIV), the virus that causes AIDS. HIV infects the subclass of T lymphocytes called T helper cells. The eventual result is the death and depletion of this subclass of cells. As briefly described earlier, T helper cells are central to the function of both the humoral and the cellular arms of acquired immunity. The interaction of these cells with B lymphocytes is necessary for both antibody production by these cells and their proliferation. The T helper cell is also required for activation and proliferation of the CD8+ cytotoxic T cells.

As AIDS progresses in the individual, the T-helper subclass becomes increasingly depleted. As a result, both the cellular and humoral immune systems become progressively less functional. The person becomes more susceptible to opportunistic organisms in the environment and eventually succumbs to any of a wide variety of diseases.

In rare congenital cases, only certain aspects of the immune system are nonfunctional. These often tragic examples serve to illustrate the role of various cells within the host defense. For example, children with B-cell deficiencies suffer from repeated bacterial infections, while yeast and viral infections rarely result in problems. Children in whom the thymus fails to develop (DiGeorge or Nezelof syndromes), however, suffer from repeated viral infections but rarely from bacterial infections.

Severe combined immunodeficiency syndrome (SCID) affects approximately one out of every 150,000 live births. This genetic disorder is the result of a lack of the enzyme adenosine deaminase (ADA), which ultimately causes a lack of functioning T cells. For years, patients with this disorder had been doomed to living in sterile bubble environments and would die at a young age because of their inability to fight even the mildest infection. Bone marrow transplants for patients with compatible donors can sometimes strengthen the immune system; however, this option is not available for everyone.

In 1990, two unrelated girls with SCID, four and nine years old, were the subject of the first clinical trial of gene therapy. T cells in their blood were isolated and cultured, and normal copies of the ADA gene were introduced into the cells. The genetically engineered T cells were then infused back into the patients over a period of approximately two years. Both girls showed remarkable improvement, with near normal levels of ADA and functioning immune systems, and were thereafter able to lead normal lives. These positive results remained several years after cessation of the actual gene therapy, indicating that this first clinical trial of gene therapy was a success. The door is now open for using gene therapy on other disorders, including those of the immune system.

Host defenses are also utilized within the homeostatic process, which can be defined as maintaining the status quo. An example of such a process is the role of the immune system in protecting humans against various forms of cancer. Although immunosuppressed individuals appear to be at no greater risk for most cancers than normal persons, certain types of skin cancers, as well as certain types of B-cell lymphomas, arise more frequently in these persons. Thus, it is likely that the immune system plays at least some role in protecting the individual from certain forms of cancer. Artificial stimulation of the immune system has, however, been utilized in an attempt to treat sundry forms of advanced cancers. The process involves the removal of immune cells from the patient and the incubation of those cells with a form of interferon generally secreted by T helper cells during their regulation of the immune response. The cells are then returned to the patient. The theory is that, by nonspecifically stimulating cytotoxic cells, some of those cells may serve to destroy the cancer. In some instances, patients have shown improvement.

Clearly, the immune system functions by means of a complex process of cellular interactions. The initial encounter with a foreign infectious agent utilizes an innate system that serves as a first line of defense. Then, through a type of learning process, a specific immune response is generated that provides a more rapid, more efficient means of generating protection.

PERSPECTIVE AND PROSPECTS

Manipulating the host's immune system in order to protect against disease dates back more than a thousand years. In order to protect themselves against smallpox, the Chinese carried out a practice called variolation, in which dried crusts obtained from the pocks of mild cases were inhaled. The practice was copied by early Arabic physicians and eventually made its way to eighteenth century Europe. In the late eighteenth century, an English country physician, Edward Jenner, observed that dairy maids who had recovered from a mild disease called cowpox rarely exhibited the scars associated with smallpox. Jenner reasoned that a person who had been exposed to the cowpox agent would be protected against smallpox. Jenner tested his theory and was proved correct. Smallpox became the first disease that could be prevented by vaccination.

Competition between French and German scientists during the late nineteenth century resulted in much of the existing basic knowledge of host defenses. A Russian, Élie Metchnikoff, working with Louis Pasteur in Paris during the 1880's, developed the views of cellular immunity that are still current. In that same period, the work of Emil von Behring and Paul Ehrlich in Berlin established the role of humoral immunity in protecting against disease.

Active immunization remains the primary method by which an individual may be protected from disease, but the process lends itself to a variety of problems. Not all antigenic determinants of the bacterium or parasite in question are equally important. A response to some antigens may actually hinder the immune response to more important determinants. Furthermore, some individuals react inappropriately to some vaccines, resulting in severe allergic reactions.

For these reasons, much research involves the attempt to isolate only the desired antigen for the vaccine. This has taken several approaches. Purified components, rather than the entire organism, have been used in some vaccines. In some cases, the gene that encodes the desired antigen has been isolated and spliced into the genetic material of a harmless organism. Such an approach has been used to produce a modified hepatitis B vaccine. The gene encoding the surface antigen of the virus has been spliced into the genome of vaccinia, long used for vaccination against smallpox. When the individual is vaccinated, the hepatitis gene is expressed (though no virus can be made), and the person becomes immune to the disease. In theory, whole cocktails of vaccines can be prepared in a similar manner.

New illnesses and other environmental hazards that affect host defenses continue to arise. AIDS may be unusually lethal, but as a previously unknown disease, it is by no means unique. Nevertheless, the ability of the host immune system to respond to new infectious agents remains a bulwark for maintaining the health of an individual.

—Richard Adler, Ph.D.;
updated by Karen E. Kalumuck, Ph.D.

See also Bacterial infections; Bacteriology; Blood and blood disorders; Cells; Glands; Immune system; Immunization and vaccination; Immunology; Immunopathology; Infection; Skin; Urinary system; Viral infections.

FOR FURTHER INFORMATION:

Adelman, Daniel C., et al., eds. *Manual of Allergy and Immunology.* Philadelphia: Lippincott Williams & Wilkins, 2002. Examines research developments and the clinical diagnosis and treatment of allergies and immune disorders. Topics include asthma, disorders of the eye, diseases of the lung, anaphylaxis, insect allergies, drug allergies, rheumatic diseases, transplantation immunology, and immunization.

Bibel, Debra. *Milestones in Immunology.* Madison, Wis.: Science Tech, 1988. A compendium of historic articles related to the development of immunology. In association with each original article is an outline explaining the significance of the material. The book presents the evolution of thought in the field in a clear manner, illustrating how knowledge builds upon previous information.

Frank, Steven A. *Immunology and Evolution of Infectious Disease.* Princeton, N.J.: Princeton University Press, 2002. Blends research from molecular biology, immunology, pathogen biology, and population dynamics to discuss how and why parasites vary to escape recognition by the immune system, vaccine design, and the control of epidemics.

Hall, Stephen S. *Commotion in the Blood: Life, Death, and the Immune System.* New York: Henry Holt, 1998. Discusses the revolution in immunotherapy, traces the story of how doctors have learned to use the immune system to develop a wide array of cutting-edge therapies, details the politics of discovery, and explains the complexities of human blood.

Murray, P. R., et al. *Medical Microbiology.* 4th ed. New York: Elsevier, 2001. Focuses on microbes that cause disease in humans. Each chapter consistently presents the etiology, epidemiology, host defenses, identification, diagnosis, prevention, and control of each disease.

Paul, William E. *Immunology: Recognition and Response.* New York: W. H. Freeman, 1991. Paul has assembled a collection of readings from *Scientific American* that deal with the indicated subject. Most of the articles are written at a level that can be understood by persons with a background in basic science.

Playfair, J. H. L. *Immunology at a Glance.* 7th ed. Boston: Blackwell Scientific, 2001. A collection of short chapters dealing with various aspects of host defense. The material, which is abbreviated, clearly defines the described subjects. The book is written in an introductory manner, though its coverage is extensive.

Roitt, Ivan. *Roitt's Essential Immunology.* 10th ed. Boston: Blackwell Scientific, 2001. A textbook written by a leading authority in the field. Though the chapters explaining the technical aspects of the subject become quite detailed, the introductory material dealing with basic host defense is clear and concise. Numerous photographs are included.

Hot flashes
Disease/disorder
Also known as: Hot flushes
Anatomy or system affected: Endocrine system, reproductive system
Specialties and related fields: Endocrinology, gynecology
Definition: Temporary sensations of warmth experienced by perimenopausal and postmenopausal women in which the upper body feels hot, the skin turns red, and sweating occurs.

Key terms:
complete hysterectomy: surgical removal of the uterus and ovaries
hormone replacement therapy (HRT): estrogen/progesterone given to postmenopausal women to alleviate symptoms associated with the menopause
natural menopause: the point at which a woman has not had her menstrual cycle for twelve consecutive months
night sweats: hot flashes that occur at night, typically during sleep
vasomotor symptoms: symptoms relating to nerves and muscles that cause blood vessels to constrict or dilate

Causes and Symptoms
Hot flashes are the most common complaint of perimenopausal and postmenopausal women, whether the menopause occurs naturally as a function of age or is artificially induced, either surgically (by complete hysterectomy) or chemically (using chemotherapy or medication that interferes with ovarian function). Hot

---

Information on Hot Flashes

Causes: Vasomotor response to decreased levels of estrogen with menopause
Symptoms: Elevated temperature in face and upper body, red skin, sweating, palpitations, anxiety, irritability
Duration: Temporary
Treatments: Lifestyle factors (cool room temperatures, light blankets at night, cool clothing, relaxation techniques, regular exercise, avoidance of smoking, cold beverages, limited intake of caffeine, alcohol, or spicy foods; hormone replacement therapy; alternative medicine (soy, phytoestrogens)

flashes are a vasomotor response to decreased levels of estrogen circulating in the bloodstream. When hot flashes occur, skin temperature rises, causing the face and upper body (or in some cases the entire body) to become hot, red, and sweaty. Flushing may also be accompanied by feelings of palpitations, anxiety, and irritability.

While the underlying physiology of hot flashes is not fully understood, it is believed to involve a disturbance in thermoregulation. Normally, the thermoregulatory mechanism in the brain, called the hypothalamus, responds to any increase in body temperature above approximately 100 degrees by sweating in order to cool off. Postmenopausal women instead sweat in response to any rise in temperature, even if it is from 96 to 97 degrees while sleeping. It appears that with declining circulating estrogen levels, norepinephrine levels rise in the brain, resulting in a downward resetting of the normal thermoregulatory set point, falsely causing women to believe that they are overheating. In response, blood vessels dilate, producing the vasomotor symptoms experienced as hot flashes.

TREATMENT AND THERAPY

Women suffering from hot flashes should wear cool clothing; keep room temperatures cool; sleep with light blankets; drink cold beverages; limit intake of caffeine, alcohol, and spicy foods; avoid smoking; use relaxation techniques; and get regular exercise.

If these measures do not alleviate hot flashes, then medical treatment is available. The most effective treatment involves estrogen (or estrogen/progesterone) replacement, which serves to reset the thermoregulatory mechanism to a higher (normal) level, so that hot flashes no longer occur. While hormone replacement therapy (HRT) is effective in alleviating hot flashes, recent research has shown that it may have undesirable long-term effects relating to cancer, heart disease, and cognitive function. Alternative treatments, including the use of soy and phytoestrogens, are becoming increasingly popular. Current research indicates that paroxetine, a selective serotonin reuptake inhibitor (SSRI), appears to be effective in alleviating hot flashes.

PERSPECTIVE AND PROSPECTS

Approximately 80 percent of women experience hot flashes during the menopause. Symptoms are most frequent and intense for the first two to four years following the cessation of menstruation. Ongoing research is attempting to identify effective treatment modalities that do not lead to long-term adverse effects.

—*Robin Kamienny Montvilo, R.N., Ph.D.*

See also Aging; Endocrinology; Gynecology; Hormone replacement therapy (HRT); Hormones; Menopause; Menstruation.

FOR FURTHER INFORMATION:

Budoff, Penny. *No More Hot Flashes.* New York: Warner Books, 1999.

Northrup, Christiane. *The Wisdom of Menopause.* New York: Bantam, 2003.

Stenchever, Morton A., et al. *Comprehensive Gynecology.* 4th ed. St. Louis: Mosby, 2001.

HUMAN GENOME PROJECT. *See* GENOMICS.

HUMAN IMMUNODEFICIENCY VIRUS (HIV)

DISEASE/DISORDER

ANATOMY OR SYSTEM AFFECTED: Immune system

SPECIALTIES AND RELATED FIELDS: Immunology, microbiology, virology

DEFINITION: A retrovirus that attacks cells of the immune system, leading to a loss of immune function and the development of acquired immunodeficiency syndrome (AIDS).

CAUSES AND SYMPTOMS

HIV is a human retrovirus containing two copies of a 9,749-base ribonucleic acid (RNA) molecule as its genetic material. Retroviruses make a deoxyribonucleic

---

INFORMATION ON HUMAN IMMUNODEFICIENCY VIRUS (HIV)

CAUSES: Transmission through exchange of body fluids (semen, vaginal fluid, blood, human milk)

SYMPTOMS: Flulike or mononucleosis-like symptoms upon initial transmission; later, various opportunistic infections

DURATION: Chronic, eventually fatal

TREATMENTS: Highly active antiretroviral therapy (HAART) with nucleoside or nucleotide analogues, reverse transcriptase inhibitors, protease inhibitors, inhibitors of cellular entry

acid (DNA) copy of their genome within a cell using a viral enzyme called reverse transcriptase. HIV contains reverse transcriptase within its virion. HIV inserts this DNA copy (provirus) randomly into a human chromosome. The provirus acts as a template to produce copies of the HIV RNA genome. Once the provirus has integrated, infection is irreversible. HIV falls into the subgroup of retroviruses called lentiviruses, "slow viruses" that do not cause a disease state until many years after infection. Untreated HIV infection progresses to AIDS in about ten years.

There are two forms of HIV. HIV-1, which arose in Central Africa, is the predominant form throughout most of the world, including the United States. HIV-2, a less common form found in Western Africa, is less harmful, reproduces more slowly, and takes more time to cause AIDS. These viruses evolved from related viruses in apes and monkeys, called simian immunodeficiency viruses (SIV). HIV-1 is believed to have arisen from SIV found in chimpanzees, while HIV-2 is believed to have arisen from SIV of the Sootey Mangabey monkey.

HIV is transmitted only through the exchange of body fluids, including semen, vaginal fluid, blood, and human milk. Therefore, the primary routes are sexual transmission, the use of dirty needles by intravenous drug users, and HIV-positive mother-to-child transmission during childbirth or from HIV-contaminated breast milk. Transmission through dirty needles used in body piercing or tattooing may occur. Early in the AIDS epidemic, infection was also acquired through the transfusion of contaminated blood or blood products, leading to a very high rate of transmission to hemophiliacs. Today, such transmission is extremely rare, as the blood supply is routinely tested for HIV.

Treatment and Therapy

As of 2003, there was no effective vaccine to prevent infection with HIV. Although no cure existed, twenty drugs were approved by the Food and Drug Administration (FDA) to treat HIV infection, and several more were in clinical trials. These drugs fell into four categories: nucleoside or nucleotide analogues, which act as direct inhibitors of reverse transcriptase; inhibitors that indirectly inhibit reverse transcriptase by binding to the enzyme; protease inhibitors that interfere with the processing of HIV proteins and completion of the virus life cycle; and inhibitors of entry of HIV into the cell. Because the virus has a very high rate of mutation, resistance to individual anti-HIV drugs may appear quickly. Present therapy, called highly active antiretroviral therapy (HAART), involves the use of three or four anti-HIV drugs simultaneously. HAART therapy, also termed "cocktail therapy," increases efficacy and reduces the probability of developing simultaneous resistance of HIV to all three or four drugs being used.

—Ralph R. Meyer, Ph.D.

See also Acquired immunodeficiency syndrome (AIDS); Autoimmune disorders; Immune system; Immunodeficiency disorders; Immunology; Immunopathology; Sexually transmitted diseases (STDs); Viral infections.

For Further Information:

DeVita, Vincent T., Jr., Samuel Hellman, Steven A. Rosenberg, James Curran, Max Essex, and Anthony S. Fauci, eds. *AIDS: Etiology, Diagnosis, Treatment, and Prevention.* 4th ed. Philadelphia: Lippencott-Raven, 1997.

Fan, Hung, Ross F. Conner, and Luis P. Villarreal. *The Biology of AIDS.* 4th ed. Sudbury, Mass.: Jones & Bartlett, 2000.

Matthews, Dawn D., ed. *AIDS Sourcebook.* 3d ed. Detroit: Omnigraphics, 2003.

Stine, Gerald J. *AIDS Update 2003.* Upper Saddle River, N.J.: Prentice Hall, 2003.

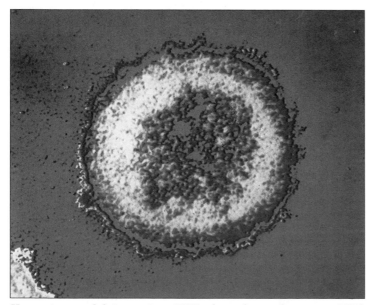

Human immunodeficiency virus (HIV), the pathogen that causes AIDS. (PhotoDisc)

HUNTINGTON'S DISEASE

DISEASE/DISORDER

ALSO KNOWN AS: Huntington's chorea

ANATOMY OR SYSTEM AFFECTED: Brain, nerves, nervous system

SPECIALTIES AND RELATED FIELDS: Biotechnology, genetics, neurology, psychiatry, psychology

DEFINITION: In this autosomal dominant genetic neurodegenerative disease, patients have uncoordinated movements as a result of neuron degeneration.

CAUSES AND SYMPTOMS

The mutated gene responsible for Huntington's disease is located on one arm of chromosome 4 and produces the protein huntingtin. The gene contains repeats of the triplet nucleotide sequence CAG. Normal individuals have between nine and thirty-five (on average eighteen or nineteen) CAG repeats in their genes; affected individuals have forty or more repeats, with an average of forty-six repeats. Individuals with between thirty-six and thirty-nine repeats may or may not develop Huntington's disease. The disease always occurs if the expansion is forty or more repeats. The larger the number of repeats above forty, the earlier the onset of the disease. The disease-causing gene is dominant, so those who inherit the mutated gene develop the disease and have a 50 percent chance of passing the defective gene on to their children.

The triplet CAG codes for the amino acid glutamine. Mutant forms of the huntingtin proteins have forty or more glutamines in the protein. Huntington's disease appears to be caused by a mutation involving a gain of function, in which the expanded polyglutamine region makes the mutant huntingtin protein toxic. Aggregates of mutant huntingtin are observed in the neurons of those who died from Huntington's disease. Normal huntingtin appears to keep neurons alive by stopping programmed cell death.

The neuropathology of Huntington's disease is primarily the degeneration of neurons of the striatum (part of the basal ganglia) and the motor cortex. Clinical manifestations of Huntington's disease typically begin in midlife (thirties and forties), with characteristic motor abnormalities such as uncoordinated movements (chorea) and loss of muscle control (dystonias), personality changes, a gradual loss of cognition, and eventually, death. Huntington's disease primarily affects the central nervous system, but most patients actually die of heart or respiratory complications from long confinement to bed or from head injuries caused by frequent falls.

INFORMATION ON HUNTINGTON'S DISEASE

CAUSES: Genetic protein defect

SYMPTOMS: Uncoordinated movements (chorea), loss of muscle control (dystonias), personality changes, gradual loss of cognition, death

DURATION: Progressive, eventually fatal

TREATMENTS: Tricyclic antidepressants for psychological problems and neuroleptics for chorea

---

TREATMENT AND THERAPY

The present treatment for Huntington's disease is the use of drugs such as tricyclic antidepressants to control psychological problems and neuroleptics to treat the associated chorea. In 2003, clinical trials were examining the effects of implanting fetal neurons into the brains of Huntington's disease patients.

PERSPECTIVE AND PROSPECTS

In 1872, George Huntington first reported this hereditary disease that he observed in a Long Island, New York, family. Because of the uncoordinated movements of patients, he termed the condition "chorea," from the Greek word for "dance." In 1981, Nancy Wexler began to study a large extended family with Huntington's disease in an isolated village on Lake Maracaibo, Venezuela. Studies of this family aided the work of localizing the gene responsible for this disease. In 1993, that gene was identified by the collaborative work of fifty-eight scientists, led by James R. Gusella and Francis S. Collins.

—*Susan J. Karcher, Ph.D.*

See also Brain; Brain disorders; Genetic diseases; Motor neuron diseases; Nervous system; Neuralgia, neuritis, and neuropathy; Neurology; Neurology, pediatric; Tics.

FOR FURTHER INFORMATION:

Cattaneo, Elena, Dorotea Rigamonti, and Chaiara Zuccato. "The Enigma of Huntington's Disease." *Scientific American* 287 (December, 2002): 92-97.

Lewis, Ricki. *Human Genetics: Concepts and Applications.* 5th ed. Boston: McGraw-Hill Higher Education, 2003.

Nussbaum, Robert L., Roderick R. McInnes, and Huntington F. Willard, eds. *Thompson and Thompson*

Genetics in Medicine. 6th ed. Philadelphia: W. B. Saunders, 2001.

Rubinsztein, David C. "Lessons from Animal Models of Huntington's Disease." *Trends in Genetics* 18 (April 4, 2002): 202-209.

HYDROCELECTOMY
PROCEDURE
ANATOMY OR SYSTEM AFFECTED: Genitals, reproductive system

SPECIALTIES AND RELATED FIELDS: General surgery, urology

DEFINITION: The removal of a hydrocele, a collection of fluid between the lining membranes protecting the testicle in the scrotum.

INDICATIONS AND PROCEDURES

Hydrocelectomy is primarily indicated for hydroceles in adults which produce discomfort, objectionable scrotal enlargement, or an uncertainty regarding underlying testicular abnormalities upon scrotal ultrasound or physical examination. The presence of a hydrocele does not necessarily require surgical intervention, drainage, or other intervention; it must be accompanied by some significant abnormality to require surgery.

Hydroceles occur in 1 percent of adult males. In patients between the ages of eighteen and thirty-five, the presence of an underlying testicular tumor must be ruled out. Accurate diagnosis can be carried out through physical examination. A hydrocele is a smooth, cystlike mass completely surrounding the testicle such that only the mass can be palpated; the testis, inside, cannot be felt. Hydroceles do not involve the spermatic cord. When a light is shined through the cyst, the light is readily transmitted. If the hydrocele is large or tense and the testis cannot be examined, ultrasound examination can eliminate the diagnosis of a testicular abnormality.

Surgical excision is the most effective method for treatment and can be done on an outpatient basis. A 5.0- to 7.6-centimeter (2.0- to 3.0-inch) incision is made in the scrotum, and the wall of the hydrocele is identified and dissected free. The hydrocele sac is removed and its edges sewn or cauterized to eliminate bleeding. The testis is then returned to the scrotum, and the incision is closed. For large hydroceles, a small drainage tube is introduced into the scrotum to limit swelling.

USES AND COMPLICATIONS

The most frequent complication of hydrocele surgery is scrotal swelling, which may continue for eight weeks.

Most patients return to full activity within seven to ten days of surgery, however, and recurrences are rare.

In addition to surgical removal, other treatment options include needle aspiration and aspiration with the injection of sclerosing agents. Needle aspiration is rarely effective and increases infection risk. Fluid usually reaccumulates within three months of aspiration. Aspiration with the injection of sclerosing agents such as tetracycline is successful in fewer than 50 percent of patients and usually requires multiple treatments.

—Culley C. Carson III, M.D.

See also Abscess drainage; Cyst removal; Reproductive system; Testicular surgery.

FOR FURTHER INFORMATION:
Glenn, James F., ed. *Glenn's Urologic Surgery.* 5th ed. Philadelphia: J. B. Lippincott, 1998.

Kay, K. W., R. V. Clayman, and P. H. Lange. "Outpatient Hydrocele and Spermatocele Repair Under Local Anesthesia." *Journal of Urology* 130, no. 2 (August, 1983): 269-271.

Sherwood, Lauralee. *Human Physiology: From Cells to Systems.* 4th ed. Belmont, Calif.: Wadsworth, 2001.

HYDROCEPHALUS
DISEASE/DISORDER
ALSO KNOWN AS: "Water on the brain"

ANATOMY OR SYSTEM AFFECTED: Brain, head, nervous system, psychic-emotional system

SPECIALTIES AND RELATED FIELDS: Critical care, general surgery, neonatology, neurology, perinatology

DEFINITION: A collection of excessive amounts of cerebrospinal fluid (CSF) within the cranial cavity, which can cause increased pressure within the brain and skull, leading to brain tissue damage and, in infants, enlargement of the skull.

KEY TERMS:

cerebrospinal fluid (CSF): the fluid that bathes and nourishes the inner and outer surfaces of the brain and spinal cord

shunt: a tube that is surgically inserted to drain excess fluid away from an area such as the brain

"water on the brain": a common term for hydrocephalus

CAUSES AND SYMPTOMS

Frequently referred to as "water on the brain," hydrocephalus is a disorder most commonly seen in new-

INFORMATION ON HYDROCEPHALUS

CAUSES: Congenital defect, head injury, infection, brain hemorrhage, tumor
SYMPTOMS: Enlarged head, lethargy, vomiting, irritability, epilepsy, rigidity of legs, loss of normal reflexes
DURATION: Typically chronic
TREATMENTS: Surgery

borns and infants but sometimes occurring in older children and adults. The water is actually a relatively small amount (about 10 cubic centimeters for every kilogram of body weight) of cerebrospinal fluid (CSF), which surrounds and cushions the brain and spinal cord on both the inside and the outside. Within the brain are four CSF-filled spaces called ventricles. The CSF is continuously formed here and then moves down through the central canal, a tube that runs the length of the spinal cord. From the base of the spine, the fluid moves upward on the outside of the spinal cord, returning to the skull, where it covers the outer surfaces of the brain. Here it is absorbed by the brain's outer lining. If interference occurs in any part of this process, CSF continues to accumulate in the brain. This usually causes increased pressure to develop within the skull. Abnormally high pressure can lead to permanent brain damage and even death. In the infant, this accumulation also causes the skull to enlarge, since the growth regions of the skull have not yet become firm.

Excessive CSF may develop due to overproduction of fluid in the brain, a blockage of the fluid's circulation, or a blockage of fluid reabsorption on the brain's surface. Hydrocephalus can be congenital or may develop as a result of a head injury, infection, brain hemorrhage, or tumor. Congenital hydrocephalus and most hydrocephalus that begins in infancy are characterized by an enlarged head, which continues to grow at an abnormally rapid pace.

Symptoms and signs that accompany congenital hydrocephalus include lethargy, vomiting, irritability, epilepsy, rigidity of the legs, and the loss of normal reflexes. If left untreated, the condition causes drowsiness, seizures, and severe brain damage, leading to death possibly within days or weeks. Hydrocephalus is also often associated with other anomalies of the brain and nervous system, such as spina bifida.

When hydrocephalus develops in older children and adults, the head size will not increase since the growth lines in the bones of the skull have hardened. If the CSF pressure increases, resulting symptoms include headaches, vomiting, vision problems, problems with muscle coordination, and a progressive decrease in mental activity.

TREATMENT AND THERAPY

Diagnosis of hydrocephalus and related nervous system defects sometimes can be made before birth, either by fetal ultrasound or by testing for the presence of an abnormal amount of a brain-associated protein, alpha-fetoprotein, in the pregnant woman's blood. However, even with early diagnosis and surgical intervention promptly after birth, the prognosis is guarded.

Older children and adults suspected of having hydrocephalus should be examined by a neurologist. A computed tomography (CT) scan or magnetic resonance imaging (MRI) of the brain can visualize the structure of the brain and the extent of the hydrocephalus.

Surgical correction is the primary treatment for hydrocephalus. The excess pressure must be drained from within the brain, or a balance between the production and elimination of CSF must be established. In some cases, a combination of surgery and medication is successful. For example, the drugs furosemide (Lasix)

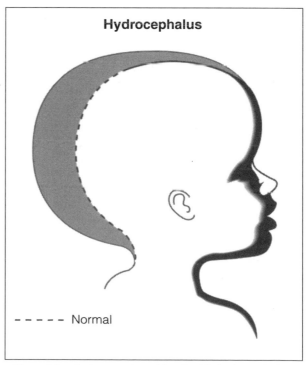

Normal head size vs. size of head with hydrocephalus.

and acetazolamide (Diamox), when used for increased CSF pressure from brain hemorrhage, may reduce the amount of CSF fluid produced and thereby decrease the amount of swelling.

Relieving the CSF pressure within the brain is generally achieved by the surgical insertion of a tube, called a shunt, through brain tissue into one of the cerebral ventricles. A one-way valve is attached to the tube; this allows CSF to escape from the skull cavity when the pressure exceeds a certain level. The tubing is then passed beneath the skin into either the right side of the heart or the abdominal cavity, where the excessive CSF can be absorbed safely. Complications of this procedure are fairly common and include repeated infections, septicemia, peritonitis, or meningitis.

PERSPECTIVE AND PROSPECTS

The outcome of treated patients with hydrocephalus has improved over the years, but the condition is still associated with long-term problems. A modest percentage of newborns with congenital hydrocephalus will survive and achieve normal intelligence.

—*Cynthia Beres*

See also Birth defects; Brain; Brain disorders; Childbirth complications; Critical care, pediatric; Fetal surgery; Meningitis; Mental retardation; Neonatology; Nervous system; Neurology, pediatric; Pediatrics; Shunts; Spina bifida; Spinal cord disorders; Surgery, pediatric.

FOR FURTHER INFORMATION:

Behrman, Richard E., et al. *Nelson Textbook of Pediatrics.* 17th ed. New York: Elsevier, 2003. Text covering all medical and surgical disorders in children, with authoritative information on genetics, endocrinology, aetiology, epidemiology, pathology, pathophysiology, clinical manifestations, diagnosis, prevention, treatment, and prognosis.

Clayman, Charles B., ed. *The American Medical Association Encyclopedia of Medicine.* New York: Random House, 1994. A concise presentation of numerous medical terms and illnesses. A good general reference.

Hydrocephalus Association, The. http://www.hydro assoc.org/. A Web site that provides information and resources, support, and educational help to patients with hydrocephalus.

Merenstein, Gerald B., and Sandra L. Gardner. *Handbook of Neonatal Intensive Care.* 5th ed. New York: Elsevier, 2002. A text covering clinical issues such as nutritional and metabolic support and diseases of the neonate.

Nixon, Harold, and Barry O'Donnel. *The Essentials of Pediatric Surgery.* 4th ed. Boston: Butterworth Heinemann, 1992. Describes in accessible terms the surgical treatment of many congenital abnormalities, including birth injuries, imperforate anus, spina bifida, hydrocephalus, pyloric stenosis, birthmarks, cleft lip and palate, and hernias.

Professional Guide to Diseases. 7th ed. Springhouse, Pa.: Springhouse, 2001. A comprehensive yet concise medical reference covering more than six hundred disorders.

Toporek, Chuck, and Kellie Robinson. *Hydrocephalus: A Guide for Patients, Families, and Friends.* Sebastopol, Calif.: O'Reilly & Associates, 1999. Provides clear advice on living with hydrocephalus.

HYDROTHERAPY

PROCEDURE

ANATOMY OR SYSTEM AFFECTED: All

SPECIALTIES AND RELATED FIELDS: Alternative medicine, physical therapy, rheumatology, sports medicine

DEFINITION: Exercise in warm water, which can aid in the treatments of several disorders.

INDICATIONS AND PROCEDURES

Hydrotherapy is one of the oldest therapies still in use. A procedure with origins in ancient Greece has today found a place in alternative medicine. In many hospitals across the United States, physicians advocate hydrotherapy, or water treatment.

One use of hydrotherapy is as an alternative method of exercising for patients with chronic heart failure, since the buoyancy effect reduces loading. Exercises to improve mobility, strength, and cardiovascular fitness can be provided easily in water. Immersion in warm water has been used in bathing resorts in Europe since the beginning of the twentieth century to reduce heart failure symptoms as well as to enhance heart function.

Systemic diseases such as diabetes mellitus, peripheral heart disease, neuropathy, steroid dependence, and venous stasis are major contributing factors to form chronic wounds. The consequence is a non-healing wound with hypoxia, infection, edema, and metabolic abnormalities. Patients with such wounds, in need of extensive debridement, are usually advised to be immersed in a full-body whirlpool. The reason behind whirlpool therapy is that whirling and agitation of the water, with injected air, removes contaminants and toxic debris and dilutes bacterial contents. The common therapeutic protocol is a twenty-to-thirty-minute session, three to four times per week. Typically, this regimen is continued for a brief period.

Physical therapists have always recommended hydrotherapy to relieve extreme pain. Therefore it is not surprising that it has found a place in providing relief for patients with fibromyalgia.

Another area where hydrotherapy has found popularity is in labor and childbirth. Studies indicate using hydrotherapy for relief of rapid pain and anxiety in labor. Subjective maternal responses to bathing in labor have been favorable. No maternal or infant infections have been attributed to bathing with intact or ruptured membranes. Maternal bathing in labor does not appear to affect Apgar scores or stress hormones at birth.

A recent study indicates that hydrotherapy has proven to be beneficial in treating Rett's syndrome. An eleven-year-old girl with stage III Rett's syndrome was treated with hydrotherapy in a swimming pool twice a week for eight weeks. In conclusion, after the application of hydrotherapy, stereotypical hand movements had decreased and purposeful hand functions and feeding skills had increased.

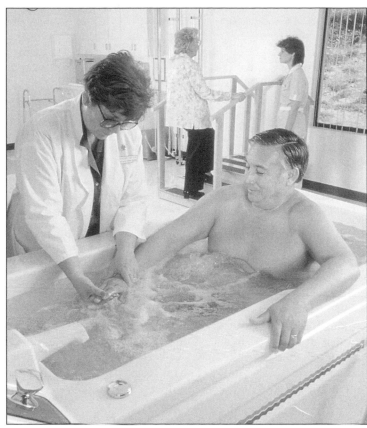

A patient receives a therapeutic bath. (Digital Stock)

PERSPECTIVE AND PROSPECTS

Ancient Greek literature contains a considerably large volume of published articles concerning different types of baths and hydrotherapy. These topics were addressed for preventive, hygienic, or therapeutic purposes. These Greek baths were classified in two categories: cold water baths and hot water baths. Cold water baths were said to slow down blood circulation; decrease the amount of sweat; increase muscular strength, the ability to work, and a sense of well-being; and improve physical, mental, and moral balance. The hot water baths were reported to be relaxing, antispasmodic, and beneficial for treating nervous disturbances.

—*Giri Sulur, Ph.D.*

See also Alternative medicine; Cardiac rehabilitation; Childbirth; Colon therapy; Exercise physiology; Fibromyalgia; Healing; Heart failure; Pain management; Physical rehabilitation; Sports medicine.

FOR FURTHER INFORMATION:

Buchman, Dian Dincin. *The Complete Book of Water Healing.* 2d ed. New York: McGraw-Hill/Contemporary Books, 2001.

Ruoti, Richard G., David M. Morris, and Andrew J. Cole, eds. *Aquatic Rehabilitation.* Philadelphia: Lippincott, 1997.

Ryrie, Charlie. *The Healing Energies of Water.* North Clarendon, Vt.: Charles Tuttle, 1999.

HYPERADIPOSIS

DISEASE/DISORDER

ALSO KNOWN AS: Severe obesity, extreme obesity
ANATOMY OR SYSTEM AFFECTED: All
SPECIALTIES AND RELATED FIELDS: Biochemistry, endocrinology, family practice, genetics, nutrition
DEFINITION: Having excess body fat; exceeding 200 percent of standard body weight as defined on a height-weight table.

CAUSES AND SYMPTOMS

Obesity results from consuming more calories than the body uses. Severe obesity accounts for less than 1 percent of all obesity in the United States but is linked to a large number of deaths each year, many of them due to heart disease or diabetes. Genetics, socioeconomic status, and emotional disturbances may all contribute to severe obesity.

One leading theory proposes that body weight is regulated by a set point in the hypothalamus (a section of the brain), similar to a thermostat setting. A higher-than-normal set point would explain why some people are obese and why losing weight and maintaining weight loss are difficult for them. It is also well established that an increase in the size and/or number of fat cells adds to the amount of fat stored by the body. Those who become obese during early childhood may have up to five times as many fat cells as people of normal weight. Because the number of cells cannot be reduced, weight loss can come about only by decreasing the amount of fat stored in each cell.

Accumulation of excess fat below the diaphragm and in the chest wall places pressure on the lungs, leading to shortness of breath and difficulty in breathing, even with minimal exertion. This may also seriously interfere with sleep. Low back pain and osteoarthritis, especially in the hips, knees, and ankles, may be seen, and skin disorders are common, owing to moisture retention in the folds of the fatty skin. Because of a low ratio of surface area to body weight in severe obesity, the body has a hard time getting rid of excess body heat, leading to excessive sweating and fluid accumulation in the ankles and feet.

Fat tends to accumulate in the abdomen in males, and in the thighs and buttocks in females. Abdominal obesity in particular is linked with a high incidence of coronary artery disease, high blood pressure, adult onset diabetes, hyperlipidemia, and gallbladder disease. In addition, an increase in menstrual disorders and in breast, uterine, and ovarian cancer is seen in women. Men have higher rates of colorectal and prostate cancer.

TREATMENT AND THERAPY

Self-help and nonclinical weight loss programs rarely work in individuals with severe obesity. Clinical programs that combine supervised weight loss, behavior modification, and exercise have shown good results. Drugs such as amphetamines (ephedrine) have questionable value in cases of severe obesity. Total fasting produces a risk of ketonemia and electrolyte imbalances, leading to cardiac arrhythmias.

Surgery has become an increasingly popular form of treatment. Vertical banded gastroplasty (stomach stapling) and gastric bypass are the most common procedures. Both produce satiety with small food intake and, if coupled with exercise, can result in weight losses approximating one-half of the excess weight (80 to 160 pounds). Jejunoileal bypass is also effective but produces a permanent malabsorption syndrome that may lead to other metabolic problems. Liposuction, where a small incision is made and fatty deposits are suctioned out, produces only moderate results in the severely obese. Because of potential risks to blood vessels and nerves, only a small amount of fat can be removed from each location.

Leptin, the protein hormone product of the ob gene, has been suggested as a useful new treatment for severe obesity. However, only about 5 percent of obese individuals fail to produce leptin on their own, and in those individuals either daily injections of leptin or gene therapy to correct the chromosomal defect would be required. Neither is currently considered a practical solution.

PERSPECTIVE AND PROSPECTS

Since 1900, the incidence of severe obesity in the United States has more than doubled, despite the fact that the average number of calories consumed per day has decreased by 10 percent. The most likely explanation is a decrease in physical activity among the population at large. While everyone needs to be conscious of dietary intake and exercise needs, parents of young children in particular need to be careful not to use food as either reward or punishment, as the early years of de-

---

INFORMATION ON HYPERADIPOSIS

CAUSES: Sedentary lifestyle, genetic predisposition, diet, emotional disorders
SYMPTOMS: Shortness of breath, difficulty breathing, sleep disruption, low back pain, osteoarthritis, skin disorders, excessive sweating, fluid accumulation in the ankles and feet
DURATION: Often chronic
TREATMENTS: Clinical programs combining supervised weight loss, behavior modification, and exercise; surgery if needed

velopment appear to be most crucial in setting the stage for later obesity.

—*Kerry L. Cheesman, Ph.D.*

See also Bariatric surgery; Eating disorders; Glands; Leptin; Malnutrition; Nutrition; Obesity; Weight loss and gain; Weight loss medications.

FOR FURTHER INFORMATION:

American Obesity Association. http://www.obesity .org/. A comprehensive Web site with information on the disease, research resources, advocacy, disability issues, community action, personal stories, among many other topics.

Bennett, J. Claude, et al., eds. *Cecil Textbook of Medicine.* 21st ed. Philadelphia: W. B. Saunders, 2000. This textbook offers a brief review of all aspects of the problem of obesity by a recognized authority in the field.

Bjorntorp, Per, ed. *International Textbook of Obesity.* New York: Wiley, 2001. Text that examines the epidemiology, causes, and current research and management.

Brownell, Kelly D., and Katherine Battle Morgen. *Food Fight: The Inside Story of America's Obesity Crisis and What We Can Do About It.* New York: McGraw-Hill, 2003. A critical examination of the United States' "toxic environment" of obesity. Explores the roots of the obesity epidemic and its impact on the country's health and productivity.

Consensus Development Conference Panel. "Gastrointestinal Surgery for Severe Obesity: Consensus Development Conference Statement." *Annals of Internal Medicine* 115, no. 12 (1991): 956-961. Describes a consensus reached by leading surgeons, gastroenterologists, endocrinologists, psychiatrists, and nutritionists on the status of surgical procedures for the treatment of severe and intractable obesity.

Ravussin, Eric, and Albert J. Stunkard. *Handbook of Obesity Treatment.* New York: Guilford Press, 2002. A comprehensive text that examines the epidemiology, prevalence, and health consequences of obesity. Topics include binge-eating disorder and night-eating syndrome, energy metabolism, genetics, exercise, behavioral weight control, drug and surgical treatment, and treatment in minorities and children.

Smith, J. Clinton. *Understanding Childhood Obesity.* Tuscaloosa: University of Mississippi Press, 1999. A handbook explaining the basic body pro- cesses and the research underway to combat childhood obesity.

HYPERCHOLESTEROLEMIA
DISEASE/DISORDER

ANATOMY OR SYSTEM AFFECTED: Blood, blood vessels, circulatory system, heart, liver

SPECIALTIES AND RELATED FIELDS: Cardiology, hematology, nutrition, pharmacology, vascular medicine

DEFINITION: A high level of cholesterol in the bloodstream, which is considered a major risk factor for heart attack or stroke.

CAUSES AND SYMPTOMS

It has been difficult for the medical profession to establish a clear, causal connection between high cholesterol in the blood and heart disease. Only by studying a large number of patients over an extended time, as was done at Framingham, Massachusetts, was it possible to establish a now widely accepted statistical correlation between high cholesterol and cardiovascular problems. Cholesterol is a fatty material similar to animal fats, which are called lipids. In the bloodstream, cholesterol lipids combine with proteins to form either a low-density lipoprotein (LDL) or high-density lipoprotein (HDL). LDL transports cholesterol from the liver and intestines to other parts of the body where it is needed. HDL transports excess cholesterol back to the liver, where it is metabolized and excreted. HDL prevents excess fat from being deposited on the walls of arteries and therefore is commonly called the

---

INFORMATION ON HYPERCHOLESTEROLEMIA

CAUSES: Diet, high levels of low-density lipoproteins (LDLs) and low levels of high-density lipoproteins (HDLs)

SYMPTOMS: Plaque buildup on artery walls and possible blockage, causing stroke or heart attack

DURATION: Chronic

TREATMENTS: Dietary changes (increase in vegetables, fruits, and grains and decrease in red meat, egg yolks, and high-fat dairy products); increased physical exercise; medications (Zocor, Lipitor)

"good" cholesterol. Research has established that LDL in blood should be less than 200 milligrams per deciliter, whereas HDL should be greater than 50 milligrams per deciliter, with a ratio of LDL to HDL of preferably four or less. A person is not aware of having high cholesterol. If the condition is not treated, however, then the likelihood of plaque buildup on artery walls and a possible blockage, causing a stroke or heart attack, is increased.

TREATMENT AND THERAPY

The first step to reduce excess cholesterol in the bloodstream is a change in diet. As a general guideline, the consumption of vegetables, fruits, and grains should be increased, while red meat, egg yolks, and high-fat dairy products should be decreased. Vegetable oils made from corn, olives, or soybeans, which are low in saturated fats, are preferable to butter and animal fats. The next step is to increase physical exercise, which generally raises HDL, the good cholesterol. Several prescription medications, such as Zocor or Lipitor, have been shown to be effective in lowering LDL. A physician needs to monitor a patient's liver function to verify that no harmful side effects are occurring.

PERSPECTIVE AND PROSPECTS

The 1985 Nobel Prize in Medicine was awarded to Drs. Michael Brown and Joseph Goldstein for their study of cell-surface receptors that control the entry of LDL into cells. They showed that some people have a deficiency of these receptors. As a result, LDL does not enter cells at the normal rate but continues to circulate in the bloodstream, where it then can adhere to artery walls. In the future, it may be possible to produce drugs that stimulate the body to make more LDL receptors, which would remove excess LDL from the bloodstream.

—*Hans G. Graetzer, Ph.D.*

See also Arteriosclerosis; Blood and blood disorders; Cholesterol; Heart disease; Hyperlipidemia; Lipids; Steroids.

FOR FURTHER INFORMATION:

Clayman, Charles B., ed. *American Medical Association Family Medical Guide*. New York: Random House, 1994.

Cooper, Kenneth H. *Controlling Cholesterol the Natural Way*. New York: Bantam Books, 1999.

Kowalski, Robert E. *The Eight-Week Cholesterol Cure*. New York: Harper & Row, 1987.

HYPERLIPIDEMIA

DISEASE/DISORDER

ANATOMY OR SYSTEM AFFECTED: Blood

SPECIALTIES AND RELATED FIELDS: Family practice, hematology, internal medicine, serology, vascular medicine

DEFINITION: The presence of abnormally large amounts of lipids (fats) in the blood.

CAUSES AND SYMPTOMS

Although elevated triglyceride levels have been implicated in clinical ischemic diseases, most investigators believe that cholesterol-rich lipids are a more significant risk factor. Although measurements of both cholesterol and triglyceride levels have been used to predict coronary disease, studies suggest that the determination of the alpha-lipoprotein/beta-lipoprotein ratio is a more reliable predictor. Because the alpha-lipoprotein has a higher density than the beta-lipoprotein, they are more often designated as high-density lipoprotein (HDL) and low-density lipoprotein (LDL), respectively. HDL is often referred to as "good cholesterol," and LDL is referred to as "bad cholesterol." The latter is implicated in the development of atherosclerosis.

Atherosclerosis is a disease that begins in the innermost lining of the arterial wall. Its lesions occur predominantly at arterial forks and branch openings, but they can also occur at sites where there is injury to the arterial lining. The initial lesion usually appears as fatty streaks or spots, which have been detected even at birth. With passing years, more of these lesions appear, and they may develop into elevated plaques that obstruct the flow of blood in the artery. The lesions are rich in cholesterol derived from beta-lipoproteins in the plasma. In addition to elevated blood lipids, other risk factors associated with atherosclerosis include hypertension, faulty arterial structure, obesity, smoking, and stress.

TREATMENT AND THERAPY

The treatment of hyperlipidemia involves both dietary and drug therapies. Although studies in nonhuman primates indicate that the reduction of hyperlipidemia results in decreased morbidity and mortality rates from arterial vascular disease, studies in humans are less conclusive. Initial treatment involves restricting the dietary intake of cholesterol and saturated fat. Drug therapy is instituted when further lowering of the serum lipids is desired. Among the drugs that have been used as antihyperlipidemic agents are lovastatin and its analogs, clofibrate and its analogs (particularly gemfibrozil), nicotinic acid, D-thyroxine, cholestyramine, probucol, and heparin. A simplified diagram of the endogenous biosynthesis and biotransformation of cholesterol is given below.

acetate → C acetyl SCoA → HMGCoA → MVA → squalene → desmosterol → cholesterol → bile acids

Lovastatin blocks the synthesis of cholesterol by inhibiting the enzyme (HMGCoA reductase) that catalyzes the conversion of beta-hydroxy-beta-methyl glutaryl coenzyme A (HMGCoA) to mevalonic acid (MVA), the regulatory step in the biosynthesis of cholesterol. Both lovastatin and MVA are beta, delta-dihydroxy acids, but lovastatin has a much more lipophilic (fat-soluble) group attached to it. Clofibrate and gemfibrozil block the synthesis of cholesterol prior to the HMGCoA stage. For this reason, they are likely to inhibit triglyceride formation as well. Nicotinic acid inhibits the synthesis of acetyl coenzyme A (acetyl SCoA) and thus would be expected to block the synthesis of both cholesterol and the triglycerides. To be effective in lowering the serum level of lipids, nicotinic acid must be taken in large amounts, which often produces an unpleasant flushing sensation in the patient. A way to inhibit the synthesis of cholesterol at the post-MVA stages has also been sought. Agents such as triparanol, which inhibit biosynthesis near the end of the synthetic sequence, have been developed. Although they are effective in lowering serum cholesterol, they had to be withdrawn from clinical use because of their adverse side effects on the muscles and eyes. Moreover, the penultimate product in the biosynthesis of cholesterol proved to be atherogenic. Investigations are being conducted on the inhibition of cholesterol synthesis at both the immediate presqualene and immediate post-squalene stages. The effects of such inhibitors on the production of steroid hormones and ubiquinones, as well as on cholesterol and triglycerides, are expected to be of considerable interest.

INFORMATION ON HYPERLIPIDEMIA

CAUSES: Hypertension, faulty arterial structure, obesity, smoking, stress
SYMPTOMS: Development of atherosclerosis
DURATION: Varies; often chronic
TREATMENTS: Dietary changes, drug therapy

D-thyroxine promotes the metabolism of cholesterol in the liver, transforming it into the more hydrophilic (water-soluble) bile acids, thereby facilitating its elimination from the body. An approach to reducing the serum level of cholesterol by a process involving the sequestering of the bile acids utilizes the resin cholestyramine as the sequestrant. The sequestered bile acids cannot be reabsorbed into the enterohepatic system and are eliminated in the feces. Consequently, more cholesterol is oxidized to the bile acids, resulting in the reduction of the serum level of cholesterol. Unfortunately, a large quantity of cholestyramine is required. Sequestration of cholesterol with beta-sitosterol prevents both the absorption of dietary cholesterol and the reabsorption of endogenous cholesterol in the intestines. Here, too, a large quantity of the sequestrant needs to be administered.

Probucol is an antioxidant. Because, structurally, it is a sulfur analog of a hindered hydroquinone, it acts as a free radical scavenger. Evidence suggests that the antihyperlipidemic effect of probucol is attributable to its ability to inhibit the oxygenation of LDL. The oxygenated LDL is believed to be the atherogenic form of LDL. Heparin promotes the hydrolysis of triglycerides as it activates lipoprotein lipase, thereby reducing lipidemia. Because of its potent anticoagulant properties, however, its use in therapy must be closely monitored. Cholesterol that is present in atherosclerotic plaques is acylated, generally by the more saturated fatty acids. The enzyme catalyzing the acylation process is acyl-CoA cholesterol acyl transferase (ACAT). The development of regulators of ACAT and the desirability of reducing the dietary intake of saturated fatty acids are based on this rationale.

Cholesterol within the cell is able to inhibit further synthesis of cholesterol by a feedback mechanism. Cholesterol that is associated with LDL is transported into the hepatic cell by means of the LDL receptor on the surface of the cell. In individuals who are afflicted with familial hypercholesterolemia, an inherited disorder that causes death at an early age, the gene that is responsible for the production of the LDL receptor is either absent or defective. Studies in gene therapy have shown that transplant of the normal LDL receptor gene to such an individual results in a dramatic decrease in the level of the "bad cholesterol" in the serum. Cholesterol derivatives that are oxygenated at various positions have also been found to regulate the serum level of cholesterol by either inhibiting its synthesis or promoting its catabolism. More studies need to be done, however, in order to demonstrate their effectiveness in humans and to establish that they themselves do not induce atherosclerosis.

—Leland J. Chinn, Ph.D.

See also Arteriosclerosis; Blood and blood disorders; Cholesterol; Heart disease; Hypercholesterolemia; Hypertension; Insulin resistance syndrome; Metabolic syndrome; Metabolism; Obesity.

FOR FURTHER INFORMATION:

Anderson, J. W. "Diet First, Then Medication for Hypercholesterolemia." *JAMA: The Journal of the American Medical Association* 290, no. 4 (July 23, 2003): 531-533. Examines the therapeutic use of anticholesteremic agents and diet therapy as treatment for hyperlipidemia.

Ball, Madeleine, and Jim Mann. *Lipids and Heart Disease: A Guide for the Primary Care Team.* 2d ed. Oxford, England: Oxford University Press, 1994. Topics include the function of lipids, plasma lipids and coronary heart disease, atherosclerosis, and hyperlipidemia.

Farnier, Michel, and Jean Davignon. "Current and Future Treatment of Hyperlipidemia: The Role of Statins." *The American Journal of Cardiology* 82, no. 4B (August 27, 1998): 3J-10J. Hyperlipidemia is recognized as one of the major risk factors for the development of coronary artery disease and progression of the atherosclerotic lesions. Dietary therapy together with hypolipidemic drugs is central to the management of hyperlipidemia.

Haffner, Steven M. "Diabetes, Hyperlipidemia, and Coronary Artery Disease." *The American Journal of Cardiology* 83, no. 9B (May 13, 1999): 17F-21F. Type 2 diabetes is associated with a marked increase in the risk of coronary artery disease. Dyslipidemia is believed to be a major source of this increased risk.

Hirsch, Anita. *Good Cholesterol, Bad Cholesterol: An Indispensable Guide to the Facts About Cholesterol.* New York: Avalon, 2002. Examines the facts on all the varieties of cholesterol, including HDL, LDL, and VDL. Also discusses how to determine what your blood cholesterol test results mean and how to manage cholesterol levels through diet, exercise, and stress management.

McGowan, Mary P., and Jo McGowan Chopra. *Fifty Ways to Lower Cholesterol.* New York: McGraw-Hill, 2002. Provides explanations of both "good" and "bad" cholesterol and the latest information on key treatments, medication, and lifestyle issues.

Rifkind, Basil M., ed. *Drug Treatment of Hyperlipidemia.* New York: Marcel Dekker, 1991. Discusses such topics as hyperlipoproteinemia and antilipemic agents. Includes bibliographical references and an index.

Safeer, Richard S., and Cynthia L. Lacivita. "Choosing Drug Therapy for Patients with Hyperlipidemia." *American Family Physician* 61, no. 11 (June 1, 2000): 3371-3382. Almost thirteen million American adults require drug therapy to meet the low-density lipoprotein goals set by the National Cholesterol Education Program.

Witiak, D. T., H. A. I. Newman, and D. R. Feller, eds. *Antilipidemic Drugs: Medicinal, Chemical, and Biochemical Aspects.* Amsterdam: Elsevier, 1991. Discusses such topics as antilipemic agents, lipids, and lipoproteins. Includes bibliographical references.

HYPERPARATHYROIDISM AND HYPOPARATHYROIDISM

DISEASE/DISORDER

ANATOMY OR SYSTEM AFFECTED: Endocrine system, glands, musculoskeletal system, neck

SPECIALTIES AND RELATED FIELDS: Endocrinology

DEFINITION: Excessive, uncontrolled secretion (hyperparathyroidism) or reduced secretion (hypoparathyroidism) of parathyroid hormone.

CAUSES AND SYMPTOMS

The precise regulation of calcium is vital to the survival and well-being of all animals. Approximately 99 percent of the calcium in the body is found in bones and teeth. Of the remaining 1 percent, about 0.9 percent is packaged within specialized organelles inside the cell. This leaves only 0.1 percent of the total body calcium in blood. Approximately half of this calcium is either bound to proteins or complexed with phosphate. The other half of blood calcium is free to be utilized by cells. For this reason, it is critical that calcium inside the cell be rigorously maintained at extremely low concentrations. Even a slight change in calcium outside the cell can have dramatic consequences.

The function and regulation of calcium. Calcium plays a vital role in many different areas of the body. For example, the entry of calcium into secretory cells, such as nerve cells, triggers the release of neurotransmitters into the synapse. A fall in blood calcium results in the overexcitability of nerves, which can be felt as a tingling sensation and numbness in the extremities. Similarly, calcium entry into cells is essential for muscle contraction in both heart and skeletal muscle.

Free calcium is thus one of the most tightly regulated substances in the body. The key player in the moment-to-moment regulation of calcium is parathyroid hormone (PTH). PTH is synthesized in the parathyroid glands, a paired gland located in the neck, and released in response to a fall in blood calcium. PTH serves several functions: to increase blood calcium, to decrease blood phosphate, and to stimulate the conversion of vitamin D into its active form, which can then stimulate the uptake of calcium across the digestive tract. Together these actions result in an increase in free calcium, which returns calcium concentrations in the blood to normal.

PTH binds to specific receptors located primarily in bone and kidney tissue. Since most calcium is stored in bone, it serves as a bank for withdrawal of calcium in times of need. Activation of a PTH receptor on osteoclasts, or bone-cutting cells, results in the production of concentrated acids that dissolve calcium from bone, thereby making more free calcium available to the blood supply. PTH also acts on the kidney, where it

> **INFORMATION ON HYPERPARATHYROIDISM AND HYPOPARATHYROIDISM**
>
> **CAUSES:** Endocrine disorder, aging, disease, accidental removal of parathyroid gland or damage to its blood supply
> **SYMPTOMS:** Osteoporosis, muscle weakness, nausea, kidney stones, peptic ulcers, muscle cramps, seizures, paranoia, depression
> **DURATION:** Often chronic
> **TREATMENTS:** Drug therapy, hormonal therapy (*e.g.*, estrogen), surgery, vitamin D supplements, calcium restriction or supplements

stimulates calcium uptake from the urine while promoting phosphate elimination. As a result, more calcium is made available to the blood and less phosphate is available to form complexes with the free calcium.

By exerting these effects on its target organs, PTH can restore low calcium concentrations in the blood to

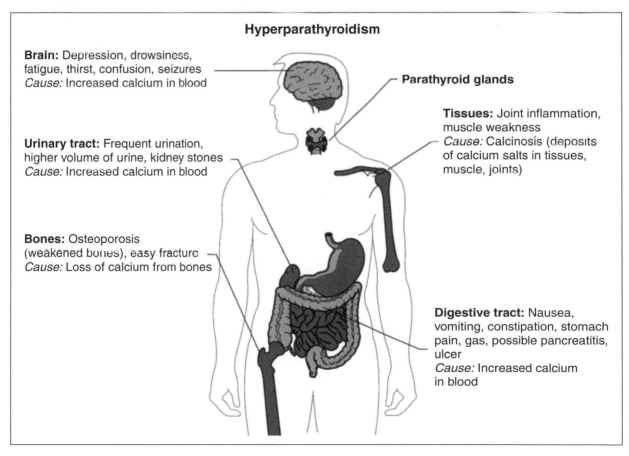

Hyperparathyroidism

Brain: Depression, drowsiness, fatigue, thirst, confusion, seizures
Cause: Increased calcium in blood

Parathyroid glands

Tissues: Joint inflammation, muscle weakness
Cause: Calcinosis (deposits of calcium salts in tissues, muscle, joints)

Urinary tract: Frequent urination, higher volume of urine, kidney stones
Cause: Increased calcium in blood

Bones: Osteoporosis (weakened bones), easy fracture
Cause: Loss of calcium from bones

Digestive tract: Nausea, vomiting, constipation, stomach pain, gas, possible pancreatitis, ulcer
Cause: Increased calcium in blood

normal. Once calcium has returned to a particular set point, PTH secretion is slowed dramatically. If PTH release is not controlled, however, the imbalance in calcium can lead to life-threatening situations. These conditions are termed hyperparathyroidism and hypoparathyroidism.

Hyperparathyroidism. This disorder is defined as the excessive and uncontrolled secretion of PTH. The release of a closely related substance, PTH-related protein, from cancer cells can also cause this condition. Hyperparathyroidism is found in 0.1 percent of the population and is more common in the elderly, who have an incidence rate of approximately 2 percent.

There are two types of hyperparathyroidism, primary and secondary. Primary hyperparathyroidism is caused by disease or damage to the parathyroid glands. For example, cancer of the parathyroid gland can result in the uncontrolled release of PTH and is characterized by an increase in blood calcium. The symptoms associated with primary hyperparathyroidism include osteoporosis, muscle weakness, nausea, and increased incidence of kidney stones and peptic ulcers. These symptoms can all be linked to the presence of excess calcium, which is a result of the oversecretion of PTH.

Secondary hyperparathyroidism often results when PTH cannot function normally, such as in kidney failure or insensitivity of target tissues to PTH. Secondary hyperparathyroidism is usually characterized by an overall decrease in blood calcium levels, even though there is a marked increase in the amount of PTH being released. Its symptoms may include muscle cramps, seizures, paranoia, depression, and, in severe cases, tetany (the tonic spasm of muscles). These symptoms are a direct result of the decline in available calcium.

Hypoparathyroidism. Less common than hyperparathyroidism, hypoparathyroidism is defined by a reduction in the secretion of PTH. This condition is normally characterized by low calcium levels and elevated phosphate levels in response to the lack of PTH. Not only are calcium levels unusually low, but phosphate levels are unusually high as well, which complicates this condition because phosphate ties up some of the free calcium.

Hypoparathyroidism can also have primary and secondary causes. Primary hypoparathyroidism is known to have two separate origins. The most common is a decrease in PTH release caused by accidental removal of the parathyroid gland. The other is damage of the blood supply around the parathyroid glands. Both occur after there has been some type of surgery or other medical procedure in the neck area. Consequently, the decline in PTH results in low calcium and elevated phosphate concentrations.

Secondary hypoparathyroidism is a frequent complication of cirrhosis and is characterized by a decrease

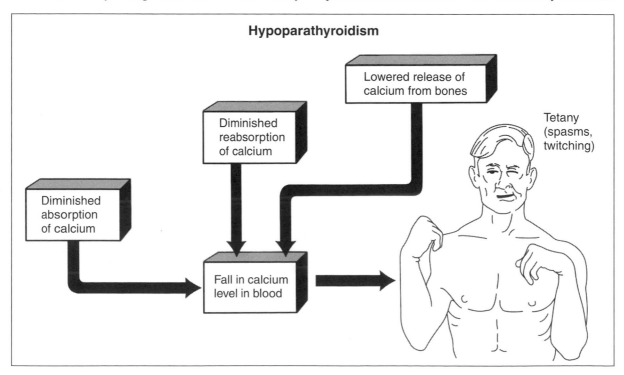

Hypoparathyroidism

Lowered release of calcium from bones

Diminished reabsorption of calcium

Diminished absorption of calcium

Fall in calcium level in blood

Tetany (spasms, twitching)

in both calcium and magnesium concentration. Because magnesium is essential for the release of PTH, this condition can be corrected with magnesium replacement.

Complications associated with all types of hypoparathyroidism include hyperventilation, convulsions, and in some cases tetany of the muscle cells.

TREATMENT AND THERAPY

The treatments for primary hyperparathyroidism vary and are dependent on the severity of the condition. Specific drugs can be prescribed that lower elevated blood calcium. Hormone therapy, which includes the administration of estrogen, also acts to restore calcium to normal. Other treatments include dietary calcium restriction and/or surgery to remove the abnormal parathyroid tissue.

Treatment of secondary hyperparathyroidism often involves correcting the problems associated with kidney failure. This can be done by administration of a dietary calcium supplement to restore plasma calcium levels or, in more severe cases, by kidney transplantation. Vitamin D therapy has also been attempted for those patients diagnosed in the early stages of renal failure.

Hypoparathyroidism is usually treated with dietary calcium and vitamin D supplementation. Both of these treatments promote calcium absorption and decrease calcium loss. The duration of the treatment depends on the severity of the condition and may last a lifetime.

Jeffrey A. McGowan and Hillar Klandorf, Ph.D.

See also Endocrine disorders; Endocrinology; Endocrinology, pediatric; Glands; Hashimoto's thyroiditis; Hormones; Osteoporosis; Stones; Vitamins and minerals.

FOR FURTHER INFORMATION:

Al Zarani, Ali, and Michael A. Levine. "Primary Hyperparathyroidism." *The Lancet* 349, no. 9060 (April 26, 1997): 1233-1238. The authors discuss primary hyperparathyroidism (PHP), a common endocrine disorder characterized by excessive secretion of parathyroid hormone and consequent hypercalcemia.

Brooks, S. J., and Robert S. Bar. *Early Diagnosis and Treatment of Endocrine Disorders.* Totowa, N.J.: Humana Press, 2003. Reviews the early signs and symptoms of common endocrine diseases, surveys the clinical testing needed for a diagnosis, and presents recommendations for therapy.

Burch, Warner M. *Endocrinology.* 3d ed. Baltimore: Williams & Wilkins, 1994. A handbook of endocrine diseases designed for the house officer. Includes bibliographical references and an index.

Gardner, David, and Francis Greenspan. *Basic and Clinical Endocrinology.* East Norwalk, Conn.: Appleton & Lange, 2000. This resource superbly reviews contributions of molecular biology to endocrinology and the practical implications of these advances. Each chapter includes advances in molecular biology and the diagnosis and management of the various syndromes.

Neal, J. Matthew. *Basic Endocrinology: An Interactive Approach.* Oxford, England: Blackwell Science, 1999. Meant to supplement existing textbooks, this guide to the basic clinical principles and physiology of clinical endocrinology is for medical students, residents, and others needing a review of clinical endocrinology.

Ruggieri, Paul. *A Simple Guide to Thyroid Disorders: From Diagnosis to Treatment.* Omaha, Nebr.: Addicus Books, 2003. A user-friendly guide that covers how the thyroid gland works, and explains common disorders. Special attention is given to how thyroid diseases affect specific populations such as women, children, and the elderly.

Wilson, Jean D. *Wilson's Textbook of Endocrinology.* 10th ed. New York: Elsevier, 2003. Text that covers the spectrum of information related to the endocrine system, including thyroid disorders, diabetes, endocrinology and aging, female reproduction and fertility control, sexual function and dysfunction, kidney stones, and endocrine hypertension.

HYPERTENSION

DISEASE/DISORDER

ANATOMY OR SYSTEM AFFECTED: Blood vessels, brain, circulatory system, heart, kidneys, urinary system

SPECIALTIES AND RELATED FIELDS: Cardiology, family practice, internal medicine

DEFINITION: An abnormally high blood pressure, an often silent cardiovascular condition that may lead to heart attack, stroke, and major organ failures.

KEY TERMS:

cardiovascular: of, relating to, or involving the heart and blood vessels

cerebrovascular: of, or involving, the cerebrum (brain) and the blood vessels supplying it

diastolic blood pressure: the pressure of the blood within the artery while the heart is at rest

hypertension: abnormally high blood pressure, especially high arterial blood pressure; also the systemic condition accompanying high blood pressure

peripheral vascular: of, relating to, involving, or forming the vasculature in the periphery (the external boundary or surface of a body); usually referring to circulation not involving cardiovascular, cerebrovascular, or major organ systems

side effect: a secondary and usually adverse effect (as of a drug); also known as an adverse effect or reaction

sphygmomanometer: a device that uses a column of mercury to measure blood pressure force; pressure is measured in millimeters of mercury

systolic blood pressure: the pressure of the blood within the artery while the heart is contracting

CAUSES AND SYMPTOMS

Hypertension is a higher-than-normal blood pressure (either systolic or diastolic). Blood pressure is usually measured using a sphygmomanometer and a stethoscope. The stethoscope is used to hear when the air pressure within the cuff of the sphygmomanometer is equal to that in the artery. When taking a blood pressure, the cuff is pumped to inflate an air bladder secured around the arm; the pressure produced will collapse the blood vessels within. As cuff pressure decreases, a slight thump is heard as the artery snaps open to allow blood to flow. At this point, the cuff pressure equals the systolic blood pressure. As the cuff pressure continues to fall, the sound of blood being pumped will continue but become progressively softer. At the point where the last sound is heard, the cuff pressure equals the diastolic blood pressure.

In hypertension, both systolic and diastolic blood pressures are usually elevated. Blood pressures are reported as the systolic pressure over the diastolic pressure, such as 130/80 millimeters of mercury. It is important to recognize there are degrees of seriousness for hypertension. The higher the blood pressure, the more

---

INFORMATION ON HYPERTENSION

CAUSES: Stress, genetic factors, obesity, diabetes mellitus, physiological factors
SYMPTOMS: Often asymptomatic
DURATION: Often long-term
TREATMENTS: Drug therapy (diuretics, beta-blockers, calcium-channel blockers, ACE inhibitors); lifestyle changes (weight reduction, alcohol restriction, regular exercise)

---

rigorous the treatment may be. When systolic pressures are in the high normal range, the individual should be closely monitored with annual blood pressure checks. Persistently high blood pressures (greater than 140-159/90-99 millimeters of mercury) require closer monitoring and may result in a decision to treat the condition with medication or other types of intervention.

The blood pressure in an artery is determined by the relationship among three important controlling factors: the blood volume, the amount of blood pumped by the heart (cardiac output), and the contraction of smooth muscle within blood vessels (arterial tone). To illustrate the first point, if blood volume decreases, the result will be a fall in blood pressure. Conversely, the body cannot itself increase blood pressure by rapidly adding blood volume; fluid must be injected into the circulation to do so.

A second controlling factor of blood pressure is cardiac output (the volume of blood pumped by the heart in a given unit of time, usually reported as liters per minute). This output is determined by two factors: stroke volume (the volume of blood pumped with each heartbeat) and the heart rate (beats per minute). As heart rate increases, output generally increases and blood pressure may rise as well. If blood volume is low, such as with excessive bleeding, the blood returning to the heart per beat is lower and could lead to decreased output. To compensate, the heart rate increases to prevent a drop in blood pressure. Therefore, as cardiac output changes, blood pressure does not necessarily change.

Last, a major controlling factor of blood pressure is arterial tone. Arteries are largely tubular, smooth muscles that can change their diameter based on the extent of contraction (tone). This contraction is largely under the control of a specialized branch of the nervous system called the sympathetic nervous system. An artery with high arterial tone (contracted) will squeeze the blood within and increase the pressure inside. There is also a relaxation phase that will allow expansion and a decrease in blood pressure. Along with relaxation, arteries are elastic to allow some stretching, which may further help reduce pressure or, more important, help prevent blood pressure from rising.

There are two general types of hypertension: essential and secondary. Secondary hypertension is attributable to some underlying identifiable cause, such as a tumor or kidney disease, while essential hypertension has no identifiable cause. Therefore, essential hypertension is a defect that results in excessive arterial pressure

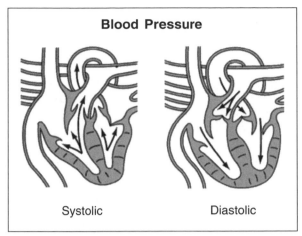

Blood Pressure

Systolic   Diastolic

Blood pressure is measured in two numbers: systolic pressure (the pressure of the blood as it flows out when the heart contracts) over diastolic pressure (the pressure of the blood within the artery as it flows in when the heart is at rest). Readings greater than 140 systolic over 90 diastolic indicate the presence of hypertension.

secondary to poor regulation by any one of the three controlling factors discussed above. Each factor can serve as a focal point for treatment with medications.

The negative consequences of hypertension are mainly manifested in the deteriorating effect that this condition has on coronary heart disease (CHD). Cardiovascular risk factors for CHD are described as two types, unmodifiable and modifiable. Unmodifiable risk factors cannot be changed. This group includes gender, race, advanced age, and a family history of heart disease (hypertensive traits can be inherited). The modifiable risk factors are cigarette smoking (or other forms of tobacco abuse), high blood cholesterol levels, control over diabetes, and perhaps other factors not yet discovered. For example, additional factors are now recognized for their adverse effects on hypertension, including obesity, a lack of physical activity, and psychological factors.

There is no definitive blood pressure level at which a person is no longer at risk for CHD. While any elevation above the normal range places the person at increased risk for CHD, what are considered high normal blood pressures were previously defined as normal. (Looking back at older data, researchers noted that persons able to maintain pressures at or below 139/89 millimeters of mercury had less severe CHD.) The definition of "normal" blood pressure may change again in the future as new information is discovered. There is a practical

limit as to how low pressure can be while maintaining day-to-day function.

In coronary heart disease, the blood supply to the heart is reduced and the heart cannot function well. The common term for arteriosclerosis, "hardening of the arteries," indicates the symptom of reduced blood flow, which is a major component of CHD. When the heart cannot supply itself with the necessary amount of blood (a condition known as ischemia), a characteristic chest pain called angina may be produced. The hardening aspect of this disease is the result of cholesterol deposits in the vessel, which decrease elasticity and make the vessel wall stiff. This stiffness will force pressures in the vessel to increase if cardiac output rises. As pressures advance, the vessel may develop weak spots. These areas may rupture or lead to the development of small blood clots that may clog the vessel; either problem will disrupt blood flow, making the underlying CHD worse. Eventually, if the blood supply is significantly reduced, a myocardial infarction (heart attack) may occur. Where the blood supply to the heart muscle itself is functionally blocked, that part of the heart will die.

Besides contributing to an increased risk of heart attack and coronary heart disease, hypertension is a major risk for other vascular problems, such as stroke, kidney failure, heart failure, and visual disturbances secondary to the effects on the blood vessels within the eye. Hypertension is a major source of premature death in the United States and by all estimates affects more than sixty million Americans. Forty percent of all African Americans and more than half of those over the age of sixty are affected. Public awareness of hypertension is increasing, yet less than half of all patients diagnosed are treated. More important, only one in five identified hypertensives have the condition under control. This

BLOOD PRESSURE AND HYPERTENSION	
Status	*Systolic/Diastolic*
Normal (maximum)	130/85
High normal	131-139/86-89
Stage I hypertension (mild)	140-159/90-99
Stage II (moderate)	160-179/100-109
Stage III (severe)	180-209/110-119
Stage IV (very severe)	210/120+

IN THE NEWS: DIURETICS VERSUS ACE INHIBITORS

The Antihypertensive and Lipid-Lowering Treatment to Prevent Heart Attack Trial (ALLHAT), a large clinical study sponsored by the National Heart, Lung, and Blood Institute (NHLBI), one of the National Institutes of Health, began in 1994 and continued for eight years. The antihypertensive portion of the study compared the effects of a diuretic with three newer, more expensive blood pressure-lowering drugs: an angiotensin-converting enzyme (ACE) inhibitor, a calcium-channel blocker, and an alpha-adrenergic blocker. Although all four drugs lower blood pressure, they had previously been tested against a placebo and not against one another. The study was designed to find which drug would be most effective for the initial treatment of high blood pressure. Study of the alpha-adrenergic blocker was stopped early because patients taking that drug had significantly more cardiovascular problems as compared to those on the diuretic.

ALLHAT's conclusions, reported in the December 18, 2002, issue of the *Journal of the American Medical Association*, were that the diuretic was most effective at lowering blood pressure and at preventing stroke and some types of heart disease, including heart attack and heart failure. Thus, ALLHAT recommended that it be the initial drug of choice. Beta-blockers were recommended as an initial option for those younger than sixty who do not suffer from diabetes or peripheral artery disease, although beta-blockers were not included in the study. For patients requiring more than one drug, ALLHAT advised that one be a diuretic; for those unable to tolerate diuretics, a calcium-channel blocker or ACE inhibitor was recommended.

ALLHAT's findings were challenged by three hypertension experts in the May, 2003, issue of the *American Journal of Hypertension*. Among other criticisms, they claimed that ALLHAT showed no significant differences in fatal and nonfatal coronary events and that the study failed to identify different types of hypertension. In particular, they cited a clinical trial reported in the February 13, 2003, *New England Journal of Medicine* that compared ACE inhibitors and diuretics in treating hypertension in the elderly. Researchers in that study chose ACE inhibitors because agents that inhibit the renin-angiotensin system seemed to provide benefits beyond the mere reduction of blood pressure. Both drugs had similar effects on blood pressure, but their data suggest that ACE inhibitors may result in fewer cardiovascular events or deaths among the elderly and may be particularly beneficial for men, who are statistically more prone to heart disease.

—*Sue Tarjan*

nervous activity (part of the autonomic nervous system), which promotes arterial contraction; overproduction of an unidentified soidium-retaining hormone or chronic high sodium intake; inadequate dietary intake of potassium or calcium; an increased or inappropriate secretion of renin, a chemical made by the kidney; deficiencies of arterial dilators, such as prostaglandins; congenital abnormalities (birth defects) of resistance vessels; diabetes mellitus or resistance to the effects of insulin; obesity; increased activity of vascular growth factors; and altered cellular ion transport of electrolytes, such as potassium, sodium, chloride, and bicarbonate.

The kidneys are greatly responsible for blood pressure control. They have a key role in maintaining both blood volume and blood pressure. When kidney function declines, secondary to problems such as a decrease in renal blood flow, the kidney will release renin. High renin levels result in activation of the renin-angiotensin-aldosterone system. The resulting chemical cascade produces angiotensin II, a potent arterial constrictor. Another chemical released is aldosterone, an adrenal hormone which causes the kidney to retain water and sodium. These two actions add to blood volume and increase arterial tone, resulting in higher blood pressure. Normally, the renin-angiotensin-aldosterone system protects kidney function by raising blood pressure when it is low. In hypertensives, the controlling forces seem to be out of balance, so that the system does not respond appropriately. The renin-angiotensin-aldosterone system has a negative effect on bradykinin, a chemical which protects renal function by producing vasodilating prostaglandins that help maintain adequate renal blood flow. This protection is especially im-

lack of control is particularly important when one considers the organs influenced by hypertension, most notably the brain, eyes, kidneys, and heart.

Although causative factors of hypertension cannot be identified, many physiological factors contribute to hypertension. They include increased sympathetic

portant in elderly individuals, who may depend on this system to maintain renal function. The system can be inhibited by medications such as aspirin or ibuprofen, resulting in a recurrence of hypertension or less control over the existing disease.

Arteries are largely smooth muscles under the control of the autonomic nervous system, which is responsible for organ function. Yet there is often no conscious control of organs; for example, one can "tell" the lungs to take a breath, but one cannot "tell" the heart to beat. The autonomic nervous system has two branches, sympathetic and parasympathetic, that essentially work against each other. The sympathetic system exerts much control over blood pressure. Many chemicals and medicines, such as caffeine, decongestants, and amphetamines, affect blood pressure by mimicking the effects of increased sympathetic stimulation of arteries.

Numerous factors associated with blood pressure elevations will affect one or more of the key determinants of blood pressure; they affect one another as well. An example will show the extent of their relationship. Sodium and water retention will increase blood volume returning to the heart. As this return increases, the heart will increase output (to a point) to prevent heart failure. This higher cardiac output may also raise blood pressure. If arterial vessels are constricted, pressures may be even higher. This elevated pressure (resistance) will force the heart to try to increase output to maintain blood flow to vital organs. Thus, a vicious cycle is started; hypertension can be perceived as a merry-go-round ride with no exit.

TREATMENT AND THERAPY

Blood pressure reduction has a protective effect against cardiovascular disease. Generally, as blood pressure decreases, arteries are less contracted and are able to deliver more blood to the tissues, maintaining their function. Further, this decreased blood pressure will help reduce the risk of heart attack in the patient with heart disease. With lower pressures, the heart does not need to work as hard supplying blood to itself or the rest of the body. Therefore, the demand for cardiac output to supply blood flow is less. This reduced workload lowers the incidence of angina.

Treatment of hypertensive patients may involve using one to four different medications to achieve the goal of blood pressure reduction. There are many types of medications from which to choose: diuretics, sympatholytic agents (also known as antiadrenergic drugs), beta-blockers (along with one combined-action alpha-beta blocker), calcium-channel blockers, peripheral vasodilators, angiotensin-converting enzyme inhibitors, and the newest class, angiotension receptor inhibitors. The list of available drugs is extensive; for example, there are fourteen different thiazide-type diuretics and another six diuretics with different mechanisms of action. So many choices may present the physician with a confusing set of alternatives.

Patients prone to sodium and water retention are treated with diuretics, agents that prevent the kidney from reabsorbing sodium and water from the urine. Diuretics are usually added to other medications to enhance those medications' activity. Research into thiazide-type diuretics has shown that these agents possess mild calcium-channel blocking activity, aiding their ability to reduce hypertension.

Beta-blocking agents are used less often than when they were first developed. They work by decreasing cardiac output through reducing the heart rate. Although they are highly effective, the heart rate reduction tends to produce side effects. Most commonly, patients complain of fatigue, sleepiness, and reduced exercise tolerance (the heart rate cannot increase to adapt to the increasing demand for blood in tissues and the heart itself). These agents are still a good choice for hypertensive patients who have suffered a heart attack. Their benefit is that they reduce the risk of a second heart attack by preventing the heart from overworking.

Calcium-channel blockers were originally intended to treat angina. These agents act primarily by decreasing arterial smooth muscle contraction. Relaxed coronary blood vessels can carry more blood, helping prevent the pain of angina. When calcium ions enter the smooth muscle, a more sustained contraction is produced; therefore, blocking this effect will produce relaxation. Physicians noted that this relaxation also produced lower blood pressures. The distinct advantage to these agents is that they are well tolerated; however, some patients may require increasing their fiber intake to prevent some constipating effects.

Peripheral vasodilators have been a disappointment. Theoretically, they should be ideal since they work directly to cause arterial dilation. Unfortunately, blood pressure has many determinants and patients seem to become "immune" to direct vasodilator effects. Peripheral vasodilators are useful, however, when added to other treatments such as beta-blockers or sympatholytic medications.

The sympatholytic agents are divided into two broad categories. The first group works within the brain to decrease the effects of nerves that would send signals to blood vessels to constrict (so-called constrict messages). They do this by increasing the relax signals coming out of the brain to offset the constrict messages. The net effect is that blood vessels dilate, reducing blood pressure. Many of these agents have fallen into disfavor because of adverse effects similar to those of beta-blockers. The second group of sympatholytics works directly at the nerve-muscle connection. These agents block the constrict messages of the nerve that would increase arterial smooth muscle tone. Overall, these agents are well tolerated. Some patients, especially the elderly, may be very susceptible to their effect and have problems with low blood pressure; this issue usually resolves itself shortly after the first dose.

The renin-angiotensin-aldosterone system is a key determinant of blood pressure. Angiotensin-converting enzyme inhibitors (ACE inhibitors) work by blocking angiotensin II and aldosterone and by preserving bradykinin. They have been found quite effective for reducing blood pressure and are usually well tolerated. Some patients will experience a first-dose effect, while others may develop a dry cough that can be corrected by dose reductions or discontinuation of the medication. The angiotension receptor inhibitors work, instead, by blocking the effects of this substance on the target cells of the arteries themselves. They are proving to be excellent substitutes for people who cannot tolerate the related class of ACE inhibitors.

Unfortunately, and contrary to popular belief, no one can reliably tell when his or her own blood pressure is elevated. Consequently, hypertension is called a "silent killer." It is extremely important to have regular blood pressure evaluations and, if diagnosed with hypertension, to receive treatment.

From 1950 through 1987, as advances in understanding and treating hypertension were made, the United States population enjoyed a 40 percent reduction in coronary heart disease and a more than 65 percent reduction in stroke deaths. (By comparison, noncardiovascular deaths during the same period were reduced little more than 20 percent.)

It is evident that blood pressure can be reduced without medications. Research in the 1980's led to a nonpharmacologic approach in the initial management of hypertension. This strategy includes weight reduction, alcohol restriction, regular exercise, dietary sodium restriction, dietary potassium and calcium supplementation, stopping of tobacco use (in any form), and caffeine restriction. Often, these methods can produce benefits without medication being prescribed. Using this approach, medication is added to the therapy if blood pressure remains elevated despite good efforts at nonpharmacologic control.

Other aspects of hypertension and hypertensive patients have been identified to help guide the clinician to the proper choice of medication. With this approach, the clinician can focus therapy at the most likely cause of the hypertension: sodium and water retention, high cardiac output, or high vascular resistance. This pathophysiological approach led to the abandonment of the rigid step-care approach described in many texts covering hypertension. The pathophysiological approach to hypertension management is based on a series of steps that are taken if inadequate responses are seen (see figure).

By far, the best strategy for controlling hypertension is to be informed. Each person needs to be aware of his or her personal risk for developing hypertension. One should have regular blood pressure evaluations, avoid eating excessive salt and sodium, increase exercise, and reduce fats in the diet. Maintaining ideal body weight may be a key control factor. Studies have shown that pa-

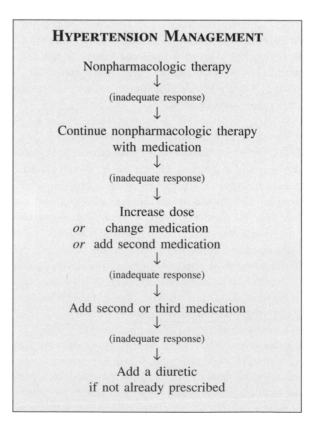

HYPERTENSION MANAGEMENT

Nonpharmacologic therapy
↓
(inadequate response)
↓
Continue nonpharmacologic therapy
with medication
↓
(inadequate response)
↓
Increase dose
or change medication
or add second medication
↓
(inadequate response)
↓
Add second or third medication
↓
(inadequate response)
↓
Add a diuretic
if not already prescribed

tients who have been successful at losing weight will require less stringent treatment. The benefits could be a need for fewer medications, reduced doses of medications, or both.

—*Charles C. Marsh, Pharm.D.;*
updated by Connie Rizzo, M.D.

See also Angina; Arteriosclerosis; Cardiology; Cholesterol; Circulation; Claudication; Embolism; Heart; Heart attack; Heart disease; Hyperadiposis; Hypercholesterolemia; Hyperlipidemia; Insulin resistance syndrome; Kidney disorders; Kidneys; Metabolic syndrome; Phlebitis; Physical examination; Preeclampsia and eclampsia; Pulmonary hypertension; Strokes; Thrombolytic therapy and TPA; Thrombosis and thrombus; Vascular medicine; Vascular system.

FOR FURTHER INFORMATION:

American Society of Hypertension. http://www.ash-us.org/. A group dedicated to promoting and encouraging the development, advancement, and exchange of scientific information in all aspects of research, diagnosis, and treatment of hypertension and related cardiovascular diseases.

McGowan, Mary P., and Jo McGowan Chopra. *The Hypertension Sourcebook*. New York: McGraw-Hill, 2001. An excellent guide to living with and managing hypertension.

Messerli, Franz H., ed. *Cardiovascular Disease in the Elderly*. 3d ed. Boston: Kluwer Academic, 1993. An excellent book for detailed discussions regarding cardiovascular disease in older persons. Issues such as aging, multiple illnesses, and the social challenges seen in the elderly are discussed.

_____. *The Heart and Hypertension*. New York: Yorke Medical Books, 1987. An excellent reference work edited by one of the most distinguished clinicians and researchers in hypertension. This text's strength is its discussion of the pathophysiology of hypertension.

Piscatella, Joseph, and Barry Franklin. *Take a Load Off Your Heart: 109 Things You Can Do to Prevent or Reverse Heart Disease*. New York: Workman, 2002. Easy-to-follow guide that details such preventive measures as managing stress, improving diet, and exercising and offers more than one hundred practical tips for preventing, stabilizing, and reversing heart disease.

Rowan, Robert L. *Control High Blood Pressure Without Drugs: A Complete Hypertension Handbook*. Rev. ed. New York: Simon & Schuster, 2001. A revised edition of a well-known book that details advances in medical research, guidelines for coping with it if it occurs, and ways to lower your blood pressure through inexpensive natural means. Includes a list of Web sites and a fully updated bibliography.

Seeley, Rod R., Trent D. Stephens, and Philip Tate. *Anatomy and Physiology*. St. Louis: Mosby Year Book, 2001. A well-illustrated, easy-to-read basic reference text for the general reader. The text's obvious strengths are its discussions of the heart, arteries, and veins and their roles in cardiovascular function.

Tierney, Lawrence M., Stephen J. McPhee, and Maxine Papadakis, eds. *Current Medical Diagnosis and Treatment 2004*. 43d ed. Stamford, Conn.: Appleton & Lange, 2003. This text, updated yearly, is the point of reference for physicians and other health care practitioners. It incorporates each year's biomedical research discoveries that have immediate, relevant, and applicable use for the patient.

HYPERTHERMIA AND HYPOTHERMIA
DISEASE/DISORDER

ANATOMY OR SYSTEM AFFECTED: All

SPECIALTIES AND RELATED FIELDS: Anesthesiology, critical care, emergency medicine, environmental health, internal medicine

DEFINITION: Hyperthermia is the elevation of the body core temperature of an organism, while hypothermia is a decrease in that temperature; both conditions are medical emergencies when not intentionally induced, and both can be useful when applied to surgical and treatment techniques.

KEY TERMS:

ambient temperature: the temperature of the surrounding environment

body temperature: the temperature that reflects the level of heat energy in an animal's body; a consequence of the balance between the heat produced by metabolism and the body's exchange of heat with the surrounding environment

frostbite: injury that results from exposure of skin to extreme cold, most commonly affecting the ears, nose, hands, and feet

hibernation: a condition of dormancy and torpor that occurs in poikilotherm vertebrates and invertebrates; as the environmental temperatures drop, the inner core temperature of such animals also drops to decrease the metabolic rate and physiological functions

homeotherms: animals, such as birds and mammals, that have the ability to maintain a high body core temperature despite large variations in environmental temperatures

CAUSES AND SYMPTOMS

Body temperature reflects the level of heat energy in the body of an animal or human being. It is the consequence of the balance between the heat generated by metabolism and the body's heat exchange with the surrounding environment (ambient temperature). Generally, animal life can be sustained in the temperature range of 0 degrees Celsius (32 degrees Fahrenheit) to 45 degrees Celsius (113 degrees Fahrenheit), but appropriate processes can store animal tissues at much lower temperature. Homeotherms, such as birds and most mammals, have the ability to maintain their high body core temperature despite large variations in environmental temperatures. Poikilotherms have slow metabolic rates at rest and, as a result, difficulty in maintaining their inner core temperatures. Such a form of thermal regulation is called ectothermic ("outer heated") and is directly affected by the uptake of heat from the environment; such organisms are often termed cold-blooded. On the other hand, homeotherms are endothermic ("inner heated") and depend largely on their fast and controlled rates of heat production; such organisms are termed warm-blooded. Thus, the lizard, an example of ectotherm, maintains its body temperature by staying in or out of shade and by assuming a posture toward the sun that would maximize the adjustment for its body heat. At night, the lizard burrows, but its body temperature still drops considerably until the next morning, when it increases with the rising sun.

Body core temperatures vary considerably among mammals and birds. For example, the sparrow's inner core temperature is about 43.5 degrees Celsius (110.3 degrees Fahrenheit), the turkey's 41.2 degrees Celsius (106.2 degrees Fahrenheit), the cat's 36.4 degrees Celsius (97.5 degrees Fahrenheit), and the opossum's 34.7 degrees Celsius (94.5 degrees Fahrenheit). In humans, although the temperature of the inner organs varies by only 1 to 2 degrees Celsius (1.8 to 3.6 degrees Fahrenheit), the skin temperature may vary 10 to 20 degrees Celsius (18 to 36 degrees Fahrenheit) below the core temperature of 37 degrees Celsius (98.6 degrees Fahrenheit), depending on the ambient temperature. This is possible because the cells of the skin, muscles, and blood vessels are not as sensitive as are those of the vital organs.

An elevation in core temperature of homeotherms above the normal range is called hyperthermia, while a corresponding decrease is called hypothermia. Both can be brought about by extremes in the environment. Although the human body can withstand a lack of food for a number of weeks and that of water for several days, it cannot survive a lack of thermoregulation, which is the maintaining of the inner core temperature. The core temperature has to be kept within strict limits; otherwise, the brain and heart will be compromised and death will result. Clinically, the inner core temperature can be monitored by recording the temperature of the rectum, the eardrum, the mouth, and the esophagus. In elderly people, the body's ability to cope with extreme temperatures may be impaired. Exposure to even mildly cold temperatures may lead to accidental hypothermia that can be fatal if not detected and treated properly.

All animals produce heat by oxidation of substrates to carbon dioxide. On the average, about 75 percent of food energy is converted to heat during adenosine triphosphate (ATP) formation and its transfer to the functional systems of the cells. In defense against heat, sweating is the primary physiological mechanism in mammals. Dogs, cats, and other furred carnivores increase evaporative heat loss by panting, while small rodents spread saliva. Human beings have two to three million glands that can produce up to 23 liters of sweat per hour for a short period of time.

Fever may occur for at least four main reasons. Infection by microorganisms is the most familiar because of its large variety of causes. Such an infection may be bacterial (as with septicemia and abscesses), viral (in measles, mumps, and influenza), protozoal (in malaria), or spichaetal (in syphilis). Fever can also take place because of immunological conditions, such as drug allergies and incompatible blood transfusions. The last two reasons are malignancy, which can lead to Hodgkin's disease and leukemia, and noninfective inflammation, which results in gout and thrombophlebitis.

Antipyretics are medicines whose consumption results in the lowering of fever. The bark of trees provides antipyretics such as spiraeic acid and its derivatives (aspirin). The mechanism of action of the nonnarcotic antipyretics remains a subject of research. Two hypotheses are considered to justify the suppression of fever. One involves inhibition of the formation of arachidonic acid metabolites, which leads to the formation of pain-reducing substances. The other postulates that a modification of the physiological membrane properties

Information on Hyperthermia and Hypothermia

Causes: Extended exposure to heat or cold

Symptoms: For hyperthermia, headache, nausea, dizziness, heat exhaustion or stroke, cessation of perspiration, hot and dry skin, rapid pulse, quick and shallow breathing; for hypothermia, tingling, pain, numbness, sometimes frostbite on nose, ears, hands, and feet

Duration: Acute

Treatments: For hyperthermia, cooling of body, replacement of body fluids, treatment of shock, emergency resuscitation; for hypothermia, warm water on affected body part, hospitalization in intensive care unit

takes place, with subsequent incorporation of drug molecules into the tertiary structure of proteins.

Temperature regulation involves the brain and spinal cord, which monitor the difference between the internal and peripheral (skin and muscle) temperature, with physiological and psychological adjustments to maintain a constant internal temperature. The brain records the various body temperatures via specialized nerve endings called thermal receptors. Heat transfer occurs between the skin surface and the environment via conduction (which takes place by means of physical contact) or convection (which occurs through the movement of air).

During cold weather, hikers and climbers are particularly at risk for hypothermia; in extreme cases, body functions are depressed to the extent that victims may be mistaken for dead. Injuries that result from skin exposure to extreme cold are described as frostbite. Frostbite most commonly affects outer organs such as the nose, ears, hands (especially the fingertips), and feet, which first turn unusually red and then unnaturally white. Early symptoms include feelings of coldness, tingling, pain, and numbness. Frostbite takes place when ice crystals form in the skin and (in the most serious cases) in the tissue beneath the skin. If not treated, frostbite may lead to gangrene, the medical term for tissue death. The freezing-thawing process causes mechanical disruption (from ice), intracellular and extracellular biochemical changes, and the disruption of the blood corpuscles. Frostbite treatment involves the use of warm water to restore blood circulation and heat to the affected body part.

There are several types of hypothermia. Immersion hypothermia occurs when a person falls into cold water. Any movement of the body leads to loss of heat, and the drastic temperature change may trigger a heart attack. Generally, a person can withstand immersion in water that is 10 degrees Celsius (50 degrees Fahrenheit) for about ten minutes before succumbing to death. Divers are equipped with wet suits to minimize heat loss, but they cool themselves rapidly when they move in cold water and, at the same time, breathe dry air mixtures. Submersion hypothermia is actual drowning in cold water. Although a person cannot last more than a few minutes without oxygen, drowning in cold water is more survivable than in water of other temperatures. As the cold water enters the lungs and bathes the skin, the body's metabolic rate decreases, which allows the individual (especially a child) up to forty-five minutes of oxygen debt before death occurs.

Clinical reports also indicate hypothermia in alcohol-intoxicated individuals. Shivering, which is common to people suffering from hypothermia, is a sequence of skeletal muscle contractions which lead to coordinated movements and produce a maximum amount of heat. Other conditions of heat loss that deteriorate the already hypothermic person include tight and wet clothing, injury causing hemorrhage, fatigue, and even psychosis.

Treatment and Therapy

Nature protects poikilotherm vertebrates and invertebrates in winter by means of hibernation. Hibernation, which is a condition of dormancy and torpor, occurs when the body temperatures of such animals drop in response to a decrease in environmental temperatures. Animals such as bears, raccoons, badgers, and some birds become drowsy in winter because ambient temperature drops of a few degrees considerably decrease their metabolic rates and physiological functions. For example, the body temperature of a bear is 35.5 degrees Celsius (96 degrees Fahrenheit) at an air temperature of 4.4 degrees Celsius (40 degrees Fahrenheit) and only 31.2 degrees Celsius (88 degrees Fahrenheit) at an air temperature of 31.2 degrees Celsius (25 degrees Fahrenheit).

In humans, however, a significant decrease in body temperature is always a medical emergency requiring immediate attention. The treatment for mild cases of hypothermia may consist only of covering the head and offering the victim a warm drink. More serious cases may involve immersing the victim in a warm bath. Severe hypothermia requires hospitalization in an intensive care unit, where the body temperature is returned to normal by placing the patient under special heat-reflecting blankets, by injecting warm fluid into the abdominal cavity, or by bypassing the circulating blood through a machine to heat it.

Hyperthermia is often termed heat stroke, while mild elevations in temperature can produce heat exhaustion. Heat stroke is a serious condition treated with emergency procedures. The victim is wrapped naked in a cold, wet sheet or blanket or sponged with cold water and fanned constantly. Salt tablets or a weak salt solution is given to conscious patients.

Both hyperthermia and hypothermia can be used medically. Although cancer treatment consists primarily of radiation therapy, surgery, and chemotherapy, experimental approaches include immunotherapy and hyperthermia. In the latter case, heat is used to destroy cancer cells. In all cases, except surgery, the tumor cells have to be killed in situ, meaning that their reproductive ability has to be inhibited without affecting irreversibly the normal tissues.

A study of cell exposure to high temperatures has demonstrated that the circulation of blood decreased as temperature treatment at 42.5 degrees Celsius (108.5 degrees Fahrenheit) continued. The electron microscope showed that after about three hours, a vascular collapse (seen as cloudiness) took place in most of the located vessels. At that point, the high-temperature treatment ended and the cells were cooled down to 33.5 degrees Celsius (92.3 degrees Fahrenheit). Two days later, the central areas displayed an extensive degree of necrosis (tissue death), while the periphery was largely unaffected.

There are indications that malignant tumor cells are more thermosensitive than the surrounding normal cells from which the malignant cells have probably developed. Although some scientists believe that brain neurons are damaged by temperature greater than 42 degrees Celsius (107.6 degrees Fahrenheit), in most cases neurons can tolerate temperatures in the range of 42.5 to 43 degrees Celsius (108.5 to 109.4 degrees Fahrenheit) for up to thirty minutes. Chemotherapy has been found to be much more potent upon exposure of the tumor cells to higher temperatures. Although the mechanisms responsible are not fully understood, there are several possible explanations. Some scientists believe that hyperthermia may increase the drug uptake by cancer cells, alter the intracellular distribution of the drug, or even alter the metabolism of the drug.

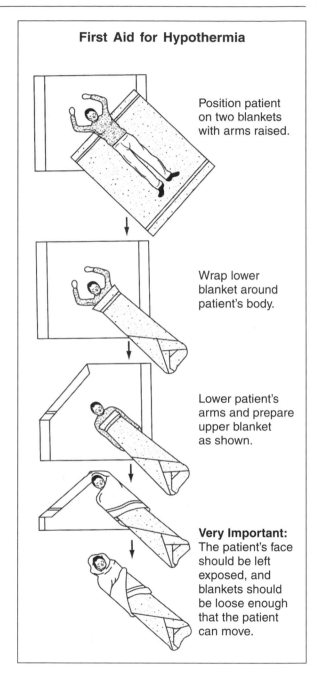

First Aid for Hypothermia

Position patient on two blankets with arms raised.

Wrap lower blanket around patient's body.

Lower patient's arms and prepare upper blanket as shown.

Very Important: The patient's face should be left exposed, and blankets should be loose enough that the patient can move.

In brain cancer patients, it was common practice to induce brain hyperthermia by means of whole body hyperthermia, but this method has been substituted by several others. Isolated perfusion of the appropriate artery and vein has produced excellent results. Radiofrequency capacitive heating (in which paddle-shaped transmitters are placed next to the exposed brain) and interstitial radiofrequency (in which a gold-plated brass electrode provides tumor temperatures of 44 degrees

Celsius while holding the surroundings at 42 degrees Celsius) are also extensively used. Microwave hyperthermia, magnetic loop induction, and ferromagnetic seeds (which are surgically implanted into the tumor and later heated by external radiofrequency of 300 to 3,000 megahertz) are also applied to brain cancer patients.

Ultrasonic irradiation, which uses a thin, stainless steel tube to induce hyperthermia, is believed to be the promising technique of the future. The heat generated by the energy produced improves the local blood supply by dilating the blood vessels. This dilation, together with an acceleration of enzyme activity, helps cells to obtain fresh nutrients and, at the same time, rid themselves of waste products. The other advantage of ultrasonic irradiation is the vibrations that it creates. In a hardened and calcified brain tumor, for example, these vibrations can crush the tumor, which can then be removed via vacuum.

Hypothermia began to be used extensively in modern surgery in the 1970's and 1980's. In certain operations, the patient's body temperature is lowered by wrapping the already anesthetized patient in a rubber blanket that contains coils through which cold water is circulated. When the temperature is sufficiently low, as determined by an electrical rectal thermometer, general anesthesia is discontinued. As a result, much less bleeding occurs in both brain and heart surgery. Under conditions of hypothermia, breathing is slower and shallower, and the brain requirements for blood and oxygen are drastically reduced. This situation allows an intentional stoppage of the heart for prolonged periods of time in order to complete the surgical repairs of that organ.

There is a point, however, below which the human body temperature cannot be lowered. In cold-blooded animals, the loading and unloading of oxygen can be carried out adequately only within a certain temperature range; thus an octopus's blood becomes fully saturated with oxygen at 0 degrees Celsius but little oxygen is unloaded by hemoglobin, which results in the animal's oxygen starvation. In humans, little oxygen is delivered to the tissues at 20 degrees Celsius (68 degrees Fahrenheit), which sets a natural limit to the possibility of lowering body temperature during surgical procedures. The lack of dissociation of oxyhemoglobin at low temperature accounts for the red color of ears and noses on cold days.

PERSPECTIVE AND PROSPECTS

Both hypothermia and hyperthermia have had a commanding role in medicine. An Egyptian papyrus roll which can be dated back to 3000 B.C.E. describes the treatment of a breast tumor with hyperthermia. Heat has been used as a therapeutic agent since the days of Hippocrates (c. 460-c. 370 B.C.E.), who stated that a patient who could not be cured by heat was actually incurable. In the seventeenth century, the Japanese performed hyperthermia to treat syphilis, arthritis, and gout, using hot water to increase the body temperature to about 39 degrees Celsius.

The medical use of hyperthermia owes much of its modern-era development to Georges Lakhovsky (1880-1942), a Russian Jew who had a brilliant physics background and did most of his work in Paris, France. Although he is not generally given the credit for it, he was the first person to design and build a "short wave diathermy" machine, which created artificial fever for the first time in 1923. His work was done primarily on patients with malignant tumors at the Hospital de la Salpetriere and the Hospital Saint-Louis. The first machine that he developed used frequencies from 0.75 megahertz to 3,000 megahertz, a range very much in use in today's clinical hyperthermia. In 1931, he started using a new machine that emitted radio waves of multiple wavelengths. He had partial success with his treatment, as reported to the Pasteur Institute and the French Academy of Sciences. Other scientists in this field include the German physicians W. Busch and P. Bruns, who applied it to erysipelas infection in 1886, and the Swedish gynecologist N. Westermark, who applied it with partial success to nonoperable carcinomas of the cervix uteri in 1898. The combination of hyperthermia and immunotherapy was applied by William B. Coley, a New York surgeon who managed to cause complete regression of malignant melanoma in patients by inducing artificial fever created by inoculation of infected erysipelas cells.

The application of hyperthermia to serious cases of cancer will take a gigantic leap once it is firmly established that the cancer cells have a greater thermosensitivity than normal cells. At this time, it is generally used in combination with surgery and radiation. Hyperthermia is applied to the cancer cells left behind following surgery, and it can kill those cells that tend to be radioresistant. Unlike radiation, hyperthermia has no known cumulative toxicity, and it can be safely reapplied to recurrent lesions. Ultrasound-induced hyperthermia has produced encouraging results, and it is hoped to be as useful as ultrasound is to the removal of kidney stones.

The application of hyperthermia in cases of acquired immunodeficiency syndrome (AIDS) has not yet provided decisively positive results. The process has involved circulating the patient's blood through a chamber heated to approximately 10 degrees Fahrenheit higher than the body temperature. Although the AIDS virus is killed, many of the patients' other enzymes are found to lose their activity. Consequently, United States health officials have opposed and criticized blood-heating therapy for this disease until more convincing results are produced.

The role of hyperthermia in treating metastatic cancer, in combination with radiation and drugs that are heat and radiation cell sensitizers, is increasing. This technique has been made feasible by the technological advancements in deep-heating machines, such as the Magnetrode and the BSO annular array, which allow the sequential regional hyperthermia of large body regions such as the thorax and the abdomen.

Hypothermic brain operations have the great advantage of reduced swelling. As a result, during the surgery the brain rarely bulges out of the opening in the skull, which is not the case when the operation is performed at room temperature. This advantage has led to reduced hospital stays and faster recovery times. The requirements of the tissues for oxygen and the rate at which they produce waste products fall as temperature drops.

—*Soraya Ghayourmanesh, Ph.D.*

See also Anesthesia; Anesthesiology; Critical care; Critical care, pediatric; Emergency medicine; Fever; Frostbite; Gangrene; Heat exhaustion and heat stroke; Surgery, general.

FOR FURTHER INFORMATION:

Ballester, J. Michael, and Fred P. Harchelroad. "Hyperthermia: How to Recognize and Prevent Heat-Related Illness." *Geriatrics* 54, no. 7 (July, 1999): 20-24. Older patients are predisposed to heat illness secondary to factors such as impaired thermoregulation, reduced sweating response to thermal stress, cardiovascular disease, diabetes, medications, and impaired mobility.

Bicher, Haim I., J. R. McLaren, and G. M. Pigliucci, eds. *Consensus on Hyperthermia for the 1990s.* New York: Plenum Press, 1989. A series of research papers presented at the Twelfth International Symposium on Clinical Hyperthermia in Rome in 1989. Topics include the clinical use and instrumentation for hyperthermia types (including ultrasound) and applications in liver, brain, and ovarian cancer.

Bloomfield, Molly M. *Chemistry and the Living Organism.* 6th ed. New York: John Wiley & Sons, 1996.

An excellent allied health text. Perspective 9-2 discusses hypothermia and death.

Forgey, William W. *Hypothermia.* Old Saybrook, Conn.: Globe Pequot Press, 1999. Written for outdoor adventurers, explains how to protect oneself from core heat loss while outdoors, to recognize the physiological effects of the cold, to distinguish between rapid onset and slow onset hypothermia, and to use the most efficient techniques to re-warm and treat a hypothermia victim.

Gautherie, Michel, ed. *Biological Basis of Oncologic Thermotherapy.* Berlin: Springer-Verlag, 1990. An advanced treatise on cancer thermotherapy that discusses heat transfer to tissues, types of hyperthermia treatment, mechanisms of heat and radiosensitization action in the killing of cells, and temperature distribution in tumors.

Gierach, John. "The Life Threatening Cold: Hypothermia." *Sports Afield* 223, no. 4 (April, 2000): 84. Gierach discusses the perils of hypothermia, a condition in which one's core body temperature drops below the body's ability to bring itself back up to normal. Provides tips for raising core temperature.

Hickey, Robert W., et al. "Hypothermia and Hyperthermia in Children After Resuscitation from Cardiac Arrest." *Pediatrics* 106, no. 1 (July, 2000): 118-122. In experimental models of ischemic-anoxic brain injury, changes in body temperature after the insult have a profound influence on neurologic outcome.

Tilton, Buck. *Backcountry First Aid and Extended Care.* 4th ed. Old Saybrook, Conn.: Globe Pequot Press, 2002. A small, portable guide to the myriad emergencies and medical problems encountered in the wilderness, including hypothermia.

Tredget, Edward E., ed. *Thermal Injuries.* Philadelphia: W. B. Saunders, 2000. Examines wounds, such as burns and frostbite, and their surgical treatments.

HYPERTROPHY

BIOLOGY

ANATOMY OR SYSTEM AFFECTED: All

SPECIALTIES AND RELATED FIELDS: Endocrinology, family practice, internal medicine

DEFINITION: The growth of a tissue or organ as the result of an increase in the size of the existing cells within that tissue or organ; this process is responsible for the growth of the body as well as for increases in organ size caused by increased workloads on particular organs.

KEY TERMS:

atrophy: the wasting of tissue, an organ, or an entire body as the result of a decrease in the size and/or number of the cells within that tissue, organ, or body

compensatory hypertrophy: an increase in the size of a tissue or an organ in response to an increased workload placed upon it

growth: the increase in size of an organism or any of its parts during the developmental process; caused by increases in both cell numbers and cell size

hyperplasia: the increase in size or growth of a tissue or an organ as a result of an increase in cell numbers, with the size of the cells remaining constant

PROCESS AND EFFECTS

The growth and development of the human body and all its parts requires not only an increase in the number of body cells as the body grows, a process known as hyperplasia, but also an increase in the size of the existing cells, a process known as hypertrophy. It is true that as humans grow, they increase the number of cells in their bodies, resulting in an increase in the size of tissues, organs, systems, and the body. For some tissues, organs, and systems, however, the number of cells is genetically set; therefore, the number of cells will increase minimally if at all after birth. Thus, if growth is to occur in those tissues, organs, and systems, it must take place by means of an increase in the size of the existing cells.

The process of hypertrophy occurs in nearly all tissues in the body but is most common in those tissues in which the number of cells is set at the time of birth. Among such tissues are adipose tissue, which is composed of fat cells, and nervous tissue, which is found in the brain, in the spinal cord, and in skeletal muscle tissue. Other tissues, such as cardiac tissue and smooth muscle tissue, also show the ability to undergo hypertrophy.

It is generally true that the number of fat cells within the human body is set at birth. Therefore, an increase in body fat is thought to result primarily from an increase in the amount of fat stored within the fat cells. An increase in the amount of fat consumed in the diet increases the amount of fat that is placed inside a fat cell, resulting in an increase in the fat cell's size.

The number of nerve cells within the brain and spinal cord also is set at birth. The cerebellum of the human brain, however, increases in size about twentyfold from birth to adulthood. This increase is brought about by an increase in the size of the existing nerve cells, and particularly by an increase in the number of extensions protruding from each nerve cell and the length to which the extensions grow. Furthermore, there is an increase in the number of the components within the cell. Specifically, there is an increase in the number of mitochondria within the cell, which provide a usable form of energy so that the cell can grow.

The number of skeletal muscle cells is also, in general, preset at the time of birth. The skeletal muscle mass of the human body increases dramatically from birth to adulthood. This increase is accomplished primarily by means of individual skeletal muscle cell hypertrophy. This increase in the diameter of the individual muscle cells is brought about by increases in the amounts of the contractile proteins, myosin and actin, as well as increases in the amount of glycogen and the number of mitochondria within individual cells. As each muscle cell increases in size, it causes an increase in the size of the entire muscle of which it is a part.

Each of the above-mentioned examples occurs naturally as part of the growth process of the human body. Some tissues, however, are capable of increasing in size as the result of an increased load or demand being placed upon them. This increased load or demand is usually brought about by an increased use of the muscle. This increase in the size of cells in response to an increased demand or use is called compensatory hypertrophy. The most common tissues that show the phenomenon of compensatory hypertrophy are the skeletal, cardiac, and smooth muscles.

Skeletal muscle is particularly responsive to being utilized. This response, however, is dependent upon the way in which the skeletal muscle is used. It is well known that an increase in the size of skeletal muscle can be brought about by such exercises as weight lifting. Lifting heavy weights or objects requires strong contractions of the skeletal muscle that is doing the lifting. If this lifting continues over a long period of time, it eventually results in an increase in the size of the existing muscle fibers, leading to an increase in the size of the exercised muscle. Because the strength of a muscle is dependent upon its size, the increase in the muscle's size results in an increase in its strength. The extent to which the size of the muscle increases is dependent upon the amount of time spent lifting the objects and the weight of the objects. The size that a muscle can reach is, however, limited.

Unlike exercises such as weight lifting, endurance types of exercise, such as walking, jogging, and aerobics, do not result in larger skeletal muscles. These types of exercise do not force the skeletal muscles to contract forcibly enough to produce muscle hypertrophy.

In the same way that an increased load or use will cause compensatory hypertrophy in skeletal muscle, a decreased use of skeletal muscle will result in its shrinking or wasting away. This process is referred to as muscle atrophy. This type of atrophy commonly occurs when limbs are broken or injured and must be immobilized. After six weeks of the limb being immobilized, there is a marked decrease in muscle size. A similar type of atrophy occurs in the limb muscles of astronauts, since there is no gravity present in space to provide resistance against which the muscles must work. If the muscles remain unused for more than a few months, there can be a loss of about one-half of the muscle mass of the unused muscle.

Cardiac muscle, like skeletal muscle, can also be caused to hypertrophy by increasing the resistance against which it works. Although endurance exercise does not cause hypertrophy in skeletal muscle, it does result in an increased size of the heart because of the hypertrophy of the existing cardiac muscle cells in this organ. In fact, the heart mass of marathon runners enlarges by about 40 percent as a result of the increase in endurance training. This increase occurs because the heart must work harder to pump more blood to the rest of the body when the body is endurance exercising. Only endurance forms of exercise result in the hypertrophy of the cardiac muscle. Weight lifting, which causes hypertrophy of skeletal muscle, has no effect on the cardiac muscle.

Smooth muscle also is capable of compensatory hypertrophy. Increased pressure or loads on the smooth muscle within arteries can result in the hypertrophy of the muscle cells. This in turn causes a thickening of the arterial wall. Smooth muscle, however, unlike skeletal and cardiac muscle, is capable of hyperplasia as well as hypertrophy.

COMPLICATIONS AND DISORDERS

Hypertrophy also occurs as a result of some pathological and abnormal conditions. The most common pathological hypertrophy is enlargement of the heart as a result of cardiovascular disease. Most cardiovascular diseases put an increased workload on the heart, making it work harder to pump the blood throughout the body. In response to the increased workload, the heart increases its size, a form of compensatory hypertrophy.

The left ventricle of the heart is capable of hypertrophying to such an extent that its muscle mass may increase four- or fivefold. This increase is the result of improper functioning of the valves of the left heart. The valves of the heart work to prevent the backflow of blood from one chamber to another or from the arteries back to the heart. If the valves in the left heart are not working properly, the left ventricle contracts and blood that should leave the ventricle to go out to the body instead returns to the left ventricle. The enlargement of the left ventricle increases the force with which it can pump the blood out to the body, thus reducing the amount of blood that comes back to the left ventricle despite the damaged heart valves. There is, however, a point at which the enlargement of the left ventricle can no longer help in keeping the needed amount of blood flowing through the body. At that point, the left ventricle finally tires out and left heart failure occurs.

The same type of hypertrophy can and does occur in the right side of the heart as well. Again, this is the result of damaged valves that are supposed to prevent the backflow of blood into the heart. Should the valves of both sides of the heart be damaged, hypertrophy can occur on both sides of the heart.

High blood pressure, also known as hypertension, may also lead to hypertrophy of the ventricles of the heart. With high blood pressure, the heart must work harder to deliver blood throughout the body because it must pump blood against an increased pressure. As a result of the increased demand upon the heart, the heart muscle hypertrophies in order to pump more blood.

The hypertrophy of the heart muscle is beneficial in the pumping of blood to the body in individuals who have valvular disease and hypertension; however, an extreme hypertrophy sometimes leads to heart failure. One of the reasons this may occur is the inability of the blood supply of the heart to keep up with the growth of the cardiac muscle. As a result, the cardiac cells outgrow their blood supply, resulting in the loss of blood and thus a loss of oxygen and nutrients needed for the cardiac cells to survive.

Smooth muscle, like cardiac muscle, may also hypertrophy under the condition of high blood pressure. Smooth muscle makes up the bulk of many of the arteries and smaller arterioles found in the body. The increased pressure on the arterial walls as a result of high blood pressure may cause the hypertrophy of the smooth muscles within the walls of the arteries and arterioles. This increases the thickness of the walls of the arteries and arterioles but also decreases the size of the hollow spaces within those vessels, which are known as the lumina. In the kidneys, the narrowing of the lumina of the arterioles may result in a decreased blood supply to these organs. The reduced blood flow to the kidneys may eventually cause the kidneys to shut down, leading to renal failure.

Smooth muscle may also hypertrophy under some unique conditions. During pregnancy, the uterus will undergo a dramatic hypertrophy. The uterus is a smooth muscle organ that is involved in the housing and nurturing of the developing fetus during pregnancy. Immediately prior to the birth of the fetus, there is marked hypertrophy of the smooth muscle within this organ. This increase in the size of the uterus is beneficial in providing the strong contractions of this organ that are needed for childbirth.

Skeletal muscle also may be caused to hypertrophy in some diseases in which there is an increase in the secretion of male sex hormones, particularly testosterone. Men's higher levels of testosterone, a potent stimulator of muscle growth, are responsible for the fact that males have a larger muscle mass than do females. Furthermore, synthetic testosterone-like hormones have been used by some athletes to increase muscle size. These synthetic hormones are called anabolic steroids. The use of these steroids does result in the hypertrophy of skeletal muscle, but these steroids have been shown to have harmful side effects.

Obesity is another condition that results largely from the hypertrophy of existing fat cells. In children, however, obesity is thought to result not only from an increase in the size of fat cells but also from an increase in their number. In adults, when weight is lost, it is the result of a decrease in the size of the existing fat cells; the number of fat cells remains constant. Thus, it is important to prevent further weight increases in overweight children to prevent the creation of fat cells that will never be lost.

In the onset of diseases that result in muscle degeneration, such as muscular dystrophy, there is a hypertrophy of the affected muscles. This hypertrophy differs from other forms of muscle hypertrophy in that the muscle cells do not increase in size because of an increase in the contractile protein, mitochondria, or glycogen, but because the muscle cells are being filled with fat. As a result of the contractile protein being replaced with fat, the affected muscles are no longer useful.

PERSPECTIVE AND PROSPECTS

The exact mechanisms that bring about and control the hypertrophy of cells and tissues are not well understood. During the growth and developmental periods, however, the hypertrophy of many tissues is thought to be under the control of blood-borne chemicals known as hormones. Among these hormones is one that promotes growth and is thus called growth hormone. Growth hormone brings about an increase in the number and size of cells. Growth hormone causes the hypertrophy of existing cells by increasing the protein-making capability of these cells. Thus, there is an increase in the number of organelles, such as mitochondria, within the cell, which leads to an increase in cell size.

Growth hormone also causes the release of chemicals known as growth factors. There are several different growth factors, but one of particular importance is nerve growth factor. Nerve growth factor is involved with the increase in number of cell processes of single nerve cells. Such chemicals have been shown to enhance the growth of damaged nerve cells in the brains of animals. As a result, it is possible that nerve growth factor could be used in the treatment of nerve damage in humans by causing the nerves to grow new cell processes and form new connections to replace those that were damaged. This may be of great importance for the treatment of those suffering from brain or spinal cord damage.

Other hormones may have similar effects on tissues other than nervous tissue. For example, the hypertrophy of the smooth muscle in the uterus is thought to be brought about hormonally. Immediately prior to birth, when the hypertrophy of the uterus is occurring, there is an increased amount of estrogen, the primary female hormone, in the blood. It is this increase in estrogen that is thought to lead to the great enlargement of the uterus during this time. Some hormones have the effect of preventing or inhibiting the hypertrophy of body tissues. The enlargement of the uterus prior to birth is brought about not only by an increase in estrogen but also as a result of a decrease in another hormone known as progesterone. Progesterone levels are high in the blood throughout pregnancy. Immediately prior to birth, however, there is a dramatic decrease in the level of progesterone in the blood. Thus, it is believed that the high level of progesterone prevents or inhibits the hypertrophy of the smooth muscle cells in the uterus, since the hypertrophy of this organ will not occur until estrogen levels are high and progesterone levels are low.

It has been suggested that compensatory hypertrophy, such as that which occurs in skeletal, smooth, and cardiac muscle, occurs as a result of the stretching of muscle. Some studies have shown that the stretching of skeletal, cardiac, and smooth muscle does lead to hypertrophy. American astronauts and Russian cosmonauts, however, showed a loss in muscle mass even though they exercised and stretched their muscles as much as three hours per day, seven days per week. This suggests that mechanisms other than the stretching of muscles may be involved in compensatory muscle hypertrophy.

Through an understanding of the mechanisms involved in muscle hypertrophy, it may one day be possible to prevent the atrophy that occurs during space flights, prolonged bed rest, and immobilization necessitated by the injury of limbs. Furthermore, the understanding of the mechanisms that control hypertrophy may help to alleviate the effects of disabling diseases such as muscular dystrophy by reversing the effects of muscle atrophy.

—*David K. Saunders, Ph.D.*

See also Endocrinology; Endocrinology, pediatric; Exercise physiology; Growth; Hormones; Muscles; Muscular dystrophy; Obesity; Pregnancy and gestation; Steroid abuse; Steroids.

FOR FURTHER INFORMATION:

Guyton, Arthur C., and John E. Hall. *Textbook of Medical Physiology.* 10th ed. Philadelphia: W. B. Saunders, 2000. An easily read textbook that provides much information on compensatory hypertrophy and other forms of hypertrophy. Provides an in-depth look at hypertrophy and the mechanisms that bring it about, particularly the effects of exercise on the hypertrophy of skeletal and cardiac muscle.

Hole, John W., Jr. *Essentials of Human Anatomy and Physiology.* 7th ed. Dubuque, Iowa: Wm. C. Brown, 1999. An introductory college anatomy and physiology text that is easily read and understood. Provides a good general overview of the processes of hypertrophy and atrophy.

Marieb, Elaine N. *Human Anatomy and Physiology.* 6th ed. Redwood City, Calif.: Benjamin/Cummings, 2003. Provides an in-depth look at how obesity occurs as a result of both hypertrophy and hyperplasia. Also provides an overview of the hormones that can cause hypertrophy and the mechanisms by which they bring about changes in size.

Shostak, Stanley. *Embryology: An Introduction to Developmental Biology.* New York: HarperCollins, 1991. Provides an introduction to the growth and development of the human body. It provides a good discussion of the role that hypertrophy plays in the development of the human body. It also points out those tissues that grow primarily by hypertrophy rather than by hyperplasia.

Tortora, Gerard J., and Sandra R. Grabowski. *Principles of Anatomy and Physiology.* 10th ed. New York: John Wiley & Sons, 2003. This textbook does a good job of explaining hypertrophy in skeletal, cardiac, and smooth muscle. It provides several examples of pathological conditions in which hypertrophy occurs and may be harmful.

Wilson, Jean D. *Wilson's Textbook of Endocrinology.* 10th ed. New York: Elsevier, 2003. Text that covers the spectrum of information related to the endocrine system, including thyroid disorders, human growth, diabetes, endocrinology and aging, female reproduction and fertility control, sexual function and dysfunction, kidney stones, and endocrine hypertension.

HYPERVENTILATION
DISEASE/DISORDER

ANATOMY OR SYSTEM AFFECTED: Lungs, respiratory system

SPECIALTIES AND RELATED FIELDS: Emergency medicine, pulmonary medicine

DEFINITION: Breathing at a faster rate than what is needed for metabolism, resulting in the exhalation of carbon dioxide faster than it is produced.

CAUSES AND SYMPTOMS

Hyperventilation is rapid deep or quick shallow breathing, both of which can result in a dramatic decrease in carbon dioxide levels and an increase in the pH of the blood. While its purpose is an attempt to get more oxygen, hyperventilation can actually result in feeling breathless or dizzy and, in extreme cases, fainting.

There are several possible causes or reasons for hyperventilation, including anxiety, panic attacks, agoraphobia (fear of open spaces), depression, anger, and overconsumption of caffeine. Hyperventilation can also be a symptom of an underlying disease process such as an infection, bleeding, or heart and lung disorder, as well as a response to altitude exposure. Hyperventilation syndrome (HVS) can be manifested either acutely or chronically.

Chronic HVS can cause a variety of physical problems involving respiratory, cardiac, neurologic, or gastrointestinal (GI) systems. Aerophobia, a fear of fresh air, brings on the GI problems such as flatulence, bloating, and belching. Besides rapid breathing, hyperventilation can cause a fast pulse, shortness of breath, chest

INFORMATION ON HYPERVENTILATION

CAUSES: Anxiety, panic attacks, fear, depression, anger, caffeine overconsumption

SYMPTOMS: Rapid deep or quick shallow breathing causing shortness of breath, fast pulse, chest pain or tightening, dry mouth, numbness around lips and hands, blurred vision, seizures, loss of consciousness

DURATION: Acute or chronic

TREATMENTS: Reassurance, removal of cause of anxiety; for severe, recurrent cases, antidepressants, beta-blockers, stress management classes, breathing retraining

pain or tightening, dry mouth (from mouth breathing), numbness around the lips and hands, and, in more severe cases, blurred vision, seizures, and loss of consciousness. The chest pain resembles typical angina but does not usually respond to nitroglycerine. Changes in the patient's electrocardiogram (ECG) are common, including ST segment elevation or depression, T-wave inversion, or a prolonged QT interval. Patients with mitral valve prolapse are particularly susceptible to HVS. On occasion, hyperventilation can also be manifested with extreme agitation, tingling in the extremities, or painful hand and finger spasms. The chief characteristic of chronic HVS is multiple complaints without supporting physical evidence. Hence, classic hyperventilation is not readily apparent, but frequent sighing may be evidenced, along with chest wall tenderness, numbness, and tingling sensations. To rule out more serious conditions, arterial blood gases, toxicology screens, and chest X rays are suggested.

Hyperventilation is a technique purposefully used by swimmers and deep-sea divers to enable prolonged breath-holding. Many drownings have been related to this practice, however, because it can cause delayed unconsciousness underwater and subsequent death.

TREATMENT AND THERAPY

Contrary to popular belief, breathing into a paper bag to slow down respiration and retain carbon dioxide is not recommended as a treatment for hyperventilation because of the potential life-threatening aggravation of a more serious medical problem such as hypoxia, a myocardial infarction (heart attack), pneumothorax, or pulmonary embolism.

After life-threatening causes of hyperventilation are eliminated, the most successful treatment for hyperventilation is reassurance, discussion of how hyperventilation is causing the patient's symptoms, and removal of the cause of the anxiety, if possible. Instructions from a respiratory therapist on proper abdominal diaphragmatic breathing are also helpful. A patient who faints should be placed flat on the floor with legs elevated. For more severe recurrent cases, antidepressants, beta-blockers, stress management classes, or breathing retraining have all been proven effective in reducing hyperventilation episodes.

—*Bonita L. Marks, Ph.D.*

See also Altitude sickness; Anxiety; Asphyxiation; Choking; Dizziness and fainting; Lungs; Numbness and tingling; Panic attacks; Pulmonary medicine; Pulmonary medicine, pediatric; Respiration; Resuscitation; Unconsciousness.

FOR FURTHER INFORMATION:

Callaham, M. "Hypoxic Hazards of Traditional Paper Bag Rebreathing in Hyperventilating Patients." *Annals of Emergency Medicine* 18, no. 6 (1989): 622-628.

Cowley, D. S., and P. P. Roy-Byrne. "Hyperventilation and Panic Disorder." *American Journal of Medicine* 83, no. 5 (1987): 929-937.

Gardner, W. N. "The Pathophysiology of Hyperventilation Disorders." *Chest* 109, no. 2 (1996): 516-534.

McArdle, W. D., F. I. Katch, and V. L. Katch. *Exercise Physiology: Energy, Nutrition, and Human Performance.* 4th ed. Baltimore: Williams & Wilkins, 2001.

HYPNOSIS

PROCEDURE

ANATOMY OR SYSTEM AFFECTED: Brain, nervous system, psychic-emotional system

SPECIALTIES AND RELATED FIELDS: Alternative medicine, anesthesiology, immunology, psychiatry, psychology

DEFINITION: The induction of an altered state of consciousness.

KEY TERMS:

hypnotherapy: a therapeutic method in which hypnosis works in conjunction with the psychotherapeutic process

hypnotic depth: a state frequently measured by the degree of suggestibility possessed by a presumably hypnotized individual *hypnotic induction:* the production of hypnosis by means of precise rules and patterns (formal) or rules and patterns that permit limited flexibility (informal)

operator: the person who induces a hypnotic state; synonymous with "hypnotist" and "suggestor"

suggestion: a communication that evokes a nonvoluntary response reflecting the ideational content of the communication

INDICATIONS AND PROCEDURES

The term "hypnosis" comes from the Greek word *hypnos*, meaning sleep. While scientists and researchers do not understand the exact nature of hypnosis, theorists agree that it is an altered state of consciousness occurring on a continuum of awareness. Hypnosis may occur naturally and spontaneously, as in the case of a daydream. The daydreamer is alert and awake but focuses attention inward rather than outward.

The trance state, often synonymous with the hypnotic state, is characterized by an altered psychological state and minimal motor functioning. A trance can be recognized by the individual's glassy-eyed stare, lack of mobility, and unresponsiveness to external stimuli. A person in a trance state has a heightened receptivity to suggestion. Hypnosis, then, is a natural state that can be induced by another or by oneself (self-hypnosis) for a specific purpose. As a method of treatment, hypnosis, which is often used in conjunction with other approaches to alter psychophysiological states, promotes an understanding that allows for creative problem solving.

In the hypnotic state, the subject is not necessarily docile or submissive and may, because of unconscious processes, reject a suggestion given by even the most expert hypnotist. Four basic types of suggestion have been described: verbal, which includes words and any kind of sound; nonverbal, which applies to body language and gestures; intraverbal, which relates to the intonation of words; and extraverbal, which utilizes the implications of words and gestures that facilitate the acceptance of ideas. Suggestions are also described as being direct or indirect. Suggestibility is a behavior that is not hindered by the individual's logical processes but is enhanced by the subject's motivation, expectation, and trust in the operator as well as by the frequency and manner in which a suggestion is given.

Typically, prior to hypnosis, a subject is seated comfortably opposite or alongside the operator. The operator and subject generally have already discussed what will occur during the hypnotic process. The subject is encouraged to talk about his or her attitudes regarding hypnosis and the operator, as well as any previous experience with hypnosis. If the situation is a clinical one, a full psychiatric history and evaluation will already have been completed. For a positive hypnotic experience to emerge, a comfortable and trusting relationship between subject and operator must exist. There must be a willingness to undergo the experience on the part of the subject and a sensitive, observant, and supportive attitude on the part of the operator. Not all subjects are hypnotizable, but it is believed that most individuals, under appropriate circumstances, can respond to simple suggestions.

The induction process can be one of many types, ranging from directing the subject to close his or her eyes and think of a peaceful scene to having the subject gaze at a particular spot, shiny object, or swinging pendulum until the subject's eyes become heavy and close. Focusing on an object or scene leads the subject to redistribute his or her attention so as to withdraw it from the general surroundings and focus it on a circumscribed area. In the meantime, the subject is encouraged to relax and to allow events to unfold naturally. This induction procedure is sometimes followed, or even replaced, by what are described as deepening techniques. The direction is given to imagine gradually descending a staircase or elevator, or drifting on a boat past a slowly disappearing landscape. Counting forward or backward is another deepening or induction technique. Throughout this procedure, the operator offers comments or suggestions in a slow, repetitive, monotonous voice, exhorting the subject to feel relaxed and calm or to float and drift.

After a period generally lasting from one to several minutes, the operator gives the subject motor and sensory suggestions. For example, the operator may ask the subject to concentrate on the feelings in his or her fingers and hand, to feel the small muscles in the fingers begin to twitch and the arm and forearm begin to feel light. The operator states that these muscles will eventually feel so light that they will lift up off the armrest of the chair and, continually floating upward, ultimately reach the side of the subject's face. The operator might add that the higher the hand floats, the deeper the hypnosis will become, and the deeper the hypnosis becomes, the higher the hand will float. The operator then adds that when the hand reaches the side of the face, the subject will be deeply hypnotized.

When this point is reached, and the hand and arm have "levitated," the operator assumes that the subject is well hypnotized and then adds suggestions that are appropriate to the situation. Not all subjects, however, respond to hypnosis to the same extent or at the same rate.

There is no evidence to support the view that the operator in hypnosis is able to control the experience and behavior of the subject against the latter's wishes. It is the subject's motivation to behave in accordance with the wishes and directions of the operator that creates that erroneous impression. Moreover, there is no evidence to support the idea that a hypnotized subject can transcend his or her normal volitional capacity because of the hypnosis; despite persuasive clinical reports of altered somatic structures in hypnosis, no physiological changes uniquely associated with hypnosis have been demonstrated. Hypnosis is not so much a way of manipulating behavior as of creating increased perception and memory.

USES AND COMPLICATIONS

Because the mind, body, and emotions are interdependent, factors that influence one influence the others as well. The roles of the mind and emotions in functional or psychophysiological (psychosomatic) illness are widely recognized, but in cases of organic illness, their importance is often underestimated.

Regardless of etiology (causes), there are physical and psychological components to all illness. Emotional states that continue over extended periods can produce physiological changes. The fear, resentment, or depression that often accompanies illness may prolong or exacerbate it and interfere with a patient's willingness or ability to participate in treatment. Addressing such issues through hypnosis can greatly improve the overall medical management of a patient, from the initial diagnosis through all forms of treatment, including the treatment of unconscious and critically ill patients.

One advantage of modern clinical hypnosis is that it requires the practitioner to approach the patient as a whole person rather than as a collection of parts, one or more of which may be diseased. For the physician using hypnosis, a medical history goes beyond a list of past illnesses, allergies, and hospitalizations. A more comprehensive picture is developed that includes an understanding of a patient's personality, present state of mind, and life history and the positive aspects as well as the stresses and strains of the patient's present environment.

The use of hypnosis in most, if not all, medical specialties has been well documented. Hypnosis can be used alone or in combination with other approaches to overcome a variety of habit disorders. While some problems, such as thumb-sucking, can be resolved relatively quickly, others, such as overeating, sometimes require extended treatment or a multidimensional approach. Smoking and bed-wetting are examples of habit disorders that can be managed through hypnosis.

There is much evidence that children as a group are more responsive to hypnosis than adults, and that infants and young children frequently experience hypnosis as a natural part of their lives. Children can often be helped in a remarkably short period of time. Hypnosis has been used with children in the treatment of such diverse ailments as bed-wetting, soiling, asthma, epilepsy, learning difficulties, some behavioral and delinquency problems, stuttering, and nailbiting.

Hypnosis has been used effectively as an adjunct to the treatment of numerous problems with autonomic (internal) nervous system components. For example, there have been many controlled studies and successful case reports on the use of hypnosis in the treatment of asthma, which is the most common of the psychophysiological respiratory disorders. Through hypnosis, a patient can be helped to break the vicious cycle in which anxiety and emotional upsets can trigger an acute asthma attack, which in turn can produce anxiety and fear of other attacks.

Hypnosis has also been used effectively in the control and relief of pain. Because pain is experienced psychologically as well as physiologically, hypnosis can help people alter the perception of pain. A patient can learn to block pain to specific areas of the body, lessen the sensation of pain, or move pain from one area of the body to another. This ability is useful in the management of many types of pain, including chronic back pain, postoperative pain, and the pain associated with illness, migraine headache, burns, childbirth, and medical procedures.

In addition to being used to treat chronic conditions such as hypertension, hypnosis has been used to provide symptomatic relief of other chronic conditions, such as musculoskeletal disorders (for example, rheumatoid arthritis, osteoarthritis, fractures, and bursitis) and hemophilia.

Hypnosis has been used in dentistry for the relief of anxiety as well as pain and has been found to be helpful in teeth grinding (bruxism) and gagging. Modern hypnodontics is not primarily concerned with producing a surgical hypoanalgesia except in rare instances in which chemical anesthesia cannot be tolerated. The dentist is concerned with making visits to his or her office more tolerable and less threatening.

In obstetrics and surgery, hypnosis has been used to induce relaxation and relieve anxiety and to reduce the amount of anesthetic necessary. Occasionally, no anesthetic is required. This is sometimes desirable in childbirth, when the mother prefers to be aware of the birth process, or in other surgical procedures in which a minimum of anesthetic is desirable.

Hypnosis has also been utilized by the police in what has been termed "investigative hypnosis." Witnesses to crimes are interrogated in an effort to improve their memory retrieval.

Hypnosis has also been helpful in increasing athletic effectiveness. It has been utilized by both team and individual athletes to increase self-confidence and other factors such as self-image and the ability to assess the competition. Hypnosis thus applied to maximize performance in sports has been very effective, but the principles involved are essentially no different from those applied to other areas of living, such as increasing the efficiency of performance in the home, school, or workplace.

Since the mid-1970's, there has been much research into immune system functioning. Studies of the effects of stress on immune system functioning are lending scientific support to anecdotal reports that indicate that hypnosis may be effective in altering the disease process in cancer and AIDS patients. Researchers have found that unless treatments for these illnesses are based on the premise that the mind, body, and emotions are all striving to achieve health, physical intervention alone (radiation or chemotherapy, for example) will not be effective.

PERSPECTIVE AND PROSPECTS

Although medical hypnosis is considered to have had its beginnings with the Viennese physician Franz Anton Mesmer (1733-1815) in the latter half of the eighteenth century, hypnosis, or something very similar to it, has been practiced by religious and other healers in various ways for centuries in most cultures. The earliest evidence of its existence was found among shamans, who were also referred to as "witch doctors," "medicine men," or "healers."

In preparation for healing, a shaman adhered to certain practices that allowed his or her powers of concentration to be heightened. Placing himself or herself in isolation, the shaman began a descent into the "lower world." This often meant visualizing an opening in the

earth and a journey downward into that opening. The journey was frequently accompanied by rhythmic drumming, chanting, singing, or dancing. The monotonous rhythm and constancy allowed the shaman's subconscious mind to become strongly focused, seek out the sick spirit of the patient, make it whole, and bring it back to the patient. The shaman actually engaged in a powerful process of visualization and suggestion during which the shaman willed the sick person to be healed.

In the eighteenth century, Mesmer recognized this ancient healing phenomenon and incorporated it into a theory of animal magnetism. Mesmer believed that a "cosmic fluid" could be stored in inanimate objects, such as magnets, and transferred to patients to cure them of illness.

Mesmer dressed flamboyantly. His consulting rooms were dimly lit and hung with mirrors, and he kept soft music playing in the background. The doctor's patients sat in a circle around a vat that contained such elements as powdered glass or iron filings. Then the patients grasped iron rods that were immersed in the vat and were believed to transmit a curing force.

Mesmer's first success was with a twenty-nine-year-old woman who suffered from a convulsive malady, a condition commonly called a "nervous disorder." Her symptoms consisted of blood rushing to her head and a tremendous pain in her ears and head. This state was followed by delirium, rage, vomiting, and fainting. During one of the woman's attacks, Mesmer applied three magnets to the patient's stomach and legs while she concentrated on the positive effects of the "cosmic fluid." In a short time, her symptoms subsided. When her symptoms resurfaced the next day, Mesmer gave her another treatment and achieved similar results. Mesmer believed that the "cosmic fluid," stimulated by the magnets, was directed through his patient's body. Her energy flow was restored, and as a result she regained her health.

Eventually Mesmer discarded the magnets. He began to regard himself as a magnet through which a fluid life force could be conducted and then transmitted to others as a healing force. This is what Mesmer described as "animal magnetism."

Despite the fact that no scientific evidence supported the existence of Mesmer's "cosmic fluids" or the concept of "animal magnetism," he had a tremendous rate of success. Thousands flocked to him for treatment. The only explanation for his success is that his patients were literally "mesmerized" into the belief and expectation that they would be cured. "Mesmerism" was a forerunner of the concept of hypnotic suggestion.

During this same period, a new slant on Mesmer's theories was introduced by one of his disciples, the Marquis de Puységur. He believed that the "cosmic fluid" was not magnetic but electric. This electric fluid was generated in all living things—in plants as well as animals. Puységur used the natural environment to fill his patients with the healing electric fluid that was expected to end their suffering. His clinic was held outdoors, where the sick were received under an elm tree in the center of the village green. Puységur believed that the tree had an innate healing power and that the force would travel through the trunk and branches to cords that he hung from the tree. At the foot of the tree, patients sat in a circle on stone benches with the cords wrapped around the diseased parts of their bodies. They were "connected" to one another when they touched their thumbs together, which made it possible for the "fluid" to circulate from person to person and to heal.

During this activity, Puységur noticed a strange phenomenon. Some of the patients entered a state of deep sleep as a result of being mesmerized. In this state, the patient could still communicate and be lucid and responsive to the suggestions of the mesmerist. The marquis had discovered the hypnotic trance but had not identified it as such.

In the mid-1800's, the hypnotic trance was used to relieve pain. An eminent London physician, John Elliotson (1791-1868), reported 1,834 surgical operations performed painlessly. In India, a Scottish surgeon named James Esdaile (1808-1859) performed many major operations, such as amputation of limbs, using mesmerism (or, as he called it, "magnetic sleep") as the sole anesthetic. One procedure involved conditioning the patient weeks prior to surgery. This was accomplished by inducing a trance state in the patient and offering posthypnotic suggestions to numb the part of the body on which the surgery was to be performed. In a second method, the hypnotist attended to the patient in the operating room, inducing a trance state and suggesting disassociation from any pain. It was possible for the patient to be completely lucid during this state and also to be oblivious to pain, as though completely anesthetized.

Mesmerism continued to provoke new theories and uses. During the late nineteenth century, an English physician, James Braid (1795-1860), gave mesmerism a scientific explanation. He believed mesmerism to be a "nervous sleep" and coined the word "hypnosis,"

which was derived from the Greek word *hypnos*, meaning sleep. Braid showed that hypnotized subjects are often abnormally susceptible to impressions on the senses and that much of the subjects' behavior was caused by suggestions made verbally.

Soon, other theories began to emerge. Jean Martin Charcot (1825-1893), a neurologist who taught in Paris, explained hypnosis as a state of hysteria and categorized it as an abnormal neurological activity.

In France, Auguste Ambroise Leibeault (1823-1904) and Hippolyte Bernheim (1837-1919) were the first to regard hypnosis as a normal phenomenon. They asserted that expectation is the most important factor in the induction of hypnosis, that increased suggestibility is its essential symptom, and that the hypnotist works on the patient by means of mental influences.

As hypnosis began to receive serious study and could be explained rationally, it began to gain acceptance in the scientific community. It was no longer relegated to the realm of the bizarre.

Sigmund Freud became interested in hypnosis at this same time and visited Leibeault and Bernheim's clinic to learn their induction techniques. As Freud observed patients enter a hypnotic state, he began to recognize the existence of the unconscious. Although he was not the first to make this observation, he was the first to recognize the unconscious as a major source of psychopathology. Early in his research, however, Freud rejected hypnosis as the tool to unlock repressed memories, favoring instead his technique of free association and dream interpretation. With the rise of psychoanalysis in the first half of the twentieth century, hypnosis declined in popularity.

Then, however, a reversal occurred. During World War II, interest in hypnosis was regenerated by the need for short-term therapy (it was often applied in cases of "battle fatigue") and by the combination of hypnosis and more traditional analytic approaches. Mind control and "brainwashing" techniques that surfaced during the Korean War again sparked interest in the power of suggestion, especially when the subject was under duress. In the late 1960's and early 1970's, with the rise of public interest in alternative forms of mental health (Transcendental Meditation, biofeedback, yoga) and ways of coping with the stress of the modern world, hypnosis experienced a rebirth. Researchers found new and potent uses for it in therapy, and the trance state began to be recognized as a highly effective tool for modifying behavior and for healing.

—Genevieve Slomski, Ph.D.

See also Alternative medicine; Anesthesia; Anesthesiology; Anxiety; Asthma; Bed-wetting; Brain; Meditation; Pain management; Psychiatry; Psychosomatic disorders; Stress; Stress reduction.

For Further Information:

Brown, Peter. *The Hypnotic Brain*. New Haven, Conn.: Yale University Press, 1994. This scholarly work examines how communication in human beings arose, the importance of nonverbal communication, the rise in oral cultures, and evidence for the common "everyday" trance.

Burrows, Graham D., et al., eds. *International Handbook of Clinical Hypnosis*. New York: Wiley, 2001. Takes a practical approach in explaining both the scientific and clinical aspects of hypnosis and providing information on a range of available psychological and physical treatments.

Forrest, Derek, and Anthony Storr. *The Evolution of Hypnotism*. Forfar, England: Black Ace Books, 1999. This book offers a history of hypnotism and its predecessor, mesmerism. Traces the major figures of mesmerism, leading up through Sigmund Freud and hypnotism's influence in the twentieth century.

Hadley, Josie, and Carol Staudacher. *Hypnosis for Change*. 3d ed. New York: Ballantine Books, 2000. This popular account provides step-by-step details on the practice of self-hypnosis. It also offers a brief historical sketch of hypnosis, explores all facets of induction, and examines various aspects of hypnotic communication. Includes a bibliography.

Yapko, Michael D. *Trancework: An Introduction to the Practice of Clinical Hypnosis*. 3d ed. Washington, D.C.: Taylor & Francis, 2003. Describes what hypnosis is and why it works in a clinical setting, surveys a broad range of hypnotic methods and techniques, and provides several trance scripts.

Zahourek, Rothlyn P., ed. *Clinical Hypnosis and Therapeutic Suggestion in Patient Care*. New York: Brunner/Mazel, 1990. Representing a variety of disciplines, the contributors to this book argue that hypnosis is a natural, noninvasive tool that can be of use in patient care.

Hypochondriasis
Disease/disorder

Also known as: Hpochondriacal neurosis or hychondriacal reaction

Anatomy or system affected: Psychic-emotional system, all bodily systems

Specialties and related fields: Psychiatry, psychology

Definition: Unwarranted belief about or anxiety over having a serious disease which is based on one's subjective interpretation of physical symptoms or sensations; the belief or anxiety is maintained in spite of appropriate medical assurances that there is no serious disease.

Key terms:

defense mechanisms: automatic, unconscious mental processes that become activated in the presence of emotional distress and anxiety; these processes work to maintain inner harmony by preventing mental awareness of that which would be otherwise too emotionally painful to endure

hypochondria: an earlier term for hypochondriasis; from classical Greek, it means the abdominal region of the body below the rib cage, from which black bile was believed to cause melancholy and yellow bile was believed to cause ill-temper

hypochondriacal neurosis: an earlier, but still-used, term for hypochondriasis; because experts have disagreed about what "neurosis" means precisely, the term is considered less descriptive than "hypochondriasis"

hypochondriacal reaction: another earlier term for hypochondriasis; experts who still prefer this term view hypochondriasis as a transient reaction to life stress and tend not to see it as a mental-emotional disorder in its own right

primary hypochondriasis: hypochondriasis as a disorder in its own right, and not accompanied by another psychiatric disorder such as generalized anxiety or panic

secondary hypochondriasis: the experience of hypochondriacal symptoms as part of an underlying, causal condition such as panic disorder, generalized anxiety disorder, schizophrenia, or major depression with psychotic features

somatization disorder: the somatoform disorder most similar to hypochondriasis; in somatization, the preoccupation is primarily with symptoms that one experiences and not with a disease that one is fearful of getting, an important distinction when these conditions are treated

somatoform disorders: the grouping of disorders that includes hypochondriasis; these disorders feature symptoms that suggest physical disease but that are actually caused by psychological upset

CAUSES AND SYMPTOMS

With hypochondriasis, the real problem is the patient's excessive worry and mental preoccupation with having or developing a disease, not the disease about which the patient is so worried. While concern about contracting a serious disease is common and normal, and may even make one more prudent, excessive worry, endless rumination, and obsessive interpretation of every symptom and sensation can disable and prevent effective functioning. A diagnosis of hypochondriasis is made when the patient's dread about the disease or diseases impairs normal activity and persists despite appropriate medical reassurances and evidence to the contrary. Even though hypochondriacs can acknowledge intellectually the possibility that their fears might be without rational foundation, the acknowledgment itself fails to bring any relief.

Researchers estimate that a low of 3 percent to a high of 14 percent of all medical (versus psychiatric) patients have hypochondriasis. Just how prevalent it is in the population as a whole is unknown. What is known is that the disorder shows up slightly more in men than in women, starts at any age but most often between twenty and thirty, shows up most often in physicians' offices with patients who are in their forties and fifties, and tends to run in families.

Most clinicians believe that hypochondriasis has a primary psychological cause or causes but that, in general, hypochondriacs have only a vague awareness that they are doing something that perpetuates and worsens their hypochondriacal symptoms. Hypochondriacs do not feign illness; they genuinely believe themselves to be sick, or about to become so.

Clinicians usually favor one of four hypotheses about how hypochondriasis starts. The hypotheses are based on anecdotal, clinical experience with patients who have gotten better when treated specifically for hypochondriasis. Researchers have rarely studied hypochondriasis using strict experimental methods. Nevertheless, the anecdotal evidence is important, because it gives clinicians a way to think about how to treat the condition.

The most popular view among mental health professionals sees hypochondriacs as essentially angry, but deep down inside. Because their life experience is of hurt, disappointment, rejection, and loss, they engage in a two-stage process to make up for their sad state of affairs. Though they believe themselves unlovable and unacceptable as they are, they solicit attention and caring by presenting themselves either as ill or as dangerously close to becoming ill. Their fundamental anger

> ### INFORMATION ON HYPOCHONDRIASIS
>
> **CAUSES:** Psychological disorders
> **SYMPTOMS:** Excessive worry, endless rumination, and obsessive interpretation of symptoms and sensations; impaired normal activity; chronic persistance despite appropriate medical reassurances and contrary evidence
> **DURATION:** Chronic, although at times temporary
> **TREATMENTS:** Psychotherapy, limited drug therapy

fosters their development of an interpersonal pattern in which they bite the emotional hands which seek to feed them. Endless worry and rumination soon render ineffective others' concern. No amount of reassurance allays their preoccupation and anxiety. In this way, those moved to show concern tire, grow impatient, and finally give up their efforts to help, proving to the worried hypochondriacs that no one really does care about them after all. Meanwhile, the hypochondriacs remain sad and angry.

This view often assumes that hypochondriasis is actually a form of defense mechanism which transfers angry, hostile, and critical feelings felt toward others into physical symptoms and signs of disease. Because hypochondriacs find it too difficult to admit that they feel angry, isolated, and unloved, they hide from the emotional energy associated with these powerful feelings and transfer them into bodily symptoms. This process seems to occur most often when hypochondriacal people harbor feelings of reproach because they are bereaved and lonely. In effect, they are angry at being left alone and left uncared for, and they redirect the emotion inwardly as self-reproach manifested in physical complaints.

Others hypothesize that hypochondriasis enables those who either believe themselves to be basically bad and unworthy of happiness or feel guilty for being alive ("existential guilt") to atone for their wrongdoings and, thereby, undo the guilt that they are always fighting not to feel. The mental anguish, emotional sadness, and physical pain so prevalent in hypochondriasis make reparation for the patients' real, exaggerated, or imagined badness.

A third view is sociological in orientation. Health providers who endorse it see hypochondriasis as society's way of letting people who feel frightened and overwhelmed by life's challenges escape from having to face those challenges, even if temporarily. Hypochondriacs take on a "sick role" which removes societal expectations that they will face responsibilities. In presenting themselves to the world as too sick to function, they also present themselves as excused from doing so. A schoolchild's stomachache on the day of a big test provides a relatively common and potentially harmless example of this role at work. Non-physically disabled adults who seek refuge from life stress by staying in bed, and who find themselves with true physical paralysis years later, provide a more serious and regrettable example.

A fourth view utilizes some experimental data which suggest that hypochondriacal people may have lower thresholds for (and lower tolerances of) emotional and physical pain. The data suggest that hypochondriacs experience physical and/or emotional sensations that are a magnification of what is normal experience. Thus, a sensation that would be sinus pressure for most people would be experienced as severe sinus headache in the hypochondriac. Hypersensitivity (lower threshold) to bodily sensations keeps hypochondriacs ever on watch for these upsetting, intense sensations because of how amplified the physical and emotional experiences are. What seems to most people an exaggerated concern with symptoms is simply prudent, self-protective vigilance to hypochondriacs.

Regardless of why the disorder develops, the majority of hypochondriacs go to their physicians with concerns about stomach and intestinal problems or heart and blood circulation problems. These complaints are usually only part of broader concerns about other organ systems and other anatomical locations. The key clinical feature of the disorder of hypochondriasis, however, is not where and how many bodily complaints there are but the patients' belief that they are seriously sick, or are just about to become so, and that the disease has yet to be detected. Laboratory tests that reveal healthy organs, physician reassurances that they are well, and long periods in which the dreaded disease fails to manifest itself are not reassuring at all. In fact, before the hypochondriasis itself is treated psychologically, it seems that nothing can stop the frantic rumination and accompanying nervousness, even the patients' acknowledgment that they may be exaggerating their reaction to their heartbeat, headache, diarrhea, morning cough, or perspiration. Hypochondriacs seem genuinely unable not to worry.

Hypochondriacs typically present their medical history in great detail and at great length. Often, they have an elaborate, exotic, and complex pathophysiological theory to explain how they acquired the disease and what it is doing, or will soon do, to them. At times, they cite recent research and give great importance to other causes, tests, or treatments that they and their health providers have not yet tried. Because their actual problem is not, strictly speaking, medical (or not only medical) and because they usually frustrate professional caretakers such as physicians, as well as nonprofessional caretakers such as family and friends, breakdown in the helping process is common. Worried patients tax physicians' time and resources, while busy physicians feel increasingly drained for what they believe is no good reason. The hypochondriacal patients sense that their concerns are not respected or taken seriously; they start to sense resentment. Phone calls to physicians' offices go unreturned for longer and longer periods. The perceived lack of access to their health providers makes the hypochondriac worry even more frenetically. The physicians increasingly believe that these patients are unappreciative—that they are, in fact, healthy and that they are not cooperating with treatment goals. Instead, these hypochondriacal patients are seen as excessively demanding. Anger builds on both sides, relationships deteriorate, and the hypochondriacs begin to "doctor-shop," while the physicians lose them as patients.

Although hypochondriasis is usually chronic, with periods in which it is more and less severe, temporary hypochondriacal reactions are also commonly seen. Such reactions most often occur when patients have experienced a death or serious illness of someone close to them or some other major life stressor, including their own recovery from a life-threatening illness.

When these reactions persist for less than six months, the technical diagnosis is a condition called "somatoform disorder not otherwise specified," and not hypochondriasis. When external stressors cause the reaction, the hypochondriacal symptoms usually remit when the stressors dissipate or are resolved. The important exception to this rule occurs when family, friends, or health professionals inadvertently reinforce the worry and preoccupation through inappropriate amounts of attention. In effect, they reward hypochondriacal behavior and increase the likelihood that it will persist: A mother may never have received more support and help at home than following breast cancer surgery; a father may never have felt his children's affection as much as when he recuperated from having a heart attack; an employee may have never obtained special allowances on the job or received so many calls from coworkers as when recovering from herniated disk surgery; or a student may never have gotten as special treatment or as many gifts from teammates as when treated for rheumatic fever. What began as a transient hypochondriacal reaction can become chronic, primary hypochondriasis.

The life of hypochondriacs is unhappy and unrewarding. Nervous tension, depression, hopelessness, and a general lack of interest in life mark the fabric of the hypochondriacs' daily routines. Actual clinical, depressive disorders can easily coexist with hypochondriasis, to the point that even antidepression medications will simultaneously alleviate hypochondriacal symptoms.

Hypochondriasis often accompanies physical illness in the elderly. As a group, the elderly have declining health, experience diminished physical capacities, and are at increased risk for contracting and developing disease. Sometimes, earlier tendencies toward hypochondriasis simply intensify with age. Sometimes, old age is simply when it first appears. Hypochondriasis is not, however, a typical or expected aspect of normal aging; most elderly people are not hypochondriacal. In those who are, however, hypochondriasis is most likely a symptom of depression, abandonment, or loneliness, and these are the conditions that should first be treated.

TREATMENT AND THERAPY

The most important aspect of treating hypochondriasis is assessing whether true organic disease exists. Many diseases in their early stages are diffuse and affect multiple organ systems. Neurologic diseases (such as multiple sclerosis), hormonal abnormalities (such as Graves' disease), and autoimmune/connective tissue diseases (such as systemic lupus) can all manifest themselves early in ways that are difficult to diagnose accurately. The frantic and obsessive reporting of hypochondriacal patients can just as easily be the worried and detailed reporting of patients with early parathyroid disease; both report symptoms that are multiple, vague, and diffuse. The danger of hypochondriasis lies in its being diagnosed in place of true organic disease, which is exactly the kind of event hypochondriacs fear will happen.

Of course, there is nothing to prevent someone with true hypochondriasis from getting or having true physical illness. Worrying about illness neither protects from nor prevents illness. Moreover, barring a sudden, lethal accident or event, every hypochondriac is bound to develop organic illness sooner or later. Physical illness can coexist with hypochondriasis—and does so when attitudes, symptoms, and mental and emotional states are extreme and disproportionate to the medical problem at hand.

The goal in treating hypochondriasis is care, not cure. These patients have ongoing mental illness or chronic maladaptation and seem to need physical symptoms to justify how they feel. Neither surgical nor medical interventions will ameliorate a psychological need for symptoms. The best treatments (when hypochondriasis cannot itself be the target of treatment, which is most of the time) are long term in orientation and seek to help patients tolerate and accommodate their symptoms while health providers learn to understand and adapt to these difficult-to-treat patients.

Medications have proved useful in treating hypochondriasis only when accompanied by pharmacotherapy-sensitive conditions such as major depression or generalized anxiety. When hypochondriasis coexists with either mental or physical disease, the latter must be treated in its own right. Secondary hypochondriasis means that the primary disorder warrants primary treatment.

The course of hypochondriasis is unclear. Clinicians' anecdotal experience tends to endorse the perception that these people are impossible as patients. Outcome studies, however, belie the pessimism. The research suggests that many who are treated get better, and the more the following conditions are present, the better the outcome is likely to be: coexisting anxiety or depressive disorder, rapid onset, onset at a younger age, higher socioeconomic status, absence of organic disease, and absence of a personality disorder.

A fifty-six-year-old married male, for example, recounted his history as never having been in really good health at any time in his life. He made many physician office visits and had, over the years, seen many physicians, though without ever feeling emotionally connected to them. Over the past several months, he felt increasingly concerned that he was having headaches "all over" his head and that they were caused by an undetected tumor in the middle of his brain, "where no X ray could detect it." He had read about magnetic resonance imaging (MRI) in a health letter to which he subscribed and said that he wanted this procedure performed "to catch the tumor early." Various prescribed medications for his headache usually brought no relief.

While productive at work and promoted several times, he had been passed over for his last promotion because, he believed, his superiors did not like him. He also stated that he believed that many on the job saw him as cynical and pessimistic but that no one appreciated the "pain and mental anxiety" he endured "day in and day out."

His spouse of thirty-two years had advanced significantly at a job she had begun ten years earlier, and she seemed to him to be closer to their three children than he was. She was increasingly involved with outside voluntary activities, which kept her quite busy. She reported that she often asked him to join her in at least some of her activities but he always said no. She said that when she arrived home late, he was often in a state of physical upset, but for which she could never seem to do the "right thing to help him." In their joint interview, each admitted often feeling angry at and frustrated with the other. She could never determine why he was sick so often and why her efforts to help only seemed to make his situation worse. He could not understand how she could leave him all alone feeling as physically bad as he did. He believed that she never seemed to worry that something might happen to him while she was out being "a community do-gooder." The husband was suffering from a classic case of hypochondriasis.

PERSPECTIVE AND PROSPECTS

Both the concept and term "hypochondriasis" have ancient origins and reflect a view that all persons are subject to their own humoral ebb and flow. Humors were once thought to be bodily fluids that maintained health, regulated physical functioning, and caused certain personality traits. In classical Greek, *hypochondria*, the plural of *hypochondrion*, referred to both a part of the anatomy and the condition known today as hypochondriasis. *Hypo* means "under," "below," or "beneath," and *chondrion* means literally "cartilage" but in this case refers specifically to the bottom tip of cartilage at the breastbone (the xiphoid or, more formally, xiphisternum). Here, below the breastbone but above the navel, two humors were thought to flow in excess in the hypochondriacal person. The liver, producing black bile, made people melancholic, depressed, and depressing; the spleen, producing yellow bile, made people bilious, cross, and cynical. This view, or a variant of it, persisted until the middle to late eighteenth century.

Sigmund Freud and other psychiatrists treated hypochondriacal symptoms with some success while approaching the disorder as a defense mechanism rather than as an excess of bodily fluids. Their treatment for the first time cast a psychological role for what had been seen as a physical problem. Mental health professionals whose theoretical orientation is psychoanalytic or psychodynamic continue to deal with hypochondriasis as they deal with other defense mechanisms.

In the 1970's, some researchers began to suggest that hypochondriasis was being incorrectly applied to describe a discrete disorder, when it was really only an adjective that described a cluster of nonspecific behaviors. They argued that hypochondriasis is not a real diagnosis. Other researchers disagreed and argued for differentiating between primary and secondary hypochondriasis. Their view has proved to have significant pragmatic utility in treating the wide range of patients who exhibit symptoms of hypochondriasis, and it remains the prevailing view.

Given the general unwillingness of patients with hypochondriasis to admit that they have a psychological problem and not some yet-to-be-found organic condition, the interpersonal difficulties that often arise between health providers and these patients, and the serious potential of concurrent organic disease, it is not surprising why hypochondriasis continues to challenge both persons afflicted with this disorder and those who treat them.

—*Paul Moglia, Ph.D.*

See also Anxiety; Bipolar disorder; Depression; Factitious disorders; Midlife crisis; Neurosis; Obsessive-compulsive disorder; Panic attacks; Phobias; Psychiatric disorders; Psychiatry; Psychiatry, child and adolescent; Psychiatry, geriatric; Psychosomatic disorders; Stress; Stress reduction.

FOR FURTHER INFORMATION:

Asmundson, Gordon J. G., et al., eds. *Health Anxiety: Clinical and Research Perspectives on Hypochondriasis and Related Conditions*. New York: Wiley, 2001. Assembles a wealth of information from the fields of medicine and psychology on the causes, assessment, and treatment of health anxiety related disorders.

Barsky, Arthur J. "Somatoform Disorders." In *Comprehensive Textbook of Psychiatry VI*. Vol. 1, edited by Harold I. Kaplan and Benjamin J. Sadock. 6th ed. Baltimore: Williams & Wilkins, 1995. While Kaplan and Sadock's book remains the standard psychiatric reference for psychiatrists and nonpsychiatric physicians alike, Barsky's chapter includes an excellent discussion of hypochondriasis that is readily intelligible to laypeople.

Ben-Tovim, David I., and Adrian Esterman. "Zero Progress with Hypochondriasis." *The Lancet* 352, no. 9143 (December 5, 1998): 1798-1799. Despite behavioral research on patients suffering from hypochondriasis, no acceptable treatment for this condition has been discovered. It is important for doctors to adequately examine these patients, however, because even hypochondriacal patients can fall ill.

De Jong, Peter J., Marie-Anne Haenen, Anton Schmidt, and Birgit Mayer. "Hypochondriasis: The Role of Fear-Confirming Reasoning." *Behaviour Research and Therapy* 36, no. 1 (January, 1998): 65-74. This article investigates whether hypochondriacal patients are prone to selectively search for danger-confirming information when asked to judge the validity of conditional rules in the context of general and health threats.

Hill, John. *Hypochondriasis: A Practical Treatise.* New York: AMS Press, 1992. Originally published in 1766, this well-regarded and readable work presents the world of the hypochondriac in ways that challenge stereotypical and biased views of them.

Starcevic, Vladen. *Hypochondriasis: Modern Perspectives on an Ancient Malady.* New York: Oxford University Press, 2000. Provides an integrative overview of hypochondriasis as a mental disorder with diverse manifestations.

HYPOGLYCEMIA
DISEASE/DISORDER

ANATOMY OR SYSTEM AFFECTED: Blood, endocrine system, glands

SPECIALTIES AND RELATED FIELDS: Endocrinology, family practice, hematology, internal medicine, serology

DEFINITION: The condition in which concentration of glucose in the blood is too low to meet the needs of key organs, especially the brain; this condition limits treatments for diabetes mellitus.

KEY TERMS:

fasting hypoglycemia: hypoglycemia that occurs when no food is available from the intestinal tract; usually caused by failure of the neural, hormonal, and/or enzymatic mechanisms that convert stored fuels (primarily glycogen) into glucose

glucagon: a pancreatic hormone which signals an elevated concentration of glucose in the circulation

gluconeogenesis: the synthesis of molecules of glucose from smaller carbohydrates and amino acids

glucose: a simple sugar, readily converted to metabolic energy by most cells of the body and essential for the welfare of brain cells

glycogen: a storage form of carbohydrate, composed of many molecules of glucose linked together; found in many tissues of the body and serves as a major source of circulating glucose

glycogenolysis: the cleavage of glycogen into its constituent molecules of glucose

hypoglycemic unawareness: the occurrence of hypoglycemia without the warning symptoms of trembling, palpitations, hunger, or anxiety

hypoglycemic unresponsiveness: inadequate recovery of the circulating glucose concentration after an episode of hypoglycemia

insulin: a pancreatic hormone which signals a reduced concentration of glucose in the circulation

neuroglycopenia: abnormal function of the brain, caused by an inadequate supply of glucose from the circulation

reactive hypoglycemia: hypoglycemia that occurs within a few hours after ingestion of a meal

CAUSES AND SYMPTOMS

The condition known as hypoglycemia exists when the concentration of glucose in the bloodstream is too low to meet bodily needs for fuel, particularly those of the brain. Ordinarily, physiological compensatory mechanisms are called into play when the circulating concentration of glucose falls below about 3.5 millimoles. Activation of the sympathetic nervous system and the secretion of glucagon are especially important in promoting glycogenolysis and gluconeogenesis. Symptoms of sympathetic nervous activation normally become apparent with glucose concentrations that are less than about 3 millimoles. Brain function is usually demonstrably abnormal at glucose concentrations below about 2 millimoles; sustained hypoglycemia in this range can lead to permanent brain damage.

Some of the symptoms of hypoglycemia occur as by-products of activation of the sympathetic nervous system. These symptoms include trembling, pallor, palpitations and rapid heartbeat, sweating, abdominal discomfort, and feelings of anxiety and/or hunger. These symptoms are not dangerous in themselves; in fact, they may be considered to be beneficial, as they alert the individual to obtain food. Meanwhile, the sympathetic nervous system signals compensatory mechanisms. The manifestations of abnormal brain function during hypoglycemia include blunting of higher cogni-

---

INFORMATION ON HYPOGLYCEMIA

CAUSES: Endocrine disorder, malnutrition, advanced stages of cancer, inherited metabolic disorders, severe infections (including overwhelming bacterial infection and malaria), certain drugs

SYMPTOMS: Trembling, pallor, palpitations and rapid heartbeat, sweating, abdominal discomfort, feelings of anxiety and/or hunger, disturbed thoughts, confusion, loss of normal control of behavior, headache, lethargy, impaired vision, abnormal speech

DURATION: Temporary to long-term

TREATMENTS: Drugs inhibiting secretion of insulin, hormonal therapy

---

tive functions, disturbed mentation, confusion, loss of normal control of behavior, headache, lethargy, impaired vision, abnormal speech, paralysis, neurologic deficits, coma, and epileptic seizures. The individual is usually unaware of the appearance of these symptoms, which can present real danger. For example, episodes of hypoglycemia have occurred while individuals were driving motor vehicles, leading to serious injury and death. After recovery from hypoglycemia, the patient may have no memory of the episode.

There are two major categories of hypoglycemia: fasting and reactive. The most serious, fasting hypoglycemia, represents impairment of the mechanisms responsible for the production of glucose when food is not available. These mechanisms include the functions of cells in the liver and brain that monitor the availability of circulating glucose. Additionally, there is a coordinated hormonal response involving the secretion of glucagon, growth hormone, and other hormones and the inhibition of the secretion of insulin. The normal consequences of these processes include the addition of glucose to the circulation, primarily from glycogenolysis, as well as a slowing of the rate of utilization of circulating glucose by many tissues of the body, especially the liver, skeletal and cardiac muscle, and fat. Even after days without food, the body normally avoids hypoglycemia through breakdown of stored proteins and activation of gluconeogenesis. There is considerable redundancy in the systems that maintain glucose concentration, so that the occurrence of hypoglycemia often reflects the presence of defects in more than one of these mechanisms.

The other category of hypoglycemia, reactive hypoglycemia, includes disorders in which there is disproportionately prolonged and/or great activity of the physiologic systems that normally cause storage of the glucose derived from ingested foods. When a normal person eats a meal, the passage of food through the stomach and intestines elicits a complex and well-orchestrated neural and hormonal response, culminating in the secretion of insulin from the beta cells of the islets of Langerhans in the pancreas. The insulin signals the cells in muscle, adipose tissue, and the liver to stop producing glucose and to derive energy from glucose obtained from the circulation. Glucose in excess of the body's immediate needs for fuel is taken up and stored as glycogen is or utilized for the manufacture of proteins. Normally, the signals for the uptake and storage of glucose reach their peak of activity simultaneously with the entry into the circulation of glucose from the food undergoing digestion. As a result, the concentration of glucose in the circulation fluctuates only slightly. In individuals with reactive hypoglycemia, however, the entry of glucose from the digestive tract and the signals for its uptake and storage are not well synchronized. When signals for the cellular uptake of glucose persist after the intestinally derived glucose has dissipated, hypoglycemia can result. Although the degree of hypoglycemia may be severe and potentially dangerous, recovery can take place without assistance if the individual's general nutritional state is adequate and the systems for activation of glycogenolysis and gluconeogenesis are intact.

DIAGNOSIS AND TREATMENT

The diagnostic evaluation of an individual who is suspected of having hypoglycemia begins with verification of the condition. Evaluation of a patient's symptoms can be confusing. On one hand, the symptoms arising from the sympathetic nervous system and those of neuroglycopenia may occur in a variety of nonhypoglycemic conditions. On the other hand, persons with recurrent hypoglycemia may have few or no obvious symptoms. Therefore, it is most important to document the concentration of glucose in the blood.

To establish the diagnosis of fasting hypoglycemia, the patient is kept without food for periods of time up to seventy-two hours, with frequent monitoring of the blood glucose. Should hypoglycemia occur, blood is taken for measurements of the key regulatory neurosecretions and hormones, including insulin, glucagon, growth hormone, cortisol, and epinephrine, as well as general indices of the function of the liver and kidneys. If there is suspicion of an abnormality in an enzyme involved in glucose production, the diagnosis can be confirmed by measurement of the relevant enzymatic activity in circulating blood cells or, if necessary, in a biopsy specimen of the liver.

Fasting hypoglycemia may be caused by any condition that inhibits the production of glucose or that causes an inappropriately great utilization of circulating glucose when food is not available. Insulin produces hypoglycemia through both of these mechanisms. Excessive circulating insulin ranks as one of the most important causes of fasting hypoglycemia, most cases of which result from the treatment of diabetes mellitus with insulin or with an oral drug of the sulfonylurea class. If the patient is known to be taking insulin or a sulfonylurea drug for diabetes, the cause of hypoglycemia is obvious; appropriate modification of the treatment should be made. Hypoglycemia caused by oral sulfonylureas is particularly troublesome because of the prolonged retention of these drugs in the body. The passage of several days may be required for recovery, during which time the patient needs continuous intravenous infusion of glucose.

Excessive insulin secretion may also result from increased numbers of pancreatic beta cells; the abnormal beta cells may be so numerous that they form benign or malignant tumors, called insulinomas. The preferred treatment of an insulinoma is surgery, if feasible. When the tumor can be removed surgically, the operation is often curative. Unfortunately, insulinomas are sometimes difficult for the surgeon to find. Magnetic resonance imaging (MRI), computed tomography (CT) scanning, ultrasonography, or angiography may help localize the tumor. Some insulinomas are multiple and/or malignant, rendering total removal impossible. In these circumstances, hypoglycemia can be relieved by drugs that inhibit the secretion of insulin.

Malignant tumors arising from various tissues of the body may produce hormones that act like insulin with respect to their effects on glucose metabolism. In some cases, these hormones are members of the family of insulin-like growth factors, which resemble insulin structurally. Malnutrition probably has an important role in predisposing patients with malignancy to hypoglycemia, which tends to occur when the cancer is far advanced.

Fasting hypoglycemia can be caused by disorders affecting various parts of the endocrine system. One such disorder is adrenal insufficiency; continued secretion of cortisol by the adrenal cortex is required for maintenance of normal glycogen stores and of the enzymes of glycogenolysis and gluconeogenesis. Severe hypothyroidism also may lead to hypoglycemia. Impairment in the function of the anterior pituitary gland predisposes a patient to hypoglycemia through several mechanisms, including reduced function of the thyroid gland and adrenal cortices (which depend on pituitary secretions for normal activity) and reduced secretion of growth hormone. Growth hormone plays an important physiologic role in the prevention of fasting hypoglycemia by signaling metabolic changes that allow heart and skeletal muscles to derive energy from stored fats, thereby sparing glucose for the brain. Specific replacement therapies are available for deficiencies of thyroxine, cortisol, and growth hormone.

Hypoglycemia has occasionally been reported as a side effect of treatment with medications other than those intended for treatment of diabetes. Drugs which have been implicated include sulfonamides, used for treatment of bacterial infections; quinine, used for treatment of falciparum malaria; pentamidine isethionate, given by injection for treatment of pneumocystosis; ritodrine, used for inhibition of premature labor; and propranolol or disopyramide, both of which are used for treatment of cardiac arrhythmias. Malnourished patients seem to be especially susceptible to the hypoglycemic effects of these medications, and management should consist of nutritional repletion in addition to discontinuation of the drug responsible. In children, aspirin or other medicines containing salicylates may produce hypoglycemia.

Alcohol hypoglycemia occurs in persons with low bodily stores of glycogen when there is no food in the intestine. In this circumstance, the only potential source of glucose for the brain is gluconeogenesis. When such an individual drinks alcohol, its metabolism within the liver prevents the precursors of glucose from entering the pathways of gluconeogenesis. This variety of fasting hypoglycemia can occur in persons who are not chronic alcoholics: It requires the ingestion of only a moderate amount of alcohol, on the order of three mixed drinks. Treatment involves the nutritional repletion of glycogen stores and the limitation of alcohol intake.

Severe infections, including overwhelming bacterial infection and malaria, can produce hypoglycemia by mechanisms that are not well understood. Patients with very severe liver damage can develop fasting hypoglycemia, because the pathways of glycogenolysis and gluconeogenesis in the liver are by far the major sources of circulating glucose in the fasted state. In such cases, the occurrence of hypoglycemia usually marks a near-terminal stage of liver disease. Uremia, the syndrome produced by kidney failure, can also lead to fasting hypoglycemia.

Some types of fasting hypoglycemia occur predominantly in infants and children. Babies in the first year of life may have an inappropriately high secretion of insulin. This problem occurs especially in newborn infants whose mothers had increased circulating glucose during pregnancy. Children from two to ten years of age may develop ketotic hypoglycemia, which is probably related to insufficient gluconeogenesis. These disorders tend to improve with time. Fasting hypoglycemia is also an important manifestation of a variety of inherited disorders of metabolism characterized by the abnormality or absence of one of the necessary enzymes or cofactors of glycogenolysis and gluconeogenesis or of fat metabolism (which supplies the energy for gluconeogenesis). Most of these disorders become evident in infancy or childhood. If there is a hereditary or acquired deficiency of an enzyme of glucose production, the problem can be circumvented by provision of a continuous supply of glucose to the affected individual.

There are several other rare causes of fasting hypoglycemia. A few individuals have had circulating antibodies that caused hypoglycemia by interacting with the patient's own insulin, or with receptors for insulin on the patient's cells. Although the autonomic (involuntary) nervous system has an important role in signaling recovery from hypoglycemia, diseases affecting this branch of the nervous system do not usually produce hypoglycemia; presumably, hormonal mechanisms can substitute for the missing neural signals.

Reactive hypoglycemia can occur with an unusually rapid passage of foodstuffs through the upper intestinal tract, such as may occur after partial or total removal of the stomach. Persons predisposed to maturity-onset diabetes may also have reactive hypoglycemia, probably because of the delay in the secretion of insulin in response to a meal. Finally, reactive hypoglycemia need not indicate the presence of any identifiable disease and may occur in otherwise normal individuals.

Diagnosis of reactive hypoglycemia is made difficult by the variability of symptoms and of glucose concentrations from day to day. Adding to the diagnostic uncertainty, circulating glucose normally rises and falls after meals, especially those rich in carbohydrates. Consequently, entirely normal and asymptomatic individuals may sometimes have glucose concentrations at or below the levels found in persons with reactive hypoglycemia. Therefore, the glucose tolerance test, in which blood samples are taken at intervals for several hours after the patient drinks a solution containing 50 to 100 grams of glucose, is quite unreliable and should not be employed for the diagnosis of reactive hypoglycemia. Proper diagnosis of reactive hypoglycemia depends on careful correlation of the patient's symptoms with the circulating glucose level, preferably measured on several occasions after ingestion of ordinary meals. Some persons develop symptoms such as weakness, nausea, sweating, and tremulousness after meals, but without a significant reduction of circulating glucose. This symptom complex should not be confused with hypoglycemia.

When rapid passage of food through the stomach and upper intestine causes reactive hypoglycemia, the administration of drugs that slow intestinal transit may be helpful. When reactive hypoglycemia has no evident pathological cause, the patient is usually advised to take multiple small meals throughout the day instead of the usual three meals and to avoid concentrated sweets. These dietary modifications can help avoid hypoglycemia by reducing the stimulus to secrete insulin.

Two rare inherited disorders of metabolism can produce reactive hypoglycemia after the ingestion of certain foods. In hereditary fructose intolerance, the offending nutrient is fructose, a sugar found in fruits as well as ordinary table sugar. In galactosemia, the sugar responsible for hypoglycemia is galactose, a major component of milk products. Management of these conditions, which usually become apparent in infancy or childhood, consists of avoidance of the foods responsible.

PERSPECTIVE AND PROSPECTS

Fasting hypoglycemia is uncommon, except in the context of treatment of diabetes mellitus. The most serious public health problem associated with hypoglycemia is that it limits the therapeutic effectiveness of insulin and sulfonylurea drugs. Evidence suggests that elevation of the circulating glucose concentration (hyperglycemia) is responsible for much of the disability and premature death among patients with diabetes. In many of these patients, therapeutic regimens consisting of multiple daily injections of insulin or continuous infusion of insulin through a small needle placed under the skin can reduce the average circulating glucose to normal. Frequent serious hypoglycemia is the most important adverse consequence of such regimens. Persons with diabetes seem to be at especially high risk for dangerous hypoglycemia for two reasons. First, there is often a failure of the warning systems that ordinarily cause uncomfortable symptoms when the circulating glucose concentration declines, a situation termed hypoglycemic unawareness. As a consequence, when a patient with diabetes attempts to control his or her blood sugar with more frequent injections of insulin, there may occur unheralded episodes of hypoglycemia that can lead to serious alterations in mental activity or even loss of consciousness. Many patients with diabetes also have hypoglycemic unresponsiveness, an impaired ability to recover from episodes of hypoglycemia. Also, diabetes can interfere with the normal physiologic responses that cause the secretion of glucagon in response to a reduction of circulating glucose, thus eliminating one of the most important defenses against hypoglycemia. If both hypoglycemic unawareness and hypoglycemic unresponsiveness could be reversed, intensive treatment of diabetes would become safer and more widely applicable.

Reactive hypoglycemia, although seldom a clue to serious disease, has attracted public attention because of its peculiarly annoying symptoms. These symptoms, which reflect activation of the sympathetic nervous system, resemble those of fear and anxiety. The symptoms are not specific, and many patients with these complaints do not have hypoglycemia.

In summary, hypoglycemia indicates defective regulation of the supply of energy to the body. When severe or persistent, hypoglycemia can lead to serious behavioral disorder, obtunded consciousness, and even brain damage. Fasting hypoglycemia may be a clue to significant endocrine disease. Reactive hypoglycemia, while annoying, usually responds to simple dietary measures. The study of hypoglycemia has led to many important insights into the regulation of energy metabolism.

—*Victor R. Lavis, M.D.*

See also Blood and blood disorders; Diabetes mellitus; Endocrine disorders; Endocrinology; Endocrinology, pediatric; Hormones; Metabolism; Obesity; Pancreas; Pancreatitis; Vitamins and minerals.

FOR FURTHER INFORMATION:

Chow, Cheryl, and M. D. Chow. *Hypoglycemia for Dummies.* New York: Wiley, 2003. Part of the popular "Dummies" series, provides a wide range of expert information on diagnosis, risk factors, treatment options, diet and exercise regimens, advice on finding the right doctor, and setting up a support network.

Cryer, Philip E. "Glucose Homeostasis and Hypoglycemia." In *Williams Textbook of Endocrinology*, edited by Jean D. Wilson and Daniel W. Foster. 9th ed. Philadelphia: W. B. Saunders, 1998. A complete and definitive chapter. Delineates especially well the coordination of the nervous and hormonal systems in physiologic defense against hypoglycemia, as well as the special problems of hypoglycemia in patients with diabetes mellitus.

Davidson, Mayer B. "Hypoglycemia." In *Diabetes Mellitus: Diagnosis and Treatment.* 8th ed. New York: John Wiley & Sons, 1986. The author has made an important contribution to the study of diabetes and metabolism. The chapter offers clear explanations of the physiological abnormalities in hypoglycemia and emphasizes the importance of fasting hypoglycemia as an index of serious illness.

Hypoglycemia Support Foundation, The. http://www.hypoglycemia.org/main.htm. Provides diet information, self tests for the disease, and helpful Internet links.

Kahn, Ronald C., and Gordon C. Weir, eds. *Joslin's Diabetes Mellitus.* 14th ed. Philadelphia: Lea & Febiger, 2002. The definitive American textbook of diabetes. Covers all causes of hypoglycemia, not simply those related to diabetes.

Lincoln, Thomas A., and John A. Eaddy. *Beating the Blood Sugar Blues: Proven Methods and Wisdom for Controlling Hypoglycemia.* New York: McGraw-Hill, 2001. The authors, both type I diabetes patients, provide a thorough guide to understanding, preventing, and treating hypoglycemia, and intersperse the narrative with personal stories from doctors and patients.

Parker, James N., and Philip M. Parker, eds. *The 2002 Official Patient's Sourcebook on Hypoglycemia.* San Diego, Calif.: Icon Health, 2002. Draws from public, academic, government, and peer-reviewed research to provide a wide-ranging handbook for adult patients with hypoglycemia.

HYPOPARATHYROIDISM. *See* HYPERPARATHYROIDISM AND HYPOPARATHYROIDISM.

HYPOSPADIAS REPAIR AND URETHROPLASTY

PROCEDURE

ANATOMY OR SYSTEM AFFECTED: Genitals, reproductive system

SPECIALTIES AND RELATED FIELDS: General surgery, urology
DEFINITION: Urethroplasty is any plastic surgery performed on the urethra; one of these procedures is the repair of hypospadias, the presence of an abnormal opening in the male urethra.

INDICATIONS AND PROCEDURES

Urethroplasty is performed to correct defects of the urethra, the tube leading from the bladder to the outside of the body through which urine exits the body. Hypospadias is a congenital defect of the distal end of the urethra in which it opens on the underside of the penis instead of at the tip. Less commonly, the opening can occur lower down on the underside of the penis or in the scrotum. Hypospadias is also associated with abnormalities in the kidneys.

The correction of hypospadias involves a technique known as a "flip-flap" repair: Two incisions on the undersurface of the glans and shaft of the penis are made, and skin from the glans is fashioned into an opening that is anatomically normal. The operation is usually done under general anesthesia.

The lines for both incisions are drawn and incisions carefully made to avoid damaging adjacent structures and erectile tissue. The prepuce is released from the body of the penis. A V-shaped flap is cut from the skin immediately below the hypospadias. The flap is rotated, and one side is sutured into one of the incisions made in the glans. The other side is similarly inserted into the other incision and sutured in place, forming a tube that extends the urethra. Excess skin from the prepuce is removed; the prepuce is sutured back into position on the shaft of the penis. The skin from the underside of the penis is brought together over the repaired urethra and sutured together. A catheter is frequently (but not universally) placed in the urethra and kept in place for up to three weeks. Some surgeons believe that the presence of a catheter helps to establish the new urethra. Others think that it only contributes to postoperative holes (fistulas) and do not use it, allowing the patient to urinate immediately through the newly constructed tube. The patient returns to the surgeon's office in a week for a postoperative check and the removal of sutures.

Another type of urethroplasty is the surgical repair of a discontinuity in the male urethra. Most commonly, this defect occurs on the underside of the penis and is attributable to the incomplete closure of the skin portions that normally fuse over the urethra during embryonic development. The technique is similar to that described above. Under general anesthesia, skin is removed from the prepuce of the penis and is sutured in place over the defect, closing the opening. A catheter may or may not be inserted. The patient returns to the surgeon's office in a week for a postoperative check and the removal of sutures.

USES AND COMPLICATIONS

The techniques associated with urethroplasty are used to repair congenital defects. Complications from these procedures are unusual, but they may include infection and stricture. Such problems can be avoided with careful attention to the finer details of the surgery.

The need for urethroplasty and hypospadias repair is unlikely to disappear. From a psychological standpoint, it benefits the patient to repair a hypospadias as early in life as possible, preferably before the age of three.

—*L. Fleming Fallon, Jr., M.D., Ph.D., M.P.H.*

See also Fistula repair; Genital disorders, male; Neonatology; Pediatrics; Reproductive system; Surgery, pediatric; Urinary system; Urology; Urology, pediatric.

FOR FURTHER INFORMATION:

Berkow, Robert, and Andrew J. Fletcher, eds. *The Merck Manual of Diagnosis and Therapy.* 17th ed. Rahway, N.J.: Merck Sharp & Dohme Research Laboratories, 1999.

Ferrari, Mario. *Renal and Genitourinary Disorders.* New York: Elsevier, 2002.

Hadidi, Ahmed T., and A. F. Azmy. *Hypospadias Surgery: Art and Science.* New York: Springer-Verlag, 2003.

Montague, Drogo K. *Disorders of Male Sexual Function.* Chicago: Year Book Medical, 1988.

Swanson, Janice M., and Katherine A. Forrest. *Men's Reproductive Health.* New York: Springer, 1984.

HYPOTHERMIA. *See* HYPERTHERMIA AND HYPOTHERMIA.

HYSTERECTOMY

PROCEDURE

ANATOMY OR SYSTEM AFFECTED: Reproductive system, uterus

SPECIALTIES AND RELATED FIELDS: Endocrinology, general surgery, gynecology, oncology

DEFINITION: The removal of the uterus and sometimes the ovaries and surrounding tissues, which is performed for a variety of indications, including uterine cancer and fibroids that cause symptoms.

KEY TERMS:

adenomyosis: a noncancerous disorder in which cells resembling the lining of the uterus are found within the muscle layer of the uterus, leading to abnormal vaginal bleeding and pain

estrogen: the female sex hormone produced by the ovaries and the adrenal gland that is responsible for the development of female secondary sex characteristics; the three types naturally produced by the body are estradiol, estrone, and estriol

Fallopian tubes: the structures located between the uterus and ovaries that are responsible for the transport of the egg; also called the oviducts

fibroid: a noncancerous tumor of the uterus, also known as leiomyoma; when large, these tumors can cause heavy menstrual bleeding leading to anemia or cause pressure symptoms in the pelvis

laparoscopy: a minimally invasive surgical procedure in which an instrument equipped with a small camera, called a laparoscope, is inserted through a small incision in the abdomen to visualize the pelvis or abdomen; surgical manipulation may be carried out during this procedure

menorrhagia: unusually heavy menstrual bleeding; when severe, it can lead to anemia

progesterone/progestin: a hormone produced in the ovaries that sustains pregnancy; birth control pills are composed primarily of progesterone, which works by suppressing ovulation

INDICATIONS AND PROCEDURES

The term "hysterectomy" comes from the Greek *hystera,* meaning "uterus," and *ektome,* meaning "to cut out." While hysterectomy refers to the removal of the uterus and, most commonly, the attached Fallopian tubes, there are several types of hysterectomies. Total hysterectomy, contrary to popular belief, does not mean that the ovaries are removed with the uterus. Rather, the term indicates the removal of the uterus and cervix. Subtotal, or partial, hysterectomy is the excision of the uterus above the cervix; the cervix is left in place. Either one or both ovaries may be removed with the uterus (unilateral oophorectomy or bilateral oophorectomy). Salpingo-oophorectomy refers to the removal of one of the Fallopian tubes along with the accompanying ovary, while bilateral salpingo-oophorectomy refers to the removal of both Fallopian tubes and ovaries.

Indications for hysterectomy can be divided into noncancerous and cancerous conditions. Within the noncancerous category, the most common indication for hysterectomy is symptomatic fibroids. Many women have fibroids, and the majority of fibroids do not cause symptoms and can be left alone. Symptomatic fibroids are those which are large enough to cause pressure symptoms in the pelvis, compress the bladder or rectum, or cause pain or discomfort during intercourse. Another type of symptomatic fibroids are those which cause excessively heavy menstrual bleeding and, when severe, anemia.

A hysterectomy is indicated in these situations if the patient fails to respond to less conservative therapy for symptomatic fibroids. Examples of conservative therapy for heavy bleeding include high-dose estrogen or birth control pills. A hysterectomy is usually performed only when childbearing is no longer desired, since removal of the uterus precludes pregnancy. Prior to hysterectomy, large fibroids may be shrunk with a course of a hormone called gonadotropin-releasing hormone. Unfortunately, this treatment results in menopausal symptoms, including hot flushes and bone density depletion, and therefore cannot be used for prolonged periods of time. More recently, treatments such as uterine artery embolization, in which the arteries feeding the uterus are blocked off using foreign particles such as gel foam, have been tried as an alternative to hysterectomy, in an attempt to preserve the uterus and avoid major surgery.

Another indication for hysterectomy is in patients who have had recurrent fibroids after myomectomy. A myomectomy is the surgical removal of isolated fibroids, rather than removal of the uterus itself. The benefit is that the uterus can be preserved, although the downside is that fibroids may regrow. Hysterectomy is the definitive treatment for uterine fibroids.

Another noncancerous indication for hysterectomy is adenomyosis, a painful condition whereby the cells of the uterine lining are abnormally embedded in the uterine muscle. No good treatments exist for this condition besides hysterectomy. Another indication for hysterectomy occurs in cases of abnormal uterine bleeding in which the bleeding is refractory to management with nonsurgical treatments, such as birth control pills or procedures that ablate the uterine lining. Other less common indications for hysterectomy are uterine prolapse (in which the uterus descends into the vaginal canal, causing discomfort or urinary incontinence), chronic pelvic pain (refractory to more conservative

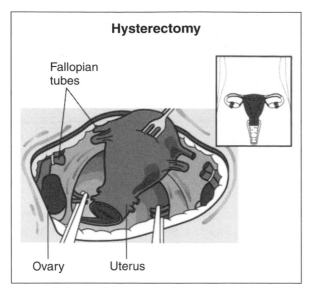

Hysterectomy

Fallopian tubes

Ovary   Uterus

The uterus, and sometimes such accompanying organs as the ovaries and Fallopian tubes, may be removed to treat disease conditions or as a contraceptive measure; the inset shows the location of the uterus.

management), and large infections of the uterus and pelvis that are unresponsive to antibiotics. Hysterectomy may also be performed as part of a cesarean section if the surgeon encounters uncontrollable bleeding after delivery of the infant.

Uterine cancer is a clear indication for hysterectomy. Often, the cancer causes abnormal uterine bleeding. Prior to hysterectomy, the cancer has usually been confirmed on biopsy of the uterine lining. If the cancer is small and localized to a small area of the uterus, then removal of the uterus alone may be curative. More often, however, uterine cancer may have spread more deeply into the uterine wall or even grown beyond the uterus. In these cases, hysterectomy may be accompanied by more extensive surgery that includes removing lymph nodes or other pelvic structures.

Most frequently, hysterectomy is accomplished through a 6- to 8-inch midline incision running either down from the navel or across the lower abdomen near or below the hairline (known as a "bikini incision"). This procedure is referred to as an abdominal hysterectomy. Vaginal hysterectomy is the removal of the uterus through the vaginal canal, rather than through a surgical opening in the abdomen. This procedure is most often performed to resolve prolapse (because the uterus has already descended into the vaginal canal) or when the uterus is not massively enlarged and can be pulled down and out through the vagina. If the hysterectomy is

performed because of large fibroid tumors, then the abdominal approach is usually used. On rare occasions, a vaginal hysterectomy may be facilitated using laparoscopy. In these cases, laparoscopy enables visualization and manipulation of the uterus via small incisions in the abdomen to assist in removal of the uterus through the vaginal canal.

During the hysterectomy, the patient is almost always under general anesthesia. The patient lies on her back for abdominal hysterectomies. In vaginal hysterectomies, the patient's legs are placed in stirrups and the knees are spread apart to enable the gynecologist to gain access to the vaginal canal. The actual removal of the uterus involves clamping, transecting, and suture ligating the blood vessels that feed the uterus and the tissues that anchor the uterus in the pelvic cavity. Care is taken by the surgeon to avoid the ureters, the tubes carrying urine from the kidney to the bladder. The ureters are very close to the lower part of the uterus and can be damaged easily. If the entire uterus is removed, then the top end of the vagina, called the cuff, is sutured closed. If the cervix is left in place, then the top of the cervix is sutured closed.

After the surgery, the patient receives narcotic pain medication and antibiotics to prevent infection and is monitored carefully to confirm that vital signs are stable and recovery is appropriate. Laboratory tests may be performed to ensure that the patient is not unusually anemic and that important organs such as the kidneys are functioning properly. Until a patient is able to walk, a catheter (a rubber tube attached to a collecting bag) will be used to pass urine. Patients may initially take liquids by mouth. When they can tolerate liquids, indicating no apparent injury to the bowels, patients may begin to take solid food. A patient may be hospitalized for two to four days after the hysterectomy, although hospital stays in general have been shortening in length. On the whole, patients who receive vaginal hysterectomies have shorter hospital stays than patients receiving abdominal hysterectomies, assuming that no complications arise. Patients can usually resume normal sexual functioning six weeks after the surgery.

Uses and Complications
Hysterectomy can be used to provide relief from pressure, pain, and bleeding from the uterus. It may also be curative in the early stages of uterine cancer and can increase survival in later stages. For women who are finished with childbearing and whose lifestyles or respon-

sibilities do not allow them to try more conservative treatments, many of which require several months to take effect, hysterectomy can provide definitive relief from symptoms within the defined time period needed to undergo scheduled surgery. In cases of life-threatening uterine hemorrhage, hysterectomy can save a woman's life.

The common complications of hysterectomy are those which are common to many major surgeries. One complication is excessive blood loss. The average blood loss during a hysterectomy is estimated at between 400 and 500 cubic centimeters (about a pint). When removal of the uterus is difficult, for instance because of the position of large fibroids, increased blood loss is likely to occur. When excessive blood loss is of concern, the patient's blood levels may be checked during the procedure. A patient who is significantly anemic may receive blood transfusions to avoid poor oxygenation of the major organs and to increase blood volume, and hence avoid shock. The number of transfusions depends on the amount of blood estimated to be lost. If a blood vessel continues to bleed after the patient leaves the operating room, then the patient may need to return to the operating room to have the bleeding vessel identified and sutured.

Another common complication of hysterectomy is infection. Even when aseptic techniques are followed, an infection may develop several days after the surgery. This is particularly true in vaginal hysterectomies, where the surgeon works through the vaginal canal, considered a clean but contaminated field. For this reason, patients are given antibiotics immediately prior to surgery in order to prevent against infection. A patient who shows signs of infection after the surgery may be placed on an extended course of antibiotics. The source of these infections can range from the vaginal cuff site to the peritoneum (the lining of the pelvic and abdominal cavity) and the urinary tract.

The third major complication that can occur with hysterectomy is inadvertent damage to internal organs. The urinary tract and the bowels are particularly at risk during hysterectomy because of their proximity to the uterus. The ureters can be occluded inadvertently by the misplacement of a suture. If discovered early, this damage can be repaired. If the problem is not recognized, however, then a damaged ureter can result in kidney malfunction. For this reason, kidney function is carefully followed after the hysterectomy through blood tests. Since the bladder sits on the bottom half of the uterus, it is a common organ that can be damaged during a hysterectomy. If the bladder is accidentally entered using the scalpel during surgery, then it can usually be repaired during the procedure. Postsurgery, the patient may need prolonged catheterization of the bladder to enhance bladder recovery. The large and small intestines are another common site of surgical injury. They can be accidentally cut or sutured. Sometimes, this problem is not detected until after the patient has left the operating room, and the problem becomes apparent when normal bowel function does not return in a timely fashion postoperatively. The patient may experience nausea, vomiting, and abdominal distension and discomfort and may not be able to pass gas from the rectum.

Another complication that can occur after surgery is the formation of blood clots, particularly in the leg veins, as a result of the patient's immobility during and after surgery. These clots can be dangerous when they break off from their source and move into the lungs, a condition called pulmonary embolism. Large pulmonary emboli can be life-threatening. Pulmonary emboli can be prevented using warm compression stockings during and after surgery to promote blood flow. Early ambulation (walking) after surgery can also decrease the chances of developing leg vein clots and pulmonary emboli.

Long-term complications of hysterectomy also include scar formation in the pelvis, called adhesions, which can interfere with bowel function or cause pelvic pain. Some patients may experience the prolapse of the remaining pelvic organs (such as the bowels and bladder) into the space formerly occupied by the uterus. Procedures may be employed during the hysterectomy to anchor the vaginal cuff and close any spaces where prolapse might occur.

In rare cases, removal of the uterus can inadvertently decrease blood supply to any remaining ovaries, leading to ischemia and loss of ovarian function. In these cases, the patient may experience the symptoms of estrogen deficiency, also known as menopausal symptoms. They include hot flushes, vaginal dryness, and, when estrogen deficiency is prolonged, bone density loss. In women whose hysterectomies included removal of the ovaries, the hot flushes may become apparent a few days after surgery. In these cases, estrogen therapy or other medications may be of benefit.

The impact of a hysterectomy on a woman's psychological state varies from woman to woman. In women who have been suffering a great deal from their symptoms, be it pressure and pain or abnormal bleeding, a hysterectomy can be a relief and enable them to return to their activities of daily living. Hysterectomy can improve sexual function in many cases. In other women, a hysterectomy can trigger a sense of loss and represent the end of the woman's fertility, which is often associated with youth and vitality.

PERSPECTIVE AND PROSPECTS

In ancient times, the complaints of women and the illnesses of the female organs were viewed as coming from an "unhappy uterus." It was believed that the uterus had the primary purpose of childbearing and that, when the uterus was not occupied with this function, it might show its wrath by abnormal bleeding and pain. These beliefs prevailed for centuries; early medical history indicates that women's gynecologic complaints were largely ignored. Moreover, no safe surgical procedures had been developed.

A noteworthy event in early American medical history was the operation attempted and documented by a frontier physician and surgeon, Ephraim McDowell. In 1809 in Danville, Kentucky, this daring young doctor carried out experimental surgery on a middle-aged woman to remove a huge ovarian tumor. Without the benefit of anesthesia and a sterile technique, he performed successful abdominal surgery on four out of five other patients.

Myomectomy, or removal of a fibroid tumor of the uterus, was the next procedure to be performed—first in France and later (about 1850) in Massachusetts by Washington Atlee. The first hysterectomy was successfully performed by Walter Burnham in the same decade, but he lost twelve of his next fifteen hysterectomy patients. In the text *Operative Gynecology* (1898), Howard A. Kelly of Baltimore describes one hundred hysterectomies that he performed in the late nineteenth century, all done because of pelvic infection. He lost only four patients, though convalescence for some survivors was prolonged.

Remarkable medical progress occurred in the twentieth century in abdominal and vaginal surgical techniques. In the 1850's, Marion Sims of South Carolina was the first to perform vaginal surgery in the United States. He successfully repaired a vesicovaginal fistula, an abnormal opening between the bladder and the vagina through which urine escapes into the vagina. In the late nineteenth century, the "Manchester" operation for uterine prolapse was performed by A. Donald in Manchester, England. Prior to this procedure, uterine pro-

lapse was treated with a pessary, a device inserted into the vagina to hold the uterus in place.

In the early part of the twentieth century, hysterectomy was considered a relatively dangerous procedure; many of the medical advances necessary for its success (such as anesthesia, asepsis, antibiotics, and blood banks) were not yet available or were fraught with problems. Hysterectomy has now become one of the safer surgical procedures; mortality figures have dropped to between 0.2 and 0.5 percent, usually resulting from pulmonary embolism (a blood clot in the lungs), a complication common to almost all major surgeries.

In the 1930's, N. Sproat Heany of Chicago devised the present-day technique of vaginal hysterectomy. Vaginal (as opposed to abdominal) hysterectomy, it was believed, resulted in a less complicated procedure with shorter convalescence and more cosmetically pleasing results for most patients. For some time, vaginal hysterectomy was viewed as superior to abdominal hysterectomy. In the 1970's, between 25 and 40 percent of all hysterectomies were accomplished vaginally, depending on the age of the woman at the time of surgery. In 1981, however, a landmark study published by the U.S. Congress, weighing the costs, risks, and benefits of hysterectomy, stated that women undergoing vaginal hysterectomy are more likely to have postoperative fever and to receive antibiotic treatment. Moreover, vaginal hysterectomy patients may undergo further surgery at a rate as high as 5 to 10 percent.

By the late 1980's and early 1990's, the trend among many gynecologists had shifted away from hysterectomy to more conservative treatments, when possible. Physicians began to question whether hysterectomies were, in some or even in most cases, medically necessary. As more information became available to women regarding alternatives to hysterectomy (a major revenue-producing surgical procedure in the United States), many women became more apt to question their physicians when told that hysterectomy was the only possible solution to their gynecological problems.

—*Genevieve Slomski, Ph.D.;*
updated by Anne Lynn S. Chang, M.D.

See also Cancer; Cervical, ovarian, and uterine cancers; Contraception; Dysmenorrhea; Ectopic pregnancy; Endometriosis; Ethics; Genital disorders, female; Gynecology; Hormone replacement therapy (HRT); Hormones; Menorrhagia; Oncology; Reproductive system; Sex change surgery; Sterilization; Tubal ligation.

FOR FURTHER INFORMATION:

Clark, Jan. *Hysterectomy and the Alternatives: How to Ask the Right Questions and Explore Other Options.* London: Vermilion, 2000. Discusses the treatment of uterine fibroids and menstrual disorders and offers alternatives to radical hysterectomy.

Dennerstein, Lorraine, Carl Wood, and Ann Westmore. *Hysterectomy: New Options and Advances.* 2d ed. New York: Oxford University Press, 1995. This popular work on hysterectomy addresses all aspects of the procedure. Includes a bibliography and an index.

Stenchever, Morton A., et al. *Comprehensive Gynecology.* 4th ed. St. Louis: Mosby, 2001. One of the definitive textbooks in the field of gynecology. It outlines in an objective and complete manner the indications for hysterectomy and the various types of hysterectomy. Also describes appropriate postoperative care and alternatives to hysterectomy.

Way, Lawrence W., and Gerard M. Doherty, eds. *Current Surgical Diagnosis and Treatment.* 11th ed. New York: Lange Medical Books/McGraw-Hill, 2003. Provides concise summaries of gynecologic problems which could lead to hysterectomy.

Iatrogenic disorders

Disease/disorder

Anatomy or system affected: All
Specialties and related fields: All
Definition: Health problems caused by medical treatments.

Causes and Symptoms

Iatrogenic disorders may be attributable to inefficient or uncaring physicians or to the risks inherent in medical procedures that are necessary to prevent death or crippling disease. Such disorders are usually divided into those caused by medications, surgery, and medical misdiagnosis.

The average patient of any age expects physicians and the medical infrastructure to deliver perfect cures for all diseases. This is not possible because some diseases have no cure and because medical treatment always involves some potential risk to the persons being treated. In fact, a percentage—usually a small one—of the patients treated for any disease develop unexpected health problems (adverse reactions) which can be diseases themselves.

The term "iatrogenic disorder" is a catchall used to encompass the many different adverse reactions that accompany the practice of modern medicine. The number of such problems has grown as medical science has become more sophisticated. They are often blamed entirely on physicians and other medical staff involved in cases producing iatrogenic disorders.

This blame is correctly directed in instances where a physician and other staff involved are uncaring, inattentive, careless, or incompletely educated. However, iatrogenic disorders often result from the nature of modern medicine. Doctors frequently attempt therapeutic methods (such as surgery) that are innovative efforts which cure serious diseases but have some inherent risk of failure. They may also use therapeutic drugs that are powerful agents for cure of specific disease processes but that have side effects causing other health problems in some people who take them. In addition, doctors will very often utilize complicated overall therapy having adverse consequences that patients may not acknowledge despite physicians' attempts to explain them orally and with consent forms.

Treatment and Therapy

Despite careful efforts of most physicians—who are informed, caring, and efficient—iatrogenic disorders accompany many medical procedures. Public attention is, however, focused most on the effects of therapeutic agents, drugs and vaccines, because patients are often unaware that no therapeutic agent in use is ever perfectly safe. Even a clear physician description of the dos and don'ts associated with such therapy may be flawed by biological variation among patients, causing problems in one individual but not others. Furthermore, the explosion of new diseases and new versions of old diseases since the late 1980's has led to much more complex treatment regimens. Consequently, iatrogenic disorders occur much more often.

This has become particularly germane in treatment of the aged, acquired immunodeficiency syndrome (AIDS) patients, and the very young. Hence, several rules must be followed concerning therapeutic agents. First, wherever possible, these medications should be used only after other means fail and the benefits to be gained clearly outweigh the risks entailed. Second, therapy should begin with the lowest possible effective dose, and all dose increases should be accompanied by frequent symptom relief and toxicity monitoring. Third, patients and responsible family members must be made aware of all possible adverse symptoms, how to best counter them, and the foods or other medications to be avoided to diminish iatrogenic potential. Such problems, in the aged, are due to biochemical changes which alter their tolerance for many medications.

Many iatrogenic disorders are caused by the presence of bacterial contamination in wounds and the fact that surgical maintenance of sterility is not absolutely perfect. For example, iatrogenesis occurs after 30 percent of surgical procedures carried out at heavily contaminated surgical sites (such as emergency surgery of abdominal wounds). In addition, the use of antibiotics can be problematic. In many cases, the large doses of these therapeutic agents required to fight primary bacterial infection will cause superinfection by other microbes, such as fungi. Furthermore, wide antibiotic

---

Information on Iatrogenic Disorders

Causes: Inherent medical risk, misdiagnosis, physician malpractice, medication error, surgical error
Symptoms: Wide ranging
Duration: Varies from acute to fatal
Treatments: Depends on circumstances

use in hospitals has led to the creation of antibiotic-resistant bacteria.

For these reasons, treatment of surgical sites requires individualized attention. Clean wounds can be closed up immediately without high risk of infection, but deep wounds known to be contaminated prior to surgery are often best handled by closing up interior tissues and leaving skin and subcutaneous tissues open until it is clear that infection is under control. Many patients are frightened by such procedures and the pain involved, not understanding that it is in their best interest. Hence, they may resist treatment and accuse conscientious physicians of causing iatrogenic disorders. Such treatment is most crucial in the aged and in young children. In elderly patients the cause is diminution of body defenses against infection (for example, the immune system). It has been reported that the elderly experience a doubled or tripled chance of experiencing postoperative complications that may be seen as iatrogenic by their families. Young children are also more at risk than postpubertal individuals and "younger" adults, for reasons related to their incompletely developed immune systems.

Iatrogenesis resulting from misdiagnosis is too complicated an issue to be considered in depth here. In some cases, it is caused by physician inadequacy, but more often such problems are attributable to the great difficulty in diagnosing any disease absolutely.

It is essential for patients and physicians to communicate effectively. Such interaction lowers the occurrence of iatrogenic disorders because patients can decide to forgo treatment or to learn how to comply exactly with complex treatment protocols. Patients who do not receive adequate answers to questions posed to physicians should seek treatment elsewhere. Physicians should completely explain potential problems associated with therapeutic procedures by oral communication, informative consent forms, and well-educated counselors.

Because of the many iatrogenic disorders associated with medical therapy, physicians often believe that the best course of treatment—where a symptom is unclear and severe danger to patients is not imminent—is to allow nature to take its course so as to do no harm. This approach is often misunderstood by patients. To clarify the issue and to satisfy them, it should be explained—by the physician—that treatment can often be more dangerous than a perceived health problem.

It is hoped that the continued development of medical science, careful and complete therapy explanations by medical staffs, and better medical understanding and better treatment compliance by patients will decrease the incidence of iatrogenic disorders.

—Sanford S. Singer, Ph.D.

See also Antibiotics; Bacterial infections; Ethics; Hospitals; Law and medicine; Malpractice; Nausea and vomiting; Surgery, general; Surgical procedures; Wounds.

FOR FURTHER INFORMATION:

Apfel, Roberta J., and Susan M. Fisher. *To Do No Harm: DES and the Dilemmas of Modern Medicine.* New Haven, Conn.: Yale University Press, 1992. The book is well written and has a glossary of medical terms, twenty pages of footnotes, a bibliography of four hundred references, and an index, all of which enhance its usefulness.

Carroll, Paula. *Life Wish: One Woman's Struggle Against Medical Incompetence.* Alameda, Calif.: Medical Consumers, 1986. This personal narrative of a woman struggling to overcome breast cancer offers warnings of malpractice and surgical errors.

Farmer, Paul. *Infections and Inequalities: The Modern Plagues.* Berkeley: University of California Press, 2001. Physician-anthropologist Farmer examines why infectious diseases such as AIDS and tuberculosis target the poor. Uses public-health case studies of the pathogenic effects of poverty and other social conditions such as access to health care.

Levy, Stuart B. *The Antibiotic Paradox: How the Misuse of Antibiotics Destroys Their Curative Powers.* Cambridge, Mass.: Perseus, 2001. A leading researcher in molecular biology explores a modern-day massive evolutionary change in bacteria due to misuse of antibiotics. He argues that a build-up of new antibiotic-resistant bacteria in individuals and in the environment is leading medicine into a dangerous territory where "miracle" drugs may be obsolete.

Preger, Leslie, ed. *Iatrogenic Diseases.* 2 vols. Boca Raton, Fla.: CRC Press, 1986. Offers helpful advice on diagnosing iatrogenic diseases. Includes bibliographical references and an index.

Sharpe, Virginia F., and Alan I. Faden. *Medical Harm: Historical, Conceptual, and Ethical Dimensions of Iatrogenic Illness.* New York: Cambridge University Press, 1998. Of the many seekers after a healthier life or of relief from suffering who rightfully expect benefit from the health care system, some are more harmed than helped. This book deals mostly with harmful medical events which happen in hospitals.

Vincent, Charles, Maeve Ennis, and Robert J. Audley, eds. *Medical Accidents*. Oxford, England: Oxford University Press, 1993. Covers such topics as diagnostic errors, iatrogenic disease, and medical malpractice. Also discusses liability insurance.

Wilson, Michael, Brian Henderson, and Rod McNab. *Bacterial Virulence Mechanisms*. New York: Cambridge University Press, 2002. Basing their discussion on research advances in microbiology, molecular biology, and cell biology, the authors describe the interactions that exist between bacteria and human cells both in health and during infection.

ILEOSTOMY AND COLOSTOMY

PROCEDURES

ANATOMY OR SYSTEM AFFECTED: Abdomen, gastrointestinal system, intestines

SPECIALTIES AND RELATED FIELDS: Gastroenterology

DEFINITION: Surgical procedures that reroute the intestines to a hole, or stoma, in the abdomen after the removal of all or part of the colon.

KEY TERMS:

anastomosis: the surgical connection of one tubular organ to another

appliance: any device for collecting or removing stool from a stoma

colon: the last section of the intestines, where most fluids are absorbed, located between the ileum and the rectum; also called the large bowel or intestine

ileum: the lower third of the small intestine, which joins with the colon

ostomy: a popular term for any operation that results in a stoma

rectum: the intestinal storage area for feces between the colon and anus

stoma: a surgically created passage between the intestines and the outer skin

stool: the waste matter of digestion excreted from the body through the anus or stoma

INDICATIONS AND PROCEDURES

Despite great advances in drugs and nonsurgical procedures, doctors can cure some disabling or life-threatening diseases of the intestines only on the operating table. Common procedures of this type are the colostomy and ileostomy, both of which replace the anus with a stoma on the abdominal wall. Such surgery stresses patients considerably, and, in the aftermath, when they must entirely relearn the once-simple act of defecation, some drift into depression, despair, and withdrawal as their bowel functions consume their attention and disturb their social lives. Even for the large majority who adjust, and for whom the procedures are a life-lengthening boon, their postsurgical body, in most cases, requires a permanent, profound change in habits and a complete reliance on technology.

Colostomy and ileostomy are medical terms compounding *stoma* (from Greek, "mouth") and a prefix identifying the section of gut that ends in the newly created "mouth." If a portion of the colon is retained and ends in a stoma, the operation constructing it is called a colostomy. If the entire colon is removed and the lower section of the small bowel, or ileum, ends in a stoma, the operation constructing it is called an ileostomy. Nonmedical support groups for patients commonly use the back-formation "ostomy" to refer to any operation that creates a stoma (including a urostomy, in which a stoma is created for the excretion of urine) and to such patients as "ostomates," although neither term belongs to medical technical vocabulary.

Physicians determine that an ileostomy or a colostomy is necessary after inspecting the damaged intestinal segments by endoscopy, by imaging, or during surgery. In consultation with a surgeon, the patient agrees to undergo the procedure. The patient fasts before the surgery and receives laxatives and enemas (except in the case of obstructions or severe ulcerative colitis) to clean as much feces from the intestines as possible and thus reduce the chance of infection during surgery. The surgeon, often with the advice of an enterostomal therapist (ET), examines the patient's abdomen carefully, checking where the skin naturally folds and stretches when the patient assumes various common body positions, and a spot for the stoma is selected that is convenient for the patient and free of stress from muscles and skin tension. That place is marked. An area to the right and below the navel is the usual location for an ileostomy. The left side is commonly chosen for a colostomy.

In ileostomy, the surgeon makes the opening incision to the left of the navel, starting a few centimeters above it and continuing to the pelvic area. After the abdominal cavity is exposed, the tissues connecting the colon to surrounding structures are severed, starting at the cecum; the blood supply is cut and tied off; and clamps are placed over the ileum and rectum. Then the colon is cut free of the small intestine and rectum and is removed. If the operation is a "subtotal" procedure, the rectum is sutured shut and left in place or the open end is pulled through the abdominal wall as a "mucous

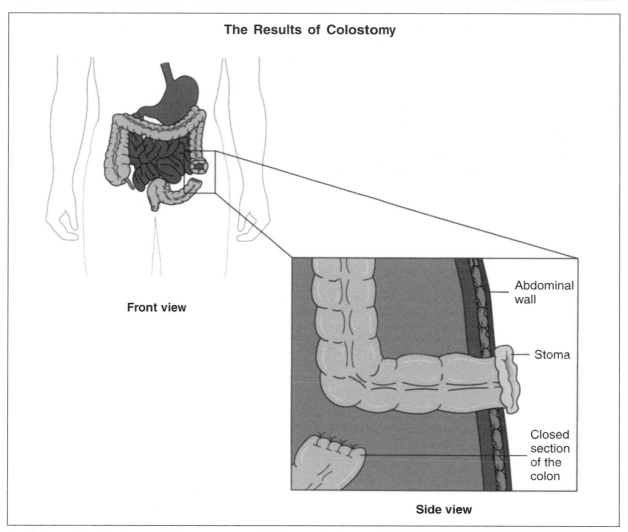

The Results of Colostomy

Front view

Abdominal wall

Stoma

Closed section of the colon

Side view

In colostomy, the colon is severed, the uppermost end of the intestine is extended through the abdominal wall to create a stoma through which fecal matter will be expelled, and the remaining section of the colon is closed off with sutures.

stoma." (Such a second stoma is sometimes fashioned because the surgeon plans to connect the ileum and rectum in a later operation.) If the surgeon performs a proctocolectomy, the rectum is removed after the stoma is made and the anus is sutured shut.

The stoma is built by cutting a small round opening first in the skin and then in the abdominal wall and pulling the end of the ileum through the hole. The end sticks above the skin, is folded back over itself, and is sutured to the edges of the hole, leaving the stoma protruding two to three centimeters. This basic ileostomy is called a Brooke ileostomy, after the English surgeon Bryan Brooke.

Variations on this basic procedure are employed depending on the wishes and health of the patient. A

Kock pouch, named after its inventor, Nils Kock of Sweden, can be fashioned just behind the stoma in the abdominal cavity to act as an artificial rectum, collecting liquid waste until the ostomate wishes to void it; because this arrangement gives the patient control over defecation, it is called a continent ileostomy. The surgeon uses about 45 centimeters of ileum to form the pouch and adjusts the stoma so that it acts as a valve until a tube is inserted for drainage. In other procedures, the surgeon operates twice more on the ostomate, first detaching the ileum and closing the stoma and then reconnecting the bowel either to the rectum or to the anus.

If the ileum and rectum are joined, the procedure is called an ileorectal anastomosis. The rectum resumes its old job as a feces reservoir, and the patient defecates normally through the anus. This arrangement is seldom employed for ulcerative colitis patients, however, since the disease usually persists in the rectum. If the ileum is sutured directly to the anus, the procedure is called an ileoanal anastomosis. Because there is no rectum to collect feces, the surgeon must construct one. The pouch is made from loops of ileum that are slit along their length and stitched together. If not enough ileum remains from which to make a pouch, the surgeon pulls the end through the rectum and ties it directly to the anus, a procedure called an endorectal ileal pull-through. The anastomosis procedures require two operations—one for the temporary stoma and construction of the pouch, one to connect the pouch and the rectum, or anus—to give the artificial rectum a chance to heal properly and so prevent leaking.

Colostomies feature somewhat more variety of stoma placement than ileostomies, but since removal of the rectum, sigmoid colon, or both are the most common reasons for the creation of the stoma, it is usually placed on the lower left of the abdomen, near the hipbone. If more of the colon is removed, the stoma may be higher up toward the rib cage. The operation begins much as for an ileostomy, except that only the portion of the colon from the damaged or diseased area to the anus is removed; and the initial incision begins near that damaged section. The remaining, healthy colon is pulled through holes in the abdomen and skin, and its end is rolled back and fastened. The stoma protrudes out about two to three centimeters, so that an appliance for storing waste, if needed, can be attached.

There are three varieties of colostomy. The first, a single-barreled end colostomy, is the classical configuration. The rectum and anus are removed, and a single circular stoma, about 25 millimeters in diameter, is the permanent exit for stool. If, however, the surgeon believes that the colon and rectum can be rejoined, the rectum is left intact and closed. Either of two procedures can be used to give the colon a rest period between the removal of the diseased section and reconnection to the rectum. A double-barreled colostomy involves slicing through the colon and making side-by-side stomas from the ends. In a loop colostomy, the colon is not cut through; instead, a slit is made in one side, which is pulled through the skin and made into an oval stoma, usually larger than other stomas. In both cases, the upper colon discharges stool, and the lower length passes mucus.

USES AND COMPLICATIONS

Both colostomy and ileostomy are last-resort or emergency treatments. When a wound, such as one caused by a knife or gunshot, punctures the intestines, waste matter, full of bacteria, spills into the abdominal cavity. The severe infection that is sure to follow can kill a patient in days; thus, an emergency operation is required. The surgeon pulls healthy bowel through the abdominal wall and forms a temporary stoma (so that no more waste can leak out of the intestines), cleans out the spillage, and repairs the damaged bowel. In many cases, it is possible to reconnect the healthy bowel to the damaged portion after the wound has healed; at the same time, the stoma is closed, and the patient resumes defecation through the anus.

Emergency operations, however, account for only a small percentage of colostomies and ileostomies. About two-thirds of surgeries to form stomas are colostomies, most of which follow operations removing cancer (usually in the lower colon or rectum) or an obstruction. Diverticulitis, the inflammation of little pouches in the colon wall, may also require a colostomy; the diversion of wastes allows the inflammation to subside and the colon wall to heal, after which the stoma may be removed and the colon reconnected. Additionally, repair of some rare birth defects may entail a colostomy.

Ileostomies account for about one-quarter of stoma-creating procedures. Most are performed to eradicate ulcerative colitis, a chronic inflammation of the colon that begins in the rectum and may spread upward until the whole colon is involved. No drug or dietary treatment cures ulcerative colitis; when the condition becomes too unbearable for a patient to endure, an ileostomy removes the source of trouble: the colon itself. Long-standing ulcerative colitis is particularly likely to become cancerous, and the colon may be removed for that reason alone. Likewise, familial polyposis, a hereditary disease which dots the colon with toadstool-shaped lumps that are likely to become cancerous, may require removal of the colon and ileostomy.

Wounds, diverticulitis, familial polyposis, and birth defects, while not particularly rare, are the reasons for relatively few stomas. Together, colorectal cancer (particularly in the elderly) and ulcerative colitis (commonly disabling patients in their twenties) lead to hundreds of thousands of stoma operations yearly in the United States. As the average age of the population increases, so does the incidence of colon cancer and the need for ostomies.

Recovery from stoma surgery is prolonged. Surgery shocks the intestines, and several days pass before the gut resumes the wavelike contractions (called peristalsis) that enable digestion and push wastes toward the stoma. In the meantime, patients live on intravenous fluid nourishment. When bowel motion restarts and wastes begin coming through the stoma, the ileostomate must develop new habits to cope with the flow of wastes (which are always fluid because the ileum does not remove sufficient water to solidify the waste matter) by learning to attach and empty appliances and to keep the stoma clean. Colostomates, especially those who have lost only their sigmoid colon, can look forward to passing firm stools and may eventually be able to live without an appliance, but months of diarrhea occur before the bowel regains full operation.

Many complications can plague the new anatomy, some of which require surgical correction. The most serious include intestinal obstruction, scar adhesions that distort the shape of the bowel, retraction of the stoma, abscesses, prolapse (more of the bowel pushing out of the body), and kidney stones (which form because persistent diarrhea can dehydrate ostomates). Less threatening, but demanding attention, are offensive odors, diarrhea, skin irritation, and bowel inflammation. Steady advances in surgical technique have lowered the complication rates, and few patients die because of the surgery.

Ostomates often must live with the stoma for the rest of their lives. Feces exit through the stoma, rather than the anus, forcing patients to "toilet train" themselves all over again. Some stomas are continent; that is, they hold back wastes until the patient is ready to defecate by draining them with a tube. Many, however, are not, and stool and gas steadily seep through the opening, where the waste matter is collected in an appliance, usually a plastic bag that seals over the stoma.

Having a plastic bag of stool on the abdomen and needing to empty it periodically to prevent it from leaking, instead of defecating by sitting down on a toilet, proves a difficult adjustment for some patients, both physically and psychologically. Several aid resources help new ostomates adjust. Specially trained registered nurses called enterostomal therapists teach patients how to manage their new stomas and how to attach appliances or insert catheters to drain continent stomas; they also help care for the stomas after the operation and periodically review their patients' progress. Gastroenterologists, physicians who specialize in the intestinal tract, can provide medical guidance and directly inspect the bowel wall behind the stoma through an endoscope, a flexible fiber-optic tube, should trouble develop. For those ostomates who feel isolated and depressed because of the stoma, the United Ostomy Association, a support group with branches throughout the United States, organizes social events and provides information and encouragement, often sending representatives to meet patients soon after surgery.

It is unfortunate that the widely felt repugnance for surgery involving the intestines and the social taboo against discussing defecation and excrement in polite conversation have obscured the triumph of stoma procedures. Much riskier and less rehabilitating surgeries, such as cardiac bypasses and organ transplantations, occupy the limelight, while ileostomies and colostomies, which prolong or improve more lives, receive scant popular attention. Medical journalists report that many patients, when told that they need a colostomy, know little or nothing of the procedure. After the doctor explains, they typically are dismayed and horrified. Nevertheless, few refuse the operation. On the other hand, potential ileostomates who suffer from ulcerative colitis are almost always better informed and look forward to the operation as the end to years of intense abdominal distress and fears about cancer.

Out of the hospital, ostomates literally face a new and different life. As well as learning to handle appliances or irrigate artificial rectums, they must face the fact that a major organ of their bodies is changed. The need for the stoma may anger or depress them, and this fixation on the change, if unalleviated, can evolve into loss of self-esteem and attendant social withdrawal. Many ostomates experience guilt in the belief that the disease and stoma, as well as the effects of the stoma on their families, are somehow their own fault.

These reactions require social and psychological therapy, extending care well beyond that afforded by the surgeon and the hospital. Support groups and the enterostomal therapist supply the majority of this care, but occasionally professional psychological help is required. The repulsion that patients feel for stomas and the consequent chance of morbid psychological reactions have encouraged surgeons to prefer anastomoses to stomas when possible, even though anastomoses are more difficult, have higher failure rates, and require a longer recovery period.

Moreover, the impression lingers, encouraged by popular accounts of research linking diet to disease, that most serious intestinal maladies (cancer in particular) result solely from poor eating habits. This type of reasoning sometimes leads to the insinuation that a stoma amounts to a kind of punishment for those habits, which is a hasty and erroneous conclusion that can worsen the guilt some ostomates feel. More often, factors over which people may have no control, such as genetic susceptibility and environmental toxins, contribute to the diseases that make stomas necessary.

Fortunately, the great majority of ostomates do adjust to their new lives; they seldom have any other alternative. Providing that the original need for surgery has been eliminated—the cancer has been removed, for example—they can look forward to an undiminished life span and few if any restrictions upon appetite, sexual function, or exercise. About 95 percent of ostomates recover completely, returning to their previous occupations after recovery, and of these the majority believe themselves to be in good or excellent health. Without the operations, all of them would have led drastically impaired lives, and many would have died. The high success rate places the ileostomy and colostomy procedures among the ranks of surgical interventions that rescue the seriously ill from otherwise incurable organic diseases.

PERSPECTIVE AND PROSPECTS

Although drastic techniques requiring much skill from surgeons and stamina from patients, ostomies did not originate with modern medicine and its sophisticated technology for sustaining patients during operations. Some colostomies date from the last quarter of the eighteenth century. In the nineteenth century, the number of operations creating a stoma—then called "artificial" or "preternatural" anus—increased, although without antiseptic conditions or anesthesia a patient's chances for survival were not good. Surgeons sometimes placed the stomas on the back instead of the abdomen. In 1908, William Ernest Miles conducted the first operation to remove a cancerous rectum; since the patient's intestines were still moving waste matter, which needed an exit, Miles created a stoma, thereby establishing one of the most common surgeries of the twentieth century.

Still, colostomies and ileostomies did not proliferate until after World War II. Since then, refinements in surgical techniques and postoperative care have steadily reduced the chance of complications and the length of the recovery period. At the same time, several variations of permanent and temporary stomas have been developed.

Like many other extreme surgical interventions, the ileostomy and colostomy testify to the limits of bio-medical knowledge: Most of these surgeries are performed because other remedies fail. Until researchers discover the mechanisms causing cancer, ulcerative colitis, and other deadly lower bowel diseases and develop nonsurgical cures, ileostomies and colostomies will remain common, especially among the elderly.

—*Roger Smith, Ph.D.*

See also Bypass surgery; Cancer; Colitis; Colon and rectal surgery; Colon cancer; Crohn's disease; Digestion; Diverticulitis and diverticulosis; Gastrectomy; Gastroenterology; Gastroenterology, pediatric; Gastrointestinal disorders; Gastrointestinal system; Intestinal disorders; Intestines.

FOR FURTHER INFORMATION:

Adrouny, Richard. *Understanding Colon Cancer.* Jackson: University Press of Mississippi, 2002. An excellent lay guide to the disease, offering information on topics such as diagnosis, prognosis, treatment, demographics, high-risk conditions, the sequence from bowel polyps to cancer, the warning signs, the stages of the disease, and theories of how colon cancer spreads.

Brandt, Lawrence J., and Penny Steiner-Grossman, eds. *Treating IBD: A Patient's Guide to the Medical and Surgical Management of Inflammatory Bowel Disease.* Reprint. New York: Raven Press, 1996. Although devoted to inflammatory bowel disease (IBD) in general, this book contains a section on surgical cures for ulcerative colitis and Crohn's disease. Types of ileostomy and anastomosis are described thoroughly in lay terms, and drawings and photographs depict the bowel reconstructions.

Bub, David S., et al. *One Hundred Questions and Answers About Colorectal Cancer.* Sudbury, Mass.: Jones and Bartlett, 2003. Provides authoritative answers to questions about treatment options, posttreatment quality of life, and sources of support.

Fries, Colleen Farley. "Managing an Ostomy." *Nursing* 29, no. 8 (August, 1999): 26. Ostomies are used to assist patients with conditions like ulcerative colitis and bowel obstruction. The selection of an ostomy should be based on the patient's needs and is available in one- or two-piece devices and a number of sizes.

Kalibjian, Cliff. *Straight from the Gut: Living with Crohn's Disease and Ulcerative Colitis.* Cambridge, Mass.: O'Reilly and Associates, 2003. Shares numerous personal stories from those suffering from colitis and offers advice on all aspects of living with the disease.

Mullen, Barbara Dorr, and Kerry Anne McGinn. *The Ostomy Book: Living Comfortably with Colostomies, Ileostomies, and Urostomies*. Rev. ed. Palo Alto, Calif.: Bull, 1992. An amusingly written, inspirational account of the most typical of ostomy cases: a colostomy necessitated by rectal cancer. It is Mullen's own story, and she relates her emotional turmoil with candor, making her account invaluable reading for anyone who must undergo a colostomy.

Parker, James N., and Philip M. Parker, eds. *The 2002 Official Patient's Sourcebook on Ulcerative Colitis*. San Diego, Calif.: Icon Health, 2002. Draws from public, academic, government, and peer-reviewed research to provide a wide-ranging reference about the causes, treatments, and risk factors of colitis.

United Ostomy Association. http://www.uoa.org/. A support group for ostomy patients that stresses education, information, support, and advocacy.

Way, Lawrence W., and Gerard M. Doherty, eds. *Current Surgical Diagnosis and Treatment*. 11th ed. Norwalk, Conn.: Appleton & Lange, 2003. A reference work on general surgery for physicians, this tome is nevertheless comprehensible to laypersons familiar with medical terminology. Presents succinct overviews of the stoma procedures and their potential complications and contains finely detailed illustrations.

IMAGING AND RADIOLOGY

PROCEDURE

ANATOMY OR SYSTEM AFFECTED: All

SPECIALTIES AND RELATED FIELDS: Nuclear medicine, radiology

DEFINITION: Medical imaging uses radiation that passes through the body to construct images of the insides of the body.

KEY TERMS:

computed tomography (CT): a scanning procedure using X rays

fluoroscope: a machine that uses a fluorescent screen instead of photographic film to display X-ray images

magnetic resonance imaging (MRI): an imaging method using radio waves

positron emission tomography (PET): a scanning procedure using gamma rays from injected radioactive pharmaceuticals

single photon emission computed tomography (SPECT): a scanning procedure using gamma rays from injected radioactive pharmaceuticals

tomography: a method to produce a three-dimensional image of the internal structure of the body by observing and recording radiation transmitted, reflected, or emitted by structures inside the body; observations are made of sections, or slices, of the body that are assembled to form the final image

ultrasound: an imaging method using high-frequency sound

INDICATIONS AND PROCEDURES

Before the advent of radiology, physicians were forced to rely on visual clues, palpation (examination by touch), and exploratory surgery to discover what lay beneath a patient's skin. X rays provided the first path around this limitation and allowed physicians to peer beneath the skin without surgery. X rays are electromagnetic radiation similar to visible light, but they have much higher energies than visible light, which makes them more penetrating.

Circumstances under which a doctor needs to "see" inside the body and might use X rays to do so include a patient who has fallen and now experiences localized pain and swelling in the leg (possible broken bone); a patient with severe pain in the lower back who passes blood in the urine (possible kidney stone); a patient who experiences intermittent and squeezing chest pain, nausea, and shortness of breath (possible constricted arteries in the heart); and a patient with a history of localized stomach pain and heartburn, also called acid reflux (possible inflamed esophagus, hiatal hernia, or ulcer).

All medical imaging devices require a source of radiation, a detector, and a way to position the patient. For X rays, the patient stands in front of a film holder or lies on a table over a film holder while X rays from an X-ray tube pass through the patient and cast the patient's shadow onto the film. The film must be as large as the body part being examined. Dense constituents such as bones show up as white on X-ray negatives, while various other body tissues show up as shades of gray depending upon the fraction of the X rays that they block.

X-ray film has been developed to have excellent resolution and contrast, and an X ray is a permanent record. It is not easy to take several X rays in quick succession, however, as might be done to examine the upper gastrointestinal tract. An alternative is to use fluoroscopy, in which a screen coated with special compounds is used in the place of film. These compounds fluoresce when struck by X rays. Advantages are that the image is immediate (no film to develop) and moving images can

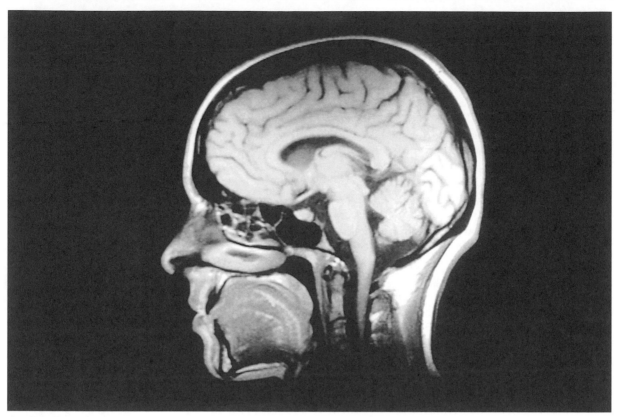

An MRI allows physicians to visualize soft tissues inside the body, such as the brain and nasopharyngeal tissues. (Digital Stock)

be viewed. The image can be made brighter by an image intensifier—a television camera-like device that amplifies the image—and a permanent record can be made by photographing this final image.

An ultrasound unit adapts sonar to medical purposes. The unit consists of a probe; electronics to generate, receive, and analyze signals; and a monitor to display the results. Such a device is relatively inexpensive compared with other types of scanners, and at the intensities used, ultrasound waves do not harm the body. The ultrasound probe contains a transducer, a crystal that can change electrical signals into sound waves and can also act as a receiver changing sound waves into electrical signals. During the examination, a gel is spread over the patient's skin in the area of interest. The gel provides good acoustical coupling between the probe and the patient's body tissue. In order to create an image of structures as small as 1 millimeter, ultrasound frequencies between 3 and 7 megahertz are used. The crystal inside the probe emits sound waves while rapidly rocking back and forth, producing a wedge of sound pulses. The crystal then becomes a receiver and picks up sound echoes that form as the sound passes from one type of tis-

sue into another. Distance can be determined from the time elapsed between sending a pulse and receiving the echo. Combining this distance information with the direction and intensity of the echo allows a computer to build an image of the structures inside the body.

This image is displayed on a monitor screen and can also be printed for a permanent record. The probe is moved around to provide the least obstructed view of the target. Since ultrasound waves pass easily through soft tissues such as the liver and fluid-filled organs such as the gallbladder or the uterus during pregnancy, ultrasound is particularly useful to examine these organs. Ultrasound does not penetrate bone or gas, and the latter property makes it difficult to examine the digestive tract with ultrasound.

Like ultrasound, magnetic resonance imaging (MRI), uses no potentially harmful radiation, but it is the most expensive of the imaging techniques. MRI uses a very large, superconducting magnet. Once the magnetic field is established, superconducting magnets require very little electrical power. In order to be superconducting, the magnet is wound with niobium-titanium wire and maintained at liquid helium temperature (about 4

Kelvins above absolute zero). The magnet itself is in the form of a very large, hollow cylinder into which the patient can be inserted. The magnetic field inside the cylinder is uniform and very strong, typically 0.5 to 2.0 tesla; for comparison, the strength of the earth's magnetic field is only about 0.00005 tesla near the surface. There are also three sets of much smaller (.0018 to .0027 of a tesla) "gradient" magnets, which are used to tweak the magnetic field at pinpoint locations during the scan. Hydrogen atoms are among the most abundant atoms in soft tissue. In a strong magnetic field, the spin axis of hydrogen nuclei (protons) precesses about magnetic field lines. The exact frequency with which it precesses depends on the proton's surroundings, or the type of tissue in which it is found.

The patient rests on a table that moves into the tunnel formed by the magnet. The magnetic field causes no noticeable sensation, but claustrophobic patients may become anxious. To combat this effect, newer machines have wider tunnels or have one side open. An insulated wire coil may be placed on the patient over the area to be examined, or coils mounted on the magnet may be used. A brief pulse of radiofrequency waves is broadcast from the coil at the same time that the gradient magnets adjust the magnetic field to the right value in a narrow slice of the patient. If the radiofrequency is at the precession frequency, then those protons with which it resonates will absorb energy. After the radiofrequency pulse, the protons produce an echo that radiates energy back to the coil. Analysis of this energy allows the identification of the type of tissue, which, along with location information from the gradient magnets, allows a computer to construct an image of the internal tissues of the patient. The image can be either two-dimensional or three-dimensional, as needed. Two-dimensional slices can be vertical, horizontal, or in any plane desired.

A scan of the brain and spinal column can detect areas of damage to the myelin (insulating sheath) surrounding nerve fibers that is the hallmark of multiple sclerosis. MRI scans are also used in diagnosing tumors, infections of the brain, strokes, torn ligaments, and many other conditions. As with X rays, contrast agents may be injected into the patient to make certain tissues or systems stand out. For example, the blood vessels in the heart may be examined in this fashion. Depending upon the size of the region to be scanned, the procedure takes from twenty to ninety minutes, and the patient must remain as still as possible during this time. Currents in the gradient magnets produce loud thumping sounds. These may be masked by providing the patient with music through earphones during the examination.

Physicians now depend so much on MRI investigations that more than 60 million are performed each year around the world. Underscoring this importance, the 2003 Nobel Prize in Medicine or Physiology was awarded to Paul C. Lauterbur and Sir Peter Mansfield for their work leading to the development of the MRI technique.

A nuclear medicine scan, also called nuclear radiology or isotope study, uses radioactive pharmaceuticals that have been injected into or ingested by the patient. The radiation dose to the patient is strictly controlled and is the least possible for the procedure to be effective. The radioactive isotopes used emit gamma rays—essentially high-energy X rays—which easily pass through the body and are observed by an array of gamma detectors. The patient lies on a table while the detector array is positioned near the target organ. In some applications, the array slowly scans a region. A computer receives information on the location and intensity of the detected gamma rays and constructs an image from this information. The image is fuzzy and lacks the fine detail that can be seen with X rays or ultrasound, but it shows directly how well the target organ functions.

To be useful for this purpose, radioactive isotopes must emit penetrating gamma rays, have a short half-life, and either be taken up by the target organ or be capable of being attached to a molecule that is taken up by the target organ. A short half-life is desirable to ensure that the isotope will cease to be radioactive not too long after it has served its purpose. Technetium-99m is frequently used because it is taken up by the thyroid and salivary glands (if those are the targets), it can be used to tag other biologically active molecules, and its half-life is only 6.01 hours.

For a thyroid study, the patient may be given a drink or a pill containing iodine-123 (13.1 hour half-life). About twenty-four hours later, the gamma emission from the thyroid is measured. This procedure shows how well the thyroid works in general. The patient may then be injected with technetium-99m and several scans made over the next hour. This provides another measure of the thyroid's functioning. It also allows a measure of the thyroid's size and shape. Any area of inactivity suggests a blockage or damage, while an unusual area of activity suggests an abnormally high tissue growth rate such as a tumor. In general, a region of rapidly growing tissue shows up as a hot spot on a nuclear medicine scan, which makes it possible to see a healing bone fracture that an X ray might miss.

A positron emission tomography (PET) scan is a special type of nuclear medicine scan that capitalizes on a property of the gamma rays emitted during positron annihilation. Positrons are positively charged and are the electron's antiparticle. Since they are oppositely charged, positrons and electrons are strongly attracted to each other, and as soon as they touch, they mutually annihilate, converting their energy into two gamma rays emitted at precisely 180 degrees to each other.

A gantry houses a large ring of gamma ray detectors arranged like a doughnut on its side. The patient rests on a movable table that carries the patient into, and perhaps through, the detector ring. Depending upon the purpose of the examination, one of several radioactive pharmaceuticals is administered. For example, fluorine-18 (half-life 109.8 minutes) is attached to glucose molecules and used to monitor the brain's metabolism. Since active areas of the brain draw the most glucose, a PET scan can watch the brain at work. When a fluorine nucleus emits a positron, the positron encounters an electron almost at once and is annihilated. The gamma ray detectors continually register hits from natural background radiation, but if two detectors located 180 degrees around the ring from each other record gamma rays of the right energy (0.511 million electron volts) and within a few nanoseconds of each other, it is virtually certain that they originated from a positron annihilation in the patient. A computer then draws a straight line between the two detectors and through the patient. Where two or more lines intersect is the location of the activity.

A single photon emission computed tomography (SPECT) scan is similar to a PET scan, but it detects only one photon at a time instead of a pair. In order to define the direction of a gamma ray photon, a collimator is placed in front of the detector array. The collimator is a slab of 5-centimeter-long lead straws pointing at the patient so that a gamma ray can reach the detector only by traveling up a straw. Such a collimator and detector array is called an Anger camera. A ring of cameras around the patient allows a computer to construct a three-dimensional image of the target organ. SPECT combines the organ function information of nuclear medicine with some of the resolution of a computed tomography (CT) scan.

The CT apparatus consists of a movable table on which the patient rests and a gantry that houses the X-ray equipment. A doughnut hole in the gantry is large enough for the patient and table to pass through. An X-ray tube is mounted in the doughnut, and an array of X-ray detectors are mounted in the doughnut directly opposite from the X-ray source. As the doughnut rotates all the way around, the X-ray beam is sent through a narrow "slice" of the patient. Instead of the normal X-ray silhouette of the patient as illuminated from one direction, silhouettes from all directions are obtained, but only as numbers, not yet as images.

The information available consists of where the detector was when it picked up the signal and how strong the signal was. As the scan continues, the computer uses this information to construct an image of that slice of the patient. While the doughnut carries the X-ray tube and detectors around and around the patient, the table advances slowly and continuously until the whole body (or the desired segment) has been scanned. Blood clots and ruptured vessels in the brain are easily detected, as well as tumors in soft tissues such as the liver.

USES AND COMPLICATIONS

Bones, bone breaks, and some tumors show up well on an X ray, but soft tissue images may require additional techniques. For examination of the upper gastrointestinal tract, the patient is given a barium solution to drink while standing in front of the X-ray detector. Barium blocks X rays and coats the esophagus and stomach lining, thereby outlining them in detail on the X ray. In the "barium swallow," a quick series of X rays are taken to follow the progress of the barium into the stomach. Constrictions in the esophagus, the action of the stomach valve, and the presence of a hiatal hernia (the upper part of the stomach bulging through a weakened diaphragm) become visible. As the barium proceeds, a stomach ulcer may stand out in outline.

To check for kidney stones and to examine the kidneys, ureters, and urinary bladder, an intravenous pyelogram (IVP) is performed. First, a contrast solution (based on iodine, which blocks X rays) is injected into the patient's vein. The patient may feel a brief warm flush as the body reacts to the iodine, but this reaction passes quickly. The solution used soon passes through the patient's system: through the kidneys, through the ureters, and to the bladder. A series of X rays are then taken in which kidney stones may be revealed; any swelling of a kidney or blockage of a ureter will show up, if present.

The angiogram, a similar but more extensive procedure, is used to examine the blood vessels of the heart or other location. In this procedure, a catheter (fine plastic tube) is inserted into the femoral artery at the groin or into a blood vessel in the upper arm. The patient is given medication for pain and anxiety. Using a fluoroscope monitor, the physician maneuvers the catheter to the desired location and then injects the contrast solution through the catheter. Several X rays are taken from various angles, and any blockages or constrictions are generally apparent. The catheter is then withdrawn, and the patient is required to rest.

CT scanning represents a major step forward in X-ray technology. A patient might suffer a sudden loss of muscle control and feeling in part of the body (possible stroke). The doctor would like to X-ray the brain for signs of a ruptured or blocked blood vessel, but contrast agents are not useful for the brain. Without them, internal organs and tissues appear only as faint ghosts in an X ray. A CT scan uses computer technology to convert special X-ray images into clear views of the organs.

While prudence dictates that radiation exposure be kept to a minimum, the medical benefit of procedures using radiation generally outweigh the risks. Provided that a radiation dose is not overwhelmingly massive, the body has amazing recuperative properties and is able to repair most radiation damage. Everyone is exposed daily to background radiation from naturally occurring trace amounts of radioactive elements and from cosmic rays. The accompanying table compares typical radiation doses received in several medical procedures to the whole body dose received from natural background and to the maximum whole body dose allowed per year for radiation workers. No discernable harm occurs to radiation workers at the maximum allowed level. The table shows that none of these procedures approaches the maximum limit, but it should be noted that a medical procedure may expose the target organ to many times the average body dose.

A typical X-ray image shows different types of tissue as various shades of gray. Recent advances in medical imaging include digitizing any image and using powerful computer programs to enhance the subtle differences between different types of tissue, even coloring them so that they are immediately obvious to the physician. Three-dimensional images can be constructed and rotated so that they can be examined from every angle. A physician can see exactly what problems will be encountered in removing a tumor. Computers can scan X rays used to screen for breast cancer, called mammograms, and draw the radiologist's attention to any questionable regions. Finally, computers can merge images from complementary techniques such as PET (shows functionality of the organ) with MRI (shows high-resolution detail) to give a more complete view.

PERSPECTIVE AND PROSPECTS

November 8, 1895, was a Friday. That evening, Wilhelm Conrad Röntgen was quite late for dinner, he ate little and quickly returned to his laboratory. That af-

COMPARISON OF RADIATION DOSES FOR VARIOUS PROCEDURES

Procedure	Natural Background Equivalent	Maximum Allowed for Radiation Workers
Ultrasound scan	none	none
MRI	none	none
Chest X ray	10 days	1 day
Thyroid iodine uptake (whole-body dose)	8 months	2 weeks
Thyroid scan Tc-99m (whole-body dose)	1 year, 7 months	1 month
Whole-body PET scan with fluorine-tagged glucose	2 years	6 weeks
Chest CT scan	2 years, 8 months	2 months
Whole-body CT scan	3 years, 4 months	10 weeks

ternoon, he had made an astounding and disquieting discovery. Many scientists of the day, including Röntgen, were studying cathode rays. The required apparatus was an evacuated glass tube with electrodes sealed inside at either end. When a high voltage was placed across the electrodes, cathode rays (electrons) streamed from the cathode, and where they struck the glass tube, the glass fluoresced.

Röntgen covered the tube with black paper and darkened the room, but still a fluorescent screen some distance away from the tube glowed whenever he operated the tube. Since cathode rays cannot travel far through air, Röntgen deduced that some unknown type of radiation must be coming from the tube. He called it X radiation (X for unknown). Placing bits of wood or metal between the tube and the screen cast shadows on the screen, some darker and some lighter. The key moment came when Röntgen held up a small lead disk. The expected shadow of the lead appeared, but holding the disk, Röntgen saw the shadows of his finger bones. He opened his hand, and the shadowy skeleton hand opened. Röntgen wondered if he could be hallucinating. In those days, some people believed that dreaming about or imagining seeing a skeleton was a premonition of one's impending death. Röntgen was concerned that others might think him crazy if he were to describe what he had seen, so he needed proof.

In the ensuing weeks, Röntgen made an intense study of the properties of X rays. Three days before Christmas, he placed photographic film in a black paper package and had his wife, Bertha, place her hand on it while he exposed it with X rays for fifteen minutes. The photograph showed the bones of Bertha Röntgen's hand, with a ring on her finger. Röntgen sent a copy of the photograph along with an explanation to a friend, but it soon found its way into newspapers all over the world. Only four months after the public announcement, Thomas Edison's company began marketing "complete outfits for x-ray work." While some considered looking at skeletons while people were still using them revoltingly indecent, the medical usefulness of X rays was immediately apparent. The first Nobel Prize in Physics ever awarded went to Röntgen in 1901 for his discovery of X rays.

In spite of the obvious medical advantages, relatively few doctors used X rays at first, but the public found them a source of entertainment. Edison built a fluoroscope for use at amusement parks. Looking through a hooded visor, spectators placed their hands between an X-ray tube and a fluorescent screen and watched their bones wiggle as they moved their hands. Casual exposure to X rays continued into the 1950's with the use of fluoroscopes by shoe stores to see how well shoes fit.

The widespread use of medical X rays was hampered by the lack of trained operators and proper equipment. This situation changed with World War I, when X-ray teams were trained and equipped by the hundreds. Marie Curie was a prime force in establishing such teams for the French and Belgian militaries. From this modest beginning, the various imaging techniques have evolved to provide the physician with "magic eyes" that can peer inside the body.

—*Charles W. Rogers, Ph.D.*

See also Angiography; Angioplasty; Computed tomography (CT) scanning; Magnetic resonance imaging (MRI); Mammography; Noninvasive tests; Nuclear medicine; Nuclear radiology; Positron emission tomography (PET) scanning; Radiation sickness; Radiation therapy; Radiopharmaceuticals; Ultrasonography.

FOR FURTHER INFORMATION:

Giger, Maryellen L., and Charles A. Pelizzari. "Advances in Tumor Imaging." *Scientific American* 275, no. 3 (September, 1996): 110-112. Describes how combining images from complementary techniques such as MRI and PET is particularly helpful, as is forming three-dimensional color images. Computer-aided diagnosis provides an automatic second opinion.

Mould, Richard F. *A Century of X-Rays and Radioactivity in Medicine.* Philadelphia: Institute of Physics, 1993. A treasure trove of historical photographs and basic explanations outlining the development of X rays and nuclear medicine.

Raichle, Marcus E. "Visualizing the Mind." *Scientific American* 270, no. 4 (April, 1994): 58-64. Discusses how PET and CT scans are used to provide images of the brain in action.

Ter-Pogossian, Michel M., Marcus E. Raichle, and Burton E. Sobel. "Positron-Emission Tomography." *Scientific American* 243, no. 4 (October, 1980): 170-181. A good basic explanation of the PET technique, including the equipment and how it is used.

IMMUNE SYSTEM

BIOLOGY

ANATOMY OR SYSTEM AFFECTED: Blood, cells, circulatory system, glands, liver, lymphatic system, spleen

SPECIALTIES AND RELATED FIELDS: Cytology, hematology, immunology, microbiology, preventive medicine, serology

DEFINITION: A system—including the spleen, thymus, lymphatic system, and specialized cells—that protects the body from foreign substances.

KEY TERMS:

antibody: any of the proteins produced in the body during an immune response; recognizes and attacks foreign antigen substances

antigen: a substance within the human body recognized as foreign either by antibodies or by special immune cells; the cause behind the stimulation of the immune response

autoimmunity: an abnormal immune reaction against antigens

immunosuppression: a decrease in the effectiveness of the immune system

pathogen: any disease-causing organism, including a virus, bacterium, protozoan, mold or yeast, or other parasite

STRUCTURE AND FUNCTIONS

The immune system is capable of recognizing and identifying many different substances foreign to the human body. To function properly, this system must receive, interpret, and transmit large amounts of information about invaders from outside or within the body. These constant and ever-changing threats to the body must be met and destroyed by one complex system—namely, the human immune system. Many organs and parts of the body play a major role in maintaining resistance; some have more important roles than others, but all parts must work in unison. The circulatory and lymphatic systems, along with specific organs, are of primary importance in the overall workings of the immune system.

Blood. Besides the outer protective layer of the skin and mucous membranes, the first line of defense in the immune system includes the blood in the circulatory system. About 50 percent of human blood is made up of a fluid called plasma, which contains water, proteins, carbohydrates, vitamins, hormones, and cellular waste. The other half of blood is composed of white cells, red cells, and platelets. The red blood cells, called erythrocytes, are responsible for moving oxygen from the lungs to the other parts of the body. The special platelet cells, called thrombocytes, enable the blood to form clots, thus preventing severe bleeding. An unborn child produces red and white blood cells in the spleen and liver, while a newborn makes blood in the center of bones, called the marrow. After maturity, all red and most white blood cells are produced in the bone marrow. Although the red cells and platelets are vital, it is the white cells that play a major role in the immune system.

In a broad sense, white blood cells surround and engulf foreign matter and adjacent dying cells in a process called phagocytosis. The function is possible since the white blood cells can move, unlike red corpuscles, by pushing their bodies out and pulling forward. Red corpuscles move because of the flow of the blood within the circulatory system. White blood cells move in the lymph vessels, where they work to defend the body against disease, but are also transported through the blood. Bacteria and other foreign material can remain alive within a white corpuscle, but sometimes the corpuscle dies from the toxins produced by the bacteria. The resulting formation of pus is actually an accumulation of dead white blood cells. At other times, the white corpuscles win and the foreign matter is destroyed.

Three major types of white blood cells, known collectively as leukocytes, are involved in immune responses. All three—granulocytes, monocytes, and lymphocytes—arise from areas in either bone marrow, the spleen, or the liver.

The granulocytes, each of which is about twice the size of a red blood cell, originate from red bone marrow and live only about twelve hours. Under the classification of granulocytes, distinct cells have different structures, sizes, and shapes. These specialized granulocytes include the neutrophils, eosinophils, and basophils. None of these cells has a specific memory for future immune responses. The neutrophil granulocyte eats and digests small foreign matter with the help of special enzymes. Between 40 and 75 percent of the white blood cells in the human body are neutrophils. When these highly mobile neutrophil cells arrive at an injury site, they burst, releasing their enzymes and melting away the surrounding tissues. Eosinophils are similar to neutrophils but seem to be specialized in fighting infection caused by parasites, because of the seven toxic proteins that they use to fight. They are also effective against fungal, bacterial, viral, or protozoan infections. Basophils, which are smaller in size, move from the bone marrow through the body and act as a control by preventing overreactions during an immune response. Basophils prevent coagulation, but they cannot destroy foreign matter. These cells account for less than 1 percent of the white blood cells found in the blood.

The second group of leukocytes includes the monocytes, the largest cells found in the blood. Monocytes are two to three times as large as red cells, yet they are not very numerous, making up 3 to 9 percent of all the leukocytes in the blood. After only a few days in the blood, they move to areas between tissues. Over the course of months or years, the monocytes enlarge ten times in size in order to specialize in phagocytosis. After this growth, they are called macrophages. They are also referred to as terminal cells since they cannot divide, and thus do not reproduce.

The third type of leukocyte, and the most sophisticated of the white blood cells, are called lymphocytes because they come from the lymph system as well as bone marrow. The T lymphocytes, which are primarily responsible for immunity, can change into helper, killer, and suppressor cells. Besides being able to recognize foreign matter precisely, they can live freely in the blood, grow larger and divide, and then change back to their original form after working against the invader. Lymphocytes circulate throughout the body, moving from the bloodstream through the lymph fluid and back into the blood. The two major types of lymphocytes are T lymphocytes (also called T cells) and B lymphocytes (also called B cells). Both T and B cells can recognize foreign matter and hook onto it. Some of these special "memory" cells remain in the body for life, preventing a specific invader from causing illness when it is encountered again in the future. These specialized cells must have a way to travel through the body; one of these transport systems is the lymphatic system.

The lymphatic system. This system is a closed network of vessels that help in circulating fluids from the body and returning them to the bloodstream. The lymphatic system also defends against disease-causing foreign materials, known as antigens. The smallest components of the lymph system are the lymphatic capillaries that run parallel to the blood capillaries. The fluid inside these capillaries, which has come across the thin wall membrane from tissues all across the body, is called lymph. These capillaries merge into larger lymphatic vessels, which then merge into a type of collecting area called a lymph node. The lymph fluid is drained into trunks that join one of two collecting ducts. The larger left thoracic duct collects lymph from the upper arm, head, and neck of the left side of the body before emptying into a vein near the neck and shoulder. The right lymphatic duct does the same for the right side of the body. After leaving the collecting ducts, the lymph fluid becomes part of the blood plasma in the veins and returns to the right atrium of the heart. Lymph does not flow like blood in veins and arteries; instead, it is controlled by muscular activity.

The spleen. This largest lymphatic organ is located in the upper left part of the abdominal cavity, behind the stomach and under the diaphragm. The hollow spaces within the spleen are filled with blood, making it soft and elastic. The white blood cells in the lining of these hollow cavities engulf and destroy foreign materials, as well as damaged red blood cells that pass through the spleen.

The thymus. This gland is located between the lungs and above the heart, just behind the upper part of the breastbone. It contains large numbers of white cells; some are inactive, but others develop and leave the thymus to become functional in the immune system.

The liver. Located in the upper right part of the abdominal cavity below the diaphragm, the liver is well protected by the ribs. Since it is the largest gland in the body, it plays a major role in metabolism while also aiding the body's ability to clot blood. In addition, various liver cells, called macrophages, help in destroying damaged red blood cells. The liver's connection to the immune system is its ability to also destroy foreign substances through phagocytosis.

Bone marrow. Marrow is located in the center of bones. It can be divided into two types, red or yellow marrow. It is the red marrow that aids in the formation of white and red blood cells. The yellow marrow stores fat and is not involved in producing blood cells. Some white blood cells come from bone marrow cells. They are released into the blood and are carried to the thymus gland, where they undergo special processing that changes them into T lymphocytes (the letter T shows that they came from the thymus gland). The other lymphocytes that do not reach the thymus after leaving the bone marrow are named B lymphocytes (B because they came from bone marrow). These B lymphocytes are abundant in lymph nodes, the spleen, bone marrow, secretory glands, intestinal lining, and in the reticuloendothelial tissue.

THE RESPONSES OF THE IMMUNE SYSTEM

Failures of the immune system can lead to devastating diseases, either because the immune system attacks itself or because it fails to defend against outside foreign antigen matter. An antigen can be any substance that stimulates the body to fight, ranging from a bacterial infection to the virus that causes acquired immunodeficiency syndrome (AIDS).

When the body fights against an antigen, the immune system can produce two types of response, either a cellular immune response or a humoral immune response. The cellular response involves specific types of cells that recognize, attack, and destroy the invading antigen. The humoral immune response is actually the body's main defense against a bacterium, virus, or fungus in the blood or body fluids. This response involves various chemicals in the bloodstream that fight against the invaders.

Another way of looking at how the body fights to keep itself healthy is to separate the immune responses into either primary or secondary responses. The second time that a given antigen enters the body, the immune system attacks with what is called the secondary immune response stored in special immune memories, making it faster and more extensive than the primary response that occurred when the antigen was first encountered. This immune memory must be built for each antigen before the body becomes immune to the wide variety of diseases and conditions to which one is exposed on a daily basis.

The body begins to build this memory prior to birth by making an inventory of all the molecules within the body. Foreign substances not in this memory are considered to be antigens, which will activate an immune response. When an antigen is first encountered, the primary response occurs, producing lymphocytes that are sensitized to the invader. Many types of lymphocytes can respond in order to create the appropriate antibody molecules, which are then released into the lymph and transported to the blood. This process may last several weeks. During this primary immune response, the B cells and T cells serve as memory cells. Because a memory for the antigen has been stored, if this antigen is encountered in the future the memory cells can react more quickly and effectively. In this secondary immune response, the antibodies are ready to react by attaching themselves to the surfaces of the antigens. There must be a specific type of antibody produced for every type of antigen. These new antibodies may survive only a few months, but the memory cells live much longer.

There are four main ways that an antibody can bind to an antigen. The antibody can pull together clusters of invading organisms to prevent the antigens from spreading. Another possibility is for this special component of the blood to punch a hole in the invader and destroy it. The antibody can also combine with the antigen, which makes it easier to destroy. In the case of a virus or a toxin, the antibody can neutralize the harmful activity by covering the outside of the antigen. With so many ways for an antibody to attach to an antigen, it is equally important for the antibody memory to be established. It is this special memory that leads to future immunity.

These memory cells are responsible for the four different types of immunity, two of which are acquired actively and two of which are acquired passively. The first type is naturally acquired active immunity, which results after the body is exposed to a live pathogen and develops the disease. The second type is artificially acquired active immunity, such as that gained after a vaccination. The immune response is triggered after an injection of weakened or dead pathogens is received, but the body does not suffer the severe symptoms of the disease. An example would be a smallpox vaccination. The third type of immunity is artificially acquired passive immunity, gained through an injection of prepared antibodies. This method is considered passive since the antibodies, called gamma globulin, were made by another person. This type of immunity usually does not last more than a few weeks, and the person will be susceptible to that pathogen in the future. Naturally acquired passive immunity occurs when the antibodies pass to the fetus from the mother, but it includes only those antibodies available in the blood of the mother. This process gives an infant certain short-term immunities for the first year of life.

These types of immunity are usually desirable, but there are occasions when an immune response is not wanted, such as after an organ transplant. When tissue or organs are transplanted from one person to another, the body may reject the foreign tissue, triggering an immune response and possibly destroying the new organ. Consequently, attempts are made to match the tissue between recipient and donor. In an effort to halt the immune response, immunosuppressive drugs are given to interfere with the recipient's ability to form antibodies, and drugs can be administered to destroy the lymphocytes that produce these antibodies. Unfortunately, the recipient is often left unprotected against infections, since the immune system is not functioning normally.

PERSPECTIVE AND PROSPECTS

In the same way that the discovery of penicillin shocked the world, immunology has created endless possibilities in medicine. When surgeons found that they could transplant an organ from one person to another, the interest in immunology exploded.

This field of medicine has discovered that the immune system's power and effectiveness can be lessened because of several factors. Improper diet, stress, disease, and excessive physical activity levels can depress the immune system. Other factors that can modify immunity include age, genetics, and metabolic and environmental factors. The anatomical, physiological, and microbial factors are shown in the susceptibility of the young and the very old to infections. For the young, the system is immature, while the aged have suffered a lifetime of assaults from pathogens. The impact of psychological stress is difficult to measure, yet it holds the potential for negatively affecting the immune system.

Before immunology can be fully understood, more knowledge must be gained about how antibodies are made and how they develop memories. Lymphocytes must be examined to discover what role they play in the immune response. Studies must look at not only the whole picture of the immune system but also its smaller parts—the organs and how each participates. Such studies could lead to better success in transplanting these organs. Unanswered questions remain about how the immune system relates to other body systems. The relationships among the brain and nervous system, hormones, and the respiratory system leave many areas ripe for further study.

Recent research has identified the significant importance of Class I major histocompatibility proteins (I-MHCPs) in the cellular immune system. When disease-associated proteins occur in a cell, they are broken into pieces by the cell's proteolytic machinery. Cell proteins become attached to antigen fragments and transport them to the surface of the cell, where they are "presented" to the body's defense mechanisms. I-MHCPs are these transport molecules. The I-MHCPs holding an antigen fragment can attach to certain immature T cells. Once such a T cell and I-MHCP-antigen complex hook up, the T cell reproduces many times. This important link between the cellular immune system and I-MHCPs has been shown in recent times by the epidemic of diseases like AIDS, which kills T cells. Class II MHCPs (II-MHCPs) interact similarly in antibody production by the humoral immune system. Understanding of the genes used in production of the I-MHCPs and the II-MHCPs has led to great hope for methods to control their production, possibilities for eventual cure of AIDS, emerging cancer treatments, and better understanding of the production of antibodies.

Additional information is needed on defects in the system, as are explanations for its dysfunctions. With greater knowledge of immunology, it may be possible to conquer AIDS, allergies, and asthma and to develop birth control methods based on the immune response. Doctors may be able to cure cancer, diabetes, herpes, infertility, multiple sclerosis, and rheumatoid arthritis. The possibilities are endless and could also include perfecting transplants of organs and skin grafts and preventing birth defects and even obesity. Through human gene therapy, those at risk for genetic disorders could be diagnosed and those with existing genetic conditions could be treated. Genetically engineered drugs and gene replacement therapy could relieve the stress on the human immune system. Until these methods become feasible, however, individuals must protect the natural immunity supplied by their bodies.

—*Maxine M. Urton, Ph.D.*

See also Acquired immunodeficiency syndrome (AIDS); Allergies; Antioxidants; Autoimmune disorders; Blood and blood disorders; Bone marrow transplantation; Cells; Chemotherapy; Circulation; Cytology; Cytopathology; Dialysis; Endocrinology; Endocrinology, pediatric; Glands; Healing; Hematology; Hematology, pediatric; Histiocytosis; Homeopathy; Hormones; Host-defense mechanisms; Human immunodeficiency virus (HIV); Immunization and vaccination; Immunodeficiency disorders; Immunology; Immunopathology; Infection; Liver; Lymphatic system; Multiple chemical sensitivity syndrome; Oncology; Preventive medicine; Serology; Severe combined immunodeficiency syndrome (SCID); Skin; Stress reduction; Systems and organs; Transfusion; Transplantation; Wiskott-Aldrich syndrome.

FOR FURTHER INFORMATION:

Adelman, Daniel C., et al., eds. *Manual of Allergy and Immunology.* Philadelphia: Lippincott Williams & Wilkins, 2002. Examines research developments and the clinical diagnosis and treatment of allergies and immune disorders. Topics include asthma, disorders of the eye, diseases of the lung, anaphylaxis, insect allergies, drug allergies, rheumatic diseases, transplantation immunology, and immunization.

Frank, Steven A. *Immunology and Evolution of Infectious Disease.* Princeton, N.J.: Princeton University Press, 2002. Blends research from molecular biology, immunology, pathogen biology, and population dynamics to discuss how and why parasites vary to escape recognition by the immune system, vaccine design, and the control of epidemics.

Immune Web. http://www.immuneweb.org/. A mailing list and resource center for people with chronic fatigue syndrome, multiple chemical sensitivities, lupus, allergies, environmental illness, fibromyalgia, candida, and other immune system disorders.

Janeway, Charles A., et al. *Immunobiology: The Immune System in Health and Disease.* 5th ed. Washington, D.C.: Taylor & Francis, 2001. An excellent text that provides a lucid and comprehensive examination of the immune system, covering such topics as immunobiology and innate immunity, the recognition of antigen, the development of mature lymphocyte receptor repertoires, the adaptive immune response, and the evolution of the immune system.

Kuby, Janis. *Immunology.* 5th ed. New York: W. H. Freeman, 2003. Excellent text that gives an overview of the immune system and its role with cells and organs, and discusses such topics as the generation of B-cell and T-cell responses, immune effector mechanisms, and the immune system in health and disease.

Life, Death, and the Immune System. New York: W. H. Freeman, 1994. This comprehensive collection of articles from *Scientific American* provides basic information and research directions on AIDS, autoimmune disorders, and allergies, as well as an excellent discussion of the immune system in general.

Marieb, Elaine N. *Essentials of Human Anatomy and Physiology.* 7th ed. Redwood City, Calif.: Benjamin/Cummings, 2003. This introductory anatomy and physiology textbook, easily accessible to those with little science background, is richly illustrated with diagrams and photographs, which help to illuminate body systems and processes.

Roitt, Ivan. *Roitt's Essential Immunology.* 10th ed. Boston: Blackwell Scientific, 2001. Written by a leading author in the field, the text provides a fine description of immunology.

Tortora, Gerard J., and Sandra R. Grabowski. *Principles of Anatomy and Physiology.* 10th ed. New York: John Wiley & Sons, 2003. An outstanding textbook of human anatomy and physiology.

IMMUNIZATION AND VACCINATION
PROCEDURE

ANATOMY OR SYSTEM AFFECTED: Blood, cells, immune system

SPECIALTIES AND RELATED FIELDS: Immunology, microbiology, preventive medicine, public health

DEFINITION: Immunization is the process by which exposure to an infectious agent or chemical confers an organism with resistance to that agent; vaccination involves the injection of a killed or attenuated microorganism, with the intention of inducing immunity.

KEY TERMS:

active immunity: immunity resulting from antibody production following exposure to an antigen

antibody: a protein secreted by lymphocytes in response to antigen stimuli, such as bacteria or viruses; also referred to as immunoglobulin

antigen: any chemical substance that stimulates the production of antibodies

attenuation: the weakening or elimination of the pathogenic properties of a microorganism; ideally, the organism is rendered harmless

passive immunity: immunity resulting from the introduction of preformed antibodies

serotype: a subgroup member within a larger species that is similar, but not identical, to other members of the species

toxoid: a toxin that has been chemically treated to eliminate its toxic properties but that retains the same antigens as the original

vaccinia: a virus which causes a poxlike illness in cattle (cowpox) and serves as smallpox vaccine in humans because of its similarity to the smallpox virus

THE FUNDAMENTALS OF IMMUNIZATION

The major day-to-day function of the immune response is to protect the body from infection. Exposure to foreign antigens such as infectious agents results in the stimulation of either of two components of the immune system: the humoral (or antibody) immune response or the cellular immune response. Although no clear division exists between these two facets of the immune system, the antibody response deals primarily with organisms such as bacteria that live outside the cell. The cellular response deals primarily with microbes that live within a cell, such as intracellular bacteria or viral-infected cells.

A specialized class of white cells called B lymphocytes carries out the production of antibodies. Stimulation of these cells results from a complicated interaction between a variety of cells, including antigen-presenting cells (macrophage and dendritic cells) and both T and B lymphocytes. The response is specific in that each type of T or B cell can interact with only a single antigen. The B cell that produces antibodies against a particular characteristic or shape on the surface of a bacterium reacts only with that particular determinant. In turn, the antibodies secreted by that B cell can interact only with specific determinants.

Antibodies secreted by B cells are themselves inert proteins. A variety of effects can result, however, when an antibody binds an antigen. The specific results depend on the nature of the antigen. For example, binding of an antibody to a toxin results in the neutralization of that substance. If the antigen is on the surface of a bacterial cell, the antibody can act as a flag that attracts other chemicals circulating in the blood. The techni-

IN THE NEWS: IMMUNIZATIONS AND BIOTERRORISM

The unprecedented terrorist attacks on the World Trade Center and the Pentagon on September 11, 2001, increased an awareness and discussion of preparedness for terrorist attacks involving the release of disease-causing organisms. Many experts believe that the primary threat is smallpox, which was declared eradicated from the world in 1980, despite being stored in a frozen state at various sites. The possibility of a terrorist group having access to these frozen stocks is disturbing. The anthrax attacks in the fall of 2001 added more urgency to the situation. Immunization provides an obvious defensive strategy against such attacks, but for the civilian population, the issue is complex: Since the vaccination process itself is associated with a small health risk, experts question who should be vaccinated. The American military added anthrax and smallpox to the list of standard immunizations given to its troops.

In late 2002, President George W. Bush debated about whether to vaccinate all U.S. citizens against smallpox and eventually settled on a plan to vaccinate 500,000 health care workers who would be at most risk in the case of a smallpox outbreak. However, by February 2003, it was reported that only a small fraction of this number actually received the vaccinations because some hospitals and individuals refused to participate in the program. *The New York Times* reported in June, 2003, that more than 450,000 military recruits had been vaccinated against smallpox. Of the recruits who were vaccinated, it was reported that ten individuals experienced heart inflammation, but all recovered. *The New England Journal of Medicine* reported in April, 2002, that smallpox vaccine stored since the 1970's was still effective even if diluted ten-fold from the original dose.

Anthrax has also proven to be a major terror agent. It can be made into a deadly weapon using a powder form that can be inhaled. The anthrax vaccine available in 2003 involved a series of six shots, which is an unusually high number. In September, 2003, the San Diego biopharmaceutical company VaxGen was awarded an $80 million government contract to develop an improved anthrax vaccine. The U.S. government also awarded a $71 million contract to Great Britain's Avecia to make three million doses of a new kind of genetically engineered anthrax vaccine. It is likely that health care workers as well as the military will continue to be immunized against these new weapons of terror.

—*Craig M. Story, Ph.D.*

The cellular immune system also reacts in a specific manner. A subclass of T lymphocytes called cytotoxic T cells reacts with specific antigenic determinants on the surface of infected cells. When the T cells bind to a target, the result is the local release of toxic chemicals that ultimately kill the target.

The development of vaccines against specific infectious microbial agents resulted in the control or elimination of many diseases caused by these agents. The first formal vaccine developed for the prevention of disease was that used by Edward Jenner against smallpox during the 1790's. Another century would pass before the molecular basis for vaccine function would begin to be understood.

Immunity to an antigen or disease may be induced using either of two methods. If preformed antibodies produced in another human or animal are inoculated into an individual, the result is passive immunity. Passive immunity can be advantageous in that the recipient achieves immunity in a short period of time. For example, if a person has been exposed to a toxin or has come into contact with an infectious agent, passive immunity can provide a rapid, short-term protection. Yet, since the individual does not generate the capacity to produce that antibody and the preformed antibodies are gradually removed from the body, no long-range protection is achieved.

The stimulation of antibody production through exposure to antigens, such as those found in a vaccine, results in active immunity. Development of effective active immunity requires a time span of several days to several weeks. The immunity is long-term, however, often lasting for the life span of the individual. Furthermore, each additional exposure to that same antigen, either through a vaccine booster or through natural exposure, results in

cal term for an antibody bound to a bacterium is an opsonin. The antibody-bacterium complex becomes much more likely to be ingested and destroyed by a specialized cell called a phagocyte than if the antibody were not present. Likewise, if the antigen is an extracellular virus particle, binding of the antibody may inhibit the ability of the virus to infect a cell.

a more rapid, greater response than those achieved previously. This increased rate of reaction is referred to as an anamnestic response.

The actual material utilized in a vaccine is variable, depending on the form of antigen. The earliest vaccine, that utilized by Jenner against smallpox, consisted of a virus that caused a disease in cattle called cowpox. The word "vaccination" is itself derived from this use; *vacca* is the Latin word for cow. While cowpox is distinct from the disease smallpox, the viruses that cause the two diseases contain similar antigenic determinants. Jenner made this observation. He exploited the fact that exposure to the cowpox virus results in active immunization against smallpox.

The use of attenuated strains of bacteria or viruses applies the same principle of cross-reaction. Attenuated organisms are mutants that have lost the ability to cause disease but that retain the antigenic character of the virulent strain. The most notable application of attenuation is the Sabin oral poliovirus vaccine (OPV). By testing hundreds of virus isolates for the ability to cause polio in monkeys, Albert Sabin was able to isolate certain strains that did not cause disease. These strains formed the basis for his vaccine. Similar testing resulted in the development of attenuated virus vaccines against a wide variety of agents, including those against measles, mumps, and rubella. Likewise, the Bacillus Calmette-Guerin (BCG) strain of *Mycobacte-*

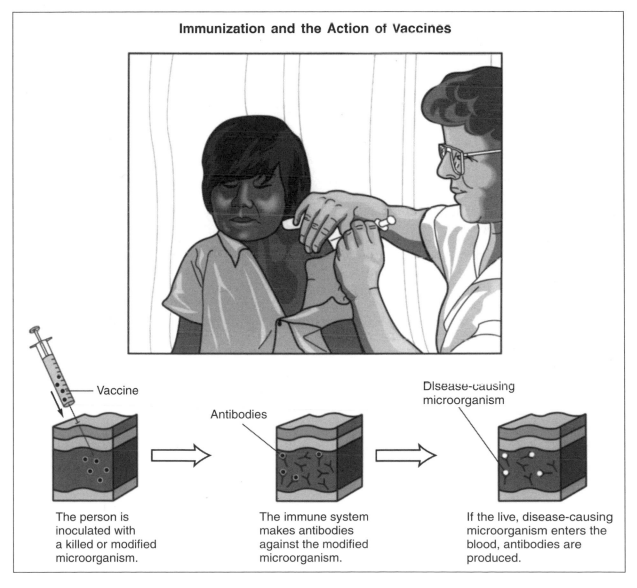

Immunization and the Action of Vaccines

Vaccine

Antibodies

Disease-causing microorganism

The person is inoculated with a killed or modified microorganism.

The immune system makes antibodies against the modified microorganism.

If the live, disease-causing microorganism enters the blood, antibodies are produced.

rium tuberculosis serves as a vaccine against the agent that causes tuberculosis. Unfortunately, the vaccine does not always result in immunity for the recipient. It is not used in the United States.

In some cases, the isolation of attenuated strains of microorganisms has proved difficult. For this reason, inactivated or killed microorganisms often serve as the basis for vaccine production. The Salk inactivated poliovirus vaccine represents the best-known example. By treating poliovirus with a solution of the chemical formalin, Jonas Salk was able to inactivate the organism. The virus retained its antigenic potential and served as an effective vaccine. A similar process has resulted in vaccines to protect against other bacterial diseases, such as bubonic plague, cholera, and pertussis (whooping cough), and against viral influenza.

In some cases, the vaccine is not directed against the etiological agent itself but against toxic materials produced by the agent. This is the case with diphtheria and tetanus. The vaccines are produced by treating the diphtheria and tetanus toxins secreted by these bacteria with formalin. The toxoids that result are antigenically similar to the actual toxins and so are able to induce immunity. They are incapable, however, of causing the deleterious effects of the respective diseases.

Only those determinants of a virus or bacterium that stimulate neutralizing antibodies are necessary in most vaccines. For this reason, the use of genetically engineered vaccines was begun in the 1980's. The first example put into use was the production of a vaccine against the hepatitis B virus (HBV). The gene that encodes the surface antigen of HBV was isolated and inserted into a piece of genetic material within the yeast *Saccharomyces*. The HBV antigen produced by the yeast was purified and subsequently found to be as effective in a vaccine as the whole virus. Since no live virus is involved, there is no danger of an attenuated strain reverting to its virulent parent. Recently, similar technology has been applied to produce vaccines that protect against chickenpox and hepatitis A virus.

Recommended Childhood Immunization Schedule (2004)

	Birth	1 mo.	2 mos.	4 mos.	6 mos.	12 mos.	15 mos.	18 mos.	4-6 yrs.	11-12 yrs.	13-18 yrs.
Hepatitis B	Dose 1	Dose 1									
			Dose 2			Dose 3					
Diphtheria, pertussis, tetanus (DPT)			Doses 1, 2, 3				Dose 4		Dose 5	Tetanus and Diphtheria Booster	
H. influenzae type B (HiB)			Doses 1, 2, 3			Dose 4					
Polio			Doses 1, 2			Dose 3			Dose 4		
Measles, mumps, rubella (MMR)						Dose 1				Dose 2	
Chickenpox (Varicella)						Dose 1					
Pneumococcal vaccine (PCV)			Doses 1, 2, 3			Dose 4					

Approved by the Advisory Committee on Immunization Practices, the American Academy of Pediatrics, and the American Academy of Family Physicians.

HISTORY AND MAJOR SUCCESSES

Since the first use of vaccination by Edward Jenner in the 1790's for the prevention of smallpox, immunization techniques have been developed for protection against most major infectious illnesses. The term "vaccination" was originally applied to immunization against smallpox, but its definition has long been expanded to include most immunization techniques. "Vaccination" and "immunization" are used interchangeably, although there are technical differences in the definitions of the words.

The nineteenth century improvements in public health measures, combined with the passage of laws for compulsory vaccination, resulted in a steady decrease in the number of smallpox cases in the United States and most countries of Europe. Even as late as 1930, however, approximately 49,000 cases were reported in the United States. In the 1950's, large numbers of cases were still being reported in areas of Africa and Asia. At that time, the World Health Organization (WHO) of the United Nations decided on a plan for the elimination of smallpox based on the fact that humans served as the sole reservoir for the smallpox virus; animals are not naturally infected with smallpox. Through the use of mass immunization techniques, the plan was to isolate areas of infection into smaller and smaller pockets.

Ironically, the origins of the vaccine in use during the 1960's are unknown. The original strain of cowpox used by Jenner was lost sometime during the nineteenth century. The strain used in the vaccine during the twentieth century, called vaccinia virus, may have originated from an isolate obtained during the Franco-Prussian War in the 1870's.

The plan for the elimination of smallpox developed by WHO ultimately proved completely successful. There are actually two different forms of smallpox. The last known natural case of variola major was reported in Bangladesh in 1974. The last known case of variola minor was reported in Somalia in 1976. Although an outbreak of smallpox resulting from a laboratory accident was reported in Great Britain, there were no additional naturally caused cases of smallpox. In 1978, WHO declared the world to be free of smallpox.

Although vaccination was effective in immunizing most persons against smallpox, use of the vaccine itself was associated with some risk. Serious complications were rare but did occasionally occur. With the disappearance of the disease, the need for routine immunization lessened, and, in 1971, compulsory vaccination of children in the United States was discontinued. In 1976, the routine vaccination of hospital employees was also discontinued. By the 1990's, the only known sites of existence of smallpox virus were freezers in four laboratories. The September 11, 2001, terrorist attacks at the World Trade Center and the Pentagon introduced a new era in which the fear of terrorists' use of biological agents has prompted renewed discussions about the reintroduction of the smallpox vaccine.

The use of vaccines for the elimination of poliomyelitis represents another success story. Although sporadic outbreaks of polio occurred in earlier centuries and probably as long ago as the time of ancient Egypt, the first epidemics appeared in the late nineteenth century. Ironically, this increase in the incidence of polio was caused by improvements in public health. Poliovirus is easily transmitted through a fecal-oral route, but the majority of cases, particularly in young children, are without symptoms, or asymptomatic. With improvements in sanitation, the first exposure to polio was often delayed until later childhood or, as in the case of President Franklin Delano Roosevelt, in the adult years. Under these circumstances, the disease is often more severe.

In 1955, the inactivated poliovirus vaccine developed by Jonas Salk was introduced for general use; in 1961, Albert Sabin's oral poliovirus vaccine was licensed for use. By the 1990's, polio had been eliminated from the Western Hemisphere and from developed countries elsewhere. Nevertheless, WHO estimated that 250,000 cases of polio occurred yearly throughout developing countries of the world. For this reason, the American Academy of Pediatrics (AAP) recommends that children receive immunizations by their first birthday and boosters at eighteen months of age and again prior to starting school. Adults who plan to travel to areas of the world in which polio is found should also be immunized.

The WHO campaign to eliminate polio has been largely successful in the Western Hemisphere. New cases are still being reported in parts of Asia and Africa. Money to fund the program has been a problem. Civil strife has prevented medical teams from entering some areas and providing immunizations.

The most significant advancement in twentieth century health care in the United States has been the elimination of most major childhood diseases. In addition to poliovirus immunization, children routinely receive a variety of early immunizations. Measles, mumps, and rubella (MMR) vaccines are administered in a single preparation at fifteen months of age. All three contain live attenuated viruses. The measles vaccine was first introduced in 1966 and resulted in a decline in reported measles cases of nearly 99 percent by the 1980's. Beginning about 1986, however, increasing numbers of cases of measles were reported among young adults who had been previously immunized. For this reason, the AAP recommends that children receive boosters of measles vaccine prior to entering high school, at approximately eleven to twelve years of age. A series of the diphtheria, pertussis, and tetanus (DPT) vaccine is administered at two, four, six, and eighteen months, with tetanus and diphtheria boosters recommended at ten-year intervals throughout the remainder of life.

With the elimination of most other major childhood illnesses, *Hemophilus influenzae* type B infections moved into the dubious position of being among the most significant causes of illness and death among young children. In 1985, a vaccine developed from the outer coat of the bacterium was licensed for use. The vaccine worked poorly in children under the age of two, the major population at risk. Consequently, an improved vaccine was developed and licensed by 1987. The second vaccine consisted of a portion of the influenza coat joined to diphtheria toxoid. It was found to immunize children effectively at eighteen months of age; immunization with the vaccine is recommended by the age of fifteen months.

By 1991, a total of nineteen vaccines had been licensed in the United States by the Food and Drug Administration (FDA) for uses in either children or adults. Aside from the eight previously described vaccines for children, eleven vaccines (five viral and six bacterial) are recommended for special circumstances. For example, in 1986, a genetically engineered hepatitis B virus vaccine was developed and licensed. The gene that encodes the virus surface antigen was placed in a small piece of deoxyribonucleic acid (DNA), a plasmid, and inserted into the common baker's yeast *Saccharomyces cerevisiae*. The antigen that is produced is used in a three-dose series to immunize individuals at risk for the disease: health care workers, institutional staff persons, and anyone else who is likely to come into contact with the virus.

Although routine vaccination of children has worked virtually to eliminate most health-threatening infectious disease from that population, immunization of adults against preventable diseases has not been as successful. It was estimated that, in the late twentieth century, 50,000 to 70,000 adults died yearly from diseases that were preventable through immunization, such as pneumococcal pneumonia, influenza, and hepatitis B.

Historically, pneumococcal pneumonia, caused by the bacterium *Streptococcus pneumonia*, has been a killer of adults. In the 1990's, an estimated 40,000 persons, primarily the elderly, died from this disease. The available vaccine is a polysaccharide vaccine, representing serotypes for twenty-three of the major strains of the bacterium. When administered by the age of fifty, the vaccine provides a significant degree of protection against the organism.

Between 1957 and 1993, nineteen influenza epidemics each resulted in more than 10,000 deaths from the disease in the United States alone. Two of the epidemics each resulted in more than 40,000 deaths. Most of these deaths were in elderly adults. Although the usefulness of vaccination among the elderly is limited, immunization against influenza will often lessen the severity of the disease, even if it fails to prevent infection.

Some specialized vaccines are recommended only for international travelers. Both killed and live attenuated oral vaccines against typhoid are licensed. The ease of administration of an oral vaccine has made this form the preferred choice. In addition, vaccines against cholera, dengue fever, plague, and yellow fever may be used in appropriate circumstances.

Although active immunization in most circumstances remains the preferred method of protection through vaccination, situations occur in which passive immunization may provide therapeutic treatment. Individuals may be immunosuppressed or lack a functional immune system. This condition may result from infection (acquired immunodeficiency syndrome, or AIDS), medical intervention (chemotherapy), or congenital reasons (severe combined immunodeficiency disease, or SCID). Whatever the cause, active immunization does not develop. In addition, there are circumstances in which the necessary time for the development of immunity through active immunization is not available, such as with exposure to tetanus toxin, the hepatitis virus, or rabies. For passive immunization or replacement therapy in immunodeficiency disorders, immunoglobulin is usually prepared from pools of plasma obtained from large numbers of blood donors. Specific immunoglobulins, directed against specific targets such as rabies or tetanus, are prepared from plasma containing high concentrations of these antibodies.

PERSPECTIVE AND PROSPECTS

The elimination of smallpox represents the classic ex-

In December, 2002, the U.S. Food and Drug Administration (FDA) approved a multicomponent vaccine containing diphtheria and tetanus toxoids, acellular pertussis adsorbed (DtaP), hepatitis B (HepB; recombinant), and inactivated poliovirus (IPV) components. This vaccine, manufactured by GlaxoSmithKline Biologics in Belgium, is called DtaP-HepB-IPV combined vaccine, or Pediarix. It is intended to be given to infants in three injections, one each at two, four, and six months of age. Pediarix provides protection against diphtheria, tetanus, pertussis (whooping cough), hepatitis B, and poliomyelitis in a series of only three injections instead of the nine injections previously given to infants. Thus, for patients and practitioners alike, it provides benefits such as saved office visits and decreased costs. Most important, the shorter injection series makes it much easier for parents, increasing the likelihood that parents will have their children immunized against these serious diseases.

The Pediarix vaccine has been subjected to numerous worldwide clinical trials to evaluate its safety and immunogenicity, or impact on the immune system. Data indicate that the vaccine is both safe and effective, with no significant adverse effects being reported. In these trials, the immunogenicity of each of the components in the combined vaccine was not shown to differ significantly from the immunogenicity of the components administered separately. These studies, involving more than seven thousand infants, reported minor adverse affects, including injection-site soreness (pain, redness, or swelling), fever, and irritability. The Pediarix vaccine has been associated with a greater frequency of fever in comparison to the separately administered vaccine components. Infants who are hypersensitive to any component of the vaccine, including yeast, neomycin, and polymyxin B, should not be given the vaccine. The Advisory Committee on Immunization Practices (ACIP), the Committee on Infectious Diseases of the American Academy of Pediatrics, and the American Academy of Family Physicians all have recommended this vaccine for routine use.

—*Steven A. Kuhl, Ph.D.*

killed 400,000 persons each year and caused more than one-third of all cases of blindness. It has also been estimated that smallpox or other diseases killed approximately 85 percent of the American Indians who died during colonial periods, certainly far more than the number who died from bullet wounds.

The principle of immunization in prevention did not originate with Edward Jenner, the English physician credited with development of the smallpox vaccine in the 1790's. A practice called variolation was well known in China and parts of the Middle East for centuries prior to Jenner. Variolation consisted of the inhalation of dried crust prepared from the pocks obtained from individuals suffering from mild cases of smallpox. A variation involved removing small amounts of fluid from an active smallpox pustule and scratching the liquid into the skin of children. Lady Mary Wortley Montagu, wife of the British ambassador to the Ottoman Empire, introduced the practice of variolation into Great Britain during the early eighteenth century. Use of variolation was empirical: The practice was often successful. The possibility remained, however, that immunization might actually introduce the disease.

ample in which the efficacy of a vaccine resulted in the eradication of disease. Smallpox was an ancient disease, with origins as early as the twelfth century B.C.E. It appeared in the Middle East in the sixth century C.E., with subsequent dissemination into northern Africa and southern Europe as a result of the Arab invasions from the sixth to the eighth centuries. The disease spread throughout Europe with the return of the Crusaders during the eleventh and twelfth centuries and reached the Americas as a result of the African slave trade in the sixteenth century. It has been estimated that, at its peak during the eighteenth century, smallpox

Born in 1749, Jenner first became aware of the protective effects of cowpox from the story of a local dairymaid who had been exposed to the disease. After years of study and observation, he became convinced of the story's validity. In 1796, he immunized an eight-year-old boy with material from a cowpox lesion. No ill effects were seen. Further immunizations supported the theory that cowpox protected against smallpox. Jenner called this material variolae vaccinae. Richard Dunning, a Plymouth physician, in an 1800 analysis of the procedure, was the first to use the term "vaccination."

Wider application of the principle of vaccination followed from Louis Pasteur's studies during the 1870's and 1880's. With his attenuation of the bacterium that caused chicken cholera, Pasteur demonstrated that one could manipulate the virulence of a microorganism. This practice soon led to his development of vaccines against both anthrax and rabies. It is ironic that no clinical trials have ever been conducted to test rabies vaccine.

The twentieth century saw the development of effective vaccines against most major childhood diseases. Use of the DPT toxoid became routine in the United States about 1945. Development of the oral Sabin vaccine and inactivated Salk vaccines during the 1950's resulted in the complete elimination of poliomyelitis from the Western Hemisphere by the 1990's. The use of genetic engineering, in which only the genes necessary to synthesize specific antigens are utilized, was first applied to the hepatitis B vaccine. It has recently been applied successfully to create vaccines against chickenpox and hepatitis A virus. A vaccine against hepatitis C virus is under development. This technology provides the potential for manufacturing vaccine "cocktails," or combinations of such genes from a variety of infectious agents in a single vaccine.

In 2000, the FDA approved conjugate pneumococcal vaccine (Prevnar) for use in children under the age of two years for the prevention of pneumococcal infections. The AAP recommended Prevnar for use in all children twenty-three months of age and younger. The AAP also recommended Prevnar for all immunocompromised children twenty-four to fifty-nine months of age who are at high risk for invasive pneumococcal infection. Prevnar may be administered in a series of four inoculations given at two, four, six, and twelve to fifteen months of age. Pneumococcal infections are a major cause of meningitis and septicemia in infants and children.

Many experts are trying to develop a vaccine to protect against AIDS. This is difficult because the very mechanism that has been exploited by other vaccines, namely the stimulation of T cells to produce antibodies that protect a recipient, is nonfunctional in AIDS. The successful development of a vaccine against AIDS will require scientific ingenuity.

—Richard Adler, Ph.D.; updated by
L. Fleming Fallon, Jr., M.D., Ph.D., M.P.H.
See also Acquired immunodeficiency syndrome (AIDS); Anthrax; Antibiotics; Bacterial infections; Bacteriology; Chickenpox; Childhood infectious diseases;

Cholera; Diphtheria; Disease; Environmental health; Hepatitis; Host-defense mechanisms; Immune system; Immunology; Influenza; Measles; Microbiology; Mumps; Pathology; Plague; Poliomyelitis; Preventive medicine; Rubella; Smallpox; Tuberculosis; Viral infections; Whooping cough; World Health Organization.

FOR FURTHER INFORMATION:

Behbehani, Abbas. *The Smallpox Story in Words and Pictures*. Kansas City: University of Kansas Medical Center, 1988. The book includes the history of Edward Jenner and his use of cowpox in the first smallpox vaccine. The drawings and photographs are of particular interest.

Bittle, J. L., and F. A. Murphy, eds. *Vaccine Biotechnology*. San Diego, Calif.: Academic Press, 1989. A discussion of the use of techniques in molecular biology and genetic engineering in vaccine development. The style and depth of coverage is appropriate to anyone with basic knowledge of biology.

Brock, Thomas D., ed. *Microorganisms: From Smallpox to Lyme Disease*. New York: W. H. Freeman, 1990. A collection of readings from *Scientific American* magazine. Included is a section on the role of vaccines in the prevention of disease, including their role in the elimination of smallpox. Also found are articles on synthetic vaccines and vaccination in Third World countries.

Plotkin, Stanley A., and Edward Mortimer, Jr., eds. *Vaccines*. 4th ed. New York: Elsevier, 2003. An excellent description of the role of vaccines in the prevention of disease. The book begins with a history of immunization practices. Each subsequent chapter deals with a specific disease and the role and history of vaccine production in its prevention. While enough detail is provided to interest someone in the field, the text is appropriate for nonscientists.

Roitt, Ivan. *Roitt's Essential Immunology*. 10th ed. Boston: Blackwell Scientific, 2001. An excellent textbook on the subject of immunology. Much of the book is detailed and requires some background in biology. Nevertheless, the chapters which deal with infection and immunization are clear and contain much that will interest nonscientists. Numerous graphs illustrate material from the text.

Rosario, Diane. *Immunization Resource Guide: Where to Find Answers to All Your Questions About Childhood Vaccinations*. Burlington, Iowa: Patter, 2001. Provides parents with information on all sides of the controversial vaccination issue and resources to make informed decisions. Includes reviews of over 90 books covering all aspects of childhood vaccinations and detailed listings of more than 130 vaccine and health organizations, periodicals, and publishers.

Vaccine Page, The. http://www.vaccines.com. Site provides access to current news about vaccines and an annotated database of vaccine resources on the Internet.

IMMUNODEFICIENCY DISORDERS
DISEASE/DISORDER

ANATOMY OR SYSTEM AFFECTED: Immune system

SPECIALTIES AND RELATED FIELDS: Genetics, immunology

DEFINITION: Genetic or acquired disorders that result from disturbances in the normal functioning of the immune system.

KEY TERMS:

antibody: protein immunoglobulin secreted by B lymphocytes; the production of antibodies is induced by specific foreign invaders, and they combine with and destroy only those invaders

B lymphocytes: also referred to as B cells; white cells of the immune system that produce antibodies; produced within the bone marrow

phagocytes: white cells of the immune system that destroy invading foreign bodies by engulfing and digesting them in a nonspecific immune response; includes macrophages and neutrophils

stem cells: multipotential precursor cells within the bone marrow that develop into white cell populations, including lymphocytes and phagocytic cells

T lymphocyte: a type of immune cell that kills host cells infected by bacteria or viruses and secretes chemicals (interleukins) that regulate the immune response

CAUSES AND SYMPTOMS

The defense of the body against foreign invaders is provided by the immune system. In nonspecific immunity, phagocytic cells engulf and destroy invading particles. Specific immunity consists of very specialized cell types that are synthesized in response to a particular type of foreign invader. Self-replicating stem cells within the bone marrow give rise to lymphocytes, which mediate specific immunity. Lymphocytes establish self-replacing colonies within the thymus, spleen, and lymph nodes. The various categories of T lymphocytes are derived from the thymus colonies, while B lymphocytes develop and mature within the bone marrow. B lym-

> ### INFORMATION ON IMMUNODEFICIENCY DISORDERS
>
> **CAUSES:** Genetic disorders, infections, damage from drug or radiation treatments, environmental factors
>
> **SYMPTOMS:** Varies; can include recurrent infections, scaly inflammation of skin, chronic inflammations of internal organs and bones, fever, fatigue
>
> **DURATION:** Often chronic
>
> **TREATMENTS:** Typically targeted at source of deficiency; can include antibody injections, antifungal medications, bone marrow transplantation, drug cocktails, alternative medicine (acupuncture, herbal medicine, meditation, homeopathy)

phocytes secrete highly specific antibodies that attack bacteria and some viruses. T lymphocytes do not secrete antibodies but instead either attack the body cells that have been infected with a bacterium or virus or produce chemical compounds that aid other types of T cells in destroying the infected cells. In immunodeficiency disorders, some or all of these defenses are compromised, which can have life-threatening consequences. Less commonly, immunodeficiency diseases are the result of genetic abnormalities and are present from birth; others are acquired through infection or exposure to damaging drug or radiation treatments.

The most severe immunodeficiency disorder is attributable to the absence of stem cells, which results in a total lack of both B and T lymphocytes. This rare genetic condition is referred to as severe combined immunodeficiency syndrome (SCID). Affected infants show a failure to thrive from birth and can easily die from common bacterial or viral infections. The most common cause of SCID is a deficiency in the enzyme adenosine deaminase. This deficiency disrupts the normal deoxyribonucleic acid (DNA) synthesis in the stem cells. A variant of SCID is Swiss-type agammaglobulinemia, in which the thymus is absent and few lymph nodes exist.

Major syndromes that involve defects specific to the T lymphocyte population are characterized by recurrent viral and fungal infections. DiGeorge syndrome results from improper development of the thymus, which in turn results in insufficient production of T lymphocytes, often accompanied by other structural abnormalities in the infant. Death usually results prior to age two from overwhelming viral infections.

The most common disorders affecting B lymphocytes are forms of hypogammaglobulinemia. This condition is characterized by insufficient levels of antibody. The cause is generally associated with increased rates of antibody breakdown or loss in the urine secondary to kidney malfunction. Bruton's agammaglobulinemia is a rare, sex-linked form of the condition, in which B cells fail to mature properly. Severe bacterial infections are the most common symptom. When the disorder is left untreated, infants generally die of severe pneumonia prior to six months of age.

Several immunodeficiency disorders may be the result of partial defects in the production and/or function of B and T lymphocytes. Wiskott-Aldrich syndrome is a genetically inherited disease manifested by recurrent infections and an itchy, scaly inflammation of the skin. Certain classes of antibodies are absent or scarce. Chronic mucocutaneous candidiasis is characterized by chronic fungal infection of the skin and mucous membranes; reduced levels of T cells are responsible for this disfiguring disorder.

Immunodeficiency disorders may also be the result of defects in phagocytic cells; the underlying cause of most of these disorders is ill-defined but often involves deficiencies in hydrolytic enzymes. In chronic granulomatosis, an inherited enzyme deficiency prevents the immune system from destroying bacteria that have been phagocytized. Infants affected by this disorder develop severe infections and chronic inflammations of internal organs and bones. The bacteria responsible for these infections are generally common flora that are not considered pathogens in healthy individuals.

Most of the disorders that affect the immune system are not inherited but develop sometime during the person's life. They are either the result of an infection or a consequence of another disease or its treatment. The use of corticosteroids to treat inflammations, or the illicit use of them in muscle-building, can interfere with the proper production and function of T lymphocytes. Other immunosuppressive drugs used to diminish the possibilities of graft or transplant rejection, or in the treatment of autoimmune diseases, can severely depress antibody production. Chemotherapeutic agents used in the treatment of cancer can affect DNA replication and severely compromise the entire immune system. Whole-body radiation can damage or destroy bone marrow stem cells.

Major trauma, surgery, and burns all lead to an increased risk of infection. These experiences result in depressed function of both the nonspecific and specific immune responses. The effect is temporary, however, and immune responses generally return to normal during the recuperative process. Advanced malignancies (cancer) are frequently associated with a depressed immune response, perhaps because of tumor proliferation and interference with the development and maturation of B and T lymphocytes.

Acquired immunodeficiency syndrome (AIDS) is caused by the human immunodeficiency virus (HIV). HIV specifically infects one type of regulatory T lymphocyte, resulting in severe immune depression. The virus may be harbored in an individual for years without symptoms. Initial symptoms may be quite mild but generally progress so that the affected individual becomes susceptible to a host of unusual bacterial and fungal infections, including a rare form of cancer called Kaposi's sarcoma. AIDS produces neurological damage in about one-third of infected individuals. HIV is transmitted primarily through unprotected sexual contact, sharing of needles for intravenous drug use, transfusion with contaminated blood products, or other contact with contaminated body fluids.

Treatment and Therapy

Treatment of immunodeficiency disorders is targeted at the source of the deficiency. For example, in DiGeorge syndrome, characterized by the congenital absence of the thymus, fetal thymus transplants may correct the problem, with improvement in lymphocyte levels seen within hours after the transplants. The use of thymus extracts has also been beneficial. Syndromes such as hypogammaglobulinemia can be managed by injection with mixtures of antibodies. Drug therapy to substitute for some absent immune components of Wiskott-Aldrich syndrome has been shown to have variable effects. The most effective treatment for chronic mucocutaneous candidiasis is aggressive antifungal medication to eradicate the causative organism; treatment must continue for several months because fungal infections are slow to respond to therapy and frequently recur. Chronic granulomatosis is notoriously difficult to treat, and the most effective therapy has been antibiotic and antifungal agents used aggressively during an overt infection.

Because of the magnitude of the defects, many inherited immunodeficiency disorders are difficult to treat successfully and are commonly fatal early in life. Chronic granulomatosis is usually fatal within the first few years of life, and only about 20 percent of patients reach the age of twenty. SCID is a serious disorder in which affected infants can die before a proper diagnosis is made. For individuals with these and other serious immunodeficiency disorders, maintenance in an environment free of bacteria, viruses, and fungi, such as a sterile "bubble," has been the best means to prevent life-threatening infections. Such an approach, however, precludes the possibility of a normal life. The most effective treatment for individuals with severely compromised immune systems is bone marrow transplantation. In this procedure, bone marrow from a compatible individual is introduced into the bone marrow of the patient. If the procedure works—and the success rate is high—in approximately one to six months the transplant recipient's immune system will be reconstituted and functional. Bone marrow transplantation is a permanent cure for these disorders, since the transplanted marrow will contain stem cells that produce all the cell types of the immune system. The difficulties in transplantation include finding a compatible donor and preventing infections during the period after the transplant. Individuals are particularly susceptible to infection prior to the activation of the transplanted bone marrow. Such patients are frequently kept in sterile bubbles to limit the possibility of infection.

Drug therapy for AIDS utilizes treatments that interfere with replication of the virus. The first drug to be approved for use was zidovudine (formerly AZT), a DNA analogue, but its success was somewhat limited, as it was associated with severe side effects and the creation of resistant virus. More recent treatments utilize drug "cocktails," combinations of drugs that act at different stages of viral replication. Vaccines and antibiotic therapy are used to prevent or treat the opportunistic illnesses that accompany AIDS. Various drugs may also help to ease symptoms of AIDS such as appetite disturbances, nausea, pain, insomnia, anxiety, depression, fever, and diarrhea. A combination of therapies has been shown to increase life expectancy in AIDS patients. Many patients choose to participate in clinical trials of experimental drugs not approved for general use in the hope that the new drug will be more effective at alleviating the disease. Others seek out alternative or nontraditional medical treatments that have a long history of use in Western cultures. These treatments include acupuncture, herbology, meditation, and homeopathy. An important aspect of therapy for AIDS patients is maintaining mental health through support groups and supportive caregivers.

Illicit use of corticosteroids can seriously compromise the immune system and may lead to permanent damage. The best therapy for this type of acquired immunodeficiency is prevention—that is, to not misuse the drugs. In their supervised use to control inflammation or other disease symptoms, normal immune function will return after treatment has been completed. A huge risk to cancer patients who are being treated with chemotherapy and/or radiation therapy is the depression of the immune system, which can lead to a host of infections being contracted and not easily fought off by the body's compromised immune system. These individuals should avoid exposure to infectious agents when possible and be attentive to lifestyle modifications that can strengthen the immune system and encourage its speedy recovery, including a nutritious diet, plenty of rest, and avoidance of stress. Close monitoring for any signs of infection facilitates rapid antibiotic therapy, which can prevent serious complications.

PERSPECTIVE AND PROSPECTS

Prior to the gains in scientific knowledge about the mechanics of the immune system, individuals with genetic immunodeficiency disorders would die of serious infections during their first few years of life. Even when it was finally realized that these individuals suffered from defects of the immune system, little could be done for most of the disorders, except to treat infections as they developed and to avoid contact with potential disease-causing organisms—a near impossibility if one is to lead a normal life. Housing persons with SCID in sterile bubbles was uncommon because of the expense and impracticality. During the 1970's, bone marrow transplants were first developed; by the 1990's they had progressed to a greater than 80 percent success rate. As a result of improved transplant-rejection drugs, transplants from donors with less-than-perfect tissue matches are now possible. Bone marrow transplantation has been a source of cure for many individuals with immune disorders.

Bone marrow transplantation is not suitable or possible in every case of immunodeficiency disorder, and scientists have long sought a means to cure the genetic defects themselves. In 1992, French Anderson of the National Institutes of Health conducted the first gene therapy trial on a young girl suffering from SCID. Some of the girl's bone marrow cells were removed from her body and exposed to an inactivated virus containing a normal gene for ADA, the defective enzyme. Some of the stem cells in the marrow incorporated the healthy gene, and the engineered cells were returned to her body. The cells lodged in her bone marrow, where they produced healthy immune cells. The procedure was repeated successfully in three other children shortly afterward.

Gene therapy is being considered for a variety of immunodeficiency conditions. In the future, bone marrow cells may be engineered to be resistant to chemotherapy and radiation therapy; therefore, patients could be given more frequent dosages of cancer-fighting therapies without destroying their ability to fight infections. Bone marrow cells may also be engineered for resistance to infection by the AIDS virus; in this way, individuals with AIDS may be given a population of cells that will reverse the immunodeficiency associated with AIDS. Aging individuals develop depressed immune systems, and medical research is searching for ways to prevent this decline. These efforts toward curing immunodeficiency diseases with the tools of contemporary molecular biology are promising.

—Karen E. Kalumuck, Ph.D.;
updated by Richard Adler, Ph.D.

See also Acquired immunodeficiency syndrome (AIDS); Allergies; Arthritis; Asthma; Autoimmune disorders; Blood and blood disorders; Bone marrow transplantation; Cells; Cytology; Cytopathology; DiGeorge syndrome; Gene therapy; Hematology; Hematology, pediatric; Host-defense mechanisms; Human immunodeficiency virus (HIV); Immune system; Immunology; Immunopathology; Serology; Wiskott-Aldrich syndrome.

For Further Information:

Abbas, Abdul K., and Andrew K. Lichtman. *Basic Immunology: Functions and Disorders of the Immune System.* New York: Elsevier, 2001. Provides introductory text to the basics of immunology and describes the primary disorders that impair its function. Illustrations, case studies, review questions, key point summaries, and a glossary are included.

Bartlett, John G., and Ann K. Finkbeiner. *The Guide to Living with HIV Infection.* 5th ed. Baltimore: Johns Hopkins University Press, 2001. This informative book developed at The Johns Hopkins University AIDS Clinic is a great resource for information about the disease and a guide for patients and caregivers in living with the disease.

Dwyer, John M. *The Body at War: The Story of Our Immune System.* 2d ed. New York: Penguin Books, 1993. This easy-to-read text is an excellent introduc-

tion to the functions of the immune system and such related topics as immune disorders, allergies, and immunology research.

Emini, Emilio A., ed. *The Human Immunodeficiency Virus: Biology, Immunology, and Therapy.* Princeton, N.J.: Princeton University Press, 2002. Collects in one volume information from specialized journals on HIV research, examining such topics as the virus life cycle, epidemiology, genetics, protease and reverse transcriptase inhibitors, receptor and co-receptor interactions, therapeutic targets, clinical treatment, immunobiology, and vaccines.

Frank, Steven A. *Immunology and Evolution of Infectious Disease.* Princeton, N.J.: Princeton University Press, 2002. Blends research from molecular biology, immunology, pathogen biology, and population dynamics to discuss how and why parasites vary to escape recognition by the immune system, vaccine design, and the control of epidemics.

Immune Web. http://immuneweb.org/. A site that offers good articles on several immunodeficiency disorders, "safe" product lists, and annotated links to other Internet sites, among other features.

Life, Death, and the Immune System. New York: W. H. Freeman, 1994. This comprehensive collection of articles from *Scientific American* provides basic information and research directions on AIDS, autoimmune disorders, and allergies, as well as an excellent discussion of the immune system in general.

Parker, James N., and Philip M. Parker, eds. *The Official Parent's Sourcebook on Primary Immunodeficiency.* San Diego, Calif.: Icon Health, 2002. Draws from public, academic, government, and peer-reviewed research to provide a wide-ranging handbook for parents whose children suffer from primary immunodeficiency.

Petrow, Steven, ed. *HIV Drug Book.* Rev. ed. New York: Pocket Books, 1998. This book was produced by Project Information, the leading community-based AIDS treatment information and advocacy organization in the United States. Its user-friendly guide provides information on the most-used HIV/AIDS treatments.

Roitt, Ivan. *Roitt's Essential Immunology.* 10th ed. Boston: Blackwell Scientific, 2001. A thorough introduction to the science of immunology. Well illustrated. Includes an extensive section on immunodeficiency disorders.

Sticherling, Michael, and Enno Christophers. *Treatment of Autoimmune Disorders.* New York: Springer-

Verlag, 2002. Explores the basic mechanisms of autoimmune disorders; neurological, gastrointestinal, ophthalmological, and skin diseases; and current and future therapeutic options.

Stine, Gerald J. *AIDS Update: 2003*. Upper Saddle River, N.J.: Prentice Hall, 2002. An overview of AIDS, its cause, and methods of treating it. Included are sections outlining the immunodeficiency disorders that are sequelae to HIV infection.

IMMUNOLOGY
SPECIALTY
ANATOMY OR SYSTEM AFFECTED: Blood, cells, immune system

SPECIALTIES AND RELATED FIELDS: Cytology, hematology, microbiology, preventive medicine, serology

DEFINITION: The study of the immune system, its protection of the body from foreign agents, and its malfunction in autoimmune diseases, in which the body's defenses react against the body's own cells or tissues.

KEY TERMS:

antibody: a protein produced by lymphocytes in response to an antigen; binds only to a specific antigen

antigen: any substance perceived by immunological defenses to be foreign and against which antibody is produced; generally a protein

autoantibody: an antibody produced against tissue antigens within a host—that is, self-antigens

complement: a series of about twenty serum proteins that, when sequentially activated by immune complexes, may trigger cell damage

determinant: a region on the surface of an antigen capable of creating an immune response or of combining with an antibody produced by an immune response

Hashimoto's disease: thyroiditis; among the earliest characterized autoimmune diseases

lupus: systemic lupus erythematosus; a chronic inflammatory disease characterized by an arthritic condition and a rash

lymphocyte: a small white blood cell constituting about 25 percent of all blood cells; two basic types are B cells (antibody production) and T cells (cellular immunity)

tolerance: the state in which an organism does not normally react against its own tissue

SCIENCE AND PROFESSION
The field of immunology deals with the ability of the immune system to react against an enormous repertoire of stimulation by antigens. In most instances, these antigens are foreign infectious agents such as viruses or bacteria. Inherent in this process is the ability to react against nearly any known determinant, whether natural or artificially produced. The most reactive antigenic determinants are proteins, though to a lesser degree, other substances such as carbohydrates (sugars), lipids (fats), and nucleic acids may also stimulate a response.

In general, the body exhibits tolerance during the constant exposure to its own tissue. The precise reasons behind tolerance are vague, but the basis for the lack of response lies in two major mechanisms: the elimination during development of immunological cells capable of responding to the body's own tissue and the active prevention of existing reactive cells from responding to self-antigens. When this regulation fails, autoimmune disease may result.

There are two major types of immunological defense: humoral immunity and cell-mediated immunity. Humoral immunity refers to the soluble substances in blood serum, primarily antibody and complement, while cellular immunity refers to the portion of the immune response that is directly mediated by cells. Though these processes are sometimes categorized separately, they do in fact interact with and regulate each other.

Antibodies are produced by cells called B lymphocytes in response to foreign antigens. These proteins bind to the antigen in a specific manner, resulting in a complex that can be removed readily by phagocytic white blood cells. More important in the context of autoimmunity, antibody-antigen complexes also activate the complement pathway, a series of some twenty enzymes and serum proteins. The end result of activation is the lysis of the antigenic targets. In general, the targets are bacteria; in autoimmune disease, the target may be any cell in the body.

The cellular response utilizes any of several types of cytotoxic cells. These can include a specialized lymphocyte called the T cell (so named because of its development in the thymus) or another unusual type of large granular lymphocyte called the natural killer (NK) cell. NK and cytotoxic T cells function in a similar manner—by binding to the target and releasing toxic granules in apposition to its cell membrane.

Though autoimmune diseases differ in scope, they do tend to exhibit certain common factors. The pathologies associated with most of these illnesses result in part from the production of autoantibodies, which are antibodies produced against the body's own cells or tissues. If the antibody binds to tissue in a particular organ, complement is activated in the tissue, causing the destruction of those regions of the organ. For example, Goodpasture's syndrome is characterized by the deposition of autoantibodies directed against the membrane of the glomerulus in the kidneys. Complement activation can result in severe organ pathology and subsequent kidney failure.

If the autoantibody binds to soluble material in blood serum, the resultant antibody-antigen complexes are carried along in the circulation, and there is the possibility that they will lodge in various areas of the body. For example, systemic lupus erythematosus (SLE, or lupus) results from the production of autoantibodies against soluble nucleoprotein, which is released from cells as they undergo normal death and lysis. The immune complexes frequently lodge in the kidney, where they can cause renal failure.

This is not to say that all autoimmune diseases result solely from autoantibody production. Though a precise role for either cytotoxic T cells or NK cells in human autoimmune disease has not been fully confirmed, several observations make such an association likely. First, large numbers of T cells are found in certain organ-specific diseases, including thyroiditis and pernicious anemia. Second, animal models of similar diseases show a specific role for such cells in the pathology of these diseases. Thus, it is likely that these cells do participate in the organ destruction.

Autoimmune disorders can be categorized in the form of a disease spectrum. At one end of the spectrum one can place organ-specific diseases. For example, Hashimoto's disease is an autoimmune thyroid disorder characterized by the production of autoantibodies against thyroid antigens. The extensive infiltration and proliferation of lymphocytes is observed (although, as described above, their roles are unproved), along with the subsequent destruction of follicular tissue.

Likewise, diabetes mellitus, Type I (formerly called juvenile-onset diabetes) may be an organ-specific autoimmune disease. In this case, however, autoantibodies are directed against the beta cells of the pancreas, which produce insulin. In pernicious (or megaloblastic) anemia, antibodies are produced against intrinsic factor, a molecule necessary for uptake of vitamin B_{12}. Subsequent pathology results from lack of absorption of the vitamin. Addison's disease, from which U.S. president John F. Kennedy suffered, is a potentially life-threatening condition resulting from antibody production against the adrenal cortex. Myasthenia gravis is characterized by severe heart or skeletal muscle weakness caused by antibodies directed against neurotransmitter receptors on the muscle. In fact, cells from any organ may be potential targets for production of an autoantibody.

Certain organ-specific autoimmune diseases in the spectrum are characterized not by antibodies directed against any specific organ, but by cellular infiltration triggered in some manner by less specific autoantibodies. For example, biliary cirrhosis, an inflammatory condition of the liver, is characterized by the obstruction of bile flow through the liver ductules. Though extensive cellular infiltration is observed, serum antibodies are directed against mitochondrial antigens, which are found within all cells. Certain types of chronic hepatitis also exhibit an analogous situation.

In some cases, antibodies may be directed against circulatory cells. Antibodies directed against red blood cells may cause subsequent lysis of the cells, leading to hemolytic anemia. Often, these are temporary conditions that have resulted from the binding of a pharmacologic chemical such as an antibiotic to the surface of the cell, which triggers an immune response. A more serious condition is hemolytic disease of the newborn (HDN), one example being erythroblastosis fetalis, or Rh disease. In this case, a mother lacking the Rh protein on her blood cells may produce an immune response against that protein, which is present in the blood of the fetus she is carrying during pregnancy. Prior to 1967, when an effective preventive measure became available, HDN was a serious problem for many pregnancies. Antibodies directed against blood platelets can cause a reduction in the number of those cells, resulting in thrombocytopenia purpura. An analogous situation can be seen with other cell types.

At the other end of the autoimmune spectrum are those diseases that are not cell- or organ-specific but result in widespread lesions in various parts of the body. Lupus received its name from the butterfly rash often seen on the faces of patients, which resembles a wolfbite (*lupus* is Latin for "wolf"). Pathologic changes can be found at various sites in the body, however, including the kidneys, joints, and blood vessels. Likewise, rheumatoid arthritis is characterized by the production of rheumatoid factor, an antibody molecule directed against other antibodies in blood serum. The resultant immune complexes lodge in joints, causing the joint pain and destruction associated with severe arthritis.

In most cases, the specific reason for the production of autoantibodies is unknown. Genetic factors are certainly involved, since some autoimmune diseases run in families. Some may be triggered by bacterial or viral infections. Viral antigens may be expressed on the surfaces of certain cells or the virus itself may be attached to the cell. Heart muscle appears to express antigenic determinants in common with certain streptococcal bacteria. A mild "strep throat" may be followed several weeks later by severe rheumatic fever.

The binding of drugs to cell surfaces may trigger an immune response. For example, penicillin may bind to the surfaces of red blood cells, triggering a hemolytic anemia. Likewise, sedormid may bind to the membrane of platelets.

Most cases of autoimmune disease, however, are triggered by no apparent cause. They may "simply" involve a breakdown of the normal regulatory mechanisms associated with the immune response.

DIAGNOSTIC AND TREATMENT TECHNIQUES

The regulation of self-reactive lymphocytes is necessary for the maintenance of tolerance by the immune system. When regulation breaks down or is otherwise defective, either humoral or cellular immunity is generated against the cells or tissues. The resultant pathology may be simply a painful nuisance or may have potentially fatal consequences. The difference relates to the extent of damage to particular organs, in the case of organ-specific autoimmune reactions, or to the level of tissue damage in systemic disease.

Despite differences in pathology, the mechanisms of tissue damage are similar in most autoimmune diseases. Most involve the formation of immune complexes. Either antibodies bind to cell surfaces or immune complexes form in the circulation. In either case, the result is complement activation. Components of the complement pathway, in turn, can either directly damage cell membranes or trigger the infiltration of a variety of cytotoxic cells.

Because the damage associated with most autoimmune diseases results from parallel processes, methods of treatment vary little in theory from one illness to another. Most involve the treatment of resultant symptoms; for example, the use of aspirin to reduce minor inflammation and, when necessary, the use of steroids to reduce the level of the immune response.

The treatment of autoimmune diseases does not eliminate the problem. The disease remains, but under ideal conditions, it is held under control. At the same time, there exists the danger of side effects of treatment. For example, most methods that reduce the level of the immune response are nonspecific; reducing the severity of the autoimmune disease may cause the patient to become more susceptible to infections by bacteria or viruses.

Certain approaches have been successful in the palliative treatment of some forms of autoimmune disease. For example, patients with myasthenia gravis (MG) exhibit significant muscle weakness. A myasthenia gravis patient may have difficulty breathing and may experience extreme fatigue, in severe cases being unable to open his or her mouth or eyelids. Associated with the disease are autoantibodies produced against the receptor for the neurotransmitter acetylcholine (ACh), the chemical utilized by nerves in regulating movement by the muscle. By blocking the ACh receptor, these antibodies inhibit the ability of nerves to control muscle movement. In effect, the patient loses control of the muscles.

Patients with myasthenia gravis often exhibit abnormalities of the thymus, the gland associated with T-cell production. In addition, there is evidence that the thymus contains ACh receptors that are particularly antigenic (perhaps exacerbating the illness). Removal of the thymus, even in adults, often aids in reducing the symptoms of the disease. The thymus, though not superfluous in adults, carries out its main functions during the early years of life, through adolescence. Thus, its removal generally has few major implications.

Often, MG will respond to more conventional forms of treatment. Steroid treatment will often reduce symptoms. Metabolic controls may also aid in reducing symptoms. For example, during normal nerve transmission of ACh, the enzyme cholinesterase is present to break down ACh, thereby regulating muscle movement. The use of anticholinesterase drugs to prolong the presence of ACh at the site of the receptor on the muscle has also been of benefit to some patients.

Systemic lupus erythematosus is among the most common of systemic autoimmune diseases. The disease usually strikes women in the prime of life, between the ages of twenty and forty. It is characterized by a butterfly rash over the facial region, weakness, fatigue, and often a fever. In many respects, the symptoms are those of severe arthritis. As the disease progresses, tissue or organ degradation may occur in the kidney or heart.

The specific cause of the symptomology is the formation of immune complexes, which consist of antibodies against cell components such as DNA or nucleoprotein. Complexes in the kidney have been large enough to observe with the electron microscope, particularly when the complexes contain cell nuclei. Similar complexes have been observed in regions of the skin characterized by inflammation and a rash. The immune complexes are sometimes ingested (phagocytized) by scavenger neutrophils, which make up the largest proportion (65 percent) of white blood cells. The presence of these so-called LE cells, white cells with ingested antibody-bound nuclei, was at one time used for the diagnosis of lupus.

As is true for many autoimmune diseases, the control of lupus often involves the use of steroids as immunosuppressive drugs. These have included drugs such as cyclosporin, which blocks T-cell function, and antimitotic drugs such as azathioprine or methotrexate, which block the proliferation of immune cells. Generalized immunosuppression as a side effect is a concern. Often, using combinations of steroids and immunosuppressives makes it possible to use lower concentrations of each, increasing the drugs' effectiveness and reducing the danger of toxicity.

Other palliative treatments of symptomology can increase patient comfort. For example, aspirin may be used to reduce inflammation or joint pain. Topical steroids can reduce the rash. Since lupus may significantly increase the photosensitivity of the skin, staying out of direct sunlight, or at least covering the surface of the skin, may reduce skin lesions. It should be emphasized again that these treatments deal only with symptoms; none will cure the disease.

Since some systemic diseases result from immune complex disorders, a reduction of the levels of such complexes has been found to be beneficial to some patients. Treatment involves a process called plasmapheresis. Plasma, the liquid portion of the blood, is removed from the patient (a small proportion at a time), after which the immune complexes are separated from the plasma. Though a temporary measure, since additional complexes continue to form, the process does prove useful.

Rheumatoid arthritis is another common autoimmune disorder. As is true of most autoimmune diseases, rheumatoid arthritis is primarily a disease of women. Symptomology results from the lodging of immune complexes in joints, resulting in the inflammation of those joints. Many cases result from the formation of antibodies directed against other antibody molecules— a case of the immune system turning against itself. Pathology results both from complement activation and from the infiltration of a variety of cells into the joint; the result is damage to both cartilage and bone.

Medical treatment usually begins with the anti-inflammatory drug of choice: aspirin. Other common treatments are those that increase patient comfort: rest, proper exercise, and weight loss, if necessary. In severe cases, steroids may be prescribed.

In general, autoimmune diseases are characterized by alternating periods of symptomology and remission. Treatments are generally similar in their approach of reducing inflammation as the first line of intervention, with the use of immunosuppression being the last resort. Since the precise origin of most of these disorders is unknown, prevention remains difficult.

PERSPECTIVE AND PROSPECTS

During the 1950's, F. Macfarlane Burnet published his theory of clonal selection. Burnet believed that antibody specificity was predetermined in the B cell as it underwent development and maturation. Selection of the cell by the appropriate antigen resulted in proliferation of that specific cell, a process of clonal selection.

Burnet also had to account for tolerance, however, the inability of immune cells to respond against their own antigens. Burnet theorized that during prenatal development, exposure to self-antigens, or determinants, resulted in the abortion of any self-reactive cells. Only those self-reactive immune cells that were directed against sequestered antigens survived.

Though Burnet's theories have reached the level of dogma in the field of immunology, they fail to account for certain autoimmune disorders. In the "correct" circumstances, the body does react against itself. Though they were not recognized at the time as such, autoimmune disorders were recognized as early as 1866. In that year, W. W. Gull demonstrated the link between chilling and a syndrome called paroxysmal hemoglobinuria. When external tissue such as skin is exposed to cold, large amounts of hemoglobin are discharged into the urine. In 1904, Karl Landsteiner established the autoimmune basis for the disease by demonstrating the role of complement in the lysis of red blood cells, causing the release of hemoglobin and the symptomology of the disorder. Further, he demonstrated that one could cause the lysis of normal cells by mixing them with sera from hemoglobinurics.

Hashimoto's disease was among the first organ-specific autoimmune diseases to be described. The disease was first described in 1912 by Hakaru Hashimoto, a Japanese surgeon, and the immune basis for the disease was established independently by Ernest Witebsky and Noel Rose in the United States, and by Deborah Doniach and Ivan Roitt in Great Britain, in 1957.

Since the 1950's, dozens of autoimmune disorders have been described. Treatment of these disorders remains, for the most part, nonspecific. Research in the area, in addition to attempts to define the precise trigger for autoimmune disease, has attempted to develop ways to suppress specifically those immune reactions responsible for the symptomology. Successes have been associated with vaccines directed against components involved with the reactions under investigation. For example, since the production of autoantibodies is the basis for some forms of disease, the generation of additional antibody molecules directed against determinants on the autoantibodies at fault could serve to neutralize the effects of those components. This procedure could be likened to a police department that arrests its own dishonest officers. There is a precedent for such an operation. Newborn children of mothers suffering from myasthenia gravis synthesize just such antibodies against the inappropriate MG antibodies that have crossed the placenta. Synthesis does seem to ameliorate the symptoms of the disease.

There is no question that autoimmune disorders represent an aberrant form of immune response. Nevertheless, an understanding of the underlying mechanism will shed light on exactly how the immune system is regulated. For example, it remains unclear how antibody production is controlled following a normal immune response. In the presence of an antigen, antibody levels increase for a period of days to weeks, reach a plateau, and then slowly decrease as additional production comes to a halt. The means by which the shutdown takes place remains nebulous.

Tolerance does not result solely from an absence of T or B cells that respond to antigens; it involves an active suppression of the process. A more detailed understanding of the process will lead to a more thorough understanding of the immune system in general.

—*Richard Adler, Ph.D.*

See also Acquired immunodeficiency syndrome (AIDS); Allergies; Autoimmune disorders; Blood and blood disorders; Bone marrow transplantation; Cells; Chemotherapy; Circulation; Cytology; Cytopathology; Dialysis; Endocrinology; Endocrinology, pediatric; Glands; Healing; Hematology; Hematology, pediatric; Histiocytosis; Homeopathy; Hormones; Host-defense mechanisms; Human immunodeficiency virus (HIV); Immune system; Immunization and vaccination; Immunodeficiency disorders; Immunopathology; Infection; Liver; Lymphatic system; Multiple chemical sensitivity syndrome; Myasthenia gravis; Oncology; Serology; Severe combined immunodeficiency syndrome (SCID); Skin; Transfusion; Transplantation; Wiskott-Aldrich syndrome.

FOR FURTHER INFORMATION:

Dwyer, John M. *The Body at War: The Story of Our Immune System*. 2d ed. London: J. M. Dent, 1993. Dwyer provides a basic discussion of the immune system for the layperson. Though their coverage is not particularly detailed, topics include the basis for immune tolerance and autoimmunity. Clearly written and accessible to the nonscientific public.

Fettner, Ann G. *Viruses: Agents of Change*. New York: McGraw-Hill, 1990. Though argumentative in her approach, Fettner provides a simple discussion of the role of viruses in disease. Included are sections on autoimmunity and the possible roles played by viruses.

Frank, Steven A. *Immunology and Evolution of Infectious Disease*. Princeton, N.J.: Princeton University Press, 2002. Blends research from molecular biology, immunology, pathogen biology, and population dynamics to discuss how and why parasites vary to escape recognition by the immune system, vaccine design, and the control of epidemics.

Janeway, Charles A., et al. *Immunobiology: The Immune System in Health and Disease*. 5th ed. Washington, D.C.: Taylor & Francis, 2001. An excellent text that provides a lucid and comprehensive examination of the immune system, covering such topics as immunobiology and innate immunity, the recognition of antigen, the development of mature lymphocyte receptor repertoires, the adaptive immune response, and the evolution of the immune system.

Kuby, Janis. *Immunology*. 5th ed. New York: W. H. Freeman, 2003. Excellent text that gives an overview of the immune system and its role with cells and organs, and discusses such topics as the generation of B-cell and T-cell responses, immune effector mechanisms, and the immune system in health and disease.

Parkham, Peter. *The Immune System*. Washington, D.C.: Taylor & Francis, 2002. A basic immunology text that details how cells and molecules work together in defending the body against invading microorganisms, describes situations in which the immune system cannot control disease, and examines what happens when the immune system overreacts.

Roitt, Ivan. *Roitt's Essential Immunology.* 10th ed. Boston: Blackwell Scientific, 2001. A textbook written by a leading authority in the field. Several chapters deal specifically with immune disorders. Concise, with a large number of illustrations, but does require a basic knowledge of biology.

Rose, Noel R., and I. R. Mackay, eds. *The Autoimmune Diseases.* 3d ed. San Diego, Calif.: Academic Press, 1998. A well-written textbook containing thorough discussions of autoimmune disorders. Primarily for those with a background in immunology, but does provide much basic information.

Immunopathology

Specialty

Anatomy or system affected: All

Specialties and related fields: Forensic medicine, immunology, pathology

Definition: The medical field that studies hypersensitivity reactions or tissue damage resulting from an immune response against one's own tissues.

Science and Profession

Immunopathology is the subdiscipline of immunology that deals with diseases resulting from the body reacting against itself. In its mildest form, immunopathology may deal with allergies that, while a nuisance, are rarely life-threatening. In more severe forms, hypersensitivity to tissue antigens may result in damage to one's own cells or organs. The process may result in a wide variety of autoimmune diseases, including arthritis, lupus erythematosus, or rheumatic fever. Physicians who deal with such disorders are trained in immunology and/or pathology. In general, the tendency toward developing an autoimmune disease has a genetic basis; in turn, exposure to a particular environmental antigen may trigger the phenomenon in the susceptible individual.

Diagnostic and Treatment Techniques

Autoimmune disease falls into four major categories: immediate hypersensitivities (allergies), antibody-dependent autoimmune reactions (transfusion reactions), immune complex disease (lupus), and delayed hypersensitivities (poison ivy). Treatment is determined by the specific form of the disease. In its simplest form, treatment consists of avoidance or removal of the allergen. In some cases, the injection of small quantities of the material into the patient may result in desensitization. In more severe situations, involving autoimmune or immune complex disease, treatment may consist of steroid derivatives that decrease the activity of immune cells. Since such inhibition is of a general nature, there exists the danger that the person may become increasingly susceptible to infection by common environmental microbes. Treatment may also be directed against the inflammatory process that leads to pathology, such as the use of aspirin in limiting the pain or inflammation of arthritis.

Perspective and Prospects

Immunopathology studies immunologically mediated reactions against one's own tissue. A better understanding of the reasons behind such a loss of tolerance to "self" antigens is necessary for prevention of the phenomenon. Such understanding will allow the development of treatments aimed either at reestablishing self-tolerance or at controlling the immune response in a manner that does not leave the individual as vulnerable to other forms of infection.

—*Richard Adler, Ph.D.*

See also Allergies; Arthritis; Autoimmune disorders; Blood and blood disorders; Bone marrow transplantation; Cells; Chemotherapy; Cytology; Cytopathology; Endocrinology; Endocrinology, pediatric; Glands; Healing; Hematology; Hematology, pediatric; Homeopathy; Hormones; Host-defense mechanisms; Immune system; Immunization and vaccination; Immunology; Lupus erythematosus; Lymphatic system; Myasthenia gravis; Oncology; Rheumatic fever; Serology; Severe combined immunodeficiency syndrome (SCID); Skin; Transfusion; Transplantation; Wiskott-Aldrich syndrome.

For Further Information:

Dabbs, David J. *Immunopathology.* New York: Harcourt Health, 2002.

Dwyer, John M. *The Body at War: The Story of Our Immune System.* 2d ed. London: J. M. Dent, 1993.

Eales, Lesley-Jane. *Immunology for Life Scientists.* New York: Wiley, 2003.

Kuby, Janis. *Immunology.* 5th ed. New York: W. H. Freeman, 2003.

Life, Death, and the Immune System. New York: W. H. Freeman, 1994.

Nilsson, Lennart. *The Body Victorious.* New York: Delacorte Press, 1987.

IMPETIGO

DISEASE/DISORDER
ANATOMY OR SYSTEM AFFECTED: Skin
SPECIALTIES AND RELATED FIELDS: Bacteriology, dermatology, immunology, microbiology
DEFINITION: One of several severe skin infections caused by bacteria.

INFORMATION ON IMPETIGO

CAUSES: Bacterial infection
SYMPTOMS: Skin inflammation, blisters, itchiness, scabbing
DURATION: Acute
TREATMENTS: Injection of antibiotics (penicillin, erythromycin)

CAUSES AND SYMPTOMS

The most common form of impetigo begins as a small inflamed region on the skin, which becomes a small blister as much as 0.5 inch in diameter. The blister eventually becomes pustular and ruptures. A thick, yellow, encrusted scab develops. The lesions are superficial and painless, but they itch. Most cases of impetigo are caused by *Streptococcus pyogenes*, but a few cases are caused by *Streptococcus agalactiae*. Approximately 20 percent of women carrying *S. agalactiae* transmit it to their newborn babies. A few babies develop impetigo from the bacteria; others develop neonatal meningitis.

Bullous impetigo of the skin is characterized by large pustules about 1 inch in diameter surrounded by reddish, inflamed zones. The pustules contain a clear, yellowish fluid. The dried lesions develop a crust. This form of impetigo is caused by certain strains of *Staphylococcus aureus* that produce an exfoliative toxin. *S. aureus* accounts for approximately 10 percent of all impetigo cases. Bullous impetigo is an extremely contagious disease that is spread by direct contact or contact with contaminated objects. *S. aureus* is carried by up to 40 percent of all humans in the nose. Hospital outbreaks of *S. aureus* are common in infant nurseries, in burn units, and among patients recovering from surgery.

TREATMENT AND THERAPY

Impetigo caused by streptococci is treated most effectively with injected penicillin or erythromycin. Oral antibiotics are not as effective against streptococci as injected drugs. An ointment called mupirocin has been found to be as effective as oral penicillin or erythromycin. Bullous impetigo can be treated effectively with oral penicillin, cephalosporin, or erythromycin.

PERSPECTIVE AND PROSPECTS

Impetigo is generally associated with young children between two and five years of age. Untreated impetigo caused by streptococci may lead to a serious kidney disease called acute glomerulonephritis. In about 1 percent of children with impetigo, many different antibodies develop against the bacteria. Some of the antibodies may cross-react with kidney tissue or simply accumulate in the kidney. These antibodies activate complement, a group of proteins that normally kill bacteria. Activated complement in the kidneys damages these organs, leading to renal failure and death. Prompt treatment of impetigo with injected penicillin or erythromycin and topical mupirocin has been very effective in preventing acute glomerulonephritis in infants and children.

—*Jaime S. Colomé, Ph.D.*

See also Antibiotics; Bacterial infections; Dermatology; Dermatology, pediatric; Kidney disorders; Kidneys; Rashes; Renal failure; Skin; Skin disorders; Streptococcal infections.

FOR FURTHER INFORMATION:

Biddle, Wayne. *Field Guide to Germs*. 2d ed. New York: Henry Holt, 2002.

Finegold, Sydney M., and William J. Martin. *Bailey and Scott's Diagnostic Microbiology*. 6th ed. St. Louis: C. V. Mosby, 1998.

Middlemiss, Prisca. *What's That Rash? How to Identify and Treat Childhood Rashes*. London: Hamlyn, 2002.

Parker, James N., and Philip M. Parker, eds. *The Official Patient's Sourcebook on Streptococcus Pneumoniae Infections*. San Diego, Calif.: Icon Health, 2002.

Pelczar, Michael J., Jr., E. C. S. Chan, and Noel R. Krieg. *Microbiology: Concepts and Applications*. New York: McGraw-Hill, 1999.

Schlegel, Hans G. *General Microbiology*. 7th ed. Cambridge, England: Cambridge University Press, 1993.

Turkington, Carol. *Encyclopedia of Skin and Skin Disorders*. New York: Facts on File, 2002.

Weedon, David. *Skin Pathology*. 2d ed. New York: Harcourt, 2002.

IMPOTENCE. *See* **SEXUAL DYSFUNCTION.**

IN VITRO FERTILIZATION

PROCEDURE

ANATOMY OR SYSTEM AFFECTED: Cells, reproductive system, uterus

SPECIALTIES AND RELATED FIELDS: Embryology, genetics, gynecology

DEFINITION: A procedure whereby eggs and sperm are combined in the laboratory to achieve fertilization, usually followed by the introduction of the resulting embryos into the uterus.

KEY TERMS:

chromosome: a structure found in the cell nucleus that is composed of deoxyribonucleic acid (DNA) and associated proteins; chromosomes are responsible for carrying genetic information and can be visualized under a microscope

clomiphene: a synthetic estrogenic substance used to induce ovulation in women who do not ovulate regularly; it is taken orally as a medication

endometriosis: a condition whereby cells of the uterine lining are found in abnormal locations, such as the pelvic cavity or ovary; endometriosis can lead to pelvic pain and the development of scars that can block the Fallopian tubes

Fallopian tube: one of two structures that conduct the egg, as it is released from the ovary, into the uterus

follicle: a spherical mass of cells and fluid within the ovary, from which the mature egg is produced

implantation: the process in which an embryo attaches and burrows into the lining of the uterus

in vitro: a Latin term used to indicate a process that has taken place outside of an organism, such as in a laboratory test tube or petri dish

ovulation: the process whereby the egg is released from the ovary and can be fertilized by sperm; this event occurs approximately at the middle portion of a woman's menstrual cycle

semen analysis: analysis of a recently ejaculated semen specimen, which includes a sperm count and an estimate of the percentage of motile sperm

zygote: the single cell formed after fertilization that is the result of the fusion of egg and sperm; it can develop into a new individual organism

INDICATIONS AND PROCEDURES

The purpose of fertilization is to create a new organism or individual that has the same number of chromosomes as the parent individuals but which has a unique mixing of genetic traits from both the mother and the father. In animals, this is accomplished by the fusion of egg and sperm cells. Both egg and sperm contain half the number of chromosomes needed to produce a healthy individual. The fusion of egg and sperm results in a zygote, or fertilized egg, which can develop into an individual organism.

Eggs and sperm are both gametes, cells which are specialized to carry out reproductive functions. The sperm cells are produced in the testicles of the male. Sperm production is continuous in the male, and millions of sperm are made within the testicles each day. Sperm cells contain genetic material within their head and are equipped with a flagellum, or whiplike tail, to enable them to swim within a liquid medium. The egg, or ovum, is about .01 millimeter in size and hundreds of times larger than the sperm. It is produced in the ovaries of females and contains cytoplasm, the cellular substance and specialized cell structures that are needed for the zygote to form and grow. In women, a single mature egg is usually made with each menstrual cycle and is released from the follicle contained in one of the ovaries. As women age, their ovaries become depleted of follicles, and eventually at the menopause, ovulation no longer occurs. Therefore, a woman's age can contribute significantly to her ability to conceive. Other causes of ovarian failure which may lead to infertility include the use of chemotherapeutic agents and premature ovarian failure syndrome.

In natural, or in vivo, fertilization, sperm from the male are deposited in the vaginal canal of the female during sexual intercourse. The sperm are contained in nutritive fluid, called semen. The sperm are able to swim up the cervical canal (the lower part of the uterus) only during and around the time of female ovulation, as the cervical mucus becomes permeable to sperm at this time. Once within the uterine cavity, the sperm make their way up into the Fallopian tubes, where they can meet the egg and proceed with fertilization.

Several steps lead to fertilization. The egg is surrounded by a layer of cells called the corona radiata. This layer is loose and easily penetrated by sperm. The next layer is the zona pellucida, which is a critical barrier in fertilization. One of the sugar-coated proteins in the zona pellucida, ZP3, captures a sperm cell by binding to its head. This causes a structure on the head of the sperm, called an acrosome, to release enzymes. This process is called the acrosomal reaction. These enzymes then digest the coat on the head of the sperm cell and digest a path for the sperm through the zona pellucida. After this, the sperm reaches the membrane of the egg, and the sperm and egg cells fuse. The chromosomes of the sperm and egg join, thus completing the process of fertilization. Subsequently, the fertilized egg travels back into the uterus and implants into the lining of the uterus, where it continues to develop as an embryo and then as a fetus.

When the natural anatomy or physiology of the reproductive system is abnormal, infertility can result. For instance, endometriosis in women can cause severe scarring of the pelvic cavity, leading to occluded Fallopian tubes or ovaries that are completely encased in scar tissue. In these cases, the egg may have difficulty reaching the Fallopian tube canal and hence is unable to meet sperm to achieve fertilization. Another cause of pelvic scarring is pelvic inflammatory disease (PID), which can be caused by sexually transmitted diseases (STDs) or ruptures in the gastrointestinal tract.

In vitro fertilization (IVF) is indicated when a couple experiences infertility. Infertility is defined as the lack of conception after one year of unprotected intercourse. There are many causes of infertility, which may be attributable to either the male or the female partner. Usually when an infertile couple seeks medical attention, they are asked to give a detailed history and receive physical examinations by the physician. Depending on the findings, the couple will be asked to undergo testing to better identify the cause of the infertility. Men will be asked to give a semen sample. The sample will be analyzed in the laboratory to ensure that adequate numbers of sperm are present and that they are able to move appropriately, a procedure called semen analysis. Women may be assessed for anatomic defects, such as whether the Fallopian tubes are blocked or large fibroid tumors in the uterus may prevent sperm from entering the Fallopian tubes. This assessment may be accomplished using a technique called a hysterosalpingogram, in which dye is introduced into the uterine cavity and an X-ray picture is taken. If a woman's Fallopian tubes are blocked, then no dye will spill into the pelvic cavity. If a woman's tubes are open, then dye will be seen spilling into the pelvic cavity. In addition, women may also undergo assessments regarding their ovarian function and ability to produce eggs. Blood tests may be drawn to assess for appropriate hormone levels.

If the cause of infertility is found to be blocked Fallopian tubes, then IVF is indicated. Sometimes, women with irregular menstrual cycles who do not ovulate at predictable intervals may be treated with a medication called clomiphene, in order to induce ovulation. If a woman fails to achieve spontaneous conception after several months of clomiphene therapy, then the physician may proceed with in vitro fertilization as the next step in the attempt to achieve conception.

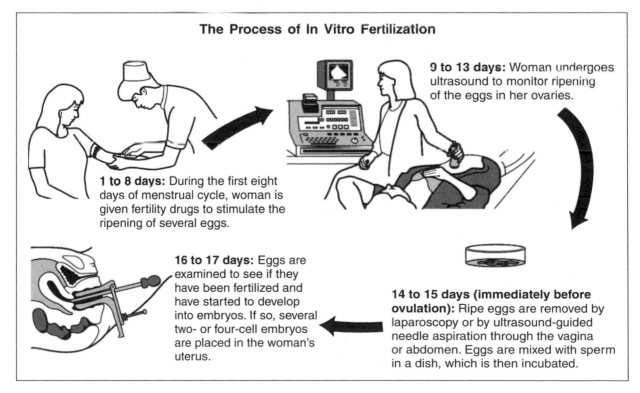

The Process of In Vitro Fertilization

1 to 8 days: During the first eight days of menstrual cycle, woman is given fertility drugs to stimulate the ripening of several eggs.

9 to 13 days: Woman undergoes ultrasound to monitor ripening of the eggs in her ovaries.

14 to 15 days (immediately before ovulation): Ripe eggs are removed by laparoscopy or by ultrasound-guided needle aspiration through the vagina or abdomen. Eggs are mixed with sperm in a dish, which is then incubated.

16 to 17 days: Eggs are examined to see if they have been fertilized and have started to develop into embryos. If so, several two- or four-cell embryos are placed in the woman's uterus.

Another example of when IVF is indicated is in cases where the sperm are defective. For instance, some men may have sperm that have difficulty swimming appropriately or penetrating the egg. In such cases, the sperm may need to be injected artificially into the egg to achieve fertilization, a procedure call intracytoplasmic sperm injection (ICSI). In order to perform this procedure, eggs must be harvested from the woman. The eggs are then placed in a petri dish, where they are injected with the sperm. Because fertilization is occurring outside the body in this situation, this procedure is also a type of in vitro fertilization. After the eggs have matured for a few days in the laboratory, the healthiest-looking zygotes are placed into the woman's uterus, a procedure called embryo transfer.

Another example in which intracytoplasmic sperm injection might be used is when the couple's infertility is caused by the man's inability to ejaculate sperm. This might occur, for instance, with a lack or occlusion of the vas deferens, the tubes that carry sperm from the testicles to the urethra where the sperm can exit the body. To obtain sperm for IVF in these cases, the male partner may undergo testicular sperm extraction, in which sperm are removed from the testicles. The sperm are then injected into the ova to achieve fertilization in vitro.

The procedures for IVF involve the induction of ovulation in the woman using hormones that stimulate the ovaries. These are usually hormones which are similar to endogenous follicle-stimulating hormone (FSH), which is responsible for follicle growth within the ovary. These exogenous hormones lead to the development of multiple follicles within both ovaries. The size and number of these follicles is observed by ultrasound, and when the appropriate number and size is achieved, the ovum harvest is performed. This procedure involves taking the woman to the operating room, where she is given anesthesia and placed on her back with her legs in stirrups and knees apart. A needle attached to a vacuum device is carefully introduced into the vaginal canal with ultrasound guidance. With the ultrasound helping to locate the ovaries and follicles precisely, the needle is inserted into the follicle through the posterior vagina. The fluid within the follicle is aspirated, and the egg usually is suctioned out of the follicle along with the follicular fluid and placed into a test tube. The same procedure is repeated until a sufficient number of eggs have been harvested or the follicles have been depleted. The eggs are then taken to the laboratory, where they are examined under a microscope.

A sperm sample is then collected from the male partner, and the sample is washed and analyzed to ensure that the sperm appear healthy and able to fertilize the eggs. The sperm are then introduced to the eggs within a petri dish containing tissue culture fluid. If intracytoplasmic sperm injection is to be performed, then single sperm are taken up into a glass needle and injected into individual eggs at this time. The petri dish is placed in an incubator for a few days. Once the embryos have developed sufficiently, a few healthy ones are chosen to be introduced into the woman's uterus through embryo transfer. This involves picking up the embryos into a semiflexible tube. The tube is then inserted carefully through the cervical canal into the uterine cavity, where the embryos are released. Embryos that are not transferred into the woman's uterus can be frozen using cryopreservation for future use.

USES AND COMPLICATIONS

IVF enables couples who suffer from infertility to conceive and bear children. Specifically, IVF is most helpful for couples whose infertility is caused by blocked Fallopian tubes or the inability of sperm to reach and penetrate the egg. In couples where the woman is unable to produce her own eggs, donor eggs from another woman may be used in IVF. If a man is unable to produce his own sperm, then sperm donors may be used in IVF.

Recent technology has enabled early prenatal diagnosis for inheritable conditions using cells taken from the early embryo during the six-to-eight-cell stage, called blastomere biopsy. Inheritable diseases caused by single gene defects, such as cystic fibrosis, Duchenne's muscular dystrophy, sickle cell disease, hemophilia, and Tay-Sachs disease, have been detected using preimplantation diagnosis. This type of prenatal diagnosis is possible only through the IVF process, as the early embryo would not be accessible to the physician in cases of spontaneous conception. Procedures such as blastomere biopsy are far from common, however, given the technical difficulty and economic costs of such procedures.

The complications associated with the IVF process include a condition called ovarian hyperstimulation syndrome. This situation can occur when a woman receives hormones to stimulate ovulation. In these cases, the follicles within the ovary become excessively stimulated and grossly enlarge the ovary. When this condition is severe, the woman can suffer abdominal pain, fluid imbalances, electrolyte imbalances, abnormal kidney function, and an accumulation of fluid in the abdominal cavity or lungs. Her blood may have an abnormal tendency to form clots, and her blood pressure may become dangerously low. These patients are monitored carefully and require hospitalization, as severe ovarian hyperstimulation syndrome can be fatal.

Other complications of the IVF process can occur during the ovum harvest procedure. These include the risks of anesthesia and infection (because the needle is a foreign body introduced through the vagina, a nonsterile field). Another risk involves bleeding. Although the needle for harvesting the eggs is under ultrasound guidance, the risk of the needle inadvertently puncturing neighboring blood vessels still exists. In addition, the ovaries themselves may bleed when punctured, as they are highly vascular organs. Bleeding that is severe and life-threatening may require abdominal or pelvic surgery to identify the location of the bleeding and to stop the bleeding with sutures. If the patient becomes significantly anemic from the bleeding, she may require a blood transfusion.

Other risks of IVF are incurred during the embryo culture process. During this process, the petri dishes containing the embryos may become contaminated with microorganisms. In addition, problems with the tissue culture medium or with the incubation process may lead to poor embryo development and the lack of any viable embryos to transfer into the woman. Another risk is the fact that embryos transferred into the uterus may not implant themselves in the lining.

The rate of achieving pregnancy after IVF is directly related to the number of embryos transferred into the uterus. When multiple embryos are transferred back into the uterus, however, the woman is at risk for a multiple gestation pregnancy. Multiple gestation pregnancies lead to an increased risk of spontaneous abortion (miscarriage) and preterm birth, as well as other pregnancy complications such as low birth weight, growth restriction in utero, increased risk of congenital anomalies, placental abnormalities, preeclampsia (a hypertensive disease of pregnancy), umbilical cord accidents and malpresentations (when the fetus is not lying in the uterus with the head down, making vaginal birth difficult). More long-term risks of in vitro fertilization are the increased risk for complications during pregnancy. For instance, women whose pregnancies were a result of assisted reproductive technologies such as IVF are at increased risk for preterm birth, when compared to age-matched women whose pregnancies were a result of spontaneous conception.

In addition, the long-term outcomes of children conceived using IVF is unknown, as the first children born as a result of this technique are beginning to enter middle age. Whether they will live normal life spans is unknown. Whether they will have normal reproductive outcomes themselves remains unclear. Whether they are more prone to diseases such as cancer later in life is also unknown.

Perspective and Prospects

The first baby conceived through in vitro fertilization was Louise Brown, who was born in 1978. The English team responsible for this important breakthrough consisted of Patrick Steptoe, a surgeon from Oldham Hospital, and Robert Edwards, a reproductive physiologist from Cambridge University. In the 1960's, animal breeding programs had successfully utilized in vitro fertilization. In 1965, Edwards reported that he had successfully induced maturation of a human egg in vitro. Edwards teamed up with Steptoe and another colleague, Jean Purdy. In 1970, they reported that they had achieved in vitro fertilization and cleavage (cell division) in human eggs. The first successful birth of an IVF baby in the United States occurred in 1981 in Norfolk, Virginia. The first successful use of a previously frozen human embryo occurred in Australia in 1984; two years later, a similar procedure was employed successfully in the United States.

A couple can undergo multiple cycles of IVF. A 1996 study reported data from large centers in three countries which showed that the cumulative pregnancy rate after six cycles of IVF was approximately 60 percent. However, if a couple fails to achieve pregnancy after six cycles, then the chances of achieving pregnancy through IVF fall significantly. At that time, the infertile couple may be counseled to seek alternative means of becoming parents, such as adoption.

In vitro fertilization and its related procedures have provided opportunities to conceive for couples who would otherwise be childless. These opportunities have led to many ethical controversies as well. What should be done with frozen embryos that are not used? What are the rights of egg or sperm donors once the child is born? What are the rights of the child to know his or her parentage and family history of medical problems? What are the rights of surrogate mothers? How many embryos should be transferred back into the woman, given the fact that multiple gestations are at increased risk for poor outcomes such as premature delivery? Is there a certain age at which women should not attempt pregnancy? Some countries such as Australia, Norway,

Spain, and the United Kingdom have responded to some of these questions by passing legislation regulating IVF. Other countries have been slower to respond, leaving decisions related to IVF to physicians, the patients themselves, and the court system.

As more couples delay childbearing, the prevalence of infertility and the need for IVF and other assisted reproductive technologies is likely to increase. Human reproduction is not an efficient process, and the older the female partner becomes, the less likely it is that natural conception will occur. For instance, a 1986 survey in the United States reported that the percentage of married women who were infertile between the ages of twenty and twenty-four was only 7 percent. By the ages of forty to forty-four, this percentage became 28 percent. This statistic is partly attributable to the fact that the total length of time during which conception is possible is less in older women, as older women ovulate less frequently than do younger women.

—*Anne Lynn S. Chang, M.D.*

See also Assisted reproductive technologies; Conception; Embryology; Ethics; Gamete intrafallopian transfer (GIFT); Genetic engineering; Gynecology; Hormones; Infertility in females; Infertility in males; Multiple births; Obstetrics; Pregnancy and gestation; Reproductive system.

FOR FURTHER INFORMATION:

Bonnicksen, Andrea L. *In Vitro Fertilization: Building Policy from Laboratories to Legislature.* New York: Columbia University Press, 1989. An excellent discussion of the history of in vitro fertilization and the ethical questions raised. An appendix includes a detailed but concise description of the technique.

Sher, Geoffrey, Virginia Marriage Davis, and Jean Stoess. *In Vitro Fertilization.* Rev. ed. New York: Facts On File, 1998. Dr. Sher and his clinical associates describe for patients in words and line drawings the process of evaluating patients and the procedures involved in IVF. The book also includes a glossary and an index.

Speroff, Leon, Robert H. Glass, and Nathan G. Kase. *Clinical Gynecologic Endocrinology and Infertility.* 6th ed. Baltimore: Lippincott Williams & Wilkins, 1999. A comprehensive textbook that outlines the evaluation and treatment of infertility, including in vitro fertilization. Also discusses the biology behind reproductive processes.

Stenchever, Morton A., et al. *Comprehensive Gynecology.* 4th ed. St. Louis: Mosby, 2001. The definitive gynecologic textbook, it offers well-written chapters on prenatal diagnosis, reproductive endocrinology, and infertility.

Wisot, Arthur, and David Meldrum. *Conceptions and Misconceptions.* Vancouver: Harley and Marks, 1997. Written by two leading fertility experts, this book is an excellent guide through the maze of in vitro fertilization and other assisted reproductive techniques. Includes an excellent discussion of the basic physiology of conception and reproduction.

INCONTINENCE

DISEASE/DISORDER

ANATOMY OR SYSTEM AFFECTED: Abdomen, bladder, gastrointestinal system, urinary system

SPECIALTIES AND RELATED FIELDS: Family practice, geriatrics and gerontology, gynecology, internal medicine, obstetrics, pediatrics, psychiatry, urology

DEFINITION: Involuntary loss of urine or feces, primarily a social and hygienic problem that particularly affects the older population.

KEY TERMS:

atonic bladder: a bladder characterized by weak muscles

enuresis: bed-wetting

frequency: urination at short intervals; a common problem accompanying incontinence

micturition: the act of urinating

nocturia: nighttime urination

sphincter: a ring-shaped muscle that surrounds a natural opening in the body and can open or close it by expanding or contracting

urge incontinence: a strong desire to urinate followed by leakage of urine

urgency: a strong desire to void urine immediately

CAUSES AND SYMPTOMS

Continence is skill acquired in humans by the interaction of two processes: socialization of the infant and maturation of the central nervous system. Without society's expectation of continence, and without broadly accepted definitions of appropriate behavior, the concept of "incontinence" would be meaningless. There are many causes for urinary incontinence. Three broad (interrelated and often overlapping) categories are physiologic voiding dysfunction, factors directly influencing voiding function, and factors affecting the individual's capacity to manage voiding.

The causes of physiologic voiding dysfunction involve an abnormality in bladder or sphincter function, or both. The bladder and sphincter have only two functions:

INFORMATION ON INCONTINENCE

CAUSES: Neurological disease, bladder inflammation, obstruction, prostate gland enlargement, urinary tract infection, diuretics, endocrine disorders (*e.g.*, diabetes mellitus, thyroid disorders), aging, pregnancy and childbirth

SYMPTOMS: Frequent urination, straining to void, poor urinary stream, feeling of urgency with resulting leakage

DURATION: Ranges from acute to chronic

TREATMENTS: Drug therapy, surgery, bladder training

to store urine until the appropriate time for urination and then to empty it completely. Voiding dysfunction involves the failure of one or both of these mechanisms. Four basic types of voiding dysfunction can be distinguished: detrusor instability, genuine stress incontinence, outflow obstruction, and atonic bladder.

Detrusor instability is a condition characterized by involuntary bladder (detrusor muscle) contraction during filling. While all the causes of bladder instability are not fully understood, it can be associated with the following: neurologic disease (brain and spinal cord abnormalities), inflammation of the bladder wall, bladder outlet obstruction, stress urinary incontinence, and idiopathic (spontaneous or primary) dysfunction. Detrusor instability usually causes symptoms of frequency, urgency, and possibly nocturia or enuresis.

Genuine stress incontinence is caused by a failure to hold urine during bladder filling as a result of an incompetent urethral sphincter mechanism. If the closure mechanism of the bladder outlet fails to hold urine, incontinence will occur. This is usually manifested during physical exertion or abdominal stress (such as coughing or sneezing). It can occur in either sex, but it is more common in women because of their shorter urethra and the physical trauma of childbirth. Men can experience stress incontinence following traumatic or surgical damage to the sphincter.

Obstruction of the outflow of urine during voiding can produce various symptoms, including frequency, straining to void, poor urinary stream, preurination and posturination dribbling, and a feeling of urgency with resulting leakage (urge incontinence). In severe cases, the bladder is never completely emptied and a volume of residual urine persists. Overflow incontinence can result. Common causes of bladder outlet obstruction

are prostatic enlargement, bladder neck narrowing, or urethral obstruction. Functional obstruction occurs when a neurologic lesion prevents the coordinated relaxation of the sphincter during voiding. This phenomenon is termed detrusor-sphincter dyssynergia.

An atonic bladder—one with weak muscle walls—does not produce a sufficient contraction to empty completely. Emptying can be enhanced by abdominal straining or manual expression, but a large residual volume persists. The sensation of retaining urine might or might not be present. If sensation is present, frequency of urination is common because only a small portion of the bladder volume is emptied each time. Sensation is often diminished, and the residual urine volume can be considerable (100 to 1,000 milliliters). Overflow incontinence often occurs.

An acute urinary tract infection can cause transient incontinence, even in a fit, healthy young person who normally has no voiding dysfunction. Acute frequency and urgency with disturbed sensation and pain can result in the inability to reach a toilet in time or to detect when incontinence is occurring. If an underlying voiding dysfunction is also present, an acute urinary tract infection is likely to cause incontinence.

Many drugs can also disturb the delicate balance of normal functioning. The most obvious category consists of diuretics, those drugs which increase urinary discharge; a large, swift production of urine will give most people frequency and urgency. If the bladder is unstable, it might not be able to handle a sudden influx of urine, and urge incontinence can result. Sedation can affect voiding function directly (for example, diazepam can lower urethral resistance) or can make the individual less responsive to signals from the bladder and thus unable to maintain continence. Other commonly prescribed drugs have secondary actions on voiding function. Not all patients, however, will experience urinary side effects from these drugs.

Various endocrine disorders can upset normal voiding function. Diabetes can cause polydypsia (extreme thirst), requiring the storage of a large volume of urine. Glycosuria (sugar in the urine) might encourage urinary tract infection. Thyroid imbalances can aggravate an overactive or underactive bladder. Pituitary gland disorders can result in the production of excessive urine volumes because of an antidiuretic hormone deficiency. Estrogen deficiency in postmenopausal women causes atrophic changes in the vaginal and urethral tissues and will worsen stress incontinence and an unstable bladder.

Several bladder pathologies can also cause incontinence by disrupting normal functioning. A patient with a neoplasm (abnormal tissue growth), whether benign or malignant, or a stone in the bladder occasionally experiences incontinence as a symptom. These are infrequent causes of incontinence.

Often it takes something else in addition to the underlying problem to tip the balance and produce incontinence. This is especially true for elderly and disabled persons who are delicately balanced between continence and incontinence. For example, immobility—anything that impedes access—is likely to induce incontinence. Immobility can be the result of the gradual worsening of a chronic condition, such as arthritis, multiple sclerosis, or Parkinson's disease, until eventually the individual simply cannot reach a toilet in time. The condition may be acute—an accident or illness that suddenly renders a person immobile might be the start of failure to control the bladder.

In the case of children, most daytime wetting persists until the child reaches school age. It is less common than bed-wetting (enuresis), and the two often go together. One in ten five-year-old children, however, still wets the bed regularly. With no treatment, this figure gradually falls to 5 percent of ten-year-olds and to 2 percent of adults. It is twice as common in boys as in girls, has strong familial tendencies, and is associated with stressful events in the third or fourth year of life. A urinary tract infection is sometimes the cause.

Fecal, as opposed to urinary, incontinence is generally caused by underlying disorders of the colon, rectum, or anus; neurogenic disorders; or fecal impaction. Severe diarrhea increases the likelihood of having fecal incontinence. Some of the more common disorders that can cause diarrhea are ulcerative colitis, carcinoma, infection, radiation therapy, and the effect of drugs (for example, broad-spectrum antibiotics, laxative abuse, or iron supplements). Fecal incontinence tends to be a common, if seldom reported, accompaniment.

The pelvic floor muscles support the anal sphincter, and any weakness will cause a tendency to fecal stress incontinence. The vital flap valve formed by the anorectal angle can be lost if these muscles are weak. An increase in abdominal pressure would therefore tend to force the rectal contents down and out of the anal canal. This might be the result of congenital abnormalities or of later trauma (for example, childbirth, anal surgery, or direct trauma). A lifelong habit of straining at stool might also cause muscle weakness.

The medulla and higher cortical centers of the brain have a role in coordinating and controlling the defecation reflex. Therefore, any neurologic disorder that impairs the ability to detect or inhibit impending defecation will probably result in a tendency to incontinence, similar in causation to the uninhibited or unstable bladder. For example, the paraplegic can lose all direct sensation of and voluntary control over bowel activity. Neurologic disorders such as multiple sclerosis, cerebrovascular accident, and diffuse dementia can affect sensation or inhibition, or a combination of both. Incontinence occurs with some demented people because of a physical inability to inhibit defecation. With others, it occurs because the awareness that such behavior is inappropriate has been lost.

Severe constipation with impaction of feces is probably the most common cause of fecal incontinence, and it predominates as a cause among the elderly and those living in extended care facilities. Chronic constipation leads to impaction when the fluid content of the feces is progressively absorbed by the colon, leaving hard, rounded rocks in the bowel. This hard matter promotes mucus production and bacterial activity, which causes a foul-smelling brown fluid to accumulate. If the rectum is overdistended for any length of time, the internal and external sphincters become relaxed, allowing passage of this mucus as spurious diarrhea. The patient's symptoms usually include fairly continuous leakage of fluid stool without any awareness of control.

Most children are continent of feces by the age of four years, but 1 percent still have problems at seven years of age. More boys than girls are incontinent, suggesting that developmental factors can be relevant because boys mature more slowly. Fecal incontinence or conscious soiling in childhood (sometimes referred to as encopresis) has, like nocturnal enuresis, long been regarded as evidence of a psychiatric or psychologic disorder in the child. The evidence, however, does not support the claim that most fecally incontinent children are disturbed.

Such children usually have fastidious, overanxious parents who are intent on toilet training. The child is punished for soiling, so defecation tends to be inhibited, both in the underwear and in the toilet. When toilet training is attempted, the child may be repeatedly seated on the toilet in the absence of a full rectum and be unable to perform. The situation becomes fraught with anxiety, and bowel movements become associated with unpleasantness in the child's mind. The child therefore retains feces and becomes constipated. Defecation then becomes difficult and painful as well.

Treatment and Therapy

The two primary methods of treating urinary incontinence involve medical and surgical intervention (drug therapy and surgery) and bladder training.

Many drugs can be prescribed to help those with urinary incontinence. Often the results are disappointing, although some drugs can be useful for carefully selected and accurately diagnosed patients. Drugs are often used to control detrusor instability and urge incontinence by relaxing the detrusor muscle and inhibiting reflex contractions. This therapy is helpful in some patients. Sometimes when the drug is given in large enough doses to be effective, however, the side effects are so troublesome that the therapy must be abandoned. Drugs that reduce bladder contractions must be used cautiously in patients who have voiding difficulty, since urinary retention can be precipitated. Careful assessment must be made of residual urine. Drug therapy is also used with caution in patients with a residual volume greater than 100 milliliters. Some drugs are used in an attempt to prevent stress incontinence by increasing urethral tone. Phenylpropanolamine and ephedrine, those most often used, are thought to act on the alpha receptors in the urethra.

Drug therapy can also be used to relieve outflow obstruction. Phenoxybenzamine is most commonly used, but this drug can have dangerous side effects, such as tachycardia (an abnormally fast heartbeat) or postural hypotension. If the bladder does not contract sufficiently to ensure complete emptying, drug therapy can be attempted to increase the force of the voiding contractions. Carbachol, bethanechol, and distigmine bromide have all been used with some success. Other drugs might be useful in treating factors affecting incontinence— for example, antibiotics to treat a urinary tract infection or laxatives to treat or prevent constipation.

Many drugs can exacerbate a tendency to incontinence. For those who are prone to incontinence, medications and dosage schedules are chosen that will have a minimal effect on bladder control. For example, a slow-acting diuretic, in a divided dose, can help someone with urgency and weak sphincter tone to avoid incontinence. An analgesic might be preferable to night sedation for those who need pain relief but who wet the bed at night if they are sedated.

Turning to surgical intervention, none of the several surgical approaches that have been used in an attempt to treat an unstable bladder has gained widespread use. Cystodistention (stretching the bladder under general anesthesia) and bladder transection, for example, are presumed to act by disturbing the neurologic pathways that control uninhibited contractions. Many vaginal and suprapubic procedures are available to help correct genuine stress incontinence in women. Surgery can also be used to relieve outflow obstruction—for example, to remove an enlarged prostate gland, divide a stricture, or widen a narrow urethra.

In cases of severe intractable incontinence, major surgery is an option. For those with a damaged urethra, a neourethra can be constructed. For those with a nonfunctioning sphincter, an artificial sphincter can be implanted. In some patients, a urinary diversion with a stoma (outlet) is the only and best alternative for continence. Although a drastic solution, a urostomy might be easier to cope with than an incontinent urethra, because an effective appliance will contain the urine.

Urinary incontinence is occasionally the result of surgery, usually urologic or gynecologic but sometimes a major pelvic or spinal procedure. Such iatrogenic incontinence can be caused by neurologic or sphincter damage, leading to various dysfunctional voiding patterns.

Several different types of bladder training or retraining are distinguishable and can be used in different circumstances. The most important element for success is that the correct regimen be selected for each patient and situation. A thorough assessment identifies those patients who will benefit from bladder training and determines the most appropriate method. Other factors that contribute to the incontinence should also be treated (for example, a urinary tract infection or constipation), because ignoring them will impair the success of a program.

Bladder training is most suitable for people with the symptoms of frequency, urgency, and urge incontinence (with or without an underlying unstable bladder) and for those with nonspecific incontinence. The elderly often have these symptoms. Patients with voiding dysfunction, other than an unstable bladder, are unlikely to benefit from bladder training.

The aim of bladder training is to restore the patient with frequency, urgency, and urge incontinence to a more normal and convenient voiding pattern. Ultimately, voiding should occur at intervals of three to four hours (or even longer) without any urgency or incontinence. Drug therapy is sometimes combined with bladder training for those with detrusor instability.

Bladder training aims to restore an individual's confidence in the bladder's ability to hold urine and to reestablish a more normal pattern. Initially, a patient keeps a baseline chart for three to seven days, recording how often urine is passed and when incontinence occurs. This chart is reviewed with the program supervisor, and an individual regimen is developed. The purpose is to extend the time between voiding gradually, encouraging the patient to practice delaying the need to void, rather than giving in to the feeling of urgency. Initially, the times chosen can be at set intervals throughout the day (for example, every one or two hours) or can be variable, according to the individual's pattern as indicated by the baseline chart. When the baseline chart reveals a definite pattern to the incontinence, it might be possible to set voiding times in accordance with and in anticipation of this pattern.

A pattern of voiding is set for patients throughout the day (timed voiding). Usually no pattern is set at night, even if nocturia or nocturnal enuresis is a problem. Patients are instructed to pass urine as necessary during the night. Sometimes the provision of a suitable pad or appliance helps to increase confidence and means that, if incontinence does occur, the results will not be disastrous. If urgency is experienced, patients are taught to sit or stand still and try to suppress the sensation rather than to rush immediately to the toilet. A normal fluid intake is encouraged because the goal is to have the patient continent and able to drink fluids adequately.

As patients achieve the target intervals without having to urinate prematurely or leaking, the intervals can gradually be lengthened. The speed of progress depends on the individual and on other variables, such as the initial severity of symptoms, motivation, and the amount of professional support. Patients usually remain at one time interval for one to two weeks before it is increased by fifteen to thirty minutes for another two weeks. Once the target of three- to four-hour voiding without urgency has been achieved, it is useful to maintain the chart and set times for at least another month to prevent relapse.

Some people find that practicing pelvic muscle exercises helps to suppress urgency. Any weakness in the pelvic floor muscles will cause a tendency not only to urinary incontinence but also to fecal stress incontinence. Mild weakness can respond to pelvic muscle exercises similar to those used in alleviating the symptoms of stress incontinence, but with a concentration on the posterior rather than the anterior portion of the pelvic muscles. Rectal tone is assessed by digital examination, during which the patient is instructed to squeeze. Regular contractions on the posterior portion of the pelvic muscles are then practiced often for at least two months (usually in sets of twenty-five, three times a day).

In cases of fecal impaction, a course of disposable phosphate enemas—one or two daily for seven to ten days, or until no further return is obtained—is the treatment of choice. A single enema is seldom efficient, even if an apparently good result is obtained, because impaction is often extensive: The first enema merely clears the lowest portion of the bowel. If fecal incontinence persists once the bowel has been totally cleared (a plain abdominal X ray can be helpful in confirming this), the condition is assumed to be neurogenic in origin rather than caused by the impaction.

PERSPECTIVE AND PROSPECTS

Historically, most health professionals have been profoundly ignorant of the causes and management of incontinence. Incontinence was often regarded as a condition over which there was no control, rather than as a symptom of an underlying physiologic disorder or as a symptom of a patient with a unique combination of problems, needs, and potentials. The unfortunate result of such limited understanding was passive acceptance of the symptom of incontinence. Incontinence, often viewed as repulsive, is often a condition that is merely tolerated. As public recognition of the implications of incontinence has increased, however, the stigma associated with it has slowly decreased. It has become common knowledge that millions of Americans suffer from incontinence, and most pharmacies and supermarkets have a section for incontinence products.

At one time, incontinence was primarily regarded as a "nursing" problem, with nurses providing custodial care—keeping the patient as clean and comfortable as possible and preventing pressure ulcers from developing. Gradually, nurses were not alone in acknowledging that incontinence was a symptom requiring investigation and intervention; those in other health professions also began to realize this need. In the 1980's, research dollars began to be allocated for the study of incontinence. In 1988, U.S. Surgeon General C. Everett Koop estimated that 8 billion dollars was being spent by the federal government on incontinence in the United States annually.

As incontinence began to be recognized by the public as a health problem rather than as an inevitable part of aging, more people admitted having the symptoms of incontinence and sought medical attention. It has been estimated that, of all cases of incontinence, more than one-third can be cured, another one-third can be dramatically improved, and most of the remainder can be significantly improved.

—Genevieve Slomski, Ph.D.

See also Bed-wetting; Constipation; Diarrhea and dysentery; Digestion; Sphincterectomy; Stone removal; Stones; Urinary disorders; Urinary system; Urology; Urology, pediatric.

FOR FURTHER INFORMATION:

Dierich, Mary, and Felecia Froe. *Overcoming Incontinence: A Straightforward Guide to Your Options.* New York: John Wiley & Sons, 2000. The authors present no-nonsense, practical advice on incontinence. Readers will learn how the urinary system works and how and when to seek professional help.

Gartley, Cheryle, ed. *Managing Incontinence.* Ottawa, Ill.: Jameson Books, 1985. An overview of the basic treatment options for urinary incontinence, including surgical and nonsurgical methods. Although somewhat technical, this work is accessible to the general reader. Includes a bibliography.

Jeter, Katherine, et al., eds. *Nursing for Continence.* Philadelphia: W. B. Saunders, 1990. This work, written by a group of nurses, addresses the diagnosis, treatment, and management of incontinence in all age groups and in special populations and circumstances in a practical, thorough, and sensitive manner.

Lucas, Malcolm, Simon Emery, and John Beynon, eds. *Incontinence: A Pelvic Team Approach.* Malden, Mass.: Blackwell Scientific, 1999. This book's editors are consultant surgeons at Swansea NHS Trust, and they have combined their expertise in this volume, in which they describe the various operations they perform to counteract urinary and fecal incontinence.

Nathanson, Laura Walther. *The Portable Pediatrician: A Practicing Pediatrician's Guide to Your Child's Growth, Development, Health, and Behavior from Birth to Age Five.* 2d ed. New York: HarperCollins, 2002. An engaging, easy-to-read guide for parents to assess their child's development, medical symptoms, and behavioral problems, including bed wetting.

National Association for Incontinence. http://www.nafc.org/site2/index.html. This is a clearinghouse for information and services related to incontinence and assistive devices. Provides education, advocacy, and support on the causes, prevention, diagnosis, treatment, and management alternatives for persons with incontinence.

Newman, Diane Kaschack. *Managing and Treating Urinary Incontinence.* Baltimore: Health Professions Press, 2002. A comprehensive resource to incontinence, covering everything from the causes of incontinence to evaluation and therapy. Includes excellent practical information such as self-care practices that will minimize urinary symptoms, tools for health professionals that can be used to train staff and educate patients, and appendices on diet habits, bladder retraining, and mechanical devices used to reduce incontinence.

Parker, William, et al. *The Incontinence Solution: Answers for Women of All Ages.* New York: Simon & Schuster, 2002. A consumer-oriented guide to incontinence with an accessible question-and-answer format. Covers causes and diagnosis, treatments, childbirth and incontinence, interstitial cystitis, and defining and diagnosing prolapse.

Raz, Sholomo, ed. *Female Urology.* 2d ed. Philadelphia: W. B. Saunders, 1996. The book begins with fundamentals of the female genitourinary tract, then analyzes the dynamics of continence mechanisms. Female urinary incontinence is treated as a multifaceted subject.

INFORMATION ON INDIGESTION

CAUSES: Varies; may include acid reflux disease, ulcers, lactose intolerance, celiac sprue, irritable bowel syndrome (IBS)

SYMPTOMS: Burning, fullness, gaseousness, and gnawing sensation in abdomen

DURATION: Temporary, often recurrent

TREATMENTS: Avoidance of food triggers (*e.g.*, dairy products, wheat) or spicy foods; change in eating habits (slower eating, frequent small meals); over-the-counter drugs (magnesium, bismuth mixtures, antacids)

INDIGESTION

DISEASE/DISORDER

ALSO KNOWN AS: Functional dyspepsia

ANATOMY OR SYSTEM AFFECTED: Gastrointestinal system

SPECIALTIES AND RELATED FIELDS: Family medicine, gastroenterology, internal medicine

DEFINITION: Discomfort in the abdomen following meals.

CAUSES AND SYMPTOMS

Indigestion is a nonspecific term used to describe a variety of sensations. Burning, fullness, gaseousness, and gnawing sensation in the abdomen are all symptoms that patients may describe as indigestion. While some people who complain of indigestion have acid reflux disease or ulcers, these are by no means the only causes. Fullness or bloating following the ingestion of milk, cheese, or other dairy products may be symptoms of lactose intolerance. This is one of the few cases of indigestion that is truly a problem in the digestive process, namely in the breakdown of milk sugars. Abdominal discomfort associated with alternating bouts of diarrhea and constipation may signal irritable bowel syndrome (IBS). More rare causes of similar discomfort include diffuse esophageal spasm, in which the food pipe contracts abnormally, and inflammation in the gallbladder.

Since the term "indigestion" is so vague, care must be taken to distinguish it from cardiac pain (angina). Psychiatric causes of abdominal pain must also be considered, especially when other etiologies have been ruled out.

TREATMENT AND THERAPY

Since the causes of indigestion are so varied, it is useful to arrive at a more precise diagnosis before offering treatment. Prior to embarking on a lengthy workup, however, some simple measures should be attempted. If symptoms resolve entirely with these measures, then no further investigation or treatment is usually required. Any particular foods that appear to worsen symptoms should be eliminated from the diet. This is especially true for dairy products and wheat, which are offensive factors in lactose intolerance and celiac sprue, respectively. Patients should also try avoiding spicy foods for a period of time. Eating slowly and having frequent small meals is good practice for people with indigestion. Some people find relief with over-the-counter remedies such as magnesium or bismuth mixtures. Antacids can also be tried, especially if acid reflux is suspected.

If symptoms persist, or if they are accompanied by trouble swallowing, vomiting, weight loss, or a change in bowel movements, then more thorough investigation is needed. This is often done through blood tests, X rays, or endoscopy.

—*Ahmad Kamal, M.D.*

See also Abdomen; Abdominal disorders; Acid reflux disease; Constipation; Crohn's disease; Diarrhea and dysentery; Digestion; Gallbladder diseases; Gastroenterology; Gastroenterology, pediatric; Gastrointestinal disorders; Gastrointestinal system; Heartburn; Intestinal disorders; Nausea and vomiting; Nutrition; Stress; Ulcer surgery; Ulcers.

FOR FURTHER INFORMATION:

Berkow, Robert, and Mark H. Beers, eds. *The Merck Manual of Diagnosis and Therapy.* 17th ed. Whitehouse Station, N.J.: Merck Research Laboratories, 1999.

Braunwald, Eugene, et al., eds. *Harrison's Principles of Internal Medicine.* 15th ed. New York: McGraw-Hill, 2001.

Peikin, Steven R. *Gastrointestinal Health.* New York: HarperCollins, 1999.

INFARCTION, MYOCARDIAL. *See* HEART ATTACK.

INFECTION
DISEASE/DISORDER

ANATOMY OR SYSTEM AFFECTED: All
SPECIALTIES AND RELATED FIELDS: Bacteriology, family practice, hematology, internal medicine, virology
DEFINITION: Invasion of the body by disease-causing organisms such as bacteria, viruses, fungi, and parasites; symptoms of infection may include pain, swelling, fever, and loss of normal function.

KEY TERMS:

antibiotic: a substance that destroys or inhibits the growth of microorganisms, such as bacteria

antibody: a small protein secreted from specialized white blood cells which binds to and aids in the destruction of pathogens

antigen: a substance found on pathogens to which the antibodies bind; also, any substance considered foreign by the body

bacteria: small microorganisms; some bacteria found normally in and on the body have helpful functions, while others that invade the body or disrupt the normal bacteria are harmful and often infectious

edema: an abnormal accumulation of fluid in the body tissues; tissue with edema is swollen in appearance

infectious: referring to a microorganism which is capable of causing disease, often with the ability to spread from one person to another

inflammation: a tissue reaction to injury which may or may not involve infection; pain, heat, redness, and edema are the usual signs of inflammation

pathogen: a microorganism or substance capable of producing a disease, such as a bacterium causing an infection

phagocytosis: the ingestion and destruction of a pathogen or abnormal tissue by specialized white blood cells known as phagocytes *virus:* a very small organism which is dependent upon a host cell to meet its metabolic needs and to reproduce

PROCESS AND EFFECTS

Healthy people live with potential pathogens; that is, people have on and in their bodies non-disease-causing bacteria. They live in harmony with these organisms and in fact benefit from their presence. For example, some of the bacteria found in the intestinal tract supply vitamin K, which is important in blood-clotting reactions.

The human body has several features which prevent disease-causing organisms from inducing an infection. These features include anatomical barriers, such as unbroken skin, and the mucus in the nose, mouth, and lungs, which can trap pathogens. Another defense is the acid within the stomach, and even bacteria that are normally present in certain areas of the body can force out more harmful bacteria. The immune system is specially developed to ward off intruders.

Immune cells and factors secreted from these cells provide the next line of defense against invading organisms. Antibodies are secreted from specialized white blood cells known as plasma cells. These antibodies are very specific for the recognition of pathogens. For example, one antibody will recognize a particular strain of bacteria but not another. Antibodies attach themselves to the part of the bacterium called the antigen. Once bound to the antigen, they aid in the destruction of the pathogen. In addition to plasma cells, other white blood cells help in combating infections. These include the phagocytes called macrophages and neutrophils. Both of these immune cells have the ability to eat and digest pathogens such as bacteria in a process known as phagocytosis.

Microorganisms that cause disease must, in some way, overwhelm the body's natural defenses and immune system. Bacteria capable of causing infections may even be naturally occurring organisms that have left their normal environment and overcome the elements that normally hold them at bay. For example, some normal bacteria that reside in the mouth may cause pneumonia (inflammation of the lungs) if they gain access to the lungs.

Other infections can be caused by pathogens that do not normally reside in the body. One can "catch" a cold or the flu, or even a sexually transmitted disease. These kinds of infections are called communicable or transmissible infections. Similarly, a physician treating someone who has been bitten by a bat, skunk, or dog will want to know whether the animal has rabies. Rabies is a viral infection which is transmitted via a bite which breaks the skin and contaminates the wound with infectious saliva.

No matter what the route of infection, the body must mount a response to the intruding microorganism. Often the signs and symptoms one observes are not caused by the direct action of the infecting pathogen, but rather reflect the immune system's response to the infection. The most frequent signs and symptoms include inflammation and pain at the site of infection, as well as fever.

The inflammatory response is a nonspecific defense that is triggered whenever body tissues are injured, as in the case of infection. The goal of the inflammatory response is to prevent the spread of the infectious agent to nearby tissues, destroy the pathogens, remove the damaged tissues, and begin the healing process.

The signs of inflammation include redness, edema (tissue swelling), heat, pain, and loss of normal function. At first glance, these reactions do not appear to be beneficial to the body, but they do help fight the infection and aid in the healing process. The redness is attributable to an increase in blood flow to the area of infection. This increase in blood to the site of infection helps provide nutrients to the tissue, as well as removing some of the waste products that develop as the immune system fights the infection. With this increase in blood flow comes an increase in the temperature and the amount of blood that leaks out of blood vessels into the tissue spaces, causing edema at the site of infection. Some of the blood that leaks into the site of infection contains clotting proteins that help form a clot around the infected area, thereby reducing the chances that the pathogen could escape into the bloodstream or uninfected tissue nearby. Pain is present when the damaged tissue releases waste products and the pathogen releases toxins. The swelling of the injured area and the pain associated with infections keep the patient from

---

INFORMATION ON INFECTION

CAUSES: Exposure to bacteria, viruses, fungi, or parasites

SYMPTOMS: Pain, swelling, fever, fatigue, loss of normal function

DURATION: Acute to chronic

TREATMENTS: Drug therapy (antibiotics, antiviral agents, antifungal agents, etc.)

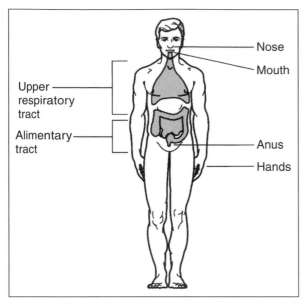

Common sites for entry of infection into the body; in addition, a break in the skin anywhere on the body is an invitation to infection.

using that area of the body and thus aid in healing. It is interesting to note that while some painkillers such as aspirin reduce the inflammatory reaction by stopping the production of some of the chemicals released during inflammation, the aspirin-like drugs do nothing to harm the pathogen, only the body's response to the microorganism.

Some of the same chemicals that are found in inflamed tissues also cause fever. This abnormally high body temperature represents the body's response to an invading microorganism. The body's thermostat, located in a region of the brain known as the hypothalamus, is set at 37 degrees Celsius (98.6 degrees Fahrenheit). During an infection, the thermostat is reset to a higher level. Chemicals called pyrogens are released from white blood cells called macrophages. Once again, aspirin-like drugs can be used to reduce the fever by inhibiting the action of some of these chemicals in the hypothalamus.

The body responds to viral infections in a similar way. Virally infected cells, however, secrete interferon, exerting an antiviral action which may provide protection to uninfected neighboring cells. It appears that interferon acts to inhibit the virus from replicating. Therefore, cells that are already infected must be destroyed to rid the body of the remaining virus.

In addition to being part of the inflammatory response, certain white blood cells play an important role in attempting to remove the pathogen. Soon after inflammation begins, macrophages already present at the site of infection start to destroy the microorganism. At the same time, chemicals are being released from both the damaged tissue and the macrophages, which recruit other white blood cells such as neutrophils. The neutrophils, like the macrophages, are effective at attacking and destroying bacteria but, unlike the macrophages, they often die in the battle against infection. Dead neutrophils are seen as a white exudate called pus.

Other manifestations of infection include systemic (whole-body) effects in addition to changes at the site of infection. As noted, fever is a systemic effect mediated by chemicals from the site of infection. Some of these same factors have the ability to act on the bone marrow to increase the production of white blood cells. Physicians look for fever and an increase in white blood cell number as a sign of infection. If the infection is severe, the bone marrow may not be able to keep up with the demand and an overall decrease in white blood cell number is found.

COMPLICATIONS AND DISORDERS

Physicians and other health care workers must use patient history, signs and symptoms, and laboratory tests to determine the type of infection and the most appropriate treatment. Patient history can often tell the examiner how and when the infection started. For example, the patient may have cut himself or herself, been exposed to someone with an infectious disease, or had intimate contact with someone carrying a sexually transmitted disease. Signs of infection—edema, pain, fever—are usually rather easy to detect, but some symptoms may be rather vague, such as feeling tired and weak. These general signs and symptoms may indicate to a physician that the patient has an infection, but they will not provide information about the type of microorganism causing the infection. Nevertheless, some microorganisms do cause specific symptoms. For example, the varicella-zoster virus that causes chickenpox or the paramyxovirus that causes measles leave characteristic rashes.

When the microorganism does not have a characteristic sign, physicians must use laboratory tests to determine the pathogen involved. Diagnosis of the disease relies on identifying the causative pathogen by microscopic examination of a specimen of infected tissue or body fluid, by growing the microorganism using culture techniques, or by detecting antibodies in the blood that have developed against the pathogen.

Once the physician determines what type of microorganism has caused the infection, he or she will have to determine the best treatment to eradicate the disease. Drug therapy usually consists of antibiotics and other antimicrobial agents. The selection of the appropriate drug is important, as certain pathogens are susceptible only to certain antibiotics. Unfortunately, few effective antiviral drugs are available for many infectious viruses. In these cases, drugs can be used to treat symptoms such as fever, pain, diarrhea, and vomiting rather than to destroy the virus.

Anti-infective drugs are commonly used by physicians to treat infections. Agents that kill or inhibit the growth of bacteria are known as antibiotics and can be applied directly to the site of infection (topical), given by mouth (oral), or injected. The latter two modes of administration allow the drug to be carried throughout the body by way of the blood. Some antibiotic drugs are effective against only certain strains of infectious bacteria. Antibiotics that act against several types of bacteria are referred to as broad-spectrum antibiotics. Some bacteria develop resistance to a particular antibiotic and require that the physician switch agents or use a combination of antibiotics. Antibiotic therapy for the treatment of infections should be used when the body has been invaded by harmful bacteria, when the bacteria are reproducing at a more rapid rate than the immune system can handle, or to prevent infections in individuals with an impaired immune system.

Some serious common bacterial infections include gonorrhea, which is sexually transmitted and treatable with penicillin; bacterial meningitis, which causes inflammation of the coverings around the brain and is treatable with a variety of antibiotics; pertussis (or whooping cough), which is transmitted by water droplets in air and treatable with erythromycin; pneumonia, which causes shortness of breath, is transmitted via the air, and can be treated with antibiotics; tuberculosis, which infects the lungs and is treatable with various antibiotics; and salmonella (or typhoid fever), which is transmitted in food or water contaminated with fecal material, causes fever, headaches, and digestive problems, and is treated with antibiotics. It should be noted that antibiotics are not effective in viral infections; only bacterial infections are treated with antibiotics.

Antiviral drugs such as acyclovir, amantadine, and zidovudine (formerly known as azidothymide, or AZT) are used in the treatment of infection by a virus. These drugs have been difficult to develop. Most viruses live within the cells of the patient, and the drug must in some way kill the virus without harming the host cells. In fact, antiviral agents cannot completely cure an illness, and infected patients often experience recurrent disease. Nevertheless, they do reduce the severity of these infections.

There are several common viral infections. Human immunodeficiency virus (HIV) infection, which causes acquired immunodeficiency syndrome (AIDS), is transmitted by sexual contact or contaminated needles or blood products; it is often treated with zidovudine but remains lethal. Chickenpox (varicella-zoster virus), which is transmitted by airborne droplets or direct contact, is treated with acyclovir. The common cold is caused by numerous viruses that are transmitted by direct contact or air droplets and has no effective treatment other than drugs that reduce the symptoms. Hepatitis is transmitted by contaminated food, sexual contact, and blood; it causes flulike symptoms and jaundice (a yellow tinge to the skin caused by liver problems) and may be helped with the drug interferon. Influenza viruses ("the flu") are transmitted by airborne droplets; the only treatment for the flu is of its symptoms. Measles is transmitted by virus-containing water droplets and causes fever and a rash; treatment consists of alleviating the symptoms. Mononucleosis is transmitted via saliva and causes swollen lymph nodes, fever, a sore throat, and generalized tiredness; a patient with mononucleosis can only receive treatment for the symptoms, as no cure is available. Poliomyelitis (polio) is transmitted by fecally contaminated material or airborne droplets and can eventually cause paralysis; no treatment is available. Rabies is caused by a bite from an infected animal, as the virus is present in the saliva; the major symptoms include fever, tiredness, and spasms of the throat, and there is no effective treatment for rabies after these symptoms have appeared. Rubella is transmitted by virus-containing air droplets and is associated with a fever and rash; there is no treatment other than for the symptoms.

A major problem with infectious diseases is that there is almost always lag time between when the microorganism has entered the body and the onset of signs and symptoms. This gap may last from a few hours or days to several years. A patient without noticeable symptoms is likely to spread the pathogen. Thus a cycle is set up in which individuals unknowingly infect others who, in turn, pass on the disease-causing agent. Large numbers of people can quickly become infected.

One way to prevent the spread of infectious agents is to vaccinate patients. Diseases such as diphtheria, measles, mumps, rubella, poliomyelitis, and pertussis are rare in the United States because of an aggressive immunization program. When a patient is vaccinated, the vaccine usually contains a dead or inactive pathogen. After the vaccine is administered (usually by injection), the immune system responds by making antibodies against the antigens on the microorganism. Since the pathogen in the vaccine is unable to cause disease, the patient has no symptoms after immunization. The next time that the person is exposed to the infectious agent, his or her immune system is prepared to fight it before symptoms become evident.

In addition to immunization to prevent infection, individuals can largely avoid serious infectious diseases through good hygiene with respect to food and drink, frequent washing, the avoidance of contact with fecal material and urine, and the avoidance of contact with individuals who are infected and capable of transmitting the disease. When such avoidance is impractical, other protective measures can be taken.

Sexually transmitted diseases are usually preventable by using barrier contraceptives and practicing "safe sex." The most common of these diseases include chlamydial infections, trichomoniasis, genital herpes, and HIV infections. Prevention is particularly important in the viral infections of herpes and HIV, as there are no known cures.

Some infections can be acquired at birth, including gonorrhea, genital herpes, chlamydial infections, and salmonella. These microorganisms exist in the birth canal, and some infectious agents can even pass from the mother to the fetus via the placenta. The more serious infections transmitted in this manner are rubella, syphilis, toxoplasmosis, HIV virus, and the cytomegalovirus. The risk of transmitting these infections can be reduced by treating the mother before delivery or performing a cesarean section (surgical delivery from the uterus), thereby avoiding the birth canal.

PERSPECTIVE AND PROSPECTS

The ancient Egyptians were probably the first to recognize infection and the body's response to the introduction of a disease-causing microorganism: Some hieroglyphics appear to represent the inflammatory process. Sometime in the fifth century B.C.E., the Greeks noted that patients who had acquired an infectious disease and survived did not usually contract the same illness a second time.

More solid scientific evidence about infections was provided in the nineteenth century by Edward Jenner, an English physician and scientist. Jenner was able to document that milkmaids seemed to be protected against smallpox because of their exposure to cowpox. With this knowledge, he vaccinated a boy with material from a cowpox pustule. The boy had a typical inflammatory response, and he showed no symptoms of smallpox after being injected with the disease a few months later. His immune system protected him from the virus. Since that time, scientists have reached a much better understanding of how the body deals with infection.

Many scientists are focusing their attention on how pathogens are transmitted from the source of infection to susceptible individuals. Epidemiology is the study of the distribution and causes of diseases that are prevalent in humans. Since some infectious diseases are communicable (transmittable), epidemiologists gather data when an outbreak occurs in a population. These data include the source of infectious agents (the tissues involved), the microorganisms causing the disease, and the method by which the pathogens are transmitted from one person to another. Physicians and other health care workers help in the battle against infections by identifying susceptible individuals; developing and evaluating sources, methods, and ways to control the spread of the pathogens; and improving preventive measures, which usually include extensive educational efforts for the general population. With this knowledge, scientists and physicians attempt to eradicate the disease.

While scientists and physicians have made great advances in the understanding of infection, many problems remain. The spread of certain diseases, such as sexually transmitted diseases, is difficult to control except by modifying human behavior. The most difficult to treat are viral illnesses in which the drugs that are used are ineffective in completely eradicating the virus, and bacterial diseases in which the bacteria have developed drug resistance. Because these microorganisms evolve rapidly, new strains continually emerge. When a new infectious agent develops, it is often years before scientists can devise an effective drug or vaccine to treat the disease. In the meantime, large numbers of patients may become ill and even die. Perhaps the most effective way to combat infection is to use preventive measures whenever practical.

—*Matthew Berria, Ph.D.*

See also Arthropod-borne diseases; Bacterial infections; Bites and stings; Childhood infectious diseases; Disease; Ear infections and disorders; Fever; Fungal infections; Iatrogenic disorders; Inflammation; Lice, mites, and ticks; Parasitic diseases; Prion diseases;

Staphylococcal infections; Streptococcal infections; Viral infections; Zoonoses; *specific diseases*.

FOR FURTHER INFORMATION:

Biddle, Wayne. *Field Guide to Germs*. 2d ed. New York: Anchor Books, 2002. This comprehensive book is easily accessible to the nonspecialist and includes a discussion of nearly every virus, bacterium, and fungus known to cause human and nonhuman animal disease. The history of the microbe and the treatment of diseases are included.

Clayman, Charles B., ed. *The American Medical Association Encyclopedia of Medicine*. New York: Random House, 1994. Covers, in alphabetical order, medical terms, diseases, and medical procedures. Lists all major infectious illnesses, with their causes and treatments. Does an excellent job of explaining rather complex medical subjects for a nonprofessional audience.

Frank, Steven A. *Immunology and Evolution of Infectious Disease*. Princeton, N.J.: Princeton University Press, 2002. Blends research from molecular biology, immunology, pathogen biology, and population dynamics to discuss how and why parasites vary to escape recognition by the immune system, vaccine design, and the control of epidemics.

Gorbach, Sherwood L., John G. Bartlett, and Neil R. Blacklow, eds. *Infectious Diseases*. 3d ed. Philadelphia: W. B. Saunders, 2003. A thorough discussion of infectious diseases. Included is a brief history, an account of the mechanisms of disease and immunity, and a concise discussion of a broad range of infectious agents.

Shaw, Michael, ed. *Everything You Need to Know About Diseases*. Springhouse, Pa.: Springhouse Press, 1996. This well-illustrated consumer reference, compiled by more than one hundred doctors and medical experts, describes five hundred illnesses and conditions, their causes, symptoms, diagnosis, treatment, and prevention. A valuable reference book for everyone interested in health and disease. Of particular interest is chapter 19, "Infection."

Sompayrac, Lauren. *How Pathogenic Viruses Work*. 5th ed. Sudbury, Mass.: Jones and Bartlett, 2002. Engaging exploration of the basics of virology. The author uses twelve of the most common viral infections to demonstrate how viruses "devise" various solutions to stay alive.

Timmreck, Thomas C. *An Introduction to Epidemiology*. 3d ed. Boston: Jones and Bartlett, 2002. A book in the Jones and Bartlett series in health sciences. Discusses epidemiological methods. Includes a bibliography and an index.

Wilson, Michael, Brian Henderson, and Rod McNab. *Bacterial Virulence Mechanisms*. New York: Cambridge University Press, 2002. Basing their discussion on research advances in microbiology, molecular biology, and cell biology, the authors describe the interactions that exist between bacteria and human cells both in health and during infection.

INFERTILITY IN FEMALES

DISEASE/DISORDER

ANATOMY OR SYSTEM AFFECTED: Genitals, reproductive system, uterus

SPECIALTIES AND RELATED FIELDS: Endocrinology, gynecology

DEFINITION: The inability to achieve a desired pregnancy as a result of dysfunction of female reproductive organs.

KEY TERMS:

cervix: the bottom portion of the uterus, protruding into the vagina; the cervical canal, an opening in the cervix, allows sperm to pass from the vagina into the uterus

endometriosis: a disease in which patches of the uterine lining, the endometrium, implant on or in other organs

follicles: spherical structures in the ovary that contain the maturing ova (eggs)

hormone: a chemical signal that serves to coordinate the functions of different body parts; the hormones important in female reproduction are produced by the brain, the pituitary, and the ovaries

implantation: the process in which the early embryo attaches to the uterine lining; a critical event in pregnancy

ovaries: the pair of structures in the female that produce ova (eggs) and hormones

oviducts: the pair of tubes leading from the top of the uterus upward toward the ovaries; also called the Fallopian tubes

ovulation: the process in which an ovum is released from its follicle in the ovary; ovulation must occur for conception to be possible

pelvic inflammatory disease: a general term that refers to a state of inflammation and infection in the pelvic organs; may be caused by a sexually transmitted disease

uterus: the organ in which the embryo implants and grows

vagina: the tube-shaped organ that serves as the site for sperm deposition during intercourse

CAUSES AND SYMPTOMS

Infertility is defined as the failure of a couple to conceive a child despite regular sexual activity over a period of at least one year. Studies have estimated that in the United States 10 percent to 15 percent of couples are infertile. In about half of these couples, it is the woman who is affected.

The causes of female infertility are centered in the reproductive organs: the ovaries, oviducts, uterus, cervix, and vagina. The frequency of specific problems among infertile women is as follows: ovarian problems, 20 percent to 30 percent; damage to the oviducts, 30 percent to 50 percent; uterine problems, 5 percent to 10 percent; and cervical or vaginal abnormalities, 5 percent to 10 percent. Another 10 percent of women have unexplained infertility.

The ovaries have two important roles in conception: the production of ova, culminating in ovulation, and the production of hormones. Ovulation usually occurs halfway through a woman's four-week menstrual cycle. In the two weeks preceding ovulation, follicle-stimulating hormone (FSH) from the pituitary gland causes follicles in the ovaries to grow and the ova within them to mature. As the follicles grow, they produce increasing amounts of estrogen. Near the middle of the cycle, the estrogen causes the pituitary gland to release a surge of luteinizing hormone (LH), which causes ovulation of the largest follicle in the ovary.

Anovulation (lack of ovulation) can result either directly—from an inability to produce LH, FSH, or estrogen—or indirectly—because of the presence of

---

INFORMATION ON INFERTILITY IN FEMALES

CAUSES: Endometriosis, cervical problems, anovulation, hormonal imbalance, abnormally shaped uterus or vagina, pelvic inflammatory disease

SYMPTOMS: Often asymptomatic; can include lack of menstrual periods, blocked Fallopian tubes, abdominal pain with endometriosis

DURATION: Short-term to chronic

TREATMENTS: Fertility drugs, surgery, fertility procedures (*e.g.,* in vitro fertilization)

---

other hormones that interfere with the signaling systems between the pituitary and ovaries. For example, the woman may have an excess production of androgen (testosterone-like) hormones, either in her ovaries or in her adrenal glands, or her pituitary may produce too much prolactin, a hormone that is normally secreted in large amounts only after the birth of a child.

Besides ovulation, the ovaries have another critical role in conception since they produce hormones that act on the uterus to allow it to support an embryo. In the first two weeks of the menstrual cycle, the uterine lining is prepared for a possible pregnancy by estrogen from the ovaries. Following ovulation, the uterus is maintained in a state that can support an embryo by progesterone, which is produced in the ovary by the follicle that just ovulated, now called a corpus luteum. Because of the effects of hormones from the corpus luteum on the uterus, the corpus luteum is essential to the survival of the embryo. If conception does not occur, the corpus luteum disintegrates and stops producing progesterone. As progesterone levels decline, the uterine lining can no longer be maintained and is shed as the menstrual flow.

Failure of the pregnancy can result from improper function of the corpus luteum, such as an inability to produce enough progesterone to sustain the uterine lining. The corpus luteum may also produce progesterone initially but then disintegrate too early. These problems in corpus luteum function, referred to as luteal phase insufficiency, may be caused by the same types of hormonal abnormalities that cause lack of ovulation.

Some cases of infertility may be associated with an abnormally shaped uterus or vagina. Such malformations of the reproductive organs are common in women whose mothers took diethylstilbestrol (DES) during pregnancy. DES was prescribed to many pregnant women from 1941 to about 1970 as a protection against miscarriage; infertility and other problems occurred in the offspring of these women.

Conception depends on normal function of the oviducts (or Fallopian tubes), thin tubes with an inner diameter of only a few millimeters; they are attached to the top of the uterus and curve upward toward the ovaries. The inner end of each tube, located near one of the ovaries, waves back and forth at the time of ovulation, drawing the mature ovum into the opening of the oviduct. Once in the oviduct, the ovum is propelled along by movements of the oviduct wall. Meanwhile, if intercourse has occurred recently, the man's sperm will be moving upward in the female system, swimming

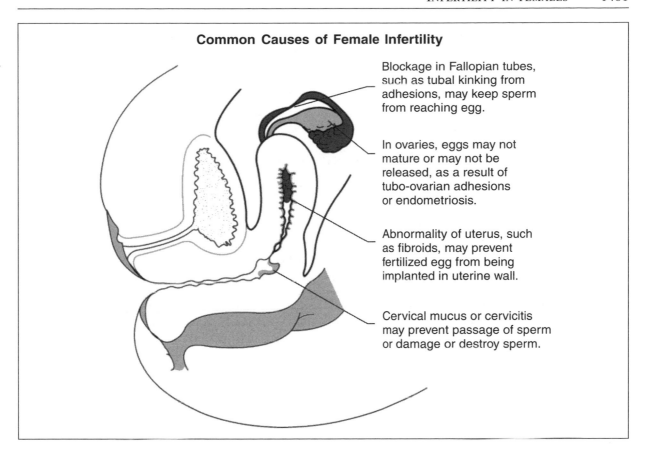

Common Causes of Female Infertility

Blockage in Fallopian tubes, such as tubal kinking from adhesions, may keep sperm from reaching egg.

In ovaries, eggs may not mature or may not be released, as a result of tubo-ovarian adhesions or endometriosis.

Abnormality of uterus, such as fibroids, may prevent fertilized egg from being implanted in uterine wall.

Cervical mucus or cervicitis may prevent passage of sperm or damage or destroy sperm.

through the uterus and the oviducts. Fertilization, the union of the sperm and ovum, will occur in the oviduct, and then the fertilized ovum will pass down the oviduct and reach the uterus about three days after ovulation.

Infertility can result from scar tissue formation inside the oviduct, resulting in physical blockage and inability to transport the ovum, sperm, or both. The most common cause of scar tissue formation in the reproductive organs is pelvic inflammatory disease (PID), a condition characterized by inflammation that spreads throughout the female reproductive tract. PID may be initiated by a sexually transmitted disease such as gonorrhea and chlamydia. Physicians in the United States have documented an increase in infertility attributable to tubal damage caused by sexually transmitted diseases.

Damage to the outside of the oviduct can also cause infertility, because such damage can interfere with the mobility of the oviduct, which is necessary to the capture of the ovum at the time of ovulation. External damage to the oviduct may occur as an aftermath of abdominal surgery, when adhesions induced by surgical cutting are likely to form. An adhesion is an abnormal scar tissue connection between adjacent structures.

Another possible cause of damage to the oviduct, resulting in infertility, is the presence of endometriosis. Endometriosis refers to a condition in which patches of the uterine lining implant in or on the surface of other organs. These patches are thought to arise during menstruation, when the uterine lining (endometrium) is normally shed from the body through the cervix and vagina; in a woman with endometriosis, for unknown reasons, the endometrium is carried to the interior of the pelvic cavity by passing up the oviducts. The endometrial patches can lodge in the oviduct itself, causing blockage, or can adhere to the outer surface of the oviducts, interfering with mobility.

Endometriosis can cause infertility by interfering with organs other than the oviducts. Endometrial patches on the outside of the uterus can cause distortions in the shape or placement of the uterus, interfering with embryonic implantation. Ovulation may be prevented by the presence of the endometrial tissues on the surface of the ovary. Yet the presence of endometriosis is not always associated with infertility. Thirty percent to forty percent of women with endometriosis cannot conceive, but the remainder appear to be fertile.

Another critical site in conception is the cervix. The cervix, the entryway to the uterus from the vagina, represents the first barrier through which sperm must pass on their way to the ovum. The cervix consists of a ring of strong, elastic tissue with a narrow canal. Glands in the cervix produce the mucus that fills the cervical canal and through which sperm swim en route to the ovum. The amount and quality of the cervical mucus change throughout the menstrual cycle, under the influence of hormones from the ovary. At ovulation, the mucus is in a state that is most easily penetrated by sperm; after ovulation, the mucus becomes almost impenetrable.

Cervical problems that can lead to infertility include production of a mucus that does not allow sperm passage at the time of ovulation (hostile mucus syndrome) and interference with sperm transport caused by narrowing of the cervical canal. Such narrowing may be the result of a developmental abnormality or the presence of an infection, possibly a sexually transmitted disease.

Treatment and Therapy

The diagnosis of the exact cause of a woman's infertility is crucial to successful treatment. A complete medical history should reveal any obvious problems of previous infection or menstrual cycle irregularity. Adequacy of ovulation and luteal phase function can be determined from records of menstrual cycle length and changes in body temperature (body temperature is higher after ovulation). Hormone levels can be measured with tests of blood or urine samples. If damage to the oviducts or uterus is suspected, hysterosalpingography will be performed. In this procedure, the injection of a special fluid into the uterus is followed by X-ray analysis of the fluid movement; the shape of the uterine cavity and the oviducts will be revealed. Cervical functioning can be assessed with the postcoital test, in which the physician attempts to recover sperm from the woman's uterus some hours after she has had intercourse with her partner. If a uterine problem is suspected, the woman may have an endometrial biopsy, in which a small sample of the uterine lining is removed and examined for abnormalities. Sometimes, exploratory surgery is performed to pinpoint the location of scar tissue or the location of endometriosis patches.

Surgery may be used for treatment as well as diagnosis. Damage to the oviducts can sometimes be repaired surgically, and surgical removal of endometrial patches is a standard treatment for endometriosis. Often, however, surgery is a last resort, because of the likelihood of the development of postsurgical adhesions, which can further complicate the infertility. Newer forms of surgery using lasers and freezing offer better success because of a reduced risk of adhesions.

Some women with hormonal difficulties can be treated successfully with so-called fertility drugs. There are actually several different drugs and hormones that fall under this heading: Clomiphene citrate (Clomid), human menopausal gonadotropin (HMG), gonadotropin-releasing hormone (GnRH), bromocriptine mesylate (Parlodel), and menotropins (Pergonal) are commonly used, with the exact choice depending on the woman's particular problem. The pregnancy rate with fertility drug treatment varies from 20 percent to 70 percent. One problem with some of the drugs is the risk of multiple pregnancy (more than one fetus in the uterus). Hyperstimulation of the ovaries, a condition characterized by enlarged ovaries, can be fatal as a result of severe hormone imbalances. Other possible problems include nausea, dizziness, headache, and general malaise.

Artificial insemination is an old technique that is still useful in various types of infertility. A previously collected sperm sample is placed in the woman's vagina or uterus using a special tube. Artificial insemination is always performed at the time of ovulation, in order to maximize the chance of pregnancy. The ovulation date can be determined with body temperature records or by hormone measurements. In some cases, this procedure is combined with fertility drug treatment. Since the sperm can be placed directly in the uterus, it is useful in treating hostile mucus syndrome and certain types of male infertility. The sperm sample can be provided either by the woman's partner or by a donor. The pregnancy rate after artificial insemination is highly variable (14 percent to 68 percent), depending on the particular infertility problem in the couple. There is a slight risk of infection, and, if donated semen is used, there may be no guarantee that the semen is free from sexually transmitted diseases or that the donor does not carry some genetic defect.

Another infertility treatment is gamete intrafallopian transfer (GIFT), the surgical placement of ova and sperm directly into the woman's oviducts. In order to be a candidate for this procedure, the woman must have at least one partially undamaged oviduct and a functional uterus. Ova are collected surgically from the ovaries after stimulation with a fertility drug, and a semen sample is collected from the male. The ova and the sperm are introduced into the oviducts through the same abdominal incision used to collect the ova. This procedure is useful in certain types of male infertility, if the woman produces an impenetrable cervical mucus, or if the ovarian ends of the oviducts are damaged. The range of infertility problems that may be resolved with GIFT can be extended by using donated ova or sperm. The success rate is about 33 percent overall, but the rate varies with the type of infertility present.

In vitro fertilization is known colloquially as the "test-tube baby" technique. In this procedure, ova are collected surgically after stimulation with fertility drugs and then placed in a laboratory dish and combined with sperm from the man. The actual fertilization, when a sperm penetrates the ovum, will occur in the dish. The resulting embryo is allowed to remain in the dish for two days, during which time it will have acquired two to four cells. Then, the embryo is placed in the woman's uterine cavity using a flexible tube. In vitro fertilization can be used in women who are infertile because of endometriosis, damaged oviducts, impenetrable cervical mucus, or ovarian failure. As with GIFT, in vitro fertilization may utilize either donated ova or donated sperm, or extra embryos that have been produced by one couple may be implanted in a second woman. The pregnancy rate with this procedure varies from 15 percent to 25 percent.

Embryo freezing is a secondary procedure that can increase the chances of pregnancy for an infertile couple. When ova are collected for the in vitro fertilization procedure, doctors try to collect as many as possible. All these ova are then combined with sperm for fertilization. No more than three or four embryos are ever placed in the woman's uterus, however, because a pregnancy with a large number of fetuses carries significant health risks. The extra embryos can be frozen for later use, if the first ones implanted in the uterus do not survive. This spares the woman additional surgery to collect more ova if they are needed. The freezing technique does not appear to cause any defects in the embryo.

Some women may benefit from nonsurgical embryo transfer. In this procedure, a fertile woman is artificially inseminated at the time of her ovulation; five days later, her uterus is flushed with a sterile solution, washing out the resulting embryo before it implants in the uterus. The retrieved embryo is then transferred to the uterus of another woman, who will carry it to term. Typically, the sperm provider and the woman who receives the embryo are the infertile couple who wish to rear the child, but the technique can be used in other circumstances as well. Embryo transfer can be used if the woman has damaged oviducts or is unable to ovulate, or if she has a genetic disease that could be passed to her offspring, because in this case the baby is not genetically related to the woman who carries it.

Some infertile women who are unable to achieve a pregnancy themselves turn to the use of a surrogate, a woman who will agree to bear a child and then turn it over to the infertile woman to rear as her own. In the typical situation, the surrogate is artificially inseminated with the sperm of the infertile woman's husband. The surrogate then proceeds with pregnancy and delivery as normal, but relinquishes the child to the infertile couple after its birth.

In Western societies, couples are often advised to seek fertility treatment if one year of unprotected sexual intercourse has failed to produce a pregnancy. However, in 2002, the findings of a study conducted in Europe noted that even couples in their late thirties have a 91 percent chance of getting pregnant naturally within two years. This finding led some doctors to suggest healthy younger couples—women who do not experience menstrual abnormalities or men who have appropriate sperm counts, for example—wait two years before consulting fertility specialists.

Perspective and Prospects

One of the biggest problems that infertile couples face is the emotional upheaval that comes with the diagnosis of the infertility. Bearing and rearing children is an experience that most women treasure. When a woman is told that she is infertile, she may feel that her femininity and self-worth are diminished. In addition to the emotional difficulty that may come with the recognition of infertility, more stress may be in store as the couple proceeds through treatment. The various treatments can cause embarrassment and sometimes physical pain, and fertility drugs themselves are known to cause emotional swings. For these reasons, a couple with an infertility problem is often advised to seek help from a private counselor or a support group.

Along with the emotional and physical trauma of infertility treatment, there is a considerable financial burden as well. Infertility treatments, in general, are very expensive, especially the more sophisticated procedures such as in vitro fertilization and GIFT. Since the chances of a single procedure resulting in a pregnancy are often low, the couple may be faced with submitting to multiple procedures repeated many times. The cost over several years of treatment—a realistic possibility—can be staggering. Many health insurance companies in the United States refuse to cover the costs of such treatment and are required to do so in only a few states.

Some of the treatments are accompanied by unresolved legal questions. In the case of nonsurgical embryo transfer, is the legal mother of the child the ovum donor or the woman who gives birth to the child? The same question of legal parentage arises in cases of surrogacy. Does a child born using donated ovum or sperm have a legal right to any information about the donor, such as medical history? How extensive should governmental regulation of infertility clinics be? For example, should there be standards for ensuring that donated sperm or ova are free from genetic defects? In the United States, some states have begun to address these issues, but no uniform policies have been set at the federal level.

The legal questions are largely unresolved because American society is still involved in religious and philosophical debates over the proprieties of various infertility treatments. Some religions hold that any interference in conception is unacceptable. To these denominations, even artificial insemination is wrong. Other groups approve of treatments confined to a husband and wife, but disapprove of a third party being involved as a donor or surrogate. Many people disapprove of any infertility treatment to help an individual who is not married. The basic problem underlying all these issues is that these technologies challenge the traditional definitions of parenthood.

—Marcia Watson-Whitmyre, Ph.D.

See also Assisted reproductive technologies; Conception; Contraception; Ectopic pregnancy; Endocrinology; Endometriosis; Gamete intrafallopian transfer (GIFT); Gynecology; Hormones; Hysterectomy; In vitro fertilization; Infertility in males; Menopause; Menstruation; Miscarriage; Obstetrics; Ovarian cysts; Pelvic inflammatory disease (PID); Pregnancy and gestation; Sexual dysfunction; Sperm banks; Sterilization; Stress; Tubal ligation.

FOR FURTHER INFORMATION:

Berger, Gary S., et al. *The Couple's Guide to Fertility.* 3d ed. New York: Broadway Books, 2001. Surveys fertility treatment options, including hormone therapies, surgery, in vitro fertilization, sperm injection, egg and sperm donors, adoption, surrogate motherhood, and alternative therapies.

Harkness, Carla. *The Infertility Book: A Comprehensive Medical and Emotional Guide.* Rev. ed. Berkeley, Calif.: Celestial Arts, 1992. Written as a guide for the infertile couple, this book offers emotional support as well as medical information. The text is augmented by firsthand accounts of individuals' reactions to their infertility and the treatments.

International Council on Infertility Information Dissemination. http://www.inciid.org/. INCIID's mission is to provide on-line resources of comprehensive, consumer-targeted infertility information that cover cutting-edge technologies and treatments. Provides fact sheets of treatments, an interactive area for member participation, library and glossary, and a comprehensive professional directory of clinics and doctors who specialize in infertility.

Phillips, Robert H., and Glenda Motta. *Coping with Endometriosis: A Practical Guide to Understanding, Treating and Living with Chronic Endometriosis.* New York: Putnam, 2000. Educates the reader on current research and addresses the psychological and emotional concerns brought on by a diagnosis.

Quilligan, Edward J., and Frederick P. Zuspan, eds. *Current Therapy in Obstetrics and Gynecology.* 5th ed. Philadelphia: W. B. Saunders, 1999. This excellent handbook provides detailed information on procedures for various infertility causes and treatments, arranged alphabetically amid other gynecological subjects.

Speroff, Leon, Robert H. Glass, and Nathan G. Kase, eds. *Clinical Gynecologic Endocrinology and Infertility.* 6th ed. Baltimore: Williams & Wilkins, 1999. A good basic textbook that can help the reader understand the normal functioning of the female reproductive system and the events associated with infertility.

Turkington, Carol, and Michael M. Alper. *Encyclopedia of Fertility and Infertility.* New York: Facts On File, 2001. Offers a wide range of information on infertility for the general reader, including causes and remedies, treatment options, medical advances, and birth control techniques. Appendices give resources for further information and support from organizations, periodicals and Web sites, and fertility clinics.

Weschler, Toni. *Taking Charge of Your Fertility.* Rev. ed. New York: HarperPerennial, 2001. This book encourages women to become responsible consumers of their own reproductive health. Includes excellent discussions of infertility, natural birth control, and achieving pregnancy.

Wisot, Arthur, and David Meldrum. *Conceptions and Misconceptions.* Vancouver: Harley and Marks, 1997. Written by two leading fertility experts, this book is an excellent guide through the maze of in vitro fertilization and other assisted reproductive techniques. Includes an excellent discussion of the basic physiology of conception and reproduction.

Zouves, Christo. *Expecting Miracles: On the Path of Hope from Infertility to Parenthood.* New York: Berkley, 2003. Provides the human side of reproductive medicine by telling several personal stories and giving an in-depth look at the options, decisions, and unexpected twists, turns, and disappointments that infertile couples experience.

INFERTILITY IN MALES
DISEASE/DISORDER

ANATOMY OR SYSTEM AFFECTED: Genitals, reproductive system

SPECIALTIES AND RELATED FIELDS: Endocrinology, urology

DEFINITION: The inability to achieve a desired pregnancy as a result of dysfunction of male reproductive organs.

KEY TERMS:

antibody: a chemical produced by lymphocytes (blood cells) that enables these cells to destroy foreign materials, such as bacteria

cryopreservation: a special process utilizing cryoprotectants that enables living cells to survive in a frozen state

cryoprotectant: one of several chemicals that enables living cells to survive in a frozen state; some cryoprotectants are made by animals that survive freezing

epididymis: an organ attached to the testis in which newly formed sperm reach maturity (that is, become capable of fertilizing an egg)

infertility: the inability to produce a normal pregnancy after one year of intercourse in the absence of any contraception; it may be caused by male and/or female factors

insemination: the placement of semen in the female reproductive tract, which may occur naturally as a result of sexual intercourse or artificially as a result of a medical procedure

testis: either of two male gonads that are suspended in the scrotum and produce sperm

varicocele: a swollen testicular vein in the scrotum occurring as a result of improper valvular function

CAUSES AND SYMPTOMS

To create a baby requires three things: normal sperm from a man, a normal egg from a woman, and a normal,

---

> ## INFORMATION ON INFERTILITY IN MALES
>
> **CAUSES:** Low sperm count, infection, blockage of sperm ducts (from swollen tissue or tumor), premature release of sperm from epididymis, improper scrotal temperature, varicoceles
> **SYMPTOMS:** Typically asymptomatic
> **DURATION:** Short-term to chronic
> **TREATMENTS:** Surgery, hormonal therapy, fertility procedures (*e.g.*, artificial insemination)

mature uterus. Anything that blocks the availability of the sperm, egg, or uterus can cause infertility. Infertility can be thought of as an abnormal, unwanted form of contraception.

Many different factors may be responsible for infertility. In general, these factors may be infectious, chemical (from inside or outside of the body, such as illegal drugs, pharmaceuticals, or toxins), or anatomical. Genetic factors may be responsible as well, since genes control the formation of body chemicals (such as hormones and antibodies) and body structures (one's anatomy). The way that these factors work is illustrated by male infertility.

The process by which sperm are made begins in a man's testis (or testicle). Because the transformation of testis cells into sperm is controlled by genes and hormones, abnormalities can cause infertility. Sperm released from the testis become mature in the epididymis. Sperm travel from the testis to the epididymis through ducts (tubes) in the male reproductive tract. A blockage of these ducts or premature release of sperm from the epididymis can cause infertility.

A blockage of reproductive ducts can occur as a result of a bodily enlargement, such as swollen tissue, a tumor, or cancer. An infection usually causes tissue swelling and can leave ducts permanently scarred, narrowed, or blocked. Infection can have a direct detrimental effect on the production of normal sperm. Cancer and the drugs or chemicals used to treat cancer can also damage a man's reproductive tract.

Another factor that may be important to male fertility is scrotal temperature. The temperature in the scrotum, the sac that holds the testes, is somewhat cooler than body temperature. The normal production of sperm seems to be dependent upon a cool testicular environment.

The leading cause of male infertility may be varicoceles, which occur when one-way valves fail in the veins that take blood away from the testicles. When these venous valves become leaky, blood flow becomes sluggish and causes the veins to swell. Many men with varicoceles are infertile, but the exact reason for this association is unknown. The reasons sometimes given are increased scrotal temperature and improper removal of materials (hormones) from the testis.

Mature sperm capable of fertilizing an egg are normally placed in the female reproductive tract by the ejaculation phase of sexual intercourse. The sperm are accompanied by fluid called seminal plasma; together, they form semen. A blockage of the ducts that transport the semen into the woman or toxic chemicals, including antibodies, in the semen can cause infertility.

For conception to take place—that is, for an egg to be fertilized after sperm enters the female tract—a normal egg must be present in the portion of the tract called the Fallopian tube, and sperm must move through the female tract to that egg. If the egg is absent or is abnormal, or if normal sperm cannot reach the egg, female infertility will result. The female factors that determine whether sperm fertilize an egg are the same as the male factors: anatomy, chemicals, infection, and genes.

In Western societies, couples are often advised to seek fertility treatment if one year of unprotected sexual intercourse has failed to produce a pregnancy. However, in 2002, the findings of a study conducted in Europe noted that even couples in their late thirties have a 91 percent chance of getting pregnant naturally within two years. This finding led some doctors to suggest healthy younger couples—women who do not experience menstrual abnormalities or men who have appropriate sperm counts, for example—wait two years before consulting fertility specialists.

For those that seek help with fertility issues, there are many methods available. Female infertility may be treated, depending upon the cause, by surgery, hormone therapy, or in vitro fertilization. Treatment of male infertility may be by surgery, hormone therapy, or therapeutic (artificial) insemination. Therapeutic insemination is often performed when the couple is composed of a fertile woman and an infertile man.

The first step for therapeutic insemination is for a physician to determine when an egg is ovulated or released into the Fallopian tube of the fertile woman. At the time of ovulation, semen is placed with medical instruments in the woman's reproductive tract, either on her cervix or in her uterus.

The semen used by the physician is obtained through masturbation by either the infertile man (the patient) or a fertile man (a donor), depending on the cause of the man's infertility. The freshly produced semen from either source usually undergoes laboratory testing and processing. Tests are used to evaluate the sperm quality. An effort may be made to enhance the sperm from an infertile patient and then to use these sperm for therapeutic insemination or in vitro fertilization. Other tests evaluate semen for transmissible diseases. During testing, which may require many days, the sperm can be kept alive by cryopreservation. Freshly ejaculated sperm remains fertile for only a few hours in the laboratory if it is not cryopreserved.

There are several processes that might enhance sperm from an infertile man. If the semen is infertile because it possesses too few normal sperm, an effort can be made to eliminate the abnormal sperm and to increase the concentration of normal sperm. Sperm may be abnormal in four basic ways: They may have abnormal structure, they may have abnormal movement, they may be incapable of fusing with an egg, or they may contain abnormal genes or chromosomes. Laboratory processes can often eliminate from semen those sperm with abnormal structure or abnormal movement. These processes usually involve replacing the seminal plasma with a culture medium. Removing the seminal plasma gets rid of substances that may be harmful to the sperm. After the plasma is removed, the normal sperm can be

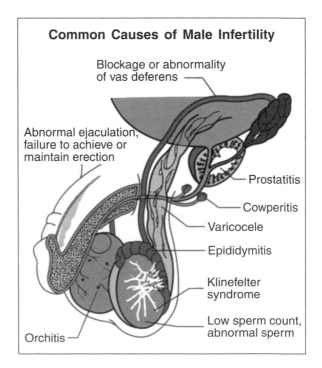

Common Causes of Male Infertility

Blockage or abnormality of vas deferens

Abnormal ejaculation, failure to achieve or maintain erection

Prostatitis

Cowperitis

Varicocele

Epididymitis

Klinefelter syndrome

Low sperm count, abnormal sperm

Orchitis

collected and concentrated. Pharmacologic agents can be added to the culture medium to increase sperm movement.

Testing for transmissible diseases is especially important if donor semen is used; these diseases may be genetic or infectious. There are many thousand genetic disorders. Most of these disorders are very rare and can be transmitted to offspring only if the sperm and the egg both have the same gene for the disorder. It is impossible, therefore, to test a donor for every possible genetic disorder; he is routinely tested only for a small group of troublesome disorders that are especially likely to occur in offspring. Tests for other disorders that the donor might transmit can be performed at the woman's request, usually based upon knowledge of genetic problems in her own family.

Much of the genetic information about a person is based on family history. Special laboratory procedures allow the genetic code inside individual cells to be interpreted. For this reason, it is important to store a sample of donor cells, not necessarily sperm, for many years after the procedure. These cells provide additional genetic information that might be important to the donor's offspring but not known at the time of insemination.

Semen can also be the source of infectious disease. Syphilis, gonorrhea, and acquired immunodeficiency syndrome (AIDS) are examples of venereal or sexually transmitted diseases (STDs). Tests for STDs can be done on blood and semen from a donor. These tests must be conducted in an approved manner, and the results must be negative before donor semen can be used therapeutically. In some cases, a test must be repeated in order to verify that the semen is not infectious.

Cryopreservation of sperm is important to therapeutic insemination for two major reasons. First, it gives time to complete all necessary testing. Second, it allows an inventory of sperm from many different donors to be kept constantly available for selection and use by patients. Sperm properly cryopreserved for twenty years, when thawed and inseminated, can produce normal babies.

Cryopreservation involves treating freshly ejaculated sperm with a cryoprotectant pharmaceutical that enables the sperm to survive when frozen; the cryoprotectant for sperm is usually glycerol. Survival of frozen sperm is also dependent upon the rate of cooling, the storage temperature, and the rate of warming at the time of thawing. Sperm treated with a cryoprotectant have the best chance of survival if they are cooled about 1 degree Celsius per minute and stored at a temperature of −150

degrees Celsius or colder. An environment of liquid nitrogen is often used to attain these storage temperatures. The storage temperature must be kept constant to avoid the damaging effects of recrystallization. When sperm are to be thawed, survival is enhanced if they are warmed at 10 to 100 degrees Celsius per minute.

The cryopreservation procedure involves the actual formation of ice, although the ice is confined to the extracellular medium. Intracellular ice is lethal. Ice formation during cryopreservation causes the cells to lose water and to shrink. The cryoprotectant seems to replace intracellular water and thereby maintain cell volume.

An alternative process for low-temperature preservation of sperm is called vitrification. Vitrification uses temperatures as cold as cryopreservation, but it avoids ice formation altogether. Instead of using one cryoprotectant, vitrification uses a mixture of several. It employs a much slower cooling rate and a much faster warming rate. Technically, vitrification is more difficult to perform; therefore, it is seldom used by clinical sperm banks.

Human sperm can be shipped to almost any location for therapeutic insemination. Sperm is usually cryopreserved before shipment and thawed at the time of insemination.

TREATMENT AND THERAPY

The use of therapeutic insemination to treat two kinds of male infertility will be considered here. The first example is male infertility that cannot be treated by other means. The second example is a fertile man at high risk for becoming infertile because of his lifestyle or because he is receiving treatment for a life-threatening disease.

The first example might occur when a heterosexual couple, having used no contraception for a year or longer, has been unsuccessful in conceiving a baby. In 40 percent of infertility cases, the woman has the major, but not necessarily the only, problem preventing the pregnancy. In 40 percent of the cases, the man is the major factor. In 20 percent, each person makes a substantial contribution to the problem. Therefore, both partners must deal with the infertility and be involved in the treatment.

The solution to a couple's infertility involves evaluation and therapy. The couple will be evaluated in regard to their present sexual activity and history, such as whether either one has ever contributed to a pregnancy. The medical evaluation of both partners will include a physical examination, laboratory tests, and even imaging techniques such as X rays, ultrasonography, or magnetic resonance imaging (MRI). For the man, the physical examination will include a search for the presence of varicoceles, and the laboratory tests will include a semen analysis. About 15 to 30 percent of couples entering an infertility program achieve pregnancy during the evaluation phase of the program, before any therapy is begun.

Varicoceles are probably the most readily detected problem that may cause male infertility. They are three times more common in infertile men than in men with proved fertility. This association does not prove that varicoceles cause infertility, however, because surgery that corrects a varicocele does not always correct infertility.

If the medical evaluation determines that the female partner has a normal reproductive tract and is ovulating on a regular basis, and if it determines that the male partner has too few normal sperm to make a pregnancy likely, the couple may be asked to consider adopting a baby or undergoing therapeutic insemination. With therapeutic insemination, the woman actually becomes pregnant, and half of the baby's genes come from the mother. The other half of the genes come from the sperm donor, usually a person unknown to the couple. The physician performing therapeutic insemination may provide the couple with extensive information on several possible donors. Such information might include race, ethnic origin, blood type, physical characteristics, results of medical and genetic tests, and personal information, but the donor usually remains anonymous. The semen from each donor has undergone laboratory testing and cryopreservation. The frozen semen is thawed at the time of insemination.

Although the idea of therapeutic insemination is simple, it usually involves some very complicated emotions. Although a couple may be very happy about all other aspects of their lives together, they are usually deeply disturbed to learn of the man's infertility. It may be extremely difficult for them to discuss his infertility with anyone else. Some people ridicule infertile men as being less virile or even being impotent. (This is not the case: The majority of infertile or sterile men have normal sex lives.) These feelings will influence the couple's selection of a sperm donor. Later, they must decide whether to tell the child about the circumstances of his or her birth. Sometimes, a child who originated through therapeutic insemination will try to learn the identity of the donor.

The donor must be considered as well. In a typical sperm bank, persons are subjected to a variety of tests before they are accepted as donors. Sperm donors are typically in their second decade of life, but some are older. These men are primarily, but not solely, motivated to be sperm donors by financial compensation. Payment effectively maintains donor cooperation for a period of several years. In addition to payment, the donor usually wants an assurance that he will not be held responsible, financially or legally, for the offspring produced by his semen. As a donor grows older, however, his attitude about his donation may change: He may wonder about the children he has helped to create.

Although male-factor infertility is the situation that benefits most from insemination and semen cryopreservation procedures, these procedures might be requested by a fertile couple that is at risk for male-factor infertility. Such couples may fear that the man's lifestyle, such as working with hazardous materials (solvents, toxins, radioisotopes, or explosives), may endanger his ability to produce sperm or may harm his genetic information. The man could be facing medical therapy that will cure a malignancy, such as Hodgkin's disease or a testicular tumor, but may render him sterile. A man facing such a situation may benefit from having some of his semen cryopreserved for his own future use, in the event that he actually becomes infertile.

Therapeutic insemination with a husband's semen is usually not as effective as with donor semen, especially when cryopreservation is involved. Although cryopreservation keeps cells alive in the frozen state, not all the cells survive. Men selected to be semen donors have sperm that survive freezing much better than the sperm of most men (although the reason for this ability is unknown). If a man undergoing medical treatment is already sick at the time that the decision is made to store his sperm, his concentration of functioning sperm may be less than normal.

There are ways to compensate for decreased semen quality. The semen may be processed in ways to increase the concentration of normal sperm. The processed semen may be placed directly into the woman's uterus (intrauterine insemination) rather than on her cervix, or in vitro fertilization may be used. In this procedure, the sperm and eggs are mixed in a laboratory and the resulting embryo is implanted in the woman. All these techniques have proved helpful to infertile couples wanting children.

PERSPECTIVE AND PROSPECTS

It has been estimated that infertility affects 8 to 15 percent of American marriages, which means that three to nine million American couples would like to, but cannot, have children without medical assistance. By the early 1990's, therapeutic insemination produced more than thirty thousand American babies yearly. This procedure advanced in the United States during the latter half of the twentieth century in large measure because of changes in attitudes, not because of new medical knowledge.

The medical knowledge to treat male infertility has been available for several centuries, even when the biological basis for pregnancy was not understood. The importance of sexual intercourse in reproduction was probably recognized by prehistoric humans. The Bible records stories of patriarchal families that knew the problem of infertility (Abraham and Sarah, Jacob and Rachel) and even indicates, in the story of Onan and Tamar (Genesis 38:9), that semen was understood to be important to reproduction. The possibility of therapeutic insemination was mentioned in the fifth century Talmud. Arabs used insemination in horse breeding as early as the fourteenth century, and Spaniards used it in human medicine during the fifteenth century.

The presence of sperm in semen was first observed by Antoni van Leeuwenhoek in the seventeenth century, but their importance and function in the fertilization process was not recognized until the nineteenth century. In 1824, Jean Louis Prévost and J. A. Dumas correctly guessed the role of sperm in fertilization, and in 1876, Oskar Hertwig and Hermann Fol proved that the union of sperm and egg was necessary to create an embryo.

Therapeutic insemination became an established but clandestine procedure in the late nineteenth century in the United States and England. Compassionate physicians pioneering therapeutic insemination encouraged secrecy to protect the self esteem of the infertile man, his spouse, the offspring, and the donor. In an uncertain legal climate, the offspring might have been viewed as the illegitimate product of an adulterous act. Even by the beginning of the twenty-first century, many Americans continued to stigmatize masturbation and therapeutic insemination. Social attitudes, especially machismo, have limited the acceptability of therapeutic insemination to many infertile couples worldwide.

Cryopreservation of sperm became practical with the discovery of chemical cryoprotectants, reported in 1949 by Christopher Polge, Audrey Smith, and Alan Parkes of England. In 1953, American doctors R. G. Bunge and Jerome Sherman were the first to use this procedure to produce a human baby. Cryopreservation made possible the establishment of sperm banks; prior to this development, sperm donors had to provide the physician with semen immediately before insemination was to take place.

Recent research has shown a few promising new techniques: intracytoplasmic injection, which involves the placement of sperm into the ovum itself, and electroejaculation, which involves electrical stimulation of the penis to promote ejaculation. Intracytoplasmic injections are useful when the sperm are immotile or the woman's own immune system aggressively rejects the man's sperm. It is not always successful, however, and is affected by age and cycle. Electroejaculation has been successfully used in men with vascular compromise, as might be caused by diabetes mellitus, or with spinal cord injuries. It is also helpful in cases where men are unable to ejaculate for psychological reasons.

Researchers continue to theorize about new fertility-enhancing techniques using sperm. In 2003, scientists discovered that sperm has a type of chemical sensor that causes the sperm to swim vigorously toward concentrations of a chemical attractant. While researchers long have known that chemical signals are an important component of conception, the 2003 findings were the first to demonstrate that sperm will respond in a predictable and controllable way. The findings provided strong evidence that the egg signals its location to the sperm and the sperm responds by swimming toward the egg, a process which could prove promising for future contraception and infertility research. Scientists note that these findings might allow specific tests to be developed to determine if the egg is making the attractant or if the sperm has the receptor, thus helping in identifying those couples who are infertile because of poor signaling between the sperm and egg.

Therapeutic insemination and other alternative means of reproduction give rise to thorny issues of personal rights of various "parents" (social, birth, and genetic) and their offspring. In the United States, a few states have addressed these issues by enacting laws, usually to grant legitimacy to offspring of donor insemination. In the United Kingdom, Parliament established a central registry of sperm and egg donors. Offspring in the United Kingdom have access to nonidentifying donor information; these children are even able to learn whether they are genetically related to a prospective marriage partner.

—Armand M. Karow, Ph.D.;
updated by Paul Moglia, Ph.D.

See also Assisted reproductive technologies; Conception; Gamete intrafallopian transfer (GIFT); Genital disorders, male; In vitro fertilization; Infertility in females; Pregnancy and gestation; Reproductive system; Sexual dysfunction; Sperm banks; Sterilization; Stress; Testicular surgery; Vasectomy.

FOR FURTHER INFORMATION:

Baran, Annette, and Reuben Pannor. *Lethal Secrets.* New York: Warner Books, 1993. The authors, medical social workers, discuss possible consequences of secrecy in donor insemination using a series of case histories.

Berger, Gary S., et al. *The Couple's Guide to Fertility.* 3d ed. New York: Broadway Books, 2001. Surveys fertility treatment options, including hormone therapies, surgery, in vitro fertilization, sperm injection, egg and sperm donors, adoption, surrogate motherhood, and alternative therapies.

Doherty, C. Maud, and Melanie M. Clark. *Fertility Handbook: A Guide to Getting Pregnant.* Omaha, Nebr.: Addicus Books, 2002. The authors, a reproductive endocrinologist and a former infertility patient, combine their experiences to explore current infertility options and treatments. Addresses the causes, getting diagnoses, choosing a fertility specialist, and utilizing new assisted reproductive technology.

Glover, Timothy D., and C. L. R. Barratt, eds. *Male Fertility and Infertility.* New York: Cambridge University Press, 1999. The editors have assembled a collection of essays by experts in the field. Includes bibliographical references and an index.

International Council on Infertility Information Dissemination. http://www.inciid.org/. INCIID's mission is to provide on-line resources of comprehensive, consumer-targeted infertility information that cover cutting-edge technologies and treatments. Provides fact sheets of treatments, an interactive area for member participation, library and glossary, and a comprehensive professional directory of clinics and doctors who specialize in infertility.

Schover, Leslie R., and Anthony J. Thomas. *Overcoming Male Infertility: Understanding Its Causes and Treatments.* New York: John Wiley & Sons, 2000. Clinical psychologist Schover has long worked with infertile couples, as urologist Thomas has with male infertility. Their combined skills and knowledge make this a valuable book. Patient-oriented, it conveys a vast amount of information understandably and maintains an underlying sense of humor.

Taguchi, Yosh, and Merrily Weisbord, eds. *Private Parts: An Owner's Guide to the Male Anatomy.* Toronto: McClelland & Stewart, 2003. A guide to male genital and sexual health, covering topics such as prostate trouble, erectile dysfunction, infertility, cancer, sexually transmitted diseases, vasectomies, and artificial insemination.

Warnock, Mary. *A Question of Life.* New York: Basil Blackwell, 1993. This report, commissioned by the British Parliament, discusses medical procedures for alleviating infertility and social issues of family formation and inheritance.

INFLAMMATION

DISEASE/DISORDER

ANATOMY OR SYSTEM AFFECTED: All

SPECIALTIES AND RELATED FIELDS: Family practice, internal medicine, pathology, rheumatology

DEFINITION: The reaction of blood-filled living tissue to injury.

In inflammation, the following changes are seen locally: redness, swelling, heat, pain, and loss of function. These changes are chemically mediated. Inflammation may be caused by microbial infection; physical agents such as trauma, radiation, and burns; chemical toxins; caustic substances such as strong acids or bases; decomposing or necrotic tissue; and reactions of the immune system. Acute inflammation is of relatively short duration (from a few minutes to a day or so), while chronic inflammation lasts longer. The local changes associated with inflammation include the outflow of fluid into the spaces between cells and the inflow or migration of white blood cells (leukocytes) to the area of injury. Chronic inflammation is characterized by the presence of leukocytes and macrophages, as well as by the proliferation of new blood vessels and connective tissue.

Inflammation is a protective mechanism for the body. Redness is attributable to increased blood flow to the injured area. Swelling is caused by the flow of fluid into the spaces between cells. Heat is produced by a combination of increased blood flow and chemical reactions in the local area. Pain results from the presence of two main chemicals found in the bloodstream: prostaglandins and bradykinin. Loss of function is a result of pain (the body limits movement to reduce discomfort) and swelling (interstitial fluid limits movement).

Acute inflammation. Many chemicals are involved in acute inflammation. Mediators of inflammation originate from blood plasma and from both damaged and normal cells. Vasoactive amines are a class of chemicals that increase the permeability of blood vessel and cell walls. The most well studied of these are histamine and serotonin. Histamine is stored in granules in mast cells that are found in both tissue and basophils, the latter being a type of cell found in the blood. Serotonin is found in mast cells and platelets; it is another type of cell found in the bloodstream. These substances cause vasodilation (expansion of the walls of blood vessels) and increased vascular permeability (leakage through the walls of small vessels, especially veins). Histamine and serotonin can be released by trauma or exposure to cold. Other chemicals that circulate in the blood can release histamine. Two of these are part of the complement system; another is called interleukin-1. The effects of histamine diminish after approximately one hour.

Plasma proteases comprise three interrelated systems that explain much that is known about inflammation: the complement, kinin, and clotting systems. The complement system is composed of twenty different proteins involved in reactions against microbial agents that invade the body. The various chemicals act in a cascade, similar to falling dominoes: Each one sets off another in sequence. The result of these chemical actions is to increase vascular permeability, promote chemotaxis (the attraction of living cells to specific chemicals), engulf invading microorganisms, and destroy pathogens through a process called lysis.

The kinin system is responsible for releasing bradykinin, a chemical substance that causes contraction of smooth muscle tissue, dilation of blood vessels, and pain. The duration of action for bradykinin is brief because it is inactivated by the enzyme kininase. Bradykinin does not promote chemotaxis.

The clotting system is made up of a series of chemicals that result in the formation of a solid mass. The most commonly encountered example is the scab that forms at the site of a cut in the skin. Like the complement system, the clotting system is a cascade of thirteen different chemicals. In addition to producing a solid mass, the clotting system also increases vascular permeability and promotes chemotaxis for white blood cells.

Other substances are involved in acute inflammation. Among the most important of these is a class called prostaglandins. Several different prostaglandin molecules have been isolated; they are derived from the membranes of most cells. Prostaglandins cause pain, vasodilation, and fever. Aspirin counteracts the effects of prostaglandins, which explains the antipyretic (fever-reducing) and analgesic (pain-reducing) properties of the drug.

Another group of substances involved in acute inflammation are leukotrienes. The primary sources for these molecules are leukocytes, and some leukotrienes are found in mast cells. This group promotes vascular leakage but not chemotaxis. They also cause vasoconstriction (a decrease in the diameter of blood vessels) and bronchoconstriction (a decrease in the diameter of air passageways in the lungs). The effect of these leukotrienes is to slow blood flow and restrict air intake and outflow. A different type of leukotriene is found only in leukocytes. This type enhances chemotaxis but does not contribute to vascular leakage. In addition, leukotrienes cause white blood cells to stick to damaged tissues, speeding the removal of bacteria and promoting healing.

Other chemical substances are known to be involved with inflammation: platelet-activating factor, tumor necrosis factor, interleukin-1, cationic (positively charged) proteins, neutral proteases (enzymes that break down proteins), and oxygen metabolites (molecules resulting from reactions with oxygen). The sources of these are generally leukocytes, although some are derived from macrophages. They reinforce the effects of prostaglandins and leukotrienes.

There are four different outcomes for acute inflammation. There may be complete resolution in which the injured site is restored to normal; this outcome usually follows a mild injury or limited trauma where there has been only minor tissue destruction. Healing with scarring may occur, in which injured tissue is replaced with scar tissue that is rich in collagen, giving it strength but at the cost of normal function; this outcome follows more severe injury or extensive destruction of tissue. There may be the formation of an abscess, which is characterized by pus and which follows injuries that become infected with pyogenic (pus-forming) organisms. The fourth outcome is chronic inflammation.

Chronic inflammation. Acute inflammation may be followed by chronic inflammation. This reaction occurs when the organism, factor, or agent responsible for the acute inflammation is not removed or when the normal processes of healing fail to occur. Repeated episodes of acute inflammation may also lead to chronic inflammation, in which the stages of acute inflammation seem to remain for long periods of time. In addition, chronic inflammation may begin insidiously, such as with a low-grade infection that does not display the usual signs of acute inflammation; tuberculosis, rheumatoid arthritis, and chronic lung disease are examples of this third alternative.

Chronic inflammation typically occurs in one of the following conditions: prolonged exposure to potentially toxic substances such as asbestos, coal dust, and silica that are nondegradable; immune reactions against one's own tissue (autoimmune diseases such as lupus and rheumatoid arthritis); and persistent infection by an organism that is either resistant to drug therapy or insufficiently toxic to cause an immune reaction (such as viruses, tuberculosis, and leprosy). The characteristics of chronic inflammation are similar to those of acute inflammation but are less dramatic and more protracted.

—*L. Fleming Fallon, Jr., M.D., Ph.D., M.P.H.*

See also Abscess drainage; Abscesses; Arthritis; Burns and scalds; Bursitis; Disease; Healing; Infection; Wounds; *specific diseases.*

FOR FURTHER INFORMATION:

Challem, Jack. *The Inflammation Syndrome: The Complete Nutritional Program to Prevent and Reverse Heart Disease, Arthritis, Diabetes, Allergies, and Asthma.* New York: Wiley, 2003. Explores the cumulative effect of low-grade inflammation that grows into chronic, debilitating diseases, including heart disease, diabetes, Syndrome X, obesity, arthritis, allergies, and asthma. Covers anti-inflammatory drugs and the impact of nutrition.

Eggs, William Joel, and Carol Svec. *The Inflammation Cure.* New York: McGraw-Hill, 2003. Examines recent research linkages between inflammation and heart disease, as well as diseases associated with aging including arthritis, Alzheimer's disease, osteoporosis, and some cancers. Covers causes, treatments, and lifestyle changes to promote wellness.

Gallin, John I., Ira M. Goldstein, and Ralph Snyderman, eds. *Inflammation: Basic Principles and Clinical Correlates.* 3d ed. New York: Raven Press, 1999. This well-written book is for the reader who wants to know about inflammation in great detail.

Gorski, Andrzej, et al., eds. *Inflammation.* Boston: Kluwer, 2001. A series of papers review current understanding of inflammatory processes and responses, from allergies to life-threatening sepsis, and evaluate therapeutic strategies aimed at combating inflammatory diseases.

Majno, Guido, Ramzi Cotran, and Nathan Kaufman, eds. *Current Topics in Inflammation and Infection.* Baltimore: Williams & Wilkins, 1982. This specialized monograph provides extensive details on the subject. It assumes that the reader is familiar with the basics of inflammation.

Robbins, Stanley L., Ramzi S. Cotran, and Vinay Kumar, eds. *Robbins' Pathologic Basis of Disease.* 6th ed. Philadelphia: W. B. Saunders, 1999. A widely used pathology text which contains a good discussion of inflammation. Written for health professionals, but the serious nonspecialist will find a wealth of material.

INFLUENZA

DISEASE/DISORDER

ANATOMY OR SYSTEM AFFECTED: Lungs, respiratory system

SPECIALTIES AND RELATED FIELDS: Epidemiology, family practice, internal medicine, public health, virology

DEFINITION: Any one of a group of commonly experienced respiratory diseases caused by viruses, responsible for many major, worldwide epidemics.

KEY TERMS:

antibody: a protein substance produced by white blood cells (lymphocytes) in response to an antigen; combats bacterial, viral, chemical, or other invasive agents in the body

antigen: a chemical substance, often on a bacterial or viral surface, containing substances that activate the body's immune response

pneumonia: a respiratory tract infection that can be caused by bacteria or viruses; it is the major complication of influenza and the major cause of influenza deaths

ribonucleic acid (RNA): the material contained in the core of many viruses that is responsible for directing the replication of the virus inside the host cell

Causes and Symptoms

Epidemics of what scientists believe was influenza have been reported in Europe and Asia for at least one thousand years. Epidemics of what could have been influenza were reported by ancient Greek and Roman historians. Influenza epidemics still occur, striking isolated societies, entire nations, or, as with pandemics, the entire world. Among the great plagues that have afflicted the world over the centuries, influenza is the one that remains active today. Smallpox has been conquered, and bubonic plague (the Black Death), yellow fever, and typhus no longer erupt every few years as they once did. Cholera still breaks out, but rarely as a major epidemic. Before acquired immunodeficiency syndrome (AIDS), influenza was called "the last of the great plagues."

The term "influenza" is from the Italian and refers to the fact that some early scientists thought that the disease was caused by the malevolent influence of the planets, stars, and other heavenly bodies. To others, this "influence" was a miasma or poisonous effluvium carried in the air—a theory which is closer to the truth.

In the eighteenth and nineteenth centuries, there were about twenty major epidemics of influenza in Europe and America. They were of varying severity—some mild, some harsh. In 1918, a pandemic of influenza became one of the worst afflictions ever endured by humankind. It came in three waves, the first in the spring of 1918. This wave was relatively mild and mortality rates were low, and it spread evenly through all age groups of the population. The second wave came in the fall, and it was the most devastating outbreak of disease seen since the great plagues of the Middle Ages. Up to 20 percent of its victims died, and about half the deaths were of people in the prime of life, twenty to forty years of age. The last wave came in the winter and was not as severe. By the time that the pandemic was

over, more than 20 million people worldwide had died from it, with more than 500,000 deaths in the United States alone.

In 1918, scientists understood enough about microbiology to realize that a microorganism caused influenza, but they originally thought that it was a bacterium, *Haemophilus influenzae*, because this organism was isolated from some of the victims. *H. influenzae* causes many diseases, but influenza is not among them, as researchers found when infection from it failed to produce influenza symptoms in test subjects. It soon became apparent that the organism responsible for influenza was unlike any bacterium that science had yet encountered. Bacteria were easily seen in the microscope and could be collected in filters. Whatever it was that caused influenza was invisible to the microscope, and it could not be trapped in filters. So, scientists postulated that the influenza pathogen was far smaller than bacteria. They used the term "filtrable virus" to describe it—an interesting locution, because what they meant was that the organism could *not* be filtered by the devices that they were using. "Filter-passing virus," another term used at the time, is more accurate.

It was not until 1931, thirteen years after the great pandemic, that the first influenza virus was isolated. It was found in swine, and the methods used to discover it formed the basis for the techniques used to isolate the human influenza virus, a major event in microbiology that occurred in 1933.

It was later found that there were not one but three kinds of human influenza virus: type A, which is the major cause of severe influenza outbreaks; type B, which also causes influenza epidemics but less often and which is usually less severe than type A; and the rarest, type C, which causes a mild, coldlike illness.

Further, it was discovered that there are different strains of virus within type A and type B, subtypes that are not identical to one another but that are related. Within each subtype there are variants. As these subtypes and variants began to appear, it became clear that the virus was capable of mutation. This was a critical discovery because it meant that influenza infection of one type would not necessarily immunize the victim against influenza of another type. This ability to mutate means that new influenza virus strains are constantly being developed—and are constantly threatening new waves of disease.

For example, in 1957, a new strain of influenza virus called the Asian flu came out of China and started a pandemic. Asian flu, or variants of it, caused the flu ep-

---

Information on Influenza

Causes: Viral infection

Symptoms: Fever, malaise, headache, muscle pain (particularly in back and legs), coughing, nasal congestion, shivering, sore throat

Duration: Acute

Treatments: Typically alleviation of symptoms; sometimes antiviral drugs (*e.g.*, ribavirin)

idemics in the years from 1957 to 1968, but immunity to it spread so that the severity of the epidemics was gradually reduced. Then the Hong Kong flu, another new strain from the Far East, appeared. People had no immunity to it, so it caused another major pandemic. Hong Kong flu and its variants caused the epidemics that occurred in the next nine years. Then, in 1977, still another pandemic arose from a newer strain, also from Eastern Asia.

In 1976, another type, swine flu, appeared in the United States. This virus infects pigs and humans and is apparently a distant descendant of the virus that caused the 1918 pandemic. It was evidently not as hardy as the 1977 virus, because that one replaced it and swine flu disappeared, although some experts predict its return.

The reason that the influenza virus can mutate readily is related to its physiological structure. The virus is usually spherical, but the shape can vary. It is extremely small, about 0.0001 millimeter in diameter. Its surface is covered with spikes of protein, hemagglutinin and neuraminidase. They are the two major antigens that trigger the body's immune system to repel the virus and provide immunity against future infection. Hemagglutinin (H) causes red blood cells to agglutinate, or clump together. Neuraminidase (N) is an enzyme.

Inside the core of the virus are two additional antigens that trigger the production of antibodies, but these antibodies do not protect against future infection. Also in the core is a feature unique to influenza virus: Instead of a single strand of ribonucleic acid (RNA), there are eight individual strands, each one a single gene. Genes are said to be "encoded" to produce specific characteristics within an organism. When the virus invades a host cell, the RNA directs a process of replication in which components of the cell are used to make new viruses. The new viruses are then released to enter other cells and continue replicating.

The H and N antigens mutate gradually over the years because of changes in the RNA genes that encode for them. This process is called antigenic drift, and it refers to slight variations that appear in the influenza virus and account for minor and localized epidemics of the disease. When a particular strain of virus has been prevalent for some time, a "herd immunity" develops in the populations exposed to it, and incidence of disease from it declines. When the H or N antigen changes radically, the process is called antigenic shift. It creates a new subtype of the virus, one that can cause a major pandemic because there is no immunity to it. There are at least thirteen variants of H (labeled H1 to H13) and at least nine variants of N (labeled N1 to N9).

Before 1968, most influenza A viruses in circulation had H2N2 antigens on their surfaces. This type of virus was the Asian flu; it had been around for some years, so the world population had become relatively immune to it. Then, in 1968, a new virus appeared in Southeast Asia, with a combination of H3N2. The H antigen had changed completely, while the N antigen remained the same, but the combination was essentially a new virus; it gave rise to the worldwide epidemic of the Hong Kong flu.

It is known that influenza viruses from animals influence the structure of the human viruses and contribute the varia-

An enlarged view of the influenza virus. (Digital Stock)

tions that become new strains capable of causing pandemics. There is an interesting theory of how the 1957, 1968, and 1977 pandemics that came out of China developed. The Chinese people not only eat an enormous amount of duck but also keep large flocks to eat insects that attack rice crops. Ducks carry a wide variety of influenza viruses in their intestines, and they live in close proximity to humans. This theory suggests that the influenza viruses from duck droppings modified the human influenza virus and created the new strains that caused the pandemics that emanated from China. Other animals, such as pigs, which gave the world swine flu, also harbor influenza viruses that can interact with the human influenza virus.

To cause disease, the virus must be inhaled, which is why the "influence" of poisonous effluvium carried in the air is a more correct attribution of the actual cause of the disease than the influence of heavenly bodies. Inside the upper respiratory tract, there is a layer of cilia-bearing cells (cells with small, hairlike filaments) that acts as a barrier against infection. Ordinarily, the tiny cilia spread a layer of mucus over respiratory tissues. The mucus collects infectious organisms and carries them to the stomach, where they are destroyed by stomach acids. The influenza virus causes the cilia-bearing cells to disintegrate, exposing a layer of cells beneath. The virus invades these and other host cells in the respiratory tract and begins replicating. Invasion and replication by the virus destroy the host cells. Destruction of the cells starts the inflammatory process that causes the symptoms of disease.

Influenza infection grows rapidly, and symptoms can appear in only a few hours, although the incubation period in most people is two days or so. Fever, malaise, headache, muscular pain (particularly in the back and legs), coughing, nasal congestion, shivering, and a sore throat are common symptoms. The disease can spread quickly among populations because the virus is airborne. There is good reason to believe that the virus can remain infective in the air for long periods of time. It has been reported that the crew members on a ship sailing past Cuba during an epidemic there were infected with the disease, presumably from virus-laden particles carried from shore by the wind.

The major complication of influenza is pneumonia, which can be caused by the influenza virus itself (primary influenza viral pneumonia), by infection from bacteria (secondary bacterial pneumonia), or by mixed viral and bacterial infection. Pneumonia is the major cause of death from influenza. In the severe pandemic of 1918, up to 20 percent of patients developed pneumonia and, of these, about half died.

Primary influenza viral pneumonia can come on suddenly, and it often progresses relentlessly with high fever, rapidly accumulating congestion in the lungs, and difficulty in breathing. Pneumonia caused by secondary bacterial infection can be caused by a large number of pathogens. In nonhospitalized patients, both children and adults, the common causes are pneumococci, streptococci, and *Haemophilus influenzae*. In older, infirm, or hospitalized patients, the common causes are pneumococci, staphylococci, and *Klebsiella pneumoniae*.

When influenza B is the pathogen, Reye's syndrome can develop, most often in children under eighteen. This disease, which causes brain and liver damage, is fatal in about 21 percent of cases.

TREATMENT AND THERAPY

There are two main goals of therapy for the patient with influenza: treatment and preventing the spread of the disease. The first aim of therapy is to keep the patient comfortable, address the symptoms of the disease that can be treated, and deal with any complications that may arise. Bed rest is recommended, particularly during the most severe stages of the disease. Exertion is to be avoided, in order to prevent excessive weakness that could encourage further infection. Aspirin, acetaminophen, and other drugs are given for fever, and painkillers are given to relieve aches and pains. Cough suppressants and expectorants can relieve the hacking coughs that develop. Drinking large amounts of liquids is advised to replace the fluids lost as a result of high fever and sweating.

Amantadine hydrochloride is sometimes given to patients with influenza A infection. It reduces fever and relieves respiratory symptoms. An analogue of amantadine, rimantadine, works similarly. In severe cases of influenza caused by either A or B virus, an antiviral drug called ribavirin can be administered as a mist to be breathed in by the patient. Ribavirin shortens the duration of fever and may alleviate primary influenza viral pneumonia.

Primary influenza viral pneumonia is usually treated in the intensive care unit of a hospital, where the patient is given oxygen and other procedures are used to give respiratory and hemodynamic support. Secondary bacterial pneumonia must be treated with appropriate antibiotics. Identifying the precise bacterium will help the physician decide which antibiotic to prescribe. This identification is not always feasible, however, in which case broad-spectrum antibiotics will be used. They are effective against the most common bacteria that cause these secondary infections: *Streptococcus pneumoniae, Staphylococcus aureus,* and *Haemophilus influenzae.*

In preventing the spread of influenza, the first line of defense is to isolate the patient from susceptible persons and to initiate a program of vaccination. Because the influenza virus is constantly mutating, vaccines are regularly reformulated to confer immunity to the current pathogens. For the most part, the differences are not great between one year's virus and the one causing the next year's disease. Current vaccines may confer immunity or may require adjustment. If a major antigenic mutation has occurred, however, immunity cannot be conferred unless a new vaccine is developed against the new strain. Because it can take months to develop a new vaccine, there is the danger that the epidemic will have run its course and infected entire populations by the time that the vaccine is ready. Fortunately, major pandemics of influenza usually start slowly, so researchers have the time to identify the new strain, create a vaccine, and disseminate it.

The usual recommendation is to vaccinate people who are at highest risk of complications from the disease. These people include those over sixty-five years of age; residents of nursing homes or other patients with chronic medical conditions; adults and children with chronic pulmonary or cardiovascular diseases, including children with asthma; adults and children who have been hospitalized during the previous year for metabolic disorders, such as diabetes mellitus, or for renal diseases, blood disorders, or immunosuppression; teenagers and children who are receiving long-term aspirin therapy (who may be at risk of developing Reye's syndrome as a result of influenza infection); and pregnant women whose third trimester occurs in winter.

When a family member brings influenza into the household, other members should be vaccinated. After vaccination, it usually takes about two weeks for immunity to develop. Amantadine may protect against influenza A in the meantime; it can be discontinued after immunity has been achieved. If, for any reason, a person cannot be vaccinated, amantadine should be given throughout the entire length of the epidemic, which may last six to eight weeks.

A history of influenza vaccine development beginning with the identification of the virus in 1933 illustrates how constant vigilance is required to combat the disease. Various influenza vaccines were developed from 1935 to 1942, but they were all unsatisfactory.

Building on the work that had gone before them, Thomas Francis and Jonas Salk (who later developed the first polio vaccine) produced a vaccine in 1942 that conferred immunity against the current strains of both influenza A and influenza B. Intensive animal testing and human trials showed that the vaccine was effective for about a year.

In 1947, however, many people who had been vaccinated came down with the disease: A new strain of influenza A virus had surfaced. The old vaccine had no effect on it, and a new vaccine had to be developed. This pattern has been repeated constantly: The original vaccine of 1942 was effective until a new strain appeared and a new vaccine had to be developed. That one was satisfactory until the next new strain, the Asian flu, appeared in 1957, and the process had to be repeated to find a vaccine that would protect against it. Similarly, in 1968 and in 1977, new vaccines had to be developed, and these have had to be modified to match the changes in the virus.

In 1999, the Food and Drug Administration approved for general use two new anti-influenza medications: Relenza (zanamivir) and Tamiflu. Both drugs act in a similar manner, by inhibiting the activity of the viral neuraminidase, an enzyme on the surface of the virus which is necessary for spread from an infected cell. Tamiflu, manufactured by Roche Laboratories, can be taken as a capsule; Relenza, produced by GlaxoSmithKline, is used as an inhalant.

Though each of the drugs has been found effective in shortening the duration and severity of influenza in some patients, their usefulness is limited. Both must be taken within forty-eight hours of the onset of symptoms, and treatment must continue for about five days. In 2001, the FDA approved a nasal mist for protection against influenza and the accompanying ear infections often seen as a complication. FluMist has proven to be more than 90 percent effective in protecting children against flu variants not found in current vaccines.

The World Health Organization (WHO) maintains reference laboratories around the world to keep up with the mutations of the influenza viruses. Their vigilance discovers new varieties as they appear. The new variants are studied, and vaccines are prepared to immunize against those strains that seem likely to cause extensive epidemics. This activity blunts the force of new pandemics and saves millions of lives.

PERSPECTIVE AND PROSPECTS

Researchers are constantly working to prevent the recurrent epidemics and pandemics of influenza, or at least to make them less severe. The fact that vaccines have to be modified periodically, and new ones developed from time to time, will probably not change.

It is theoretically possible for a pandemic of the severity of 1918 to occur. If a new subtype of the influenza virus were to arise and its initial spread were rapid, it could rage around the globe before an effective vaccine could be developed and made available. Mass devastation and death could result.

Another major concern is the enormous number of influenza virus strains that are living in animals. Hundreds of different types of influenza virus have been isolated from birds alone. These strains have the potential of causing mutations in the human influenza virus, as the Chinese ducks did in causing the Asian flu, the Hong Kong flu viruses, and the virus that caused the pandemic of 1977. In 2004, infections spread by chickens in China resulted in a number of deaths and renewed concerns about mutations.

So far, medical science has been able to produce vaccines capable of protecting against the new mutant viruses as they arise. Even when a significant portion of any society is vaccinated, however, some people still become infected and there are no agents available that can kill the influenza virus. Furthermore, there are few therapeutic measures that can do any more than alleviate individual symptoms. Basically, the body's own immune system is the best therapy currently available.

Chemoprophylaxis (prevention of a disease by the use of a drug) with amantadine is effective in limiting the spread of disease caused by influenza A, but amantadine has some undesirable side effects, and the drug seems to have no effect on the virus itself. Rimantadine, a closely related compound, is equally effective as a chemoprophylactic agent and seems to be better tolerated. It is still considered an experimental drug, however, and it has not been licensed.

No chemotherapeutic agent (a drug capable of curing a disease) has yet been developed that will kill an influenza virus in the same way that an antibiotic destroys bacteria and other microorganisms. The search for antiviral agents is among the most urgent activities in medical science, and the problems are enormous. Yet the science is young. As researchers learn more about the structure, physiology, and activities of viruses, they will also develop means of controlling them.

When an agent is discovered that is safe and effective against influenza virus, it could be subject to the same limitations as the vaccines; that is, it may have to be modified periodically to remain effective against the new strains of influenza virus that are continually developing, and it may be necessary to develop new agents to deal with radically new mutants.

—C. Richard Falcon

See also Antibiotics; Bacterial infections; Centers for Disease Control and Prevention (CDC); Epidemiology; Fever; Lungs; Microbiology; Nausea and vomiting; Noroviruses; Pneumonia; Pulmonary diseases; Pulmonary medicine; Pulmonary medicine, pediatric; Respiration; Reye's syndrome; Viral infections; World Health Organization; Zoonoses.

For Further Information:

Biddle, Wayne. *Field Guide to Germs*. 2d ed. New York: Henry Holt, 2002. This comprehensive book is easily accessible to the nonspecialist and includes a discussion of nearly every virus, bacterium, and fungus known to cause human and nonhuman animal disease. The history of the microbe and the treatment of diseases are included.

Giesecke, Johan. *Modern Infectious Disease Epidemiology*. 2d ed. London: Hodder Arnold, 2001. Divided into two sections, the first covers the tools and principles of epidemiology from an infectious disease perspective. The second covers the role of contact pattern from an assessment angle, exploring such topics as infectivity, incubation periods, seroepidemiology, and immunity.

Kimball, Chad. *Colds, Flu and Other Common Ailments*. New York: Omnigraphics, 2002. A comprehensive guide for general readers covering treatment issues and controversies surrounding common ailments and injuries. Includes discussions on ailments of the nose, throat, lungs, ears, eyes, and head; common injuries; alternative therapies; choosing a doctor; and buying drugs and finding health information online.

Kiple, Kenneth F., ed. *The Cambridge World History of Human Disease*. New York: Cambridge University Press, 1993. The section on influenza gives a useful account of the epidemics and pandemics of influenza throughout the years.

Kolata, Gina. *Flu: The Story of the Great Influenza Pandemic of 1918 and the Search for the Virus That Caused It*. New York: Farrar, Straus and Giroux, 1999. Kolata's book vividly describes how the 1918 influenza outbreak, the most deadly pandemic the United States has ever faced, affected society. It not only offers an apocalyptic vision of the course of the disease but also details the ongoing efforts to track down its source.

Larson, David E., ed. *Mayo Clinic Family Health Book*. 3d ed. New York: William Morrow, 2003. A good general medical text for the layperson. The section on influenza is short but thorough.

Sahelian, Ray, and Victoria Dolby Toews. New York: Avery, 1999. *The Common Cold Cure: Natural Remedies for Colds and Flu*. The miseries of the common cold are many, and while a definitive medical cure remains elusive, its most annoying symptoms can certainly be addressed and, as Sahelian and Toews maintain, its duration shortened without the use of over-the-counter pharmaceuticals.

Tyrrell, David A., and Michael Fielder. *Cold Wars: The Fight Against the Common Cold*. New York: Oxford University Press, 2002. Traces the history of the common cold from ancient Egypt to the modern age and examines advances in its treatment.

Wagner, Edward K., and Martin Hewlett. *Basic Virology*. 2d ed. Boston: Blackwell, 2003. A very readable undergraduate text covering issues of virology and viral disease, properties of viruses and virus-cell interaction, working with viruses, and replication patterns of specific viruses.

INSECT BITES. *See* BITES AND STINGS.

INSOMNIA. *See* SLEEP DISORDERS.

INSULIN RESISTANCE SYNDROME
DISEASE/DISORDER

ALSO KNOWN AS: Syndrome X, Deadly Quartet, metabolic syndrome

ANATOMY OR SYSTEM AFFECTED: All

SPECIALTIES AND RELATED FIELDS: Cardiology, endocrinology, internal medicine, nutrition

DEFINITION: A reduced sensitivity to the action of insulin, which brings glucose into body tissues to be used as a source of energy.

KEY TERMS:

glucose: blood sugar

insulin: a peptide hormone secreted by the pancreas; it helps the body by promoting glucose utilization, protein synthesis, and the formation and storage of neutral lipids by regulating the sugar metabolism

syndrome: a cluster of symptoms

CAUSES AND SYMPTOMS

Normally, after a meal, the body digests food, nutrients are absorbed into the blood, and the level of glucose (sugar) in the blood rises. Glucose is then quickly transported into cells for use, as glucose is the principal energy source in the human body. Most tissues, particularly skeletal muscle tissue, require insulin action to transport glucose into cells. Insulin, a hormone secreted by the pancreas, helps transport glucose into cells by binding with receptors on cells as a key would fit into a lock. Once the key—insulin—has fitted into the lock and unlocked the door, the cell allows the entry of glucose, and the glucose can pass from the bloodstream into the cell. Inside cells, glucose is either used for energy or stored for future use in the form of glycogen in liver or muscle cells.

Insulin resistance occurs when the normal amount of insulin secreted by the pancreas is not able to unlock the door for glucose entering into cells. In some cases, the pancreas secretes additional insulin to maintain a normal blood glucose level. In other cases, when the body cells do not respond to even higher levels of insulin, glucose builds up in the blood resulting in a high blood glucose (sugar) level, or Type II diabetes (non-insulin-dependent diabetes). Thus, the consequences of insulin resistance include decreased insulin function throughout the body, and hyperinsulinemia (a high insulin level in the blood).

However, insulin resistance does not occur alone. People with insulin resistance often have some other abnormalities, including an increased level of triglycerides (blood fat), a decreased level of high-density lipoprotein (HDL) cholesterol (good cholesterol), hypertension (high blood pressure), and obesity (overweight). This cluster of abnormalities, together with hyperinsulinemia and hyperglycemia (high blood glucose), is called insulin resistance syndrome, which is also known as Syndrome X or Deadly Quartet. The

---

INFORMATION ON INSULIN RESISTANCE SYNDROME

CAUSES: Unclear, possibly genetic disorders; aggravated by obesity and physical inactivity

SYMPTOMS: Often asymptomatic; can include hypertension and obesity

DURATION: Typically long-term

TREATMENTS: Lifestyle changes (caloric restriction, weight loss, exercise); drug therapy (metformin, troglitazone)

syndrome is a cluster of risk factors for heart disease, and insulin resistance may be the common factor linking other risk factors.

The cause of insulin resistance is still not clear as of today. Some scientists believe that a defect in specific genes may result in insulin resistance and Type II diabetes. What is currently known is that insulin resistance is aggravated by obesity and physical inactivity.

As a consequence of hyperinsulinemia, additional fat is stored in the body, because the body is trying to protect itself by turning excess insulin into triglyceride. High insulin levels in the blood also contribute to high levels of low-density lipoprotein (LDL) cholesterol (so-called bad cholesterol), low levels of high-density lipoprotein (HDL) cholesterol, and hypertension. Obesity, associated with insulin resistance, often shows as upper body obesity.

Because insulin resistance syndrome does not have any outward physical signs, 20 to 25 percent of the "healthy" population may be insulin resistant but are not aware of it. Almost all individuals with Type II diabetes and many with hypertension, cardiovascular disease, and obesity are insulin resistant.

TREATMENT AND THERAPY

Insulin resistance often goes unrecognized until later in life when metabolic abnormalities develop. Thus, the first step of the treatment for this disorder is to identify those who may be at risk, including those who are overweight, have a parent or sibling with Type II diabetes, and have high blood pressure. Women who had diabetes during pregnancy also have a higher risk for this disorder. To diagnose this disorder, the oral glucose tolerance test can be used.

It is possible to reduce insulin resistance by caloric restriction, weight loss, exercise, and drug therapy. The multiple risk factor intervention treatment is usually recommended, aiming aggressively at reducing all cardiac risk factors that may exist. The key of this multiple risk factor intervention treatment is the modification of lifestyle. Lowering calorie intake can reduce insulin resistance within a few days. A diet low in saturated fat (less than 10 percent of total calories) and more moderate in total fat content (less than 40 percent of total calories) is beneficial. Concentrated sweets should be cut down. Weight loss, maintenance of ideal body weight, and regular exercise are essential. This kind of behavioral intervention is recommended for all those who have hypertension, high cholesterol, simple obesity, heart disease, diabetes, or insulin resistance syndrome.

If medical treatment is necessary, a variety of drugs are available, such as metformin and troglitazone. Metformin is a drug which enhances insulin sensitivity without affecting insulin secretion (not effective in the absence of insulin). It lowers glucose by decreasing glucose production in the liver. In addition, metformin decreases blood pressure, induces weight loss, and has a beneficial effect on lowering LDL cholesterol and triglyceride levels. Metformin has several gastrointestinal side effects, including diarrhea, nausea, and anorexia. These symptoms often improve with dosage reduction. Metformin also impairs absorption of vitamin B_{12} and folic acid but rarely causes clinical symptoms. In patients with kidney or heart disease, the use of metformin can increase the risk of lactic acidosis.

Troglitazone increases glucose transport. The treatment effect from troglitazone may not occur until two to three weeks after initiation of the drug. Troglitazone decreases the concentration of blood glucose and triglycerides, but increases HDL cholesterol. Some clinical trials have also shown that troglitazone decreases blood pressure. One important side effect of troglitazone is liver dysfunction. Thus, the liver function should be checked each month for the first six months of therapy, every two months for the next six months, and periodically thereafter. Often a combined therapy (using two or more drugs) plus behavioral intervention are used together for the treatment of insulin resistance.

PERSPECTIVE AND PROSPECTS

No data are currently available to determine if long-term drug therapy aimed at reducing insulin resistance can prevent the development of diabetes and, consequently, heart disease. To investigate this issue, the Diabetes Prevention Program was recently initiated. This large randomized trial will compare four treatment groups—intensive lifestyle intervention, metformin, or troglitazone with standard diet and exercise, and a control group—to determine the effectiveness of these interventions on the prevention of Type II diabetes among high-risk people with insulin resistance. The United Kingdom Prospective Diabetes Study is a multicenter, prospective, randomized intervention trial, in which the combination effect of diet and drug therapy is being evaluated.

Insulin resistance syndrome is more common in well-developed countries, such as the United States, where the population is becoming more sedentary and more obese. As both physical inactivity and obesity aggravate insulin resistance, more effective prevention and treatment of obesity should have a major impact on reducing the development of the Deadly Quartet.

—Kimberly Y.-Z. Forrest, Ph.D., M.P.H.

See also Diabetes mellitus; Endocrine disorders; Endocrinology; Endocrinology, pediatric; Gestational diabetes; Hormones; Metabolic syndrome; Obesity.

FOR FURTHER INFORMATION:

Brook, Charles G. D., and Nicholas J. Marshall. *Essential Endocrinology.* Rev. 4th ed. Cambridge, Mass.: Blackwell Scientific, 2001. This text addresses the field of endocrinology, describing the physiology of the endocrine glands and the hormones that they produce. Includes an index.

Henry, Helen L., and Anthony W. Norman, eds. *Encyclopedia of Hormones.* 3 vols. San Diego, Calif.: Academic Press, 2003. A comprehensive overview of the role of hormones, the major physiological systems in which they operate, and the biological consequences of an excess or deficiency of a particular hormone.

Orgel, Stephen C., et al. *Insulin Resistance and Insulin Resistance Syndrome.* London: Routledge, 2002. Explores the cellular and whole body pathogenic mechanisms and phenotypic expressions in various models of insulin resistance.

Reaven, Gerald M., Terry Kristen Strom, and Barry Fox. *Syndrome X, the Silent Killer: The New Heart Disease Risk.* New York: Simon & Schuster, 2001. Examines the diet-related causes of Syndrome X.

Romaine, Deborah S., and Jennifer B. Marks. *Syndrome X: Managing Insulin Resistance.* New York: HarperCollins, 2000. An accessible book that looks at causes, risk factors, treatments, and changes in lifestyle to promote wellness.

The Wound Care Institute, Inc., for the Advancement of Wound Healing and Diabetic Foot Pathology. http://www.woundcare.org. Users can search this site for a variety of articles on insulin resistance syndrome.

INTENSIVE CARE. *See* CRITICAL CARE; CRITICAL CARE, PEDIATRIC.

INTERNAL MEDICINE
SPECIALTY

ANATOMY OR SYSTEM AFFECTED: Abdomen, bladder, gallbladder, gastrointestinal system, glands, heart, intestines, kidneys, liver, lungs, pancreas, reproductive system, respiratory system, spleen, stomach, urinary system, uterus

SPECIALTIES AND RELATED FIELDS: Cardiology, endocrinology, gastroenterology, gynecology, nephrology, proctology, pulmonary medicine

DEFINITION: The field of medicine concerned with the diagnosis and treatment of disease of the body's inner organs and structures, usually including surgery on these organs.

KEY TERMS:

acute: referring to a short-term disease process

cellular biology: the study of the processes that take place within a cell

chronic: referring to a long-term disease process

inflammation: redness, pain, and heat resulting from trauma or infection; often the first step in the body's self-healing process

molecular biology: study of the interactions that occur among the molecules that make up living organisms

pathogen: any microorganism that can cause disease, including bacteria, viruses, fungi, yeasts, and parasites

trauma: physical injury to bodily tissue

SCIENCE AND PROFESSION

Internists, or practitioners of internal medicine, are skilled in the diagnosis and treatment of disease conditions that can occur virtually anywhere within the human body. They must be expert in human biology and anatomy and in pathophysiology (that is, the study of the processes that lead to disease conditions). By its nature, internal medicine embraces many other medical specialties, such as cardiology or gastroenterology. In fact, many internists become certified in related specialties.

The original model for the modern internist was Sir William Osler (1849-1919), a Canadian physician who practiced in the United States for much of his life. Osler was deeply beloved and respected for his compassion and humanity as well as his extraordinary skills in anatomy and diagnosis and in effecting cures for his patients. In his long career as physician and teacher of medicine, Osler formulated many of the guiding principles in the practice of internal medicine.

Knowledge of many scientific disciplines is required of internists. They must understand the physical and biological basis of disease. This involves knowledge of genetics, cellular biology, immunology, and the activities and nature of the various microorganisms that cause disease, such as bacteria, viruses, fungi, yeasts, and parasites.

Internists must understand the components and role of each type of cell in the human body and know how the cell functions. Human cells are not simple entities, but complex miniature organisms with many activities going on simultaneously, particularly metabolic processes. Just as important, internists must understand what happens within and outside of the cell in the disease process. For example, they must know how individual bacteria cause infection and how viruses invade cells, use them for their replication, and then destroy them. Internal medicine involves all the body's organ systems and structures, such as the heart and circulatory system, the gastrointestinal system, the genitourinary system, the respiratory system, the skin, the brain, and the skeletal system.

Internists must also be able to examine patients and diagnose the presence or absence of disease. This process involves a wide variety of techniques and procedures. It usually begins with an introductory interview, followed by physical examination of the patient. Pain is the most common symptom of disease, and manifestation of it is investigated thoroughly.

DIAGNOSTIC AND TREATMENT TECHNIQUES

Internists understand the intricate pathways of pain throughout the body and know that proper explanation of a pain will often lead directly or indirectly to a correct diagnosis of the underlying disorder. Much of the diagnostic skill of the internist, however, is in the understanding that pain may be ambiguous. Headache can point to the possibility of many disorders, ranging from sinusitis to severe pathologies within the brain. Pain in the chest can be caused by upper respiratory tract infection or heart disease. Pain in the limbs and/or joints may indicate physical trauma as a result of accidents or overexercising, or it may be attributable to arthritic or rheumatic disease or other causes. Abdominal pain can be present in literally dozens of different conditions. Similarly, back and neck pain can be caused simply by physical exertion or may point to a serious underlying disease.

Blood pressure and pulse are checked in the physical examination, and the doctor listens to heart and chest sounds through a stethoscope. The ears, mouth, and nose are examined. Body temperature is an important diagnostic consideration. Excess body heat or fever often accompanies infection and may also be present in other disease conditions. The doctor also checks for enlargement of lymph nodes and other signs that might suggest infection or other disorders.

Blood or urine samples are often taken for laboratory analysis. The internist will specify the tests he or she wants in the laboratory workup. These will include standard assays to give the internist a general picture of the patient's health and may include special tests for individual functions that the doctor may suspect are impaired.

Changes in the function of different body systems can lead the physician through the process of diagnosis. For example, such symptoms as dizziness; fainting; numbness; vision, speech, or hearing disturbances; or coma may be caused by dysfunction of the nervous system or may point to heart disease or other disorder. Abnormalities in respiratory function have specific meaning to the internist and may lead to a diagnosis ranging from a common cold to a more serious respiratory disease or a disease of other organs, such as the heart. Alterations in the skin may indicate a dermatological disorder or may suggest some internal condition.

Sometimes, a diagnosis is easy to make: The presenting symptoms are obvious signs of a specific disease. Sometimes, a group of symptoms, called a syndrome, may be ambiguous and could be related to any of a number of conditions. If the exact nature of a disease or its cause is uncertain, the internist will conduct a differential diagnosis in which possible causes of the disease are investigated in order to eliminate those that are not candidates and to pinpoint the actual cause.

Internists treat a wide variety of disorders. Among the most significant are the infectious diseases. They must study the pathogenesis (from *pathos*, meaning "disease" and *genesis*, meaning "origin" or "source") of infectious diseases in order to know how to diagnose and treat them. Harmful bacteria cause disease in different ways, but one way or another, they damage and destroy body cells and tissue. Some cause infection at the point where they enter the body, such as at the site of a wound, or in the respiratory tract when they are breathed into the body. Sometimes, bacteria are carried from their site of entry to other parts of the body, where they colonize and cause infection.

The range of bacterial infections is enormous, but one thing that they often have in common is inflammation. Inflammation is the beginning of the immune process by which the body defends itself against invading pathogens. It starts when the body recognizes that the invading organism is a foreign entity by detecting foreign antigens (substances on the surfaces of invading organisms such as bacteria and viruses). The body then releases certain white blood cells, called leukocytes, that are specific for producing antibodies that can destroy the organism. Once the body has identified a foreign organism and created antibodies for it, the immune system will retain a memory of the organism and destroy it whenever it enters the body again.

When confronted with bacterial infection, internists may recognize the organism that causes it from the patient's symptoms, or they may have to take specimens from the site of inflammation and test them in order to identify the organism involved. Sometimes, the organism is identified by microscopic examination, often using a dye that stains certain bacteria. Sometimes, it is necessary to grow the organism in a culture medium in order to identify it. The organism may also be identified by its antigen or by the type of antibody that the immune system produces to fight it.

The signs of viral infection are often exactly the same as those of bacterial infection. The main difference is that the causative organism cannot be isolated and identified as easily. Unlike bacteria, viruses cannot be seen through a microscope or otherwise identified by many of the methods used for bacteria. They can be cultured, however, or antigens or antibodies may be detectable.

In addition to infectious diseases, internists are called on to treat dysfunction in all parts of the body. They treat many patients suffering from heart disease, the major killer of Americans. The heart is actually subject to a wide range of disorders, the most common and the most deadly of which is coronary artery disease. Internists have many means of both diagnosing heart diseases and, often, predicting them. The patient's presenting symptoms and an analysis of the patient's lifestyle will often suggest the possibility of heart disease. Various in-office and laboratory procedures will inform the internist of the precise status of the patient's heart function and help direct the course of therapy.

Cancer, the second most common cause of mortality in the United States, is often seen by internists. Lung cancer is the leading cause of cancer death, followed by cancer of the colon or rectum, breast, prostate gland, urinary tract, and uterus. The lymph system, blood, mouth, pancreas, skin, stomach, and ovary are also common sites. The term "cancer" describes a large number of disorders. What all cancers have in common is that the cells of an organ multiply uncontrollably. As the cancer cells proliferate, they crowd out other cells and interfere with organ function. Sometimes cancer cells from one organ spread to neighboring organs or are carried to other parts of the body. This process is called metastasis, and it can indicate that the cancer

has spread or is spreading throughout the body. Internists may be responsible for treating cancer patients throughout the disease process or may refer them to oncologists, or cancer specialists.

Diseases of the respiratory system are major concerns of the internist. In addition to bacterial and viral infections, there are many acute and chronic respiratory conditions. One major example is asthma. Its cause is unknown, but it is believed to be at least partially attributable to allergy. When an asthma attack occurs, airways in the lungs swell and constrict. Mucus builds up and airflow is restricted, causing the patient to wheeze and gasp for air. Many internists have become skilled in helping asthmatic patients, alleviating symptoms, and preventing attacks.

All parts of the body harbor the potential for disease, infectious and otherwise. They are all, to some degree, the province of internists. The kidneys and the urinary system, the gastrointestinal system, the immune system, the endocrine glands, the brain and the nervous system, and the skeletal system are all within the internist's broad purview. Often disorders in these various organs and systems can be treated fully by internists. When they believe that a patient needs a physician with greater knowledge in a particular area of medicine, however, internists will refer the patient to an appropriate specialist.

In addition to their diagnostic skills, internists must possess a wide knowledge of modern treatment modalities. Surgery is rarely among the procedures mastered by the internist, so surgical procedures are routinely referred to surgeons specializing in the particular techniques involved.

Primary among the internist's tools for fighting infectious diseases are the antibiotics. These are the mainstays of therapy for infections caused by bacteria and other nonviral microorganisms. Since the first antibiotics were developed in the 1930's and 1940's, literally hundreds more have been developed. Scores of these are in use, and new agents are constantly being introduced.

It is vital for internists to keep abreast of new antibiotics because disease-causing organisms are often able to develop resistance against antibiotic agents that have been in use for a long time. For example, many strains of bacteria that were susceptible to penicillin have developed the ability to counteract its antibiotic effect. Other agents had to be found to destroy these resistant strains. This phenomenon occurs across virtually the entire range of the available antibiotics: Prolonged use of a given agent often allows the target organism to develop resistance to it. Internists must also be skilled in the proper use of antibiotics. Knowing which agent or combination of agents to prescribe, in what amounts, and for how long are important considerations in developing the patient's treatment plan. Antibiotics are not useful for treating viral infections, but there are a limited number of antiviral agents available for treating certain diseases.

Immunization against infectious diseases can be an important concern of the internist. The most extensive immunization programs in the United States are directed toward the vaccination of children and thus are generally carried out by pediatricians and family practitioners. Internists are often responsible, however, for the immunization of adult patients. Immunization against influenza is recommended for the elderly, particularly when a new strain of influenza virus arises. It is also recommended that elderly hospitalized patients be vaccinated against pneumococcal pneumonia. Internists are a primary avenue of immunization against hepatitis B, particularly among high-risk target populations, such as medical personnel, intravenous drug abusers, and adult male homosexuals. Internists are also involved in immunizing patients who require special vaccinations because of exposure to disease or for travel to foreign countries.

Patients who require long-term or lifelong therapy for noninfectious diseases include individuals with heart diseases, high blood pressure, diabetes, cancer, respiratory disorders, and a host of other conditions. The challenge to the internist is to develop a regimen that is both efficacious and safe. Drug therapy is prominent in the internist's treatment armamentarium. In either short-term or long-term drug therapy, problems may arise. The patient may develop significant side effects or adverse reactions. The drug may lose its effectiveness after months or years of therapy. The condition may change and require dosage adjustments, additional medications, or a complete change of regimen.

Consistent monitoring of the patient's condition is an important part of therapy. The internist wants to ensure that the prescribed regimen is working and that the therapy is comfortable for the patient. For example, the earliest agents for high blood pressure, or hypertension, often had such disagreeable side effects that patients would stop taking them. Hypertension has virtually no symptoms. After the patient started taking medication, however, he or she could experience loss of energy, list-lessness, impotence, dream disturbances, and many other unwelcome effects. Similarly, diabetes patients who are dependent on regular insulin injections sometimes neglect their therapy. They may balk against sticking themselves with needles three or four times a day, and they may not monitor their blood sugar adequately. Preventing the devastating and potentially fatal consequences of diabetes depends on rigorous compliance with all aspects of the diabetes regimen, including diet, insulin, and monitoring.

Thus, patient compliance with therapy becomes one of the major tasks of the internist and virtually any other physician: If the patient does not cooperate with the regimen that the doctor prescribes, the therapy is not likely to be effective. For this reason, many internists now make patient counseling part of their practice. The modern internist recognizes that patients must understand their therapeutic goals, why they are being given certain medicines, and what these drugs can be expected to accomplish. Further, many internists find that it is wise to alert their patients to possible adverse reactions, although they understand the necessity of not frightening the patient. Some internists find the time to discuss their therapeutic regimens thoroughly with their patients. Others use nursing staff or other health care workers to educate patients.

Treatment modalities change constantly, and internists are required to be aware of the latest advances in order to modify their therapy programs to take advantage of improvements in drugs or procedures. Not only are new drugs constantly being approved for use, but modern medical science is continually learning new facts about old diseases as well, and these new insights often radically alter the way a given disease is treated. A good example is a stomach ulcer. For years, it was thought that certain ulcers in the stomach were caused by erosion of the stomach wall by gastric juices. A group of investigators found, however, that a significant number of ulcer patients were also infected with the bacterium *Helicobacter pylori*. It has been suggested that infection may play a role in the development of these ulcers and that, therefore, therapy should be amended to include an antibacterial agent that is effective against *H. pylori*.

Furthermore, the internist's patient load is changing. Most internal medicine practices are treating increasing numbers of elderly patients, who have special needs. Internists must be aware of the constant advances in geriatric medicine in order to modify therapy for older patients.

PERSPECTIVE AND PROSPECTS

In the last decades of the twentieth century, internal medicine became somewhat fragmented as more and more physicians elected to practice in narrower specialties, such as cardiology, gastroenterology, hematology, or oncology, among many others. Specialties are still very much needed, but the practice of medicine seems to be headed back to the broader range of the internist.

As in the past, internists are at the forefront of progress in treatment. Recent generations have seen a far-reaching revolution in an understanding of the basic chemistry of life. As scientists elucidate the activities that occur at the molecular level of physical processes, insights are gained into exactly how the body works, as well as how antagonistic pathogens function. From this knowledge, new treatments have been devised for managing disease states.

A good example is the treatment of hypertension, one of the most common conditions seen by internists. Years ago, the only medications for high blood pressure were essentially sedatives and diuretics. It was not fully understood exactly what occurred at the cellular and molecular level that caused vasoconstriction, which is the main physical characteristic of hypertension. Researchers discovered complex biochemical activities that contributed to vasoconstriction and other aspects of high blood pressure. They were then able to develop agents that could treat the condition more effectively than anything available before. Internists now have a wealth of antihypertensive agents with which to work. Some reduce blood pressure by reducing heart activity, some dilate blood vessels by direct action, and some interfere with the biochemical processes that cause vasoconstriction. In addition, most of the agents that internists and other physicians use for hypertension cause many fewer side effects and adverse reactions than their predecessors.

In the fight against infectious diseases, new research is combining genetics with molecular biology to elucidate the exact biochemical processes by which pathogenic organisms invade and damage body cells and tissues. This research is having an enormous impact on the understanding of bacteria and viruses: how they work, how they mutate, and, perhaps most important, in what ways they are vulnerable. With increased knowledge comes increased capability to design more efficient antibiotics and to find agents that will inhibit the pathogen's ability to develop resistant strains. Internists are among the leaders in the application of these technologies. Because they see such a wide range of

disease conditions, internists often function as the main channel by which new medications and treatments reach the patient.

—*C. Richard Falcon*

See also Abdomen; Abdominal disorders; Angina; Arrhythmias; Arteriosclerosis; Bacterial infections; Beriberi; Bleeding; Bronchitis; Candidiasis; Cardiology; Cardiology, pediatric; Cholecystitis; Cirrhosis; Colitis; Colonoscopy and sigmoidoscopy; Constipation; Coughing; Crohn's disease; Diabetes mellitus; Dialysis; Diarrhea and dysentery; Digestion; Diverticulitis and diverticulosis; *E. coli* infection; Emphysema; Endocarditis; Endoscopy; Gallbladder diseases; Gangrene; Gastroenterology; Gastroenterology, pediatric; Gastrointestinal disorders; Gastrointestinal system; Glands; Guillain-Barré syndrome; Gynecology; Heart; Heart attack; Heart disease; Heart failure; Heartburn; Hepatitis; Hernia; Incontinence; Indigestion; Influenza; Intestinal disorders; Intestines; Ischemia; Kidney disorders; Kidneys; Legionnaires' disease; Leprosy; Liver; Liver disorders; Lungs; Mitral insufficiency; Multiple sclerosis; Nephritis; Nephrology; Nephrology, pediatric; Palpitations; Pancreas; Pancreatitis; Parasitic diseases; Peristalsis; Peritonitis; Pneumonia; Proctology; Pulmonary medicine; Pulmonary medicine, pediatric; Renal failure; Reproductive system; Reye's syndrome; Rheumatic fever; Rheumatoid arthritis; Roundworms; Scarlet fever; Schistosomiasis; Staphylococcal infections; Stone removal; Stones; Streptococcal infections; Tapeworms; Tumor removal; Tumors; Ulcer surgery; Ulcers; Urinary system; Urology; Urology, pediatric; Viral infections; Whooping cough; Worms.

FOR FURTHER INFORMATION:

Braunwald, Eugene. *Harrison's Principles of Internal Medicine.* 15th ed. New York: McGraw-Hill, 2001. A standard text on internal medicine. Includes bibliographical references and an index.

Frank, Steven A. *Immunology and Evolution of Infectious Disease.* Princeton, N.J.: Princeton University Press, 2002. Blends research from molecular biology, immunology, pathogen biology, and population dynamics to discuss how and why parasites vary to escape recognition by the immune system, vaccine design, and the control of epidemics.

Kiple, Kenneth, ed. *The Cambridge World History of Human Disease.* New York: Cambridge University Press, 1993. This text is useful for tracing the progress in medical practice through the years.

Larson, David E., ed. *Mayo Clinic Family Health Book.* 3d ed. New York: William Morrow, 2003. This text from the world-renowned medical facility was written for the layperson. Its coverage of medical practice in general and the diseases treated by the internist are clear and thorough.

Wagman, Richard J., ed. *The New Complete Medical and Health Encyclopedia.* 4 vols. New York: Facts On File, 2002. A good general medical reference work for the layperson. Its coverage of internal medicine is useful for clarifying the nature of the internist's practice and contrasting it with the subspecialties often practiced by internists.

INTERNET MEDICINE

SPECIALTY

ALSO KNOWN AS: Telehealth, telemedicine, e-medicine

ANATOMY OR SYSTEM AFFECTED: All

SPECIALTIES AND RELATED FIELDS: All

DEFINITION: The use of World Wide Web-based and other electronic long-distance communication technologies for health information, assessment, service delivery, training, and public health administration.

KEY TERMS:

anonymous: of unknown authorship, unidentified by a singular identity

assessment: a thorough physical and/or psychiatric examination; a process of systematically collecting comprehensive information about health care behavior, physical and psychiatric conditions, and general well-being for the purpose of diagnosis or treatment planning

clinical trials: scientifically based research examinations of new treatment procedures, techniques, devices, or pharmaceuticals that are considered state of the art in the treatment of diseases and other medical disorders

confidential: a situation distinguished by the willing disclosure of intimate information because of assurances that the information will be protected from general distribution or unauthorized disclosure; information which, if disclosed, has the potential to be damaging or dangerous to the patient's reputation, status, or associates

diagnosis: a process of distinguishing knowledge about symptoms and problems that leads to the rendering of conclusions about physical and psychiatric illness; a label used to communicate specific health information among professionals, researchers, health systems, and insurance providers; a label which informs the process of treatment

Internet: a worldwide electronic system connecting individual computer users, computer networks, Web sites, and computer facilities for business, government, and organizational purposes

privacy: the state of being free from unwanted or unauthorized observation or other intrusion

professional licensing: state-granted privileges to health care and other professionals allowing them to deliver services or to participate in certain activities; a privilege that is revokable and subject to censure; a privilege usually granted only after thorough examination of the skill and practice of a person seeking licensure

profiling: the collection of data to summarily categorize and track the behavior of individual users or types of users, through electronic or other tracking systems, to learn more about their behavior, usually for the purpose of prediction, done either with or without the knowledge or consent of the user

screening: a triage process; a process of asking a few questions of an individual, as opposed to an assessment, in order to determine whether there is sufficient risk of a problematic condition being present to justify completing a detailed evaluation or, instead, to justify assigning that individual to a category of lesser or no risk

Web site: a location on the Internet that has an individual address and that presents information, usually in the form of individual pages, or Web pages, that the owner of the Web site wishes to make available to Internet users

SCIENCE AND PROFESSION

The Internet is a computer-based tool that is facilitating communication among vast numbers of individuals, groups, businesses, and governments. In addition to facilitating purely social and business-related ventures, the Internet is proving to be a valuable tool for improving the state of public health. This is because a new type of medical care and medical services has developed. These services, typically called telehealth, telemedicine, and e-medicine, use the Internet as a key tool in their dispensation, organization, and evaluation of health care services. Such services have taken the form of a variety of health care-related Web sites that provide services once available only through a face-to-face visit with a doctor or other health or social services professional. The Web sites are valuable in that they provide almost instantaneous information and other communications assistance to patients, their families, treatment professionals, trainers, trainees in the health care and social service professions, and medical researchers.

In terms of assisting patients, Internet-based medical approaches provide a variety of services to individual Internet users. First, they provide a wealth of information on different symptoms and medical conditions. They also allow for screening of such conditions to see if they warrant further attention from medical professionals and advice on how to handle minor health ailments and medical emergencies. They also help consumers to find medical advice, health care providers, self-help or support groups, and therapy over the Internet, all of which may or may not be supervised by medical professionals. Finally, they can give patients and their families information on different treatment options, including common procedures, the latest in alternative medicine, and even current clinical trials information.

Internet medicine can also be very helpful for family members of individuals having medical problems. Often, family members do not know how best to help their significant others in times of medical need. To meet this need, Web sites may post a wide variety of information that can help people understand the conditions, the requirements of treatment, the limits of treatment, and things they can do to be helpful to the ill family member. Additionally, Web sites sometimes offer online support for family members through mechanisms such as e-mail and e-mail lists, also known as listservs, or other ongoing support groups in settings such as Internet chat rooms.

Health care and social service providers also find the Internet beneficial for their work. For some, it might be as simple as using the Internet to schedule appointments, or to communicate test results, reminder information about treatment procedures, or appointment reminders via e-mail with clients. For others, it might involve using special Web sites to conduct assessments of clients for the purpose of tracking their treatment success or progress. Professionals may also use telemedicine in order to learn about new treatments and procedures, or to learn about new drugs and other pharmaceutical products. In addition, health care and social service providers may benefit their general practice by using the Internet to keep abreast of new clinical trials to test state-of-the-art treatments, changes in licensing laws affecting their practice, and the development of new health care databases for tracking, triage, and communication with insurance companies. Finally, some providers are actually using the Internet for health services delivery.

Health care providers in training and their trainers also benefit greatly from telemedicine. To trainees living in remote areas or those who might be highly mobile, such as those in the armed forces, the Internet provides immediate access to large online libraries, knowledgeable online teachers, and databases full of important medical information. Both long-established and new institutions interested in telemedicine increasingly are translating typical face-to-face training approaches into distance-based training programs utilizing the Internet. Encyclopedias, descriptions of techniques, pictures of what different conditions might look like both inside and outside the body, and even video of actual procedures are available online. Similarly, instruction in the use of such material is available online through training programs that lead to certificates of training and actual accredited degrees, ranging from bachelor's to doctoral degrees and postdoctoral training. In addition to helping individuals who are at remote locations, such material also can be used to reach a larger number of trainees than might typically be able to observe or attend such training. The increased ability to teach, show procedures, or give supervision at a distance using pictorial, written, oral, and video information greatly facilitates continuing education and improvement of general health care practice. It also helps to facilitate the evaluation of those practices and training sessions. Since all of the work takes place over the Internet, different aspects of the work can be monitored and evaluated electronically.

Much of the evaluation of this kind of information is done by researchers who are studying client, trainer, provider, or even health care system behavior and organization. This is done by evaluating information, also known as data, in individual sessions or visits to Web sites, as well as by examining data that is collected over time, across multiple visits. For instance, a person might first go to a Web site for information on a specific medical condition and then, at a later time or times, come back and look up different treatment approaches, or visit online discussion groups. What they do from time to time would be evaluated by researchers to see how individuals use the site, how long they stay on it, or what things they try searching for which may not yet be on the site. The process of watching behavior over time is called tracking. Tracking allows researchers to pro-

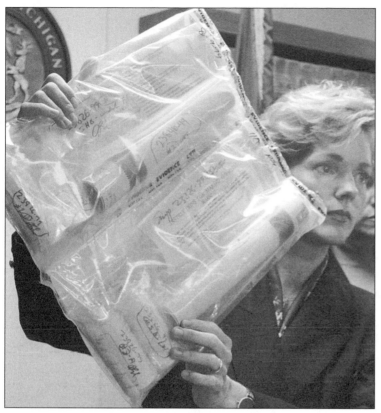

One disadvantage of the Internet is the ease with which illegal or dangerous substances, such as this home manufacturing kit for "date rape" drug gamma hydroxybutrate (GHB), can be distributed. (AP/Wide World Photos)

file the users of Web sites to learn more about their behavior, usually for the purpose of predicting their behavior and response to treatment. By creating tracking databases of what happens with Web site users, the information gathered can be used to improve services and to decrease long-term health care service, training, and administration costs on a continuing basis.

Because of all the data being collected on how individuals are using different Web sites or other Internet-based services, there has been some concern over the individual's right to privacy and the protection of the information collected. For instance, some people have been concerned that if they are searching for information related to the human immunodeficiency virus (HIV) or substance use, they might be identified as being at risk for having that condition whether they do or not. Further, many individuals do not want that information linked to their identities or medical records. On one hand, they may be wishing to avoid solicitation of business from sellers of medical services or products because of their association with the condition; they do

not want their personal information sold for that purpose to the providers of such products or services. On the other hand, they may also wish to maintain privacy and keep their information confidential so as to avoid having any threat to their future insurability or their ability to get health care coverage. As an example, if a health care provider such as a health maintenance organization (HMO) tracked users' information on a Web site and discovered, through the database, that someone who was now applying for coverage had certain medical conditions, that person might have a greater risk of being refused coverage if his or her time on the Web site was not completely anonymous. In sum, given these concerns, users of Internet medicine need to understand that there are differences between the terms privacy, confidentiality, and anonymity, as well as in the legal issues and protections one can exercise when using this type of medicine. Each Web site may be operating under different constraints, and so it is always important for users of these services to be sure they understand how the Web sites handle privacy. Finding out how a Web site protects or does not protect the privacy of its users is the only way users can determine how safe it is to reveal confidential information when they use a specific Web site.

DIAGNOSTIC AND TREATMENT TECHNIQUES
One of the biggest opportunities offered by Internet medicine is that of increasing the ability of individuals to do self-screening for medical conditions to see if they need medical assistance. Likewise, the ability of service providers to do screening and assessment for a larger number of people is increased relative to what can be done in person. This is because the assessments can be administered via the computer, saving valuable provider time. Additionally, assessments can be completed online and sent to providers in advance for immediate evaluation. While it may be some time before conclusive diagnoses can be offered via online technology, such advances are not far off; the differences between online and in-person assessments are being studied.

Intervention via the Internet is also much improved because large quantities of information can be dispensed electronically, printed out by clients or their families, or distributed to large numbers of individuals. Such informational interventions can be important for facilitating proper compliance with medical prescription regimens, helping clients to avoid bad drug interactions, or providing reminders about other things needed to facilitate wellness. Informational interventions can also be used for primary prevention, or preventing problems from happening in the first place. By providing suggestions for problem prevention, much suffering could be spared and many health care dollars can be saved. This is especially true for teenagers and college-age populations, who are often savvy Internet users.

Treatment also takes place on the Internet via simultaneous online interactions such as in chat rooms, communicating via videoconferencing as in a normal conversation but using video cameras, and simple asynchronous e-mail between the client and the provider. Generally this type of treatment is a complement to face-to-face treatment. For instance, some HMOs use online support groups as additional treatment for persons already receiving therapy. Others are using programs such as self-guided online courses that clients can work through to benefit their health. In general, practitioners are permitted to do this so long as they are properly licensed. This usually requires being licensed by the state in which they are practicing and/or where the client is receiving the services.

PERSPECTIVE AND PROSPECTS

The Internet continues to grow on a daily basis, with an increasing number of computer owners and Web sites taking advantage of its capabilities. Communications technologies are also improving constantly, allowing for almost instant individual communication of written, oral, and visual information at distances and speeds that were inconceivable in the past. As a result of these developments, as well as increases in health care costs and the potential economic and health benefits provided by Internet medicine, this specialty area is here to stay. Commitments by governments to examine such developments in health care underscore this likelihood. In 1998, for example, the Health Resources and Service Administration of the United States Department of Health and Human Services established the Office for the Advancement of Telehealth. This office is devoted to advancing the use of telehealth and Internet-based medicine to facilitate improvement in the state of pub-

lic health and research on public health. The ability of such approaches to provide more services with streamlined administrative procedures and decreased costs holds much promise for improving the state of public health.

—*Nancy A. Piotrowski, Ph.D.*

See also Allied health; Alternative medicine; Clinical trials; Education, medical; Family practice; Health maintenance organizations (HMOs); Herbal medicine; Noninvasive tests; Nursing; Pharmacology; Pharmacy; Physical examination; Screening; Self-medication.

FOR FURTHER INFORMATION:

Armstrong, Myrna L. *Telecommunications for Health Professionals: Providing Successful Distance Education and Telehealth.* New York: Springer, 1998. Provides strategies for using distance education and resources. Legal and ethical issues are discussed to inform patients, providers, students, and legislators.

Bauer, Jeffrey C., and Marc A. Ringel. *Telemedicine and the Reinvention of Healthcare.* New York: McGraw-Hill, 1999. History as well as technical, social, and policy-oriented issues are reviewed in this book that discusses telemedicine as a revolution in a series of scientific advances affecting health care.

Coiera, Enrico. *Guide to Medical Informatics, the Internet, and Telemedicine.* New York: Oxford University Press, 1997. The boundaries of appropriate communication of medical information via the Internet are outlined in this book tailored to the general reader, student, or trainer of health care provision.

Darkins, Adam William, and Margaret Ann Cary. *Telemedicine and Telehealth: Principles, Policies, Performance, and Pitfalls.* New York: Springer, 2000. Defines and examines telemedicine, discussing how it is organized, provided, and managed, along with its medical, social, economic, and cultural significance.

Davis, James B., Maureen Lynch, and Kathryn Swanson. *Health and Medicine on the Internet 2003.* Los Angeles: Health Information Press, 2002. Provides an annual guide for individuals interested in Internet-based health care.

Goldstein, Douglas E. *E-Healthcare: Harness the Power of the Internet, e-Commerce, and e-Care.* Gaithersburg, Md.: Aspen, 2000. An easy to understand resource, for patients, service providers, and entrepreneurs interested in online health care, describing the types of services provided and important legal issues. Helpful CD-ROM included.

Kinsella, Audrey. *Home Telehealth in the Twenty-first Century: A Resource Book About Improved Services That Work*. Kensington, Md.: Information for Tomorrow, 2000. Provides an in-depth discussion of how telemedicine can help with chronic medical concerns.

Maheu, Marlene, Ace Allen, and Pamela Whitten. *E-Health, Telehealth, and Telemedicine: A Guide to Startup and Success*. New York: Wiley, 2001. A resource guide for health organizations that want to use communication technologies to expand and transform their organizations. Covers topics such as program development, technical options, and ethical, legal, and regulatory issues.

Office for the Advancement of Telehealth. http://tele health.hrsa.gov/index.htm. An organization devoted to advancing the use of telehealth and Internet-based medicine to facilitate improvement in the state of public health and research on public health.

Price, Joan. *Complete Idiot's Guide to Online Medical Resources*. Indianapolis: Que, 2000. Provides information on traditional and alternative medicine approaches, helping readers evaluate Internet-based information so as to avoid bad or unreliable advice or recommendations.

Interstitial pulmonary fibrosis (IPF)

Disease/disorder

Also known as: Idiopathic pulmonary fibrosis, cryptogenic fibrosing alveolitis

Anatomy or system affected: Heart, lungs

Specialties and related fields: Emergency medicine, internal medicine, pulmonary medicine

Definition: An inflammatory disease that results in the scarring and fibrosis of the lung alveolar tissue (air sacs).

Causes and Symptoms

Interstitial pulmonary fibrosis (IPF) is a chronic lung disease that causes scarring of the tissue between the air sacs (interstitium). It may be the result of a variety of causes, such as occupational exposure to silica or asbestos, drugs, radiation, and diseases such as sarcoidosis or connective tissue diseases (systemic lupus erythematosus, rheumatoid arthritis). When no known cause can be ascertained, the disease is known as idiopathic pulmonary fibrosis. It affects both sexes equally, with the highest incidence between the ages of forty and sixty.

The disease is characterized by an initial inflammation of the alveoli attributable to a known or unknown injury-causing agent, followed by healing by scarring and fibrosis of the interstitium. This results in a decreased transfer of oxygen to the blood, causing symptoms of increasing shortness of breath (dyspnea) and chest pain. The symptoms of the disease appear insidiously, with the patient noticing a dry cough and increasing shortness of breath, initially on exertion and eventually at rest. As the disease progresses, the patient is unable to perform daily activities and may require long-term oxygen therapy. Clubbing of the fingers and blueness of the extremities can be observed in these patients. Death is usually the result of respiratory failure, right-sided heart failure, a blood clot (embolism) in the lungs, stroke, or heart attack.

Diagnosis of IPF is made by correlating a chest X ray, a computed tomography (CT) chest scan, lung function tests, bronchoscopy, and a measurement of blood oxygen content. Lung biopsy and microscopic examination of the tissue is the only confirmatory test that would also show the extent of damage and help determine the prognosis of the disease.

Treatment and Therapy

Treatment must be initiated as soon as the diagnosis is made. Because of the chronic nature of the disease, most patients require lifelong treatment. Treatment modalities differ with age and the stage of the disease, but all aim at reducing the inflammation and stopping the fibrosis. Drugs are the mainstay of treatment, with

---

Information on Interstitial Pulmonary Fibrosis (IPF)

Causes: Various; may include occupational exposure to silica or asbestos, drugs, radiation, diseases (sarcoidosis, lupus erythematosus, rheumatoid arthritis)

Symptoms: Scarring of lung tissue, shortness of breath, chest pain, dry cough, clubbing of fingers, blue extremities; death may come from respiratory failure, heart failure, blood clot, stroke, heart attack

Duration: Progressive, eventually fatal

Treatments: Drugs (prednisone, cyclophosphamide); oxygen therapy; physical therapy and exercise; lung transplantation

prednisone (a corticosteroid) and cyclophosphamide being the most commonly used ones. Oxygen therapy improves the blood oxygen level in patients with severe breathlessness, and physical therapy and exercise also help in improving muscle strength and breathing. Patients with severe fibrosis require lung transplantation, the success rate of which is about 60 percent.

—*Rashmi Ramasubbaiah, M.D.,
and Venkat Raghavan Tirumala, M.D., M.H.A.*

See also Lungs; Occupational health; Oxygen therapy; Pulmonary diseases; Pulmonary medicine; Respiration.

FOR FURTHER INFORMATION:

Braunwald, Eugene, et al., eds. *Harrison's Principles of Internal Medicine*. 15th ed. New York: McGraw-Hill, 2001.

Parker, James N., and Philip M. Parker, eds. *The Official Patient's Sourcebook on Idiopathic Pulmonary Fibrosis*. San Diego, Calif.: Icon Health, 2002.

Rakel, Robert E., ed. *Textbook of Family Practice*. 6th ed. Philadelphia: W. B. Saunders, 2002.

INTESTINAL CANCER. *See* STOMACH, INTESTINAL, AND PANCREATIC CANCERS.

INTESTINAL DISORDERS
DISEASE/DISORDER

ANATOMY OR SYSTEM AFFECTED: Abdomen, anus, gastrointestinal system, intestines

SPECIALTIES AND RELATED FIELDS: Family practice, gastroenterology, internal medicine

DEFINITION: Diseases or disorders of the small intestine, large intestine (or colon), liver, pancreas, and gallbladder.

KEY TERMS:

acute: the stage of a disease or presence of a symptom that begins abruptly, with marked intensity, and subsides after a short time

chronic: the stage of a disease or presence of a symptom that develops slowly and usually lasts for the lifetime of the individual

diarrhea: the passage of approximately six loose stools within a twenty-four-hour period caused by a variety of circumstances, such as infection, malabsorption, or irritable bowel

diverticulitis: inflammation or swelling of one or more diverticula, caused by the penetration of fecal material through thin-walled diverticula and the collection of bacteria or other irritating agents there

diverticulosis: the presence of diverticula in the colon, which may lead to diverticulitis

diverticulum: an outpouching through the muscular wall of a tubular organ, such as the stomach, small intestine, or colon

electrolytes: elements or compounds found in blood, interstitial fluid, and cell fluid that are critical for normal metabolism and function

peristalsis: the involuntary, coordinated, rhythmic contraction of the muscles of the gastrointestinal tract that forces partially digested food along its length

stricture: an abnormal narrowing of an organ because of pressure or inflammation

villi: folds within the small intestine that are important for the absorption of nutrients into the blood

PROCESS AND EFFECTS

Intestinal diseases and disorders are sometimes included with those of the digestive system. For the sake of clarity, this article makes the distinction between the structures of the digestive and intestinal tracts. The entire digestive tract, which includes the intestinal tract and is approximately 7.6 to 9.1 meters in length in adults, begins in the mouth and ends with the anus. It includes organs specific to digestion, such as the esophagus and stomach and their substructures. The intestinal tract, which constitutes the major part of the digestive tract, includes the small intestine, the large intestine (also known as the colon), and the organs that branch off these structures (the liver, pancreas, and gallbladder). The function of the small and large intestines is to

---

INFORMATION ON
INTESTINAL DISORDERS

CAUSES: Infection by bacteria or parasites, obstruction, cancer or tumor of rectum and colon, polyps

SYMPTOMS: Varies; can include persistent diarrhea, abdominal cramping or bloating, pain, swelling, fever, fatigue, constipation, nausea and vomiting, loss of appetite

DURATION: Acute or chronic

TREATMENTS: Surgery, anti-inflammatory and antidiarrheal medications, antibiotics, chemotherapy and/or radiation therapy

break down food, absorb its nutrients into the bloodstream, and carry off waste products of digestion as feces.

The small intestine is approximately 6.1 meters long and 3.8 centimeters in diameter and is made up of the duodenum, the jejunum, and the ileum. It is where the process of digestion begins in full. The smaller products broken down by the stomach are received by the small intestine, where they are absorbed into the bloodstream through its lining by villi combined with bile (from the liver) and pancreatic juices.

Almost all food nutrients are absorbed in the small intestine. What passes into the large intestine is a mix of unabsorbed nutrients, water, fiber, and electrolytes. Most of the moisture from this process is removed as the mix passes through the large intestine, leaving solid waste products. Before excretion as feces, approximately 90 percent of the liquid that entered the large intestine has been reabsorbed. This reabsorption is necessary for health because the liquid contains sodium and water.

The large intestine is approximately 1.5 meters long and connected to the small intestine at the ileocecal valve. Waste products from the digestive process pass through this valve into a large holding area of the large intestine called the cecum. The appendix is attached to this structure. The large intestine consists of the ascending colon (which begins on the right side of the abdomen and moves up toward the liver), the transverse colon (which crosses the abdomen), and the descending colon (which moves down the left side of the abdomen). The sigmoid colon is an S-shaped structure which connects to the descending colon and joins the rectum, a tube 12 to 20 centimeters long that leads to the anus. Small microorganisms in the large intestine break down waste products not broken down by the stomach and small intestines, resulting in gas (also known as flatus).

COMPLICATIONS AND DISORDERS

Diseases and disorders of the intestinal tract constitute a major health problem affecting many individuals at one point or another in their lives. The common diseases and disorders that affect the intestinal tract are those of acute inflammatory disorders (appendicitis), diverticular disorders (diverticulosis and diverticulitis), chronic inflammatory bowel disease (Crohn's disease and ulcerative colitis), intestinal infections (intestinal parasites and bacterial infections with *Salmonella*, *Shigella dysenteriae*, and *Escherichia coli*), intestinal

obstructions, cancers or tumors of the rectum and colon, and polyps.

The most common acute inflammatory disorder is appendicitis. Its symptoms usually affect individuals between the ages of ten and thirty and include abdominal pain and tenderness, nausea and vomiting, loss of appetite, rapid heart rate, fever, and an elevated white blood cell count. Normally, the appendix, whose function is not clearly understood, fills and empties with food as regularly as does the cecum, of which it is a part. It sometimes becomes inflamed because of either kinking or obstruction, producing pressure and initiating symptoms. The most common major complication associated with appendicitis is perforation, which causes severe pain and an elevation of temperature. In these cases, a physician must be notified immediately. Treatment consists of surgical removal of the appendix.

Diverticular disorders include diverticulosis and diverticulitis. Diverticulosis is the presence of diverticula without any inflammation or symptoms. Diverticulitis is the result of an inflammation or infection of the intestine produced when food or bacteria are retained in a diverticulum. Signs of diverticulosis include cramplike pain in the left lower part of the abdomen, bowel irregularity, diarrhea, constipation, and thin stools. There may be some intermittent rectal bleeding with diverticulitis.

Inflammatory bowel disease (IBD) of unknown cause is most common in whites (usually female) between the ages of fifteen and thirty-five, occurring most frequently in the American Jewish population. The two types of IBD are Crohn's disease, which is also known as regional enteritis, and ulcerative colitis. The disorders are considered to be separate diseases with similar characteristics.

Crohn's disease may affect any part of the intestinal tract but often affects the small intestine. The inflammation usually involves the entire thickness of the intestinal wall. Treatment for Crohn's disease depends on the presence or absence of symptoms. If there are no symptoms, treatment is not necessary. If there is evidence of inflammation, however, anti-inflammatory medication may be prescribed. Vitamin and mineral replacement may be given because of the problems of absorption associated with this disease. Surgery may be required at some point in the disease process because of its associated complications, such as obstruction.

Ulcerative colitis is characterized by tiny ulcers and abscesses in the inner lining of the colon, where it is usually confined. There is a tendency for these ulcerations to bleed, causing bloody diarrhea. The chronic nature of inflammatory bowel disease may cause a stricture, which can result in an obstruction requiring surgical intervention. As with Crohn's disease, the treatment for ulcerative colitis depends on the type of symptoms and may consist of medication, nutrition, or surgery. Anti-inflammatory drugs are used for flare-ups of the disease. Liquid food supplements may be given to compensate for nutrients lost in diarrhea. Intravenous therapy may be prescribed if the colon is considered too diseased to tolerate food.

There are many types of infections that affect the intestinal tract. The most common bacterial infections are caused by microorganisms such as *Salmonella* and *Shigella*. *Salmonella* bacteria are commonly found in meats, fruits (through contaminated fertilizer), poultry, eggs, dairy products, and contaminated marijuana. Pet turtles are also a source of this bacteria. The source of infections for *Shigella* bacteria is feces from an infected person, with the route of transmission being oral-fecal—for example, changing the soiled diaper of an infant, or having a bowel movement, and then eating or preparing food without properly washing the hands.

Intestinal parasites may also cause infection. The most common of these parasites, *Giardia lamblia*, is present where water supplies are contaminated by raw sewage. The primary treatment for these conditions consists of replacement of lost fluids and essential electrolytes. Although not normally used because they may interfere with the elimination of the causative agent, antidiarrheal medications may be prescribed.

Intestinal obstruction occurs when the normal flow of the intestine is partially or totally impeded because of an accumulation of contents, gas, or fluid. It may also be caused by the intestine's inability to propel contents along the intestinal tract in the process called peristalsis. Peristalsis may be obstructed by scars that bind together two normally separate anatomic surfaces (adhesions), hernias, or tumors. Another cause may be a paralytic ileus, a paralysis of the peristaltic movement of the intestinal tract caused by the effect of trauma or toxins on the nerve endings that regulate intestinal movement. Conservative treatment consists of decompression of the bowel using a nasogastric tube. Surgical treatment may be indicated if the bowel is completely obstructed.

While tumors of the small intestine are rare, tumors of the colon are common. Cancer of the colon and rectum is the second most common type of cancer in the United States (with lung cancer being the

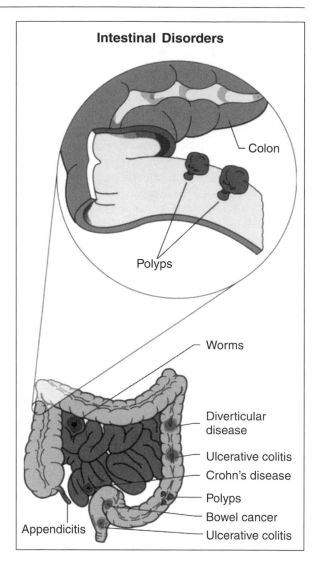

Intestinal Disorders

Colon

Polyps

Worms

Diverticular disease

Ulcerative colitis

Crohn's disease

Polyps

Bowel cancer

Ulcerative colitis

Appendicitis

most common). The majority of intestinal tumors are benign (noncancerous) and discovered between the ages of forty and sixty. There are several types of benign tumors, which do not spread. They include lipomas, leiomyomas, angiomas, and adenomas. A small percentage of tumors of the small intestine is malignant (cancerous). The most common are adenocarcinomas, leiomyosarcomas, carcinoid tumors, and lymphomas. The symptoms of these tumors include weight loss, abdominal pain, nausea and vomiting, and bleeding. Treatment is dependent upon the stage and location of the tumor. Surgical removal of the tumor may be coupled with chemotherapy and/or radiation therapy.

Polyps are benign tumors of the large intestine and are common to individuals over the age of sixty. They arise from the lining of the colon and are usually found during tests to diagnose other conditions. Polyps include several different varieties, the most common of which is a hyperplastic polyp. Hyperplastic polyps are less than one-half of a centimeter in diameter and do not pose a health risk. Juvenile polyps can occur in childhood, and inflammatory polyps are believed to result from injury or inflammation, such as after an episode of ulcerative colitis. Neither of these conditions poses a health risk. There is a major category of polyps known as adenomas, however, which have the potential for malignancy. These types of polyps are generally removed to prevent the development of cancer.

Rectal cancer and colon cancer are two types of cancer common among both men and women. Factors that predispose an individual to these types of cancer include family history or a prior history of adenomatous colon polyps, colon cancer, or ulcerative colitis. The precise cause of these cancers is unknown, but diet is believed to play a significant role, specifically diets low in fiber and high in animal fat. One of the key symptoms of these conditions requiring immediate attention (especially for individuals over the age of forty) is rectal bleeding. Treatment consists of surgery to remove the affected part of the colon. The physician may prescribe additional treatment in the form of chemotherapy and/or radiation therapy.

PERSPECTIVE AND PROSPECTS

Problems associated with the intestinal tract are characterized by a variety of symptoms and treatments. These problems may be temporary in nature or may be manifestations of more serious underlying conditions interfering with the normal functions of absorption, fluid and electrolyte balance, and elimination. Symptoms are signs of malfunction and should not be ignored or go untreated.

Preventing problems associated with the intestinal tract may not always be possible because the causes of some intestinal diseases and disorders are unknown. Nevertheless, there has been substantial research related to intestinal diseases and disorders to support a strong correlation between nutrition and intestinal tract health. For example, there is evidence to support the relationship between the consumption of sugars, high amounts of animal protein and fat, and cholesterol and cancer-causing agents in the intestinal tract. Stress and its resulting influence on stomach acidity also contribute to intestinal ill health. Smoking and lack of regular exercise may also negatively influence normal peristalsis.

The prevention of these and other problems related to intestinal health are important not only to general health but also to work productivity. In the United States, for example, intestinal problems account for a large percentage of lost work time. Education about intestinal health and health issues beginning early in one's life will lower the incidence of some of the more common intestinal diseases and disorders.

—*John A. Bavaro, Ed.D., R.N.*

See also Abdomen; Abdominal disorders; Appendectomy; Appendicitis; Bacterial infections; Bypass surgery; Celiac sprue; Cholecystitis; Cirrhosis; Colic; Colitis; Colon and rectal polyp removal; Colon and rectal surgery; Colon cancer; Colon therapy; Colonoscopy and sigmoidoscopy; Constipation; Crohn's disease; Diarrhea and dysentery; Digestion; Diverticulitis and diverticulosis; Enemas; Enterocolitis; Fistula repair; Food poisoning; Gallbladder diseases; Gastroenterology; Gastroenterology, pediatric; Gastrointestinal disorders; Gastrointestinal system; Hemorrhoid banding and removal; Hemorrhoids; Hernia; Hernia repair; Hirschsprung's disease; Ileostomy and colostomy; Indigestion; Internal medicine; Intestines; Irritable bowel syndrome (IBS); Jaundice; Lactose intolerance; Liver cancer; Liver disorders; Malabsorption; Malnutrition; Nutrition; Obesity; Obstruction; Pancreatitis; Parasitic diseases; Peristalsis; Pinworms; Proctology; Renal failure; Roundworms; Soiling; Stomach, intestinal, and pancreatic cancers; Tapeworms; Tumor removal; Tumors; Worms.

FOR FURTHER INFORMATION:

Clayman, Charles B., ed. *The American Medical Association Encyclopedia of Medicine.* New York: Random House, 1994. Written in an encyclopedic format, this book is an authoritative guide to all aspects of medical and health topics. Contains many illustrations of various body systems and organs that are clearly presented and simple to understand.

Kapadia, Cyrus R., James M. Crawford, and Caroline Taylor. *An Atlas of Gastroenterology: A Guide to Diagnosis and Differential Diagnosis.* Boca Raton, Fla.: Pantheon, 2003. Provides a fully illustrated, nonspecialist understanding of myriad gastrointestinal diseases, including heartburn, dyspepsia, diarrhea, irritable bowel syndrome, and pancreatitis. Includes bibliographic references and index.

Larson, David E., ed. *Mayo Clinic Family Health Book.* 3d ed. New York: William Morrow, 2003. This comprehensive medical guide was written for the general public by experts in the field of medicine. Intestinal disorders of the abdominal cavity are discussed in sections titled "Diseases and Disorders" and "Tests and Treatments."

Payne, Wayne A., and Dale B. Hahn. *Understanding Your Health*. 7th ed. St. Louis: Mosby Year Book, 2001. An introductory textbook that is easy to read. Focuses on overall health and disease prevention. Each chapter offers a list of references and recommended readings related specifically to its content.

Peikin, Steven. *Gastrointestinal Health*. Rev. ed. New York: HarperCollins, 1999. Concerned almost wholly with the effect of nutrition on gastrointestinal (GI) maladies, the author offers a self-help guide for the afflicted. After explaining the GI tract's workings and describing common symptoms, Peikin specifies diets that he argues will relieve symptoms.

Tapley, Donald F., et al., eds. *The Columbia University College of Physicians and Surgeons Complete Home Medical Guide*. Rev. 3d ed. New York: Crown, 1995. An outstanding reference guide organized by each organ system and its function. Written in easily understandable terms and avoids the use of medical jargon. Part 3 provides in-depth information on how the body works and includes a full-color atlas showing major organ systems.

Tortora, Gerard J., and Sandra R. Grabowski. *Principles of Anatomy and Physiology*. 10th ed. New York: John Wiley & Sons, 2003. This highly readable text gives a clear and accurate description of the anatomy and physiology of the gastrointestinal system. The illustrations and diagrams are excellent. The authors include descriptions of major disorders and clinical applications.

INTESTINES

ANATOMY

ANATOMY OR SYSTEM INVOLVED: Abdomen, anus, gastrointestinal system

SPECIALTIES AND RELATED FIELDS: Gastroenterology, internal medicine

DEFINITION: The portion of the gastrointestinal tract from the lower end of the stomach to the anus, which consists of the small intestine and the colon (large intestine).

KEY TERMS:

amylase: the enzyme responsible for breaking down carbohydrates in the small intestine; amylase enters the intestinal tract from the salivary glands and the pancreas

colon: the large intestine, divided from the small intestine by the cecum (a controlled passageway) and ending at the sigmoid, which leads food waste into the rectum

fiber: food material derived from plant substances that retain the full structure of their cell walls despite the chemical effects of the digestive process

lipases: enzymes secreted by the pancreas into the small intestine; these serve to break down fatty materials (triglycerides) in the first intestinal stage of digestion

peristalsis: the muscular contraction in the walls of the intestines that propels food material forward through the bowels

STRUCTURE AND FUNCTIONS

After the initial process of digestion takes place in the stomach, food passes into the intestines, where the chemical action of several gastric juices separates out the nutritive content of fats, carbohydrates, and proteins. This nutritive material is then absorbed into the bloodstream through the walls of the intestines, while waste material is collected for excretion.

In adult humans, the small intestine and large intestine together represent a total length of about 9 meters (30 feet). Both small and large intestines are hoselike muscular organs; the former is much longer, but substantially narrower, than the latter. The two intestines are joined at the cecum, which is located in the right-lower abdominal cavity. The appendix, which is sometimes called a "blind pouch" because it is unessential to the main processes performed in the gastrointestinal tract, projects from the cecum.

The physical disposition and function of the large intestine, or colon, are distinct from those of the small intestine. As the large intestinal tube leaves the cecum, it assumes a specific shape, following horizontal and vertical lines within the abdominal cavity. This is not the case with the small intestine, whose extensive length (about 7 meters, or 23 feet) takes an intertwined "nesting" shape in the limited abdominal space available. By contrast, the colon, which is about 1.5 meters (5 feet) in length, has three easily identifiable sections: the ascending colon on the right side of the abdominal cavity, the transverse colon, and the descending colon on the left side of the abdomen. A final leftward bend in the colon at the sigmoid provides for its attachment to the rectum.

The two parts of the intestines carry out distinct functions in the overall digestive process. As food material passes from the lower end, or pylorus, of the stomach, only a part of the digestive process has occurred. Once partially digested food enters the small intestine, it is propelled through the intestine by means of a process of muscular contraction in the intestinal wall, which is called peristalsis.

As the food moves forward, different substances, some secreted from the lining of the intestine itself, and others—principally, bile and pancreatic fluid, which enter the upper intestine (duodenum) from the liver and pancreas—contribute to a further breaking down of food material.

Very small projections called villi are found along the interior surface of the small intestine. The villi absorb those portions of the food material that have been altered by the digestive process. From the villi, nutritive material is passed into the blood and lymphatic system for distribution to cells throughout the body. This process continues in the middle and end portions (jejunum and ileum, respectively) of the small intestine until, passing through the cecum, the remaining residue enters the large intestine.

The mixture of material contained in the large intestine, or colon, consists of indigestible food, bacteria, and substantial amounts of water. Most of the water is absorbed into the body through the walls of the colon, while the remaining waste material, or feces, is excreted through the rectum.

In order to understand how food materials are actually absorbed by the villi inside the small intestine and passed into the bloodstream, one must consider several chemical processes, according to the nature of the material in question.

For example, the triglyceride components of fat, chains of fatty acids attached to glycerol, are chemical compounds that do not dissolve in water (a major part of the main bloodstream). The pancreatic enzymes called lipases split the triglycerides into separate units of fatty acid. Once separated, these fatty acids become coated with bile salts secreted by the liver, a process that allows them to pass into the mucous cells lining the intestine. As this passage occurs, the coated fatty acids (micelles) resume their chainlike form as triglycerides. At this point, however, the triglycerides have assumed an altered chemical state. In this altered form, fats can be absorbed into the blood and carried throughout the body to be used as body "fuel" or, if unused, stored in fatty tissues.

Carbohydrates must be broken down into simple sugars (glucose, galactose, and fructose) before they can be absorbed by the cell linings of the small intestine. This process occurs when the more complex carbohydrates (both starches and sugars) are split by the chemical effects of the enzyme amylase, which enters the small intestine from the salivary glands and the pancreas.

Finally, proteins, which contain the amino acids so essential for the process of tissue formation in the body, must be split in several stages, the first of which occurs in the stomach itself. Here, proteins are partially broken down by the action of the gastric juices, mainly pepsin. Once protein material passes into the upper part of the small intestine, or duodenum, the process is accelerated by the influence of two main pancreatic enzymes: trypsin and chymotrypsin. These secretions cause the proteins to release amino acids in three forms: simple, dual, or triplicate bodies. It is not until these three forms are actually inside the cell walls of the small intestine that other enzymes split the dual and triplicate amino acids into their simplest single form, which can be absorbed into the veins that carry nourishment to the various organs of the body.

In the overall chemical process leading to the absorption of various body nutrients by the small and large intestines, there is a certain "absorptive specialization" in different zones of the gastrointestinal tract. Iron and calcium, for example, are absorbed in the duodenum, while proteins, fats, sugars, and all vitamins except vitamin B_{12} are absorbed in the jejunum. Finally, in the ileum, salt, vitamin B_{12}, and bile salts are processed.

DISORDERS AND DISEASES

Doctors have always known that the digestive processes of the intestines can be affected in either positive or negative ways by the nature of the food that is consumed. In the simplest terms, negative reactions are manifested by the obvious effects of indigestion and diarrhea. The control of such symptoms of improper or incomplete digestion may appear to the layperson to be a simple matter of using "over-the-counter" tablets such as laxatives or "antigas" pills. Treatment of the symptoms of indigestion, however, may provide only a superficial solution to a problem that is much more serious.

An area of important medical concern that goes beyond the general discomfort caused by imbalanced digestive functioning of the intestines involves peptic ulcers. A peptic ulcer is an open sore on the mucous membrane lining the gastrointestinal tract. The general label "peptic ulcer" was applied to this condition since the discovery, in the mid-1830's, of pepsin, the first clearly identified enzyme known to contribute to the chemical breakdown of ingested foods. Although later stages of research into the digestive process yielded much more extensive knowledge of the component elements of gastric juices, the specific name has remained attached to the general phenomenon of intestinal ulceration. The term "gastric ulcer" refers specifically to ulceration in the stomach lining.

Generally speaking, peptic ulcers occur when there is an imbalance between the task of digestion to be accomplished by the intestines and the amounts and levels of concentration of the gastric juices secreted into the gastrointestinal tract. When the amounts or concentrated strengths of gastric juices in the intestines exceed the level required for digestion (or flow into the intestine when no food has been ingested), these agents actually begin to digest the membranes of the intestine itself.

Various forms of treatment for intestinal ulcers have been developed, including both therapeutic drugs that have the capacity to counteract the corrosive effects of excessive gastric juices and, in the preventive vein, diets that contain natural combatants against intestinal disorders, especially high-fiber, unprocessed, or lightly processed foods.

In recent years, research into the causes of ulcers has extended into the field of gastrointestinal hormonal secretions originating not in the pancreas itself but in the intestine or stomach. These secretions reach the pancreas later through the bloodstream and stimulate its production of digestive juices. Such secretive processes may, if they fail to communicate properly balanced "codes" concerning the task of digestion that needs to take place in the intestines, cause an excessive supply (in volume or strength) of gastric juices, which can cause ulcerations to develop.

The most serious pathological condition that can affect the intestines is cancer of the colon. Thought to develop from a degenerative process originating in benign polyps (stem-based tumors that may develop in areas of the organism lined with mucous membrane, such as the nose, the colon, and, in females, the uterus), cancer of the colon has registered a survival rate that is statistically higher than those of cancers in other vital organs of the abdominal cavity (the liver and stomach, in particular). This is partly because—if the cancer is discovered in time—substantial areas of the colon that have been attacked by cancer can be removed surgically without endangering the continued essential functioning of the intestines.

Almost all questions relating to the pathology of the intestinal tract are somehow connected with the type of food that is eaten. Thus, medical science has turned increasingly to publicizing preventive dietary practices that can have a bearing on all functions of the intestines, from the simplest level of discomfort to the most serious level of chronic diseases.

As stated above, a relatively recent and valuable contribution to the knowledge of natural ways to aid in the absorptive work of both the small intestine and the colon—and to reduce the dangers of ulceration and/or intestinal cancer—involves the role of the fiber content of foods. Fiber is generally described as consisting of polysaccharides and lignin, two plant substances that, more than any other nutritive material, retain their natural forms as plant cell walls and are not broken down by human digestive enzymes. The plant food that is richest in these materials is wheat bran, which contains about 40 percent fiber. As fiber-rich foodstuffs such as bran pass through the gastrointestinal tract, the fiber material they contain is subject to fermentation by anaerobic bacteria in the colon. Two chemical results of this complex process seem to be the removal of deoxycholic acid from the bile and the reduction of the cholesterol saturation level of the bile. Both effects are deemed beneficial, since the reduction of deoxycholic acid and cholesterol in intestinal bile tends, at the very least, to reduce the likelihood of developing gallstones. Fiber-rich diets in combination with the reduction of excess weight became standard symbols of preventive health care by the 1990's.

By the mid-twentieth century, typical personal diets in the Western world contained commercially refined foodstuffs that were rich in sugars and syrups, which are mainly fiber depleted. In addition to the specific disease-related factors mentioned above, medical science has noted that high consumption of fiber-depleted foods results in higher levels of energy intake (absorption of Calories) during the digestive process that occurs in the intestines. In simple terms, when Calorie intake exceeds the level required by the normally exercised body, the result is weight gain that may continue to the point of obesity.

PERSPECTIVE AND PROSPECTS

Medical science began to become aware of the various digestive functions of hormonal secretions only in the first decades of the twentieth century. Although the early nineteenth century American army surgeon William Beaumont was the first doctor to discover the presence of gastric juices in the intestines, his analysis of digestive fluids remained quite elementary. Beaumont could easily identify hydrochloric acid in stomach secretions.

He also took samples of bile from the intestinal tract and performed laboratory experiments that proved the role of bile in breaking down fatty materials. What remained unsolved were the identity and origins of other components of gastric juice and an explanation for their controlled secretion from surrounding organs in the abdominal cavity into the intestines. Beaumont's view that mental concentration (including "negative mental concentration," or anxiety) induced the flow of gastric juices proved eventually to be only partially correct.

It was only in 1902 that the British doctors Ernest Henry Starling and Sir William Maddock Bayliss were able to show that, in addition to nerve "signals," certain chemical factors induced the flow of gastric juices, specifically from the pancreas into the intestinal tract. These doctors found that, in fact, the small intestine released into the bloodstream a "chemical transmitter" that, as it circulated to the other vital organs, stimulated the production and flow of the pancreatic juices necessary for digestion. They called this "chemical transmitter" secretin. To this initial agent would be added a whole category of secretions that are called "hormones," a term taken from the Greek word for "urging on."

A discovery was made in 1928 that helped to clarify the complex relationship of hormones, gastric juice secretion, and the carrying out of the digestive process by the small and large intestines. This was the discovery of pancreozymin, the second main "chemical transmitter" affecting the pancreas, by the American researcher Andrew Ivy. Pancreozymin was found to cause the release by the pancreas of an enzyme-rich fluid made up of three agents: trypsin, lipase, and amylase. Each agent proved to be an activator in the process of breaking down different nutrients (protein, fats, and carbohydrates, respectively).

Although the intestines are the ultimate destination of and seat of activity for the pancreatic juices released by command of this hormone (as well as of the last major digestion-linked hormone, gastrin, which was discovered in 1955), secretin alone has its origin in the intestines themselves. Both pancreozymin and gastrin are secreted from the stomach.

In time, researchers found that most gastrointestinal hormones are secreted by specialized cells that line the interior of the stomach. Such cells react at various levels according to the composition of the food that has been ingested, sending chemical signals, via the hormones they secrete, that determine the relative amounts and strengths of the several gastric juices that enter the intestines from the pancreas. A similar question of varied amounts and strengths of gastric juices was linked to the so-called vagus nerve function, which also activates pancreatic flow to the intestinal tract.

The functional relationship between these two activator agents—the one nervous and the other chemical—has become one of the primary interests of researchers who deal with the most common ailment attacking the intestinal organs: peptic ulceration.

—*Byron D. Cannon, Ph.D.*

See also Abdomen; Abdominal disorders; Bypass surgery; Colitis; Colon and rectal surgery; Colonoscopy and sigmoidoscopy; Digestion; Endoscopy; Enemas; Gastroenterology; Gastroenterology, pediatric; Gastrointestinal disorders; Gastrointestinal system; Hemorrhoids; Hernia; Internal medicine; Intestinal disorders; Laparoscopy; Malnutrition; Nutrition; Obstruction; Peristalsis; Proctology.

FOR FURTHER INFORMATION:

Janowitz, Henry D. *Good Food for Bad Stomachs*. New York: Oxford University Press, 1997. A popular work on indigestion and diseases of the gastrointestinal system that suggests diet therapy. Includes an index.

_____. *Indigestion: Living Better with Upper Intestinal Problems from Heartburn to Ulcers and Gallstones*. New York: Oxford University Press, 1994. Uses a scientific and "commonsense" approach to address myriad gastrointestinal disorders.

Marieb, Elaine N. *Human Anatomy and Physiology*. 6th ed. Redwood City, Calif.: Benjamin/Cummings, 2003. This introductory anatomy and physiology textbook, easily accessible to those with little science background, is richly illustrated with diagrams and photographs, which help to illuminate body systems and processes.

Scanlon, Valerie, et al. *Essentials of Anatomy and Physiology*. 4th ed. Philadelphia: F. A. Davis, 2002. A text designed around three themes: the relationship between physiology and anatomy, the interrelations among the organ systems, and the relationship of each organ system to homeostasis.

Sleisenger, Marvin H., and John S. Fordtran, eds. *Sleisenger and Fordtran's Gastrointestinal and Liver Disease: Pathophysiology, Diagnosis, Management*. 7th ed. 2 vols. Philadelphia: W. B. Saunders, 2002. A comprehensive textbook.

Tortora, Gerard J., and Sandra R. Grabowski. *Principles of Anatomy and Physiology*. 10th ed. New York: John Wiley & Sons, 2003. An outstanding textbook of human anatomy and physiology, and a good first text to consult before reading more advanced gastro-enterology texts and journal articles.

Wolfe, M. Michael, and Sidney Cohen. *Therapy of Digestive Disorders: A Companion to Sleisenger and Fordtran's Gastrointestinal and Liver Disease.* Philadelphia: W. B. Saunders, 2000. This resource is divided into sections that discuss such topics as esophageal, gastroduodenal, pancreaticobiliary, hepatic, intestinal, and miscellaneous disorders.

INTOXICATION

DISEASE/DISORDER

ALSO KNOWN AS: Inebriation

ANATOMY OR SYSTEM AFFECTED: Brain, heart, psychic-emotional, reproductive system, respiratory system

SPECIALTIES AND RELATED FIELDS: Cardiology, pathology, pharmacology, preventive medicine, psychiatry, public health, toxicology, vascular medicine

DEFINITION: a physical and mental state resulting from having consumed a psychoactive substance and characterized by maladaptive changes in physiological, psychological, mood, and/or cognitive processes.

CAUSES AND SYMPTOMS

Intoxication is a type of substance use disorder described in the *Diagnostic and Statistical Manual of Mental Disorders: DSM-IV-TR* (rev. 4th ed., 2000) by the American Psychiatric Association. Intoxication results from the consumption of substances such as alcohol, caffeine, marijuana, other illicit drugs, and even prescription drugs.

Intoxication is diagnosed via identification of the substance in the body system and the observation of characteristic symptoms in the person affected. Tests of breath and/or urine samples are used. Additionally, simply watching the individual for psychological and behavioral signs or asking the individual to perform certain tasks can help as well. For instance, police officers suspecting alcohol intoxication may request individuals to try to walk a straight line or to close their eyes and try to stand up straight. Such tests allow the officers to observe the person's balance and body sway. Loss of balance or significant body sway can indicate intoxication.

Each substance, however, has specific symptoms associated with its intoxication state. For instance, alcohol intoxication is marked by symptoms such as slurred speech, coordination problems, unsteady gait, nystagmus, impairments in memory or attention, and stupor. Nystagmus is an involuntary condition affecting the

---

INFORMATION ON INTOXICATION

CAUSES: Overconsumption of substances such as alcohol, caffeine, marijuana, or other illicit drugs, prescription drugs

SYMPTOMS: Varies; with alcohol, may include slurred speech, coordination problems, unsteady gait, impairments in memory or attention, stupor, coma

DURATION: Temporary

TREATMENTS: Detoxification

---

eyes in which they do not track the movement of objects smoothly. Stupor is a condition in which the person is in a daze and has numbed senses. With alcohol intoxication, stupor can escalate to coma. In addition to these symptoms, problematic behaviors may also manifest themselves, such as aggression, impaired judgment, mood problems, or problems interacting socially or at work.

TREATMENT AND THERAPY

Intoxication is short-lived; once a substance has been processed out of the body, the effects dissipate. Treatment usually consists of a process called detoxification, often shortened to detox. Typically, this is done in emergency rooms or inpatient units in hospitals. Symptoms are monitored closely as the person withdraws from the substance. Withdrawal varies depending on how long the person has used the substance and how much has been used. Severe withdrawal from certain substances, such as alcohol, can be lethal.

PERSPECTIVE AND PROSPECTS

Intoxication for some substances is easier to identify than for others. Increasingly, methods are being developed to identify intoxication with greater ease via objective measures. For instance, technology to assess the iris of the eye to detect marijuana intoxication or the use of patches to detect substance use, such as with drugs that may be excreted in sweat, are two recent efforts.

—*Nancy A. Piotrowski, Ph.D.*

See also Addiction; Alcoholism; Caffeine; Club drugs; Coma; Marijuana; Poisoning; Toxicology.

FOR FURTHER INFORMATION:

American Psychiatric Association. *Diagnostic and Statistical Manual of Mental Disorders: DSM-IV-TR.* Rev. 4th ed. Washington, D.C.: Author, 2000.

Julien, R. M. *A Primer of Drug Action*. Rev. and updated ed. New York: W. H. Freeman, 2001.

Weil, A., and R. Winifred. *From Chocolate to Morphine: Everything You Need to Know About Mind-Altering Drugs*. Rev. and updated ed. Boston: Houghton Mifflin, 1998.

Intraventricular hemorrhage
Disease/disorder

Anatomy or system affected: Brain, nervous system

Specialties and related fields: Neonatology, neurology

Definition: Bleeding into or around the normal fluid spaces within the brain.

Key terms:

cerebrospinal fluid (CSF): fluid produced within the ventricles of the brain that flows around the brain and spinal cord

cranial ultrasound: the use of sound waves to obtain a picture of the brain

hydrocephalus: a condition characterized by the abnormal accumulation of fluid within the cranial vault, often accompanied by enlargement of the head and damage to the brain

indomethacin: a nonsteroidal anti-inflammatory drug (NSAID) administered to preterm babies in an attempt to decrease the likelihood of developing intraventricular hemorrhage

ventricles: fluid-filled spaces within the brain

Causes and Symptoms

Intraventricular hemorrhage (IVH) occurs most commonly in premature babies, especially those weighing under 1,500 grams. IVHs have been seen as well in adults as a secondary complication of hemorrhagic stroke, leaving the individual with a poor prognosis.

IVH in premature babies is thought to occur when there is oxygen deprivation during delivery or complications following delivery. Since the blood vessels in the brain of the baby are fragile, they may rupture easily, resulting in excessive bleeding into (intraventricular) or around (periventricular) the ventricles. Generally, there are no outward symptoms. Some infants with IVH may suddenly develop seizures or anemia. IVH is usually diagnosed by cranial ultrasound routinely done on high-risk infants between three and ten days of life, since most cases occur by day three.

Intraventricular hemorrhages are categorized into four grades based on severity. Grade I involves bleed-

---

Information on Intraventricular Hemorrhage

Causes: Unknown; possibly oxygen deprivation during premature delivery or subsequent complications, leading to rupture of blood vessels in brain

Symptoms: Generally none, sometimes seizures or anemia; may result in hydrocephalus

Duration: Acute, with possible long-term consequences if severe (motor problems, developmental delay, seizures, blindness, deafness)

Treatments: Prevention through intravenous indomethacin during first three days of life, steroids given to mother prior to delivery; alleviation of symptoms; insertion of shunt for hydrocephalus

---

ing confined to the small area where it began. Grade II involves blood extending into the ventricles, with no ventricular enlargement. Grade III involves more blood extending into the ventricles, with ventricular enlargement. Grade IV has blood collecting within the brain tissue (intraparenchymal hemorrhage), reflecting injury to the brain. Hydrocephalus is a common complication of Grade III or IV bleeds.

Treatment and Therapy

Premature babies are given intravenous indomethacin once daily for the first three days of life in order to decrease the likelihood of severe IVH. Steroids given to the mother prior to delivery have also decreased the frequency of severe IVH, as have improved monitoring and care of premature babies. No specific treatment exists for IVH, except to treat symptoms and underlying health problems. If hydrocephalus develops, it can be treated with frequent lumbar punctures or ventricular taps. If the condition persists, a shunt may be placed surgically to drain the extra CSF throughout life. In adults who suffer IVH secondary to hemorrhagic stroke, fibrolytic agents (so-called clot busters) are being evaluated as a mode of treatment.

Perspective and Prospects

IVH has been reported in 35 to 50 percent of infants weighing under 1,500 grams. As gestational age increases, the likelihood of IVH decreases. Grade I IVHs rarely involve long-term problems. Those classified as Grade IV generally do result in long-term sequelae, including motor problems, developmental delay, seizures, blindness, and deafness.

—*Robin Kamienny Montvilo, R.N., Ph.D.*

See also Bleeding; Brain; Brain disorders; Hydrocephalus; Neonatology; Nervous system; Neurology; Neurology, pediatric; Perinatology; Premature birth; Shunts.

FOR FURTHER INFORMATION:

Klaus, Marshall, and A. Fanaroff, eds. *Care of the High-Risk Neonate.* 5th ed. Philadelphia: W. B. Saunders, 2001.

Victor, Maurice, and Allan H. Ropper. *Adams and Victor's Principles of Neurology.* 7th ed. New York: McGraw-Hill, 2000.

Volpe, Joseph. *Neurology of the Newborn.* 4th ed. Philadelphia: W. B. Saunders, 2001.

INVASIVE TESTS

PROCEDURES

ANATOMY OR SYSTEM AFFECTED: All

SPECIALTIES AND RELATED FIELDS: All

DEFINITION: Tests that require the passage of an instrument through the body's protective barriers.

INDICATIONS AND PROCEDURES

Skin, sphincters, and gag and cough reflex systems are some of the defenses that can be penetrated to gather important diagnostic information. Invasive tests provide medical insights that are unattainable by noninvasive or laboratory tests. Invasive tests are typically performed last in a diagnostic protocol, however, because penetration of the body defenses is not without risk. An anesthetic agent is commonly used to minimize any discomfort or pain that may arise during the tests. Although invasive, these tests often circumvent the trauma of exploratory surgery.

In general, invasive tests may be classified as those that allow the physician to obtain samples of fluid, tissue, or tumors directly from their site of origin (through aspiration, lumbar puncture, and biopsy) or those that allow direct viewing of specific areas of the body through endoscopy. Some test procedures allow both direct viewing and sample collection; bronchoscopy is one such example.

One of the more familiar aspiration tests is amniocentesis. Amniocentesis involves removing 20 to 30 milliliters of fluid from the amniotic sac for analysis. This test is used in prenatal care at weeks fifteen to eighteen in order to assess the genetic makeup of the fetus or to detect developmental abnormalities.

Fluid from effusions can also be aspirated for analysis. Effusions are collections of an abnormally large quantity of fluid within a serous or synovial cavity. While a small amount of fluid is normal in these cavities, a large amount indicates a pathology that should be identified and treated. Once an effusion is tapped, the fluid is grossly examined for color and for clarity or turbidity. Microscopic investigations of the fluids are performed to assess the types of cells present (such as immune cells or malignant cells) and to identify microorganisms that may be present. Paracentesis is the removal of fluid from effusions within the abdominal, or peritoneal, cavity. If the effusion in this region is large, it is called ascites. Removal of fluid from the lung cavity, called thoracentesis, requires penetration of the chest wall between the ribs (intercostal spaces). Common causes of effusions include infections, congestive heart failure, kidney disease, and malignancy.

Synovial fluid is most commonly aspirated from the knee, but other joints can be investigated in this manner. Red blood cells, inflammatory cells, or crystals may be identified by microscopic evaluation of the aspirated fluid. Osteoarthritis, rheumatoid arthritis, and gout are some diseases that can be diagnosed through synovial fluid aspiration.

Cerebrospinal fluid (CSF) is housed within the bony cranium and spinal column. Fluid from this space is collected by lumbar puncture (spinal tap) and is drawn when a viral, bacterial, or fungal meningitis is suspected. Lumbar puncture may also be performed when a tumor or leukemia of the central nervous system is suspected, or to determine whether a subarachnoid hemorrhage is present.

Fine needle aspiration (FNA) is a specific kind of percutaneous (through-the-skin) needle biopsy. FNA can be used to collect a sample of cells from any palpable mass. By directly inserting a needle into the mass and then washing, or flushing, the region, some cells can be eroded from the tissue surface. These cells are set adrift in the fluid, which is sucked back into the flushing syringe. Microscopic evaluation of the cells can then be performed. Breast, neck, abdominal, and lymph nodes are some of the places where FNA is utilized.

Alternative biopsy techniques include gently scraping off a small surface, as in the Papanicolaou (Pap) smear of the cervix, or removing a deeper tissue sample, as in the punch biopsy of the cervix. Biopsy can sometimes require small surgical incisions to reach a certain organ, such as muscle, skin, breast, bone, or renal (kidney) biopsy.

Tissue biopsies may be taken directly from an organ without surgical incisions; one way to do this is with endoscopy. Typically, endoscopes are flexible probing instruments fitted with fiber-optic viewing devices. Often, a tool attachment allows the use of tiny cutting and sampling devices. Small pieces of tissue can be removed from some otherwise inaccessible areas of the body. Different kinds of endoscopes are used to accommodate the unique structural features of body regions, such as the bronchi, stomach, or colon. Sterile techniques are implemented in all cases.

Bronchoscopy is utilized in diagnosing pulmonary infections and lung cancers or in locating and removing foreign objects found in the airways. Esophageal-gastroscopy is used to determine the source of upper gastrointestinal problems such as gastric or peptic ulcers, esophageal varices, esophageal reflux, or malignancy. Colonoscopy is similarly used to evaluate the origins of lower gastrointestinal problems. Colon polyps can be identified, and the mucosal lining of the colon can be evaluated for ulcerative colitis, diverticula, or adenocarcinomas.

Finally, arteriography (including angiography) and cardiac catheterization are important and frequently used invasive tests. These tests are used to evaluate the cardiovascular system. Angiography combines radiographic techniques with the injection of dyes into arteries. This combination allows the physician to determine whether an artery is blocked (occluded). Angiography is particularly useful in patients who have heart conditions, such as angina, and can be used to evaluate renal (kidney) arteries, aortic dissection, or cerebral aneurysms. The result of arteriography is a critical component in determining whether surgery or drug intervention is best for a given patient.

As a diagnostic tool, cardiac catheterization provides insight into the health of a heart. Pictures of the heart can be taken as the catheter is advanced into the right side and then the left side of the heart. A dye is injected into the heart so that the flow can be traced as the heart pumps. The heart chambers, valves, and blood vessels can be evaluated. Additionally, pressures within the heart chambers can be recorded.

Uses and Complications
The greatest health risk with any invasive test is infection. For this reason, sterile methods are used to keep infections and mortality caused by infections to a minimum. With proper care, the risks of invasive testing are surpassed by the benefits of the early and proper diagnosis that such tests provide.

—*Mary C. Fields, M.D.*

See also Amniocentesis; Angiography; Arthroscopy; Biopsy; Blood testing; Breast biopsy; Catheterization; Chorionic villus sampling; Colonoscopy and sigmoidoscopy; Cystoscopy; Endometrial biopsy; Endoscopy; Laparoscopy; Magnetic resonance imaging (MRI); Positron emission tomography (PET) scanning; Radiopharmaceuticals.

For Further Information:
Cavanaugh, Bonita Morrow. *Nurse's Manual of Laboratory and Diagnostic Tests*. 4th ed. Philadelphia: F. A. Davis, 2003. Provides information on hundreds of laboratory and diagnostic tests, with each test presented in two distinct, cross-referenced sections: "Background Information" sections provide a complete description of each test and its purposes; "Clinical Application Data" sections focus on the information nurses most commonly need while caring for clients.

Classen, Meinhard, and C. J. Lightdale. *Gastroenterological Endoscopy*. New York: Thieme Medical, 2002. Text that examines such topics as the impact of endoscopy, its history of use, diagnostic procedures and techniques, therapeutic procedures, descriptions of diseases involving the upper and lower intestine, endoscopic features of infectious diseases of the gastrointestinal tract, and pediatric endoscopy.

Dublin, Arthur B., ed. *Outpatient Invasive Radiologic Procedures: Diagnostic and Therapeutic*. Philadelphia: W. B. Saunders, 1989. Discusses such topics as radiography, radiotherapy, and diagnostic imaging. Also covers interventional radiography. Includes bibliographical references and an index.

Griffith, H. Winter. *Complete Guide to Symptoms, Illness and Surgery*. Rev. ed. New York: Berkley, 2000. Covers more than five hundred diseases and disorders and includes information about causes and risk factors, preventive techniques, and diagnostic tests.

Pagana, Kathleen Deska, and Timothy James Pagana. *Mosby's Diagnostic and Laboratory Test Reference*. 6th ed. New York: Elsevier, 2002. A clinical handbook that gives alphabetically organized laboratory and diagnostic tests for easy reference. Each listing includes such things as alternate or abbreviated test names, type of test, normal findings, possible critical values, test explanation and related physiology, and potential complications.

1442 • Irritable bowel syndrome (IBS)

Ravin, Carl E., ed. *Imaging and Invasive Radiology in the Intensive Care Unit*. New York: Churchill Livingstone, 1993. Discusses such topics as critical care medicine, diagnostic imaging, and interventional radiology. Includes bibliographical references and an index.

Sloan, John P., et al., eds. *Biopsy Pathology of the Breast*. 2d ed. New York: Oxford University Press, 2001. A practical guide to diagnosing breast pathology. Second edition examines the way in which advances in mammographic screening, more treatment options, greater involvement by pathologists in clinical management, and the expansion of molecular pathology have impacted the field.

Zaret, Barry L., ed. *Yale University School of Medicine Patient's Guide to Medical Tests: Detailed Descriptions of the Most Common Diagnostic Procedures*. Boston: Houghton Mifflin, 1998. Written and edited by Yale University School of Medicine faculty, this resource provides detailed information on types of diagnostic tests, how doctors use them, and what patients can do for themselves.

IRRITABLE BOWEL SYNDROME (IBS)

DISEASE/DISORDER

ALSO KNOWN AS: Colitis, spastic colon

ANATOMY OR SYSTEM AFFECTED: Abdomen, anus, gastrointestinal system, intestines, nervous system

SPECIALTIES AND RELATED FIELDS: Alternative medicine, gastroenterology, nutrition

DEFINITION: A common intestinal disorder characterized by abdominal pain and cramps, altered bowel habits, bloating, and nausea.

KEY TERMS:

biofeedback: the technique of making unconscious or involuntary bodily processes perceptible to the senses in order to manipulate them by conscious mental control

Crohn's disease: a disease characterized by inflammation of the intestines, whose early symptoms may resemble those of irritable bowel syndrome

defecation: passage of feces through the anus

endoscopy: the use of a small-diameter, flexible tube of optical fibers with an external light source to examine visually the interior of the body

feces: undigested food and other waste that is eliminated through the anus

gastroenterology: diagnosis and treatment of diseases and disorders of the digestive tract

lactose: a sugar found in milk and milk products; some people cannot digest lactose, causing lactose intolerance, which can produce symptoms that resemble those of irritable bowel syndrome

peristalsis: a series of muscular contractions that move food through the intestines during the process of digestion

ulcerative colitis: an inflammatory disease that causes ulcers in the large intestine

CAUSES AND SYMPTOMS

Although the causes of irritable bowel syndrome (IBS) are not understood, it is believed to result from changes in activity of the major part of the large intestine, or colon. Following food digestion by the stomach and the small intestine, the undigested material is pushed toward the rectum by peristalsis. When peristalsis becomes disrupted by IBS, the flow becomes too slow, causing constipation, or too fast, causing diarrhea.

Some foods and drinks appear more likely to trigger IBS attacks by disrupting peristalsis. Fatty foods, fried foods, milk products, chocolate, drinks with caffeine, and alcohol can exacerbate the symptoms of IBS, as well as some fruits or vegetables, such as cabbage, broccoli, cauliflower, asparagus, or brussels sprouts. In some cases, however, no specific foods cause specific symptoms, as any food intake seems to worsen symptoms. Often, IBS-aggravating foods vary from person to person.

The nervous system's links between the brain and the intestines suggest that stress may be culprit in IBS. Many IBS sufferers report symptoms following a meal when they experience stress. Female reproductive hormones are thought to trigger IBS attacks, because IBS is sometimes accentuated during menstruation.

INFORMATION ON IRRITABLE BOWEL SYNDROME (IBS)

CAUSES: Unclear; possibly changes in activity of colon resulting from dietary factors, stress, female reproductive hormones

SYMPTOMS: Abdominal pain and cramps, diarrhea or constipation, bloating, nausea

DURATION: Chronic

TREATMENTS: Dietary changes, antispasmodic drugs, psychological counseling, behavioral therapy (*e.g.*, hypnosis and biofeedback, relaxation techniques)

IBS is more commonly seen in women than in men, with up to 20 percent of the American population affected. Although it can occur at any time, IBS generally appears in the patient's teens and twenties, and it frequently is found in members of the same family.

Although symptoms vary in intensity, they do not grow steadily worse over time. Abdominal pain is always present, or discomfort associated with constipation, diarrhea, or alternating constipation with diarrhea. Other symptoms include bloating, passage of mucus, nausea, gas, an increased urge to defecate, and a feeling of incomplete rectal evacuation.

Diagnosis of IBS is an involved process that is accomplished through a standard evaluation called the Rome criteria. Symptoms present for three months of the year are considered, along with the results of physical examination, laboratory tests, stool sample, and endoscopy—all of which rule out serious diseases such as colon cancer.

TREATMENT AND THERAPY

Generally, a low-fat, high-fiber diet lessens symptoms, although the tolerance of fiber as well as of all foods varies from person to person. Dietary changes vary according to the severity of the patient's symptoms. In mild cases of IBS, known aggravating foods should be identified and avoided. Symptoms may be eased by eating smaller meals or eating smaller portions. Since no diet has been found that controls all symptoms, a diary of symptoms and food intake is valuable in determining which foods are offensive. Constipation and diarrhea can be alleviated by taking one tablespoon of Metamucil or Fiberall daily. Establishment of fixed times for meals and bathroom visits helps regulate bowel habits.

For more severe symptoms, dietary changes should be supplemented with antispasmodic drugs for abdominal pain. Psychological counseling; behavioral therapy, including hypnosis and biofeedback; and relaxation techniques are recommended to reduce anxiety and encourage learning to cope with the pain of IBS. Severe pain from IBS can be blocked with antidepressants. Moderate exercise has also been shown to be beneficial.

In addition to dietary changes prescribed by doctors, alternative practitioners advise herbal remedies such

---

IN THE NEWS: RETURN OF RISKY DRUG LOTRONEX

Lotronex (alosetron hydrochloride) was approved by the Food and Drug Administration (FDA) in February, 2000, to treat irritable bowel syndrome (IBS) in women whose major symptom is chronic diarrhea. (Men were not part of the original trial, although some men have been prescribed the drug.) It was voluntarily withdrawn from the market in November, 2000, by GlaxoSmithKline, its manufacturer, because of dangerous adverse effects experienced by some patients. Most serious were severe constipation and ischemic colitis, a potentially fatal condition in which blood stops flowing to the colon, causing bowel tissue to die. Most patients experiencing these effects required hospitalization, and several died. By April, 2001, 141 cases of severe gastrointestinal complications had been reported to the FDA.

Despite such lethal side effects, the withdrawal of Lotronex resulted in a storm of protest by patients who believed that they were helped by the drug. An FDA advisory panel recommended its return, but only with several restrictions and for women with particularly severe IBS who do not respond to other treatments. In June, 2002, Lotronex became the first prescription drug banned for safety reasons to be returned to the market. As of early 2003, however, it remained difficult to obtain, partly because of its restrictions. Lotronex can be prescribed only by physicians who enroll in a prescribing program run by GlaxoSmithKline; enrollment is based on the physicians' statements regarding their qualifications to prescribe the drug and their pledge to educate patients about its risks as well as its benefits. In addition, physicians must give patients an FDA-approved medication guide, and they must report serious adverse effects to the manufacturer. Moreover, all patients must sign a form acknowledging their awareness of the drug's dangers and return to the doctor for every refill; doctors are advised to start patients on half of the original dosage and to increase the dosage gradually. Despite these restrictions, members of the FDA watchdog group Public Citizen and others believe that the risks of taking the drug outweigh its benefits, particularly at the reduced dosage, which tested little better than a placebo during the original clinical trials.

—Sue Tarjan

as ginger and peppermint oil or the antispasmodic ingredients in chamomile, valerian, or rosemary. Aromatherapy, hydrotherapy, acupuncture, chiropractic, and osteopathy may also be useful.

PERSPECTIVE AND PROSPECTS

IBS was once believed to be a psychological disorder, but more contemporary researchers believe it is a physical disorder that has specific characteristics and causes real pain. Although there is no cure for IBS, it is not a life-threatening condition. It has not been shown to cause intestinal bleeding or inflammation, as in Crohn's disease, ulcerative colitis, or cancer. Long-term management, though frustrating, involves commitment to therapy for six months or more to find the best combinations of medicine, diet, counseling, and support for control of IBS symptoms. Recent research has discovered a genetic link to panic and anxiety that may be a link to IBS. Other studies stress a mind-body connection to assist in minimizing the symptoms of IBS.

—*Mary Hurd*

See also Abdominal disorders; Colitis; Constipation; Crohn's disease; Diarrhea and dysentery; Gastroenterology; Gastrointestinal disorders; Gastrointestinal system; Intestinal disorders; Intestines; Lactose intolerance; Peristalsis.

FOR FURTHER INFORMATION:

Darnley, Simon, and Barbara Millar. *Understanding Irritable Bowel Syndrome.* New York: Wiley, 2003. A balanced overview of the different explanations of the disease available and the range of treatments to be found. Includes information about special diets, drugs, and alternative therapies, as well as personal stories of IBS patients.

Irritable Bowel Syndrome Self Help and Support Group. http://www.ibsgroup.org/. Provides support to those who suffer from IBS or family members of an IBS patient and medical professionals who want to learn more about IBS. The IBS Support Group works to educate those who are living with IBS and to increase awareness about this and other functional gastrointestinal disorders.

Kalibjian, Cliff. *Straight from the Gut: Living with Crohn's Disease and Ulcerative Colitis.* Cambridge, Mass.: O'Reilly and Associates, 2003. Shares numerous personal stories from those suffering from colitis and offers advice on all aspects of living with the disease.

National Digestive Diseases Information Clearinghouse. http://digestive.niddk.nih.gov/. Site offers an overview of irritable bowel syndrome; information on its causes, effects, and treatments; and suggestions for further reading.

Saibil, Fred. *Crohn's Disease and Ulcerative Colitis: Everything You Need to Know.* Rev. ed. Toronto, Ont.: Firefly Books, 2003. A leading expert on IBD, Saibil covers topics such as signs and symptoms, how the gastrointestinal system works normally and how IBD affects it, procedures and instruments used to diagnose IBD, effects of diet, children and IBD, and effects on sexual activity and childbearing.

Sklar, Jill, Manual Sklar, and Annabel Cohen. *First Year—Crohn's Disease and Ulcerative Colitis: An Essential Guide for the Newly Diagnosed.* New York: Avalon, 2002. A unique guide for patients with specific gastrointestinal disorders, setting expectations and answering questions related to the first week of diagnosis, the first months, and the first year. Topics include treatment options, dietary choices, fertility issues, and holistic alternatives.

ISCHEMIA

DISEASE/DISORDER

ANATOMY OR SYSTEM AFFECTED: Blood vessels, brain, circulatory system

SPECIALTIES AND RELATED FIELDS: Cardiology, critical care, neurology, vascular medicine

DEFINITION: The interruption or temporary restriction of blood flow to a particular area of the body, such as an organ.

CAUSES AND SYMPTOMS

When a localized area of the brain does not receive enough blood, neurons and supportive tissue such as glia are deprived of the essential oxygen and glucose that keeps them alive. If the brain does not receive sufficient blood for even a few minutes, the result is an ischemic stroke.

Although it is possible for ischemia to have no detectable symptoms, when it occurs to the internal carotid, middle cerebral, or vertebral-basilar arteries, symptoms such as confusion, impaired speech, double vision, or numbness on one side of the face can be experienced. In the majority of instances, these symptoms are temporary and do not result in permanent brain damage. If blood flow is restricted to the coronary ar-

INFORMATION ON ISCHEMIA

CAUSES: Blood clots, artherosclerosis
SYMPTOMS: Depends on location; may include confusion, impaired speech, double vision, numbness on one side of face, chest pain
DURATION: May be temporary or permanent
TREATMENTS: Drug therapy (*e.g.*, aspirin, nitroglycerin); surgery (*e.g.*, angioplasty)

tery of the heart (cardiac ischemia), then the heart muscle may suffer permanent damage. Symptoms of cardiac ischemia may include chest pain.

Ischemia is commonly caused by the formation of blood clots or by artherosclerosis, in which the walls of the arteries become narrowed as a result of the buildup of fat deposits.

TREATMENT AND THERAPY

Ischemic stroke can be assessed with high-resolution ultrasound equipment or magnetic resonance angiography (MRA) to detect blood flow. It is common to use computed tomography (CT) scanning or magnetic resonance imaging (MRI) to rule out the possibility that a blood vessel has burst, leading to a hemorrhage. Drug therapies such as administering aspirin or stronger blood-thinning agents help when ischemia is caused by clotting. Nitroglycerin can quickly open up coronary arteries and reduce the chest pain experienced when the heart is affected. Drugs that lower blood pressure are also helpful treatments.

Surgery might be needed to correct an obstruction that cannot be dissolved. Angioplasty can be used to expand affected arteries, particularly when the cause is atherosclerosis.

PERSPECTIVE AND PROSPECTS

Rudolf Virchow, a nineteenth century German physician, was the first to use the term "ischemia." Since the time that ischemia was originally identified, medical advances in diagnostics have been improved through the use of echocardiograms that send out sound waves to create an image of the heart's internal structures. When the affected organ is the brain, treatment improvements have included the administration of unique drugs that can mitigate damage to surrounding nerve cells indirectly affected by the lack of blood.

Much has been learned about the need for a balanced diet, regular exercise, and controlling hypertension as

means to reduce the likelihood of suffering from an ischemic attack.

—*Bryan C. Auday, Ph.D.*

See also Angioplasty; Arteriosclerosis; Bypass surgery; Cardiology; Circulation; Claudication; Heart; Heart attack; Heart disease; Heart failure; Hyperlipidemia; Hypertension; Strokes; Thrombosis and thrombus; Transient ischemic attacks (TIAs); Vascular medicine; Vascular system.

FOR FURTHER INFORMATION:

American Heart Association. *Heart Attack Treatment, Prevention, Recovery.* New York: Time Books, 1996.

Blumenfeld, Hal. *Neuroanatomy Through Clinical Cases.* Sunderland, Mass.: Sinauer Associates, 2002.

Kalat, James W. *Biological Psychology.* 8th ed. Belmont, Calif.: Wadsworth/Thomson Learning, 2004.

Kolb, Bryan, and Ian Q. Whishaw. *Fundamentals of Human Neuropsychology.* 5th ed. New York: Worth, 2003.

Zillmer, Eric A., and Mary V. Spiers. *Principles of Neuropsychology.* Belmont, Calif.: Wadsworth/Thomson Learning, 2001.

ITCHING

DISEASE/DISORDER
ALSO KNOWN AS: Pruritus
ANATOMY OR SYSTEM AFFECTED: Skin
SPECIALTIES AND RELATED FIELDS: Dermatology, otorhinolaryngology, pharmacology, psychiatry
DEFINITION: An unpleasant sensation on or in the skin that causes a desire to scratch or rub the affected area.

CAUSES AND SYMPTOMS

Itching is elicited by the physical or chemical stimulation of nerve receptors in the skin. It can be caused by a wide variety of problems in a variety of different organ systems.

Nearly any skin lesion may itch; skin-related causes include such varied problems as eczema, psoriasis, contact dermatitis, insect bites, bacterial infections, fungal infections, sunburn, and exposure to wool. Viral infections such as chickenpox can cause intense itching. Itching of the eyes and nose are commonly associated with allergies. Itching without a skin rash may be caused by a number of internal problems. Various endocrine problems in children associated with itching include liver disease, kidney failure, thyroid disease, and diabetes. Some malignancies, particularly lymphomas, may cause itching. Hookworms and pinworms are

---

INFORMATION ON ITCHING

CAUSES: Eczema, psoriasis, contact dermatitis, insect bites, bacterial or viral infections, fungal infections, sunburn, exposure to wool, allergies, malignancies, parasites, reaction to certain drugs

SYMPTOMS: Varies; can include dry, red, or flaky skin; rashes; hives; pain and inflammation

DURATION: Acute to chronic

TREATMENTS: Hydration, moisturizing lotion, various medications (primarily antihistamines)

---

both internal causes of itching, as are certain drugs. Finally, some women experience generalized itching during pregnancy.

Certain psychiatric problems are associated with itching. Patients may scratch hard enough to create deep ulcers. The intensity of the itching seems to be related to the degree of nervous tension. In addition, patients who suffer from certain psychotic states or those who abuse drugs such as cocaine may experience a deep itching sensation that they describe as bugs crawling beneath the skin.

Itching may rarely be associated with neurologic disease in which changes in sensation are interpreted by the patient as itching. Occasionally, circulatory problems will cause itching, primarily on the legs. Both of these conditions are more common in older adults than in children or young adults.

TREATMENT AND THERAPY

Treatment should be directed toward the cause of the itching. Hydration (bathing followed by moisturizing lotion) may be helpful in providing relief. When itching is the result of an allergen such as poison ivy, however, a drying agent should be used. Various medications (primarily antihistamines) may relieve itching, but most also cause significant sleepiness.

—*Rebecca Lovell Scott, Ph.D., PA-C*

See also Allergies; Antihistamines; Athlete's foot; Bacterial infections; Bites and stings; Candidiasis; Chickenpox; Dermatitis; Dermatology; Dermatology, pediatric; Diabetes mellitus; Eczema; Endocrine system; Endocrinology; Endocrinology, pediatric; Fungal infections; Hemorrhoids; Hepatitis; Hives; Impetigo; Lice, mites, and ticks; Liver; Liver disorders; Parasitic diseases; Pinworms; Pityriasis rosea; Poisonous plants; Psoriasis; Rashes; Renal failure; Ringworm; Scabies; Sexually transmitted diseases (STDs); Skin; Skin disorders; Sunburn; Thyroid disorders; Viral infections; Worms.

FOR FURTHER INFORMATION:

Adelman, Daniel C., et al., eds. *Manual of Allergy and Immunology.* 4th ed. Philadelphia: Lippincott Williams & Wilkins, 2002.

Bernhard, Jeffrey D., ed. *Itch: Mechanisms and Management of Pruritus.* New York: McGraw-Hill, 1994.

Fleischer, Alan B., Jr. *The Clinical Management of Itching.* New York: Parthenon, 2000.

Larson, David E., ed. *Mayo Clinic Family Health Book.* 3d ed. New York: William Morrow, 2003.

Middlemiss, Prisca. *What's That Rash? How to Identify and Treat Childhood Rashes.* London: Hamlyn, 2002.

Rodale, J. I. *The Itch and What to Do Besides Scratching.* Emmaus, Pa.: Rodale Books, 1971.

Turkington, Carol. *Encyclopedia of Skin and Skin Disorders.* New York: Facts On File, 2002.

Weedon, David. *Skin Pathology.* 2d ed. New York: Harcourt, 2002.

JAUNDICE

DISEASE/DISORDER

ANATOMY OR SYSTEM AFFECTED: Blood, liver, skin

SPECIALTIES AND RELATED FIELDS: Gastroenterology, hematology, internal medicine

DEFINITION: Yellow discoloration of skin resulting from increased levels of bilirubin in the blood.

INFORMATION ON JAUNDICE

CAUSES: Excess of pigment bilirubin resulting from various liver or blood disorders, gallstones, tumors, infection (*e.g.*, hepatitis), or certain drugs

SYMPTOMS: Yellowing of skin and whites of eyes, dark urine, itchy skin

DURATION: Acute

TREATMENTS: Depends on cause; may include surgery to remove gallstones or tumors

CAUSES AND SYMPTOMS

Jaundice is not a disease per se, but rather a common sign of various disorders in the liver or the blood. Bilirubin is a pigment formed by the breakdown of hemoglobin, the oxygen-carrying molecule in red blood cells. Bilirubin is then transported to the liver, where it is processed into a water-soluble form. This process is known as conjugation. Conjugated bilirubin is secreted into the bile ducts and eventually excreted in feces. An increase in red blood cell breakdown, impairment in liver function, or blockage of the bile ducts can all result in the buildup of bilirubin. The first visible manifestation of this is often scleral icterus, a yellowing of the white part of the eyes. When levels of conjugated bilirubin are abnormally high, it may be seen in the urine as urobilinogen, which causes a darkening of the urine.

Once the bilirubin level in the blood exceeds 2.5 milligrams per deciliter, the yellow skin discoloration of jaundice can be seen. It is apparent first at the bottom of the tongue and later throughout the skin. Jaundice is sometimes associated with itching, presumably because of the deposition of bilirubin under the skin.

TREATMENT AND THERAPY

The treatment of jaundice depends on its cause. The first step is to determine whether there is an excess of conjugated bilirubin or unconjugated bilirubin. High levels of unconjugated bilirubin suggest an increase in red blood cell breakdown, known as hemolysis. This condition can be confirmed by examination of a peripheral blood smear and other laboratory studies. Most cases of hemolysis are the result of another underlying cause, such as infection or drugs. Hemolysis can also result from the body's immune system attacking its own red blood cells. Unconjugated bilirubin is also elevated in inherited disorders such as Gilbert's syndrome and Crigler-Najjar syndrome. These disorders are usually detected in early childhood.

Excess conjugated bilirubin, on the other hand, suggests a blockage in the biliary tree, which can be attributable to gallstones or, less commonly, a tumor. Gallstones can be confirmed with ultrasonography and may require surgery if they cause symptoms. Rarer causes of blockage in the biliary tree include strictures and sclerosing cholangitis. Disease of the liver itself can also result in high levels of conjugated bilirubin, but oftentimes both types of bilirubin are elevated. Such diseases include viral hepatitis (hepatitis A, B, or C), as well as alcohol and drug-induced hepatitis.

—*Ahmad Kamal, M.D.*

See also Cirrhosis; Gallbladder diseases; Hepatitis; Jaundice, neonatal; Liver; Liver disorders; Stones.

FOR FURTHER INFORMATION:

Arias, Irwin M., and James L. Boyer, eds. *The Liver: Biology and Pathobiology.* 4th ed. Philadelphia: Lippincott Williams & Wilkins, 2001.

Braunwald, Eugene, et al., eds. *Harrison's Principles of Internal Medicine.* 15th ed. New York: McGraw-Hill, 2001.

Palmer, Melissa. *Dr. Melissa Palmer's Guide to Hepatitis and Liver Disease: What You Need to Know.* New York: Putnam, 1999.

JAUNDICE, NEONATAL

DISEASE/DISORDER

ANATOMY OR SYSTEM AFFECTED: Blood, bones, brain, liver, spleen

SPECIALTIES AND RELATED FIELDS: Hematology, neonatology, neurology

DEFINITION: A yellowish coloration visible on the skin that is the most frequent physical finding in newborn infants.

KEY TERMS:

bilirubin encephalopathy: disease resulting from damage to the brain cells by bilirubin; also called kernicterus

exchange transfusion: the removal of an individual's blood and its replacement with a donor's blood

hyperbilirubinemia: a condition in which the bilirubin concentration in the blood reaches a level that is higher than that generally found in umbilical cord blood (1.5 milligrams per 100 milliliters)

hypertonia: an increase in muscle tone

hypotonia: a decrease in muscle tone

phototherapy: a treatment consisting of exposure to light from a bank of fluorescent or other types of lamps

CAUSES AND SYMPTOMS

Most jaundice found in children is neonatal nonhemolytic jaundice, a yellowish pigmentation of the skin of some infants. The term "nonhemolytic" is used to differentiate this condition from jaundice caused by blood group incompatibilities (such as Rh or ABO groups) or other enzyme abnormalities of the red blood cells.

Neonatal nonhemolytic jaundice is the result of an excess of the pigment bilirubin. Bilirubin is derived from two major sources. One source is the normal destruction of circulating red blood cells (erythrocytes). The normal life span of the erythrocytes varies from 80 to 120 days. Old erythrocytes are removed and destroyed in specific tissues in the spleen and liver, where the hemoglobin of the red blood cells is broken down and converted to bilirubin. This accounts for 75 percent of the daily production of bilirubin, and 1 gram of hemoglobin yields 35 milligrams of bilirubin. The remaining 25 percent of bilirubin is derived from ineffective erythropoiesis (red blood cell formation) in the bone marrow and other tissue heme or heme proteins from the liver.

The bilirubin formed is transported in the plasma of the blood and bound reversibly to albumin, a protein in the blood and tissues. This bilirubin-albumin complex is then transported to the liver, where it is converted into a water-soluble compound (or conjugated) by the enzyme glucuronyl transferase in the interior of the liver cells. The conjugated bilirubin is excreted into the bile capillaries and then into the intestine. Once in the small intestine, the conjugated bilirubin is converted by bacteria in the colon into a colorless compound known as urobilinogen. In the newborn infant, because of the lack of bacteria in the colon and the presence of the enzyme B-glucuronidase in the gut wall, a significant amount of the conjugated bilirubin is deconjugated and reabsorbed back into the plasma pool, a process known as the enterohepatic shunt.

Chemical hyperbilirubinemia can be defined as a serum concentration of bilirubin that exceeds 1.5 milli-

INFORMATION ON NEONATAL JAUNDICE

CAUSES: Excess of pigment bilirubin in newborns

SYMPTOMS: Typically yellowish skin; can include sleepiness, lethargy, irritability, poor feeding, vomiting, fever, high-pitched or shrill cry

DURATION: Acute

TREATMENTS: Phototherapy, exchange transfusion

grams per 100 milliliters. Visible yellowing (icterus) of the skin is caused by the combination of normal skin color, bilirubin-albumin complexes located outside the blood vessels, and precipitated bilirubin acid in the membranes of the cell walls. It first becomes visible when serum bilirubin reaches from 3 to 6 milligrams per deciliter, depending on the infant's skin texture and pigmentation and on the observer. In the neonate, jaundice is detected by blanching the skin over a bony structure with digital pressure, thus revealing the underlying color of the skin and subcutaneous tissue. Jaundice is first seen in the face and then progresses toward the trunk and extremities.

In general, infants whose jaundice is restricted to the face and trunk and does not extend below the umbilicus have serum bilirubin levels of about 12 milligrams per deciliter or less, while those whose hands and feet are jaundiced have serum bilirubin levels in excess of 15 milligrams per deciliter. A more objective way to estimate the depth of jaundice in neonates is with the use of an icterometer, a strip of transparent plastic with five transverse yellow strips in different shades. The baby's skin is blanched using pressure, and the resulting shade of yellow is matched against a color scale. In recent years, a transcutaneous bilirubinometer has been developed, which provides an electronic readout of an index that corresponds with a serum bilirubin concentration. A more precise way to judge jaundice is to draw a small amount of blood (usually less than a tablespoon) from the baby and to measure its serum concentration in a laboratory.

A transient rise in serum bilirubin concentration is almost universally seen in healthy newborns. This type of jaundice, called physiologic jaundice, may be attributable to several factors. First, this condition may result from increased bilirubin load on liver cells caused by increased red blood cell volume, decreased red blood cell survival time, increased heme from muscles, or increased enterohepatic circulation of bilirubin. Second, the condition may result from decreased liver uptake of bilirubin from plasma caused by a decrease in specific proteins in liver cells (termed Y and Z proteins) for the transport of bilirubin. Third, it may result from defective bilirubin conjugation caused by decreased enzyme activity. Fourth, physiologic jaundice can result from defective bilirubin excretion.

The serum bilirubin level in newborns reaches its peak between forty-eight and seventy-two hours after birth and then decreases, so that the yellowish pigmentation may not be visible by the fifth to seventh day. The peak level of serum bilirubin in physiologic jaundice varies from a mean of 5 to 15 milligrams per 100 milliliters. A number of factors will confound the level of serum bilirubin present with this condition. They include maternal pregnancy history, complications, drugs, gestational age, early initiation of feeding, type of feeding (breast milk or formula), and ethnicity. The heterogeneity of the human population makes it difficult to apply a particular serum bilirubin level to the definition of physiologic jaundice. No jaundice should be dismissed as physiologic, however, without at least a review of maternal and neonatal history, an examination of the infant for signs of illness, and further laboratory investigation when indicated.

In some cases, excess bilirubin can cause neurotoxicity leading to brain damage known as bilirubin encephalopathy or kernicterus. This damage can result in either neonatal death or the development of long-term abnormal neurologic findings, such as cerebral palsy, a low intelligence quotient (IQ), lower school achievement, hyperactivity, and deafness. The identification of jaundiced newborn infants at risk for kernicterus is difficult. The data suggest that healthy infants with serum bilirubin levels as high as 25 to 30 milligrams per 100 milliliters may not have adverse neurologic effects, since the bilirubin is bound to adequate albumin and the blood-brain barrier formed by cerebral blood vessels is intact in these infants. Early hospital discharge policies practiced in many maternity centers, however, make it difficult to assess the evolution of physiologic as well as pathologic jaundice, or confounding factors such as infection. Clinicians, practitioners, and home health visitors need to pay special attention to the degree of jaundice and when it is associated with danger signs such as sleepiness, lethargy, irritability, poor feeding, vomiting, fever, high-pitched or shrill cry, hypertonia or hypotonia (depending on whether the infant is asleep or awake), neck and trunk arching, dark urine, or light stools.

Treatment and Therapy

The treatment of jaundice depends on the underlying pathology. For clinical purposes, the two major types need to be separated: jaundice resulting from hemolytic disease (Rh, ABO, and other blood group incompatibilities) and nonhemolytic jaundice. Nonhemolytic jaundice may be physiologic or an accentuation of physiologic jaundice, such as jaundice caused by polycythemia (an increased number of red blood cells), cephalhematoma (the collection of blood in the scalp between the bone and bone lining), bruising, cerebral or other hemorrhages, swallowed blood, increased enterohepatic shunting (because of breast-feeding, delayed passage of stools, or gastrointestinal tract obstruction), and infection or sepsis.

Although no general consensus exists concerning the management of nonhemolytic jaundice, infants with this condition are generally treated with phototherapy when the serum bilirubin level reaches between 15 and 18 milligrams per 100 milliliters, using the upper value for uncomplicated physiologic jaundice and the lower value when the jaundice has accentuating factors. Phototherapy consists of exposure of the baby's skin to light energy from a bank of fluorescent or other special lamps. The light converts the fat-soluble bilirubin, which cannot be excreted, into a water-soluble bilirubin, which can be easily excreted in the bile, thus lowering the serum concentration of bilirubin.

When the serum bilirubin level reaches between 20 and 25 milligrams per 100 milliliter—some clinicians advocate between 25 and 30 milligrams per 100 milliliters—exchange transfusion is generally recommended. In this method, all of the baby's bilirubin-containing blood is removed and exchanged with compatible blood, without bilirubin, from a donor. Both forms of treatment, phototherapy and exchange transfusion, aim to reduce or remove bilirubin from the baby's system, thereby preventing brain injury.

Perspective and Prospects

Jaundice was identified as a major problem in newborn infants in the nineteenth century. Its association with brain injury was first described by German pathologist Johannes J. Orth in 1875. Fifty years later, brain damage was further identified with increased destruction of red blood cells because of hemolysis caused by Rh and ABO blood group incompatibilities.

It was also realized, however, that jaundice is encountered in normal newborn infants. The major problem has been to identify which infant is at risk for brain damage when bilirubin is at a particular level. Since there are multiple confounding factors, better means are being developed for identifying risks, such as laboratory methods to identify free (unbound) bilirubin and noninvasive clinical methods such as auditory evoked potential to measure brain waves in response to sound, the use of computers to analyze the shrillness of the baby's cry, and nuclear magnetic resonance (a form of X ray) to measure the energy metabolism of brain cells. In addition, methods to prevent the formation of bilirubin or to reduce its levels by decreasing the activity of the enzyme heme oxygenase are being studied.

—*Paul Y. K. Wu, M.D.*

See also Anemia; Blood and blood disorders; Cerebral palsy; Hematology, pediatric; Hemolytic disease of the newborn; Hepatitis; Jaundice; Light therapy; Liver; Liver disorders; Neonatalogy.

For Further Information:

Appleby, Julie. "Jaundice-Caused Brain Damage Is on the Rise." *USA Today*, October 26, 2000, p. D10. Because babies are being sent home from the hospital earlier, many cases of jaundice are missed. There have been eighty-eight cases of jaundice-caused brain damage in the United States since 1984, the majority since 1990.

Avery, Gordon B., Mary A. Fletcher, and Mhairi G. MacDonald, eds. *Neonatology: Pathophysiology and Management of the Newborn.* 5th ed. Philadelphia: J. B. Lippincott, 1999. A standard textbook on the pathophysiology and management of the major disease processes affecting the neonate, first published in 1975. Two coeditors have joined Avery in bringing out this edition, now with sixty-one chapters.

Behrman, Richard E., et al. *Nelson Textbook of Pediatrics.* 17th ed. New York: Elsevier, 2003. Text covering all medical and surgical disorders in children with authoritative information on genetics, endocrinology, aetiology, epidemiology, pathology, pathophysiology, clinical manifestations, diagnosis, prevention, treatment, and prognosis.

Fanaroff, Avroy A., and Richard J. Martin. *Neonatal-Perinatal Medicine: Diseases of the Fetus and Infant.* 7th ed. St. Louis: C. V. Mosby, 2001. This classic reference work is one of the most comprehensive to date and features discussions on the diverse practice of neonatal-perinatal medicine, pregnancy dis-orders and their impact on the fetus, delivery room care, provisions for neonatal care, and the development and disorder of organ systems.

Kirchner, Jeffrey T. "Clinical Assessment of Neonatal Jaundice." *American Family Physician* 62, no. 8 (October 15, 2000): 1880. Neonatal jaundice is a common condition, most often caused by normal physiologic mechanisms and not usually of significant concern. The decision to obtain a serum bilirubin level in a newborn usually is based on the child's appearance and the clinical judgment of the physician.

Jaw wiring

Procedure

Anatomy or system affected: Bones, gums, mouth, musculoskeletal system, teeth

Specialties and related fields: Dentistry, emergency medicine, nutrition, orthodontics, plastic surgery, speech pathology

Definition: A surgical procedure in which the upper and lower teeth are brought closely together and secured with wire in order to immobilize the jaw.

Key terms:

arch bar: a pliable piece of metal with small hooked attachments; one is fitted along the upper teeth, another is fitted along the lower teeth, the two pieces are connected to the teeth with wires, and other wires are looped around the hooks and brought together to prevent jaw movement

facial edema: swelling of the facial tissue

intermaxillary fixation: the medical term for jaw wiring

mandible: the lower jawbone

maxilla: the upper jawbone

oral hygiene: care of the teeth and mouth

orthognathic surgery: jaw reconstruction

reduction: the restoration of a fractured bone to its normal position

zygoma: the cheekbone

Indications and Procedures

Jaw wiring is often necessary to repair fractures in the jaw. The principles of treatment for facial fractures, in which bones need to be lined up and held in position until healing takes place, are the same as for a fractured arm or leg. Whereas an arm or leg fracture is reduced and casted to hold the bones in proper alignment, however, this method cannot be used for fractures of the face. Instead, once the fractures have been reduced (the bones have been restored to their proper positions), the jaws are wired shut to prevent the displacement of bone or bone fragments until they have healed.

Fractures of the face can involve any of the facial bones. The lower jawbone (mandible) is the most commonly fractured facial bone. Nevertheless, the upper jawbone (maxilla), the cheekbone (zygoma), the nasal bones, or the orbits (formed from bones of the cranium and face around the eyes) may also suffer fractures. A fracture may involve an individual bone or a combination of bones. One of the most common causes of facial fractures is blunt trauma. A blow to the face, the impact from an automobile or motorcycle accident, and a gunshot wound to the face are some examples of such trauma.

When considering fractures of the face, more than simply the bony structures must be evaluated. The skeletal structure encapsulates and protects organs that are vital to the functions of seeing, breathing, eating, talking, and swallowing. Early identification and treatment of fractures of the face are necessary to maintain maximum function of these delicate organs. Therefore, even though facial fractures and related injuries to soft tissue are seldom fatal, they must be treated immediately, since improper care could result in disfigurement, permanent sensory impairment, and lifelong disabilities.

In addition to facial fractures, jaw wiring is sometimes performed to correct malformations of the facial bones, certain birth defects, and acquired disfigurements as a result of trauma or growth-related imperfections. At times, jaw wiring is performed to correct malformations that have caused headaches, chewing disorders, and breathing and speech impairments. This type of surgery is referred to as orthognathic or jaw reconstruction surgery, part of which may involve jaw wiring. This procedure may also be performed as a weight-loss treatment for obese persons.

When a patient is hospitalized for elective facial surgery involving jaw wiring, or intermaxillary fixation, ample time can be given to preparing the patient for the surgical procedure and both preoperative and postoperative care. For the patient who sustains facial trauma, however, the same opportunity for surgical preparation may not be possible.

Facial fractures can often be reduced and immobilized by jaw wiring on the day of the injury. When there is marked facial edema (swelling), when other serious injuries are present, or when the person has eaten within a certain period of time prior to the trauma, however, the surgery will need to be delayed until a general anesthetic can be administered safely and the patient's condition has stabilized to the point that the surgical procedure can be tolerated.

The purpose of jaw wiring is to reduce and stabilize the fracture in such a manner that proper alignment of the bone will be maintained until it has healed. If the surgery is for jaw reconstruction, then the bone is fractured and positioned by the surgeon. These surgical fractures also require stabilization so that they will heal in the intended position. Interosseous wiring (the wiring of one portion of bone to another) using stainless steel wire may be necessary to maintain proper bone alignment. Sometimes, compression plates are used to secure the bones together. At other times, a bite block splint is inserted between the teeth to provide stabilization. This splint resembles a denture plate. An appliance called an external fixation device may be needed to keep the bones in proper alignment until they are healed.

If the patient wears dentures, then the denture plates are wired to the bone, the lower plate to the mandible, and the upper plate to the maxilla, prior to the jaw-wiring procedure. If the patient has no teeth at all, a bite block splint must be wired to the mandible and the maxilla, similar to the way in which dentures would be wired into place.

Jaw wiring is accomplished by first attaching arch bars to the base of the teeth. Arch bars are pliable pieces of metal with small hooked attachments on one side. They come in pre-cut lengths and can also be cut to fit the individual's mouth. One fits along the base of the lower dental arch, and the other fits along the base of the upper dental arch. Thin pieces of stainless steel wire are passed around the base of each tooth and brought out, then hooked around the arch bar and twisted firmly into place to secure the arch bar itself. The wires are cut, and their edges are tucked down between the teeth to prevent them from poking into gum or cheek tissue. If the patient wears dentures, the arch bar is either wired or glued to the denture plate with a special glue before the plate is wired to the bone structure.

Once the arch bars are positioned and secured, then special rubber bands are drawn around the hooked attachments from the upper to the lower bar. These bands are what actually hold the jaw tightly together. They are usually replaced with thin wires a few days after surgery, when the danger of nausea and vomiting have passed. Wire cutters need to be kept within easy reach at all times, in the event of vomiting. Should this happen, only the wires that hold the teeth together are clipped, and they will need to be reapplied by the physician.

USES AND COMPLICATIONS

Until the 1970's, orthognathic surgery carried a purely cosmetic connotation among the general public. Gradually, with surgical practice, documentation, research, and reports of the results of orthognathic surgery, people have come to understand the importance of such surgery in terms of proper physical functioning, as well as psychological and social functioning. Surgical reconstruction of the face can produce amazing results, but it also comes with a price. The process sometimes takes several years and teamwork by dentists, orthodontists, oral and/or plastic surgeons, and sometimes even psychiatrists to achieve these results. It can also be very costly because some insurance companies still consider orthodontia and corrective surgery cosmetic rather than functional and do not accept claims for these services.

Whatever the reason for jaw wiring, this process involves much more than a simple surgical procedure. Patients are usually hospitalized. Many of them are young, and others have had little hospital experience and may be anxious about the outcome. Lack of family support or financial concerns may increase this anxiety. Other injuries may be present in addition to the facial ones, some of which could be life-threatening and need to be attended to first.

Since jaw wiring usually means that the jaws are tightly wired shut, careful immediate postoperative monitoring by a nurse is needed to ensure that respiratory functioning is adequate, nausea and vomiting are controlled, mouth care is performed, nutritional intake of an all-liquid diet is satisfactory, and facial swelling and pain are reported to the surgeon, if necessary.

Before being discharged from the hospital, patients need to be shown proper mouth care techniques. Primary among them is the use of an electrical appliance that delivers pulsating jets of water, saline, or a mouth care solution to areas between the teeth and under the gum line. It rinses out food debris and harmful bacteria from the mouth. Mouth care is very important during the period of time when the jaws are wired, so that healing is promoted and dental caries (cavities) are prevented.

Good nutritional habits are also important during this time. Since the patient's diet must be liquid in form, concerns about weight loss, adequate food variations, appropriate nutrients for healing, management of food preparation, and possible nutritional supplementation need to be addressed and resolved before a patient is discharged. Patients should have a written diet plan to use at home. Medications needed for pain and nausea, vitamins, and sometimes antibiotics will also need to be obtained in liquid form. Instructions regarding how to administer emergency care, when to call the doctor, and how to cut wires if vomiting occurs must be given.

Follow-up care with the physician will be needed to evaluate progress and to arrange for the clipping of wires and the removal of the arch bars. These procedures are usually done in the physician's office.

PERSPECTIVE AND PROSPECTS

It is likely that attempts were made to treat fractures of the face from the time of the cave dwellers, but no records of such attempts were kept. The earliest known records relating to the treatment of jaw fractures are found in the Smith Papyrus, which is thought to have been written about 25 to 30 centuries B.C.E. The author advises against the treatment of compound (open) fractures but recommends that the dislocation of the mandible be treated. Definite proof of the art of dentistry was found among the Etruscans, an ancient people living in what is now Tuscany and part of Umbria, in about 600 to 500 B.C.E.: Skeletal remains with the teeth bound with gold wire have been discovered.

In the time of Hippocrates (c. 460-c. 370 B.C.E.), the Greek physician known as the Father of Medicine, writings bear evidence that facial injuries or fractures were treated with some method of wiring. A section of the Corpus Hippocraticum reads:

> If the jaw is broken right across, which rarely happens, one should adjust it in the manner described [one thumb inside the mouth and the fingers outside, for reduction]. After adjustment one should fasten the teeth together as was described above [with gold wire or, lacking that, with linen thread], for this will contribute greatly to immobility, especially if one joins them properly and fastens the ends as they should be.

The use of bandages to treat facial maladies was also practiced by some ancient cultures. Galen of Pergamum (129-c. 199 C.E.) and Soranus of Ephesus (98-138 C.E.) describe such methods. An ancient manuscript by Soranus of Ephesus illustrates the types of bandages used by the ancients to treat head and facial injuries.

Greek writings even suggested dietary practices in cases of jaw injury. When the mandible was fractured, liquid nourishment was recommended, and solid foods were withheld until bone healing was definite. Patients were also advised not to talk for a certain period of time.

In the thirteenth century, Italian surgeon Guglielmo da Saliceto (c. 1210-c. 1277), also known as William of Saliceto, performed one of the first documented cases of jaw wiring, attaching the teeth of the lower jaw to the corresponding teeth of the upper jaw. He used linen and silk thread, twisting them together and then waxing the twist to keep it in place. In the next several centuries, however, the medieval literature lacks any references to the management of facial bone fractures. Whether the work of earlier surgeons was unknown or whether such surgical practices remained standard during these years, without notable progress, remains a mystery.

It was toward the end of the nineteenth century that the development of intermaxillary fixation by wiring was developed by an American physician and dentist, Thomas Lewis Gilmer (1849-1931). Gilmer carried out the jaw wiring procedure "by twisting wires around the necks of the teeth of the upper and lower jaws, by adjusting the lower teeth to the occlusion of the upper jaw, and by twisting together the connecting upper and lower wires for stabilization."

Many great names are associated with the twentieth century contributions to improved and refined methods of jaw wiring techniques and patient care during this process. Much was learned about the nature of facial fractures themselves from the work of French physician Rene LeFort. LeFort conducted a series of experiments in the early twentieth century to study facial fracture combinations. He subjected cadaver skulls to violent blows under many conditions and at various angles and then described the outcomes.

A survey of the progress made in jaw wiring would be incomplete without recognition of the impact that antibiotic therapy, advanced anesthetic techniques, and blood replacement therapy have had on this procedure and on medical science as a whole. These achievements paved the way for open surgical procedures and internal fixation, which have led to dramatic results and remarkable changes for individuals undergoing jaw wiring.

—*Karen A. Mattern*

See also Bones and the skeleton; Dentistry; Emergency medicine; Fracture and dislocation; Fracture repair; Hyperadiposis; Nutrition; Obesity; Orthodontics; Orthopedic surgery; Orthopedics; Orthopedics, pediatric; Plastic surgery.

FOR FURTHER INFORMATION:

Fonseca, Raymond J., and Robert V. Walker, eds. *Oral and Maxillofacial Trauma*. 2d ed. Philadelphia: W. B. Saunders, 2000. This text discusses wounds and injuries to the face, mouth, and jaw, as well as therapies to treat them. Includes a bibliography and an index.

Niamtu, Joseph, III. "Cosmetic Oral and Maxillofacial Surgery Options." *The Journal of the American Dental Association* 131, no. 6 (June, 2000): 756-764. A global diagnosis and treatment plan which includes facial esthetics can enhance cosmetic dentistry and serve to frame the work of the restorative dentist.

Reyneke, Johan. *Essentials of Orthognathic Surgery*. Chicago: Quintessence, 2003. Discusses patients with dentofacial deformities, focusing on the surgical and orthodontic principles of orthognathic surgery rather than on research and treatment philosophies. Covers principles of clinical evaluation, treatment planning, and surgical procedures, and clinical cases are presented to demonstrate treatment outcomes.

Salter, Robert B. *Textbook of Disorders and Injuries of the Musculoskeletal System*. 3d ed. Philadelphia: Lippincott Williams & Wilkins, 1998. Four sections of the book—"Basic Musculoskeletal Science and Its Applications," "Musculoskeletal Disorders: General and Specific," "Musculoskeletal Injuries," and "Research"—examine the diagnosis and treatment principles of disorders and trauma of the musculoskeletal system.

Watts, V., S. Madick, J. Pepperney, and C. Petras. "When Your Patient Has Jaw Surgery." *RN* 48 (October, 1985): 44-47. This article written for health care professionals focuses on jaw surgery as a result of facial deformities rather than fractures, describing some deformities. Also includes postoperative care of the patient.

White, Raymond P., and David M. Sarver, eds. *Contemporary Treatment of Dentofacial Deformity*. New York: Elsevier, 2002. Explores the ways in which orthodontists, oral and maxillofacial surgeons, and facial plastic surgeons can work together to treat dentofacial deformities.

JOINT DISEASES. *See* ARTHRITIS.

JOINT REPLACEMENT. *See* ARTHROPLASTY; HIP REPLACEMENT.

JUVENILE RHEUMATOID ARTHRITIS
DISEASE/DISORDER

ANATOMY OR SYSTEM AFFECTED: Back, circulatory system, eyes, heart, immune system, joints, musculoskeletal system

SPECIALTIES AND RELATED FIELDS: Exercise physiology, family practice, immunology, ophthalmology, orthopcdics, pcdiatrics, psychology

DEFINITION: A usually chronic autoimmune disease of unknown cause, characterized by joint swelling, pain, and sometimes the destruction of joints.

KEY TERMS:

articular: of or relating to a joint or joints

autoimmune disease: a disease in which the body's immune system attacks itself

manifestation: an outward or visible expression

systemic: relating to the body as a whole, not limited to a particular part

CAUSES AND SYMPTOMS

Juvenile rheumatoid arthritis is an autoimmune disease of children that attacks the joints. It appears in three different subgroups that vary according to severity and type of extra-articular manifestation. Other significant variations within these subgroups include age at disease onset, the sex of affected children, genetic predisposition, and prognosis.

The first major clinical pattern is systemic disease, which includes about 20 percent of children with juvenile rheumatoid arthritis. This type has the most dramatic onset and is the least common form of the illness. It affects boys more than girls and can begin at any age. The most characteristic manifestations are high, intermittent fevers and a temporary red rash occurring during periods of fever. Occasionally, more serious complications are involved. In some cases, systemic onset is marked by polyarthritis, which affects large and small multiple joints, and moves subsequently to disease of the knee or hip with no further involvement of other joints. The systemic complaints, which are often sudden and explosive in nature, may recur months or years later. Some children with systemic onset, however, never develop lasting arthritis.

Polyarticular juvenile rheumatoid arthritis, the second subgroup, includes children in whom five or more joints have been involved in the first six months of illness. It affects more girls than boys and can begin at any age. This subgroup includes about 25 percent of children with juvenile rheumatoid arthritis and is frequently mild. Within this subgroup exists a smaller subgroup, which includes about 5 percent of children with juvenile rheumatoid arthritis and rarely begins before the eighth birthday. The arthritis is often severe, with joint destruction occurring within the first year.

Polyarthritis may involve swelling of the joints over a period of time, in which pain is not a prominent feature, or a sudden articular swelling, in which pain can be severe. Weight-bearing joints, usually knees and ankles, are often involved initially.

The third major subgroup is pauciarticular disease, which involves about 40 percent of all children with juvenile rheumatoid arthritis. In the initial episode of this type, only one joint is involved. More joints usually become involved within a few weeks or months, although occasionally involvement is restricted to one joint. Most often, the knee is the primary area, with the ankles and hips being the sites of minimal involvement.

TREATMENT AND THERAPY

The first step in treating juvenile rheumatoid arthritis is the identification of the child's problems and potential problems, which include active joint disease, disabilities, ocular disease, growth retardation, and psychosocial disability. Because the cause of chronic arthritis is not known, treatment suppresses the symptoms and does not cure the disease itself.

Drug therapy is used to relieve inflammatory pain and immobility. The major anti-inflammatory drug used for juvenile rheumatoid arthritis is aspirin. For children who cannot tolerate aspirin, a nonsteroidal anti-inflammatory drug (NSAID) may be substituted. Unfortunately, corticosteroids, the most effective anti-inflammatory drugs known, are of little benefit in treating juvenile rheumatoid arthritis because of their serious side effects. They can be used only in the treatment of severe, life-threatening systemic disease.

Physical and occupational therapy attempts to maintain strength and stamina and to preserve and increase the range of motion in the joints and in supporting muscles. All children with significant joint involvement should have a daily home program of activities and exercises directed toward the prevention and correction of disabilities which, after appropriate instruction, can be supervised by the parents. In addition to exercise, the program consists of the use of moist heat, adequate rest, and proper diet, which are aimed at maintaining strength. Children with severe disabilities may need hospitalization for intensive therapy.

Beyond physical therapy, orthopedic treatment for the joints may include splinting to preserve or repair joint motion. In the rehabilitation of older children who have suffered serious damage, the replacement of affected joints may provide good results.

INFORMATION ON JUVENILE RHEUMATOID ARTHRITIS

CAUSES: Unknown
SYMPTOMS: High, intermittent fevers; temporary red rash occurring during periods of fever; joint pain; occasionally polyarthritis
DURATION: Acute and recurrent
TREATMENTS: Alleviation of symptoms through medication (anti-inflammatory drugs), physical and occupational therapy, orthopedic treatment (*e.g.*, splinting)

Juvenile rheumatoid arthritis offers significant challenges for families. The family pediatrician or physician must act as teacher and adviser both to the patient and to family members. Other health care professionals who may be important to the care of children with juvenile rheumatoid arthritis are ophthalmologists, pediatric nurses, social workers, and psychiatrists, as well as the child's schoolteachers.

PERSPECTIVE AND PROSPECTS

Dr. George R. Still's finding in 1896 that juvenile rheumatoid arthritis includes at least three distinct joint afflictions first brought the subgroups to the attention of the medical profession and has fostered a greater understanding of the disease.

For most children with juvenile rheumatoid arthritis, early diagnosis and appropriate therapy point to a good prognosis. Of the children with systemic onset, at least 75 percent will enjoy a good outcome, whereas the rest may suffer severe arthritis, possibly resulting in disability. Between 80 and 90 percent of children with polyarthritis escape without permanent joint damage, although the disease itself may be chronic. The overall prospects for children with pauciarticular disease are not known.

Although most children suffering from juvenile rheumatoid arthritis eventually outgrow it, it is difficult for most parents to accept that accurate prediction for the ultimate outcome for their child is impossible. Nevertheless, a positive attitude, careful medical management, physical therapy, and psychologic support can improve the quality of life for all children with juvenile rheumatoid arthritis.

—Mary Hurd

See also Exercise; Massage; Musculoskeletal system; Orthopedics, pediatric.

FOR FURTHER INFORMATION:

Arthritis Foundation. http://www.arthritis.org/. Provides information on arthritis support groups, exercise classes, and other resources for persons with arthritis. Also offers information, education, and publications specific to juvenile arthritis.

Behrman, Richard E., and Robert M. Kliegman, eds. *Nelson Essentials of Pediatrics*. 4th ed. Philadelphia: W. B. Saunders, 2001. This is a great text for medical students rotating through pediatrics. It has thorough explanations of diseases and treatments.

Brewer, Earl J. *The Arthritis Sourcebook*. 3d ed. New York: McGraw-Hill, 2000. A thorough guide to information on treatments, medications, and alternative therapies for the myriad forms of arthritis.

Brewer, Earl J., Edward H. Giannini, and Donald A. Person. *Juvenile Rheumatoid Arthritis*. 2d ed. Philadelphia: W. B. Saunders, 1982. A brief study of the condition of juvenile rheumatoid arthritis. Includes bibliographical references.

Kimball, Chad T. *Childhood Diseases and Disorders Sourcebook: Basic Consumer Health Information About Medical Problems Often Encountered in Preadolescent Children*. Detroit: Omnigraphics, 2002. Offers basic facts about cancer, sickle cell disease, diabetes, and other chronic conditions in children and discusses frequently used diagnostic tests, surgeries, and medications. Long-term care for seriously ill children is also presented.

Melvin, Jeanne L., and Virginia Wright, eds. *Pediatric Rheumatic Diseases*. Vol. 3. Bethesda, Md.: American Occupational Therapy Association, 2000. Covers essential information on team treatment for various disease groups, understanding pain in children, pediatric outcome assessment, the effects of arthritis and treatment on school achievement, surgical treatment, and detailed case studies, among other topics.

Merenstein, Gerald B., et al., eds. *Handbook of Pediatrics*. 18th ed. Stamford, Conn.: Appleton & Lange, 1997. This popular handbook provides comprehensive and easily accessible information on pediatrics. A reliable source of quick information on the care of children from infancy through adolescence, this edition has been completely revised, updated, and streamlined.

Parker, James N., and Philip M. Parker, eds. *Juvenile Rheumatoid Arthritis: The Official Patient's Sourcebook*. San Diego, Calif.: Icon Health, 2002. Draws from public, academic, government, and peer-reviewed research to provide a wide-ranging handbook for patients with juvenile arthritis.

KAPOSI'S SARCOMA
DISEASE/DISORDER

ANATOMY OR SYSTEM AFFECTED: Intestines, liver, lungs, skin

SPECIALTIES AND RELATED FIELDS: Internal medicine, oncology

DEFINITION: A disease in which cancer cells are found in tissues, causing lesions on the skin and/or mucous membranes and spreading to other organs in the body.

CAUSES AND SYMPTOMS

It is uncertain whether Kaposi's sarcoma is actually cancer because, unlike cancer, it arises from several cell types. Although there is no accepted staging system for Kaposi's sarcoma, patients are grouped by the type that they have. The three types are classic, epidemic, and recurrent.

Classic Kaposi's sarcoma usually occurs in older men of Mediterranean heritage. It progresses slowly (over ten to fifteen years), with progression bringing lower limb swelling, impeded blood flow, possible spread to other organs, and other types of cancer in later life. Epidemic Kaposi's sarcoma, found in people with acquired immunodeficiency syndrome (AIDS), is a more virulent, fast-spreading, and fatal form, with symptoms of painless, either flat or raised, pink or purple plaques on the skin and mucosal surfaces. This type usually spreads to the lungs, liver, spleen, lymph nodes, digestive tract, and other internal organs. Recurrent Kaposi's sarcoma comes back after it has been treated in the original area where it started. Sometimes, it appears in another part of the body.

TREATMENT AND THERAPY

Four kinds of treatment are usually used: surgery (taking out the cancer), chemotherapy (using drugs to kill cancer cells), external beam radiation therapy (using high-dose X rays to kill cancer cells), and biological therapy (using the body's immune system to fight the cancer).

Classic Kaposi's sarcoma may be treated by radiation therapy, local excision (cutting out the lesion and some of the tissue around it), systemic chemotherapy (in which the drug enters the bloodstream, travels through the body, and kills cancer cells outside the original site), intralesional chemotherapy (in which the drug is injected into the lesion), or a combination of these treatments.

Epidemic Kaposi's sarcoma is treated by surgery, including electrodesiccation and curettage (burning the lesion and removing it with a sharp instrument) and cryotherapy (killing the tumor by freezing it). It can also be treated with chemotherapy or biological therapy.

PERSPECTIVE AND PROSPECTS

Until the early 1980's, Kaposi's sarcoma was found mainly in older male patients who had received organ transplants. The AIDS epidemic gave rise to cases that spread quickly among homosexual men and African men. Recovery depends on the type of Kaposi's sarcoma, age, general health, and whether the condition is accompanied by AIDS.

—*Patricia A. Ainsa, M.P.H., Ph.D.*

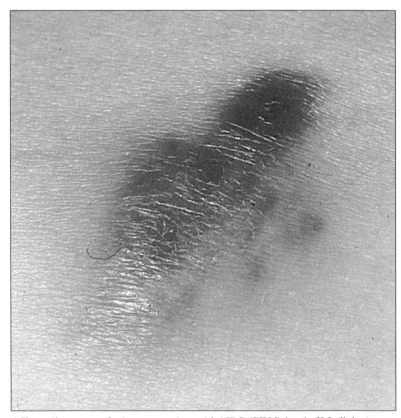

A Kaposi's sarcoma lesion on a patient with AIDS. (SIU School of Medicine)

INFORMATION ON KAPOSI'S SARCOMA

CAUSES: Unknown; epidemic type found in patients with AIDS
SYMPTOMS: Flat or raised, pink or purple plaques on the skin and mucosal surfaces; lower limb swelling, impeded blood flow
DURATION: Ranges from acute to chronic with recurrent episodes
TREATMENTS: Surgery, chemotherapy, external beam radiation therapy, biological therapy

See also Acquired immunodeficiency syndrome (AIDS); Biopsy; Cancer; Chemotherapy; Cryosurgery; Malignancy and metastasis; Oncology; Radiation therapy; Sarcoma.

FOR FURTHER INFORMATION:

Corey, Lawrence, ed. *AIDS: Problems and Prospects.* New York: W. W. Norton, 1993.

Dollinger, Malin, Ernest H. Rosenbaum, and Greg Cable. *Everyone's Guide to Cancer Therapy.* 4th rev. ed. Kansas City, Mo.: Andrews & McMeel, 2002.

Feigal, Ellen G., Alexandra M. Levine, and Robert J. Biggar. *AIDS-Related Cancers and Their Treatment.* New York: Marcel Dekker, 2000.

Gottlieb, Geoffrey J., and A. Bernard Ackerman. *Kaposi's Sarcoma: A Text and Atlas.* Philadelphia: Lea & Febiger, 1988.

Parker, James N., and Philip M. Parker, eds. *The Official Patient's Sourcebook on Kaposi's Sarcoma.* San Diego, Calif.: Icon Health, 2003.

Shepherd, Frances A. *Management of Kaposi's Sarcoma Associated with Human Immunodeficiency Virus Infection.* Ottawa: Health and Welfare Canada, 1991.

KARYOTYPING

PROCEDURE

ALSO KNOWN AS: Chromosome analysis
ANATOMY OR SYSTEM AFFECTED: Cells
SPECIALTIES AND RELATED FIELDS: Cytology, embryology, genetics, neonatology, obstetrics, oncology, pathology, perinatology
DEFINITION: The photographing of all the chromosomes of a single cell to identify extra, missing, or abnormal chromosomes.

KEY TERMS:

autosomes: all the chromosomes, except for the sex chromosomes
karyotype: a photograph of all the chromosomes in a single cell
mitosis: cell division
nondisjunction: a malfunction of mitosis, resulting in cells with an abnormal chromosome number

THE CELL AND CHROMOSOMES

Every cell in the human body—except for red blood cells—contains a nucleus with rod-shaped structures called chromosomes. The chromosomes, in turn, contain the genes, which are the units that transmit heredity from parents to offspring.

The forty-six individual chromosomes in a human cell exist as twenty-three pairs of so-called "homologues." Homologous chromosomes are similar in size and appearance. The first twenty-two pairs of homologues are referred to as autosomes, while pair number twenty-three contains two dissimilar chromosomes known as the X and Y or sex chromosomes, which determine gender. Sperm and eggs each have twenty-three chromosomes, or half the usual number. When a sperm fertilizes an egg, the normal chromosome number (forty-six) is reestablished in the first cell of life, the zygote.

Cells reproduce by mitosis, a process of simple division, the result being two identical daughter cells, each containing forty-six chromosomes. Since chromosomes contain the genetic information, it follows that mitosis must proceed with precision every time a cell divides. During the earliest stages of embryonic development, however, mistakes sometimes occur and the cells wind up with more or fewer chromosomes. This malfunction of mitosis is called nondisjunction, and the incorrect number of chromosomes is passed to all the cells in the developing embryo. This leads to a variety of abnormal conditions, all of which can be diagnosed with the procedure known as karyotyping.

PROCEDURE AND INTERPRETATION

A karyotype is a photograph of all the chromosomes in a single cell. The prefix "karyo-" refers to the nucleus, the part of the cell where chromosomes reside; the suffix "-type" means characterization. Thus, a karyotype is a characterization of a nucleus in terms of its chromosomes.

Karyotypes are performed on embryos to diagnose chromosomal abnormalities and on adults who suspect chromosomal aberrations that could be passed on to offspring. Although a karyotype can be constructed from almost any cell in the body that contains a nucleus, it is most often performed on white blood cells, which are easily harvested from a routine blood sample.

The procedure is simple. Once the blood is collected, the white cells are separated from the red. In the laboratory, the white blood cells are then stimulated to undergo mitosis. At the stage of mitosis when the chromosomes are most visible, the process is chemically halted. The chromosomes are then stained to make them more visible, after which they are photographed and the individual chromosomes cut out and rearranged as homologous pairs in descending order by size. Each pair of chromosomes is also given a number, the largest pair being designated number 1. Then another photograph is taken of the chromosomes in the rearranged format. The result is the karyotype. The entire process, from collecting the blood sample to growing the cells to preparing the karyotype, takes from one to three weeks.

Once the karyotype has been created, it is ready to be interpreted by a cytogeneticist, a person who is an expert in the study of chromosomes. The most common disorders visible with karyotyping are Down syndrome, an extra copy of chromosome number 21; Klinefelter syndrome, a male with an extra X chromosome, resulting in sterility and the development of some female features; and Turner syndrome, a female missing an X chromosome, resulting in sterility and a masculine body build.

PERSPECTIVE AND PROSPECTS

Karyotyping was first reported in the mid-1950's when chromosomes were examined in fetal cells collected from amniotic fluid. This was the beginning of the discipline of prenatal genetic diagnosis. At the time, there was no ultrasound to guide the needle through the amniotic membrane, which increased the risk of damaging the fetus. The karyotyping itself required four or five weeks of cell culture and was not always successful.

Today, karyotyping is commonly used to diagnose chromosomal abnormalities in both fetuses and already-born individuals. It is considered to be an absolutely safe procedure, the only risks being those inherent in penetrating the amniotic sac with a needle. Also, although the advent of ultrasound has greatly reduced the risk to the fetus, the possibility always exists of inadvertently collecting maternal cells when the mother's tissues are penetrated.

Karyotyping has been a fairly static procedure since its inception, having seen little innovation. Dyes are simply added to highlight the chromosomes for identification purposes. There is now, however, a new method called spectral karyotyping, which involves the use of fluorescent dyes that highlight specific regions of the chromosomes. A device called an interferometer is used to detect slight color variations invisible to the human eye and then assign visible colors to the homologous chromosomes. This method is superior to traditional karyotyping with chemical stains because it more clearly identifies chromosomes that are damaged or that contain fragments of other, nonhomologous chromosomes.

—*Robert T. Klose, Ph.D.*

See also Amniocentesis; Biopsy; Cells; Chorionic villus sampling; Cytology; DNA and RNA; Gene therapy; Genetic engineering; Genetics and inheritance; Laboratory tests.

FOR FURTHER INFORMATION:

Harris, Henry. *The Cells of the Body: A History of Somatic Cell Genetics.* Cold Spring Harbor, N.Y.: Cold Spring Harbor Laboratory Press, 1995.

Krogh, David. *Biology: A Guide to the Natural World.* 2d ed. Upper Saddle River, N.J.: Prentice-Hall, 2001.

Parker, Sybil, ed. *McGraw-Hill Concise Encyclopedia of Science and Technology.* 4th ed. New York: McGraw-Hill, 1998.

Vogel, F., and A. G. Motulsky. *Human Genetics: Problems and Approaches.* Berlin: Springer, 1997.

KERATOSES. *See* WARTS.

KIDNEY DISORDERS

DISEASE/DISORDER

ANATOMY OR SYSTEM AFFECTED: Kidneys, urinary system

SPECIALTIES AND RELATED FIELDS: Internal medicine, nephrology, urology

DEFINITION: Disorders, from structural abnormalities to bacterial infections, that can affect the kidneys and may lead to renal failure.

KEY TERMS:

creatinine: the breakdown product of creatine, a nitrogenous compound found in muscle, blood, and urine

cystinosis: a congenital disease characterized by glucose and protein in the urine, as well as by cystine deposits in the liver and other organs, rickets, and growth retardation

hematuria: the abnormal presence of blood in the urine

hydronephrosis: the cessation of urine flow because of an obstruction of a ureter, allowing urine to build up in the pelvis of the kidney; can cause renal failure

oliguria: the diminished capacity to form and pass urine, so that metabolic products cannot be excreted efficiently

reflux: the abnormal backward flow of urine

toxemia: blood poisoning

uremia: the presence of excessive amounts of urea and other nitrogenous waste products in the blood

CAUSES AND SYMPTOMS

Disorders of the kidney can occur for a variety of reasons. The cause may be congenital (present from birth) or may develop very quickly and at any age. Many of these problems and disorders can be easily treated. The main areas of kidney disorders are classified as malformations in development of the kidney, part of the kidney, or the ureter; glomerular disease; tubular and interstitial disease or disruption; vascular (other than glomerular) disease; and kidney dysfunction that occurs secondary to another disease.

The kidney frequently exhibits congenital anomalies, some of which occur during specific developmental stages. Agenesis occurs when the ureteric bud fails to develop normally. When the tissue does not develop, the ureter itself fails to form. If there is an obstruction where the ureter joins the pelvis of the kidney, there may be massive hydronephrosis (dilation). One or both kidneys may be unusually small, containing too few tubules. The kidneys may be displaced, too high or offset to one side or the other. They may even be fused. All these conditions could seriously affect the manufacture of urine, its excretion, or both.

INFORMATION ON KIDNEY DISORDERS

CAUSES: Congenital defects, bacterial infections, trauma

SYMPTOMS: Varies; can include swelling, uremia, fever, rash, renal pain, body aches, nausea, fatigue, mental dullness

DURATION: Acute to chronic

TREATMENTS: Medications (diuretics, vasodilators, calcium antagonists, oral antibiotics); short-term dialysis; hemodialysis; catheterization; surgery such as transplantation

Glomerulonephritis refers to a diverse group of conditions that share a common feature—primary involvement of the glomerulus. The significance of glomerulonephritis is that it is the most common cause of end-stage renal failure. Its features include urinary casts, high protein levels (proteinuria), hematuria, hypertension, edema (swelling), and uremia. The two forms of glomerulonephritis are primary and secondary. In the primary form, only the kidneys are affected, but in the secondary form, the lesion (affected area) is only one of a series of problems.

Nephrotic syndrome is usually defined as an abnormal condition of the kidney characterized by the presence of proteinuria together with edema and high fat and cholesterol levels. It occurs in glomerular disease, in thrombosis of a renal vein, and as a complication of many systemic diseases. Nephrotic syndrome occurs in a severe, primary form characterized by anorexia, weakness, proteinuria, and edema.

Interstitial nephritis is inflammation of the interstitial tissue of the kidney, including the kidneys. Acute interstitial nephritis is an immunologic, adverse reaction to certain drugs; drugs especially associated with it are nonsteroidal anti-inflammatory drugs (NSAIDs) and some antibiotics. Acute renal failure, fever, rash, and proteinuria are indicative signs of this condition. If the medication is stopped, normal kidney function returns. Chronic interstitial nephritis is defined as inflammation and structural changes associated with such conditions as ureteral obstruction, pyelonephritis, exposure of the kidney to a toxin, transplant rejection, or certain systemic diseases.

Kidney stones (calculi) are commonly manufactured from calcium oxalate and/or phosphate, triple phosphate, uric acid (urate), or a mixture of these. Calcium stones are not necessarily the result of high serum calcium, although they can be. Struvite calculi of magnesium ammonium (triple) phosphate mixed with calcium are bigger but softer than other types; they grow irregularly, filling much of the kidney pelvis. They arise from infection with urea-splitting organisms that cause alkaline urine. Urate stones are a complication of gout.

Those who have a tendency to develop stones may experience concomitant infection known as pyonephrosis. Pyonephrosis is a result of not only blockage at the junction of the ureter and kidney pelvis but also any constricture at this location. Bacteria from the bloodstream collect and cause an abscess to form. If the tube is completely blocked, the inflammation produces enough pus to rupture a portion of the kidney, and more of the abdominal cavity becomes involved.

Pyelonephritis is inflammation of the upper urinary tract. Acute pyelonephritis may be preceded by lower tract infection. The patient complains of lethargy, fever, and back pain. The major symptoms are fever, renal pain, and body aches accompanied by nausea and toxemia. Chronic pyelonephritis often affects the renal tubules and the small spaces within the kidney. Fibrous tissue may take over these areas and cause gradual shrinking of the functional kidney. The chronic form may also result from previous bacterial infection, reflux, obstruction, overuse of analgesics, X rays, and lead poisoning.

Obstruction may be caused by inadequate development of the renal tissue itself, closing off one or both ureters. Other malformations and certain calculi can also obstruct urine flow. Reflux may occur when the contraction of the bladder forces urine backward, up toward and into the kidney. Lesser degrees of reflux do not damage the kidney, but the greater the reflux, the more likely damage will occur. Bacterial infection is often attributable to *Escherichia coli*, but other bowel bacteria may also infect the area. They generally move upward from outside the body through the urinary organs, but they may move inward from the bloodstream.

Acute renal failure is defined as a sudden decline in normal renal function that leads to an increase in blood urea and creatinine. The onset may be fast (over days) or slow (over weeks) and is often reversible. It is characterized by oliguria and rapid accumulation of nitrogenous wastes in the blood, resulting in acidosis. Acute renal failure is caused by hemorrhage, trauma, burns, toxic injury to the kidney, acute pyelonephritis or glomerulonephritis, or lower urinary tract obstruction. Occasionally, it will progress into chronic renal failure.

Chronic renal failure may result from many other diseases. Its signs are sluggishness, fatigue, and mental dullness. Patients also display other systemic problems as a result of chronic renal failure. Almost all such patients are anemic; three-fourths of them develop hypertension. The skin becomes discolored; the muddy coloration is caused by anemia and the presence of excess melanin.

Renal symptoms suggestive of renal dysfunction include increases in frequency of urination, color changes in urine, areas of edema, and hypertension. The patient may experience only one symptom but is more likely to have a series of complaints. To determine the cause of renal disease, several diagnostic tools can be used to distinguish the type of pathogenic process affecting the kidney. The degree to which other body systems are involved determines whether the disease process is systemic or confined to the kidneys. Other valuable clues may be gathered from medical history, family history, and physical examination. The key factors, however, are renal size and renal histopathology.

Examination of the urine can reveal important data relative to renal health. Stick tests may show the abnormal presence of blood, glucose, and/or protein. Assaying the kind and amount of protein may pinpoint the cause of the disease. Urine contaminated with bacteria has always been used as an indication of some form of urinary tract infection. Microscopic examination of urine sediment may help diagnose acute renal failure. Blood tests may also indicate the source of a renal disorder. A series of blood tests might reveal rising urea and creatinine levels. The urea-to-creatinine ratio may aid in determining if and which type of acute renal failure may be present. A high red cell count might suggest kidney stones, a tumor, or glomerular disease; a high white cell count would hint at inflammation and/or infection. Cells cast from the kidney tubules may indicate acute interstitial nephritis, while red cell breakdown products may mean glomerulonephritis. The diagnostician should also be diligent in tracking down possible septic causes. Repeated cultures of blood and urine should help ascertain if there is an abscess anywhere near the kidney.

X rays can provide useful information. An abdominal X ray may show urinary stones and abnormalities in the renal outline. Ultrasound will measure renal size, show scarring, and reveal dilation of the tract, perhaps as a result of an obstructive lesion. Abdominal ultrasound has become the investigation of choice because it can be performed at the patient's bedside.

Renal biopsy can give an accurate diagnosis of acute renal failure but may be more dangerous to the patient than the condition itself. The main indications for biopsy would be suspected acute glomerulonephritis and renal failure that has lasted six weeks.

Treatment and Therapy

If glomerulonephritis is suspected or diagnosed, its treatment seeks to avoid complications of the illness. The patient is monitored daily for fluid overload; as long as the patient is retaining fluid, blood tests that measure urea, creatinine, and salt balance are also run daily. The patient should stay in bed and restrict fluid as well as potassium intake. Medications may be prescribed: diuretics, vasodilators for hypertension, and calcium antagonists. If the cause is bacterial, a course of oral antibiotics may be given. If these measures are unsuccessful, short-term dialysis may be needed. Some urinary abnormalities may last for as long as a year.

The first measure undertaken to treat acute renal failure is to rebuild depressed fluid volumes: blood if the patient has hemorrhaged, plasma for burn patients, and electrolytes for a patient who is vomiting and has diarrhea. If infection is suspected as the underlying cause, an appropriate antibiotic should be administered when blood cultures confirm the presence of bacteria. After fluid volumes have been replenished, a diuretic may be necessary to reduce swelling of tissues within the kidney.

In chronic renal failure, the major undertaking is to relieve the obstruction of the urinary tract. If the blockage is within the bladder, simple catheterization may relieve it. If a stone or some similar obstacle is blocking a ureter, however, surgery to remove it may be necessary. A tube may be inserted to allow urine drainage, and the stone will pass or be removed.

In sufferers of recurrent stones, maintaining a high urine output is important, which requires the patient to drink fluids throughout the day and even at bedtime. Those enduring intense pain may need to be hospitalized. Analgesics for pain are administered, as well as forced fluid intake to increase urine output so that the stone might be passed. If these measures do not work, surgical intervention may be necessary.

Patients suffering from progressive, incurable renal failure need medical aid managing conservation of, substitution for, and eventual replacement of nephron function. Conservation attempts to prolong kidney function for as long as possible; renal function is aided by drug treatment. Substitution means the maintenance of kidney function by dialysis, especially hemodialysis. Replacement is the restoration of renal function by a kidney transplant. By this third stage of treatment, urine formation is independent of further drug treatment, and kidney function must be achieved by other means. Patients suffering from end-stage renal failure have two options: dialysis and transplantation. A patient may go from dialysis to transplantation. In fact, if a compatible donor (preferably a sibling) is available, a transplant is advisable. For those without a suitable donor, long-term hemodialysis is the first option.

Dialysis is defined as the diffusion of dissolved molecules through a semipermeable membrane. Several types of dialysis are available. Hemodialysis filters and cleans the blood as it passes through the semipermeable membranous tube in contact with a balanced salt solution (dialysate). Hemodialysis can be performed in a dialysis unit of a hospital or at home. It must usually be done two or three times a week, with each session lasting from three to six hours, depending on the type of membranes used and the size of the patient. Hemodialysis can lead to acute neurological changes. Lethargy, irritability, restlessness, headache, nausea, vomiting, and twitching may all occur. In some patients, neurological complications occur after dialysis is terminated. Convulsions are the most common of these consequences. In continuous abdominal peritoneal dialysis, a fresh amount of dialysate is introduced from a bag attached to a permanently implanted plastic tube. Wastes and water pass into the dialysate from the surrounding organs; then the fluid is collected four to eight hours later. Peritoneal dialysis is performed by the patient. It is continuous, so the clearance rate of wastes is higher. The most important neurological complications of peritoneal dialysis are worsening of urea-induced brain abnormalities accompanied by twitching and, rarely, psychosis and convulsions.

Transplantation of a kidney is considered for patients with primary renal diseases as well as end-stage renal failure resulting from any number of systemic and metabolic diseases. Success rates are highest for those suffering from lupus nephritis, gout, and cystinosis. If a kidney is received from a close relative, there is a 97 percent one-year survival rate. Even if the organ transplant comes from a nonrelative, the survival rate is still 90 percent.

—*Iona C. Baldridge*

See also Dialysis; Edema; Genital disorders, male; Incontinence; Kidney transplantation; Kidneys; Lithotripsy; Nephrectomy; Nephritis; Nephrology; Nephrology, pediatric; Polycystic kidney disease; Pyelonephritis; Renal failure; Stone removal; Stones; Urethritis; Urinary disorders; Urinary system; Urology; Urology, pediatric.

FOR FURTHER INFORMATION:

Cameron, J. Stewart. *History of Dialysis*. New York: Oxford University Press, 2002. Traces the history of dialysis, including discussions of the concepts of diffusion and anticoagulation, early attempts of dialysis in animals and humans, and recent developments in the field.

Catto, Graeme R. D., and David A. Power. *Nephrology in Clinical Practice*. London: Edward Arnold, 1988. This book addresses health care professionals in particular. Its goal is to educate practitioners in methods of recognition and diagnosis and of treatment.

Daugirdas, John T., ed. *Handbook of Dialysis.* 3d ed. Philadelphia: Lippincott Williams & Wilkins, 2000. A practical guide that focuses primarily on the management of dialysis patients but also explores the physiologic basis for dialytic therapies and the pathophysiology of relevant disease states.

Dische, Frederick E. *Concise Renal Pathology.* 2d ed. Oxford, England: Oxford University Press, 1995. For those in training for medical fields, this book describes renal anatomy and pathology. The terminology is somewhat simplified so that the descriptions are more understandable.

Greenberg, Arthur, et al., eds. *Primer on Kidney Diseases.* 3d ed. New York: Elsevier, 2001. A publication from the National Kidney Foundation that covers such topics as fluid and electrolyte disorders, hypertension, dialysis, and renal transplantation.

Morgan, Steven H., and Jean-Pierre Grunfeld, eds. *Inherited Disorders of the Kidney: Investigation and Management.* New York: Oxford University Press, 1999. Discusses a range of kidney disorders, including cystic diseases; glomerular, tubular, and metabolic disorders; hypertension; and carcinomas. Examines the role of genetics.

National Kidney Foundation. http://www.kidney.org/. Offers thorough information on myriad kidney problems and diseases; supports patient services such as transplantation, drug banks, and educational projects; and makes referrals to local agencies.

O'Callaghan, Chris A., and Barry Brenner. *The Kidney at a Glance.* Boston: Blackwell Science, 2000. Covers a range of topics related to the kidneys, presenting text on one page and accompanying illustrations on the facing page. Covers basic anatomy and physiology and the pathologies and presentations of renal and urinary tract disease.

Parker, James N., and Philip M. Parker, eds. *The Official Patient's Sourcebook on Urinary Tract Infection.* San Diego, Calif.: Icon Health, 2002. Draws from public, academic, government, and peer-reviewed research to provide a wide-ranging handbook for patients with recurring urinary tract infections.

_____. *The 2002 Official Patient's Sourcebook on Kidney Failure.* San Diego, Calif.: Icon Health, 2002. Draws from public, academic, government, and peer-reviewed research to provide a wide-ranging reference about the causes, treatments, and risk factors of kidney disease and failure.

Schrier, Robert W., ed. *Diseases of the Kidney and Urinary Tract.* 7th ed. Philadelphia: Lippincott Williams & Wilkins, 2001. Covers full range of the biochemical, structural, and functional correlations in the kidney, as well as hereditary diseases, urological diseases and neoplasms of the genitourinary tract, acute renal failure, and nutrition, drugs, and the kidney, among many additional topics.

Tierney, Lawrence M., Stephen J. McPhee, and Maxine Papadakis, eds. *Current Medical Diagnosis and Treatment 2004.* 43d ed. Stamford, Conn.: Appleton & Lange, 2003. This reference volume covers all aspects of internal medicine. It is readable and concisely describes more than one thousand diseases and disorders, as well as their medical management.

KIDNEY REMOVAL. *See* NEPHRECTOMY.

KIDNEY STONES. *See* KIDNEY DISORDERS; STONE REMOVAL; STONES.

KIDNEY TRANSPLANTATION
PROCEDURE

ANATOMY OR SYSTEM AFFECTED: Abdomen, kidneys, urinary system

SPECIALTIES AND RELATED FIELDS: General surgery, nephrology

DEFINITION: A surgical procedure that replaces the recipient's diseased, nonfunctioning kidney with a donated one.

KEY TERMS:

end-stage renal disease: the final phase of long-standing kidney disease, characterized by a nearly complete loss of function

hemodialysis: the use of an external apparatus to filter the blood of patients with end-stage renal disease

immunosuppression: the use of a variety of drugs to depress the immune system's response to foreign tissue; lowers the probability of rejection of transplanted organs

rejection: a cellular and chemical attack by the immune system on a transplanted organ, which is recognized as foreign to the body

renal: referring to the kidneys

INDICATIONS AND PROCEDURES

Transplantation of a human kidney from a donor to a recipient has been used since the middle of the twentieth century to improve the quality and length of life for people with renal failure. While hemodialysis—or the use of an artificial kidney machine, as it is commonly known—can be used satisfactorily for years, transplantation is often the ultimate goal because it can return the patient to a near-normal life.

The kidneys play a pivotal role in maintaining a stable internal environment by controlling fluid levels, excreting waste products, and regulating the blood concentration of acids and bases and of ions such as sodium and potassium. The kidneys are also responsible for regulating blood pressure by secreting substances that constrict the blood vessels. Clearly, the derangement of such complex functions, as occurs in renal disease, is life-threatening.

There are many reasons for renal failure, but the most frequent are inherited disorders, severe infections, toxic substances, allergic reactions, diabetes mellitus, and hypertension. The latter two, which are common illnesses in the United States, result in renal damage because of long-term injury to the blood vessels. The symptoms of minimally or nonfunctioning kidneys reflect an accumulation of toxic waste products and dramatic changes in the chemical composition of the blood. Every system is affected until coma and death ensue. The process of hemodialysis is used intermittently to cleanse the blood and maintain life. Transplantation in the otherwise healthy person, however, is preferred.

An extraordinary amount of cooperation and preparation is necessary for successful kidney transplantation. The donor organ may come from a living blood relative or from a cadaver within minutes of death. The organ is removed and maintained at low temperature in a special preservative solution for up to forty-eight hours. A suitable recipient is located through a national registry that can rapidly pair a cadaver organ to a waiting patient. The chosen candidate is immediately prepared for surgery, and through an abdominal incision, the kidney is placed in the abdomen and connected to the blood supply by its artery and vein. The ureter, the urine-collecting duct, is attached to the bladder. The recipient's own diseased kidneys may or may not be removed; their presence does not interfere with the transplanted organ. Within hours, the newly transplanted organ begins to form urine.

USES AND COMPLICATIONS

All transplanted organs and tissues face both immediate and long-term rejection by the recipient's immune system. Recognizing the donated kidney as foreign, or "nonself," the immune system attacks it both physi-

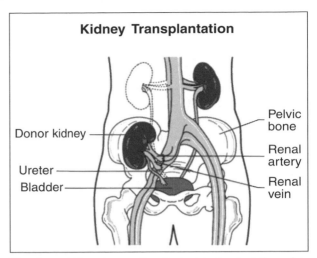

Kidney Transplantation

The donor kidney is usually attached in front of the pelvic bone, rather than in the location of the nonfunctioning kidney, which is not removed in some cases.

cally and chemically. The injury can be so severe as to result in the organ's death and the need for its surgical removal. In an attempt to prevent this reaction, certain steps are taken both before and after transplantation surgery.

Matching a donor and recipient involves careful selection that must minimize the physiological differences that exist between people. The blood types (the ABO and Rh systems) should be the same. Gene sequences on the sixth chromosome that code for immune system components are also matched as closely as possible in a process known as human leukocyte antigen (HLA) compatibility. Living, first-degree relatives, such as parents or siblings, often provide the best survival rates because of the genetic similarities between donor and recipient. The loss of one kidney in a healthy individual does not appear to affect the body.

The excellent success rates that have been achieved—nearly 80 percent—are attributable both to preoperative matching and to immunosuppression, which is begun shortly before surgery and continued for many months afterward. Potent drugs are used to inhibit the recipient's immune system, thereby protecting the new kidney from attack and significantly reducing rejection. Eventually, the drugs are tapered off and stopped, having allowed the body time to adjust to the foreign tissue and the kidney time to heal.

As can be expected in a procedure as difficult as kidney transplantation, the risks and complications are many. In the immediate postoperative period, hemorrhaging from the attached renal artery or vein, leakage from the ureter, organ malfunction, and immediate rejection can occur. Often, difficulties begin weeks or even months later, because of both rejection damage to the kidney and side effects related to severe immunosuppression. Immunosuppression leaves the body prey to bacterial, viral, and fungal infections, as well as cancer. Sometimes, a vicious cycle begins, in which life-threatening infections require the discontinuation of the immunosuppressive drugs, and the probability of organ rejection and irreparable kidney damage is heightened. Continual patient monitoring is absolutely essential to maintain the delicate balance between the risks and benefits involved in this procedure.

PERSPECTIVE AND PROSPECTS

Prior to 1962, when immunosuppressive drugs were unavailable and matching could only be based on blood type, kidney transplantation was an experimental procedure usually involving the organ of a living, first-degree relative. In the following decades, an extraordinary surge in information about the immune system and the genes that control the rejection response, as well as the discovery of powerful drugs, made transplantation a successful alternative for patients supported by hemodialysis. It also significantly increased the donor pool of organs by allowing unrelated cadaver kidneys to be used. It is in both areas, more precise matching and the development of less toxic postoperative drugs, that research continues. Contributions made in this field are readily used for research in all other organ transplantation as well.

—*Connie Rizzo, M.D.*

See also Circulation; Cysts; Dialysis; Internal medicine; Kidney disorders; Kidneys; Nephrectomy; Nephritis; Nephrology; Nephrology, pediatric; Polycystic kidney disease; Renal failure; Transplantation; Urinalysis; Urinary disorders; Urinary system; Urology; Urology, pediatric; Xenotransplantation.

FOR FURTHER INFORMATION:

American Kidney Fund. http://www.akfinc.org/. Provides financial assistance for individuals with chronic kidney failure.

Brezis, M., et al. "Renal Transplantation." In *Brenner and Rector's The Kidney*, edited by Barry M. Brenner and Floyd C. Rector, Jr. 6th ed. Philadelphia: W. B. Saunders, 1999. A chapter in a treatise which, at more than two thousand pages, is the most comprehensive and authoritative source on the normal and diseased human kidney.

Carpenter, C., and M. Lazarus. "Dialysis and Transplantation in Renal Failure." In *Harrison's Principles of Internal Medicine*, edited by Kurt Isselbacher et al. 14th ed. New York: McGraw-Hill, 1998. A chapter in a standard text on internal medicine. Includes bibliographical references and an index.

Danovitch, Gabriel. *Handbook of Kidney Transplantation*. 3d ed. Philadelphia: Lippincott Williams & Wilkins, 2000. A clinical handbook that gives a practical overview of renal transplantation and includes up-to-date coverage of topics such as immunosuppressive drugs, short- and long-term post-transplant management, complications, and ethical and legal issues.

National Kidney Foundation. http://www.kidney.org/. Offers thorough information on myriad kidney problems and diseases; supports patient services such as transplantation, drug banks, and educational projects; and makes referrals to local agencies.

Schrier, Robert W., and Carl W. Gottschalk, eds. *Diseases of the Kidney*. 7th ed. Boston: Little, Brown, 2001. Addresses the spectrum of systemic diseases and the kidney, covering malignancies, paraproteinemias, HIV, hepatitis, cryoglobulimea, sickle cell disease, sarcoidosis, and tropical diseases, in an atlas format.

KIDNEYS

ANATOMY

ANATOMY OR SYSTEM AFFECTED: Abdomen, circulatory system, urinary system

SPECIALTIES AND RELATED FIELDS: Hematology, nephrology, urology

DEFINITION: The organs that control the amount and composition of body water by separating the blood into waste products (which leave the body as urine) and nutrients (which are returned to the blood).

KEY TERMS:

Bowman's capsule: the group of renal cells that forms the cup of a nephron; fluids that seep from glomerular capillaries into the hollow wall of the capsule will be transformed into urine during their passage through the renal tubule leading from the capsule

glomerulus: a tuft or ball of capillaries contained within a Bowman's capsule

nephron: the almost-microscopic functional unit of the kidney, composed of special capillary blood vessels and of a Bowman's capsule connected to a renal tubule; each kidney has approximately 1.2 million nephrons

renal: of or relating to the kidneys

renal pelvis: the central pocket or sac of each kidney, which collects urine from all nephrons and channels it into the ureter

renal tubule: the tubular portion of a nephron that allows renal fluid to flow from the Bowman's capsule to the renal pelvis; these tubules, shaped like hairpins, are crucially important in the production of urine

ureter: the tube that transports urine from the renal pelvis to the urinary bladder

STRUCTURE AND FUNCTIONS

The normal human body has two kidneys, fist-sized organs located behind the abdomen and under the diaphragm. Each kidney, shaped like a bean, has a notch called the hilum, and the backbone separates the two kidneys. The kidneys make urine from blood. The renal artery transports blood into the kidney, while the renal vein transports blood out of the kidney. The blood vessels and the ureter connect with the kidney at its hilum.

The two kidneys are essentially identical in structure and function; consequently, kidney function can be discussed in the singular. The kidneys are a major functional unit of the circulatory system—unlike organs such as the brain, skin, or uterus, which are merely supported by that circulation. The kidney controls the environment of all cells of the body, an activity which is essential to life. That environment is salt water, and to understand the structure and function of the kidney, it is necessary to understand the nature of salt water in the body.

The human body is about 56 percent water, and the composition of this fluid is very important. One-third of this water is outside the cells; some of this extracellular fluid is between cells, and some of it is the liquid in blood vessels (blood is composed of liquid and cells). Two-thirds of the body's water is inside cells. The cell membrane surrounding each cell retains the intracellular fluid, but the water molecules move freely across the cell membrane. The size of each cell is determined by its water content. Cells swell or shrink based on the accumulation or loss of water molecules. The concentration of substances dissolved in the water determines whether water will accumulate inside or outside cells. Some of these dissolved substances are gases such as oxygen and carbon dioxide; some are minerals such as hydrogen, sodium, and calcium; some are sugars or proteins; and others are nutrients and waste products.

The amount and the composition of body water is controlled by the kidneys. Two other organs that aid in controlling the composition of body water are the lungs and the digestive tract; they can add or remove materials from the body water. The kidneys control the composition of body water primarily by removing materials from body water. Unlike the lungs and the digestive tract, however, the kidneys also regulate the amount of body water. The kidneys carry out both of these functions by acting on the blood. The kidney has three other important functions: It helps to control blood pressure, helps to control the manufacture of red blood cells, and participates in the manufacture of vitamin D. This article focuses on function of the normal kidney and what can make the kidney function abnormally.

Each kidney contains more than a million nephrons, its functional units, arranged in cones. A nephron is composed of blood vessels and a Bowman's capsule, a cup of renal cells containing the capillary tuft called a glomerulus and attached to a renal tubule.

A kidney has between eight and eighteen cones of nephrons. The base of each cone is near the surface of the kidney, and the peak of each cone is pointed at the renal pelvis, the central sac that collects and channels urine. Each nephron acts like a very sophisticated filtration system for the blood. Approximately 20 to 25 percent of all the blood in the body flows through the blood vessels of the kidneys every minute.

The action of the nephron actually begins with a porous filter, the glomerulus, that separates particles from a liquid. In this case, the liquid is blood plasma and the particles are blood cells and those protein molecules that are too large to pass through the glomerular pores. About 20 percent of the liquid in the blood seeps through the wall of glomeruli and into the inner space of Bowman's capsules. This liquid that crosses into a Bowman's capsule contains water, minerals, sugars, amino acids, and products of cell metabolism. The body needs to retain many of these substances, including water, so they must be recaptured by nephrons and returned to the blood.

The recapturing process occurs in the renal tubules. This is the process in which the nephron differs from an ordinary filter. The tubules have special cells that are capable of selectively reabsorbing those materials that must be retained by the body. These materials are passed from the liquid inside the tubules, through the tubule cells, and into blood capillaries that are laced or braided around the outside wall of the tubules. About 99 percent of the water molecules that seep into the re-

Anatomy of a Kidney

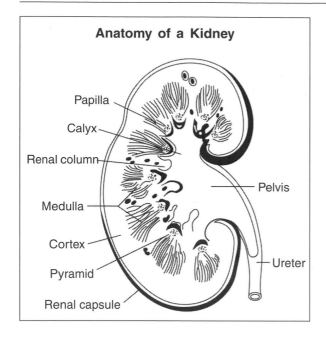

Papilla

Calyx

Renal column

Medulla

Cortex

Pyramid

Renal capsule

Pelvis

Ureter

the kidney, which contains sensing mechanisms that respond to changes in fluid composition. The kidney makes a hormone, called renin, that increases blood pressure. Other sensors that respond to changes in fluid composition are located in the brain. When these sensors detect changes that require action, the brain, acting through the pituitary gland, releases hormones, such as antidiuretic hormone (ADH), that act on the kidney. Another important hormone that controls kidney function, aldosterone, comes from the adrenal gland. The actual means by which these hormones control kidney function, however, is only partially understood.

By other mechanisms, the kidney detects whether the blood contains sufficient red blood cells (erythrocytes). Red blood cells are responsible for carrying oxygen to all the other cells in the body. When more red blood cells are needed, the kidney makes a hormone called erythropoietin, which stimulates the bone marrow and causes it to make more red blood cells.

DISORDERS AND DISEASES

The advantage of having a pair of kidneys becomes obvious if renal function becomes impaired. A person does quite well with one kidney; in fact, half of one kidney is sufficient to keep an individual alive.

A kidney problem may be suspected if an individual experiences changes in urination, such as pain on urination, changes in frequency of urination (more often or less often than usual), or changes in the urine that is formed (such as in its amount, appearance, or odor). Puffiness of the skin all over the body, but especially of the hands, feet, ankles, and face, may indicate abnormal renal function. This puffiness signifies water retention. Kidney disease can also be manifested by severe pain in the lower back, side, abdomen, or sex organs. The pain may be long-lasting or may occur with startling suddenness.

A person can be born with abnormal kidneys; this is a form of kidney disease. Normal kidneys, however, can malfunction because of a problem in the kidney itself, a problem in the blood circulation, or a problem in the flow of urine from the kidneys. Examples of abnormal kidneys at birth, abnormal urinary flow (kidney stones), and kidney infection will be discussed.

The formation of the kidneys by a fetus is quite complex and is controlled by genes. The development of the kidneys, other parts of the urinary tract (the ureters, bladder, and urethra), and the sex organs are all closely related. There are many opportunities for the developmental process to go wrong. Sometimes no kidneys

nal tubules from the glomeruli are returned to the blood. The substances that do not need to be retained by the body continue to flow through the tubules and eventually leave the kidney as urine.

The mechanism in the renal tubular cells that selectively reabsorbs substances from the tubular liquid is quite special. The membrane of each cell contains proteins that act as chemical pumps. These pump proteins pick up substances to be reabsorbed from the tubular liquid and pass those substances into and through the tubular cells, where they enter renal capillaries. The reabsorbed substances may be salts or electrolytes, such as sodium or bicarbonate, or they may be sugars or even amino acids. As these substances are reabsorbed, much of the tubular water is also reabsorbed.

The pump proteins can work in the opposite direction as well. They can move substances from the renal capillaries surrounding the tubules, through the wall of the tubules, and into the tubular liquid. This process is called tubular secretion. Substances that commonly undergo tubular secretion are potassium, ammonium, and acid.

The remarkable action of the pump proteins requires fuel—in this case, adenosine triphosphate (ATP). ATP is made by living cells from oxygen, sugar, fatty acids, and nucleic acids in the blood. Pump proteins stop working when cells are unable to make ATP.

The pressure of the blood flow through the glomeruli and the reabsorption process of the renal tubules are closely controlled. This control takes place directly in

are formed, sometimes the two kidneys are fused together, and sometimes more than one pair of kidneys is formed.

One of the most common malformations of the kidney is polycystic kidney disease, a hereditary (genetic) disorder affecting about 2 in 1,000 people. In the United States, it is ten times more common than sickle cell disease and fifteen times more common than cystic fibrosis. In polycystic kidney disease, each kidney contains numerous fluid-filled sacs, or cysts, scattered throughout the organ. The cysts are of different sizes, some very small and some the size of a grape. Polycystic kidneys are noticeably enlarged.

The cysts are caused by a malformation of the renal tubules. A cyst is formed when a renal tubule develops a branch from the main tubule. Tubules are not supposed to form branches; if this occurs, however, then the branch may become sealed off from the original tubule so that it has no entrance or exit. These sealed-off tubules are the cysts. They are capable of secretory activity because their cells contain pump proteins. The cysts enlarge as they accumulate fluid, putting pressure on the blood vessels, their capillaries, and the nephrons. The flow of blood and of urine is hindered. Patients with polycystic kidney disease often develop high blood pressure, kidney stones, and kidney infections. The disease can begin before birth, but symptoms may not occur until childhood or early adulthood. The intensity or severity of the disease varies greatly, from symptomless to life-threatening. Treatment of mild polycystic kidney disease may consist of relieving the pain, curing the infection, and controlling the blood pressure. Treatment of severe or life-threatening polycystic renal disease requires dialysis or kidney transplantation.

Stones in the urinary tract are very common. About 1 in 100 Americans have stones, and 1 in 1,000 adults experiences such severe symptoms that hospitalization is required. Kidney stones are caused by a prolonged high concentration of certain minerals in the urine, usually calcium, oxalate, or urate. The stones usually consist of crystals bound together by proteins.

The size and shape of kidney stones vary greatly. They may be microscopic or the size of a pea or even larger; they may be smooth or jagged. The stones may be passed from the urinary tract during urination, but some require removal by a urologist. Microscopic stones may not cause any symptoms, while larger stones can be very painful and may produce blood in the urine. Because stones hinder the flow of urine, their presence can allow bacteria to grow in the urinary tract, producing an infection.

Kidney stones that produce symptoms and are not passed by the patient must be removed. Some stones may be removed with a ureteroscope while the patient is under general anesthesia. A ureteroscope is a urological instrument like a hollow tube. It is inserted into the urinary tract through the external opening of the urethra and passed through the bladder and into the ureter. The tube can actually be inserted into the renal pelvis. The optical system of the ureteroscope allows the physician to see inside the urinary tract. Through the ureteroscope, kidney stones may be broken up by applying ultrasonic, laser, or electrohydraulic (acoustic shockwave) energy.

An alternative means of removing large kidney stones is extracorporeal shock-wave lithotripsy, or ESWL. ESWL is desirable because it uses shock waves to break up the stones, thus eliminating the need to insert medical instruments into the patient. In one method of ESWL, the anesthetized patient is placed in a tub of water. X-ray imaging locates and monitors the stones as shock waves crush them. The patient's tissues are not damaged, and the sandy remains of the stones are then passed with urine. The development of ESWL has offered a useful means of treating kidney stones, but it has not eliminated the need for surgical or ureteroscopic removal of these stones from some patients. Each patient and each stone is different; they require the professional evaluation of a urologist.

Urinary tract infections are common, affecting 10 to 20 percent of women at some point in their lives; they are less common in men. Pathogens usually infect the kidneys by ascending the urinary tract via the urethra, bladder, and ureters. The normal bladder is an effective barrier to these infections, but any obstruction to the flow of urine, such as enlarged prostate, renal cysts, pregnancy, or a urinary stone, will weaken this barrier. Sometimes, pathogens infect the kidneys through the blood. Most urinary tract infections can be effectively treated with antibiotics. It is important for the physician to choose an antibiotic that is effective against the causative pathogen. Each antibiotic is effective against only a few types of bacteria, and many different bacteria can cause urinary tract infections.

Infections involving the kidney are especially serious. Because the kidneys are essential to life, these infections must be treated promptly and completely. Some infections affect the kidney even after the infection is cured. The body reacts to pathogens by producing proteins called antibodies, which circulate in the bloodstream. Antibodies in the blood can coat and damage the glomerular filters in Bowman's capsules. This reduces the effectiveness of the filters, allowing blood and protein to enter the urine and causing the body to become puffy. The medical term for this serious kidney disease is glomerulonephritis. Treatment is available, but it is better to prevent the disease from occurring. If left untreated, the kidney damage may be so extensive that dialysis or transplantation is required to prevent death.

PERSPECTIVE AND PROSPECTS

The ancient Greeks seem to be the earliest people whose writings about the kidney have survived. They had no regard for the importance of this organ, mainly because their frame of reference consisted of four "humors." Even before 500 B.C.E., the Greeks were developing the doctrine of the four elements of the inanimate universe: air, fire, water, and earth. From this idea, Polybus, the son-in-law of Hippocrates, created the corollary of the four "humors" responsible for life: yellow bile (choler), blood, phlegm (pituita), and black bile (melancholia). The concept of humors dominated the thinking of Aristotle (384-322 B.C.E.) when he wrote about his study of the anatomy of kidneys in several animals, including humans. This approach delayed an understanding of even the basic concept that kidneys and urine are related, an idea finally proposed about 290 B.C.E. by Erasistratus of Ceos.

Knowledge of Erasistratus comes mainly from Galen (129-c. 199 C.E.). Galen, rather than applauding the advances of his forebears, ridiculed unfounded assertions. He conducted physiological experiments on living animals, such as observing the effect of cutting and tying one ureter while leaving the opposite one intact. His experiments yielded much information about renal physiology. The writings of Galen formed the foundation of medical knowledge for the next four hundred years. Students and teachers, rather than building upon the experimental process, accepted the proclamations of Galen as dogma.

The next great advance in renal knowledge came from the Italian anatomist Bartolommeo Eustachio (1520-1574), who, without the benefit of a microscope, discovered the renal tubules and their relationship to the renal vascular system. His descriptions and drawings of 1564 were lost in the Vatican library until 1714. In the meantime, another Italian, Lorenzo Bellini (1643-1704), independently discovered the renal tu-

bules and discerned their function. A contemporary, Marcello Malpighi (1628-1694), discovered glomeruli and their relationship to tubules.

Subsequent advances had to wait until the nineteenth century, when knowledge of all aspects of human biology and medicine began a rapid advance. Many independent advances in the nineteenth and twentieth centuries—in surgery, pharmacology, and immunology—made the transplantation of kidneys and other major organs possible. General anesthesia was developed independently by two Americans: by Crawford Long in 1842 and by William T. G. Morton in 1846. Antiseptic procedures were originated in 1867 by the Englishman Joseph Lister, and vascular surgical techniques were developed in 1902 by French surgeon Alexis Carrel and Hungarian surgeon Emerich Ullman. Anticoagulants were developed in 1914 and 1915, and systemic antibiotics were developed in the 1930's and 1940's. Blood typing was begun in Europe by Karl Landsteiner (1868-1943). Tissue immunology was first explained in 1953, and tissue typing was introduced in France and the United States in the 1960's. Immunosuppressive drugs were developed during this same period. Kidney transplantation is also possible because of extracorporeal support devices such as the dialysis machine, the heart-lung machine, and the organ perfusion machine.

The first transplant of a human kidney between identical twins was performed on December 23, 1954, by Joseph E. Murray. He later performed the first human kidney transplant between unrelated persons on April 5, 1962. By the 1990's, tens of thousands of kidney transplants were being performed in the United States every year. There are many more persons waiting for a transplant than there are kidneys available for transplantation. The solution to this problem is unclear. Transplants between living persons in the same family may be encouraged, and transplants from animals to humans may be perfected. It is even possible that a transplantable artificial kidney can be developed, but this task will be enormously difficult, considering all the functions of a natural kidney.

—*Armand M. Karow, Ph.D.*

See also Adrenalectomy; Blood and blood disorders; Circulation; Corticosteroids; Cysts; Dialysis; Internal medicine; Kidney disorders; Kidney transplantation; Laparoscopy; Lithotripsy; Nephrectomy; Nephritis; Nephrology; Nephrology, pediatric; Polycystic kidney disease; Pyelonephritis; Renal failure; Stone removal; Stones; Systems and organs; Transplantation; Urinalysis; Urinary disorders; Urinary system; Urology; Urology, pediatric.

FOR FURTHER INFORMATION:

Andreoli, Thomas E., et al., eds. *Cecil Essentials of Medicine*. 5th ed. Philadelphia: W. B. Saunders, 2001. This paperback book, written for physicians, describes diseases and their treatment in humans. Contains a good section on the kidneys.

Brenner, Barry M., and Floyd C. Rector, Jr., eds. *Brenner and Rector's Kidney*. 2 vols. 7th ed. Philadelphia: W. B. Saunders, 2003. This treatise, at more than two thousand pages, is the most comprehensive and authoritative source on the normal and diseased human kidney.

Gottschalk, Carl W., Robert W. Berliner, and Gerhard H. Giebisch, eds. *Renal Physiology: People and Ideas*. Bethesda, Md.: American Physiological Society, 1987. This collection of scholarly essays traces the historical development of renal physiology. While the work is exhaustive and comprehensive, emphasis is placed on the nineteenth and twentieth centuries.

Marieb, Elaine N. *Essentials of Human Anatomy and Physiology*. 6th ed. Redwood City, Calif.: Benjamin/Cummings, 2003. This introductory anatomy and physiology textbook, easily accessible to those with little science background, is richly illustrated with diagrams and photographs, which help to illuminate body systems and processes.

O'Callaghan, Chris A., and Barry Brenner. *The Kidney at a Glance*. Boston: Blackwell Science, 2000. Covers a range of topics related to the kidneys, presenting text on one page and accompanying illustrations on the facing page. Covers basic anatomy and physiology and the pathologies and presentations of renal and urinary tract disease.

Vander, Arthur J. *Renal Physiology*. 5th ed. New York: McGraw-Hill, 1995. This paperback book, written for medical students, describes the anatomy and physiology of the normal human kidney. Provides extensive, exhaustive information in a comprehensible format. The text may be somewhat challenging for those who have not taken introductory college-level courses in chemistry and biology.

Voet, Donald, and Judith G. Voet. *Biochemistry*. Rev. ed. New York: Wiley, 2002. A good book to use for the description and explanation of the chemical processes taking place in the kidney and other areas of the body.

KINESIOLOGY

SPECIALTY

ANATOMY OR SYSTEM AFFECTED: Brain, cells, circulatory system, heart, lungs, muscles, musculoskeletal system, nervous system, psychic-emotional system, respiratory system, spine

SPECIALTIES AND RELATED FIELDS: Cardiology, exercise physiology, orthopedics, physical therapy, psychology, sports medicine

DEFINITION: The applied science of human movement, which combines the general areas of anatomy (the study of structure) and physiology (the study of function).

SCIENCE AND PROFESSION

In 1989, the American Academy of Physical Education endorsed the term "kinesiology" to describe the entire field traditionally known as physical education, which includes the following subdisciplines: exercise physiology, biomechanics, motor control and learning, sports nutrition, sports psychology, sports sociology, athletic training programs, pedagogy, adapted physical education, cardiac rehabilitation, and physical therapy.

Exercise physiology describes the body's muscular, cardiovascular, and respiratory functioning during both short-term and long-term exercise. Research has focused on muscle fiber typing, oxygen uptake assessment, lactic acid metabolism, thermoregulation, body composition, and muscle hypertrophy. Biomechanics applies Isaac Newton's laws of physics to improve the mechanical efficiency of muscle movement patterns; using high-speed video and computer analysis, flaws in joint and limb dynamics can be assessed and changed to optimize performance. Motor control and learning pinpoint the areas of the brain and spinal cord that are responsible for the acquisition and retention of motor skills. Understanding the neurological basis of reflex and voluntary muscle movements helps to refine teaching strategies and describe the mechanisms of fatigue.

Sports nutrition describes how the body stores, circulates, and converts nutrients for aerobic and anaerobic energy production through carbohydrate loading and other strategies. Sports psychology explores the workings of the mind before, during, and after exercise and competition. Sports sociology examines aspects such as cultural, ethnic, and gender differences; dynamics in small and large groups; and the role of sports in ethical and moral development. Athletic trainers work with sports physicians and surgeons to prevent and rehabilitate injuries caused by overuse, trauma, or disease. Physical therapists use clinical exercise therapy and other modalities in a variety of rehabilitation settings.

Allied health areas under the kinesiology umbrella include pedagogy (teaching progressions for movement skills), adapted physical education (activities for the physically and mentally challenged), and cardiac rehabilitation (recovery stages for those disabled by heart disease). Professional organizations in the field of kinesiology include the American College of Sports Medicine, the American Physical Therapy Association, the National Athletic Trainers Association, the National Strength and Conditioning Association, and the American Alliance for Health, Physical Education, Recreation, and Dance.

—Daniel G. Graetzer, Ph.D.

See also Allied health; Anatomy; Cardiac rehabilitation; Exercise physiology; Muscles; Nervous system; Neurology; Physical rehabilitation; Physiology; Respiration; Sports medicine.

FOR FURTHER INFORMATION:

Brooks, George A., and Thomas D. Fahey. *Fundamentals of Human Performance.* New York: Macmillan, 1987.

McArdle, William, Frank I. Katch, and Victor L. Katch. *Exercise Physiology: Energy, Nutrition, and Human Performance.* 5th ed. Philadelphia: Lippincott Williams & Wilkins, 2001.

Oatis, Carol A. *Applied Kinesiology.* Philadelphia: Lippincott Williams & Wilkins, 2003.

Plowman, Sharon A., and Denise L. Smith. *Exercise Physiology for Health, Fitness, and Performance.* San Francisco: Benjamin/Cummings, 2002.

Powers, Scott K., and Edward T. Howley. *Exercise Physiology: Theory and Application to Fitness and Performance.* 5th ed. New York: McGraw-Hill, 2003.

Sharkey, Brian J. *Physiology of Fitness.* 3d ed. Champaign, Ill.: Human Kinetics Books, 1990.

KLINEFELTER SYNDROME

DISEASE/DISORDER

ANATOMY OR SYSTEM AFFECTED: Breasts, endocrine system, genitals, hair, psychic-emotional system, reproductive system

SPECIALTIES AND RELATED FIELDS: Embryology, endocrinology, genetics, psychology

DEFINITION: A male chromosomal disorder causing infertility and significant femaleness.

CAUSES AND SYMPTOMS

Klinefelter syndrome is caused by a variation in the number of sex chromosomes. Normal males possess one X and one Y chromosome, while females have two X chromosomes. When an embryo has two X chromosomes and one Y chromosome (XXY), normal development and reproductive function are hampered and the boy shows the symptoms of Klinefelter syndrome. These symptoms include breast development, incomplete maleness, and school or social difficulties. The major symptom is sterility or very reduced fertility. The testes remain small after puberty and produce few, if any, sperm.

In adolescence, breast tissue develops significantly in about 50 percent of all cases. In addition, normal facial and pubic hair may not develop in these boys. Although their average height is six feet, young men with Klinefelter syndrome are often unathletic and less physically strong or coordinated than their peers. Some affected individuals exhibit some degree of subnormal intelligence. Others appear passive and without self-confidence or experience difficulties learning language and speech.

TREATMENT AND THERAPY

Klinefelter syndrome is diagnosed using a karyotype, an analysis of the chromosomes from blood or cheek cells. It can determine the presence of forty-seven chromosomes, including one Y and two X. Although Klinefelter syndrome is genetic and cannot be cured, treatment in the form of a monthly injection of testosterone can be administered to supplement the usually insufficient amount produced by the boy's own testes. This therapy should enhance male physical development by increasing the size of the penis and causing pubic and facial hair growth and greater muscle bulk.

Hormone therapy cannot increase the size of the testes, however, nor can it cure sterility. It cannot reverse breast tissue development, which can only be treated by

---

INFORMATION ON KLINEFELTER SYNDROME

CAUSES: Genetic chromosomal disorder
SYMPTOMS: Infertility, breast development, small testes that produce few, if any, sperm
DURATION: Lifelong
TREATMENTS: None; hormonal therapy for symptoms

surgical removal. It may, however, increase self-esteem and a sense of maleness, thereby easing social interactions.

PERSPECTIVE AND PROSPECTS

Found in one or two of every thousand males born, Klinefelter syndrome is the most common human chromosomal variation. Described by Harry Klinefelter in 1942, its cause was discovered by Patricia Jacobs and John Strong in 1959. Affected males have normal erections and may suffer no major effects other than those mentioned above.

—*Grace D. Matzen*

See also Genetic diseases; Genetics and inheritance; Gynecomastia; Hermaphroditism and pseudohermaphroditism; Puberty and adolescence; Reproductive system; Sexual differentiation.

FOR FURTHER INFORMATION:

Bandmann, H.-J., and R. Breit, eds. *Klinefelter's Syndrome.* New York: Springer-Verlag, 1984.

Fanaroff, Avroy A., and Richard J. Martin. *Neonatal-Perinatal Medicine: Diseases of the Fetus and Infant.* 2 vols. 7th ed. New York: Elsevier, 2001.

Klinefelter Syndrome and Associates. http://www .genetic.org/.

Millunsky, Aubrey. *Genetic Disorders of the Fetus: Diagnosis, Prevention, and Treatment.* 4th ed. Baltimore: Johns Hopkins University Press, 1998.

Morales, Ralph. *Out of Darkness: An Autobiography of Living with Klinefelter Syndrome.* Louisville, Ky.: Chicago Spectrum Press, 2002.

Parker, James N., and Philip M. Parker, eds. *The Official Parent's Sourcebook on Klinefelter Syndrome.* San Diego, Calif.: Icon Health, 2002.

Theilgaard, Alice, et al. *A Psychological-Psychiatric Study of Patients with Klinefelter's Syndrome.* Aarhus, Denmark: Universitetsforlaget i Aarhus, 1971.

Wilson, Jean D. *Wilson's Textbook of Endocrinology.* 10th ed. New York: Elsevier, 2003.

Zuppinger, Klaus. *Klinefelter's Syndrome: A Clinical and Cytogenetic Study in Twenty-four Cases.* Copenhagen: Periodica, 1967.

KLIPPEL-TRENAUNAY SYNDROME
DISEASE/DISORDER

ALSO KNOWN AS: Angio-osteohypertrophy, nevus varicousus osteohypertrophicus syndrome, hemangiectasia hypertrophicans, Klippel-Trenaunay-Weber syndrome

ANATOMY OR SYSTEM AFFECTED: Blood vessels, circulatory system, gastrointestinal system, joints, lymphatic system

SPECIALTIES AND RELATED FIELDS: Genetics, internal medicine, pediatrics, vascular medicine

DEFINITION: A rare congenital syndrome characterized by hemangiomas of the vascular system that can affect bone or soft tissue throughout the body.

CAUSES AND SYMPTOMS

Klippel-Trenaunay syndrome was first described in 1900 in patients exhibiting a combination of varicose veins, multiple vascular nevi (birthmarks on the skin sometimes called port-wine stains), and excessive growth or development (hypertrophy) of limbs or soft tissue. Increased vascularity is common. At birth, a large vein may be observed running from the lower leg into the upper thigh, referred to as the Klippel-Trenaunay vein.

The molecular basis for the disease is unclear, as most cases appear as simply random occurrences. Among those few cases which appear to be heritable, it is believed that an autosomal dominant gene may be at fault, possibly linked to chromosome numbers 5 or 11. Evidence suggests that, at the molecular level, deregulation of deoxyribonucleic acid (DNA) methylation of imprinted genes may play a role.

Whichever gene may be at fault, it is believed the mutation occurs early in embryonic development. The result is that the defect appears randomly among cells as they migrate and differentiate early during embryonic stages, resulting in the seemingly haphazard distribution of the trait as the fetus develops.

Diagnosis is based upon the triad of vascular or soft tissue defects, with venous or capillary malformations

---

INFORMATION ON KLIPPEL-TRENAUNAY SYNDROME

CAUSES: Unknown, possibly genetic

SYMPTOMS: Varicose veins, port-wine stains, limb or soft tissue hypertrophy, noticeable large vein running from lower leg into upper thigh, localized tumors, excessive bleeding

DURATION: Lifelong

TREATMENTS: Alleviation of symptoms, such as compression garments and leg elevation for varicose veins, surgery for limb hypertrophy, anticoagulants

leading to localized, and often extensive, tumors. Preliminary diagnosis can be based upon any two of the characteristics. Another symptom may be excessive bleeding, especially from the rectum or detected in the urine.

Treatment and Therapy

If the disorder becomes apparent during the prenatal period, then the prognosis is generally poor. Treatment in the adult is generally symptomatic, although the possibility of internal organ involvement, as well as pulmonary embolisms, leaves the patient at risk even in the absence of symptoms.

Since varicose veins are generally apparent, the patient may wear compression garments, elevating the legs at intervals. Surgery may be necessary to correct limb hypertrophy. Because the formation of embolisms is a risk, the patient may utilize anticoagulants prophylactically, particularly prior to surgery. Corticosteroid use may help limit swelling in some cases. In the absence of significant malformations, the patient should simply be monitored on an annual basis.

Perspective and Prospects

The rare and sporadic nature of the disorder complicates routine screening. At best, proper prenatal care during pregnancy may result in diagnosis if the disorder does appear. Research into the molecular basis of the disorder may eventually determine its origins.

—*Richard Adler, Ph.D.*

See also Birthmarks; Skin; Skin disorders; Varicose veins; Vascular medicine; Vascular system.

For Further Information:

Baskerville, P. A., et al. "The Etiology of the Klippel-Trenaunay Syndrome." *Annals of Surgery* 202 (November, 1985): 624-627.

Mulliken, J. B., and A. Young, eds. *Vascular Birthmarks: Hemangiomas and Malformations*. Philadelphia: W. B. Saunders, 1988.

Telander, R. L., et al. "Prognosis and Management of Lesions of the Trunk in Children with Klippel-Trenaunay Syndrome." *Journal of Pediatric Surgery* 19 (1984): 417-422.

Kneecap removal
Procedure

Also known as: Patellectomy

Anatomy or system affected: Bones, joints, knees, legs, muscloskeletal system, tendons

Specialties and related fields: General surgery, orthopedics

Definition: The surgical removal of the kneecap.

Indications and Procedures

The kneecap, or patella, is the triangular bone at the front of the knee. It is held in position by the lower end of the quadriceps muscle, which surrounds the patella and is attached to the upper part of the tibia by the patellar tendon. The role of the kneecap is to protect the knee.

Kneecap removal surgery, or patellectomy, is performed as a result of fracture, frequent dislocation, or painful arthritis in the kneecap. Fracture is usually caused by a direct or sharp blow to the knee. Dislocation of the patella is often linked to a congenital abnormality, such as the underdevelopment of the lower end of the femur or excessive laxity of the ligaments that support the knee. Painful degenerative arthritic conditions, such as retropatellar arthritis and chondromalacia patelae, inflame and roughen the undersurface of the kneecap. Arthritic pain often worsens with the climbing of stairs or bending of the knee.

Before surgery begins, a clinical examination is conducted including blood and urine studies, and X rays of both knees. The knee is thoroughly cleansed with antiseptic soap. Anesthesia is administered either by local injection or spinal injection or by inhalation and injection (general anesthesia).

Surgery begins with an incision made around the kneecap. The skin is pulled back, exposing the muscle-covered kneecap. Surrounding muscle and connecting tendons attached to the kneecap are cut, and the kneecap is carefully removed. The remaining muscle is then sewn back together with strong suture material. Surgery is completed with the closing of the skin with sutures or clips. Full recovery takes about six weeks.

Uses and Complications

Following surgery, a scar will form along the incision. As the incision heals, the scar will recede gradually. Pain from the incision can be alleviated with heating pads. The affected leg should be elevated with pillows. Frequent movement of legs while resting in bed will decrease the likelihood of deep vein blood clots. General activity and returning to work is encouraged as soon as possible. Standing for prolonged periods of time, however, is not recommended during recovery. Following the approximate six-week recovery time, physical therapy is often used to restore strength to the knee.

Possible complications associated with kneecap removal include excessive bleeding and surgical wound infection. Additional complications can occur during recovery if general postoperative guidelines are not followed. Some loss of function can be expected.

—*Jason Georges*

See also Arthritis; Bones and the skeleton; Fracture and dislocation; Lower extremities; Orthopedic surgery; Orthopedics; Orthopedics, pediatric; Physical rehabilitation.

FOR FURTHER INFORMATION:

Bentley, George, and Robert B. Greer, eds. *Orthopaedics*. 4th ed. Oxford, England: Linacre House, 1993.

Greenfield, Lazar J., et al. *Surgery: Scientific Principles and Practice*. 3d ed. Philadelphia: Lippincott Williams & Wilkins, 2001.

Tapley, Donald F., et al., eds. *The Columbia University College of Physicians and Surgeons Complete Home Medical Guide*. Rev. 3d ed. New York: Crown, 1995.

Tierney, Lawrence M., Stephen J. McPhee, and Maxine Papadakis, eds. *Current Medical Diagnosis and Treatment 2004*. 43d ed. Stamford, Conn.: Appleton & Lange, 2003.

Way, Lawrence W., and Gerard M. Doherty, eds. *Current Surgical Diagnosis and Treatment*. 11th ed. Norwalk, Conn.: Appleton & Lange, 2003.

KNOCK-KNEES

DISEASE/DISORDER

ALSO KNOWN AS: Genu valgum

ANATOMY OR SYSTEM AFFECTED: Bones, feet, hips, joints, knees, legs, ligaments, muscles

SPECIALTIES AND RELATED FIELDS: Orthopedics, pediatrics, physical therapy

DEFINITION: A deformity in which the knees are positioned close together or turn toward each other and the tibias and ankles are apart when the feet are placed in a normal standing position.

CAUSES AND SYMPTOMS

Knock-knees, affecting both knees or occasionally only one, are a normal condition as children mature. Infants' leg bones are slightly rotated because of uterine positioning. As toddlers' legs straighten after having bowlegs, their tibias and knees often temporarily rotate toward the body's axis, causing the feet to be several inches apart. When knock-knees are not representative of normal physical development, they occur because of health conditions such as infections, obesity, or frac-

---

INFORMATION ON KNOCK-KNEES

CAUSES: Normal condition in infants; infections, obesity, or fractures in older individuals

SYMPTOMS: Altered knee positioning, imbalanced center of gravity, sometimes arthritis

DURATION: Usually temporary

TREATMENTS: None, unless pain develops or movement is impeded; may include stretching, shoe inserts, physical therapy, orthopedic braces, surgery

---

tured legs that disrupt knee growth. Knock-knees are sometimes a symptom of other conditions.

Mobility may be affected with knock-knees. Patients sometimes adjust leg and foot movement to compensate for altered knee positioning and imbalanced centers of gravity. Usually, children walk with their toes turned in for balance when they have knock-knees. Knock-kneed adults sometimes develop arthritis because of the strain on knee joints and ligaments. Knock-knees can also place stress on patients' backs and hips.

TREATMENT AND THERAPY

Medical professionals do not treat most knock-knees unless specific cases seem abnormal, cause pain, or impede movement. Growth usually corrects knee positioning. Physicians measure legs and the distance between ankles to assess the progress of natural correction. X rays are useful to detect bone problems that may exacerbate knock-knees. Photographs can document leg alignment.

Stretching the leg muscles can aid the natural resolution of knock-knees. Shoes designed with inserts can mitigate the stress on feet and manipulate patients to walk straight. Physical therapy can alleviate cartilage and joint pain associated with knock-knees.

If young patients do not outgrow knock-knees, ankle distances increase to 4 inches or more, or the condition worsens, particularly in one knee, then medical intervention often becomes necessary to ensure that patients are capable of normal movement. Physicians sometimes advise patients to wear a brace. If such efforts are unsuccessful, then the patient may undergo surgery to adjust leg bones and growth plates.

Treatment is essential for diseases or conditions in which knock-knees is a symptom. Some patients seek medical correction for aesthetic reasons.

PERSPECTIVE AND PROSPECTS

Beginning in the late nineteenth century, physicians routinely recommended therapeutic braces to treat knock-knees. During the 1950's, Soviet doctor Gavril Abramovich Ilizarov devised a fixator that encircles legs and uses tension to correct rotation problems associated with knock-knees. Italian doctor Antonio Bianchi-Maiocchi first used this device in Western countries in 1981. Dr. James Aronson brought the method to the United States in the 1980's. In that decade, Ukrainian doctor Veklich Vitaliy adapted Ilizarov's fixator for a procedure that is often used to correct severe knock-knees.

By the late twentieth century, however, physicians discouraged the use of braces to treat normal cases of knock-knees. Most advised patients to permit natural correction to occur, emphasizing that devices would not quicken that process.

—*Elizabeth D. Schafer, Ph.D.*

See also Bones and the skeleton; Growth; Lower extremities; Orthopedics; Orthopedics, pediatric.

FOR FURTHER INFORMATION:

Bianci-Maiocchi, Antonio, and James Aronson, eds. *Operative Principles of Ilizarov: Fracture Treatment, Nonunion, Osteomyelitis, Lengthening, Deformity Correction.* Baltimore: Williams & Wilkins, 1991.

England, Stephen P., ed. *Common Orthopedic Problems.* Philadelphia: W. B. Saunders, 1996.

Herring, John A., ed. *Tachdjian's Pediatric Orthopaedics.* 3d ed. 3 vols. Philadelphia: W. B. Saunders, 2002.

KWASHIORKOR

DISEASE/DISORDER

ALSO KNOWN AS: Malignant malnutrition, protein malnutrition, protein-calorie malnutrition, Mehl hrschaden

ANATOMY OR SYSTEM AFFECTED: Gastrointestinal system, muscles, skin

SPECIALTIES AND RELATED FIELDS: Family practice, nutrition, pediatrics

DEFINITION: A form of malnutrition caused by inadequate protein intake.

CAUSES AND SYMPTOMS

Kwashiorkor occurs most commonly in areas of famine, limited food supply, and low levels of education, which can lead to inadequate knowledge of diet and appropriate dietary intakes. Early symptoms are general and include fatigue, irritability, and lethargy. As protein deprivation continues, symptoms include failure to gain weight and linear growth. Other progressed symptoms include apathy, decreased muscle mass, edema, a large protuberant belly (resulting from decreased albumin in the blood), diarrhea, and dermatitis. Skin may lose pigment where it has peeled away or darken where it has been irritated or traumatized. Hair may become thin and brittle and may change color, becoming lighter or reddish. As a result of immune system damage, patients may suffer from increased numbers of infections and increased severity of what normally might be mild infections. In the final stages, shock and/or coma usually precede death.

TREATMENT AND THERAPY

A physical examination may show an enlarged liver and generalized edema. Treatment varies depending on the degree of malnutrition. Patients in shock will require immediate treatment. Often, calories are given first in the form of carbohydrates, simple sugars, and fats. Proteins are started after other caloric sources have provided increased energy. Vitamin and mineral supplements are essential. Many children will have developed intolerance to milk lactose (sugar intolerance) and will need to be supplemented with lactase (an enzyme) if they are to benefit from milk products. Adequate diet with appropriate amounts of carbohydrates, fat, and protein will prevent kwashiorkor.

PERSPECTIVE AND PROSPECTS

Kwashiorkor means "deposed child" in one African dialect, referring to a child "deposed" from the mother's

---

INFORMATION ON KWASHIORKOR

CAUSES: Protein deprivation

SYMPTOMS: Fatigue, irritability, lethargy, poor growth, apathy, edema, decreased muscle mass, large belly, diarrhea, dermatitis, loss of skin pigmentation, changes in color and texture of hair, infections; may progress to shock, coma, and death

DURATION: Progressive if untreated

TREATMENTS: Depends on degree of malnutrition; may include treatment for shock and increased calorie intake (first as carbohydrates, simple sugars, and fats, then proteins)

breast by a newborn sibling. Kwashiorkor is found largely in tropical and subtropical regions where the diet is high in starch (such as cereal grains or plantains) and low in protein. The incidence of kwashiorkor in children in the United States is extremely low, and only rare, isolated cases are seen. Treatment early in the course of kwashiorkor generally produces positive results. Treatment in later stages will improve a child's general health, but the child may be left with permanent physical ailments and intellectual disabilities. With delayed or no treatment, the condition is fatal.

—Jason A. Hubbart, M.S.

See also Edema; Food biochemistry; Malnutrition; Nutrition.

FOR FURTHER INFORMATION:

American Academy of Pediatrics. Committee on Nutrition. *Pediatric Nutrition Handbook*. Edited by Ronald E. Kleinman. 4th ed. Elk Grove Village, Ill.: Author, 1998.

Champakam, S., S. G. Srikantia, and C. Gopalan. "Kwashiorkor and Mental Development." *American Journal of Clinical Nutrition* 21 (1968): 844.

Golden, M. H. N. "Severe Malnutrition." In *Oxford Textbook of Medicine*, edited by D. J. Weatherall, J. G. G. Ledingham, and D. A. Warrell. 3d ed. New York: Oxford University Press, 1996.

KYPHOSIS

DISEASE/DISORDER

ALSO KNOWN AS: Dowager's hump
ANATOMY OR SYSTEM AFFECTED: Back, bones
SPECIALTIES AND RELATED FIELDS: Orthopedics
DEFINITION: A marked increase of the normal curvature of the thoracic vertebrae or upper back, sometimes referred to as dowager's hump because of its prevalence in elderly women.

CAUSES AND SYMPTOMS

Patients with kyphosis appear to be looking down with their shoulders markedly bent forward. They are unable to straighten their backs, their body height is reduced, and their arms therefore appear to be disproportionately long. The increased curvature of the thoracic vertebrae tilts the head forward, and the patient has to raise her head and hyperextend her neck in order to look forward. This posture increases the strain on the neck muscles and leads to discomfort in the neck, shoulders, and upper back. It limits the field of vision and increases the patient's chances of tripping over an object not directly

---

INFORMATION ON KYPHOSIS

CAUSES: Osteoporosis, tumors, infection
SYMPTOMS: Inability to straighten one's back, reduced body height, appearance of disproportionately long arms, strain on neck muscles leading to discomfort, pain
DURATION: Chronic
TREATMENTS: Hormone therapy, drug therapy (*e.g.*, Fosamax, teriparatide)

---

in the line of vision. It also shifts forward the body's center of gravity and increases the chances of falling.

In severe cases, kyphosis limits chest expansion during breathing. As a result, less air gets into the lungs, which become underventilated and prone to infections. Pneumonia is a common cause of death in these patients. In very severe cases, the curvature of the thoracic vertebrae is so pronounced that the lower ribs lie over the pelvic cavity. Patients with severe kyphosis are not able to lie flat on their backs, and many spend most of their time sitting up in a chair or in bed, propped by a number of pillows. Unless the patient changes positions frequently, the pressure exerted by the vertebrae on the skin and subcutaneous tissue may precipitate pressure sores (bed sores) on the upper back. Pressure sores may also develop on the buttocks. The sores often become infected, and the infection may spread to the blood, leading to septicemia and death.

The most common cause of kyphosis is osteoporosis, a disease in which the bone mass is reduced. As a result, the bones become mechanically weak and are unable to sustain the pressure of the body weight. The vertebrae gradually become wedged and partially collapsed, more so in the front (anteriorly) than in the back (posteriorly), thus increasing the forward curvature of the thoracic vertebrae. Sometimes, the compression of a vertebra is associated with sudden, very severe, and incapacitating pain that is usually relieved spontaneously after about four weeks. In most cases, however, the compression is a gradual process associated with slowly worsening back discomfort. The discomfort is caused by the strain imposed on the muscles on either side of the vertebrae. In rare instances, the nerves exiting the spinal cord become trapped by the wedged or collapsed vertebrae, and the patient experiences severe pain that tends to radiate to the area supplied by the entrapped nerve.

Less common causes of kyphosis include the compression of a vertebra as a result of tumors or infections.

In these cases, the angulation of the thoracic curvature is very prominent.

TREATMENT AND THERAPY

The availability of medications to treat and prevent osteoporosis should reduce significantly the prevalence of both that disease and kyphosis.

—*Ronald C. Hamdy, M.D.*

See also Bone disorders; Bones and the skeleton; Osteoporosis; Pneumonia; Safety issues for the elderly; Spinal cord disorders; Spine, vertebrae, and disks.

FOR FURTHER INFORMATION:

Byyny, Richard, and Leonard Speroff. *A Clinical Guide for the Care of Older Women*. 2d ed. Baltimore: Williams & Wilkins, 1996.

Currey, John D. *Bones: Structures and Mechanics*. Princeton, N.J.: Princeton University Press, 2002.

Heaney, Robert P. "Osteoporosis." In *Nutrition in Women's Health*, edited by Debra A. Krummel and Penny M. Kris-Etherton. Gaithersburg, Md.: Aspen, 1996.

Hodgson, Stephen F., ed. *Mayo Clinic on Osteoporosis: Keeping Bones Healthy and Strong and Reducing the Risk of Fractures*. Rochester, Minn.: Mayo Clinic, 2003.

Meredith, C. M. "Exercise in the Prevention of Osteoporosis." In *Nutrition of the Elderly*, edited by Hamish Munro and Gunter Schlierf. Nestle's Nutrition Workshop Series 29. New York: Raven Press, 1992.

Nelson, Miriam E., and Sarah Wernick. *Strong Women, Strong Bones: Everything You Need to Know to Prevent, Treat, and Beat Osteoporosis*. New York: G. P. Putnam, 2001.

Van De Graaff, Kent M., and Stuart Ira Fox. *Concepts of Human Anatomy and Physiology*. 5th ed. Dubuque, Iowa: Wm. C. Brown, 2000.

LABORATORY TESTS

PROCEDURES

ANATOMY OR SYSTEM AFFECTED: Blood, cells

SPECIALTIES AND RELATED FIELDS: Bacteriology, cytology, endocrinology, epidemiology, forensic medicine, genetics, hematology, histology, immunology, microbiology, oncology, pathology, pharmacology, serology, toxicology, virology

DEFINITION: The collection and analysis of body fluids such as blood and urine in order to establish a diagnosis or to monitor a treatment regimen.

KEY TERMS:

antibody: a protein produced in the body by the immune system that recognizes and binds selectively to foreign material (antigens) to facilitate their elimination; antibodies can be cultivated in animals or by artificial means in the laboratory and chemically altered for use as reagents in immunoassays

clinical chemistry: a chemistry specialty which deals with an analysis of the chemical components of body fluids

clinical laboratory: a general term for those areas of a medical facility where analyses of body fluids are performed

clinical microbiology: the scientific discipline involving the study of microscopic organisms (such as bacteria, fungi, and viruses) that cause disease

coagulation: the process of blood clotting, a very complicated process that can be affected by many disease states; the clotting process is inhibited for specimen collection purposes using substances called anticoagulants

hematology: the medical specialty dealing with the detection and diagnosis of blood-related diseases

immunoassay: the use of antibody-antigen recognition as the basis of a medically useful method of detecting and measuring a substance in body fluids

pathology: the medical specialty that deals with the structural and biochemical changes that are produced by disease

INDICATIONS AND PROCEDURES

Clinical laboratory testing is a vital element in diagnosis. After physical examination and the taking of the patient's medical history, the physician will often request that specific tests be performed on blood, urine, or other body fluids. Appropriate specimens are collected and forwarded to the laboratory for specimen processing.

Blood is the most common specimen submitted for testing in the clinical laboratory. In a hospital or large referral laboratory, there may be special personnel, called phlebotomists, employed to collect blood. In a small office laboratory, blood may be collected by the attending physician or nurse. Blood is collected in a syringe or in special tubes which may contain anticoagulants.

Urine is the next most common laboratory specimen and is collected as a result of a single void (random urine specimen) or for a time period of twenty-four hours or more. In the latter case, the collection container may also contain substances that act as a preservative. If a long-term urine specimen is necessary, it is very important for the patient to follow the directions regarding collection. Failure to follow these directions can lead to erroneous laboratory results.

Less commonly collected specimens include cerebrospinal fluid, gastric (stomach) fluid, and amniotic fluid. Cerebrospinal fluid is usually collected by a physician by direct sampling with a needle (lumbar puncture, or spinal tap). Gastric fluid is obtained by the insertion of a gastric collection tube. Amniotic fluid is collected by an obstetrician in the process called amniocentesis, in which a sample of the fluid surrounding the fetus is removed by the insertion of a needle through the mother's abdomen. Frequently, laboratory tests are also ordered on infectious material associated with a wound or surgical incision.

A major aspect of specimen collection is ensuring that the sample is correctly labeled and that no mix-up of specimens has occurred. Part of this process may involve checking identification armbands or asking patients or nursing staff to confirm identification. While this procedure may be exasperating to the patient or nursing personnel, it is a necessary part of detecting errors.

Immediately after the specimen is received in the laboratory, documentation of time of receipt and the tests requested is made, which is referred to as logging in the specimen. Each sample receives a special code called an accession number. The test performance and results are tracked with this number, since multiple specimens can be received on a single patient in a given day. This process is usually computerized and may utilize bar code labeling in a process very similar to that used for automatic cash-register pricing of grocery items.

In large hospital or referral laboratories, the processing center is responsible for distributing the sample to the laboratory sections, where various tests are performed. Since each test requires a specific amount of sample, specimen processing also involves determin-

IN THE NEWS: IN-HOME MEDICAL TESTING

In-home health testing has become increasingly popular as a result of its convenience, privacy, and affordability. Home tests can enable the consumer to determine the potential risk for developing a health problem even when no immediate signs or symptoms exist, or they can enable the consumer to follow a specific medical condition more accurately. Several home tests are available for over-the-counter purchase, including those that test for cholesterol levels, drugs of abuse, fecal occult blood, glucose levels, hepatitis C, human immunodeficiency virus (HIV), ovulation timing, pregnancy, prothrombin time screening, and vaginal pH. Home test kits should not be used as stand-alone measures to determine one's health care, but rather the results should be used in conjunction with proper medical advice in order to confirm the test results.

Most reports state that the test kits approved by the Food and Drug Administration (FDA) are either "about as accurate" or "fairly accurate," when compared to those that a doctor would use, provided that the instructions are carefully followed. The consumer should understand that no test is 100 percent accurate; test accuracy is improved when the consumer can read, understand, and follow the directions for test administration carefully. A home test kit will require accurate timing, specific collection materials, and typically a body fluid sample. Failure to comply with any of these factors could result in an inaccurate reading. If a product is not approved by the FDA, then the test's safety and efficacy is in question. Internet shopping for diagnostic test kits can be particularly misleading, since not all test kits available for purchase in this fashion are FDA-approved and some are illegal to sell over the Internet.

A search of the Clinical Laboratory Improvement Amendments (CLIA) database will inform the consumer if a home test has FDA approval. In order to use this search engine, the consumer must know if the test is considered a "test kit" (a consumer takes a sample, performs the test, and analyzes it, all on one's own) or a "collection kit" (a consumer takes a sample but sends it out to a laboratory for analysis). Collection kits are not currently listed on the CLIA database, although one can contact the FDA directly to find out if a kit is FDA-approved. The FDA maintains another database called Manufacturer and User Facility Device Experience (MAUDE), which lists reports on problems with kits and testing devices. The *Consumer Reports* magazine and Web site can also provide the consumer with additional product comparison information for a handful of home tests.

—*Bonita L. Marks, Ph.D.*

whole blood specimen is separated into cellular and liquid components by centrifugation. The sample is spun rapidly so that the force of the spin sediments the cells, with the serum or plasma layer on top.

Once the specimen is distributed to the pertinent laboratory sections, testing is done using a variety of analytical techniques. The testing methodology is almost as varied as the types of analyses requested. A few general statements, however, are applicable. Automation is the guiding force behind laboratory test methodology development. Routinely ordered tests are done with instruments specifically designed to perform a group or panel of tests, rather than each test being performed individually by a technologist using manual chemistry methods. Automation coupled with computerization has greatly increased laboratory efficiency, decreased turnaround time (the time required for a test to be performed and results to be reported to the physician), eliminated human errors, and allowed more tests to be performed on smaller test sample material. The latter advantage is particularly important for pediatric specimens, in which sample size is usually an important consideration. Automation also eliminates much of the technologist's contact with the specimen, considerably reducing the risk of spreading infectious diseases.

Each section of the laboratory is responsible for a specific set of tests. The chemistry section performs chemical analyses of body fluids. Panels of tests related to kidney, heart, and liver function are also done. In addition, tests to measure amounts of therapeutic drugs, hormones, blood proteins, and cancer-related proteins are accom-

ing that the correct amount of fluid has been collected and reserved for proper performance of the test.

For blood specimens, many laboratory determinations are made regarding plasma, or serum, which is the liquid component of blood that contains no cells. The

plished with immunoassay techniques. The development of antibody-related techniques has revolutionized testing in all areas of the clinical laboratory. The ability to customize antibody production and adapt it to specific analytical requirements has allowed the continual development of new tests and methodologies.

The hematology section is responsible for monitoring the level of blood cells and clotting factors. Other specialized tests to diagnose cancer of the blood cells may also be done. Blood typing and donor testing are technically hematology-related tests, but they are usually reserved for a separate section designated as blood bank or transfusion services. Transfusion service is a specialty in its own right and is almost always reserved for hospital-associated laboratories.

Microbiology is the section where body fluids are checked for infectious microorganisms. Once an organism is identified, the section can also determine which antibiotics may be useful for treatment by performing antibiotic susceptibility tests.

As the laboratory tests are performed, the results are recorded and reported to the physician. Computerization has permitted the transfer of patient results directly from the instrument performing the test to the patient's file, eliminating many tedious and error-prone clerical functions.

For hospital and reference laboratories, a laboratory director—either a physician (usually a pathologist) who specialized in laboratory medicine or a scientist with doctoral level training in a laboratory specialty—monitors the performance of the laboratory, helps physicians with the interpretation of ambiguous or complex laboratory results, and provides guidance on the introduction of new tests or instrumentation. Most laboratories also have a section supervisor or administrator who is an experienced medical technologist to oversee the daily laboratory routine.

In the United States, hospital and reference laboratories are inspected periodically by federal and state government agencies as well as professional medical societies to check the quality of the work performed. The most commonly used proficiency testing program is that administered by the College of American Pathology (CAP), which also sponsors a program of peer inspection of laboratories. Many state and federal agencies will accept CAP approval of a laboratory as a substitute for a detailed inspection by its own agency.

USES AND COMPLICATIONS

Because of the variety of laboratory testing, it is im-

practical to cover its applications in depth in a brief review. Instead, a few illustrative tests which are performed often or which are associated with familiar disorders will be presented. The most frequently ordered laboratory tests are serum glucose tests, serum electrolyte (salt) level measurements, and complete blood count (CBC) tests.

The maintenance of blood glucose (sugar) levels is essential for body activity and brain function. The laboratory measurement of blood glucose is one of the oldest known procedures performed in the clinical laboratory. It is part of the diagnostic procedures used to monitor and test for diabetes mellitus. Glucose and electrolyte testing are performed in the chemistry section of the laboratory, while a CBC takes place in hematology. Certain levels of electrolytes—sodium, chloride, potassium, and calcium—are needed for proper cardiac function. An abnormal level of these salts could also indicate possible hormonal or kidney malfunction. The CBC is a measure of the cell populations that carry oxygen (red blood cells), fight infection or invasion by foreign substances (white blood cells), and activate the blood-clotting mechanism (platelets). The white cell population is elevated in infections but also in cases of leukemia (malignant growth of a white cell population). More specialized testing is needed when leukemia is suspected. An instrument called a flow cytometer can be used to count and detect subtypes of white cells. These data, along with a pathologist's microscopic examination of a blood smear and the results of clinical examination, are used to arrive at a diagnosis of the specific type of leukemia present. The identification of the cell population causing the cancer is important for determining treatment and prognosis.

A deficiency of red cells or their oxygen-carrying hemoglobin molecule is called anemia. It can be caused by iron deficiency and other impairments of red cell production, chronic bleeding, or accelerated red cell destruction (hemolysis). Each of the causes must be either confirmed or ruled out through additional testing or by clinical examination.

Platelet deficiency is a major cause of clotting disorders, although many other causes of bleeding disorders exist. The specific defect can be determined by measuring the clotting time and by using special immunoassays to measure clotting substances in the blood.

Many hormonal (endocrine) disorders can be diagnosed through laboratory testing. For example, the thyroid, the regulator gland for body metabolism, can produce a variety of symptoms when it is not functioning properly. Thyroid testing is the most common endocrine-related laboratory procedure requested by physicians. The blood levels of thyroid hormone and of the pituitary factor that stimulates the thyroid gland are measured in the laboratory using immunoassay methods. These types of assays can also be used to monitor other hormones involved in fertility, growth, and the function of the adrenal gland (the gland that helps maintain sugar metabolism and electrolyte balance).

Immunoassay methodology has also permitted the routine laboratory testing of therapeutic drugs as well as of drugs of abuse. In the past, the technology for analyzing drugs in biological fluids involved expensive, labor-intensive techniques that were impractical for routine laboratory use. With the introduction of immunologically based testing for drugs, however, it became possible to monitor patients on antibiotics, immunosuppressive agents, cardiac drugs, and antiseizure medication. Testing has been automated so that these drug levels can be performed as routine laboratory procedures. Assay results can be used to establish an individual dosage schedule so that dosage is maintained in the therapeutic range and does not exceed the concentration threshold leading to toxic effects or decline to values too low to achieve adequate treatment (subtherapeutic levels).

A continuing research effort is directed toward developing specific diagnostic cancer tests. These tests could be used to screen patients for tumors in order to detect them early, when therapy would be most effective. Substances that appear in body fluids coincident with the growth of tumors are referred to as tumor markers. The ideal tumor marker would appear only in patients afflicted with a specific type of cancer. Its concentration would reflect the size of the tumor as well as the presence of metastasis, in which tumor cells migrate from the initial cancer site to other sites in the body.

The ideal tumor marker has not yet been discovered. Most have not been specific or sensitive enough to use as a screening tool for detecting tumors, although they have been useful for monitoring the effects of therapy. One example of a useful marker is prostate-specific antigen (PSA). The level of this protein in serum is very low when the prostate gland is normal. When prostate cancer is present, however, the serum level, as measured by immunoassay, is elevated. The test can also be used for screening, provided that any positive result is confirmed by clinical examination. It is also used following prostate surgery or radiation therapy in order to determine the completeness of tumor removal. Con-

tinually high or rising levels of PSA in the serum following treatment indicate that residual tumor is still present.

In the microbiology department, the culturing of body fluids and antibiotic susceptibility studies allow the selection of the most appropriate antibiotic for treatment. The course and duration of treatment can then be followed in the chemistry laboratory using the therapeutic drug monitoring techniques discussed above. When an infection is suspected, body fluids are cultured or incubated with media selected to grow only specific microorganisms. Antibiotic susceptibility studies are performed by culturing the organism with various antibiotics until growth is arrested. Many strains of bacteria and other microorganisms will become resistant to an antibiotic which had proven effective previously, and patients who are allergic to some antibiotics may need to be treated with an alternative regimen.

The detection and identification of viruses has become a subspecialty in microbiology with distinctly different culturing techniques. Newer immunoassay methods and other biotechnologically based methods have made virus diagnosis easier. Acquired immunodeficiency syndrome (AIDS) testing is a prime example of the application of immunoassay techniques to virology testing. A detection technique which required growth of the human immunodeficiency virus (HIV) in the laboratory would be extraordinarily difficult and tedious. It would also be prohibitively expensive and time-consuming to screen large populations such as blood donors and high-risk groups. Instead, laboratory screening for HIV utilizes an automated immunoassay technique based on the detection of patient antibodies to virus-specific antigens. Although this test is very specific, the possibility of false positives is greatly minimized by confirming all positive screening results with another antibody test called a Western blot. In this test, a serum sample from a suspected HIV-positive patient is applied to a membrane impregnated with virus proteins. The virus proteins are localized at a characteristic position determined by their migration rate when the membrane coated with virus proteins is subjected to an electric field in a process called protein electrophoresis. After the membrane has been treated with patient serum and color development reagents, the presence in the patient sample of an antibody to one or more of these proteins is revealed as a colored stripe on the membrane. A combination of the two tests is a cost-efficient and extremely accurate procedure to confirm a suspected diagnosis of HIV infection.

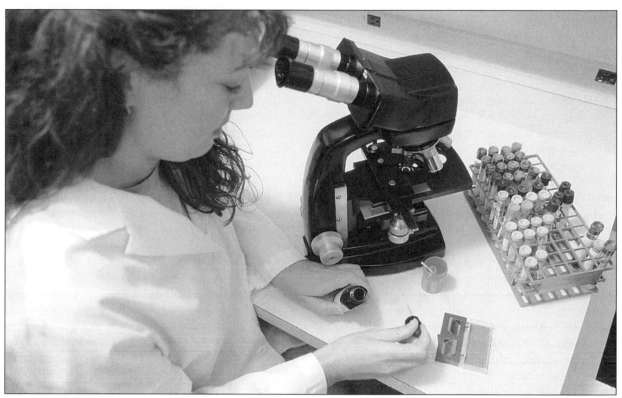

Laboratory tests are vital in the diagnosis of disease. A scientist examines samples with a microscope. (PhotoDisc)

PERSPECTIVE AND PROSPECTS

According to a study of the history of the clinical laboratory by J. Büttner, the concept of the modern hospital laboratory was first documented in 1791 when French physician and chemist Antoine-François de Fourcroy wrote that in hospitals "a chemical laboratory should be set up not far away from a ward having twenty or thirty beds." Büttner asserts that the two suppositions necessary for the creation of these laboratories were the idea that the results of laboratory examinations can be used as "chemical signs" in medical diagnosis and a new concept of disease which was the result of the "birth of the clinic" at the end of the eighteenth century.

During this phase of laboratory development, investigations were performed at patients' bedsides by physicians themselves. In the period from 1840 to 1855, clinical laboratories were established as operations distinct from hospitals and clinics. Most of these laboratories were developed in German-speaking countries and staffed by scientists who performed tests for the hospitals and taught medical students physiological chemistry. From 1855 onward, the concept of the clinical laboratory spread rapidly, with clinicians assuming directorship roles. The laboratory ultimately serving as

a model for clinical laboratories in the United States was established by the renowned pathologist Rudolf Virchow at Berlin University. As the chair for pathological anatomy, he set up a "chemical department" within the institute for pathology in 1856. This laboratory represented a center of clinical chemistry research and established the clinical laboratory as integral to pathology.

Laboratories have evolved as essential but distinctly separate specialties of medical services. Although there is little or no participation in the analytical process by the physicians ordering the tests, a major part of a physician's diagnostic skill is knowing which tests to order as a supplement to examination and medical history. Laboratory tests cost money and time and may be useless in the diagnostic process if not ordered in a judicious fashion. The old medical admonishment to "treat the patient, not the laboratory result" is still an appropriate consideration. Moreover, responsibility for the correct interpretation of the results lies with the attending physician, who has access to all the pertinent patient data.

Laboratory results are usually interpreted with the help of a reference range. Reference ranges ideally represent laboratory values characteristic of a sample population which is free of known disease. If the results lie within this range, however, the laboratory result cannot always be assumed to rule out a specific diagnosis. Since considerable biological variation exists for most laboratory values, diseased individuals can sometimes yield test values in the normal range and, conversely, healthy individuals can occasionally have low or elevated values.

In order to verify a diagnosis, all laboratory results and clinical impressions should complement one another. The detection of blood-clotting deficiencies by the hematology department could be related to a poorly functioning liver, which will also be reflected in changes in enzymes and blood proteins measured in the chemistry laboratory. Cardiac disorders are diagnosed not only by examining an electrocardiograph (EKG or ECG) but also by measuring the levels of specific cardiac-related enzymes which rise to abnormally high levels when cardiac blood supply is diminished (such as with myocardial infarction, or heart attack). In summary, the clinical laboratory provides a valuable tool for physicians, but it should never displace clinical examination and medical history as methods of determining the final diagnosis.

—*David J. Wells, Jr., Ph.D.*

See also Amniocentesis; Bacteriology; Biopsy; Blood and blood disorders; Blood testing; Breast biopsy; Cells; Cytology; Cytopathology; DNA and RNA; Endometrial biopsy; Forensic pathology; Genetic engineering; Genetics and inheritance; Gram staining; Hematology; Hematology, pediatric; Histology; Hormones; Karyotyping; Microbiology; Microscopy; Pathology; Screening; Serology; Toxicology; Urinalysis.

FOR FURTHER INFORMATION:

Bennington, James L., ed. *Saunders Dictionary and Encyclopedia of Laboratory Medicine and Technology.* Philadelphia: W. B. Saunders, 1984. An excellent reference to laboratory vocabulary and terminology. Gives detailed information about complicated procedures and topics, rather than a simple dictionary definition.

Cavanaugh, Bonita Morrow. *Nurse's Manual of Laboratory and Diagnostic Tests.* 4th ed. Philadelphia: F. A. Davis, 2003. Provides information on hundreds of laboratory and diagnostic tests, with each test presented in two distinct, cross-referenced sections: "Background Information" sections provide a complete description of each test and its purposes; "Clinical Application Data" sections focus on the information nurses most commonly need while caring for clients.

Griffith, H. Winter. *Complete Guide to Symptoms, Illness and Surgery.* Rev. ed. New York: Berkley, 2000. Covers more than five hundred diseases and disorders and includes information about causes and risk factors, preventive techniques, and diagnostic tests.

Henry, John B., ed. *Clinical Diagnosis and Management by Laboratory Methods.* 20th ed. Philadelphia: W. B. Saunders, 2001. The classic text on the clinical laboratory. Multiple authors cover all aspects of laboratory operations, including management and administration. The most recent edition should be consulted.

Pagana, Kathleen Deska, and Timothy James Pagana. *Mosby's Diagnostic and Laboratory Test Reference.* 6th ed. New York: Elsevier, 2002. A clinical handbook that gives alphabetically organized laboratory and diagnostic tests for easy reference. Each listing includes such things as alternate or abbreviated test names, type of test, normal findings, possible critical values, test explanation and related physiology, and potential complications.

Price, Christopher P., and David J. Newman, eds. *Principles and Practice of Immunoassay.* 2d ed. New York: Stockton Press, 1997. This work covers all aspects of immunoassays, including assay development, laboratory quality assurance, and test methodology.

Tietz, Norbert W. *Clinical Guide to Laboratory Tests.* 4th ed. Philadelphia: W. B. Saunders, 2001. A paperback condensation of the vital information needed for the interpretation of clinical laboratory tests. Tests are arranged alphabetically in tabular form for easy reference.

LACERATION REPAIR

PROCEDURE

ANATOMY OR SYSTEM AFFECTED: Skin

SPECIALTIES AND RELATED FIELDS: Emergency medicine, general surgery, plastic surgery

DEFINITION: The closure of an irregular skin wound.

INDICATIONS AND PROCEDURES

A laceration is a jagged, torn, mangled, or ragged wound. This type of wound is most commonly encountered in the skin, although any tissue may be lacerated. Lacerations are caused by sharp objects such as a piece of metal, glass, or a stick, or they may occur in accidents involving machinery or animals.

The first priority in laceration repair is to stop bleeding, thereby minimizing blood loss. This is usually accomplished by pressure either directly on the wound or on the injured blood vessel nearest the injury site.

The second priority with a laceration is to clean the wound, which involves the removal of any foreign material or debris. With penetrating injuries, this cleaning must be done carefully lest the removal of the object initiate bleeding. Tissue that has been destroyed beyond the body's ability to repair it must also be removed; this process is called debridement. Devitalized tissue is removed to prevent infection. The wound site is then cleaned through irrigation with saline and a disinfectant, usually a mild soap or a chemical.

Lacerations may then be treated for bacterial or other pathogenic contamination. Aqueous solutions containing an antibiotic are used with most wounds. If contamination with other pathogens is suspected, appropriate agents are used to rinse the wound. Antibiotic powders may be employed in field conditions, although this form of treatment is unusual in a hospital setting. Other than soap and water, there is no special treatment for viral contamination.

Closure of the wound is then completed. The edges are brought together and may be held in place with forceps. Sutures, or stitches, are inserted to hold the edges together while the tissue heals. On skin surfaces, these sutures are usually nonabsorbable and are later removed. The amount of time that sutures are kept in place varies with the location of the wound and the age of the patient: Mucous membranes heal more quickly than the palm, for example, and children's skin heals more rapidly than that of adults. Removable sutures are made of nylon or a similar material. Sutures that are used beneath the skin cannot be removed and are made of material that will break down within the body. Wound closure may also be accomplished with wire, staples, or adhesive tape. These materials have some advantages—durability (wire), ease of placement (staples), and minimal pain (tape)—and disadvantages—potential contamination (wire) and premature, accidental removal (tape). Lacerations should be rechecked by a physician when sutures or other means of wound closure are removed.

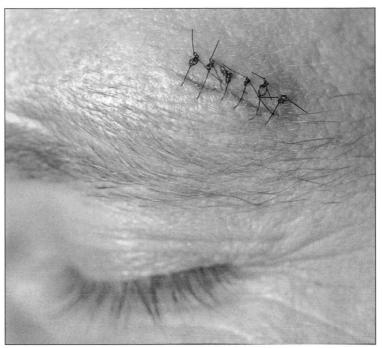

Stitches or sutures may be required to hold together the edges of lacerations that are large, deep, or ragged. (PhotoDisc)

USES AND COMPLICATIONS

The techniques of laceration repair are used on all parts of the body where such wounds occur. Plastic surgery may be required to improve the appearance of the repaired tissue and to reduce scars when the patient believes that cosmetic results are an issue. In addition to scarring, other complications that may be associated with the repair of lacerations include infection and tetanus. All these problems can be minimized through good surgical techniques, the use of antibiotics, and careful postoperative care. The repair of lacerations to exposed facial skin is especially important. Careful technique minimizes scarring, as do some new methods of wound closure.

—*L. Fleming Fallon, Jr., M.D., Ph.D., M.P.H.*

See also Bleeding; Emergency medicine; Grafts and grafting; Healing; Plastic surgery; Skin; Wounds.

FOR FURTHER INFORMATION:

Crosby, Lynn A., and David G. Lewallen, eds. *Emergency Care and Transportation of the Sick and Injured.* 8th ed. Rosemont, Ill.: American Academy of Orthopaedic Surgeons, 2002.

Greenfield, Lazar J., et al. *Surgery: Scientific Principles and Practice.* 3d ed. Philadelphia: Lippincott Williams & Wilkins, 2001.

Handal, Kathleen A. *The American Red Cross First Aid and Safety Handbook*. Boston: Little, Brown, 1992.

Thygerson, Alton L. *First Aid and Emergency Care Workbook*. Boston: Jones and Bartlett, 1987.

Weedon, David. *Skin Pathology*. 2d ed. New York: Harcourt, 2002.

LACTOSE INTOLERANCE
DISEASE/DISORDER

ANATOMY OR SYSTEM AFFECTED: Gastrointestinal system, intestines, stomach

SPECIALTIES AND RELATED FIELDS: Gastroenterology, nutrition

DEFINITION: Lactose intolerance is an inability to break down and absorb milk sugar, known as lactose, resulting in stomach pain, gas, and diarrhea if lactose is consumed.

CAUSES AND SYMPTOMS

Lactose is a complex sugar commonly found in dairy products. It is composed of two simple sugars, glucose and galactose. In babies and young children, a gene produces an enzyme called lactase that breaks down lactose into its two component sugars, which are then absorbed into the bloodstream through the intestinal wall. In many people, sometime after early childhood, the lactase gene is "turned off." It no longer synthesizes lactase, which prevents the digestion and absorption of lactose.

Normal bacterial inhabitants of the intestines synthesize lactase and break down the lactose molecules, producing large quantities of gas as a by-product. This can lead to cramping for the lactose-intolerant individual. The presence of lactose in the large intestine causes excessive amounts of water to move into the intestine, which can lead to diarrhea. Symptoms subside one to two days after the last lactose-containing food has been consumed.

TREATMENT AND THERAPY

Lactose intolerance can often be misdiagnosed as a host of gastrointestinal disorders, largely as a result of the commonness of its major symptoms, cramps and diarrhea. Typically, a dietary history must be kept. Patients with lactose intolerance will note an association between their symptoms and the consumption of milk products containing lactose. After elimination of these products from the diet, symptoms should not recur.

There is no treatment for lactose intolerance; prevention of symptoms is the general course of action. Avoidance of foods that contain lactose—including milk, ice cream, and cheese—is usually the best recourse. For those who wish to indulge in these products, over-the-counter lactase pills are available; their use usually prevents symptoms of the disorder.

PERSPECTIVE AND PROSPECTS

The vast majority of the world's population is lactose intolerant, yet this disorder was not recognized in the United States until the latter third of the twentieth century. Today, lactase supplements are available to help prevent symptoms for lactose-intolerant people who choose to consume dairy products. Alternatively, more and more dairy products are being manufactured as lactose-free; they can be consumed safely by the lactose-intolerant population.

—*Karen E. Kalumuck, Ph.D.*

See also Acid reflux disease; Diarrhea and dysentery; Digestion; Enzymes; Gastroenterology; Gastroenterology, pediatric; Gastrointestinal disorders; Gastrointestinal system; Irritable bowel syndrome (IBS); Nutrition.

FOR FURTHER INFORMATION:

Dobler, Merri Lou. *Lactose Intolerance Nutrition Guide*. Chicago: American Dietetic Association, 2002.

Gracey, Michael, ed. *Diarrhea*. Boca Raton, Fla.: CRC Press, 1991.

Greenberger, Norton J. *Gastrointestinal Disorders: A Pathophysiologic Approach*. 4th ed. Chicago: Year Book Medical, 1989.

Janowitz, Henry D. *Your Gut Feelings: A Complete Guide to Living Better with Intestinal Problems*. Rev. ed. New York: Oxford University Press, 1994.

Lactose.co.uk. http://www.lactose.co.uk/.

Parker, James N., and Philip M. Parker, eds. *The Official Patient's Sourcebook on Lactose Intolerance*. San Diego, Calif.: Icon Health, 2002.

Peikin, Steven R. *Gastrointestinal Health*. Rev. ed. New York: HarperCollins, 1999.

LAMINECTOMY AND SPINAL FUSION
PROCEDURES

ANATOMY OR SYSTEM AFFECTED: Back, bones, spine

SPECIALTIES AND RELATED FIELDS: General surgery, orthopedics

DEFINITION: Surgical procedures that join two or more vertebrae, the arching bones that make up the spine.

INDICATIONS AND PROCEDURES

Laminectomies, which are designed to relieve pressure on the spinal cord, are often performed as the initial surgery in cases of extreme back pain caused by the compression of the spinal canal. An incision is made in the patient's back to expose the laminae, the flattened portions of the vertebral arch, and one or more adjacent laminae are chipped away. On occasion, several laminae are excised.

In such cases, spinal fusion, which involves the immobilization of the spine with steel rods or bone grafts, is indicated. Spinal fusion, like laminectomy a major surgery done under general anesthesia, is performed if X rays reveal unusual motion between adjacent vertebrae.

The causes of the severe back pain that usually precedes laminectomy or spinal fusion may be related to three conditions: osteoarthritis, which causes deterioration of the spinal joints; scoliosis caused by an injury or tumor that is destroying vertebrae; or spondylolisthesis, the dislocation of facet joints. In spinal fusion, when the damaged vertebrae are exposed, joint fusion is sometimes performed by using bone chips from the patient's pelvis. Following surgery, the vertebrae are held in place with plates or screws.

USES AND COMPLICATIONS

Both laminectomy and spinal fusion usually relieve the persistent back pain that has caused patients to seek treatment. Such surgery involves distinct risks, inasmuch as the spinal cord is exposed and there is often considerable blood loss. In the hands of a seasoned orthopedic surgeon, however, the risk is minimized.

Recovery from the surgery can be slow and often involves up to six weeks of confinement in bed. After this confinement, patients are usually required to wear a plaster cast until final vertebral fusion has occurred. This process can take half a year.

Fusion sometimes places an additional burden on the rest of the spinal column. In some cases, this pressure results in renewed back pain in other areas of the spine. Additional surgery may be indicated to control this pain.

—*R. Baird Shuman, Ph.D.*

See also Bone grafting; Bones and the skeleton; Disk removal; Fracture and dislocation; Grafts and grafting; Orthopedic surgery; Orthopedics; Orthopedics, pediatric; Osteoarthritis; Scoliosis; Spinal cord disorders; Spine, vertebrae, and disks.

FOR FURTHER INFORMATION:

Cotler, J. M., and H. B. Cotler, eds. *Spinal Fusion: Science and Technique.* New York: Springer-Verlag, 1990.

Frymoyer, John W., and Sam W. Wiesel, eds. *The Adult and Pediatric Spine: Principles, Practice, and Surgery.* Philadelphia: Lippincott Williams & Wilkins, 2004.

Hitchon, Patrick W., Setti Rengachary, and Vincent C. Traynelis. *Techniques in Spinal Fusion and Stabilization.* New York: Thieme Medical, 1994.

Naraghi, Fred F., et al., eds. *Spine Secrets.* New York: Elsevier, 2002.

Szpalski, Marek, et al., eds. *Instrumental Fusion of the Degenerative Lumbar Spine: State of the Art, Questions, and Controversies.* Philadelphia: Lippincott-Raven, 1996.

Watkins, Robert G., and John S. Collis, Jr. *Lumbar Discectomy and Laminectomy.* Rockville, Md.: Aspen, 1987.

Wetzel, F. Todd, et al. *Spine Surgery: A Practical Atlas.* Norwalk, Conn.: Appleton and Lange, 2002.

Yonenobu, K., K. Ono, and Y. Takemitsu, eds. *Lumbar Fusion and Stabilization.* New York: Springer, 1993.

LAPAROSCOPY

PROCEDURE

ANATOMY OR SYSTEM AFFECTED: Abdomen, gallbladder, gastrointestinal system, intestines, kidneys, reproductive system, urinary system, uterus

SPECIALTIES AND RELATED FIELDS: Endocrinology, gastroenterology, general surgery, gynecology

DEFINITION: The examination of the abdominal organs with a laparoscope, a fiber-optic tube which can also be used to perform surgery to correct several disease conditions.

KEY TERMS:

abdomen: the area of the body between the diaphragm and the pelvis; it contains the visceral organs

cholecystectomy: the surgical removal of the gallbladder

ectopic pregnancy: the development of a fertilized egg in a Fallopian tube instead of the uterus; can be fatal to the mother unless it is corrected surgically

endometriosis: a female reproductive disease in which cells from the uterine lining (the endometrium) grow outside the uterus, causing severe pain and infertility and sometimes the need for hysterectomy

Fallopian tubes: the two tubes through which eggs pass on the way from the ovaries to the uterus

general anesthesia: anesthesia that induces unconsciousness

implant: a section of endometrial tissue found outside
the uterus

local anesthesia: anesthesia that numbs the feeling in a
body part, administered by injection or direct application to the skin

INDICATIONS AND PROCEDURES

Laparoscopy is a surgical technique for examining the
abdominal organs and for treating surgically many diseases of these organs. The instrument used is called a
laparoscope. It is a flexible tube that contains fiber optics for visualization purposes and a channel through
which physicians can pass special surgical instruments
into the abdominal cavity.

Upon insertion of a laparoscope into the abdomen
through a small surgical incision (usually near the navel), physicians can observe the liver, kidneys, gallbladder, pancreas, spleen, and exterior aspects of the intestines in both sexes. Hence the technique is useful for
detecting cirrhosis of the liver, the presence of stones
and tumors, and many other diseases of the abdominal
organs. The female reproductive organs can also be examined in this manner.

Before laparoscopy can be carried out, the patient
must fast for at least twelve hours. The patient is given a
local or general anesthetic, depending on the purpose
of the procedure. In exploratory abdominal examinations, the instrument is inserted into the abdomen
through a small incision in the abdominal wall after local anesthesia has numbed it. Often, especially when
extensive surgery is anticipated, the procedure begins
after general anesthesia produces unconsciousness.
Upon the completion of exploration or surgery, the
laparoscope is withdrawn and the incision is closed.

Laparoscopic abdominal examination is often used
to detect endometriosis, the presence of endometrial
cells outside the uterus. This procedure begins with the
administration of local anesthesia when only exploration or biopsy is planned. General anesthesia is used
when the removal of implants (endometrial tissue) is
anticipated. The entry incision is made near the navel,
and the laparoscope is inserted. The fiber-optics system
is used to search the abdominal organs for implants.
Visibility of the abdominal organs is usually enhanced
by pumping in a harmless gas, such as carbon dioxide,
to distend the abdomen. After the confirmation of
endometriosis, surgical implant removal is carried out
immediately, unless the decision is made to institute

drug therapy instead. Full recovery from this surgery
requires only a day of postoperative bed rest and a week
of curtailing activities.

Laparoscopy can also be employed for female sterilization. The patient is given a general anesthetic. After
laparoscopic visualization of the Fallopian tubes in the
gas-distended abdomen is achieved, surgical instruments for tube cauterization or cutting are introduced
and the sterilization is carried out. The entire procedure
often requires only thirty minutes, which is one reason
for its popularity. In addition, patients can go home in a
few hours and have fully recovered after a day or two of
bed rest and seven to ten days of curtailing activities.

USES AND COMPLICATIONS

Common laparoscopic surgeries are cholecystectomy
(the removal of the gallbladder), the removal of gallstones and kidney stones, tumor resection, female sterilization by cutting or blocking the Fallopian tubes, the
treatment of endometriosis through the removal of implants from abdominal organs, and the removal of biopsy samples from abdominal organs. Traditional uses
of laparoscopy in female reproductive surgery are to

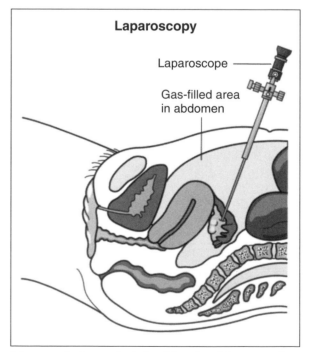

*Many surgical procedures involving the abdomen, such as
appendectomy or the removal of eggs from the ovaries for in
vitro fertilization, can be performed using laparoscopy. Gas
is pumped into the abdominal cavity, and a fiber-optic scope
and instruments are inserted through a small hole in the skin.*

identify and correct pelvic pain resulting from endometriosis, ectopic pregnancy, and pelvic tumors.

Laparoscopy has several advantages. There is rarely a need for patients on chronic drug therapy to discontinue medication before laparoscopy. In addition, the use of laparoscopy dramatically lowers surgical incision size, surgical trauma, length of hospital stay, and recovery time. Laparoscopy should be avoided, however, in cases of advanced abdominal wall cancer, severe respiratory or cardiovascular disease, or tuberculosis. Extreme obesity does not disqualify a patient from undergoing laparoscopy but makes the procedure much more difficult to perform.

As laparoscopic surgery has increased in scope, more procedures yield surgical tissues that are larger in size than the laparoscope channel (for example, the removal of gallbladders, gallstones, and ovaries). In many cases these organs and structures are cut into small pieces for removal. If potentially dangerous items are involved—such as malignancies that can spread on dissection—larger, more conventional incisions are often combined with laparoscopy.

PERSPECTIVE AND PROSPECTS

Since the 1970's, the uses of laparoscopy have constantly expanded. Once confined to the exploratory examination of the abdomen, the methodology has been applied to a large number of different types of surgery in addition to those already mentioned. Such versatility is attributable to the development of better laparoscopes, advanced instrumentation for diverse surgeries, and improved fiber-optic and video technologies.

As a consequence of these advances, many surgeons predict that most future abdominal surgery will be laparoscopic. The driving force for such innovation includes the public demand for quicker recovery times. In the United States, this desire is intensified by the requirements of insurance companies, employers, and the federal government for shorter hospital stays. Both changes are made possible by decreased severity of surgical trauma in laparoscopy when compared to traditional surgery, a result of the smaller incisions. The dramatic trend toward laparoscopy can be seen with cholecystectomies: Of those done in 1992, 70 percent were laparoscopic, compared to less than 1 percent in 1989.

—*Sanford S. Singer, Ph.D.*

See also Abdomen; Abdominal disorders; Appendectomy; Appendicitis; Biopsy; Cholecystectomy; Ectopic pregnancy; Endometriosis; Endoscopy; Gyne-

cology; Internal medicine; Sterilization; Stone removal; Stones; Tubal ligation; Tumor removal; Tumors.

FOR FURTHER INFORMATION:

Graber, John N., et al., eds. *Laparoscopic Abdominal Surgery.* New York: McGraw-Hill, 1993. A text for surgery residents and practicing surgeons wishing to gain an understanding of the theory and technique of laparoscopic surgery, written by experts in each area who were instrumental in the development of laparoscopic approaches. Abundantly illustrated with clear, detailed line drawings and color photographs.

Henderson, Lorraine, and Ros Wood. *Explaining Endometriosis.* 2d ed. St. Leonards, Australia: Allen and Unwin, 2001. Details possible causes, diagnosis, surgeries, and current treatment options for endometriosis.

Kapadia, Cyrus R., James M. Crawford, and Caroline Taylor. *An Atlas of Gastroenterology: A Guide to Diagnosis and Differential Diagnosis.* Boca Raton, Fla.: Pantheon, 2003. Provides a fully illustrated, nonspecialist understanding of myriad gastrointestinal diseases, including heartburn, dyspepsia, diarrhea, irritable bowel syndrome, and pancreatitis. Includes bibliographic references and index.

Reddick, Eddie Joe, ed. *An Atlas of Laparoscopic Surgery.* New York: Raven Press, 1993. Discusses such topics as cholecystectomy and peritoneoscopy. Includes an index.

Zollinger, Robert M., et al. *Zollinger's Atlas of Surgical Operations.* 8th ed. New York: McGraw-Hill, 2002. A comprehensive examination of surgery. Covers basic surgical anatomy and vascular, gynecologic, gastrointestinal, and miscellaneous abdominal procedures.

Zucker, Karl A. *Surgical Laparoscopy.* Philadelphia: Lippincott Williams & Wilkins, 2000. Discusses the gastrointestinal system, peritoneoscopy, and the methods of biliary tract surgery and endoscopic surgery.

LARYNGECTOMY

PROCEDURE

ANATOMY OR SYSTEM AFFECTED: Respiratory system, throat

SPECIALTIES AND RELATED FIELDS: General surgery, oncology, otorhinolaryngology

DEFINITION: The removal of all or part of the voice box, or larynx.

INDICATIONS AND PROCEDURES

Continued hoarseness and coughing can indicate laryngeal disorders. Polyps, which may be caused by excessive smoking or drinking, can form on the larynx. Children sometimes develop warts on it. Although these polyps and warts are generally benign, they should be removed and subjected to biopsy to preclude the presence of cancer.

Polyps, warts, and tumors are all detected quite easily with a laryngoscopic examination carried out by an otorhinolaryngologist with a mirror, an endoscope (a flexible fiber-optic tube), or a combination of the two. Such an examination, in addition to determining whether a growth is benign or cancerous, can detect signs of cancer in the lining of the larynx.

If cancer is detected early enough, radiation can usually control it. If the disease has advanced significantly, however, a laryngectomy may be necessary. In this surgical procedure, performed under general anesthesia, an incision is made in the neck and the larynx is removed. The windpipe directly below the larynx is then sewn to the skin around the surgical opening to form a permanent opening, or stoma, through which the patient breathes.

USES AND COMPLICATIONS

This surgery is used when cancer is sufficiently advanced that radiation therapy cannot destroy it. The major complication is that the patient's air supply is now taken through the stoma, meaning that swimming is precluded and that bathing must be undertaken with considerable caution.

A more apparent complication is that, with the loss of the larynx, one cannot speak. Through an extensive and painstaking course of speech therapy, however, esophageal speech can be achieved. This involves swallowing air and expelling it in such a way that it can be shaped by the palate, lips, and tongue into understandable words and sentences. An electronic larynx is also available. It makes a buzzing sound which, when pressed against the top of the throat, permits the patient to convert the sound into words.

—*R. Baird Shuman, Ph.D.*

See also Cancer; Endoscopy; Otorhinolaryngology; Speech disorders; Tumors; Warts.

FOR FURTHER INFORMATION:

Blom, Eric D., Mark I. Singer, and Ronald C. Hamaker. *Tracheoesophageal Voice Restoration Following Total Laryngectomy.* San Diego, Calif.: Singular, 1998.

Edels, Yvonne, ed. *Laryngectomy: Diagnosis to Rehabilitation.* Rockville, Md.: Aspen Systems, 1983.

Ferrari, Mario. *Ear, Nose and Throat Disorders.* New York: Elsevier, 2002.

Griffith, H. Winter. *Complete Guide to Symptoms, Illness and Surgery.* Rev. ed. New York: Berkley, 2000.

Montgomery, William. *Surgery of the Larynx, Trachea, Esophagus and Neck.* New York: Elsevier, 2002.

Sataloff, Robert T. *Reflux Laryngitis and Related Disorders.* San Diego, Calif.: Singular, 1999.

Serafini, I. *Restoration of Laryngeal Function After Laryngectomy.* New York: Karger, 1969.

Zollinger, Robert M., et al. *Zollinger's Atlas of Surgical Operations.* 8th ed. New York: McGraw-Hill, 2002.

LARYNGITIS

DISEASE/DISORDER

ANATOMY OR SYSTEM AFFECTED: Throat

SPECIALTIES AND RELATED FIELDS: Otorhinolaryngology, speech pathology

DEFINITION: Inflammation of the larynx (voice box), often associated with common colds, bacterial infection, or straining the voice. The throat is dry, swallowing becomes difficult, and speech is a hoarse whisper.

CAUSES AND SYMPTOMS

The larynx, located directly above the windpipe (trachea), is the short, hollow tube containing the vocal cords, two heavily lined slits in a mucous membrane. Voiced sounds, such as vowels, result when air from the lungs induces vocal fold vibration. Laryngitis occurs when the folds are obstructed or do not vibrate properly; depending on the cause, laryngitis is classified as simple, chronic, diphtheritic, tuberculous, or syphilitic.

Simple laryngitis may be caused by bacterial infection (common cold, typhoid fever), a virus (influenza), or nonbacterial irritants (chemical fumes, dust, or tobacco smoke). The primary infection site is the mucous membrane lining the larynx. It becomes red and swollen, secreting a viscous discharge that impedes vocal fold vibration. In severe cases of viral infection, the larynx may become completely obstructed, causing suffocation.

Chronic laryngitis often results from excessive smoking, alcoholism, or consistent strain or abuse of the voice. It is an occupational hazard of auctioneers, orators, singers, and those who frequently shout for long periods, such as cheerleaders. Nondisease-induced chronic laryngitis may also be instigated by hysteria, allergic reaction, remote disease of the nerves serving

Information on Laryngitis

Causes: Bacterial infection (common cold, typhoid fever, diphtheria, syphilis); viral infection (influenza); irritants (chemical fumes, dust, smoke, alcohol); consistent strain or abuse of voice

Symptoms: Red and swollen larynx; discharge; obstruction that can cause suffocation if severe; polyps, cysts, or other fibrous growths on vocal cords

Duration: Acute or chronic

Treatments: Depends on cause; may include resting the voice, antibiotics, or surgery

the voice, strong external pressure against the larynx, or irritation caused by tubes inserted down the throat to sustain breathing.

Diphtheritic laryngitis occurs when diphtheria afflicting the upper throat spreads to the larynx. The result may be a membrane of diseased cells infiltrating the mucous membrane and obstructing the vocal cords.

Tuberculous laryngitis is a secondary infection spread from the lungs. Tubular nodulelike growths are formed in larynx tissue, leaving ulcers on the surface. Starting at the vocal cords, this infection may spread over the entire larynx and eventually destroy the epiglottis and laryngeal cartilage.

Syphilitic laryngitis is one of the many complications of syphilis. Sores or mucous patches form in the larynx, eventually producing tissue destruction and scar formation. The mucous membrane becomes dry and covered with polyps (small bumps of tissue that project from the surface). These polyps distort the larynx, shorten the vocal cords, and produce persistent hoarseness.

Treatment and Therapy

Simple laryngitis is best treated by resting the voice. When it is absolutely necessary to speak, it should be with a soft, breathy voice, not a whisper. The throat should be kept well lubricated by frequent drinks of water and not cleared. Relative humidity in the recovery room should be maintained at 40 to 50 percent, and alcohol, tobacco, and decongestants should be avoided. Complete recovery usually occurs within several days.

A persistent hoarseness indicates a bacterial infection (usually curable by antibiotics) or polyps, cysts, or other fibrous growths on the vocal cords. These

growths may become ulcerated and require surgical intervention. Although cancer of the larynx is not uncommon (2 percent of malignancies), it is usually completely curable if detected sufficiently early.

Systemic diseases not localized in the larynx, such as tuberculosis and syphilis, are best treated by antibiotics.

—George R. Plitnik, Ph.D.

See also Common cold; Laryngectomy; Multiple chemical sensitivity syndrome; Nasopharyngeal disorders; Otorhinolaryngology; Pharyngitis; Sore throat; Strep throat; Tonsillectomy and adenoid removal; Tonsillitis; Voice and vocal cord disorders.

For Further Information:

Bellenir, Karen, and Peter D. Dresser, eds. *Contagious and Non-contagious Infectious Diseases Sourcebook*. Detroit: Omnigraphics, 1996.

Colton, Raymond H., and Janina K. Casper. *Understanding Voice Problems: A Physiological Perspective for Diagnosis and Treatment*. 2d ed. Baltimore: Williams & Wilkins, 1996.

Swartzberg, J. E., and S. Margen. *Wellness Self-Care Handbook*. New York: Rebus, 1998.

Tucker, Harvey M. *The Larynx*. 2d ed. New York: Thieme Medical, 1993.

Laser use in surgery

Procedure

Anatomy or system affected: Eyes, skin

Specialties and related fields: Dermatology, oncology, ophthalmology, urology

Definition: The application of laser technology to surgical procedures, such as the vaporization of blood clots or arterial plaque, the breaking up of kidney stones into small fragments, the removal of birthmarks, and the stoppage of hemorrhaging in the retina of the eye.

Key terms:

ionization: a process in which a neutral atom loses one or more of its orbital electrons because of light, heat, or electrical collisions

laser: an acronym for light amplification by stimulated emission of radiation; a laser produces a very-high-intensity light beam at a single wavelength

optical fiber: a very thin thread made of high-purity glass, plastic, or quartz; used to transmit light from a laser into the body

photon: a particle of light whose energy depends on its wavelength (that is, its color); many billions of individual photons make up a light beam

pulsed laser: a laser technique used to deliver a light beam of high power for a very short time in order to localize the heating effect without damaging surrounding tissue

shock wave: a miniature explosion caused by intense local heating with a laser beam; used to fragment stones in the kidney or gallbladder

stimulated emission of radiation: the process in a laser whereby an avalanche of photons is created, all of which are synchronized in wavelength and direction of travel

wavelength: a property used to measure colors in the spectrum of light from infrared to ultraviolet; usually expressed in units of microns (one micron is equal to one-millionth of a meter)

THE FUNDAMENTALS OF LASER TECHNOLOGY

The first successful laser was built in 1960 by Theodore H. Maiman at the Hughes Aircraft Research Laboratory in Palo Alto, California. Since then, many applications have been developed for lasers. These include the compact disc player, telephone systems with fiber optics, guidance systems for military weapons, supermarket checkout scanners, quality control in industry, entertainment with laser light shows, and numerous medical applications.

Ordinary light sources such as flashlights, flames, and the sun do not emit laser light. The individual atoms emit their light waves in a random, uncoordinated manner, in the same way that water waves spread out at random when a handful of pebbles is thrown into a pool. In contrast, a laser beam consists of light waves that are all synchronized; they all have the same wavelength and remain in step as they travel in the same direction. Synchronizing the light emission from billions of atoms in a light source is the chief difficulty in building a laser.

The key idea for solving this problem had been proposed in an article on the general theory of light absorption and emission by atoms written by the famous physicist Albert Einstein in the 1920's. When an atom absorbs a burst of light energy (a photon), an electron in the atom is raised from a lower energy level to a higher one. A short time later, the electron spontaneously falls back down to the lower energy level, emitting a photon of light in the process. Einstein's contribution was to suggest a third mechanism in addition to ordinary absorption and emission. Based on theoretical arguments of symmetry and the conservation of energy, he proposed a new process called "stimulated emission of ra-

diation." (The word "laser" is an acronym for light amplification by stimulated emission of radiation.)

To understand stimulated emission, consider an atom whose electron has been raised to a higher energy level, called an "excited state." This state is unstable, and the electron ordinarily will fall back down to the lower energy level in a short time. Suppose, however, that a photon of precisely the right energy strikes the atom while the electron is still in its temporary excited state. This photon cannot be absorbed because the electron is already in its excited state. Einstein reasoned that the incoming photon would cause the excited electron to fall to the lower energy level. A photon would then be emitted from the atom and would join the incoming photon. The two photons would be exactly synchronized in wavelength and direction.

If there were many atoms whose electrons had previously been raised to excited states, the process of stimulated emission would continue. The two photons could strike two other excited atoms and stimulate them to emit light energy, making a total of four photons. These four would trigger four more atoms, making eight photons, and so forth. Eventually, a so-called photon avalanche consisting of a huge number of synchronized light waves would be generated, which is the desired laser beam.

To make a successful laser, some additional requirements must be met. For one thing, a source of energy must be provided to raise most of the electrons to their excited states. For a gas laser, this energy is normally supplied by a high voltage. Examples of gas lasers are those using carbon dioxide, argon, or a mixture of helium and neon. A solid crystal, such as a clear ruby rod, would be excited by a bright burst of light from a device similar to a camera flash attachment. A solid-state diode laser is energized by a flow of electric current across a diode junction. In each case, it is necessary to "pump" the laser so that many atoms are in their excited state, ready and waiting to be triggered by an incoming photon to release their energy.

Another requirement for a successful laser is that the electrons must remain in their excited state for a longer-than-normal time. The problem with most materials is that electrons fall spontaneously to their lower energy level almost instantaneously, in less than one-millionth of a second. The photon avalanche effect requires that a substantial majority of the atoms be in their excited state. For very short-lived excited states, it is not possible to maintain this condition. Experimenters have no way to control the lifetime of excited states, so they must search for those atoms and molecules that already have the appropriate longer lifetime supplied by nature. It has not been possible to build a laser using hydrogen gas, for example, because hydrogen does not have any long-lived excited states. The spontaneous emission of light takes place so quickly that there is no time for a photon avalanche to develop.

Another condition for laser action is to have two parallel mirrors at the ends of the laser material. The laser beam bounces back and forth many times between the mirrors at the speed of light, gaining or maintaining its energy from the excited atoms of the laser material. One of the mirrors is made slightly less than 100 percent reflecting, so that a small portion of the laser energy is allowed to exit in a narrow beam. For most medical applications, a thin optical fiber is joined directly to the end of the laser in order to transmit the beam to the desired location in the body.

Much research has been done to develop good optical fibers. The fiber should transmit a laser beam with very little loss of energy along the way. The technology of drawing thin glass fibers with few impurities or imperfections has become quite sophisticated. A fiber must be thin and uniform so that the laser beam will be forced to travel down its center, thus avoiding the loss of light energy through the walls.

For an ultraviolet laser, glass fibers cannot be used because of absorption. (The sun's ultraviolet radiation is absorbed by ordinary eyeglasses.) Special quartz fibers with low absorption have been developed for lasers in the ultraviolet region of the spectrum. In the infrared region of the spectrum, new optical materials are still under continuing investigation.

The wavelength (color) of a laser is determined entirely by the energy levels of the atoms or molecules being used. For example, a carbon dioxide laser always has a wavelength of 10.6 microns, which is infrared. The helium-neon gas laser always produces visible red light at a wavelength of 0.63 microns. A wide range of laser wavelengths has become available as a result of extensive research efforts by physicists and optical engineers. Since 1960, lasers have become much more rugged and dependable in construction. Some lasers operate with a continuous beam, while others produce very short pulses, depending on the desired application. Also, lasers can be designed to operate at a low power level for diagnostic purposes or a high power level for surgery.

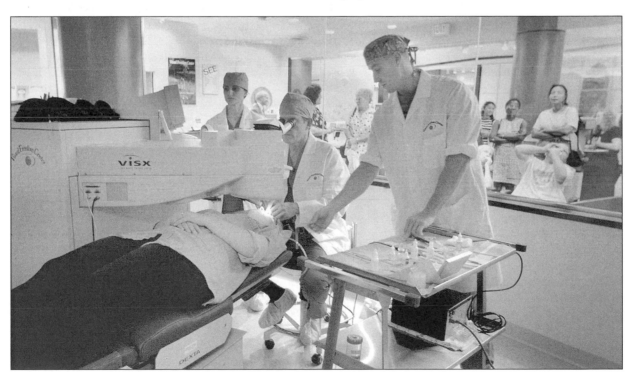

Lasers are taking a more prominent role in many procedures, especially eye surgery. Some worry that the popularity of laser vision correction—here a patient is treated at a shopping mall as spectators look on—has compromised safety. (AP/Wide World Photos)

Safety precautions must be followed when working with a laser. Not only the patient but also the surgical team must be protected from possible harmful radiation. The eyes must be protected from laser beam reflections from a shiny surface. Ultraviolet light is a special hazard because its high-energy photons can cause cell damage and genetic mutations. The great benefits of laser surgery can be negated by an inexperienced or careless surgeon.

USES AND COMPLICATIONS

The first medical use of a laser beam was for surgery on the retina of the eye, in 1963. Diabetic patients in particular frequently develop excessive blood vessels in the retina that give their eyes a typically reddish color. In advanced cases, the blood vessels can hemorrhage and eventually cause blindness. The green light of an argon laser will pass through the clear cornea and lens of the eye, but when it hits the dark brown melanin pigment of the retina, it will be absorbed and cause a tiny hot spot. The physician uses a series of laser pulses, carefully focused on affected areas of the retina, to burn away the extra blood vessels. The remarkable property of the laser beam in this procedure is that its energy penetrates to the rear of the eye, leaving the clear fluid unaffected.

In a greenhouse, light from the sun comes in through the glass but infrared radiation cannot get back out. This example illustrates that some materials, such as glass, are transparent for visible light but opaque for infrared light. Similarly, the front of the eye is transparent for visible light but absorbs infrared light. Therefore, an infrared laser such as the YAG (yttrium-aluminum-garnet) laser can be used for surgery near the front of the eye because its light energy is selectively absorbed there.

A particular problem following cataract surgery is that a secondary cataract may develop on the membrane behind the implanted artificial lens. About one-third of patients with such a lens implant require a second surgery to remove the secondary cataract. A YAG laser beam will pass through the cornea and artificial lens but can be focused to produce a hot spot at the site of the secondary cataract to destroy it. More than 200,000 such procedures are performed each year in the United States, and the result is a dramatic, almost instantaneous improvement of vision.

A third form of laser eye surgery, LASIK (laser in-situ keratomileusis), became quite popular at the end of the twentieth century; it has, in fact, become the most commonly performed surgery in the country. In LASIK surgery, the cornea of the eyeball is reshaped to help patients overcome myopia (nearsightedness), hyperopia (farsightedness), or astigmatism. The procedure is done with a cool beam laser that can be used to remove thin layers of tissue from selected sites on the cornea to change its curvature. Success rates for the surgery are high: 90 to 95 percent of the patients get 20/40 vision, and 65 to 75 percent of the patients get 20/20 vision or better. The surgery is not without its problems, however. Because of its popularity and the large fee charged for a quick and fairly simple procedure, unqualified or less experienced physicians are oftentimes performing the delicate procedure; approximately 5 percent of patients receiving LASIK surgery receive less-than-satisfactory results. Two other corrective procedures for eyesight involving lasers are Kera-Vision Intacs (intrastomal corneal rings), which involves placing a lens in the cornea, and PRK (photorefractive keratectomy), where the cornea is scraped without LASIK's actual incision into the cornea.

Another dramatic medical application of the laser is the breaking up of stones in the kidney, ureter, or gallbladder. Such calcified, hard deposits previously could be removed only by surgery. It is now possible, for example, to insert an optical fiber of less than half a millimeter in diameter through the urethra and then transmit the laser beam to the site of the stone. High-power light pulses of very short duration (less than one-billionth of a second) create a shock wave that breaks the stone into small fragments that the body can eliminate.

Another promising application of laser surgery that has received much publicity is laser angioplasty, which is used to open up a blood vessel near the heart that is partially or wholly blocked by a deposit of plaque. The hope is that the laser procedure may be able to replace heart bypass surgery, but the results are still preliminary.

Laser angioplasty involves inserting a catheter that contains a fiberscope, an inflation cuff, and an optical fiber into the artery of the arm and advancing it into the coronary artery. The fiberscope enables the physician to see the blockage, the cuff is used to stop the blood flow temporarily, and the optical fiber transmits the laser energy that vaporizes the plaque. Sometimes, the laser method is used only to open up a small channel, after which balloon angioplasty is used to stretch the walls of the blood vessel.

The main risk in using the laser beam is that the alignment of the optical fiber inside the artery may be deflected and cause a puncture of the blood vessel wall.

Improvements in the imaging system are needed. Also, further work must be done to see which light wavelengths are most effective in removing plaque and preventing recurrence of the obstruction.

The heating effect of a laser beam has been used by surgeons to control bleeding. For example, bleeding ulcers in the stomach, intestine, and colon have been successfully cauterized with laser light transmitted through an optical fiber. A similar procedure has been used to treat emphysema patients. An optical fiber is inserted through the wall of the chest, and the laser's heat is used to shrink the small blisters that are present on the surface of the lungs. Also, the heat from a laser has been used during internal surgery to seal the surrounding capillaries that contribute to bleeding.

For the preceding procedures, a carbon dioxide gas laser that emits infrared light is normally used. The reason is that water molecules in the tissue absorb the infrared wavelengths most efficiently. The optical fibers used to transmit infrared light are not as efficient and reliable as those used for visible or ultraviolet light, however, so further research on fiber materials is in progress.

One notable success of laser surgery has been the removal of birthmarks. Because of their typically reddish-purple coloration, birthmarks are commonly called port-wine stains. They can be quite unsightly, especially when located on the face of a person with an otherwise light complexion. To remove such a birthmark, the laser beam has to burn out the network of extra blood vessels under the skin. A similar procedure can be used to remove unwanted tattoos.

The color of the laser must be chosen so that its wavelength will be absorbed efficiently by the dark purple stain. What would happen if a purple laser beam were used? Its light would be reflected rather than absorbed by a purple object, and it would not produce the desired heating. Yellow or orange is most effectively absorbed by a purple object. The surgeon must be careful that the laser light is absorbed primarily by the purple birthmark without harming the normal, healthy tissue around it.

Experimental work is being done to determine whether laser surgery can be applied to cancer. Small malignant tumors in the lungs, bladder, and trachea have been treated with a technique called photodynamic therapy. The patient is injected with a colored dye that is preferentially absorbed in the tumor. Porphyrin, the reddish-brown pigment in blood, is one substance that has been known for many years to become concentrated in malignant tissue. The suspected site is irradiated with ultraviolet light from a krypton laser, causing it to glow like fluorescent paint, which allows the surgeon to determine the outline of the tumor. To perform the surgery, an intense red laser is focused on the tumor to kill the malignant tissue. Two separate optical fibers must be used for this procedure, one for the ultraviolet diagnosis and one for the red laser therapy.

The three traditional cancer treatments of surgery, chemotherapy, and radiation therapy all seek to limit damage to healthy tissue surrounding a tumor. Photodynamic surgery by laser must develop its methodology further to accomplish the same goal.

Much has already been accomplished in applying laser surgery to various body organs. Future developments are likely to emphasize microsurgery on smaller structures, such as individual cells or even genetic material in DNA molecules.

PERSPECTIVE AND PROSPECTS

Some inventions, such as the printing press, the steam engine, and the electric light bulb, were made by innovators who were trying to solve a particular practical problem of their time. Other inventions, such as the microscope, radio waves, and low-temperature superconductivity, initially were scientific curiosities arising from basic research, and their later applications were not at all anticipated. The laser belongs to this second category.

The first successful laser, built by Theodore Maiman, consisted of a small cylindrical ruby rod with shiny mirrored ends and a bright flash lamp to excite the atoms in the rod. His goal was to determine whether the separately excited atoms could be made to release their absorbed energy almost simultaneously in one coordinated burst of monochromatic (single wavelength) light.

No one could have foreseen the wide range of technological applications that resulted from Maiman's experiment. It is important to appreciate that he did not set out to improve telephone communication or eye surgery; those developments came about after the laser became available.

It is worthwhile here to summarize some of the general uses for lasers in modern technology. The tremendous advances in medical applications could not have happened without the concurrent development of new types of lasers, with a variety of wavelengths and power levels, needed for other industrial products.

Among laser applications are the following: the compact disc (CD) player, in which the laser beam replaces the LP record needle; optical fibers that can carry several thousand simultaneous telephone calls; supermarket check-out scanners, in which a laser beam reads the universal product code on each item; three-dimensional pictures, called holograms, that are displayed at many art museums; military applications, such as guided weapons and Star Wars technology; surveying, bridge building, and tunneling projects in which exact alignment is critical; and nuclear fusion research, in which high-power lasers can produce nuclear reactions that may become a future source of energy as coal and oil resources are depleted. Sophisticated advances in using lasers to control specific chemical reactions and to predict earthquakes are under development.

The future of laser technology in medicine will continue to advance as biologists, electrical and optical engineers, physicians, biophysicists, and people from related disciplines share this common interest.

—Hans G. Graetzer, Ph.D.;
updated by Cassandra Kircher, Ph.D.

See also Angioplasty; Astigmatism; Bionics and biotechnology; Bleeding; Blurred vision; Cataract surgery; Cataracts; Cervical procedures; Dermatology; Electrocauterization; Eye surgery; Eyes; Malignant melanoma removal; Myopia; Neurosurgery; Ophthalmology; Skin; Skin disorders; Skin lesion removal; Stone removal; Stones; Tattoo removal; Ulcer surgery; Ulcers.

FOR FURTHER INFORMATION:

Alster, Tina S., and Lydia Preston. *Skin Savvy: The Essential Guide to Cosmetic Laser Surgery*. New York: Cadogan, 2002. A guide that provides an overview of current laser procedures in cosmetic surgery, information on the variety of lasers used for which procedures, and practical advice on whether or not certain surgeries would be right for specific conditions.

American Society for Laser Surgery and Medicine, Inc. http://www.aslms.org/. Site offers a database for referral to a laser practitioner, and links to *Lasers in Surgery and Medicine.*

Buettner, Helmut, ed. *Mayo Clinic on Vision and Eye Health: Practical Answers on Glaucoma, Cataracts, Macular Degeneration, and Other Conditions.* Rochester, Minn.: Mayo Foundation for Medical Education and Research, 2002. A helpful handbook on all the medical, social, and emotional facets of vision impairment and the treatments available.

Ehrlich, Matthew. *How to See Like a Hawk When You're Blind as a Bat*. Venice, Fla.: Doctor's Advice Press, 1999. Ehrlich, an opthalmologist, provides a thorough description of various eye problems and whether LASIK eye surgery can be used to correct them. He draws on statistics from a group of LASIK patients to show final outcomes and the proportion of people who experience various complications.

Fitzpatrick, Richard E., and Mitchel P. Goldman. *Cosmetic Laser Surgery*. St. Louis: Mosby, 2000. Discusses methods of cosmetic surgery using lasers. Includes bibliographical references and an index.

IEEE Journal of Quantum Electronics 26, no. 12 (December, 1990). A special issue on lasers in biology and medicine. This journal is the professional publication of the Institute of Electrical and Electronic Engineers. The articles require some technical background on the part of the reader.

Narrins, Rhoda, and Paul Jarrod Frank. *Turn Back the Clock Without Losing Time: Everything You Need to Know About Simple Cosmetic Procedures*. New York: Crown, 2002. A user-friendly guide to procedures that covers laser resurfacing and includes a "frequently asked questions" section for each treatment.

Sutton, Amy, ed. *Eye Care Sourcebook: Basic Consumer Health Information About Eye Care and Eye Disorders*. 2d ed. Detroit: Omnigraphics, 2003. A complete guide to eye care that includes such topics as eye anatomy, preventive vision care, refractive disorders and eye diseases, current research and clinical trials, and a list of organizations.

Victor, Steven. *Ageless Beauty: A Dermatologist's Secrets for Looking Younger Without Surgery*. New York: Crown, 2003. Details several innovative approaches to skin care, including laser surgery.

MAGILL'S
MEDICAL GUIDE

ALPHABETICAL LIST OF CONTENTS

Entries by Anatomy or System Affected

Amniocentesis
Anthrax
Appendectomy
Appendicitis
Bariatric surgery
Bladder removal
Burping
Bypass surgery
Candidiasis
Celiac sprue
Cesarean section
Cholecystectomy
Colic
Colitis
Colon and rectal polyp removal
Colon and rectal surgery
Colon cancer
Colon therapy
Colonoscopy and sigmoidoscopy
Computed tomography (CT) scanning
Constipation
Crohn's disease
Diabetes mellitus
Dialysis
Diarrhea and dysentery
Digestion
Diverticulitis and diverticulosis
Endoscopy
Enemas
Enterocolitis
Fistula repair
Gallbladder diseases
Gastrectomy
Gastroenterology
Gastroenterology, pediatric
Gastrointestinal disorders
Gastrointestinal system
Gastrostomy
Gaucher's disease
Giardiasis
Hernia
Hernia repair
Hirschsprung's disease
Ileostomy and colostomy
Incontinence
Indigestion
Internal medicine
Intestinal disorders
Intestines
Irritable bowel syndrome (IBS)
Kidney transplantation
Kidneys
Laparoscopy

Liposuction
Lithotripsy
Liver
Liver transplantation
Malabsorption
Nephrectomy
Nephritis
Nephrology
Nephrology, pediatric
Obstruction
Pancreas
Pancreatitis
Peristalsis
Peritonitis
Pregnancy and gestation
Prostate cancer
Pyloric stenosis
Reproductive system
Roundworm
Shunts
Splenectomy
Stents
Sterilization
Stomach, intestinal, and pancreatic cancers
Stone removal
Stones
Syphilis
Tubal ligation
Ultrasonography
Urethritis
Urinary disorders
Urinary system
Urology
Urology, pediatric
Worms

ANUS
Colon and rectal polyp removal
Colon and rectal surgery
Colon cancer
Colon therapy
Colonoscopy and sigmoidoscopy
Diaper rash
Endoscopy
Enemas
Episiotomy
Fistula repair
Hemorrhoid banding and removal
Hemorrhoids
Hirschsprung's disease
Intestinal disorders
Intestines
Irritable bowel syndrome (IBS)

Soiling
Sphincterectomy

ARMS
Amputation
Bones and the skeleton
Carpal tunnel syndrome
Cornelia de Lange syndrome
Fracture and dislocation
Fracture repair
Liposuction
Muscles
Pityriasis rosea
Rotator cuff surgery
Skin lesion removal
Tendinitis
Tendon disorders
Tendon repair
Thalidomide
Upper extremities

BACK
Bone disorders
Bone marrow transplantation
Bones and the skeleton
Cerebral palsy
Chiropractic
Disk removal
Dwarfism
Gigantism
Juvenile rheumatoid arthritis
Kyphosis
Laminectomy and spinal fusion
Lumbar puncture
Muscle sprains, spasms, and disorders
Muscles
Osteoporosis
Pityriasis rosea
Sciatica
Scoliosis
Slipped disk
Spinal cord disorders
Spine, vertebrae, and disks
Spondylitis
Sympathectomy
Tendon disorders

BLADDER
Abdomen
Bed-wetting
Bladder removal
Candidiasis
Catheterization

Thyroid disorders
Thyroid gland
Thyroidectomy
Turner syndrome
Weight loss medications

EYES
Albinos
Antihistamines
Astigmatism
Auras
Batten's disease
Behçet's disease
Blindness
Blurred vision
Botox
Cataract surgery
Cataracts
Chlamydia
Color blindness
Conjunctivitis
Corneal transplantation
Cornelia de Lange syndrome
Cytomegalovirus (CMV)
Diabetes mellitus
Dyslexia
Eye surgery
Eyes
Face lift and blepharoplasty
Galactosemia
Glaucoma
Gonorrhea
Gulf War syndrome
Jaundice
Juvenile rheumatoid arthritis
Laser use in surgery
Leukodystrophy
Macular degeneration
Marfan syndrome
Marijuana
Microscopy, slitlamp
Motor skill development
Multiple chemical sensitivity
    syndrome
Myopia
Ophthalmology
Optometry
Optometry, pediatric
Pigmentation
Ptosis
Reiter's syndrome
Rubinstein-Taybi syndrome
Sense organs
Sjögren's syndrome

Strabismus
Sturge-Weber syndrome
Styes
Toxoplasmosis
Trachoma
Transplantation
Visual disorders

FEET
Athlete's foot
Bones and the skeleton
Bunions
Cornelia de Lange syndrome
Corns and calluses
Cysts
Feet
Flat feet
Foot disorders
Fragile X syndrome
Frostbite
Ganglion removal
Gout
Hammertoe correction
Hammertoes
Heel spur removal
Lower extremities
Nail removal
Nails
Orthopedic surgery
Orthopedics
Orthopedics, pediatric
Osteoarthritis
Pigeon toes
Podiatry
Rubinstein-Taybi syndrome
Sports medicine
Tendinitis
Tendon repair
Thalidomide
Warts

GALLBLADDER
Abscess drainage
Abscesses
Bariatric surgery
Cholecystectomy
Cholecystitis
Fistula repair
Gallbladder diseases
Gastroenterology
Gastroenterology, pediatric
Gastrointestinal disorders
Gastrointestinal system
Internal medicine

Laparoscopy
Liver transplantation
Malabsorption
Nuclear medicine
Stone removal
Stones
Ultrasonography

**GASTROINTESTINAL
    SYSTEM**
Abdomen
Abdominal disorders
Acid reflux disease
Allergies
Anthrax
Appendectomy
Appendicitis
Bacterial infections
Bariatric surgery
Botulism
Bulimia
Burping
Bypass surgery
Candidiasis
Celiac sprue
Childhood infectious diseases
Cholera
Cholesterol
Colic
Colitis
Colon and rectal polyp removal
Colon and rectal surgery
Colon cancer
Colon therapy
Colonoscopy and sigmoidoscopy
Constipation
Crohn's disease
Cytomegalovirus (CMV)
Diabetes mellitus
Diarrhea and dysentery
Digestion
Diverticulitis and diverticulosis
E. coli infection
Eating disorders
Ebola virus
Emotions: Biomedical causes and
    effects
Endoscopy
Enemas
Enterocolitis
Fistula repair
Food biochemistry
Food poisoning
Gallbladder diseases

Gastrectomy
Gastroenterology
Gastroenterology, pediatric
Gastrointestinal disorders
Gastrointestinal system
Gastrostomy
Giardiasis
Glands
Gulf War syndrome
Halitosis
Heartburn
Hemorrhoid banding and removal
Hemorrhoids
Hernia
Hernia repair
Hirschsprung's disease
Histiocytosis
Host-defense mechanisms
Ileostomy and colostomy
Incontinence
Indigestion
Internal medicine
Intestinal disorders
Intestines
Irritable bowel syndrome (IBS)
Klippel-Trenaunay syndrome
Kwashiorkor
Lactose intolerance
Laparoscopy
Lipids
Liver
Malabsorption
Malnutrition
Marijuana
Metabolism
Motion sickness
Muscles
Nausea and vomiting
Noroviruses
Nutrition
Obesity
Obstruction
Pancreas
Pancreatitis
Peristalsis
Pinworm
Poisoning
Poisonous plants
Polycystic kidney disease
Premenstrual syndrome (PMS)
Proctology
Protozoan diseases
Pyloric stenosis
Radiation sickness

Reiter's syndrome
Roundworm
Salmonella infection
Scleroderma
Sense organs
Shigellosis
Shunts
Soiling
Stomach, intestinal, and pancreatic
    cancers
Systems and organs
Tapeworm
Taste
Teeth
Toilet training
Trichinosis
Tumor removal
Tumors
Typhoid fever and typhus
Ulcer surgery
Ulcers
Vagotomy
Vitamins and minerals
Weaning
Weight loss and gain
Worms

GENITALS
Aphrodisiacs
Assisted reproductive technologies
Behçet's disease
Candidiasis
Catheterization
Cervical, ovarian, and uterine
    cancers
Cervical procedures
Chlamydia
Circumcision, female, and genital
    mutilation
Circumcision, male
Contraception
Culdocentesis
Cyst removal
Cysts
Electrocauterization
Endometrial biopsy
Episiotomy
Fragile X syndrome
Genital disorders, female
Genital disorders, male
Glands
Gonorrhea
Gynecology
Hemochromatosis

Hermaphroditism and
    pseudohermaphroditism
Herpes
Hydrocelectomy
Hypospadias repair and
    urethroplasty
Infertility in females
Infertility in males
Klinefelter syndrome
Masturbation
Orchitis
Pap smear
Pelvic inflammatory disease (PID)
Penile implant surgery
Prader-Willi syndrome
Reproductive system
Rubinstein-Taybi syndrome
Sex change surgery
Sexual differentiation
Sexual dysfunction
Sexuality
Sexually transmitted diseases
    (STDs)
Sperm banks
Sterilization
Syphilis
Testicles, undescended
Testicular surgery
Testicular torsion
Toilet training
Trichomoniasis
Urology
Urology, pediatric
Vasectomy
Warts

GLANDS
Abscess drainage
Abscesses
Addison's disease
Adrenalectomy
Assisted reproductive technologies
Biofeedback
Breasts, female
Contraception
Cyst removal
Cysts
Diabetes mellitus
DiGeorge syndrome
Dwarfism
Eating disorders
Endocrine disorders
Endocrinology
Endocrinology, pediatric

Gigantism
Glands
Goiter
Gynecomastia
Hashimoto's thyroiditis
Hormone replacement therapy
   (HRT)
Hormones
Hyperparathyroidism and
   hypoparathyroidism
Hypoglycemia
Internal medicine
Liver
Mastectomy and lumpectomy
Melatonin
Metabolism
Mumps
Neurosurgery
Nuclear medicine
Nuclear radiology
Obesity
Pancreas
Parathyroidectomy
Prader-Willi syndrome
Prostate gland
Prostate gland removal
Sex change surgery
Sexual differentiation
Steroids
Styes
Testicular surgery
Thyroid disorders
Thyroid gland
Thyroidectomy

GUMS
Abscess drainage
Abscesses
Cavities
Cleft lip and palate
Cleft lip and palate repair
Crowns and bridges
Dental diseases
Dentistry
Dentistry, pediatric
Dentures
Endodontic disease
Fluoride treatments
Gingivitis
Gulf War syndrome
Gum disease
Jaw wiring
Nicotine
Nutrition

Orthodontics
Periodontal surgery
Periodontitis
Root canal treatment
Scurvy
Teeth
Teething
Tooth extraction
Toothache
Wisdom teeth

HAIR
Albinos
Cornelia de Lange syndrome
Dermatitis
Dermatology
Eczema
Gray hair
Hair
Hair loss and baldness
Hair transplantation
Klinefelter syndrome
Lice, mites, and ticks
Nutrition
Pigmentation
Radiation sickness
Radiation therapy

HANDS
Amputation
Arthritis
Bones and the skeleton
Bursitis
Carpal tunnel syndrome
Cerebral palsy
Cornelia de Lange syndrome
Corns and calluses
Cysts
Fracture and dislocation
Fracture repair
Fragile X syndrome
Frostbite
Ganglion removal
Nail removal
Nails
Neurology
Neurology, pediatric
Orthopedic surgery
Orthopedics
Orthopedics, pediatric
Osteoarthritis
Rheumatoid arthritis
Rheumatology
Rubinstein-Taybi syndrome

Scleroderma
Skin lesion removal
Sports medicine
Tendinitis
Tendon disorders
Tendon repair
Thalidomide
Upper extremities
Warts

HEAD
Altitude sickness
Aneurysmectomy
Aneurysms
Angiography
Antihistamines
Botox
Brain
Brain disorders
Cluster headaches
Coma
Computed tomography (CT)
   scanning
Concussion
Cornelia de Lange syndrome
Craniosynostosis
Craniotomy
Dizziness and fainting
Electroencephalography (EEG)
Embolism
Epilepsy
Fetal tissue transplantation
Fibromyalgia
Hair loss and baldness
Hair transplantation
Head and neck disorders
Headaches
Hydrocephalus
Lice, mites, and ticks
Meningitis
Migraine headaches
Nasal polyp removal
Nasopharyngeal disorders
Neurology
Neurology, pediatric
Neurosurgery
Rhinoplasty and submucous
   resection
Rubinstein-Taybi syndrome
Seizures
Shunts
Sports medicine
Strokes
Sturge-Weber syndrome

Temporomandibular joint (TMJ)
  syndrome
Thrombosis and thrombus
Unconsciousness
Whiplash

HEART
Aneurysmectomy
Aneurysms
Angina
Angiography
Angioplasty
Anxiety
Apgar score
Arrhythmias
Arteriosclerosis
Biofeedback
Bites and stings
Blue baby syndrome
Bypass surgery
Caffeine
Cardiac rehabilitation
Cardiology
Cardiology, pediatric
Cardiopulmonary resuscitation
  (CPR)
Catheterization
Circulation
Congenital heart disease
Cornelia de Lange syndrome
DiGeorge syndrome
Electrical shock
Electrocardiography (ECG or EKG)
Embolism
Endocarditis
Exercise physiology
Fatty acid oxidation disorders
Glycogen storage diseases
Heart
Heart attack
Heart disease
Heart failure
Heart transplantation
Heart valve replacement
Hemochromatosis
Hypertension
Internal medicine
Juvenile rheumatoid arthritis
Kinesiology
Lyme disease
Marfan syndrome
Marijuana
Mitral valve prolapse
Nicotine

Pacemaker implantation
Palpitations
Prader-Willi syndrome
Respiratory distress syndrome
Resuscitation
Reye's syndrome
Rheumatic fever
Rubinstein-Taybi syndrome
Scleroderma
Shock
Sports medicine
Stents
Steroid abuse
Strokes
Thoracic surgery
Thrombolytic therapy and TPA
Thrombosis and thrombus
Toxoplasmosis
Transplantation
Ultrasonography
Yellow fever

HIPS
Aging
Arthritis
Arthroplasty
Arthroscopy
Bone disorders
Bones and the skeleton
Chiropractic
Dwarfism
Fracture and dislocation
Fracture repair
Hip fracture repair
Hip replacement
Liposuction
Lower extremities
Orthopedic surgery
Orthopedics
Orthopedics, pediatric
Osteoarthritis
Osteochondritis juvenilis
Osteoporosis
Physical rehabilitation
Pityriasis rosea
Rheumatoid arthritis
Rheumatology
Sciatica

IMMUNE SYSTEM
Acquired immunodeficiency
  syndrome (AIDS)
Allergies
Antibiotics

Antihistamines
Arthritis
Asthma
Autoimmune disorders
Bacterial infections
Bacteriology
Bites and stings
Blood and blood disorders
Bone grafting
Bone marrow transplantation
Candidiasis
Cells
Chagas' disease
Childhood infectious diseases
Chronic fatigue syndrome
Cornelia de Lange syndrome
Corticosteroids
Cytology
Cytomegalovirus (CMV)
Cytopathology
Dermatology
Dermatopathology
DiGeorge syndrome
Disseminated intravascular
  coagulation (DIC)
E. coli infection
Emotions: Biomedical causes and
  effects
Endocrinology
Endocrinology, pediatric
Enzymes
Fungal infections
Grafts and grafting
Gram staining
Guillain-Barré syndrome
Gulf War syndrome
Hashimoto's thyroiditis
Healing
Hematology
Hematology, pediatric
Histiocytosis
Hives
Homeopathy
Host-defense mechanisms
Human immunodeficiency virus
  (HIV)
Immune system
Immunization and vaccination
Immunodeficiency disorders
Immunology
Immunopathology
Juvenile rheumatoid arthritis
Leprosy
Lupus erythematosus

KIDNEYS
Abdomen
Abscess drainage
Abscesses
Adrenalectomy
Corticosteroids
Cysts
Dialysis
Fructosemia
Hanta virus
Hypertension
Internal medicine
Kidney disorders
Kidney transplantation
Kidneys
Laparoscopy
Lithotripsy
Metabolism
Nephrectomy
Nephritis
Nephrology
Nephrology, pediatric
Nuclear medicine
Nuclear radiology
Polycystic kidney disease
Preeclampsia and eclampsia
Pyelonephritis
Renal failure
Reye's syndrome
Scleroderma
Stone removal
Stones
Toilet training
Transplantation
Ultrasonography
Urinalysis
Urinary disorders
Urinary system
Urology
Urology, pediatric

KNEES
Amputation
Arthritis
Arthroplasty
Arthroscopy
Bone disorders
Bones and the skeleton
Bowlegs
Bursitis
Endoscopy
Exercise physiology
Fracture and dislocation
Kneecap removal

Knock-knees
Liposuction
Lower extremities
Orthopedic surgery
Orthopedics
Orthopedics, pediatric
Osgood-Schlatter disease
Osteoarthritis
Physical rehabilitation
Rheumatoid arthritis
Rheumatology
Sports medicine
Tendinitis
Tendon disorders
Tendon repair

LEGS
Amputation
Arthritis
Arthroplasty
Arthroscopy
Bone disorders
Bones and the skeleton
Bowlegs
Bursitis
Cerebral palsy
Cornelia de Lange syndrome
Dwarfism
Fracture and dislocation
Fracture repair
Gigantism
Hemiplegia
Hip fracture repair
Kneecap removal
Knock-knees
Liposuction
Lower extremities
Muscle sprains, spasms, and
  disorders
Muscles
Muscular dystrophy
Numbness and tingling
Orthopedic surgery
Orthopedics
Orthopedics, pediatric
Osteoarthritis
Osteoporosis
Paralysis
Paraplegia
Physical rehabilitation
Pigeon toes
Pityriasis rosea
Poliomyelitis
Quadriplegia

Rheumatoid arthritis
Rheumatology
Rickets
Sciatica
Sports medicine
Tendinitis
Tendon disorders
Tendon repair
Thalidomide
Varicose vein removal
Varicose veins
Venous insufficiency

LIGAMENTS
Flat feet
Muscle sprains, spasms, and
  disorders
Muscles
Orthopedic surgery
Orthopedics
Orthopedics, pediatric
Osteogenesis imperfecta
Physical rehabilitation
Slipped disk
Sports medicine
Tendon disorders
Tendon repair
Whiplash

LIVER
Abdomen
Abdominal disorders
Abscess drainage
Abscesses
Alcoholism
Blood and blood disorders
Circulation
Cirrhosis
Corticosteroids
Cytomegalovirus (CMV)
Edema
Fatty acid oxidation disorders
Fetal surgery
Fructosemia
Galactosemia
Gastroenterology
Gastroenterology, pediatric
Gastrointestinal disorders
Gastrointestinal system
Gaucher's disease
Glycogen storage diseases
Hematology
Hematology, pediatric
Hemochromatosis

Hemolytic disease of the newborn
Hepatitis
Histiocytosis
Internal medicine
Jaundice
Jaundice, neonatal
Kaposi's sarcoma
Liver
Liver cancer
Liver disorders
Liver transplantation
Malabsorption
Malaria
Metabolism
Niemann-Pick disease
Polycystic kidney disease
Reye's syndrome
Schistosomiasis
Shunts
Thrombocytopenia
Transplantation
Wilson's disease
Yellow fever

LUNGS
Abscess drainage
Abscesses
Allergies
Altitude sickness
Anthrax
Antihistamines
Apgar score
Apnea
Asphyxiation
Asthma
Bacterial infections
Bronchiolitis
Bronchitis
Cardiopulmonary resuscitation (CPR)
Chest
Childhood infectious diseases
Choking
Chronic obstructive pulmonary
    disease (COPD)
Common cold
Corticosteroids
Coughing
Croup
Cystic fibrosis
Cytomegalovirus (CMV)
Diphtheria
Edema
Embolism
Emphysema

Endoscopy
Exercise physiology
Fetal surgery
Hanta virus
Heart transplantation
Heimlich maneuver
Hiccups
Histiocytosis
Hyperventilation
Influenza
Internal medicine
Interstitial pulmonary fibrosis (IPF)
Kaposi's sarcoma
Kinesiology
Legionnaires' disease
Lung cancer
Lung surgery
Lungs
Marijuana
Measles
Multiple chemical sensitivity
    syndrome
Nicotine
Niemann-Pick disease
Oxygen therapy
Plague
Pleurisy
Pneumonia
Pulmonary diseases
Pulmonary hypertension
Pulmonary medicine
Pulmonary medicine, pediatric
Respiration
Respiratory distress syndrome
Resuscitation
Scleroderma
Severe acute respiratory syndrome
    (SARS)
Smoking
Sneezing
Thoracic surgery
Thrombolytic therapy and TPA
Thrombosis and thrombus
Toxoplasmosis
Transplantation
Tuberculosis
Tumor removal
Tumors
Whooping cough
Wiskott-Aldrich syndrome

LYMPHATIC SYSTEM
Angiography
Bacterial infections

Blood and blood disorders
Breast cancer
Breast disorders
Burkitt's lymphoma
Cancer
Cervical, ovarian, and uterine
    cancers
Chemotherapy
Circulation
Colon cancer
Corticosteroids
DiGeorge syndrome
Edema
Elephantiasis
Gaucher's disease
Histology
Hodgkin's disease
Immune system
Immunology
Immunopathology
Klippel-Trenaunay syndrome
Liver cancer
Lower extremities
Lung cancer
Lymphadenopathy and lymphoma
Lymphatic system
Malignancy and metastasis
Mononucleosis
Oncology
Prostate cancer
Skin cancer
Sleeping sickness
Splenectomy
Stomach, intestinal, and pancreatic
    cancers
Systems and organs
Tonsillectomy and adenoid
    removal
Tonsillitis
Tumor removal
Tumors
Upper extremities
Vascular medicine
Vascular system

MOUTH
Acid reflux disease
Behçet's disease
Candidiasis
Canker sores
Cavities
Cleft lip and palate
Cleft lip and palate repair
Cold sores

Neurology
Neurology, pediatric
Neurosurgery
Niemann-Pick disease
Nuclear radiology
Numbness and tingling
Orthopedic surgery
Orthopedics
Orthopedics, pediatric
Paget's disease
Palsy
Paralysis
Paraplegia
Parkinson's disease
Pharmacology
Pharmacy
Phenylketonuria (PKU)
Physical rehabilitation
Poisoning
Poliomyelitis
Porphyria
Precocious puberty
Preeclampsia and eclampsia
Premenstrual syndrome (PMS)
Prion diseases
Quadriplegia
Rabies
Reye's syndrome
Sciatica
Seasonal affective disorder
Seizures
Sense organs
Shingles
Shock therapy
Shunts
Skin
Sleep disorders
Sleeping sickness
Sleepwalking
Smell
Snakebites
Spina bifida
Spinal cord disorders
Spine, vertebrae, and disks
Sports medicine
Stammering
Strokes
Sturge-Weber syndrome
Stuttering
Sympathectomy
Syphilis
Systems and organs
Taste
Tay-Sachs disease

Teeth
Tetanus
Thrombolytic therapy and TPA
Tics
Touch
Tourette's syndrome
Toxicology
Toxoplasmosis
Trembling and shaking
Unconsciousness
Upper extremities
Vagotomy
Wilson's disease
Yellow fever

NOSE
Allergies
Antihistamines
Aromatherapy
Auras
Childhood infectious diseases
Common cold
Cornelia de Lange syndrome
Decongestants
Fifth disease
Halitosis
Nasal polyp removal
Nasopharyngeal disorders
Nicotine
Nosebleeds
Otorhinolaryngology
Plastic surgery
Pulmonary medicine
Pulmonary medicine, pediatric
Respiration
Rhinitis
Rhinoplasty and submucous
    resection
Rosacea
Rubinstein-Taybi syndrome
Sense organs
Sinusitis
Skin lesion removal
Smell
Sneezing
Sore throat
Taste
Viral infections

PANCREAS
Abscess drainage
Abscesses
Diabetes mellitus
Digestion

Endocrinology
Endocrinology, pediatric
Fetal tissue transplantation
Food biochemistry
Gastroenterology
Gastroenterology, pediatric
Gastrointestinal disorders
Gastrointestinal system
Glands
Hemochromatosis
Hormones
Internal medicine
Malabsorption
Metabolism
Pancreas
Pancreatitis
Polycystic kidney disease
Stomach, intestinal, and pancreatic
    cancers
Transplantation

**PSYCHIC-EMOTIONAL
    SYSTEM**
Addiction
Aging
Alcoholism
Alzheimer's disease
Amnesia
Anesthesia
Anesthesiology
Anorexia nervosa
Antidepressants
Antihistamines
Anxiety
Aphasia and dysphasia
Aphrodisiacs
Aromatherapy
Asperger's syndrome
Attention-deficit disorder (ADD)
Auras
Autism
Bariatric surgery
Biofeedback
Bipolar disorder
Bonding
Brain
Brain disorders
Bulimia
Chronic fatigue syndrome
Club drugs
Cluster headaches
Cognitive development
Colic
Coma

Concussion
Corticosteroids
Death and dying
Delusions
Dementias
Depression
Developmental stages
Dizziness and fainting
Domestic violence
Down syndrome
Dyslexia
Eating disorders
Electroencephalography (EEG)
Emotions: Biomedical causes and
    effects
Endocrinology
Endocrinology, pediatric
Factitious disorders
Failure to thrive
Fibromyalgia
Grief and guilt
Gulf War syndrome
Hallucinations
Headaches
Hormone replacement therapy
    (HRT)
Hormones
Hydrocephalus
Hypnosis
Hypochondriasis
Kinesiology
Klinefelter syndrome
Lead poisoning
Learning disabilities
Light therapy
Marijuana
Memory loss
Menopause
Mental retardation
Midlife crisis
Migraine headaches
Miscarriage
Motor skill development
Narcolepsy
Narcotics
Neurology
Neurology, pediatric
Neurosis
Neurosurgery
Nicotine
Nightmares
Obesity
Obsessive-compulsive disorder
Palpitations

Panic attacks
Paranoia
Pharmacology
Pharmacy
Phobias
Postpartum depression
Post-traumatic stress disorder
Prader-Willi syndrome
Precocious puberty
Psychiatric disorders
Psychiatry
Psychiatry, child and adolescent
Psychiatry, geriatric
Psychoanalysis
Psychosis
Psychosomatic disorders
Puberty and adolescence
Rabies
Schizophrenia
Seasonal affective disorder
Separation anxiety
Sexual dysfunction
Sexuality
Shock therapy
Sibling rivalry
Sleep disorders
Sleepwalking
Soiling
Speech disorders
Sperm banks
Stammering
Steroid abuse
Stillbirth
Stress
Strokes
Stuttering
Suicide
Tics
Toilet training
Tourette's syndrome
Weight loss and gain
Wilson's disease

REPRODUCTIVE SYSTEM
Abdomen
Abdominal disorders
Abortion
Acquired immunodeficiency
    syndrome (AIDS)
Amenorrhea
Amniocentesis
Anatomy
Anorexia nervosa
Assisted reproductive technologies

Breast-feeding
Breasts, female
Candidiasis
Catheterization
Cervical, ovarian, and uterine
    cancers
Cervical procedures
Cesarean section
Childbirth
Childbirth complications
Chlamydia
Chorionic villus sampling
Circumcision, female, and genital
    mutilation
Circumcision, male
Conception
Contraception
Culdocentesis
Cyst removal
Cysts
Dysmenorrhea
Eating disorders
Ectopic pregnancy
Electrocauterization
Endocrinology
Endometrial biopsy
Endometriosis
Episiotomy
Fetal alcohol syndrome
Fistula repair
Gamete intrafallopian transfer
    (GIFT)
Genetic counseling
Genital disorders, female
Genital disorders, male
Glands
Gonorrhea
Gynecology
Hermaphroditism and
    pseudohermaphroditism
Hernia
Herpes
Hormone replacement therapy
    (HRT)
Hormones
Hot flashes
Human immunodeficiency virus
    (HIV)
Hydrocelectomy
Hypospadias repair and
    urethroplasty
Hysterectomy
In vitro fertilization
Infertility in females

Infertility in males
Internal medicine
Klinefelter syndrome
Laparoscopy
Menopause
Menorrhagia
Menstruation
Miscarriage
Multiple births
Mumps
Myomectomy
Nicotine
Obstetrics
Orchitis
Ovarian cysts
Pap smear
Pelvic inflammatory disease (PID)
Penile implant surgery
Placenta
Precocious puberty
Preeclampsia and eclampsia
Pregnancy and gestation
Premature birth
Premenstrual syndrome (PMS)
Prostate cancer
Prostate gland
Puberty and adolescence
Reproductive system
Sex change surgery
Sexual differentiation
Sexual dysfunction
Sexuality
Sexually transmitted diseases
 (STDs)
Sperm banks
Sterilization
Steroid abuse
Stillbirth
Syphilis
Systems and organs
Testicles, undescended
Testicular surgery
Testicular torsion
Toxemia
Trichomoniasis
Tubal ligation
Turner syndrome
Ultrasonography
Urology
Urology, pediatric
Vasectomy
Von Willebrand's disease
Warts

RESPIRATORY SYSTEM
Abscess drainage
Abscesses
Altitude sickness
Amyotrophic lateral sclerosis
Antihistamines
Apgar score
Apnea
Asphyxiation
Asthma
Bacterial infections
Bronchiolitis
Bronchitis
Cardiopulmonary resuscitation
 (CPR)
Chest
Chickenpox
Childhood infectious diseases
Choking
Chronic obstructive pulmonary
 disease (COPD)
Common cold
Corticosteroids
Coughing
Croup
Cystic fibrosis
Decongestants
Diphtheria
Edema
Embolism
Emphysema
Epiglottitis
Exercise physiology
Fetal surgery
Fluids and electrolytes
Fungal infections
Halitosis
Hanta virus
Head and neck disorders
Heart transplantation
Heimlich maneuver
Hiccups
Hyperventilation
Influenza
Internal medicine
Interstitial pulmonary fibrosis (IPF)
Kinesiology
Laryngectomy
Laryngitis
Legionnaires' disease
Lung cancer
Lung surgery
Lungs
Marijuana

Measles
Monkeypox
Mononucleosis
Multiple chemical sensitivity
 syndrome
Nasopharyngeal disorders
Nicotine
Niemann-Pick disease
Otorhinolaryngology
Oxygen therapy
Pharyngitis
Plague
Pleurisy
Pneumonia
Poisoning
Pulmonary diseases
Pulmonary hypertension
Pulmonary medicine
Pulmonary medicine, pediatric
Respiration
Resuscitation
Rheumatic fever
Rhinitis
Roundworm
Severe acute respiratory syndrome
 (SARS)
Sinusitis
Sleep apnea
Smallpox
Sneezing
Sore throat
Strep throat
Systems and organs
Thoracic surgery
Thrombolytic therapy and TPA
Thrombosis and thrombus
Tonsillectomy and adenoid removal
Tonsillitis
Toxoplasmosis
Tracheostomy
Transplantation
Tuberculosis
Tumor removal
Tumors
Voice and vocal cord disorders
Whooping cough
Worms

SKIN
Abscess drainage
Abscesses
Acne
Acupressure
Acupuncture

Age spots
Albinos
Allergies
Amputation
Anesthesia
Anesthesiology
Anthrax
Anxiety
Arthropod-borne diseases
Athlete's foot
Auras
Bariatric surgery
Batten's disease
Behçet's disease
Biopsy
Birthmarks
Bites and stings
Blisters and boils
Blood testing
Burns and scalds
Candidiasis
Canker sores
Cells
Chagas' disease
Chickenpox
Cleft lip and palate repair
Cold sores
Corns and calluses
Corticosteroids
Cryotherapy and cryosurgery
Cyanosis
Cyst removal
Cysts
Dermatitis
Dermatology
Dermatology, pediatric
Dermatopathology
Diaper rash
Ebola virus
Eczema
Edema
Electrical shock
Electrocauterization
Face lift and blepharoplasty
Fifth disease
Frostbite
Fungal infections
Glands
Grafts and grafting
Gulf War syndrome
Hair
Hair loss and baldness
Hair transplantation
Hand-foot-and-mouth disease

Heat exhaustion and heat stroke
Hemolytic disease of the newborn
Histiocytosis
Hives
Host-defense mechanisms
Impetigo
Itching
Jaundice
Kaposi's sarcoma
Laceration repair
Laser use in surgery
Leishmaniasis
Leprosy
Lice, mites, and ticks
Light therapy
Lower extremities
Lupus erythematosus
Lyme disease
Malignant melanoma removal
Measles
Moles
Monkeypox
Multiple chemical sensitivity
  syndrome
Nails
Necrotizing fasciitis
Neurofibromatosis
Nicotine
Numbness and tingling
Obesity
Otoplasty
Pigmentation
Pinworm
Pityriasis alba
Pityriasis rosea
Plastic surgery
Poisonous plants
Porphyria
Psoriasis
Radiation sickness
Rashes
Reiter's syndrome
Ringworm
Rosacea
Roseola
Rubella
Scabies
Scarlet fever
Scurvy
Sense organs
Shingles
Skin
Skin cancer
Skin disorders

Skin lesion removal
Smallpox
Stretch marks
Sturge-Weber syndrome
Sunburn
Tattoo removal
Tattoos and body piercing
Touch
Umbilical cord
Upper extremities
Von Willebrand's disease
Warts
Wiskott-Aldrich syndrome
Wrinkles

SPINE
Anesthesia
Anesthesiology
Bone cancer
Bone disorders
Bones and the skeleton
Cerebral palsy
Chiropractic
Disk removal
Fracture and dislocation
Head and neck disorders
Kinesiology
Laminectomy and spinal fusion
Lumbar puncture
Marfan syndrome
Meningitis
Motor neuron diseases
Multiple sclerosis
Muscle sprains, spasms, and
  disorders
Muscles
Muscular dystrophy
Nervous system
Neuralgia, neuritis, and neuropathy
Neurology
Neurology, pediatric
Neurosurgery
Numbness and tingling
Orthopedic surgery
Orthopedics
Orthopedics, pediatric
Osteoarthritis
Osteogenesis imperfecta
Osteoporosis
Paget's disease
Paralysis
Paraplegia
Physical rehabilitation
Poliomyelitis

Quadriplegia
Sciatica
Scoliosis
Slipped disk
Spina bifida
Spinal cord disorders
Spine, vertebrae, and disks
Spondylitis
Sports medicine
Sympathectomy
Whiplash

SPLEEN
Abdomen
Abdominal disorders
Abscess drainage
Abscesses
Anemia
Bleeding
Gaucher's disease
Hematology
Hematology, pediatric
Immune system
Internal medicine
Jaundice, neonatal
Lymphatic system
Metabolism
Niemann-Pick disease
Splenectomy
Thrombocytopenia
Transplantation

STOMACH
Abdomen
Abdominal disorders
Abscess drainage
Abscesses
Acid reflux disease
Allergies
Bariatric surgery
Botulism
Bulimia
Burping
Bypass surgery
Colitis
Crohn's disease
Digestion
Eating disorders
Endoscopy
Food biochemistry
Food poisoning
Gastrectomy
Gastroenterology
Gastroenterology, pediatric

Gastrointestinal disorders
Gastrointestinal system
Gastrostomy
Halitosis
Heartburn
Hernia
Hernia repair
Indigestion
Influenza
Internal medicine
Kwashiorkor
Lactose intolerance
Malabsorption
Malnutrition
Metabolism
Motion sickness
Nausea and vomiting
Nutrition
Obesity
Peristalsis
Poisoning
Poisonous plants
Pyloric stenosis
Radiation sickness
Roundworm
Salmonella infection
Stomach, intestinal, and pancreatic
   cancers
Ulcer surgery
Ulcers
Vagotomy
Vitamins and minerals
Weaning
Weight loss and gain

TEETH
Cavities
Cornelia de Lange syndrome
Crowns and bridges
Dental diseases
Dentistry
Dentistry, pediatric
Dentures
Endodontic disease
Fluoride treatments
Forensic pathology
Fracture repair
Gastrointestinal system
Gingivitis
Gum disease
Jaw wiring
Lisping
Nicotine
Nutrition

Orthodontics
Osteogenesis imperfecta
Periodontal surgery
Periodontitis
Prader-Willi syndrome
Root canal treatment
Rubinstein-Taybi syndrome
Teeth
Teething
Temporomandibular joint (TMJ)
   syndrome
Thumb sucking
Tooth extraction
Toothache
Veterinary medicine
Wisdom teeth

TENDONS
Carpal tunnel syndrome
Cysts
Exercise physiology
Ganglion removal
Hammertoe correction
Kneecap removal
Orthopedic surgery
Orthopedics
Orthopedics, pediatric
Osgood-Schlatter disease
Physical rehabilitation
Sports medicine
Tendinitis
Tendon disorders
Tendon repair

THROAT
Acid reflux disease
Antihistamines
Auras
Bulimia
Catheterization
Choking
Croup
Decongestants
Epiglottitis
Fifth disease
Gastroenterology
Gastroenterology, pediatric
Gastrointestinal disorders
Gastrointestinal system
Goiter
Head and neck disorders
Heimlich maneuver
Hiccups
Histiocytosis

Laryngectomy
Laryngitis
Nasopharyngeal disorders
Nicotine
Nosebleeds
Otorhinolaryngology
Pharyngitis
Pulmonary medicine
Pulmonary medicine, pediatric
Quinsy
Respiration
Smoking
Sore throat
Strep throat
Tonsillectomy and adenoid removal
Tonsillitis
Tracheostomy
Voice and vocal cord disorders

URINARY SYSTEM
Abdomen
Abdominal disorders
Abscess drainage
Abscesses
Adrenalectomy
Bed-wetting
Bladder removal
Candidiasis
Catheterization
Circumcision, male
Cystitis
Cystoscopy
Cysts
Dialysis
E. coli infection
Endoscopy
Fetal surgery
Fistula repair
Fluids and electrolytes
Geriatrics and gerontology
Hermaphroditism and
    pseudohermaphroditism
Host-defense mechanisms
Hypertension

Incontinence
Internal medicine
Kidney disorders
Kidney transplantation
Kidneys
Laparoscopy
Lithotripsy
Nephrectomy
Nephritis
Nephrology
Nephrology, pediatric
Pediatrics
Penile implant surgery
Pyelonephritis
Reiter's syndrome
Renal failure
Reye's syndrome
Schistosomiasis
Stone removal
Stones
Systems and organs
Toilet training
Transplantation
Trichomoniasis
Ultrasonography
Urethritis
Urinalysis
Urinary disorders
Urinary system
Urology
Urology, pediatric

UTERUS
Abdomen
Abdominal disorders
Abortion
Amenorrhea
Amniocentesis
Assisted reproductive technologies
Cervical, ovarian, and uterine
    cancers
Cervical procedures
Cesarean section
Childbirth

Childbirth complications
Chorionic villus sampling
Conception
Contraception
Culdocentesis
Dysmenorrhea
Ectopic pregnancy
Electrocauterization
Endocrinology
Endometrial biopsy
Endometriosis
Fistula repair
Genetic counseling
Genital disorders, female
Gynecology
Hermaphroditism and
    pseudohermaphroditism
Hysterectomy
In vitro fertilization
Infertility in females
Internal medicine
Laparoscopy
Menopause
Menorrhagia
Menstruation
Miscarriage
Multiple births
Myomectomy
Obstetrics
Pap smear
Pelvic inflammatory disease (PID)
Placenta
Pregnancy and gestation
Premature birth
Premenstrual syndrome (PMS)
Reproductive system
Sex change surgery
Sexual differentiation
Sperm banks
Sterilization
Stillbirth
Tubal ligation
Ultrasonography

ENTRIES BY SPECIALTIES AND RELATED FIELDS

Anesthesia
Anesthesiology
Apgar score
Burns and scalds
Catheterization
Club drugs
Coma
Critical care
Critical care, pediatric
Electrical shock
Electrocardiography (ECG or EKG)
Electroencephalography (EEG)
Emergency medicine
Emergency medicine, pediatric
Geriatrics and gerontology
Grafts and grafting
Hanta virus
Heart attack
Heart transplantation
Heat exhaustion and heat stroke
Hospitals
Hyperthermia and hypothermia
Necrotizing fasciitis
Neonatology
Nursing
Oncology
Osteopathic medicine
Pain management
Paramedics
Psychiatry
Psychiatry, child and adolescent
Psychiatry, geriatric
Pulmonary medicine
Pulmonary medicine, pediatric
Radiation sickness
Resuscitation
Safety issues for children
Safety issues for the elderly
Severe acute respiratory syndrome
  (SARS)
Shock
Thrombolytic therapy and TPA
Toxic shock syndrome
Tracheostomy
Transfusion
Tropical medicine
Wounds

CYTOLOGY
Acid-base chemistry
Bionics and biotechnology
Biopsy
Blood testing
Cancer

Carcinoma
Cells
Cholesterol
Cytology
Cytopathology
Dermatology
Dermatopathology
E. coli infection
Enzymes
Fluids and electrolytes
Food biochemistry
Gaucher's disease
Genetic counseling
Genetic engineering
Genomics
Glycolysis
Gram staining
Healing
Hematology
Hematology, pediatric
Histology
Immune system
Immunology
Karyotyping
Laboratory tests
Lipids
Malignant melanoma removal
Metabolism
Microscopy
Mutation
Oncology
Pathology
Pharmacology
Pharmacy
Sarcoma
Sarcopenia
Serology
Stem cells
Toxicology

DENTISTRY
Abscess drainage
Abscesses
Aging: Extended care
Anesthesia
Anesthesiology
Canker sores
Cavities
Crowns and bridges
Dental diseases
Dentistry
Dentistry, pediatric
Dentures
Endodontic disease

Fluoride treatments
Forensic pathology
Fracture and dislocation
Fracture repair
Gastrointestinal system
Gingivitis
Gum disease
Halitosis
Head and neck disorders
Jaw wiring
Lisping
Nicotine
Orthodontics
Osteogenesis imperfecta
Periodontal surgery
Periodontitis
Plastic surgery
Prader-Willi syndrome
Prostheses
Root canal treatment
Rubinstein-Taybi syndrome
Sense organs
Sjögren's syndrome
Teeth
Teething
Temporomandibular joint (TMJ)
  syndrome
Thumb sucking
Tooth extraction
Toothache
Von Willebrand's disease
Wisdom teeth

DERMATOLOGY
Abscess drainage
Abscesses
Acne
Age spots
Albinos
Anthrax
Anti-inflammatory drugs
Athlete's foot
Biopsy
Birthmarks
Blisters and boils
Burns and scalds
Carcinoma
Chickenpox
Corns and calluses
Corticosteroids
Cryotherapy and cryosurgery
Cyst removal
Cysts
Dermatitis

Antidepressants
Antihistamines
Anti-inflammatory drugs
Antioxidants
Arthritis
Athlete's foot
Attention-deficit disorder (ADD)
Bacterial infections
Bed-wetting
Bell's palsy
Beriberi
Biofeedback
Birthmarks
Bleeding
Blisters and boils
Blurred vision
Bronchiolitis
Bronchitis
Bunions
Burkitt's lymphoma
Burping
Caffeine
Candidiasis
Canker sores
Chagas' disease
Chickenpox
Childhood infectious diseases
Chlamydia
Cholecystitis
Cholesterol
Chronic fatigue syndrome
Cirrhosis
Cluster headaches
Cold sores
Common cold
Constipation
Contraception
Corticosteroids
Coughing
Cryotherapy and cryosurgery
Cytomegalovirus (CMV)
Death and dying
Decongestants
Dehydration
Depression
Diabetes mellitus
Diaper rash
Diarrhea and dysentery
Digestion
Dizziness and fainting
Domestic violence
Enterocolitis
Epiglottitis
Exercise physiology

Factitious disorders
Failure to thrive
Family practice
Fatigue
Fever
Fifth disease
Fungal infections
Ganglion removal
Genital disorders, female
Genital disorders, male
Geriatrics and gerontology
Giardiasis
Grief and guilt
Gynecology
Gynecomastia
Halitosis
Hand-foot-and-mouth disease
Headaches
Healing
Heart disease
Heartburn
Heat exhaustion and heat stroke
Hemorrhoid banding and removal
Hemorrhoids
Herpes
Hiccups
Hirschsprung's disease
Hives
Hyperadiposis
Hypercholesterolemia
Hyperlipidemia
Hypertension
Hypertrophy
Hypoglycemia
Incontinence
Indigestion
Infection
Inflammation
Influenza
Intestinal disorders
Juvenile rheumatoid arthritis
Laryngitis
Leukodystrophy
Malabsorption
Maple syrup urine disease (MSUD)
Measles
Mitral valve prolapse
Moles
Mononucleosis
Motion sickness
Mumps
Münchausen syndrome by proxy
Muscle sprains, spasms, and
    disorders

Myringotomy
Nasal polyp removal
Nasopharyngeal disorders
Niemann-Pick disease
Nightmares
Nosebleeds
Nutrition
Obesity
Orchitis
Osgood-Schlatter disease
Osteopathic medicine
Otoplasty
Pain
Parasitic diseases
Pediatrics
Pharmacology
Pharmacy
Pharyngitis
Physical examination
Physician assistants
Pigeon toes
Pinworm
Pityriasis alba
Pityriasis rosea
Pneumonia
Poisonous plants
Prader-Willi syndrome
Precocious puberty
Psychiatry
Psychiatry, child and adolescent
Psychiatry, geriatric
Ptosis
Puberty and adolescence
Pyelonephritis
Quinsy
Rashes
Reflexes, primitive
Reiter's syndrome
Rheumatic fever
Ringworm
Rubella
Safety issues for children
Safety issues for the elderly
Scabies
Scarlet fever
Sciatica
Sexuality
Shingles
Shock
Sibling rivalry
Sinusitis
Sjögren's syndrome
Skin disorders
Sneezing

Sore throat
Sports medicine
Sterilization
Strep throat
Stress
Styes
Sunburn
Supplements
Temporomandibular joint (TMJ)
  syndrome
Tendinitis
Testicular torsion
Tetanus
Toilet training
Tonsillitis
Tourette's syndrome
Toxicology
Trachoma
Ulcers
Urology
Vascular medicine
Vasectomy
Viral infections
Vitamins and minerals
Von Willebrand's disease
Weaning
Weight loss medications
Whooping cough
Wounds

FORENSIC MEDICINE
Autopsy
Blood and blood disorders
Blood testing
Bones and the skeleton
Cytopathology
Dermatopathology
DNA and RNA
Forensic pathology
Genetics and inheritance
Genomics
Hematology
Histology
Immunopathology
Laboratory tests
Law and medicine
Pathology

GASTROENTEROLOGY
Abdomen
Abdominal disorders
Acid reflux disease
Amyotrophic lateral sclerosis
Anthrax

Appendectomy
Appendicitis
Bariatric surgery
Bulimia
Bypass surgery
Celiac sprue
Cholecystectomy
Cholecystitis
Cholera
Colic
Colitis
Colon and rectal polyp removal
Colon and rectal surgery
Colon cancer
Colonoscopy and sigmoidoscopy
Computed tomography (CT)
  scanning
Constipation
Critical care
Critical care, pediatric
Crohn's disease
Cytomegalovirus (CMV)
Diarrhea and dysentery
Digestion
Diverticulitis and diverticulosis
E. coli infection
Emergency medicine
Endoscopy
Enemas
Enterocolitis
Enzymes
Failure to thrive
Fistula repair
Food biochemistry
Food poisoning
Gallbladder diseases
Gastrectomy
Gastroenterology
Gastroenterology, pediatric
Gastrointestinal disorders
Gastrointestinal system
Gastrostomy
Giardiasis
Glands
Heartburn
Hemochromatosis
Hemorrhoid banding and removal
Hemorrhoids
Hernia
Hernia repair
Hirschsprung's disease
Ileostomy and colostomy
Indigestion
Internal medicine

Intestinal disorders
Intestines
Irritable bowel syndrome (IBS)
Lactose intolerance
Laparoscopy
Liver
Liver cancer
Liver disorders
Liver transplantation
Malabsorption
Malnutrition
Metabolism
Nausea and vomiting
Noroviruses
Nutrition
Obstruction
Pancreas
Pancreatitis
Peristalsis
Poisonous plants
Polycystic kidney disease
Proctology
Pyloric stenosis
Roundworm
Salmonella infection
Scleroderma
Shigellosis
Soiling
Stomach, intestinal, and pancreatic
  cancers
Stone removal
Stones
Tapeworm
Taste
Toilet training
Trichinosis
Ulcer surgery
Ulcers
Vagotomy
Von Willebrand's disease
Weight loss and gain
Wilson's disease
Worms

GENERAL SURGERY
Abscess drainage
Adrenalectomy
Amputation
Anesthesia
Anesthesiology
Aneurysmectomy
Appendectomy
Bariatric surgery
Biopsy

Bladder removal
Bone marrow transplantation
Breast biopsy
Breast surgery
Bunions
Bypass surgery
Cataract surgery
Catheterization
Cervical procedures
Cesarean section
Cholecystectomy
Circumcision, female, and genital
    mutilation
Circumcision, male
Cleft lip and palate repair
Colon and rectal polyp removal
Colon and rectal surgery
Corneal transplantation
Craniotomy
Cryotherapy and cryosurgery
Cyst removal
Disk removal
Ear surgery
Electrocauterization
Endarterectomy
Endometrial biopsy
Eye surgery
Face lift and blepharoplasty
Fistula repair
Ganglion removal
Gastrectomy
Grafts and grafting
Hair transplantation
Hammertoe correction
Heart transplantation
Heart valve replacement
Heel spur removal
Hemorrhoid banding and removal
Hernia repair
Hip replacement
Hydrocelectomy
Hypospadias repair and
    urethroplasty
Hysterectomy
Kidney transplantation
Kneecap removal
Laceration repair
Laminectomy and spinal fusion
Laparoscopy
Laryngectomy
Laser use in surgery
Liposuction
Liver transplantation
Lung surgery

Malignant melanoma removal
Mastectomy and lumpectomy
Myomectomy
Nail removal
Nasal polyp removal
Nephrectomy
Neurosurgery
Oncology
Ophthalmology
Orthopedic surgery
Otoplasty
Parathyroidectomy
Penile implant surgery
Periodontal surgery
Phlebitis
Plastic surgery
Prostate gland removal
Prostheses
Rhinoplasty and submucous
    resection
Rotator cuff surgery
Sex change surgery
Shunts
Skin lesion removal
Sphincterectomy
Splenectomy
Sterilization
Stone removal
Surgery, general
Surgery, pediatric
Surgical procedures
Surgical technologists
Sympathectomy
Tattoo removal
Tendon repair
Testicular surgery
Thoracic surgery
Thyroidectomy
Tonsillectomy and adenoid
    removal
Toxic shock syndrome
Tracheostomy
Transfusion
Transplantation
Tumor removal
Ulcer surgery
Vagotomy
Varicose vein removal
Vasectomy
Xenotransplantation

GENETICS
Aging
Albinos

Alzheimer's disease
Amniocentesis
Assisted reproductive technologies
Attention-deficit disorder (ADD)
Autoimmune disorders
Batten's disease
Bioinformatics
Bionics and biotechnology
Birth defects
Bone marrow transplantation
Breast cancer
Breast disorders
Chorionic villus sampling
Cloning
Cognitive development
Colon cancer
Color blindness
Cornelia de Lange syndrome
Cystic fibrosis
Diabetes mellitus
DiGeorge syndrome
DNA and RNA
Down syndrome
Dwarfism
Embryology
Endocrinology
Endocrinology, pediatric
Enzyme therapy
Enzymes
Failure to thrive
Fetal surgery
Fragile X syndrome
Fructosemia
Galactosemia
Gaucher's disease
Gene therapy
Genetic counseling
Genetic diseases
Genetic engineering
Genetics and inheritance
Genomics
Grafts and grafting
Hematology
Hematology, pediatric
Hemophilia
Hermaphroditism and
    pseudohermaphroditism
Huntington's disease
Hyperadiposis
Immunodeficiency disorders
In vitro fertilization
Insulin resistance syndrome
Karyotyping
Klinefelter syndrome

Mastitis
Menopause
Menorrhagia
Menstruation
Myomectomy
Nutrition
Obstetrics
Ovarian cysts
Pap smear
Pelvic inflammatory disease
  (PID)
Peritonitis
Postpartum depression
Preeclampsia and eclampsia
Pregnancy and gestation
Premenstrual syndrome (PMS)
Reiter's syndrome
Reproductive system
Sex change surgery
Sexual differentiation
Sexual dysfunction
Sexuality
Sexually transmitted diseases
  (STDs)
Sterilization
Syphilis
Toxemia
Toxic shock syndrome
Trichomoniasis
Tubal ligation
Turner syndrome
Ultrasonography
Urethritis
Urinary disorders
Urology
Von Willebrand's disease
Warts

HEMATOLOGY
Acid-base chemistry
Acquired immunodeficiency
  syndrome (AIDS)
Anemia
Bleeding
Blood and blood disorders
Blood testing
Bone grafting
Bone marrow transplantation
Burkitt's lymphoma
Cholesterol
Circulation
Cyanosis
Cytology
Cytomegalovirus (CMV)

Cytopathology
Dialysis
Disseminated intravascular
  coagulation (DIC)
Fluids and electrolytes
Forensic pathology
Healing
Hematology
Hematology, pediatric
Hemolytic disease of the newborn
Hemophilia
Histiocytosis
Histology
Hodgkin's disease
Host-defense mechanisms
Hypercholesterolemia
Hyperlipidemia
Hypoglycemia
Immune system
Immunology
Infection
Ischemia
Jaundice
Jaundice, neonatal
Kidneys
Laboratory tests
Leukemia
Liver
Lymphadenopathy and lymphoma
Lymphatic system
Malaria
Nephrology
Nephrology, pediatric
Niemann-Pick disease
Nosebleeds
Rh factor
Septicemia
Serology
Sickle cell disease
Stem cells
Thalassemia
Thrombocytopenia
Thrombolytic therapy and TPA
Thrombosis and thrombus
Transfusion
Vascular medicine
Vascular system
Von Willebrand's disease

HISTOLOGY
Autopsy
Biopsy
Cancer
Carcinoma

Cells
Cytology
Cytopathology
Dermatology
Dermatopathology
Fluids and electrolytes
Forensic pathology
Healing
Histology
Laboratory tests
Malignant melanoma removal
Microscopy
Nails
Necrotizing fasciitis
Pathology
Tumor removal
Tumors

IMMUNOLOGY
Acquired immunodeficiency
  syndrome (AIDS)
Allergies
Antibiotics
Antihistamines
Arthritis
Asthma
Autoimmune disorders
Bacterial infections
Biological and chemical weapons
Bionics and biotechnology
Bites and stings
Blisters and boils
Blood and blood disorders
Bone cancer
Bone grafting
Bone marrow transplantation
Breast cancer
Cancer
Candidiasis
Carcinoma
Cervical, ovarian, and uterine
  cancers
Childhood infectious diseases
Chronic fatigue syndrome
Colon cancer
Corticosteroids
Cytology
Cytomegalovirus (CMV)
Dermatology
Dermatopathology
DiGeorge syndrome
Endocrinology
Endocrinology, pediatric
Fungal infections

Grafts and grafting
Healing
Hematology
Hematology, pediatric
Histiocytosis
Hives
Homeopathy
Host-defense mechanisms
Human immunodeficiency virus
    (HIV)
Hypnosis
Immune system
Immunization and vaccination
Immunodeficiency disorders
Immunology
Immunopathology
Impetigo
Juvenile rheumatoid arthritis
Laboratory tests
Leprosy
Liver cancer
Lung cancer
Lupus erythematosus
Lymphatic system
Microbiology
Multiple chemical sensitivity
    syndrome
Myasthenia gravis
Nicotine
Noroviruses
Oncology
Oxygen therapy
Pancreas
Prostate cancer
Pulmonary diseases
Pulmonary medicine
Pulmonary medicine, pediatric
Rheumatology
Sarcoma
Sarcopenia
Scleroderma
Serology
Severe combined immunodeficiency
    syndrome (SCID)
Skin cancer
Stem cells
Stomach, intestinal, and pancreatic
    cancers
Stress
Stress reduction
Thalidomide
Transfusion
Transplantation
Tropical medicine

Wiskott-Aldrich syndrome
Xenotransplantation

INTERNAL MEDICINE
Abdomen
Abdominal disorders
Anatomy
Anemia
Angina
Anti-inflammatory drugs
Antioxidants
Anxiety
Arrhythmias
Arteriosclerosis
Autoimmune disorders
Bacterial infections
Bariatric surgery
Behçet's disease
Beriberi
Biofeedback
Bleeding
Bronchiolitis
Bronchitis
Burkitt's lymphoma
Burping
Bursitis
Candidiasis
Chickenpox
Childhood infectious diseases
Cholecystitis
Cholesterol
Chronic fatigue syndrome
Cirrhosis
Claudication
Cluster headaches
Colitis
Colonoscopy and sigmoidoscopy
Common cold
Constipation
Corticosteroids
Coughing
Cretinism
Crohn's disease
Cyanosis
Diabetes mellitus
Dialysis
Diarrhea and dysentery
Digestion
Disseminated intravascular
    coagulation (DIC)
Diverticulitis and diverticulosis
Dizziness and fainting
Domestic violence
E. coli infection

Edema
Embolism
Emphysema
Endocarditis
Endoscopy
Factitious disorders
Family practice
Fatigue
Fever
Fungal infections
Gallbladder diseases
Gangrene
Gastroenterology
Gastroenterology, pediatric
Gastrointestinal disorders
Gastrointestinal system
Gaucher's disease
Genetic diseases
Geriatrics and gerontology
Goiter
Gout
Guillain-Barré syndrome
Hanta virus
Headaches
Heart
Heart attack
Heart disease
Heart failure
Heartburn
Heat exhaustion and heat stroke
Hemochromatosis
Hepatitis
Hernia
Histology
Hodgkin's disease
Human immunodeficiency virus
    (HIV)
Hypercholesterolemia
Hyperlipidemia
Hypertension
Hyperthermia and hypothermia
Hypertrophy
Hypoglycemia
Incontinence
Indigestion
Infection
Inflammation
Influenza
Insulin resistance syndrome
Internal medicine
Intestinal disorders
Intestines
Ischemia
Itching

Pharmacy
Plastic surgery
Proctology
Prostate cancer
Prostate gland
Prostate gland removal
Prostheses
Pulmonary diseases
Pulmonary medicine
Radiation sickness
Radiation therapy
Radiopharmaceuticals
Sarcoma
Sarcopenia
Serology
Skin
Skin cancer
Skin lesion removal
Smoking
Stem cells
Stomach, intestinal, and pancreatic
  cancers
Stress
Sunburn
Thalidomide
Toxicology
Transplantation
Tumor removal
Tumors
Wiskott-Aldrich syndrome

OPHTHALMOLOGY
Aging: Extended care
Albinos
Anti-inflammatory drugs
Astigmatism
Batten's disease
Behçet's disease
Biophysics
Blindness
Blurred vision
Botox
Cataract surgery
Cataracts
Color blindness
Conjunctivitis
Corneal transplantation
Eye surgery
Eyes
Geriatrics and gerontology
Glaucoma
Juvenile rheumatoid arthritis
Laser use in surgery
Macular degeneration

Marfan syndrome
Microscopy, slitlamp
Myopia
Ophthalmology
Optometry
Optometry, pediatric
Prostheses
Ptosis
Reiter's syndrome
Rubinstein-Taybi syndrome
Sense organs
Strabismus
Sturge-Weber syndrome
Styes
Trachoma
Visual disorders

OPTOMETRY
Aging: Extended care
Astigmatism
Biophysics
Blurred vision
Cataracts
Eyes
Geriatrics and gerontology
Glaucoma
Myopia
Ophthalmology
Optometry
Optometry, pediatric
Ptosis
Sense organs
Styes
Visual disorders

ORGANIZATIONS AND
  PROGRAMS
Allied health
American Medical Association
  (AMA)
Blood banks
Centers for Disease Control and
  Prevention (CDC)
Clinical trials
Education, medical
Food and Drug Administration
  (FDA)
Health maintenance organizations
  (HMOs)
Hospice
Hospitals
Medicare
National Cancer Institute (NCI)
National Institutes of Health (NIH)

Sperm banks
Stem cells
World Health Organization

ORTHODONTICS
Bones and the skeleton
Dental diseases
Dentistry
Dentistry, pediatric
Jaw wiring
Nicotine
Orthodontics
Periodontal surgery
Teeth
Teething
Tooth extraction
Wisdom teeth

ORTHOPEDICS
Amputation
Arthritis
Arthroplasty
Arthroscopy
Bariatric surgery
Bone cancer
Bone disorders
Bone grafting
Bones and the skeleton
Bowlegs
Bunions
Bursitis
Cancer
Chiropractic
Craniosynostosis
Disk removal
Dwarfism
Ewing's sarcoma
Feet
Flat feet
Foot disorders
Fracture and dislocation
Fracture repair
Geriatrics and gerontology
Growth
Hammertoe correction
Hammertoes
Heel spur removal
Hip fracture repair
Hip replacement
Jaw wiring
Juvenile rheumatoid arthritis
Kinesiology
Kneecap removal
Knock-knees

Liposuction
Malignancy and metastasis
Malignant melanoma removal
Moles
Necrotizing fasciitis
Neurofibromatosis
Obesity
Otoplasty
Otorhinolaryngology
Plastic surgery
Prostheses
Ptosis
Rhinoplasty and submucous
    resection
Sex change surgery
Skin
Skin lesion removal
Sturge-Weber syndrome
Surgical procedures
Tattoo removal
Tattoos and body piercing
Varicose vein removal
Varicose veins
Wrinkles

PODIATRY
Athlete's foot
Bone disorders
Bones and the skeleton
Bunions
Corns and calluses
Feet
Flat feet
Foot disorders
Fungal infections
Hammertoe correction
Hammertoes
Heel spur removal
Lower extremities
Nail removal
Orthopedic surgery
Orthopedics
Physical examination
Pigeon toes
Podiatry
Tendon disorders
Tendon repair
Warts

PREVENTIVE MEDICINE
Acupressure
Acupuncture
Aging: Extended care
Alternative medicine

Aromatherapy
Biofeedback
Caffeine
Cardiology
Chiropractic
Cholesterol
Chronobiology
Disease
Electrocardiography (ECG or EKG)
Environmental health
Exercise physiology
Family practice
Genetic counseling
Geriatrics and gerontology
Holistic medicine
Host-defense mechanisms
Hypercholesterolemia
Immune system
Immunization and vaccination
Immunology
Mammography
Massage
Meditation
Melatonin
Noninvasive tests
Nursing
Nutrition
Occupational health
Osteopathic medicine
Pharmacology
Pharmacy
Physical examination
Phytochemicals
Preventive medicine
Psychiatry
Psychiatry, child and adolescent
Psychiatry, geriatric
Screening
Serology
Spine, vertebrae, and disks
Sports medicine
Stress
Stress reduction
Tendinitis
Tropical medicine
Yoga

PROCTOLOGY
Bladder removal
Colon and rectal polyp removal
Colon and rectal surgery
Colon cancer
Colonoscopy and sigmoidoscopy
Crohn's disease

Diverticulitis and diverticulosis
Endoscopy
Fistula repair
Gastroenterology
Gastrointestinal disorders
Gastrointestinal system
Genital disorders, male
Geriatrics and gerontology
Hemorrhoid banding and removal
Hemorrhoids
Hirschsprung's disease
Internal medicine
Intestinal disorders
Intestines
Irritable bowel syndrome (IBS)
Physical examination
Proctology
Prostate cancer
Prostate gland
Prostate gland removal
Reproductive system
Urology

PSYCHIATRY
Addiction
Aging
Aging: Extended care
Alcoholism
Alzheimer's disease
Amnesia
Amyotrophic lateral sclerosis
Anorexia nervosa
Antidepressants
Anxiety
Asperger's syndrome
Attention-deficit disorder (ADD)
Auras
Autism
Bariatric surgery
Bipolar disorder
Bonding
Brain
Brain disorders
Breast surgery
Bulimia
Chronic fatigue syndrome
Circumcision, female, and genital
    mutilation
Club drugs
Corticosteroids
Delusions
Dementias
Depression
Developmental stages

Domestic violence
Eating disorders
Electroencephalography (EEG)
Emergency medicine
Emotions: Biomedical causes and
    effects
Factitious disorders
Failure to thrive
Family practice
Fatigue
Grief and guilt
Gynecology
Hallucinations
Huntington's disease
Hypnosis
Hypochondriasis
Incontinence
Intoxication
Light therapy
Marijuana
Masturbation
Memory loss
Mental retardation
Midlife crisis
Münchausen syndrome by proxy
Neurosis
Neurosurgery
Nicotine
Nightmares
Obesity
Obsessive-compulsive disorder
Pain
Pain management
Panic attacks
Paranoia
Penile implant surgery
Phobias
Postpartum depression
Post-traumatic stress disorder
Prader-Willi syndrome
Psychiatric disorders
Psychiatry
Psychiatry, child and adolescent
Psychiatry, geriatric
Psychoanalysis
Psychosis
Psychosomatic disorders
Schizophrenia
Seasonal affective disorder
Separation anxiety
Sex change surgery
Sexual dysfunction
Sexuality
Shock therapy

Sleep disorders
Speech disorders
Steroid abuse
Stress
Stress reduction
Sudden infant death syndrome
    (SIDS)
Suicide
Toilet training
Tourette's syndrome

PSYCHOLOGY
Addiction
Aging
Aging: Extended care
Alcoholism
Amnesia
Amyotrophic lateral sclerosis
Anorexia nervosa
Anxiety
Aromatherapy
Asperger's syndrome
Attention-deficit disorder (ADD)
Auras
Bariatric surgery
Bed-wetting
Biofeedback
Bipolar disorder
Bonding
Brain
Bulimia
Cardiac rehabilitation
Cirrhosis
Club drugs
Cognitive development
Death and dying
Delusions
Depression
Developmental stages
Domestic violence
Dyslexia
Eating disorders
Electroencephalography (EEG)
Emotions: Biomedical causes and
    effects
Environmental health
Factitious disorders
Failure to thrive
Family practice
Forensic pathology
Genetic counseling
Grief and guilt
Gulf War syndrome
Gynecology

Hallucinations
Holistic medicine
Hormone replacement therapy
    (HRT)
Huntington's disease
Hypnosis
Hypochondriasis
Juvenile rheumatoid arthritis
Kinesiology
Klinefelter syndrome
Learning disabilities
Light therapy
Marijuana
Meditation
Memory loss
Mental retardation
Midlife crisis
Motor skill development
Münchausen syndrome by proxy
Neurosis
Nightmares
Nutrition
Obesity
Obsessive-compulsive disorder
Occupational health
Pain management
Panic attacks
Paranoia
Phobias
Plastic surgery
Postpartum depression
Post-traumatic stress disorder
Psychosomatic disorders
Puberty and adolescence
Separation anxiety
Sex change surgery
Sexual dysfunction
Sexuality
Sibling rivalry
Sleep disorders
Sleepwalking
Speech disorders
Sports medicine
Steroid abuse
Stillbirth
Stress
Stress reduction
Sturge-Weber syndrome
Stuttering
Sudden infant death syndrome
    (SIDS)
Suicide
Temporomandibular joint (TMJ)
    syndrome

Tics
Toilet training
Tourette's syndrome
Weight loss and gain
Yoga

PUBLIC HEALTH
Acquired immunodeficiency
  syndrome (AIDS)
Aging: Extended care
Allied health
Alternative medicine
Anthrax
Arthropod-borne diseases
Bacteriology
Beriberi
Biological and chemical weapons
Biostatistics
Blood banks
Blood testing
Botulism
Chagas' disease
Chickenpox
Childhood infectious diseases
Chlamydia
Cholera
Chronic obstructive pulmonary
  disease (COPD)
Club drugs
Common cold
Corticosteroids
Creutzfeldt-Jakob disease (CJD)
Dermatology
Diarrhea and dysentery
Diphtheria
Domestic violence
Drug resistance
E. coli infection
Ebola virus
Elephantiasis
Emergency medicine
Environmental diseases
Epidemiology
Fetal alcohol syndrome
Food poisoning
Forensic pathology
Gonorrhea
Gulf War syndrome
Hanta virus
Hepatitis
Hospitals
Human immunodeficiency virus
  (HIV)
Immunization and vaccination

Influenza
Kwashiorkor
Lead poisoning
Legionnaires' disease
Leishmaniasis
Leprosy
Lice, mites, and ticks
Lyme disease
Malaria
Malnutrition
Marijuana
Measles
Medicare
Meningitis
Microbiology
Monkeypox
Multiple chemical sensitivity
  syndrome
Mumps
Necrotizing fasciitis
Nicotine
Niemann-Pick disease
Nursing
Nutrition
Occupational health
Osteopathic medicine
Parasitic diseases
Pharmacology
Pharmacy
Physical examination
Physician assistants
Pinworm
Plague
Pneumonia
Poliomyelitis
Prion diseases
Protozoan diseases
Psychiatry
Psychiatry, child and adolescent
Psychiatry, geriatric
Rabies
Radiation sickness
Roundworm
Rubella
Salmonella infection
Schistosomiasis
Screening
Serology
Severe acute respiratory syndrome
  (SARS)
Sexually transmitted diseases
  (STDs)
Shigellosis
Sleeping sickness

Smallpox
Syphilis
Tapeworm
Tattoos and body piercing
Tetanus
Toxicology
Toxoplasmosis
Trichinosis
Trichomoniasis
Tropical medicine
Tuberculosis
Typhoid fever and typhus
Whooping cough
World Health Organization
Worms
Yellow fever
Zoonoses

PULMONARY MEDICINE
Amyotrophic lateral sclerosis
Anthrax
Asthma
Bronchiolitis
Bronchitis
Catheterization
Chest
Chronic obstructive pulmonary
  disease (COPD)
Coughing
Critical care
Critical care, pediatric
Cyanosis
Cystic fibrosis
Edema
Embolism
Emergency medicine
Emphysema
Endoscopy
Environmental diseases
Environmental health
Fluids and electrolytes
Forensic pathology
Fungal infections
Gene therapy
Geriatrics and gerontology
Hanta virus
Hyperventilation
Internal medicine
Interstitial pulmonary fibrosis
  (IPF)
Lung cancer
Lung surgery
Lungs
Nicotine

Occupational health
Oxygen therapy
Paramedics
Pediatrics
Physical examination
Pleurisy
Pneumonia
Prader-Willi syndrome
Pulmonary diseases
Pulmonary hypertension
Pulmonary medicine
Pulmonary medicine, pediatric
Respiration
Respiratory distress syndrome
Severe acute respiratory syndrome
   (SARS)
Sleep apnea
Smoking
Thoracic surgery
Thrombolytic therapy and TPA
Tuberculosis
Tumor removal
Tumors

RADIOLOGY
Angiography
Biophysics
Biopsy
Bone cancer
Bone disorders
Bones and the skeleton
Cancer
Catheterization
Computed tomography (CT)
   scanning
Critical care
Critical care, pediatric
Emergency medicine
Ewing's sarcoma
Imaging and radiology
Liver cancer
Lung cancer
Magnetic resonance imaging
   (MRI)
Mammography
Noninvasive tests
Nuclear medicine
Nuclear radiology
Oncology
Positron emission tomography
   (PET) scanning
Prostate cancer
Radiation sickness
Radiation therapy

Radiopharmaceuticals
Sarcoma
Sarcopenia
Stents
Surgery, general
Ultrasonography

RHEUMATOLOGY
Aging
Aging: Extended care
Anti-inflammatory drugs
Arthritis
Arthroplasty
Arthroscopy
Autoimmune disorders
Behçet's disease
Bone disorders
Bones and the skeleton
Bursitis
Corticosteroids
Fibromyalgia
Geriatrics and gerontology
Gout
Hip replacement
Hydrotherapy
Inflammation
Lyme disease
Orthopedic surgery
Orthopedics
Orthopedics, pediatric
Osteoarthritis
Physical examination
Rheumatic fever
Rheumatoid arthritis
Rheumatology
Rotator cuff surgery
Scleroderma
Sjögren's syndrome
Spondylitis
Sports medicine

SEROLOGY
Anemia
Blood and blood disorders
Blood testing
Cholesterol
Cytology
Cytopathology
Dialysis
Fluids and electrolytes
Forensic pathology
Hematology
Hematology, pediatric
Hemophilia

Hodgkin's disease
Host-defense mechanisms
Hypercholesterolemia
Hyperlipidemia
Hypoglycemia
Immune system
Immunology
Immunopathology
Jaundice
Laboratory tests
Leukemia
Malaria
Pathology
Rh factor
Septicemia
Serology
Sickle cell disease
Thalassemia
Transfusion

SPEECH PATHOLOGY
Alzheimer's disease
Amyotrophic lateral sclerosis
Aphasia and dysphasia
Audiology
Autism
Cerebral palsy
Cleft lip and palate
Cleft lip and palate repair
Dyslexia
Ear infections and disorders
Ear surgery
Ears
Electroencephalography (EEG)
Hearing loss
Hearing tests
Jaw wiring
Laryngitis
Learning disabilities
Lisping
Paralysis
Rubinstein-Taybi syndrome
Speech disorders
Strokes
Stuttering
Thumb sucking
Voice and vocal cord disorders

SPORTS MEDICINE
Acupressure
Anorexia nervosa
Arthroplasty
Arthroscopy
Athlete's foot

Biofeedback
Blurred vision
Bones and the skeleton
Cardiology
Critical care
Dehydration
Eating disorders
Emergency medicine
Exercise physiology
Fracture and dislocation
Fracture repair
Glycolysis
Head and neck disorders
Heat exhaustion and heat stroke
Hydrotherapy
Kinesiology
Massage
Motor skill development
Muscle sprains, spasms, and
    disorders
Muscles
Nutrition
Orthopedic surgery
Orthopedics
Orthopedics, pediatric
Oxygen therapy
Physical examination
Physical rehabilitation
Physiology
Psychiatry
Psychiatry, child and adolescent
Rotator cuff surgery
Safety issues for children
Spine, vertebrae, and disks
Sports medicine
Steroid abuse
Steroids
Tendinitis
Tendon disorders
Tendon repair

TOXICOLOGY
Biological and chemical weapons
Bites and stings
Blood testing
Botulism
Club drugs
Critical care
Critical care, pediatric
Cyanosis
Dermatitis
Eczema
Emergency medicine
Environmental diseases

Environmental health
Food poisoning
Forensic pathology
Gaucher's disease
Hepatitis
Herbal medicine
Homeopathy
Intoxication
Itching
Laboratory tests
Lead poisoning
Liver
Mold and mildew
Multiple chemical sensitivity
    syndrome
Nicotine
Occupational health
Pathology
Pharmacology
Pharmacy
Poisoning
Poisonous plants
Rashes
Snakebites
Toxicology
Toxoplasmosis
Urinalysis

UROLOGY
Abdomen
Abdominal disorders
Bed-wetting
Bladder removal
Catheterization
Chlamydia
Circumcision, male
Cystitis
Cystoscopy
Dialysis
E. coli infection
Endoscopy
Fetal surgery
Fluids and electrolytes
Genital disorders, female
Genital disorders, male
Geriatrics and gerontology
Gonorrhea
Hermaphroditism and
    pseudohermaphroditism
Hydrocelectomy
Hypospadias repair and
    urethroplasty
Incontinence
Infertility in males

Kidney disorders
Kidney transplantation
Kidneys
Lithotripsy
Nephrectomy
Nephritis
Nephrology
Nephrology, pediatric
Pediatrics
Pelvic inflammatory disease (PID)
Penile implant surgery
Polycystic kidney disease
Prostate cancer
Prostate gland
Prostate gland removal
Pyelonephritis
Reiter's syndrome
Reproductive system
Schistosomiasis
Sex change surgery
Sexual differentiation
Sexual dysfunction
Sexually transmitted diseases
    (STDs)
Sterilization
Stone removal
Stones
Syphilis
Testicles, undescended
Testicular surgery
Testicular torsion
Toilet training
Transplantation
Trichomoniasis
Ultrasonography
Urethritis
Urinalysis
Urinary disorders
Urinary system
Urology
Urology, pediatric
Vasectomy

VASCULAR MEDICINE
Amputation
Aneurysmectomy
Aneurysms
Angiography
Angioplasty
Anti-inflammatory drugs
Arteriosclerosis
Biofeedback
Bleeding
Blood and blood disorders

Bypass surgery
Catheterization
Cholesterol
Circulation
Claudication
Dehydration
Diabetes mellitus
Dialysis
Embolism
Endarterectomy
Exercise physiology
Glands
Healing
Hematology
Hematology, pediatric
Hemorrhoid banding and removal
Hemorrhoids
Histology
Hypercholesterolemia
Hyperlipidemia
Ischemia
Klippel-Trenaunay syndrome
Lipids
Lymphatic system
Mitral valve prolapse
Necrotizing fasciitis
Nicotine
Osteochondritis juvenilis
Phlebitis
Podiatry
Preeclampsia and eclampsia
Progeria
Shunts
Smoking

Stents
Strokes
Sturge-Weber syndrome
Thrombolytic therapy and TPA
Thrombosis and thrombus
Toxemia
Transfusion
Transient ischemic attacks (TIAs)
Varicose vein removal
Varicose veins
Vascular medicine
Vascular system
Venous insufficiency
Von Willebrand's disease

VIROLOGY

Acquired immunodeficiency
    syndrome (AIDS)
Biological and chemical weapons
Chickenpox
Childhood infectious diseases
Chlamydia
Chronic fatigue syndrome
Common cold
Creutzfeldt-Jakob disease (CJD)
Croup
Cytomegalovirus (CMV)
Drug resistance
Ebola virus
Encephalitis
Fever
Hanta virus
Hepatitis
Herpes

Human immunodeficiency virus
    (HIV)
Infection
Influenza
Laboratory tests
Measles
Microbiology
Microscopy
Monkeypox
Mononucleosis
Mumps
Noroviruses
Parasitic diseases
Pelvic inflammatory disease (PID)
Poliomyelitis
Pulmonary diseases
Rabies
Rheumatic fever
Rhinitis
Roseola
Rubella
Serology
Severe acute respiratory syndrome
    (SARS)
Sexually transmitted diseases
    (STDs)
Shingles
Smallpox
Tonsillitis
Tropical medicine
Viral infections
Warts
Yellow fever
Zoonoses